TRAUMA NURSING
The Art and Science

TRAUMA NURSING
The Art and Science

Janet A. Neff, RN, MN, CEN, CCRN
Trauma Coordinator
Emergency Medical Services Liaison
Stanford University Hospital
Stanford, California

Pamela Stinson Kidd, RN, PhD, CEN
Assistant Professor, College of Nursing
Critical Care Research Consultant, University Hospital
University of Kentucky
Lexington, Kentucky

with 272 illustrations

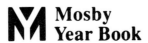
**Mosby
Year Book**

St. Louis   Baltimore   Boston   Chicago   London   Philadelphia   Sydney   Toronto

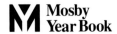
**Mosby
Year Book**
Dedicated to Publishing Excellence

Executive Editor: Don Ladig
Managing Editor: Robin Carter
Project Manager: Patricia Tannian
Senior Production Editors: Betty Hazelwood, Kathleen L. Teal
Designer: Susan Lane
Illustrator: Mark Swindle

Printed in the United States of America

Mosby–Year Book, Inc.
11830 Westline Industrial Drive
St. Louis, Missouri 63146

Library of Congress Cataloging in Publication Data

Neff, Janet A.
    Trauma nursing : the art and science / Janet A. Neff, Pamela
Stinson Kidd.
        p.   cm.
    Includes bibliographical references and index.
    ISBN 0-8016-6655-4
    1. Wounds and injuries–Nursing.   2. Emergency nursing.   I. Kidd,
Pamela Stinson.   II. Title
    [DNLM: 1. Emergency Nursing.   2. Wounds and Injuries–nursing.
WY 154 N383t]
RD93.95.N44 1992
610.73'61--dc20
DNLM/DLC
for Library of Congress

93   94   95   96   97   CL / DC   9   8   7   6   5   4   3   2   1

Contributors

■■■

Sarah D. Cohn, MSN, JD
Associate Counsel, Medicolegal Affairs
Yale-New Haven Hospital
Yale University
New Haven, Connecticut

Peggy Devney, RN, MSN
Clinical Nurse Specialist
Transplantation and Nephrology
UCSF Medical Center
San Franciso, California

Lynn E. Eastes, RN, MSN, CCRN
Trauma Coordinator
Oregon Health Sciences University
Portland, Oregon

Nancye Feistritzer, RN, MSN, CNOR
Division Director of Operating Room Services
University Hospital, University of Kentucky
Lexington, Kentucky

Jody Foss, RN, MSN
Director of the Center for Member Services
Former Assistant Director of Education
The Association of Operating Room Nurses
Denver, Colorado

Elizabeth A. Henneman, RN, MS, CCRN
Pulmonary Clinical Nurse Specialist
UCLA Intensive Care
Los Angeles, California

Philip L. Henneman, MD, FACEP
Director, Adult Emergency Department
Harbor-UCLA Medical Center
Torrance, California

S. Marshal Isaacs, MD
Emergency Medicine Attending
San Francisco General Hospital;
Assistant Director of Prehospital Division, City and
    County of San Francisco
San Francisco, California

Karen Johnson, RN, MSN, CCRN
Critical Care Clinical Nurse Specialist
Instructor, College of Nursing
University Hospital, University of Kentucky
Lexington, Kentucky

†Allen Jones, MD
Former Chief Medical Examiner
Pima County, Arizona;
Former Director
Forensic Sciences Center
Tucson, Arizona

Karma Klauber, RN, MS, CRRN
Rehabilitation Consultant
Private Practice;
Former Program Director, NeuroCare, Inc.
San Diego, California

Judy L. Larsen, RN, CEN
Head Nurse, Division of Emergency Services
Group Health Central Hospital
Seattle, Washington

Susan Engman Lazear, RN, MN, CEN
Director
Specialists in Medical Education
Honolulu, Hawaii

---

†Deceased

Karen Kidd Lovett, MDiv, AAPC

Methodist Counseling Services Pastoral Counselor
Louisville, Kentucky

Michelle Lucatorto, RN, MSN, CNRN

Neuroscience Clinical Nurse Specialist
Shadyside Hospital
Pittsburgh, Pennsylvania

Linda K. Manley, RN, BSN, CEN, CCRN

Pediatric Outreach Education Coordinator
Columbus Children's Hospital;
Flight Nurse, SKYMED
Ohio State University
Columbus, Ohio

Christine May, RN, MSN

Associate Director, Trauma Services
Children's Hospital Medical Center
Oakland, California;
Assistant Clinical Professor, School of Nursing
University of California at San Francisco
San Francisco, California

Kathleen B. McLeod, RN, MA, CEN

Trauma Program Manager
Tucson Medical Center
Tucson, Arizona

Wayne C. McLeod, RN, BA, R-EMTP, CEN

Flight Nurse, University AIRCARE
University Medical Center
Tucson, Arizona

Gail Mornhinweg, RN, PhD

Associate Professor, College of Nursing
University of Louisville
Louisville, Kentucky

Rodney Newman, RN, MSN, ANP, CCRN

Critical Care Superivsor
Mountain View Hospital
Payson, Utah

Kathleen S. Oman, RN, MS, CEN

Clinical Nurse Specialist
Surgical / Trauma Services
Denver General Hospital
Denver, Colorado

Jean A. Proehl, RN, MN, CEN, CCRN

Emergency Clinical Nurse Specialist
Broward General Medical Center
Ft. Lauderdale, Florida

Renee Semonin-Holleran, RN, PhD, CEN, CCRN

Chief Flight Nurse, University Air Care
University of Cincinnati
Cincinnati, Ohio

Diane M. Sklarov, RN, MSN

Director, Outpatient Services
Miami Heart Institute
Miami, Florida

Joan Andrews Snyder, RN, MS, CEN

Former Clinical Consultant
Sharp Healthcare Corporation
San Diego, California

Patricia A. Southard, RN, MS, JD

Trauma Director
Oregon Health Sciences University
Portland, Oregon

Joe E. Taylor, RN, PhD, CEN, CNAA

Vice President, Clinical Support Services
South Central Regional Medical Center
Laurel, Mississippi

Lori D. Taylor, RN, BSN, CEN

Deputy Coroner, Spokane County;
Trauma Program Manager
Sacred Heart Medical Center
Spokane, Washington

Judie Wischman, RN, MA

Director, Emergency Services
Group Health Central Hospital
Seattle, Washington

Preface

■■■

Trauma Nursing: The Art and Science was conceived several years ago when the editors realized that existing books did not address the nursing role in trauma care to its fullest extent. For example, prevention of injuries was rarely addressed. Nursing diagnoses were integrated but not discussed from an evolutionary perspective. Quality improvement issues were not discussed, nor were legal and forensic issues always delineated. The most blatant omissions were discussions regarding clinical controversies, integration of "cutting edge research," and questions for the reader that could be answered through future research. Because the editors and contributors have practiced in a variety of roles in trauma care— trauma resuscitation nurse, trauma nurse coordinator, clinical researcher, and trauma care educator—we are aware of the rapid changes in technology, interventions, and expected outcomes that impact trauma nursing.

Organization

Trauma Nursing: The Art and Science is organized in a logical, nursing-oriented approach that simulates the realities of trauma nursing practice. We believe by mirroring reality we provide the most practical approach to presenting this content—both for students who must learn to apply this content to practice and for practitioners who must constantly evaluate, apply, and individualize the content. We like to think of this as a common sense approach to the trauma patient.

The content is conceptually based, to be consistent with nursing's role in treating the human response to injury. Chapter subheadings in the clinical care chapters use terminology generated by the North American Nursing Diagnosis Association (NANDA) to facilitate the selection of appropriate nursing diagnoses for patients experienc-

ing injuries discussed in the chapter. We hope this will facilitate use and documentation of nursing diagnoses in your present role.

The book is organized into six major sections: Unit I, Trauma and Society; Unit II, Professional Issues in Trauma Nursing; Unit III, Nursing Care of the Trauma Patient; Unit IV, Trauma Throughout the Lifespan; Unit V, Selected Trauma Sequelae; and Unit VI, Nursing Within the Trauma Continuum.

The trauma system is addressed throughout the book. It is discussed in the greatest detail in the following chapters: Evolution of Trauma Care (Chapter 1); Legal Issues (Chapter 4); and Trauma Quality Management (Chapter 6). The trauma system is further discussed in the appendixes: trauma care resources are outlined in Appendix A, and disaster planning is discussed in Appendix B. Guidelines from the American College of Emergency Physicans (ACEP) are presented in Appendix C, and organ donation is discussed in Appendix D.

Prevention of Traumatic Injury (Chapter 2) reflects the editors' philosophy that trauma is a disease. Thus there are risk factors that indicate one's susceptibility for this disease. Alleviating risk factors is another way that trauma nurses can decrease the morbidity and mortality associated with traumatic injury.

Nursing Diagnosis (Chapter 3) explains the history of nursing diagnoses, the rationale for the present classification system, and how diagnoses can enhance, not impede, nursing practice. Diagnoses that pertain specifically to the trauma patient are discussed.

Chapter 5, Forensic Aspects, was included to increase the awareness of nursing responsibility in evidence collection. The assessment of trauma cases to determine index of suspicion and how forensic information has been used in injury prevention and detection are discussed also.

Trauma Quality Management (Chapter 6) illustrates strategies for measuring patient outcomes and the quality of a trauma system. The chapter reflects current issues in trauma care reimbursement in relation to case management.

Unit III, Nursing Care of the Trauma Patient, is organized in a uniquely functional way. This presentation differs from that of most trauma nursing books. For example, in books organized by body systems, facial injuries are usually discussed in a separate chapter or with head/ENT injuries. Since the primary nursing concern in treating a trauma patient with facial injuries is to maintain airway patency and ventilation, because of massive bleeding, edema, and unstable facial structures, in *Trauma Nursing*, facial injuries are discussed in Chapter 8, Ventilation and Gas Transport. Another example is Chapter 10, Sensory/Perceptual, which includes head and eye injuries. The eyes are frequently associated with head injuries and are examined as part of a neurologic assessment. Therefore this material is covered in the same chapter.

Tissue Integrity (Chapter 13) is addressed in a separate chapter. The correct cleaning, closure, and dressing of wounds are major priorities because of the growing incidence of sepsis and septic syndrome in trauma patients after stabilization and resuscitation. Chapter 15, Adaptation: Psychosocial and Spiritual, addresses psychosocial responses the nurse frequently encounters when caring for trauma patients. Why patients may respond in this manner and how healthcare providers can positively intervene are also discussed.

All individuals, regardless of their developmental age or state, are susceptible to traumatic injury-producing events. Thus Unit IV, Trauma Throughout the Lifespan, addresses the unique characteristics and treatment strategies associated with traumatic injury in children, pregnant women, and the elderly.

Unit V, Selected Trauma Sequelae (Chapter 19), comprises one chapter, which explains the interrelationships among trauma sequelae so the reader may obtain a greater appreciation of the consequences of hypoperfusion. Nutritional supplementation is also addressed.

The continuum of trauma care is addressed in Chapters 20 through 24: Air Transport of the Trauma Patient, Emergency Department Care of the Trauma Patient, Perioperative Care of the Trauma Patient, Critical Care of the Trauma Patient, and Rehabilitation of the Trauma Patient. Information in these chapters assists the nurse to set priorities of patient needs, based on their point on the trauma trajectory, as well as to appreciate the practice perspective of colleagues.

Special Features

This book is clinically based. Each clinical chapter begins and ends with a case study and a series of interactive review questions, with answers designed to stimulate critical thinking by applying the most important concepts discussed in the chapter. These questions can also serve as a checkpoint for the reader to determine his or her degree of familarity with chapter material or to examine retention. Objectives are presented in each chapter so the reader can anticipate major points.

Annotated bibliographies are provided at the end of each clinical chapter to assist the reader in making future reading selections. The reference lists in each chapter are comprehensive; they include classic as well as current material. For the visual learner, ample figures and tables are included to graphically illustrate information. Many of the illustrations have been newly created for this book. Because the current focus in trauma care is on patient outcomes, a Complications section is included in each clinical chapter to help focus the reader on the relationships among injury, treatment, and outcome.

Research questions are included in each chapter to stimulate each of us to approach trauma care with an inquisitive and questioning mind. We firmly believe that each one of us can contribute to generating a new knowledge base in trauma nursing. Our contribution may take various shapes and forms. Providing research questions is one way we hope to contribute and make "going back to school" a little easier.

The inclusion of competencies in the clinical chapters provides information that can be used in developing nursing evaluation and orientation forms. Continuing education sessions can be planned to address essential competencies. These serve to help delineate the "nice to know" from the "must know" material and focus on the psychomotor component of nursing.

Conclusion

Trauma Nursing: The Art and Science was written by experts across the country who have published numerous articles and books before contributing to this book. We are proud to be associated with these colleagues. Each of us can benefit from the knowledge of one another. These contributors are the "cream of the crop" in their fields. The diversity in geographic location of the contributors increases the applicability of the book's content and provides a broader perspective.

The book ends with an epilogue written by a retired emergency department nurse who provided nursing care for trauma patients over a 40-year period, before these patients were known as "trauma patients." She reminds us that the best form of nursing is based on the blending of the art and science of our discipline. How easy it is to forget the art for the sake of the science when the science is evolving so quickly! However, within each of us the art is also evolving. The epilogue leaves us with a mission that is a challenge to complete.

It is our sincere hope that you will be able to (1) find the information you need in a timely fashion, (2) understand the rationale behind strategies, (3) link important concepts together in a meaningful manner, and (4) develop a greater appreciation of your contribution to trauma patient outcomes from reading this book. We invite you to write to us in care of the publisher if you have comments on the book.

Acknowledgments

We sincerely thank Don Ladig for his vision in acquiring this work, Robin Carter for her developmental expertise and stamina, Betty Hazelwood for her meticulous and talented editing, Susan Lane for her excellent design, Mark Swindle for his highly original illustrations, the many other members of the Mosby–Year Book family who contributed to this book, and our contributors for their sustained efforts and creativity.

Janet A. Neff

Pamela Stinson Kidd

To my parents and sisters, who supported me from the
time the book was just an idea until its final form,
who patiently waited for the often-promised life
"after the book," and who were a constant source
of encouragement, keeping the goal always in sight.

To those who labor to publish and those who share
their knowledge in practice.

To the students and colleagues who challenge me with
questions of "why" and stimulate me to find
the answers.

To my other sanity-keepers:
the felines, equines, and canine.

J.A.N

J.A.N

To my parents and family, who gave me such a firm
foundation; there are no shifting sands, only new
mountains to climb.

To my "Bogs," you make a pattern out of chaos and
solving the puzzle fun.
I love you both.

To our contributors, their family, and friends,
thanks for your perserverance.
Together, we make a great team.

P.S.K.

We thank our fellow trauma nurses
for being there at all hours of the day and night,
when they are tired, understaffed, and overwhelmed.
We must continue to uphold our patient care standards,
and we must support one another in the process.

Contents in Brief

Contents

■■■■■■■■■■■■■■■■■■■■■■■■■■■■■■■■■■■

TRAUMA NURSING
The Art and Science

I

TRAUMA AND SOCIETY

1 Evolution of Trauma Care

Joan Andrews Snyder

■■■

OBJECTIVES
- ❑ Describe the historical development of trauma care delivery systems.
- ❑ Discuss the benefits of organized emergency medical systems with designated trauma centers.
- ❑ List considerations for triage of trauma patients in in the field, and describe two levels of prehospital care personnel.
- ❑ Compare the use of land and air transport for rural and urban trauma care systems.
- ❑ Outline the trauma resuscitation nurse's role, and name two areas for research related to this role.

INTRODUCTION Trauma is a serious public health problem. Traumatic injury, both accidental and intentional, is the leading cause of death in the first four decades of life. Trauma has no respect for age, presents without warning, and frequently causes profound loss of function for the persons involved. The quality of the initial assessment and management of a severely injured patient influences the trauma patient's final outcome—an organized approach affords an optimal outcome. The nature of traumatic injuries requires team members to have a broad knowledge base of treatment principles and an appreciation for the multiplicity of injury.

Each year more than 140,000 Americans die and approximately 80,000 are permanently disabled as a result of injury (National Research Council, 1985). Trauma typically involves more children and young adults (and therefore results in the loss of more productive work years) than cancer and heart disease combined. In addition to the loss of productivity, health care costs $100 billion annually. The emotional costs are immeasurable.

MORTALITY AND MORBIDITY PEAKS

If the number of fatalities caused by trauma is plotted as a function of time after injury, a trimo-dal distribution appears (Trunkey, 1983) (Figure 1-1). The first peak, approximately 50% of all trauma-related deaths, represents those patients who die instantaneously or in the first few minutes after injury. These fatalities invariably are caused by such injuries or combination of injuries as severe brain lacerations or rupture of the heart, aorta, or other large vessels. The few patients who survive such devastating injuries usually either encounter trauma close to a trauma center or present with classic symptomatology. In these instances, rapid prehospital response time and early, accurate medical diagnosis are responsible for dramatic successes. The primary way to reduce the number of victims in the immediate death category is through preventing accidents or reducing the severity of the insult, by such measures as the use of automobile restraint devices.

The second peak, which occurs within hours of injury, accounts for approximately 30% of injury fatalities and is usually the result of neurologic injury or severe blood loss from cavitary hemorrhage. A considerable number of these deaths can be prevented if there is rapid transport from the scene of the accident to a hospital fully staffed and prepared to care for such patients. Some have referred to this period as the "golden hour," when resuscitation and definitive care are

3

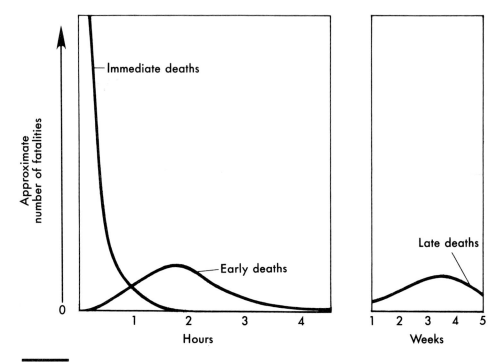

Figure 1-1   Distribution of fatalities caused by trauma as function of time after injury. Note that trimodal distribution occurs: 50% of deaths occur in first phase (immediate deaths), 30% of deaths occur in second phase (early deaths), and 20% of deaths occur in third phase (late deaths).

most effective. Resuscitation involves assuring patency of the airway, assisting with ventilation, and supporting circulation with adequate amounts of fluid or blood products. Definitive care includes timely surgical intervention and coordinated critical care management. The concept of trauma centers is built on the premise that time is vital for preserving life after a traumatic event. A trauma center is a facility that provides 24-hour, in-house coverage by surgeons and supporting staff to care for trauma patients. The integration of prehospital care, rapid transport times, aggressive resuscitation, and immediate surgical treatment within a regionalized trauma system has reduced preventable trauma deaths from the 20% to 30% range to the 2% to 9% range (Shackford, Cooper, Hollingsworth-Fridlund, & Eastman, 1986).

The third peak in trauma deaths occurs days to weeks after injury and is usually the result of infection or multiple organ failure. Reduction in late mortality depends on standardized treatment protocols, concentration of expertise, and contin-

ued research efforts focusing on the acute response to trauma.

The goal of trauma care systems is to provide an organized approach to the reduction of deaths in each of the peaks in this trimodal distribution. A structure is provided for assuring rapid transport of the victim to an appropriate trauma facility, which provides timely resuscitation and stabilization by trained personnel. A multidisciplinary team approach to definitive care and the promotion of continual research in such areas as sepsis and traumatic shock are essential.

ORIGINATION OF TRAUMA CARE

The concept of regionalized trauma systems is not a new one; many of the advances in caring for major trauma victims can be attributed to care provided during past military conflicts. Advances in field resuscitation, rapid evacuation, and aggressive treatment of casualties have led to a decline in death rates of battle casualties who reach medical facilities.

Early in the nineteenth century, Barron Larrey, who was Napoleon's chief surgeon, developed two concepts to improve the care of wounded soldiers that persisted until modern times (Dible, 1970). The first was the "flying ambulance," a cart on wheels used to evacuate patients to the rear of the battlefield. The use of this device sharply reduced the time it took to access definitive care. Before this invention the injured often remained on the battlefield for as long as 36 hours. Larrey's second contribution was the creation of a battlefield hospital zone, which allowed victims to be concentrated in one area and to be operated on as close to the front lines as possible.

During World War I the overall mortality rate was 8.5% and the time lag between injury and surgery ranged from 12 to 18 hours. This time lag was reduced during World War II to between 6 and 12 hours, and the mortality rate fell to 5.8% (Beebe & DeBakey, 1952). The reduction was attributed to (1) improvements in prehospital medical aid and (2) well-developed triage systems. The most dramatic change took place during the Korean War, when the U.S. Army Medical Corps bypassed aid stations and transported victims from the battlefield directly to a mobile army surgical hospital (MASH). Helicopters, which were primarily reserved for rescuing downed pilots, were increasingly adapted for medical transports. The average lag time from injury to definitive care was 2 to 4 hours, and the mortality rate dropped to an unprecedented 2.4% (Eiseman, 1967). Success was also related to the presence of highly trained medical teams and the availability of large quantities of whole blood. Refinement in helicopter evacuation of wounded continued during the Vietnam War, when the helicopter truly became the symbol of the war. In this period, 97.5% of the casualties who reached U.S. medical facilities survived and the mean time from field to a corps surgical hospital was only 1 hour (Heaton, 1966). In both the Korean and Vietnam conflicts, helicopters carrying trained paramedics literally brought the emergency room to the victim, dramatically increasing the victim's chance for survival. In addition, no soldier in Vietnam was more than 35 minutes away from a facility capable of delivering definitive life-saving care. Unfortunately, the same is not true regarding traffic victims in the United States today.

Experienced MASH unit veterans, military nurses, and physicians were the first to see the potential of applying the lessons learned in the jungle to domestic settings. They returned to the United States to find a dearth of written standards for competence and training of civilian ambulance attendants in comparison with armed services' medics. Emergency departments were unprepared to care for acutely injured patients. After these veterans described field rescue and survival that was unparalleled on the streets of the United States, organizations such as the American Medical Association (AMA) and the American College of Surgeons (ACS) began to question the nation's priorities in this arena.

TRAUMA SERVICES
Emergency Medical Services

Before the 1960s, little attention was given to emergency medical care. Communication between emergency vehicles and hospital emergency departments was unheard of, and acutely ill patients were "scooped and ran" (also referred to as "scooped and hauled") to the nearest emergency department, regardless of the facility's ability to handle the specific emergency. Community and political education regarding the status of emergency medical services (EMS) and trauma patient care peaked in 1966 with publication of the classic National Research Council/National Academy of Sciences white paper "Accidental Death and Disability: The Neglected Disease of Modern Society" (National Research Council, 1966). This report reflected on the gross deficiencies in prehospital care and proposed a long-range plan for changes in every facet of emergency care. This farsighted report provided the basic blueprint and building blocks for subsequent improvements in EMS programs.

The Highway Safety Traffic Act of 1966 initiated the modern era of emergency care by requiring each state to include emergency medical services as part of its highway safety program. This law authorized federal funding through the Department of Transportation for emergency medical technician (EMT) training and the purchase of ambulances. About the same time, Pantridge and Geddes (1967) demonstrated in Ireland that ventricular fibrillation could be successfully treated outside the hospital and proposed the use of mobile intensive care units. The main purpose of these units was to shorten the time from the initial onset of symptoms to the delivery of medical care. Work in several centers in the United States demonstrated that early intervention in car-

Components of an established EMS program

Provision of workforce
Training of personnel
Communications
Transportation
Facilities
Critical care units
Use of public safety agencies
Consumer participation
Accessibility of care
Transfer of patients
Standard medical record keeping
Consumer information and education
Independent review and evaluation
Disaster linkage
Mutual aid agreements

Based on EMS Act of 1973.

diac conditions could provide impressive advantages before transportation (Cobb, Baum, & Alvarez, 1975). Advanced life support (ALS) units extended the hospital's resources into the community; thus the era of "stabilize and transport" was born.

The EMS Act of 1973 was perhaps the single most important piece of legislation affecting the development of emergency and trauma systems. The act called for the creation of a "lead agency" role under the Department of Health and Welfare and identified 15 components (see box above) to assist system planners in establishing areawide or regional EMS programs (Public Law 93-154, 1973). Most of the current EMS programs were built with the infusion of these federal funds. Better equipment and skill of prehospital providers resulted in rapid transport of injured patients to hospitals closest to the scene of an accident; however, it soon became apparent that transport to the closest facility was not optimal if that hospital lacked the resources and expertise required to treat major trauma victims.

Hospital Services

The EMS Act of 1973 also called for improvements in emergency department care and staffing. Early attempts focused on categorization, or classifying the capabilities of emergency departments

to handle a broad spectrum of emergency conditions. Categorization allowed prehospital care personnel and private citizens to have advanced knowledge of the capabilities of each facility, so that each could choose the appropriate institution for treatment.

Moylan, Detmer, Rose, and Schulz (1976) investigated the relationship between categorization of emergency care and quality, finding a positive correlation between the level of categorization and acceptable care. A similar study reported no correlation between categorization and mortality rate, but concluded that although categorization was useful for establishing standards and improving care, it was inadequate for determining regional health policy or predicting patient outcomes (Detmer, Moylan, Rose, Schulz, & Duke, 1977). In response to these studies and other similar investigations, categorization was expanded to the establishment of standards for the capabilities of emergency facilities to provide care for patients with specific critical care needs.

Classification of trauma services

Optimal care of the trauma patient may require a system to have a tiered response, using several levels of available hospital resources. The American College of Surgeons (ACS) (1976) developed classification guidelines for trauma hospitals in which three levels of resources exist. Level I trauma hospitals, which are usually university-based teaching facilities, (1) provide comprehensive care with in-house specialists and (2) support medical education and research in trauma. Level II trauma hospitals, predominantly community hospitals, provide a level of clinical care similar to that of level I hospitals, using private medical physicians as in-house team leaders with backup on-call (rather than in-house) specialists. Level III trauma hospitals are small neighborhood hospitals or hospitals in rural settings and focus attention on prompt assessment and resuscitation followed by surgical treatment by on-call physicians and interhospital transfer of the most severely injured patients. Appendix A lists the 1990 criteria developed by the ACS Committee on Trauma for each level of hospital resources.

Designation of trauma facilities involves a geopolitical process and goes beyond categorization to include policy enforcement by an authorized agency, usually a governmental body. In this instance, trauma victims are typically directed within a given region to *only* those designated facilities that have undergone a rigorous evaluation process, or a verification of having met ACS criteria. Hospitals are designated "trauma centers" because they have committed resources and assembled teams of professionals with expertise to immediately and effectively treat traumatized individuals.

Trauma system impact   Clear evidence exists that designated regional trauma systems not only improve outcomes after resuscitation in life-threatening situations, but also focus attention on the prehospital arena, promoting better systems of transport to a center where definitive care can be given. West, Trunkey, and Lim (1979) compared trauma care in San Francisco County (in which all major trauma victims were brought to a single level I trauma center) with that in Orange County (in which trauma victims were transported to the closest receiving hospital). One hundred consecutive trauma fatalities from motor vehicle accidents were selected from each area, excluding field deaths and deaths occurring during transport. In Orange County, 73% of the non–central nervous system, in-hospital deaths secondary to motor vehicle trauma were judged to have been preventable, as compared with the deaths in San Francisco County, of which none were considered clearly preventable. As a result of this study, Orange County regionalized trauma care and designated five trauma centers, triaging all major trauma victims to these five facilities. A follow-up study (West, Cales, & Gazzinaga, 1983) reported a substantial reduction in the number of deaths judged preventable at 1 year after designation.

Assuming that large numbers of patients with minor injuries might skew data, reflecting better outcomes, Shackford et al., (1987) examined the impact of a trauma system on the outcome of the most severely injured, comparing observed survival with that of predicted survival, using the TRISS methodology. The observed survival rate was found to be significantly greater than that predicted for patients with severe physiologic derangement (an original Trauma Score <8; see Chapter 7), and improved survival was greatly attributed to the integration of prehospital and hospital care, as well as prompt surgical procedures. The TRISS methodology can be used to estimate the probability of survival based on the trauma

patient's age, the quantification of anatomic injury as measured by the Injury Severity Score, and the physiological status of the patient on admission as determined by the Revised Trauma Score.

Cales, Anderson, and Heilig (1985) studied the use of ambulances, emergency departments, and hospitals before and after implementation of a regional trauma system and reported short-term, insignificant changes in the use of emergency departments. Serious injuries accounted for only 1 of 1000 persons, approximately 1 of 250 emergency department visits, and 1 of 20 ambulance transports. In a regional trauma system, only 5% of all land ambulance–transported patients were redirected past emergency departments to established trauma centers and there were no significant changes in the use or referral patterns of nontrauma emergency department patients.

Regional Trauma Systems
Historical perspectives

In 1961 a pioneering clinical shock-trauma unit was established at the University of Maryland. Using a grant from the U.S. Army, this 2-bed unit was designed as a setting for research regarding the pathophysiologic and immunologic response to shock in humans. This shock-trauma program became the core of the Maryland state EMS system and was later expanded to a 107-bed facility, the only free-standing trauma hospital in the nation. Similarly, the first civilian trauma unit was established in 1966 at Cook County Hospital in Chicago and expanded in 1971 to a statewide system of trauma centers, which combined a total of 50 community hospitals and large medical centers. Three levels of trauma centers were identified, with each level holding specific functional capabilities for the care of the trauma patient. The system eventually incorporated regionalization of unique patient services, such as burn centers and acute spinal cord injury centers. These early efforts produced working models for other states and regions to examine when creating their own unique system for trauma care.

Contemporary perspectives

A regional trauma system consists of hospitals, personnel, and public service agencies that have a planned response for caring for injured patients. The plan must integrate all aspects of care from the time of the accident through the rehabilitative phase when the patient will return to the community. Special problems must be considered, such as geography, population density, community and regional resources, availability of personnel, and the costs of creating a system.

In many regions an abundance of hospitals wish to become trauma centers, and the central planning authority must determine how many hospitals should be designated. This is decided according to population densities, injury occurrence rates, and access routes to health care facilities. The central planning authority, or "lead agency," is the organizational unit responsible for trauma systems development. This role may be fulfilled by a public agency, such as the EMS division of the department of public health, or by a private, nonprofit corporation, such as a trauma foundation.

For every 1 million persons, approximately 500 to 1000 are critically injured every year who require evaluation in a trauma center (ACS, 1990). The volume of patients often determines the number of trauma centers needed in a given geographic area. Regionalization demands that special resources will be concentrated in several select hospitals and that these trauma centers will see an increased volume of seriously injured patients to maintain clinical skill levels and efficient use of specialized equipment. A landmark retrospective study of the Chicago trauma system reported a strong inverse relationship between the volume of seriously injured patients seen and mortality rates (Smith et al., 1990). The authors support configuration of trauma systems so that designated trauma centers would indeed see an increased volume of seriously injured patients. They cautioned that *not* limiting the number of trauma hospitals may have a deleterious effect on the outcome of patients in a given system.

In regard to case/procedure volume requirements for personnel, Luft, Bunker, and Enthoven (1979) reported a positive correlation between surgical patient outcome and the number of high-risk surgical procedures that were performed, indicating that an individual surgeon should manage 50 critical surgical patients per year to maintain skill level. Although a similar study has not been done for trauma patients, it is generally accepted that surgeons will be considered to have adequate experience in trauma surgery if they

treat 50 severe or urgent cases each year. This concept could also be applied to other trauma team members, implying that repeated experience with trauma patients is positively correlated with maintenance of skill levels.

Regionalization of specialized care for burns, replantation of severed limbs, spinal cord injuries, and pediatric trauma patients is often provided for in trauma system development. Regionalizing these services avoids duplication of the necessary level of skill for injuries that represent lower volumes of patients. Centralizing these specialty centers provides a concentration of technology and skill level in an effort to decrease the morbidity and mortality associated with these unique patient populations.

The guidelines for optimal care of the trauma patient in designated centers is generally focused on experience in urban settings. In rural areas few hospitals can provide professional or institutional resources to meet such requirements; therefore one of the most important considerations for a rural trauma system is developing methods for interhospital transfer. As an example, the statewide plan for Oregon incorporates unique standards for interfacility transport between rural and urban trauma centers to meet the diverse geographic needs of this state (Southard & Trunkey, 1990).

Developmental issues

Some regions of the country have learned a valuable lesson from initially creating more trauma centers than needed, which resulted in poor utilization of resources and inability to maintain skill level. Other issues that force hospitals to discontinue trauma center care are malpractice liability coverage costs and the lack of financial reimbursement for indigent trauma patients. In 1985 a network of eight trauma hospitals began to receive trauma patients in Dade County, Florida; however, by 1986 malpractice issues forced all but one hospital to drop out of the system. In the Los Angeles area, escalating financial losses forced restructuring of the trauma system, which was originally configured in 1983, with only one third of the original 25 designated hospitals remaining in the current system.

These problems are being partially addressed on the federal and state levels through the introduction of legislation supporting the development of regional systems and providing a base for un-

---

Trauma Care Systems Planning and Development Act of 1990

1. Conduct and support research, training, evaluations, and demonstration projects with respect to trauma care.
2. Foster the development of appropriate, modern systems of trauma care through the sharing of information among agencies and individuals involved in the study and provision of such care.
3. Provide technical assistance to state and local agencies.
4. Sponsor workshops and conferences.
5. Establish an advisory council on trauma care systems.
6. Establish a national clearinghouse on trauma care and emergency medical services.
7. Establish programs for improving trauma care in rural areas.
8. Develop a model plan for the designation of trauma centers and for triage, transfer, and transportation policies that may be adopted by the states.

---

compensated care. Several states have enacted various forms of legislation, such as surcharges on motor vehicle violations, motor vehicle license registration, or driver's license fees, to offer some financial support for the trauma system. California increased the tax on cigarettes threefold, with the resultant funds to be distributed to emergency medical services and trauma centers. After several years of debate, the Trauma Care System Planning and Development Act of 1990, an amendment to the Public Health Service Act, was signed into law. This act allows for $60 million of support, through grants and technical assistance, for trauma systems development on a state level (Public Law 101-590). The box above summarizes the activities outlined in this important piece of legislation.

A key concept for the establishment of a trauma center within any hospital is commitment, both personal and institutional. Hospitals that demonstrate this commitment can provide a high level of service for injured patients in their community. Optimal care means that costly equipment and experienced personnel must be immediately available 24 hours a day. A priority system must exist for access to support services, such as radiology and laboratory facilities, as well as surgical suites and critical care beds. The demands for the medical staff include availability, surgical resuscitative skill level, and continuing education (ACS, 1990).

TRAUMA CARE CONTINUUM

Hospital care for the trauma patient exists along a continuum, starting with resuscitation in the emergency department or designated area and ending with rehabilitation and discharge. Each area of the hospital contributes specific functions that are integrated into an organized system of care for the most severely injured patients. Recently, two hospital ships were christened by the U.S. Navy, evidence that military organizations have taken a renewed interest in designing systems to care for the wounded in times of war. The hospital ships, former oil tankers, resemble self-sufficient regional trauma centers, with 12 operating rooms and 80 intensive care beds per ship (Harvey, 1988). These ships, the U.S.N.S. Mercy and U.S.N.S. Comfort, were deployed to the Middle East during Operation Desert Storm in 1991 and were staffed by military trauma specialty physicians and nurses (Figure 1-2).

Trauma care systems have made great strides since the decade when medical and nursing personnel with recent battlefield experience began to organize prehospital and hospital care for the traumatically injured patient. Some of this growth, however, has been hampered by the phasing out of funding for EMS, resulting in unevenly distributed state and local trauma systems. By the mid-1980s only 2 states had comprehensive regional trauma systems (see box, p. 11) and 19 states and the District of Columbia had some system components but lacked statewide programs (West, Williams, Trunkey, & Wolferth, 1988). The remaining 29 states had yet to initiate a plan for trauma center designation. A 1985 National Research Council/National Academy of Sciences paper criticized the national neglect of what it saw as the *most* significant health problem in the United States—the epidemic of trauma (National Research Council, 1985).

Trauma care professionals must continue to pursue a solution to this dilemma to ensure the highest quality of care for trauma victims. Creating a system that provides a structure for transporting the right patient (triage) to the right facil-

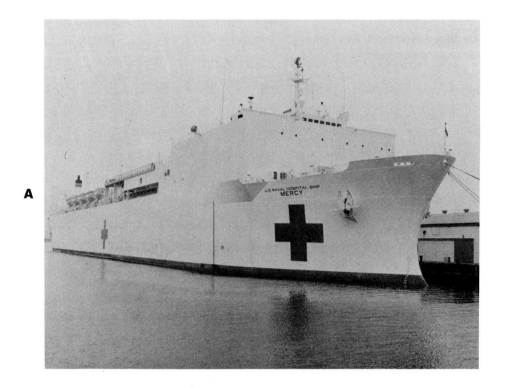

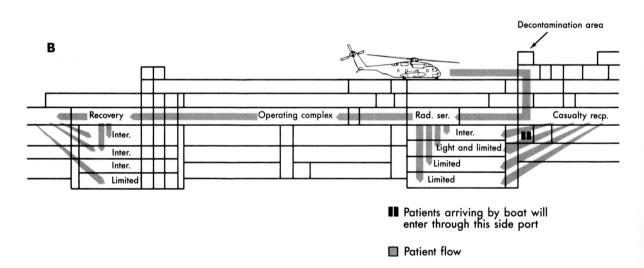

Figure I-2 **A,** One of two U.S. Naval Hospital ships deployed to Middle East during Operation Desert Storm in 1991; **B,** interior of ship. *Inter.,* Intermediate; *Rad. Ser.,* radiology service; *Casualty recp.,* Casualty reception. (Courtesy the Military Sealift Command, Pacific.)

Statewide regional trauma systems

States with all essential components of a regional trauma system

Maryland
Virginia

States that lack one or more components		States with no formal trauma system	
California	New Jersey	Alabama	Minnesota
Delaware	New Mexico	Alaska	Montana
District of Columbia	New York	Arkansas	Nebraska
Florida	North Carolina	Arizona	Nevada
Georgia	Oregon	Colorado	North Dakota
Idaho	Pennsylvania	Connecticut	Ohio
Illinois	Rhode Island	Hawaii	Oklahoma
Mississippi	South Carolina	Indiana	South Dakota
Missouri	Utah	Iowa	Tennessee
New Hampshire	West Virginia	Kansas	Texas
		Kentucky	Vermont
		Louisiana	Washington
		Maine	Wisconsin
		Massachusetts	Wyoming
		Michigan	

Note. Modified from "Trauma Systems: Current Status—Future Challenges" by J.G. West, M.J. Williams, D.D. Trunkey, and C.C. Wolferth, Jr., 1988, *Journal of the American Medical Association, 259* (24), p. 3597.

ity (designation) in the right amount of time (transportation) creates controversies in all areas of the system. The remainder of this chapter will address these components of a regional trauma system.

Prehospital Setting

Triage

Triage is the classification, or sorting, of patients in terms of medical need and disposition. During the Vietnam War, surgeons triaged incoming wounded at the field hospital, determining the order in which patients underwent surgical procedures. In trauma care systems, decisions involve the estimation of injury severity at the scene of the accident. Triage in this setting determines the type of transport used to access care, the level of prehospital transporting personnel, the level of hospital care needed, and the priority of medical intervention. Factors that must be considered in these judgments include the range of resources available and the time or distance to definitive care.

Identifying the small proportion of trauma patients who require prompt access to definitive care remains an enormous challenge, given the adverse conditions at accident scenes. Assessment of the patient's severity of injury is based on determining the extent of force that has been applied to the body, the presence of abnormal clinical signs, and the presence of preexisting medical conditions that may provide deleterious effects for patients with relatively minor trauma.

Trauma severity scoring A variety of physiologic changes occur with anatomic injury, and a number of physiologic severity scores have been developed to mathematically quantify these changes. Routine clinical measurements, such as blood pressure, respiratory rate, and level of consciousness, are used to assess the amount of injury to the vascular structures, respiratory system, and neurologic system and therefore provide an indirect guide to the severity of organ damage. Such a scale must be easy to use and must reliably and accurately predict outcomes, such as probability of death or length of hospitalization. Understandably, no such single parameter has yet to win the ultimate confidence of trauma care personnel.

However, severity indexes that correlate well with outcome are potentially valuable when

---

High-impact variables

- Falls from 20 feet or more
- High speed auto crash of 20 mph or more
    Initial speed of >40 mph
    Velocity change >20 mph
- Pedestrian struck at 5 mph or more
- Space intrusion of >1 foot
- Rear displacement of the front axle
- Rollover or ejection from vehicle
- Significant extrication time (>20 min) required
- Death of another passenger in car
- Motorcycle crash >20 mph

---

added to other observations that indicate a large amount of force applied to the victim. Because of short prehospital response times and strong compensatory mechanisms, physiologic changes may not be present on initial examination. It is therefore useful to note in the history and physical the estimated amount of force involved to properly identify those patients who are at great risk of having severe injuries. Such variables as the height of fall, the structural deformation of a vehicle, and the speed of the vehicle can be used to estimate the amount and direction of force applied to the patient's body. The box above shows variables that signify high-impact incidents and should be considered when directing trauma patients to the appropriate health care facility.

Patients who might be more susceptible to injury are those at either end of the life span, when compensatory drives are lessened. Age and the presence of preexisting medical conditions, such as cardiac disease, should heighten the trauma care provider's awareness of the increased consequences of trauma for these patients.

Until a system is developed to correctly identify all patients for appropriate levels of care, there will be a number of patients who are incorrectly triaged. *Undertriage* refers to patients who are incorrectly identified as *not* needing trauma center care and who may die because of failure to reach a system in a short time. *Overtriage* refers to patients who are incorrectly directed to trauma centers for care when retrospectively they could have been cared for in a community emergency department. The two "errors" in triage are very interde-

pendent, and a large percentage of overtriage might be necessary to keep undertriage at a safe level (West, Murdock, Baldwin, & Whalen, 1986).

The system for triage in urban environments is somewhat different from that in rural areas, where access to definitive care may involve longer distances and greater prehospital time periods. If injury occurs more than 30 minutes away from a trauma care facility, a stronger argument can be made for treating patients initially at the nearest available hospital, with secondary triage to the more distant level I or II trauma center in a timely manner.

Treatment

The supposition on which most prehospital care systems have been built is that much can be done to improve outcome before arrival at a hospital. Extending hospital capabilities in the community by using mobile intensive care units was initiated to decrease the number of cardiac arrest patients who died before reaching a hospital. Prehospital care is the first phase of trauma care but does not necessarily provide similar advantages for trauma patients, because stabilization at the scene lengthens the time to surgical intervention.

Those who emphasize the need for regional trauma systems also advocate prehospital care improvements. This includes having paramedics available in the early phase of trauma care to perform invasive resuscitative techniques, such as controlling a compromised airway, preventing aspiration, and starting intravenous infusions to limit the effects of exsanguination. Frey, Huelke, and Gikas (1969) concluded that improvements in initial care could have improved survivability in 18% of those who died before reaching a hospital. These findings were supported by a later study that attributed successful outcomes to the presence of trained paramedical personnel (West, Cales, & Gazzinaga, 1983).

Conversely, others believe that time is the enemy of the trauma patient and advanced life support (ALS) procedures do require time for execution. Proponents emphasize the importance of prompt evacuation, and time to operative intervention is considered to be the single most important factor influencing outcome. Gervin and Fischer (1982) showed that delayed transport as a result of field interventions is associated with a decrease in survival after penetrating cardiac trauma.

The "scoop and haul" versus "stay and stabilize" debate has been repeatedly examined; however, both sides readily agree that time influences outcomes for the severely injured and that a crucial task for all prehospital personnel is that of reducing the time from injury to surgical intervention. The application of advanced life support should be individualized for each situation, with early evacuation of all patients and stabilization perhaps best performed while en route to a trauma care facility.

Transportation

The goals of trauma transportation include the provision of prompt response by qualified professionals who are responsible for extrication, stabilization, and transport to the nearest appropriate trauma center. In most instances a ground unit is the first ambulance dispatched to the accident scene. In urban areas several types of response systems may be used. In a single response system, an ALS unit is dispatched to every call; it is hoped that the victim's injuries will justify its use. A more cost-effective means of providing care involves a dual response system, in which the first unit dispatched is a basic life support (BLS) unit. The BLS team initiates life-saving measures and activates an ALS unit if deemed necessary. A third option includes simultaneous dispatch of a fire department BLS unit and a transporting ALS unit.

In rural settings a single response is most often used. The ground ambulance may stabilize the patient on the scene if transport is to be longer than 30 minutes, or it may proceed to the nearest hospital where the patient can be stabilized before transport to a trauma center. ALS units are uncommon in this setting, because maintaining skill levels is too great a financial burden for most rural communities where trauma patient encounters are limited.

Air transport   The use of helicopter transport for trauma patients continues to be investigated in a variety of settings. Aeromedical transportation costs are high in comparison with ground alternatives and in many regions the impetus to use helicopters is somewhat driven by economics—primarily to generate revenue by increasing patient census rather than to meet medical needs. Other systems use air ambulances as a means to transport patients expeditiously from remote areas or past congested traffic routes. Fischer, Flynn, Miller, and Duke (1984) reported that helicopter response teams staffed by skilled physicians and flight nurses provided an invaluable service for trauma patients in large, densely populated metropolitan areas. Air transport can be used also as an extension of a regional trauma system to isolated rural areas. In this instance operative stabilization of life-threatening conditions at the local facility precedes rapid transport to the urban trauma center, and air transport is of prime importance in obtaining definitive care. Both helicopter and fixed-wing aircraft may be integral components for rural trauma care networks.

Staffing the rotorcraft with highly trained personnel creates yet another controversy. The first helicopter system in the United States used existing police helicopters to transport trauma patients, staffed only by BLS-prepared state police medic observers (Cowley, Hudson, Scanlan & Trump, 1973)—a program of basic life support techniques and rapid transport over moderate distances. In sharp contrast, Baxt and Moody (1983) reported a 52% reduction in predicted mortality for patients transported by a helicopter staffed by a physician and nurse team. The authors postulate that a decrease in mortality is partially reflective of the application of advanced treatment modalities and continuity of medical care teams. What remains undisputed is that helicopter transports significantly improve outcome by decreasing transport times, and therefore criteria for air ambulance use should be based on medical standards that optimize care at realistic cost levels. (For further information regarding helicopter transport refer to Chapter 20.)

Hospital Setting

Hospital care for the traumatically injured patient exists along a continuum, using all of the major treatment areas—from the emergency department to the rehabilitation unit. Traumatic injuries are complex, frequently involving more than one body region. Successful intervention requires aggressive, timely actions by a number of specialty personnel. Delays in care at any level of re-

Suggested personnel involved in trauma resuscitation

Trauma resuscitation team members

Trauma surgeon
Emergency physician
Anesthesiologist
Emergency department nurse
Nurse recorder
Laboratory technician
Blood bank technician
Radiology technician
Respiratory therapist

Trauma support team members

Social service staff member/chaplain
Intensive care nurse
Perioperative nurse
Security personnel
Nursing house supervisor
Clinical pharmacist

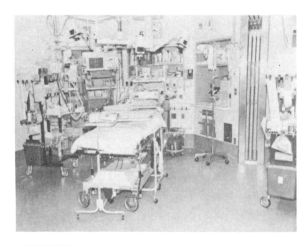

Figure 1-3 Trauma resuscitation area. (*Note.* From "Shock Trauma: The Culmination of a Dream" by B.J. Breeze, and P.C. Epifanio, 1989, *Journal of Emergency Nursing, 15* [5], p. 29A.)

suscitation can result in unnecessary morbidity and possibly death. To maximize efficiency and avoid duplication of effort, most trauma care facilities maintain a trauma response team. Suggested members for a trauma response team are listed in the box above.

Trauma team

The trauma team can be activated whenever prehospital triage indicates that a patient would benefit from rapid access to trauma care. Team members respond to a designated trauma resuscitation area and prepare for patient arrival, clarifying team roles and delegating tasks to promote a coordinated approach to stabilization. The resuscitation area should contain all equipment necessary to resuscitate and stabilize major trauma victims (Figure 1-3). Disorganization greatly decreases the acute trauma patient's chance of survival, and therefore the trauma team operates under prearranged protocols, which are usually based on the guidelines provided in the ACS Advanced Trauma Life Support course. The purpose of trauma treatment protocols is to define a priority system for trauma patients, using a uniform, highly specific set of guidelines.

The organization of trauma teams includes the identification of a team leader for optimal team interaction. The team leader must coordinate the treatment plan and collaborate efficiently with all members. The skills, knowledge base, and responsibilities of the trauma surgeon are significantly different from those of the emergency physician, and the identification of a trauma team leader has historically created "turf battles" between the two groups. Emergency physicians are skilled and practiced in the art of resuscitation and airway control, interventions that are essential for treatment of life-threatening injuries. Trauma is, however, a surgical condition, with the needs of the most severely injured patients mandating prompt surgical intervention. Many institutions recognize the value of combining both areas of expertise and have clearly outlined the areas of care that the individual specialists are responsible for. Resuscitation and early surgical involvement must be combined in such a manner to facilitate patient care rather than delay it.

In a university setting the team may include physician residents from general surgery, family practice, and emergency medicine, with varying levels of skill. Roles must be clearly delineated and identified early, with a senior resident assuming the role of team captain.

Trauma resuscitation area

The location of the trauma resuscitation area varies from setting to setting. The majority of trauma care facilities provide for trauma patient resuscitation within a defined area of the emergency department, which is stocked with specialized equipment necessary for life-saving interventions. Other facilities create a resuscitation area close to the operating room or intensive care unit, which may be a substantial distance from the emergency department (Morgan, Berger, Land, & Schwab, 1986). A small group of patients require direct admission to the operating room. Indications for operating room resuscitation include cardiac arrest after penetrating trauma, major amputation, and complex wounds with hypotension (Shackford, 1988). Roles and responsibilities for the trauma team are essentially the same regardless of where the patient is resuscitated.

Trauma resuscitation nurse

Trauma resuscitation nurses represent the core of team involvement, playing a vital role in quick assessment, preparation of equipment, and team coordination. Emergency department nurses usually assume this role, which involves complex clinical problem solving while maintaining smooth team interaction. Trauma resuscitation nurses must expeditiously combine intellectual and technical skills, adjusting clinical decisions quickly and appropriately. Often the surgeon performs a brief assessment for life- or limb-threatening injuries, and a total assessment is planned for later stages of care. The trauma nurse can follow the patient through all phases of resuscitation and continually assess the patient for life-threatening injuries, as well as subacute problems that can be treated later. The Emergency Nurses Association established the Trauma Nursing Core Course as a means to educate and to verify basic trauma nursing knowledge.

The trauma resuscitation nurse (TRN) role may also be fulfilled by a specially trained intensive care nurse, who can offer critical care expertise and continuity of care along the spectrum of trauma care (Waters & Haun, 1986). In the emergency department the TRN assumes primary responsibility for monitoring vital signs and accurately assessing the patient's response to diagnostic procedures or treatment interventions. The TRN can also (1) accompany the patient throughout special diagnostic testing, such as angiography or computerized tomography scanning, (2) continue to act as patient advocate during surgical intervention, and (3) care for the patient in the intensive care unit. The goals of this system are to maximize continuity, foster efficient communication, and provide consistent psychologic support for trauma patients and their families.

Often the TRN is the sole health care member consistently at the patient's bedside and therefore can establish trust. Trauma patients and families require continual crisis intervention and intense support through all phases of trauma care, and trauma nurses are in a unique position to meet these needs.

Another model of trauma nursing team organization involves the use of nursing personnel from the emergency department, the intensive care unit, and the operating room as collaborative members of the resuscitation team. The skills of each nurse can be combined as part of team protocols to allow for maximum benefit to the patient. The emergency nurse can provide quick assessment and rapid prioritization of team responsibilities. The intensive care nurse assumes the role of monitoring nurse, providing critical continued physical assessment and evaluating the patient's response to treatment. The surgical nurse can assist with invasive procedures and facilitate prompt transfer to the operating suite. The skills of all three areas of nursing expertise are not mutually exclusive, and the synergy of nursing action can provide a collaborative base for quality patient care.

In any facility, nursing team member roles should be carefully planned according to the staffing resources each area of the trauma center can consistently provide, and job descriptions should be clearly outlined. Team members who do not work primarily in resuscitative settings should be involved in a brief orientation course that includes an overview of the prehospital system, resuscitative protocols, equipment skill laboratories, and review of trauma resuscitation area layout. Nurses new to trauma care can be "buddied" with experienced trauma nurses for a number of resuscitations to further demonstrate role responsibilities and assist with problem solving.

Emergent care of the trauma patient often precludes providing the ideal learning environment for the trauma orientee; therefore clearly communicated roles and standardized room layout support smooth interaction among team members.

The nature of trauma care lends itself readily to prevention programs and patient education. Nurses in all areas of the trauma center can establish the trusting atmosphere needed to discuss ways that patients can avoid serious injury in the future. Patient and public education programs can be organized by the nursing staff to address such topics as alcohol or drug use while driving, the use of seat belts and infant restraint seats, and the proper use of protective gear for recreational or occupational safety.

Nursing involvement is crucial to system integration, and the designation of trauma centers has supported the growth of trauma nursing as a specialty and created opportunities for advanced nursing roles. The trauma nurse coordinator (TNC) is a registered nurse who possesses expert knowledge in the practice of trauma nursing care and is responsible for the administration of the trauma management system (Beachley, Snow, & Trimble, 1988). The TNC must collaborate with other team members to develop standards of care for trauma patients and must continually monitor the effectiveness of the trauma team through quality assurance activities. Although the role of TNC is fairly common in most designated trauma centers, two unique nursing roles have been developed in established centers to meet specific objectives. The use of nurse practitioners was introduced in a university-based tertiary care facility to provide assistance to the overburdened housestaff in response to a rapidly rising trauma patient volume (Spisso, O'Callaghan, McKennan, & Holcroft, 1990). The nurse practitioners evaluate patient progression through the hospital and recommend appropriate treatment modalities based on standard procedures. In one community hospital setting, a trauma case manager role was created to provide support for the medical team and to serve as advocate for the multidisciplinary needs of the trauma patient (Holmquist, Songne, Shaver, & Pierog, 1991). The role incorporates utilization management techniques with clinical nursing expertise and may optimize quality of care while decreasing the average length of stay for trauma patients.

TRAUMA CARE EVALUATION

The evaluation of trauma care delivery is accomplished through a variety of activities, each using explicit standards to identify problems. Medical standards of care have been defined by the American College of Surgeons and relate to the timeliness of physician response, the accuracy and timeliness of diagnosis and treatment, and the review of patient outcomes. Monitoring of these standards involves data collection, peer review, and clinical case audits.

Medical records can be used to assess trauma system care retrospectively. Data collection is usually organized in a trauma registry, a tool designed to contain detailed data related to such factors as response time intervals, vital signs, diagnostic examinations, and surgical procedures. The Major Trauma Outcome Study (MTOS) combined patient data from trauma centers throughout the country for comparison of trauma patient populations. More than 120,000 trauma patients from the United States, Canada, Australia, and the United Kingdom have been submitted to this pool of data, which was coordinated by the American College of Surgeon's Committee on Trauma (Champion et al., 1990). This national trauma patient data base was used to revise the TRISS model (see p. 127), which is still widely used for trauma hospital evaluations of patient outcome, based on predictions of trauma patient survival.

Peer review can be accomplished through morbidity and mortality conferences, daily rounds of the surgical team, and multidisciplinary case conferences. Many trauma centers use videotape recordings of trauma resuscitations as a means of team evaluation and education. Retrospective review of resuscitation tapes provides the team with opportunities to identify problems, educate new team members, and evaluate program changes that have been instituted to solve previous problems (Hoyt et al., 1988). Team members can view these tapes concurrently to analyze priority setting by the team, interaction of team members, and adherence to standardized protocols. Simply observing one's actions in a recorded trauma resuscitation may profoundly encourage needed behavioral changes.

Trauma nursing care standards have yet to be established nationally, although several trauma care facilities have created individual nursing performance standards. The Society of Trauma Nurses developed standards for trauma nursing education and designation that may provide trauma care systems with the initial means of establishing specific trauma nursing audits. Recently the Emergency Nurses' Association Trauma Committee spearheaded a collaborative effort among nursing specialty groups (National Flight Nurses' Association, American Association of Critical Care Nurses, Association of Operating Room Nurses, American Association of Nurse Anesthetists, and Association of Rehabilitation Nursing) to create a trauma nursing resource document. The nursing care guidelines, which were patterned after the ACS Optimal Resources document, outline personnel and equipment standards, as well as required nursing qualifications for those who care for trauma patients.

Because of the multidisciplinary nature of issues associated with trauma center organization and evaluation, an interdepartmental committee is usually established in trauma centers to provide periodic review of system coordination and participation in problem solving. Representatives from all ancillary departments and nursing and medical divisions should be included to provide operational direction for the actual trauma team.

Ongoing assessment of individual and trauma system performance usually includes periodic site review by a team of nationally recognized experts in trauma care. The survey team may tour the physical plant to review transport modes and availability of equipment. Review of nursing departments includes the assessment of the number of nursing staff allocated to trauma care departments and the current knowledge and skill levels of the nursing staff. In addition to reviewing prepared materials that document these skills, the reviewer often interviews nurses throughout the trauma center to validate the nursing staff's knowledge of trauma care (Hollingsworth-Fridlund, Andrews, & Hoyt, 1989). Clinical care, however, is predominantly evaluated by the survey team through review of the documentation in the trauma patients' medical records. A specified, well-designed trauma flow sheet can facilitate documentation of trauma nursing care delivered when the trauma patient's status is rapidly changing and many aspects of care are delivered at an accelerated rate (Frankel & Southard, 1989).

SUMMARY Trauma care systems provide a preplanned response for meeting the needs of seriously injured victims. An effective system involves accurate identification of major trauma victims and rapid transport to a designated trauma center where definitive care can be provided. Regionalization of trauma care requires that many interdependent components be functional and effective. Trauma nurses are involved in all aspects of trauma care delivery, providing a vital link between trauma team members and supporting continuity of care. Trauma nursing continues to be a growing specialty area and offers unique opportunities for nurses to expand their area of expertise.

RESEARCH QUESTIONS

- What nursing skills are most important for the optimal outcome of trauma patients? What basic information should be considered core level knowledge for all trauma nurses?
- Which nursing specialty area should assume primary responsibility for trauma patients during the resuscitative phase (emergency department, operating suite, or intensive care unit)?
- What methods are most effective for trauma nurses to use in maintaining continuous technical skill levels and assuring core trauma knowledge?
- What preexisting medical conditions have a pronounced effect on patient survival or outcome? What physical indicators of these conditions should be used in triage? in continuous nursing assessments?
- What is the impact of trauma center designation on nurse staffing at non–trauma care centers?
- Does designation as a trauma center aid in the recruitment and retention of nursing staff?

RESOURCES*

American Association of Automotive Medicine
40 Second Ave.
Arlington Heights, IL 60005
(708) 390-8927

American College of Surgeons, Committee on Trauma
National Advanced Trauma Life Support (ATLS)
55 E. Erie St.
Chicago, IL 60611
(312) 664-4050

---

*This list is partial; any resource not included was solely by oversight.

American Trauma Society
1400 Mercantile Lane, Suite 188
Landover, MD 20785
(301) 925-8811

Center for Injury Prevention
Trauma Foundation, Building One, Room 306
San Francisco General Hospital
San Francisco, CA 94110
(415) 821-8209

Emergency Nurses Association
Trauma Nursing Committee
Trauma Nursing Core Course (TNCC)
230 E. Ohio St., Suite 600
Chicago, IL 60611
(312) 649-0297

Foundation for Burns and Trauma, Inc.
PO Box 80055
Phoenix, AZ 85060
(602) 277-6115

Harborview Injury Prevention Center
Harborview Medical Center
325 9th Ave.
Seattle, WA 98104
(206) 223-8388

Maryland Institute for Emergency Medical Services Systems
   (MIEMSS)
22 South Greene St.
Baltimore, MD 21203
(301) 328-3156

National Highway Traffic Safety Administration
U.S. Dept. of Transportation
400 7th St. SW
Washington, DC 20590
(202) 366-0123

National Safety Council
44 N. Michigan Ave.
Chicago, IL 60611
(312) 527-4800

National Study Center for Trauma
Trauma Information Exchange Systems (TIES)
Emergency Health Services Research Center (EHSRC)
22 So. Greene St.
Baltimore, MD 21203
1-800-872-2820

Orange County Trauma Society
321 N. Rampart Ave.
Orange, CA 92668
(714) 591-0602

Oregon Trauma Research and Education Foundation
c/o Emanuel Hospital
2801 Gantenbein
Portland, OR 97227
(503) 280-4960

Pennsylvania Trauma Systems Foundation
5070 Ritter Road, Suite 100
Mechanicsburg, PA 17055
(717) 697-5512

Society of Trauma Nurses
888 17th Street NW, Suite 1000
Washington, DC 20006
(301) 328-3930

Trauma Research and Education Foundation
c/o Mercy Hospital
4077 5th Avenue
San Diego, CA 92103
(619) 295-5428

TRAUMA NURSING GRADUATE PROGRAMS*

University of Alabama School of Nursing
University Station
Birmingham, AL 35294
(205) 934-6070

University of California, San Francisco
Dept. of Physiological Nursing N611Y
San Francisco, CA 94143
(415) 476-0999

University of Maryland at Baltimore
Trauma/Critical Nursing
655 W. Lombard St.
Baltimore, MD 21201
(301) 328-6198

University of Pittsburgh School of Nursing
Univ. of Pittsburgh
Pittsburgh, PA 15261
(412) 624-2404

University of Texas Health Science Center at Houston
1100 Holcombe Blvd.
Houston, TX 77030
(713) 792-7800

University of Washington
Dept. of Physiological Nursing SM-28
Seattle, WA 98195
(206) 543-1091

Vanderbilt University School of Nursing
102 Godchaux Hall
Nashville, TN 37240
(615) 322-2815

Widener University
Graduate Nursing
Chester, PA 19013
(215) 499-4207

---

*Any trauma-related graduate nursing program excluded was solely by oversight. Many other colleges and universities offer trauma practicums or allow a student to focus on trauma care while enrolled in other nursing majors, such as critical care or medical-surgical nursing. The author advises interested parties to investigate this on an individual basis.

ANNOTATED BIBLIOGRAPHY

Beachley, M., & Snow, S. (1988). Developing trauma care systems: A nursing perspective. *Journal of Nursing Administration, 18*(4), 22-29.
  A brief review of the history of trauma care in the United States, emphasizing nursing's role and outlining nursing responsibilities for future system development. Includes discussion of the nursing department's role in the phases of individual trauma center development.

Boyd, D., Edlich, R., & Micik, S. (1983). *Systems approach to emergency medical care.* Norwalk, CT: Appleton-Century-Crofts.
  An excellent resource book documenting the experience of developed emergency medical systems in the United States. Provides an extensive review of the components of an emergency medical system including medical control, training, transport modes, and system evaluation. Discusses key clinical components including cardiac, poison, and multiple trauma–related services, such as burn, spinal, and head injuries.

Cales, R., & Heilig, R. (1986). *Trauma care systems.* Rockville, MD: Aspen Publishers.
  Addresses an organized, systematic approach to trauma care, with both administrative and clinical components, along the continuum of triage to rehabilitation. Contains appendixes of standards that provide the structure for trauma care systems.

Dunn, E., Berry, P., & Cross, R. (1986). Community hospital to trauma center. *Journal of Trauma, 26*(8), 733-737.
  A detailed review of the financial and organizational needs for building a system of trauma care within one facility. Contains a review of nursing activities related to the establishment of standardized education and clinical protocols.

West, J., Williams, M., Trunkey, D., & Wolferth, C. (1988). Trauma systems: Current status—future challenges. *Journal of the American Medical Association, 259*(24), 3597-3600.
  A discussion of the essential components of a regional trauma system and analysis of the current state of affairs in the United States related to the designation of trauma centers. Provides background information for nursing managers and staff involved in improving trauma care delivery systems.

REFERENCES

American College of Surgeons, Committee on Trauma. (1976). Optimal hospital resources for the care of the seriously injured. *Bulletin American College of Surgeons, 61*(9):15-22.

American College of Surgeons, Committee on Trauma. (1990). Resources for optimal care of the injured patient. *Bulletin American College of Surgeons, 75*(9), 20-29.

Baxt, W., & Moody, P. (1983). The importance of rotorcraft aeromedical emergency medical services on trauma mortality. *Journal of the American Medical Association, 249*(22), 3047-3051.

Beachley, M., Snow, S., & Trimble, P. (1988). Developing trauma care systems: The trauma nurse coordinator. *Journal of Nursing Administration, 18*(7), 34-42.

Beebe, G., & DeBakey, M. (1952). *Battle casualties: Incidence, mortality and logistic considerations.* Springfield, IL: Charles C. Thomas.

Cales, R., Anderson, P., & Heilig, R. (1985). Utilization of medical care in Orange County: The effect of implementation of a regional trauma system. *Annals of Emergency Medicine, 14*, 853-858.

Champion, H., Copes, W., Sacco, W., Lawnick, M., Keast, S., Bain, L., Flanagan, M., & Frey, C. (1990). The major trauma outcome study: Establishing national norms for trauma care. *Journal of Trauma, 30* (11), 1356-1365.

Cobb, L., Baum, R., & Alvarez, H. (1975). Resuscitation from out-of-hospital ventricular fibrillation: 4 year follow-up. *Circulation, 51-52* (Suppl III), 223-235.

Cowley, R., Hudson, F., Scanlan, E., & Trump, B. (1973). An economical and proved helicopter program for transporting the emergency critically ill and injured patient in Maryland. *Journal of Trauma, 13*, 1029-1038.

Detmer, D., Moylan, J., Rose, J., Schulz, R., & Duke, J. (1977). Regional categorization and quality of care in major trauma. *Journal of Trauma, 17*, 592-599.

Dible, J. (1970). *Napoleon's surgeon.* London: Heinemann Medical Books.

Eiseman, B. (1967). Combat casualty management in Vietnam. *Journal of Trauma, 7*, 53-63.

Fischer, R., Flynn, T., Miller, P., & Duke, J. (1984). Urban helicopter response to scene of injury. *Journal of Trauma, 24*(1), 946-951.

Frankel, P., & Southard, P. (1989). Trauma care documentation: A comprehensive guide. *Journal of Emergency Nursing, 15* (5), 393-398.

Frey, C., Huelke, D., & Gikas, P. (1969). Resuscitation and survival in motor vehicle accidents. *Journal of Trauma, 9*, 292-310.

Gervin, A., & Fischer, R. (1982). The importance of prompt transport in salvage of patients with penetrating heart wounds. *Journal of Trauma, 22*, 443-448.

Harvey, M. (1988). [untitled]. *UCLA Nursing, 5*(1), 12-13.

Heaton, L. (1966). Army medical services activities in Vietnam. *Military Medicine, 131*, 646-647.

Hollingworth-Fridlund, P., Andrews, J., & Hoyt, K.S. (1989). Preparing for hospital site review for trauma center designation: A survey of nurse evaluators. *Journal of Emergency Nursing, 15* (5), 405-409.

Holmquist, P., Songne, E., Shaver, T., & Pierog, L. (1991). Trauma case manager development and implementation as a nursing role in a community trauma center. *Journal of Trauma, 31* (1), 103-106.

Hoyt, D., Shackford, S., Hollingsworth-Fridlund, P., Mackersie, R., Hansbrough, J., Wachtel, T., & Fortune, J. (1988). Video recording trauma resuscitations: An effective teaching technique. *Journal of Trauma, 28* (4), 435-440.

Luft, H., Bunker, J., & Enthoven, A. (1979). Should operations be regionalized? The empirical relation between surgical volume and mortality. *New England Journal of Medicine, 301*, 1364-1369.

Morgan, T., Berger, P., Land, S., & Schwab, C. (1986). Trauma center and the operating room. *AORN Journal, 44*(3), 417-426.

Moylan, J., Detmer, D., Rose, J., & Schulz, R. (1976). Evaluation of the quality of hospital care for major trauma. *Journal of Trauma, 16*, 517-523.

National Research Council. (1966). *Accidental death and disability: The neglected disease of modern society.* Washington, DC: National Academy Press.

National Research Council. (1985). *Injury in America: A continuing public health problem*. Washington, DC: National Academy Press.

Pantridge, J., & Geddes, J. (1967). A mobile intensive care unit in the management of myocardial infarction. *Lancet*, 2, 271-273.

Public Law 93-154. (1973). *EMS Systems Act of 1973*. 93rd United States Congress.

Public Law 101-590. (1990). *Trauma Care Systems Planning and Development Act of 1990*. 101st United States Congress.

Shackford, S., Cooper, G., Hollingsworth-Fridlund, P., & Eastman, A. (1986). The effect of regionalization upon the quality of trauma care as assessed by concurrent audit prior to and after institution of a trauma system: A preliminary report. *Journal of Trauma*, 9, 812-820.

Shackford, S., Baxt, W., Hoyt, D., Baxt, W., Eastman, A., Hammill, F., Knotts, F., & Virgilio, R. (1987). The impact of a trauma system upon the outcome of severely injured patients. *Archives of Surgery*, 122, 523-527.

Shackford, S. (1988). Initial resuscitation. In University of California San Diego, Division of Trauma (Eds.), *Trauma and burn manual* (pp 10-12). San Diego: UCSD Medical Center.

Sharar, S., Luna, G., Rice, C., Valenzuela, T., & Copass, M. (1988). Air transport following surgical stabilization: An extension of regionalized trauma care. *Journal of Trauma*, 28(6), 794-797.

Smith, R., Frateschi, L., Sloan, E., Campbell, L., Krieg, R., Edwards, L., & Barrett, J. (1990). The impact of volume on outcome in seriously injured trauma patients: Two years experience of the Chicago trauma system. *Journal of Trauma*, 30 (9), 1066-1076.

Southard, P., & Frankel, P. (1989). Trauma care documentation: A comprehensive guide. *Journal of Emergency Nursing*, 15 (5), 393-398.

Southard, P., & Trunkey, D. (1990). Rural trauma: The Oregon experiment. *Journal of Emergency Nursing*, 16 (5), 321-325.

Spisso, J., O'Callaghan, C., McKennan, M., & Holcroft, J. (1990). Improved quality of care and reduction of house-staff workload using trauma nurse practitioners. *Journal of Trauma*, 30 (6), 660-663.

Trunkey, D. (1983). Trauma. *Scientific American*. 249, 28-35.

Waters, S., & Haun, M. (1986). Trauma resuscitation nurse: A career development option for the experienced critical care nurse. *Dimensions in Critical Care Nursing*, 5(6), 369-373.

West, J., Trunkey, D., & Lim, R. (1979). Systems of trauma care: A study of two counties. *Archives of Surgery*, 114, 455-460.

West, J., Cales, R., & Gazzinaga, A. (1983). Impact of regionalization: The Orange County experience. *Archives of Surgery*, 118, 740-744.

West, J., Murdock, M., Baldwin, L., & Whalen, E. (1986). A method for evaluation of field triage criteria. *Journal of Trauma*, 26, 653-659.

West, J., Williams, M., Trunkey, D., & Wolferth, C. (1988). Trauma systems: Current status, future challenges. *Journal of the American Medical Association*, 259, 3597-3600.

2 Prevention of Traumatic Injury

Pamela Stinson Kidd

OBJECTIVES
- ❏ Identify risk factors associated with traumatic injury.
- ❏ Examine the emotional and cognitive aspects of risk-taking behavior.
- ❏ Discuss sociocultural influences on driving behavior.
- ❏ Examine the role of the trauma nurse in the prevention of traumatic injury.

INTRODUCTION This chapter discusses prevention of traumatic injury from a personal and professional perspective. Risk-taking behavior is discussed to identify susceptibility factors during patient assessment. Although traumatic injuries in general are discussed, motor vehicle crashes (MVCs) are the main focus, because MVCs are the number one killer of Americans between the ages of 1 and 34 years (National Committee for Injury Prevention and Control [NCIPC], 1989). Traffic deaths cost society an average of $425,000 per fatality (Miller, Luchter, & Brinkman, 1988). It has been estimated that the total medical costs per critical injury averages $138,000 (NHTSA, 1988). Overall, 142,000 Americans died in 1985 as a result of traumatic injury. Injury is a major public health problem (Committee on Trauma Research, 1985). The discussion of injury prevention is important in a book devoted to addressing nursing care of the trauma patient. All nurses are responsible for incorporating preventive health measures as part of their general or specialized practice. Smeltzer (1988) identified a schematic model for research in trauma nursing (Figure 2-1). A phase in this model is antecedent events. She states that nursing research should concentrate on prevention of trauma by identifying (1) characteristics of patients at risk for traumatic in-

jury, (2) why they are at risk, and (3) how nursing can diminish this risk.

RISK PERCEPTIONS

The definition of risk varies from person to person. It must mean more than the number of fatalities associated with an event, since MVCs are consistently ranked lower in terms of threat than is a nuclear event. There appear to be some enduring, personality-related components to the motivational aspects of risk taking (Knowles, 1977). For instance, some individuals become involved in events that have uncertain outcomes because to those individuals the uncertainty is an essential, sought-after component of the event (Machlis & Rosa, 1990). Recreational forms of risk taking, such as hang gliding and rappelling, may fit into this category. The opposite of this may be "involuntary risk." These situations involve being in the "wrong place" at the "wrong time." Health care providers promote the perception of involuntary risk by referring to the trauma *patient* as the trauma *victim*. In reality, choices may have been made by the patient before the event that increased his or her personal vulnerability.

The perception of involuntary risk is promoted also by society's use of the term "accident" when

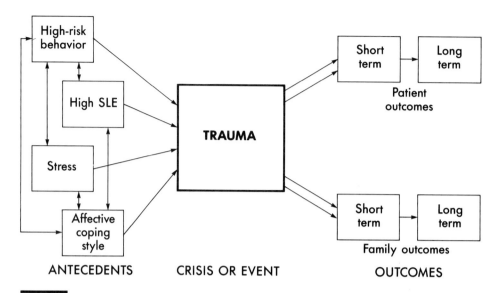

Figure 2-1   Model for trauma nursing research. This schematic model illustrates the three phases of trauma: antecedents (including high-risk behaviors, stressful life events (SLE), stress, and affective coping styles); traumatic event; and short-term and long-term outcomes related to the patient and family. This model illustrates the inter-relationships of these factors. (*Note.* Redrawn from "Research in Trauma Nursing: State of the Art and Future Directions" by S.C. O'Connell Smeltzer, 1988, *Journal of Emergency Nursing, 14* [3], p. 145.)

discussing traumatic injury and death. The World Heath Organization (WHO) defines an accident as an unpremeditated event resulting in recognizable damage (WHO, 1986). This definition is global and does not attempt to explain how one determines whether an event was unintentional or what object has sustained recognizable damage (e.g., the motor vehicle, person, or both). The use of the term *accident* does not explain why certain injury-producing events (e.g., MVCs) occur in predictable and repeatable patterns but rather assumes a random nature of occurrence (Houck, 1986). Traumatic injuries are viewed as resulting from chance or fate. Perception and acceptance of risk are based on social and cultural factors. What is considered in one society as risky may not be viewed as risky in another. Western culture encourages freedom, adventure, and courageous behavior. The differences between courageous behavior and risk taking are not clear. Society may not be willing to label certain behaviors as risky, since individuals who are not considered

deviant frequently perform these behaviors. To illustrate, involvement in a MVC is not considered deviant or socially undesirable behavior.

Most Americans feel they face more risk today than in the past, whereas the experts have the opposite view (Slovic, 1987). One tends to evaluate risks after viewing a signal of vulnerability, (e.g., airplane crash). Involvement in an injury-producing event can trigger personal reappraisal of vulnerability. Risk perceptions may form after an event occurs. For example, being involved in a MVC versus reading about a MVC in the newspaper may have a greater influence on driving. People tend to deny that their own actions are responsible for negative outcomes, as a way of maintaining self-esteem (Weinstein, 1984). If an action is viewed as controllable (e.g., driving), and a negative event occurs (i.e., MVC), a greater threat to self-esteem is experienced. Health threats viewed by the individual as controllable in nature are more likely to have a decreased admission of risk. Risk-decreasing factors, such as driving within the speed limit, may have a greater impact on comparative risk judgments than risk-increasing factors, such as drinking alcoholic beverages and driving. Therefore a person's "net" view may be that he or she has minimal driving risk because he or she drives within the speed limit while drinking alcoholic beverages. Individuals have an optimistic view of personal risk factors.

Risk-Taking Behavior

Risk-taking behavior has been linked to physiologic, cultural, and sociologic causes. In some studies, individuals who selected riskier situations had higher monoamine oxidase and testosterone levels (Farley, 1986; Zuckerman, 1979). Society's ambivalence toward risk and its tendency to reward certain forms of risk taking (i.e., heroes) facilitates risk taking. It has been hypothesized that individuals with lower mastery of other social settings (e.g., work and home) look for mastery outside these areas and engage in risk taking (Levenson, 1990).

Risk taking is usually viewed as either a cognitive or emotional activity. The cognitive perspective stresses the probability of outcomes and the amount of loss associated with an event. Risk perceptions are generated from facts. An individual examines variables (e.g., personal health values, liability, and increased insurance rates) before engaging in an activity. Cognitive theories assume that the person has access to the facts and is capable of analyzing them (Bloomquist, 1986). Adolescents may not be capable of making this analysis because of the operation of *imaginary audience* and *personal fable* (Elkind, 1984). Imaginary audience presumes that everyone is watching you and they are concerned with your actions. This belief may encourage adolescents to drive fast to "prove" they are capable. Personal fable is a phenomenon that arises from imaginary audience where the adolescent believes that "if everyone is watching me, then I must be special and different." Adolescents may believe that others may get pregnant or may die in a MVC but they will not.

Emotionally oriented theories of risk taking view risk taking as serving an important psychologic function of the individual. The person may have a need for varied, novel, complex sensations, and the person is willing to take physical and social risks for the experience (Zuckerman, 1979). Risk events may serve as signals, and am-

Table 2-1 Total motor vehicle deaths in the United States

Year	Total deaths	Deaths per 100,000 people
1979	51,093	23
1980	51,091	22
1981	49,301	21
1982	43,945	19
1983	42,589	18
1984	44,257	19
1985	43,825	18
1986	46,087	19
1987	46,390	19
1988	47,093	19
1989	45,555	18
1990	44,529	18

Note. From the Insurance Institute for Highway Safety (IIHS) Facts (1991). *Public Statistics.* Arlington, VA: Insurance Institute for Highway Safety.

plification of the signal through praise of friends or the media may increase perception of the risk associated with the event and serve as a positive reinforcer (Machlis & Rosa, 1990). Society helps to amplify perception of the risk associated with a behavior by labeling (e.g., "dead man's curve") and by rating situations (e.g., class V rapids).

Prevention Research

Despite increasing public awareness of risks, knowledge of safety precautions, and sophistication of health services, the incidence of deaths from MVCs has remained remarkably stable in the United States (Table 2-1). The mortality from traumatic injury has decreased since World War II (Doece, 1986). This fact is related to the development of the trauma care delivery system both in the community and within the hospital environment and not to the diminishing frequency of traumatic events.

Injuries can be viewed from an epidemiologic perspective. Haddon (1980) developed and expanded a matrix for classifying factors associated with injuries. In the matrix, three factors—host (ultimately the trauma patient); vector, or agent/vector (e.g., handgun or motor vehicle); and environment—interact simultaneously over time to cause injury. There are three phases to injury causation. The preinjury phase focuses on vari-

Table 2-2 Haddon's matrix

Phase	Host (human)	Vector (vehicle)	Physical environment	Socioeconomic environment

Precrash	Driver vision
	Alcohol intoxication
	Experience and
	  judgment
	Amount of travel
		Brakes, tires
		Center of gravity
		Jackknife tendency
		Speed of travel
		Ease of control
		Load characteristics
			Visibility of hazards
			Road curvature and gradient
			Surface coefficient of friction
			Divided highways, one-way
			  streets
			Intersections, access control
			Signalization
				Attitudes about alcohol
				Laws related to impaired
				  driving
				Speed limits
				Support for injury preven-
				  tion efforts

Crash	Safety belt use
	Osteoporosis
		Speed capability
		Vehicle size
		Automatic restraints
		Placement, hardness,
		  and sharpness of
		  contact surfaces
		Load containment
			Recovery areas
			Guard rails
			Characteristics of fixed objects
			Median barriers
			Roadside embankments
			Speed limits
				Attitudes about safety belt
				  use
				Laws about safety belt use
				Enforcement of child
				  safety seat laws
				Motorcycle helmet use
				  laws

Postcrash	Age
	Physical condition
		Fuel system integrity	Emergency communication
			  systems
			Distance to and quality of
			  emergency medical services
			Rehabilitation programs
				Support for trauma care
				  systems
				Training of EMS personnel

Note. From "Injury Prevention: Meeting the Challenge" by the National Committee for Injury Prevention and Control, 1989, American Journal of Preventive Medicine, 5 (Suppl 3), p.8.

ables that interact to increase susceptibility to the point of causation. The injury phase addresses variables that determine whether an injury will result from the energy dissipation. The postinjury phase encompasses variables that may affect the severity of the injury's consequences. Table 2-2 illustrates application of Haddon's matrix to the prevention of MVCs. In this example, environment has been differentiated into physical and socioeconomic aspects.

Research to date has focused on road conditions, engineering factors, personal reaction time, and addictive personalities in relation to the occurrence of traumatic injury. Life-style factors that place a person at risk for trauma have been only superficially explored. Human behavior and personal responsibility remain important in injury causation. Several reasons why these human factors are not addressed follow. First, life-style characteristics and human behavior are more difficult to measure than those characteristics related to the environment or agent/vector,

such as weather, road conditions, and traffic patterns.

Another reason is the assumption by many individuals of personal responsibility for the traumatic injury. If the individual assumes the responsibility, society may deny the problem. The trauma patient may accept blame for poor reaction time, driving too fast, or failure to yield the right-of-way, to perpetuate the illusion that control can usually be maintained over the environment, when in reality the road was poorly engineered or there were too many vehicles on that road at that time of day.

Another reason for the lack of prevention research is the number of accident and trauma services that are being developed. Trauma services in some regions generate revenue. They produce jobs and provide an arena for the marketing of products. Thus there are private interest groups in society, such as insurance companies, that financially need to perpetuate the view that "accidents will happen." When individuals accept this view,

---

Driving statistics

1. There were 39,779 fatal crashes in 1990.
2. The probability of being involved in a motor vehicle injury accident during a 75-year lifetime is greater than 86%.
3. Traffic crashes rank as the number one killer of Americans between the ages of 1 and 40 years.
4. Of motor vehicle–related deaths, 82% occur during normal weather conditions.
5. In 1986 an average of one person was killed in a traffic crash every 11 minutes.
6. The cost of all traffic deaths and injuries in the United States during 1986 was about $74.2 billion. Some of the costs were:
   - $27.4 billion in property damage
   - $16.4 billion in lost productivity
   - $4.1 billion in medical costs
7. Of the total passenger car fatalities, 92% occur in the front seat.
8. Three of every four traffic crashes happen within 25 miles of the home.

Note. Modified from the National Highway Traffic Safety Administration (NHTSA) (1988). *Public Statistics.* Washington, D.C.: National Highway Safety Administration, and Facts, 1991 Edition, Insurance Institute for Highway Safety.

---

accidents become a normal part of life, which one cannot prevent and should prepare for.

Prevention efforts aimed at decreasing morbidity and mortality from vehicular crashes have been ineffective. Previously, the majority of money allocated to "accident control" has been used for personal health services and rapid transportation of "victims" instead of environmental changes and educational programs. Theoretically, all deaths caused by MVCs are preventable (Knowles, 1977). However, costs associated with their prevention have been considered too high (e.g., placement of seat belts on schoolbuses) or chances of harm too low for our culture to insist on stronger preventive measures. MVCs are tolerated because they do not threaten the existence of the culture, since multiple fatalities from a crash do not reach catastrophic potential and enrage public outcry. The losses, although real, are insidious. The box above itemizes costs associated with MVCs. In addition to these direct financial costs are the nonquantifiable costs, such as pain, grief, and suffering of the involved person and family. Most people in modern society have a relatively low awareness of the potential for harm in their everyday activities. The growth and development of urban infrastructure have produced a need for advanced transportation systems. Road travel and its risks have become a necessary and accepted part of life.

DRIVING AS A SOCIAL PHENOMENON

The automobile was readily accepted by society. It became an extension of the family and the self as evidenced by the development of the garage (to protect the vehicle); vehicle comfort measures (plush seats and air conditioning to extend the home environment); and personalized license plates and bumper stickers (for individual expression). The person can express aggressions (driving someone off the road) and perhaps even socially unacceptable behavior (giving a nonverbal gesture) in the "safety" of the vehicle (Marsh & Collett, 1987). Driving a car implies adulthood (with a new environment to indulge in sexual gratification). Driving allows one to make decisions and to get away from home. Motor vehicles support our freedom and independence (as used in oil company advertising) and provide an opportunity for control and mastery (Hailwood, 1988).

Cars make a statement about wealth. The more expensive cars have the engine power to go faster than any tires are capable of handling (Hailwood, 1988). The vehicles cannot be driven legally as they were designed to be, yet the power is available and serves to symbolize control and success. Of North American new car buyers, 80% purchase an automobile without test driving it, another indication that cars are not purchased solely for transportation purposes (Hailwood, 1988).

Driving presents a paradox. The driver is supposed to be in control, yet "accidents" occur. Most individuals have fears about the inherent dangers associated with driving. Good luck charms are used, and prayers are offered to prevent loss of control. The tradition of placing a statue of Saint Christopher on a dashboard is just one example of symbolically protecting the self and the vehicle (Marsh & Collett, 1987).

Several variables in the literature have been associated with involvement in a MVC. These vari-

---

Variables commonly associated with involvement in a motor vehicle crash

Demographic characteristics

16 to 29 years of age
Male
Divorced marital status (2 or more divorces)
Current marital separation/disharmony
Frequent occupational change/poor work record

Philosophic outlook

Lack of self-care/fate will determine outcome
Risk-taking behavior as a way of life—impacts areas other than just physical risk (including emotional risk, e.g., infidelity)
Lack of purpose or meaning in life

Personality patterns

Immature
Irresponsible
Impulsiveness
Aggressive behavior
Hopelessness
Depression stimulated by loss of significant object/ person
Low self-esteem
Creative tendencies
Family instability (parental divorce, abuse situations)
Personal view of time (loses track of time and then needs to rush)

Physical functioning

History of chronic illness
Degree of sensory and motor proficiency
Reaction time
Fatigue
Alcohol consumption
Degree of cognitive judgment needed to operate vehicle

Environmental influences

Poor visibility
Poorly engineered roadway
Poorly maintained roadway
Weather conditions (e.g., rain, fog, dust storm)
Poorly engineered vehicle
Traffic congestion

---

havior. To illustrate, divorce may be viewed as positive or negative, depending on personal circumstances.

Risky driving has been associated with thrill seeking, aggressive tendencies, drug use, and strong peer influences (Wilson & Jonah, 1988). In one study, three subtypes of drivers were identified by personality assessment. One group was characterized by impulsivity, sensation seeking, and aggressive behavior. These individuals were deficient in impulse control. The second group had an external perception of control, were emotionally distressed, and harbored resentment against others. They were deficient in coping skills. Driving increased these individuals' perception of personal control. The third group had an internal perception of control and were assertive individuals. This group was older and had higher social positions and occupational status than the other two groups (Donovan, Umlauf, & Salzberg, 1988). It may be necessary to assess trauma patients' personality profile to provide interventions that will be meaningful.

ADOLESCENT INJURIES

Alcohol use has been associated with injuries in general. Adolescents tend to use alcohol to cope with stressors rather than to deal with peer pressure (Johnson & White, 1989). Those who drink and drive are more likely to ride with an intoxicated driver. The frequency of drinking alcholic beverages rather than the amount of intake at one time is a better predictor of a MVC (Johnson & White, 1989).

Adolescents who have experienced previous injuries that are school or sport based, come from a low socioeconomic situation, and have experienced recent stressful life events (e.g., parental unemployment, parental discord, or relocation) have a higher incidence of MVCs (Slap, Chaudhuri, & Vorters, 1991). Even though adolescents may be aware of safety precautions, they still tend to not use safety measures (e.g., fastening seat belt) (Scott & Cabral, 1988). This may be related to the operation of the personal fable phenomenon. Because some form of risk taking is culturally supported during adolescence, adolescents need to be exposed to activities that have decreased risk but are associated with feelings of mastery. The Outward Bound program is an example of an activity of this nature.

ables are organized into categories (see box above). It is important to note that it is the individual's interpretation of these variables that ultimately impacts his or her life-style and driving be-

---

Injury prevention strategies

1. Prevent the creation of the hazard.
   Example: Allow only adolescents who have at least a 2.0 grade point average to obtain a driving permit.

2. Reduce the amount of the hazard.
   Example: Produce vehicle engines that can go only 10 miles faster than the maximum legal speed limit.

3. Prevent the release of a hazard that already exists.
   Example: Make bathtubs less slippery.

4. Modify the rate or spatial distribution of the hazard.
   Example: Require motor vehicle airbags.

5. Separate, in time or space, the hazard from that which is to be protected.
   Example: Use bike paths to separate riders from drivers.

6. Separate by a material barrier the hazard from that which is to be protected.
   Example: Use electrical outlet safety covers for unused sockets.

7. Modify relevant basic qualities of the hazard.
   Example: Make crash-absorbent bumpers.

8. Make what is to be protected more resistant to damage from the hazard.
   Example: Improve the physical condition of high-risk drivers.

9. Begin to counter the damage already done by the hazard.
   Example: Require American College of Surgeons review to obtain trauma center status to maintain consistency among facilities.

10. Stabilize, repair, and rehabilitate the object of the damage.
   Example: Initiate driver rehabilitation programs before hospital discharge.

GENERAL ASSESSMENT AND INTERVENTIONS

Haddon, 1980b, developed a list of ten general strategies for injury prevention (see box above). These countermeasures were designed to prevent or interfere with the energy transfer process that results in injury. This list provides a framework for logically examining prevention strategies.

PROTECTION STRATEGIES
Passive Protection

The federal government requires that all new cars, as of 1990, provide automatic protection (passive restraint system). However, passive restraint systems do not guarantee injury prevention and many individuals fail to use their manual seat belts in addition to the automatic seat belt. Lack of use is attributed to forgetfulnesss and the false sense of security the automatic seat belt provides. The chance of being killed or injured during a MVC increases when the lap belt is not used in addition to the automatic device (University of North Carolina Highway Safety Research Center, 1990).

Drivers of cars with airbags have the lowest use rate of lap belts, usually because of the misconception that airbags provide full protection (University of North Carolina Highway Safety Research Center, 1990). In reality, airbags are designed to be effective only in frontal crashes.

Airbags inflate in less than one twenty-fifth of a second (faster than the blink of an eye). They are inflated upon contact with an object at a speed greater than 12 mph. A crash sensor activates the airbag. Sodium azide, kept in a sealed container within the airbag system, is converted to nitrogen. Nitrogen gas inflates the airbag. Figure 2-2 illustrates deployment of an airbag. Airbags are designed to last longer than the life of the vehicle, and they do not need to be checked or replaced periodically. The purpose of an airbag is to keep the occupant from hitting objects in the vehicle. An accidental inflation is rare. Because of the speed with which the bag inflates and deflates, an accidental inflation should not cause

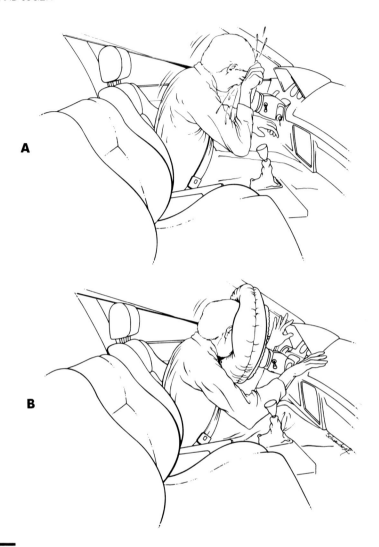

Figure 2-2 Illustration of **A,** driver thrown forward without airbag, and **B,** airbag as passive protection device. (*Note.* From *Facial injuries* [3rd ed.] by R.C. Schultz, 1988, St. Louis: Mosby–Year Book, Inc.)

the driver to lose control of the vehicle. Airbags are designed to remain inflated long enough to protect occupants in multiple collisions that occur during one traffic crash, such as the airbag-equipped vehicle hitting one object, bouncing off, and hitting a second object. They are not designed to be effective in a second separate crash that occurs later. Airbags, like seat belts, should be replaced after a MVC. The cost of airbag replacement is covered by insurance.

A few cases of injury from airbag deployment have been documented. Injuries documented in the literature include (1) chemical keratitis from airbag rupture, (2) second-degree burns to the face, chest, and arms from airbag malfunction and skin friction, and (3) one case of choroidal rupture (Rosenblatt, Freilich, & Kirsch, 1991; Shebar & Laurenzano, 1991).

Seat belt use varies with risk perceptions, which may differ based on driving conditions, weather, distance, and condition of the agent/motor vehicle. Drivers tend to use seat belts when it is "worth it." An example of increased seat belt use is on long road trips where drivers perceive that the increased travel speed and unknown roadways increase their personal vulnerability. Safety behavior is influenced by social norms and expectations, as well as personal aspiration. People may evaluate actions (driving over the speed limit) in terms of the probable direct consequences of the action (getting to work on time). Getting to work on time is culturally expected. Being involved in a MVC on the way is deemed less likely and worth the risk. Even if the individual has had a previous MVC, the fact that driving over the speed limit increases the risk of being involved in a MVC may be ignored if the personal aspiration is to arrive at work on time. A time management course may be a viable intervention for preventing MVCs with this type of driver.

Mandatory Protection

Mandatory protection presents a conflict to those who accept and assimilate the American cultural value system, which endorses freedom and independence. The literature has demonstrated that even with mandatory laws, more than one third of the population does not wear seat belts and those at greatest risk for involvement in a MVC (ages 15 to 24 years) remain least likely to use seat belts (Goldbaum, Remington, Powell, Hogelin, & Gentry, 1986). The use of seat belts is one example of a preventive strategy that has the potential of decreasing by 60% the number of serious injuries and fatalities (Goldbaum et al, 1986). Arguments to support the development of mandatory policies have focused on the assumption that society's benefits exceed society's cost from such measures (Warner, 1987). However, conclusive evidence has not been provided regarding the usefulness of mandatory self-protection in reducing society's cost, since self-protection may result in a nonfatal crash requiring long-term social resources (Peltzman, 1975). In one study, the use of manual seat belts reduced injury severity by 60%, decreased hospital admissions by 64%, and decreased hospital charges by 66% (Orsay et al., 1988).

Motorcycle fatalities are estimated to be more than 20% higher where cyclists are not required to wear helmets. The usage rate is almost 100% in areas with a mandatory helmet law versus a 50% usage rate in areas without mandatory use laws (American Trauma Society, 1990). Mandatory self-protection laws are not consistently enforced and may be repealed, depending on economic and political constraints (Weisbuch, 1987).

MEDIA

The media influence safety behavior. If peer counterforces are present and the family constraints are minimal, the media greatly influence the adolescent (Roberts, 1989). The media have a responsibility to display negative consequences of risky behavior, such as the "good guy" dying in a high-speed chase scene.

Advertisements influence driving behavior. A study in Austria demonstrated that advertisement strategies emphasizing safety had greater impact on driving behavior than speed limits and energy crisis information. When the advertisement focus changed, emphasizing sporting qualities of the vehicle, driving behavior returned to its prestudy characteristics (Schmidt, 1982).

Automobile advertisements are presented in a manner to convince the consumer that he or she has control and mastery of the vehicle. Words are used in the advertisements that suggest that the vehicle possesses human qualities: "grip the road," "body and soul," "swift reflexes." Subliminally, these suggestions may encourage drivers to be less cautious and aware of their driving, since the "car has so much control." Driving becomes an "automatized" behavior. The promotion of safety in the media may decrease injuries.

ROLE MODELING

Parents may not be aware of the negative safety behavior they are modeling. When a parent fails to use protective devices (e.g., seat belt, helmet), the child perceives that protection is not necessary. Many parents have not been exposed to the routine use of safety seats or belts. Use of restraints prevents children from roaming freely about in a moving vehicle, which causes outward displays of displeasure. This crying and acting-out behavior can deter use of restraints. Parents must be reminded that it is their duty to preserve their child's well-being. Because there has been no cultural heritage relative to the use of vehicular protective/restraint devices passed on to today's parents, children usually have to role model these behaviors for parents. It may be possible to change parental safety behavior by focusing on parental concern for the child. This approach has the dual impact of promoting injury prevention in the total family unit.

CULTURAL VIEWS

Cultural norms regarding the use of motor vehicles should be changed. For example, the perceived capacity of a car has typically consisted of as many people as can fit in the available seating space. Cultural change is necessary to redefine car capacity as the number of occupants for which seat belts are available. Changing cultural norms requires (1) providing extensive education to individuals, parents, and children, (2) providing motivation for using restraints, and (3) facilitating use by designing easily applied restraints (Foss, 1987).

EDUCATIONAL PROGRAMS

Educational programs can be designed systematically to allow evaluation of the program's effectiveness. Prevention strategies can be developed after identifying the behavior patterns and attitudes of the target population. The involvement of public agencies and community leaders assures reaching the greatest number of individuals and promotes commmunity commitment. An example of an educational program is setting up safety checkpoints, where public officials stop motorists and check seat belt usage. Motorists using seat belts may be rewarded with a prize or "seat belt salute" (i.e., salute or thumbs-up gesture). Those not using seat belts or those using restraint devices incorrectly are taught proper application and are given educational materials (University of North Carolina Highway Safety Research Center, 1991). Figure 2-3 illustrates correct use of shoulder and lap belts.

It may be diffficult to maintain or implement safety education programs during economic recession, since it is difficult to quantify the benefits of such programs. The Safety Seal program, which operates out of Providence Hospital in Anchorage, Alaska, is one example of a program that has received grant funding to expand during a depressed economy (Sloan, 1990). Grant funding lends credibility to an existing program, enhances community awareness, and promotes community involvement. Trauma nurses can be active in grant writing or serve as nursing consultants to grants that focus on injury prevention.

Courses are designed to promote safe driving behavior, such as those available from the National Safety Council. Most of these materials are targeted for specific groups and are usually job related (e.g., bus drivers, truck drivers). Driver education programs are not provided in many public education systems.

THE TRAUMA NURSE AND INJURY PREVENTION

Trauma nursing is practiced in a variety of settings. Nurses practicing in areas where the trauma patient's condition has stabilized could explore the patient's beliefs about the injury-producing event. Preinjury behavior and life-style factors, such as how the patient handles stress and anger, as well as his or her driving practices (if appropriate), could be discussed. Even though applicable to only a small proportion of individuals, the use of the motor vehicle as a way of camouflaging indirect self-destructive behavior may be discovered, and the patient can be appropriately referred (Howard & Monhaut, 1988; Tsuang, Boor, & Fleming, 1985).

Broadly based risk/safety education programs may not be effective, because people differ in their risk beliefs. People think in causal terms in relation to risk. Their terms may not fit scientific theories, but they are considered to be true by the person. Asking trauma patients what they believed caused their injury can provide insights into their risk perceptions and provide data from which to address injury prevention while the patient is still hospitalized. The trauma patient who appears to have sensation-seeking tendencies, as evidenced by past medical history or personality assessment, may need assistance to identify the negative consequences of the injury-producing event. Health care providers should not remind this person that he or she is lucky to be alive, since this may positively reward the sensation-seeking aspects of the event. Confronting the person with the link between his or her behavior and the pain, loss of transportation, and medical expenses associated with the event may have a greater impact on future safety behavior. Research is needed to test these hypotheses. Trauma assessment forms could be modified to include areas for documenting information about risk taking and safety behavior instead of simply a check box to record whether the patient was using a restraint/protection device.

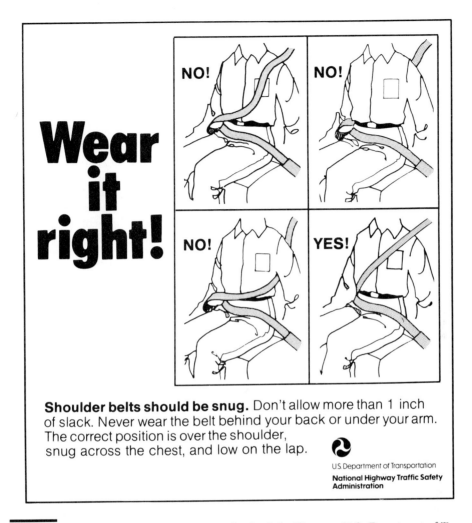

Figure 2-3   Proper use of shoulder harness and safety belt. (Courtesy U.S. Department of Transportation, National Highway Safety Administration.)

Assessment of the patient's social support system and network, recent stressful life events, and coping abilities may provide insights into the patient's degree of future injury susceptibility. Referral of the patient to psychosocial services may provide him or her with the financial and psychologic ability to enact safety behavior.

The trauma nurse should be aware of common myths associated with restraint use to effectively teach patients regarding vehicle safety. Myths and clarifications about seat belts and airbags are presented in the boxes on p. 32. Patients may be ready to discuss restraint use after they have been

involved in a MVC and recognize their personal susceptibility. Proper restraint use is illustrated in Figure 2-3. Some emergency departments display this information in waiting rooms.

Trauma nurses can help prevent injuries by viewing their nursing role from a social perspective. Professional nursing associations, as well as individual nurses, can place pressure on manufacturers to market safety aspects of their products. If as much money were placed on engineering safety as on speed and cosmetic design, perhaps injuries would decrease further. Nissan discontinued a television advertisement after one airing be-

Myths associated with restraint use

Myth: I don't need safety belts; I'm a good driver.
Answer: But you cannot control the other driver.

Myth: I might be saved if I'm thrown clear in an accident.
Answer: But your body cannot withstand hitting the ground or pavement or being hit by another vehicle.

Myth: In case of a crash, I can brace myself with my hands.
Answer: It is not possible to brace your body; the force of impact at just 10 mph is equal to catching a 200 pound bag of cement dropped from a first story window.

Myth: I just don't think I will be in an accident.
Answer: The majority of people are involved in a crash once every 10 years. You do not know what day it will happen, so be ready.

Myth: I might be trapped inside a burning car.
Answer: Less than ½ of 1% of all injury-producing crashes involve fire or submersion; but especially in these situations, a safety belt can save your life by keeping you alert and capable of escaping quickly.

Myth: You don't need to wear them in the back seat.
Answer: The overall risk of injury is reduced as much as 40% by wearing safety belts in the rear seat. An estimated 660 lives could be saved annually by wearing safety belts as rear-seated passengers.

Note. From the "Combined Accident Reduction Report (CARE)" (1989). Public information printed with Federal Highway Safety Funds and distributed through the Kentucky State Police, Frankfort, Ky.

Myths associated with airbag use

Myth: Seat belts are enough protection.
Answer: Airbags are designed to work in frontal or front-angle crashes. They do not provide adequate protection alone in lateral, rear, or rollover crashes. Shoulder belts must be used in conjunction with the airbag to provide adequate protection.

Myth: Airbags inflate without cause. I may lose control of the car.
Answer: Airbags will inflate in an impact equivalent to hitting a wall at 12 mph or greater. They will not inflate from a sudden stop, bump, or low-speed crash.

Myth: The airbag will not work when I need it.
Answer: There have been no documented cases of failure of airbags to function. They require no maintenance and will work for the life of the vehicle.

Myth: I might be injured from the airbag.
Answer: There are few documented cases of injuries sustained from airbag inflation. Airbags inflate from a chemical reaction, not an explosion. They are filled with nitrogen, a harmless gas that we breathe every day, since it comprises 78% of the air.

Note. Modified from the American Coalition for Traffic Safety, 1989.

cause of a request made by 18 health care, insurance, and law enforcement groups. The advertisement showed a chase scene with the car exceeding 140 mph (Insurance Institute for Highway Safety, 1990). Thus pressure placed on manufacturers and the media to market safety can be effective.

Nurses can support national organizations that focus on promoting safety. Mothers Against Drunk Driving (MADD) is one organization that has been politically influential in upgrading penalties for poor driving judgment (evidenced in a driving-while-intoxicated [DWI] citation). This association also supports rewarding states for pro-

active actions, such as license sanctions and offender-funded DWI programs (MADD, 1989). State implementation of preventive strategies is rewarded by the state receiving additional highway safety fund grants.

Almost half of all MVCs are alcohol related. However, the number of alcohol-related traffic fatalities has decreased since 1982. This decrease may be related to stricter state laws and their enforcement, increased public awareness and outcry, increased media attention, and educational programs.

Trauma nurses can also support insurance companies that provide discounts to motorists who attend driving courses periodically or that provide incentives for using passenger restraints. Insurance companies that reward home safety (e.g., use of home fire alarms) can also be supported. Nurses can be powerful role models for other individuals by using safety devices and being alert and aware while driving.

SUMMARY   Injuries are a major health problem. Prevention is a part of all nursing roles, yet, to date, trauma nursing has focused on the injury and postinjury phases of Haddon's matrix. Major improvements have been made in caring for the trauma patient in the areas of resuscitation, stabilization, and physical rehabilitation. It is time for trauma nurses to focus energy on injury prevention; it is hoped that they will effect major improvements in this area also.

RESOURCES

American Academy of Pediatrics (childhood injuries)
141 NW Point Blvd.
Elk Grove, IL 60009

American Coalition for Traffic Safety, Inc.
808 17th St. NW, Suite 260
Washington, DC 20006
(202) 857-0002

American Driver and Traffic Safety Education Association
239 Florida Ave.
Salisbury, MD 21801

Emergency Nurses C.A.R.E. (Cancel Alcohol Related Emergencies)
18 Lyman Street, PO Box 4571
Westborough, MA 01581
(617) 366-7591

Insurance Institute for Highway Safety
1005 N. Glebe Road
Arlington, VA 22201

Mothers Against Drunk Driving (MADD)
669 Airport Freeway, Suite 310
Hurst, TX 76053
(817) 268-6233

Motor Vehicle Occupant Protection Educational Resource List for Nurses
American Nurses Association
2420 Pershing Road
Kansas City, MO 64108

National Safety Council
444 N. Michigan Ave.
Chicago, IL 60611
(312) 527-4800

Safe Kids
National Coalition to Prevent Childhood Injury
111 Michigan Ave. NW
Washington, DC 20010
(202) 939-4993

U.S. Department of Transportation
National Highway Traffic Safety Administration (NHTSA)
400 7th St. SW
Washington, DC 20590
(202) 366-5972

U.S. Consumer Product Safety Commission
Washington, DC 20207
(301) 492-6800

University of North Carolina
Highway Safety Research Center
CB#3430
Chapel Hill, NC 27599-3430

REFERENCES

American Trauma Society. (1990). Helmet laws increase survival rate. *Journal of Trauma, 15*(2), 5.

Baker, S. (1987). The neglected epidemic: Stone lecture, 1985 America Trauma Society meeting. *Journal of Trauma, 27*, 343-348.

Bloomquist, G. (1986). A utility maximization model of driver traffic safety behavior. *Accident Analysis and Prevention, 18*, 371-375.

CARE. (1989). *The combined accident reduction report.* Washington, DC: Department of Transportation.

Committee on Trauma Research, Commission on Life Sciences, National Research Council, and Institute of Medicine. (1985). *Injury in America: A continuing public health problem.* Washington, DC: National Academy Press.

Department of Health and Human Services. (1986). *The 1990 health objectives for the Nation: A midcourse review.* Washington, DC: Public Health Service.

Doece, T. (1986). The neglected disease: An update. *Journal of American Medical Association, 255*, 1334.

Donovan, D., Umlauf, R., & Salzberg, P. (1988). Derivation of personality sub-types among high risk drivers. *Alcohol, Drugs, and Driving, 4*, 233-244.

Elkind, D. (1984). Teenage thinking! Implications for health care. *Pediatric Nursing, Nov/Dec*, 383-385.

Farley, F. (1986). The Big T in personality. *Psychology Today, 20*(5), 44-52.

Fischoff, B., Slovic, P., & Lichenstein, S. (1979). Weighing the risks. *Environment, 21*, 17-38.

Foss, R. (1987). Sociocultural perspective on child occupant protection. *Pediatrics, 80*, 886-893.

Goldbaum, G., Remington, P., Powell, K., Hogelin, G., & Gentry, E. (1986). Failure to use seat belts in the United States. *Journal of American Medical Association, 255*, 2459-2462.

Haddon, W. (1980a). Options for the prevention of motor vehicle crash injury. *Israel Journal of Medical Sciences, 16*, 45-68.

Haddon, W. (1980b). Advances in the epidemiology of injuries as a basis for public policy. *Public Health Reports, 95*, 411-421.

Haddon, W., Suchman, E., & Klein, D. (1964). *Accident Research*, New York: Harper & Row.

Hailwood, E. (1988). "Vroom at the top." *Canadian Business, 12*, 42-49.

Houck, T. (1986). Injuries are not accidents. *Public Health Reports, 124*.

Howard, J., & Monhaut, N. (1988). Behavioral issues: Suicide by vehicular crash: Recognition and early intervention. *Journal of Emergency Nursing, 14*, 230-244.

Insurance Institute for Highway Safety. (1990). Nissan ad will not run again. *Status Report, 25*(4), 1, 4.

Johnson, V., & White, H. (1989). An investigation of factors related to intoxicated driving behaviors among youth. *Journal of Studies on Alcohol, 50*, 320-330.

Knowles, J. (1977). The responsibility of the individual. *Daedalus, 30*, 358-368.

Levenson, M. (1990). Risk taking and personality. *Journal of Personality and Social Psychology, 58,* 1073-1080.

Licht, K. (1975). Safety and accidents: A brief conceptual analysis and a point of view. *Journal of School Health, XLV,* 530-534.

Machlis, G., & Rosa, E. (1990). Desired risk: Broadening the social amplification of risk framework. *Risk Analysis, 10,* 161-168.

Marsh, P., & Collett, P. (1987). Driving passion. *Psychology Today, 56*(6), 16-24.

Miller, T.R., Luchter, S., & Brinkman, C. (1988). Crash costs and safety investment. *Association for Advances in Automotive Medicine,* 69-88.

Mothers Against Drunk Driving (MADD). (1989). *Madd in Action, 8*(2), 8-10, 12.

National Committee for Injury Prevention and Control. (1989). Injury Prevention meeting: The challenge. *American Journal of Preventive Medicine, 5*(Suppl 3), 8.

National Highway Traffic Safety Administration. (1988). *Accident Facts,* Washington, DC.

Orsay, E., Turnbull, T., Dunne, M., Barrett, J., Langenberg, P., & Orsay, C. (1988). Prospective study of the effect of safety belts on morbidity and health care costs in motor-vehicle accidents. *Journal of American Medical Association, 260,* 3598-3603.

Peltzman, S. (1975). The effects of automobile safety legislation. *Journal of Political Economy, 83,* 677-721.

Roberts, D. (1989). The impact of media portrayal of risky driving on adolescents: Some speculations. *Alcohol, Drugs, & Driving, 5,* 13-20.

Rosenblatt, M., Freilich, B., & Kirsch, D. (1991). Correspondence. *New England Journal of Medicine, 325* (21), 1518-1519.

Schmidt, L. (1982). Automobile advertising and traffic safety. *Arbeiten Aus Dern Verkehrs Psychologischen Institut, 19,* 80-93.

Scott, H.D., & Cabral, R. (1988). Predicting hazardous lifestyles among adolescents based on health-risk assessment data. *American Journal of Health Promotion, 2*(4), 23-28.

Shebar, E., & Laurenzano, J. (1991). Correspondence. *New England Journal of Medicine, 325* (21), 1519.

Slap, G., Chaudhuri, S., & Vorters, D. (1991). Risk factors for injury during adolescence. *Journal of Adolescent Health, 12,* 263-268.

Sloan, K. (1990). The Safety Seal injury prevention program: A response to the epidemic of injury and death in children. *Journal of Emergency Nursing, 16*(2), 83-89.

Slovic, P. (1987). Perception of risk. *Science, A 236* (4799), 280-285.

Smeltzer, S. (1988). Research in trauma nursing: State of the art and future directions. *Journal of Emergency Nursing, 14,* 145-153.

Tsuang, M., Boor, M., & Fleming, J. (1985). Psychiatric aspects of traffic accidents. *American Journal of Psychiatry, 142,* 538-546.

University of North Carolina Highway Safety Research Center. (1990). Automatic misuse. *Highway Safety Direction, 3*(1), 2-3, 11.

University of North Carolina Highway Safety Research Center (1991). Rural community safety belt program. *Highway Safety Directions, 3*(2), 2-5.

Vezega, M., & Klein, T. (1990). Alcohol-related traffic fatalities: United States, 1982-1989. *Morbidity and Mortality Weekly Report, 39*(49), 1-2.

Warner, K. (1987). Public policy and automobile occupant restraint: An economist's perspective. *Accident Analysis and Prevention, 19,* 39-50.

Weinstein, N. (1984). Why it won't happen to me: Perceptions of risk factors and susceptibility. *Health Psychology, 3,* 431-457.

Weisbuch, J. (1987). The prevention of injury from motorcycle use: Epidemiologic success, legislative failure. *Accident Analysis and Prevention, 19,* 21-28.

Wilson, R.J., & Jonah, B. (1988). The application of problem behavior theory to the understanding of risky driving. *Alcohol, Drugs, & Driving, 4,* 173-191.

World Health Organization. (1986). *Evaluation of the Strategy of Health for All by the Year 2000. Volume 3,* Region of the Americas.

Zuckerman, M. (1979). *Sensation seeking: Beyond the optimal level of arousal.* Hillsdale, NJ: Erlbaum.

UNIT II

PROFESSIONAL ISSUES IN TRAUMA NURSING

3 *Nursing Diagnosis*

■■■

Gail Mornhinweg

OBJECTIVES

❏ *Identify the purposes of using nursing diagnosis.*

❏ *Discuss the history of nursing diagnosis and the North American Nursing Diagnosis Association (NANDA).*

❏ *Relate the use of nursing diagnosis to the practice of trauma nursing.*

❏ *Describe the process of developing a nursing diagnosis.*

❏ *Develop research ideas related to nursing diagnosis in the trauma setting.*

INTRODUCTION The emergency period affects the patient, family, and significant others in many ways. Many stress factors are associated with the admission to an emergency care facility, including the setting itself, possibility of temporary or permanent life-style changes, possible body image change, lack of control, fear of pain, fear of death, fear of the unknown, disability, loss of time from work, and the cost of medical care. The patient may show signs of anxiety in various ways, depending on the level of stress encountered.

The family and/or significant others may present with a different set of problems, such as feelings of guilt, anxiety, or depression. They may also be dealing with some of the same stressors as the injured or ill family member. These stressors often elicit feelings of fear, helplessness, hopelessness, isolation, mistrust, and abandonment. Accurate and complete identification and labeling of these problems provide the basis for designing nursing interventions to treat them.

CASE STUDY A man in his mid-20s was involved in a motor vehicle crash and was brought by ambulance to the emergency department. The EMS had radioed the following report during transport: respiratory rate 28 with coarse rales, breath sounds diminished in the right anterior chest field, O₂ per mask at 100%; BP 86/50, HR 126 and regular; pupils equal and reactive, Glascow Coma Scale—9; shortening of the right leg with edema and crepitus; bowel sounds present; multiple lacerations and abrasions on face, arms, and posterior thorax.

After assimilating the radioed information, the nurse "knows" that the patient probably has a right pneumothorax, closed head injury, and a right femoral shaft fracture. The emergency department physician assesses the patient on arrival and orders blood work, urinalysis, CT scan of the head, and chest and right leg and hip x-ray studies. In addition to the IV initiated in the field, the nurse starts a second IV, continues monitoring vital signs and level of consciousness, inserts a nasogastric tube, and maintains alignment of the right leg. The nurse notices a grimace on the patient's face when his hare traction splint is accidentally bumped. Breath sounds on the right are no longer audible, and there is no right-sided chest expansion. The physician is notified and inserts a chest tube. All physician's orders have been accomplished, the patient's vital signs are stabilized, and he is to be transferred to the intensive care unit.

To make a medical diagnosis, the physician used multiple methods to elicit data, which included physical assessment and laboratory and x-ray studies. In collaboration with the nurse's assessment of decreased breath sounds and absence of thoracic movement, the physician diagnoses a right pneumothorax. The patient's medical diagnoses also include closed fracture of the right femoral shaft and closed head injury with no evidence on the CT scan of active intra-cranial bleeding.

Before transfer, the patient arouses to verbal stimuli and opens his eyes. Within 15 minutes his Glascow coma scale rating is 13. He converses but is disoriented and has no memory of the accident. He states that he is married and has a 3-year-old daughter.

What are the patient's probable nursing diagnoses?

The nurse develops a list of the patient's problems as all of the information is considered. This includes memory or concentration problems; decreased activity; inability to work because of hospitalization; anxiety; headache; pain from the fractured femur and multiple abrasions; high risk for infection because of intravenous lines; hazards of immobility; breathing difficulties; alterations in self-concept or esteem because he may not be able to continue all the roles of husband and father; fear; and possible hopelessness. These are all *nursing* diagnoses—human responses or manifestations of the medical diagnoses of fracture, head injury, and pneumothorax.

Probable nursing diagnoses are the following:
- pain
- anxiety
- fear
- ineffective breathing pattern
- decreased cardiac output
- high risk for decreased cerebral tissue perfusion

MEDICAL VERSUS NURSING DIAGNOSIS

The word *diagnosis* has been discussed at length. It is the art or act of identifying a disease from its signs and symptoms; a concise technical description of a taxon; investigation or analysis of the cause or nature of a condition, situation, or problem; and a statement or conclusion concerning the nature or cause of some phenomenon (Webster, 1987).

The scope of medical practice is to diagnose and treat a disease or condition (e.g., appendicitis, acute myocardial infarction) or a traumatic injury (e.g., fractured femur, subdural hematoma resulting from trauma). Medicine is defined as the art and science of preventing, alleviating, and curing disease (Webster).

The scope of nursing practice is the diagnosis and treatment of actual or potential health prob-

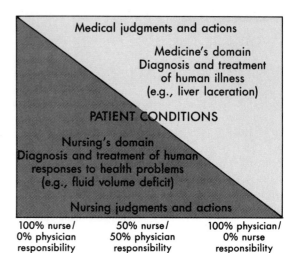

Figure 3-1 Comparison of nursing and medical judgments and actions. (*Note.* Adapted from *Classification of Nursing Diagnoses: Proceedings of the Seventh Conference* by A.M. McLane, (Ed.). (1987). St. Louis: Mosby–Year Book, Inc.

lems. This may be further described as the assessment and treatment of the manifestations of disease or injury. These manifestations may include pain, anxiety, fear, loneliness, inability to bathe or feed oneself, and inability to continue in the usual role of father or mother as the result of a traumatic injury. One of the roles of the nurse is that of diagnosing and "caring" (Figure 3-1).

Nursing diagnosis is not new. The trauma nurse has made diagnoses since first entering the emergency or trauma department. Whether at the novice or expert level, the nurse has assessed the patient and made a "diagnosis." He or she decided then which patient should be cared for first and which diagnosis should be treated first. The diagnosis can be developed either collaboratively with physicians or other health team members, or independently. Determining priorities is always first in the mind of the trauma nurse, who makes decisions based on the available information.

STANDARDS

Nursing diagnosis was formally accepted as a function of nursing practice by the American Nurses Association in its publication *Standards of Nursing Practice* (1973). The Standards provide a means for determining the quality of nursing care that a patient receives and are based on the nurs-

Standards of emergency nursing practice

Standard I: Comprehensive Triage   Triage every patient entering the emergency care system and determine priorities based on physical and psychosocial needs.

Standard II: Assessment   Initiate accurate and ongoing assessment of physical and psychosocial problems.

Standard III: Analysis   Analyze assessment data to formulate a nursing diagnosis.

Standard IV: Planning   Formulate a comprehensive nursing care plan based on nursing diagnosis, and collaborate in the formulation of the overall plan of care.

Standard V: Intervention   Implement a plan of care based on assessment, nursing diagnosis, and medical diagnosis.

Standard VI: Evaluation   Evaluate and modify the plan of care based on observable responses and attainment of outcomes and goals.

Standard VII: Human Worth   Provide care based on philosophical and ethical concepts, such as reverence of life, respect, inherent dignity, worth, autonomy, and individuality.

Standard VIII: Communication   Assure open and timely communication with emergency patients, significant others, and team members.

Note. From *Standards of Emergency Nursing Practice* (2nd ed.) Emergency Nurses Association, 1991, St. Louis: Mosby–Year Book, Inc.

ing process: assessment, diagnosis, plan of care, implementation, and evaluation. The new (1991) ANA Standards of Clinical Nursing Practice standard II states that "the nurse analyzes the assessment data in determining diagnoses." These standards were written to apply to all nursing practice settings.

The Emergency Nurses Association (ENA) also established Standards of Emergency Nursing Practice (1991). They believe that the scope of emergency nursing practice involves the assessment, diagnosis, treatment, and evaluation of perceived, actual or potential, sudden or urgent, physical or psychosocial problems that are primarily episodic or acute and that occur in a variety of settings (p. 1). They have written standards to describe practice, professionalism, education, and research (see box on left). The eight practice standards include comprehensive triage, assessment, analysis, planning, intervention, evaluation, human worth, and communication (pp. 5, 21, 35, 57, 73, 81, 95, 103). These standards apply to the individual who has been involved in trauma. The nurse must be able to adhere to these practice standards in all settings impacting emergency care, which include the acute care facility, prehospital setting, and emergency setting.

The third standard in the practice section states that the nurse shall analyze assessment data to formulate a nursing diagnosis. A nursing diagnosis, according to ENA, is a clinical judgment about an individual, family, or community response to actual and potential health problems and life processes. Nursing diagnoses provide the basis for selection of nursing interventions to achieve outcomes for which the nurse is accountable (p. 239).

In 1986 the National Flight Nurses Association (NFNA) also included nursing diagnosis in its practice standards. Comprehensive standard II states that "the nursing diagnosis is derived from analysis of the health status data." Other national organizations representing specialties involved in trauma care have also included nursing diagnosis into their practice standards. These include the American Association of Critical Care Nurses (AACN), the Association of Operating Room Nurses (AORN), and the American Association of Rehabilitation Nurses (AARN).

NURSING DIAGNOSIS

The American Nurses Association (1980) defined nursing as "the diagnosis and treatment of human responses to actual or potential health problems." In 1988 the American Nurses Association (ANA) accepted the North American Nursing Diagnosis Association's (NANDA) Taxonomy I as a tool to guide in the selection of these nursing diagnoses. During the 1990 NANDA conference the following definition of nursing diagnosis was accepted: "A nursing diagnosis is a clinical judgment about individual, family, or community responses to actual or potential health problems/life processes. Nursing diagnoses provide the basis for selection of nursing interventions to achieve outcomes for which the nurse is accountable." Although the history of nursing diagnosis is relatively brief, its impact has been widespread and controversial.

History of Nursing Diagnosis

Nursing diagnosis has been a major focus in nursing for a relatively short time, but its actual history is much longer. For many years nursing has looked for a system (although not necessarily called *nursing diagnosis*) to list, classify, and describe nursing/patient problems.

Florence Nightingale was the first nurse diagnostician, as evidenced by her identifying nutrition deficits and addressing environmental effects of light and color. More recently McManus (1950) discussed nursing diagnosis as a responsibility of nurses. Abdellah (1957) described 21 nursing problems and McCain (1965) discussed 13 functional areas for assessment. They both were early proponents of classification systems. Chambers (1962) described nursing diagnosis as an investigation of the facts and limited to the activities legally within the practice of a professional nurse. Other early proponents of nursing diagnosis (Durand & Price, 1966) stated that it is a statement of a conclusion resulting from recognition of a pattern from a nursing investigation. More recently, nursing diagnosis has been conceptually defined by various authors and theorists. Gordon (1976) described nursing diagnosis as actual or potential health problems that nurses, by virtue of their education and experience, are capable of treating and licensed to treat.

History of NANDA

The purpose of the North American Nursing Diagnosis Association (NANDA) is to develop, refine, and promote a taxonomy of nursing diagnostic terminology for use by professional nurses. The association also acts as a clearinghouse for information, such as bibliographies and research studies being conducted on individual nursing diagnoses.

In 1973 Kristine Gebbie and Mary Ann Lavin of St. Louis University invited 100 nurses from different geographic areas, employment agencies, and clinical practice areas to participate in the first National Conference for the Classification of Nursing Diagnosis. Their goals were to articulate the health problems that comprise the domain of nursing and to classify those problems into some type of system. On completion of the conference, the group had described 100 nursing diagnoses pertinent to ten physiologic systems.

Over the next 15 years, seven conferences were conducted for the continued development of nursing diagnoses and a taxonomic structure. From 1973 to 1977 the nursing diagnoses were classified alphabetically. In 1977 Sr. Callista Roy recommended that a theorist group be formed to help develop a conceptual model for the diagnoses. During the third conference (1978) the assembly recognized the work of the theorist group and developed a framework for diagnoses. Much of the work during the third and fourth conferences dealt with additions, alterations, and deletions of some of the originally stated diagnoses.

NANDA was established as a formal organization in 1982 during the fifth conference. This was partially the result of the contributions made by nurses from Canada. This first conference held since the ANA's Social Policy Statement included the function of "diagnosing" in the role of the nurse. The goal of the sixth conference was dissemination of information, so all nurses were invited and more than 450 participated. Proposed nursing diagnoses were reviewed during the seventh conference and 21 diagnoses were approved, increasing the total to 84. Also, at this conference Taxonomy I was endorsed.

The taxonomy is a means by which to classify, or order, the accepted diagnoses. It classifies the diagnoses according to the nine human response patterns developed by the theorist group. These patterns include *exchanging, communicating, relating, valuing, choosing, moving, perceiving, knowing,* and *feeling.* The numeric order assists in the conceptualization of the diagnoses from abstract to concrete. For example, *exchanging* is pattern 1. Included in pattern 1 is the nursing diagnosis *High Risk for Injury;* this has been assigned the number 1.6.1. The next diagnosis is *High Risk for Suffocation,* a less abstract or more specific type of injury, so it has been assigned a lower number, 1.6.1.1. The numbers also assist in computer programing and retrieval.

At the eighth conference (1988) the ANA accepted Taxonomy I as a tool to guide the practice of nursing. Sixteen new or revised nursing diagnoses were accepted for testing, and various changes in Taxonomy I labels were made for consistency. The most recent conference, the ninth (1990), accepted two new diagnoses: altered protection and effective breastfeeding. Taxonomy I Revised 1990 was developed on completion of this conference (see box, pp. 41-42). Various

NANDA-Approved nursing diagnostic categories

This list represents the NANDA-approved nursing diagnostic categories for clinical use and testing (1988). Changes have been made in 15 labels for consistency.

Pattern 1: Exchanging

1.1.2.1	Altered nutrition: more than body requirements
1.1.2.2	Altered nutrition: less than body requirements
1.1.2.3	Altered nutrition: potential for more than body requirements
1.2.1.1	High risk for infection
1.2.2.1	High risk for altered body temperature
1.2.2.2	Hypothermia
1.2.2.3	Hyperthermia
1.2.2.4	Ineffective thermoregulation
1.2.3.1	Dysreflexia
*1.3.1.1	Constipation
1.3.1.1.1	Perceived constipation
1.3.1.1.2	Colonic constipation
*1.3.1.2	Diarrhea
*1.3.1.3	Bowel incontinence
1.3.2	Altered patterns of urinary elimination
1.3.2.1.1	Stress incontinence
1.3.2.1.2	Reflex incontinence
1.3.2.1.3	Urge incontinence
1.3.2.1.4	Functional incontinence
1.3.2.1.5	Total incontinence
1.3.2.2	Urinary retention
*1.4.1.1	Altered (specify type) tissue perfusion (renal, cerebral, cardiopulmonary, gastrointestinal, peripheral)
1.4.1.2.1	Fluid volume excess
1.4.1.2.2.1	Fluid volume deficit (1)
1.4.1.2.2.1	Fluid volume deficit (2)
1.4.1.2.2.2	High risk for fluid volume deficit
*1.4.2.1	Decreased cardiac output
1.5.1.1	Impaired gas exchange
1.5.1.2	Ineffective airway clearance
1.5.1.3	Ineffective breathing pattern
1.6.1	High risk for injury
1.6.1.1	High risk for suffocation
1.6.1.2	High risk for poisoning

Pattern 1: Exchanging—cont'd

1.6.1.3	High risk for trauma
1.6.1.4	High risk for aspiration
1.6.1.5	High risk for disuse syndrome
†1.6.2	Altered protection
1.6.2.1	Impaired tissue integrity
*1.6.2.1.1	Altered oral mucous membrane
1.6.2.1.2.1	Impaired skin integrity
1.6.2.1.2.2	High risk for impaired skin integrity

Pattern 2: Communicating

2.1.1.1	Impaired verbal communication

Pattern 3: Relating

3.1.1	Impaired social interaction
3.1.2	Social isolation
*3.2.1	Altered role performance
3.2.1.1.1	Altered parenting
3.2.1.1.2	High risk for altered parenting
3.2.1.2.1	Sexual dysfunction
3.2.2	Altered family processes
3.2.3.1	Parental role conflict
3.3	Altered sexuality patterns

Pattern 4: Valuing

4.1.1	Spiritual distress (distress of the human spirit)

Pattern 5: Choosing

5.1.1.1	Ineffective individual coping
5.1.1.1.1	Impaired adjustment

NANDA-Approved nursing diagnostic categories—cont'd

5.1.1.1.2	Defensive coping
5.1.1.1.3	Ineffective denial
5.1.2.1.1	Ineffective family coping: disabling
5.1.2.1.2	Ineffective family coping: compromised
5.1.2.2	Family coping: potential for growth
5.2.1.1	Noncompliance (specify)
5.3.1.1	Decisional conflict (specify)
5.4	Health seeking behaviors (specify)

Note. From North American Nursing Diagnosis Association, 1990, *Taxonomy I Revised 1990.* Copyright 1990 by North American Nursing Diagnosis Association.
*Categories with modified label terminology.
†New diagnostic categories approved in 1990.

Continued.

NANDA-Approved nursing diagnostic categories — cont'd

Pattern 6: Moving

6.1.1.1	Impaired physical mobility
6.1.1.2	Activity intolerance
6.1.1.2.1	Fatigue
6.1.1.3	High risk for activity intolerance
6.2.1	Sleep pattern disturbance
6.3.1.1	Diversional activity deficit
6.4.1.1	Impaired home maintenance management
6.4.2	Altered health maintenance
*6.5.1	Feeding self-care deficit
6.5.1.1	Impaired swallowing
6.5.1.2	Ineffective breastfeeding
†6.5.1.3	Effective breastfeeding
*6.5.2	Bathing/hygiene self-care deficit
*6.5.3	Dressing/grooming self-care deficit
*6.5.4	Toileting self-care deficit
6.6	Altered growth and development

Pattern 7: Perceiving

*7.1.1	Body image disturbance
*7.1.2	Self-esteem disturbance
7.1.2.1	Chronic low self-esteem
7.1.2.2	Situational low self-esteem
*7.1.3	Personal identity disturbance
7.2	Sensory/Perceptual alterations (specify) (visual, auditory, kinesthetic, gustatory, tactile, olfactory)
7.2.1.1	Unilateral neglect
7.3.1	Hopelessness
7.3.2	Powerlessness

Pattern 8: Knowing

8.1.1	Knowledge deficit (specify)
8.3	Altered thought processes

Pattern 9: Feeling

*9.1.1	Pain
9.1.1.1	Chronic pain
9.2.1.1	Dysfunctional grieving
9.2.1.2	Anticipatory grieving
9.2.2	High risk for violence: self-directed or directed at others
9.2.3	Post-trauma response
9.2.3.1	Rape-trauma syndrome
9.2.3.1.1	Rape-trauma syndrome: compound reaction
9.2.3.1.2	Rape-trauma syndrome: silent reaction
9.3.1	Anxiety
9.3.2	Fear

methods of classifying nursing diagnoses have been proposed, including categorization by body system, by function, and by medical diagnosis. Although these methods may facilitate finding a particular nursing diagnosis, the organization suggested in Taxonomy I Revised 1990 marks the beginning of a new approach to looking at patients in an independent manner. The taxonomy committee is constantly evaluating methods for assisting in the development of a workable classification system.

This taxonomy is intended to place the nursing diagnoses in some sort of order, to reveal some degree of relationship among the diagnoses, to al-low for the insertion of new or as yet undiscovered diagnoses, and to show a logical progression (abstract to concrete).

The first number denotes the pattern (pattern 1: exchanging). For example 1.3.1.1 Constipation: belongs to pattern 1: exchanging; the second number (1.**3**.1.1) denotes that it is the third diagnosis in pattern 1; the third number (1.3.**1**.1) denotes that the diagnosis is the first type of alteration in elimination (bowel); and the fourth number (1.3.1.**1**) specifies that it is the first type of bowel elimination diagnosis in difference to 1.3.1.2, which is diarrhea (the second bowel elimination diagnosis).

NURSING DIAGNOSIS AND THE NURSING PROCESS

The emerging science of nursing is based on a broad theoretical framework. The nursing process is the means by which this framework is applied to the practice of nursing. Various models of the nursing process exist, but the most commonly used model includes the following five steps: assessment, diagnosis, planning, interventions, and evaluation. The model used by the ANA (1980) includes data collection, nursing diagnosis, planning, treatment, and evaluation.

The nursing process is to provide a systematic means of problem solving. It organizes the practice of nursing into five easily recognizable phases. The first phase, assessment, is of vital importance, because if this step is in error, the results of the process will be in error. In assessment, the nurse uses all of his or her skills and knowledge to recognize, combine, test, question, and consult with co-workers to identify the patient's needs, problems, concerns, and actual or potential human responses.

Nursing diagnoses are the conclusions that the nurse makes after critically interpreting and analyzing the assessment findings. The list of NANDA-approved nursing diagnoses is by no means all-inclusive and is continually evolving. Also, the inexperienced nurse may find it difficult to use the exact terminology of NANDA. What may be more important is that the intent of the diagnosis is understood; the approved terminology will come with experience. NANDA is changing some terminology to be more consistent with nursing clinical language.

The planning step identifies strategies to correct, prevent, or minimize the nursing diagnoses or problems identified in the assessment phase. Planning should always begin with establishing priorities of care, which are best remembered by using the ABCs of **A**irway, **B**reathing, and **C**irculation. The initiation and completion of those actions necessary to achieve the desired outcomes are described in the intervention/implementation/treatment phase. These actions, particularly in the emergency and intensive care settings, may be independent or collaborative. The selection of nursing interventions depends on the nature of the diagnosis, the research base of the intervention, the feasibility for the success of the intervention, the patient's acceptability of the intervention, and the nurse's ability to use the intervention.

The final phase in the nursing process is evaluation, which is ongoing. It is meant to assess the extent to which the intervention/treatment was successful. The nurse assesses how well the patient has responded and met clinical objectives and then initiates corrective measures as necessary. The nurse may need to set new goals and develop a new plan of care.

Application of the Nursing Process to Trauma

CASE STUDY Sam Fitzgerald, a 22-year-old graduate student, was driving home at 2 AM from a part-time job. As he passed through an intersection, a speeding pickup truck hit his car on the passenger's side. Sam's car landed against a line of trees.

The respiratory system should always be the first priority in assessment. While this is being performed, a history of the trauma should be obtained, including the events preceeding the event, all information regarding the events of the injury, and mechanisms of injury. After the initial assessment, nursing diagnoses are formulated on the basis of observing and assessing certain characteristics or cues that are typically found in each diagnosis. The characteristics that follow are typically associated with the respective diagnoses (left-hand column, p. 44).

MVA injuries often involve the nonuse of seat belts, thus the transfer of kinetic forces hitting a stationary object. The nurse combines his or her assessment skills of the present injury with knowledge of similar injuries observed previously—all experiences aid in assessing the immediate situation.

After Sam is removed from the car, the nurse assists in maintaining airway patency, stabilizing and immobilizing the cervical spine, initiating intravenous therapy, monitoring vital signs, and preparing for transport.

The next phase of the assessment typically occurs in the emergency department after the initial resuscitation phase and includes further assessment, diagnosis, and treatment. This phase reflects a more collaborative approach. Diagnostic procedures reveal fractures of ribs 4, 5, 6, and 7 on the right, probable cardiac contusion, and mild concussion. Sam's flail chest is to be managed by positive pressure ventilation. He can re-

Diagnosis	Characteristics/Cues
Ineffective breathing pattern	Dyspnea Shortness of breath Altered chest expansion Pain Anxiety
Decreased cardiac output	Position of body against steering wheel (mechanism of injury) Skin pallor Irregular pulse Restlessness Hypotension
High risk for decreased cerebral tissue perfusion	Laceration of forehead Mechanism of injury Hypotension Restlessness Inability to remember accident
Pain	Verbal complaints of chest pain Muscle guarding
High risk for cervical and thoracic spine injury	Mechanism of injury

spond appropriately by nodding his head. The cervical and thoracic spine do not appear to be injured, but there are multiple lacerations on his face caused by a shattered windshield. The ECG shows some ventricular ectopy. The nursing assessment at this time determines that the diagnoses that are shown in the column on the right are pertinent.

The characteristics/cues assist the nurse in not only identifying or assessing the nursing diagnoses but intervening appropriately. The intervention for ineffective breathing caused by fractured ribs is different from that for ineffective breathing caused by a mucus plug or anxiety.

After Sam is moved to the critical care setting, further assessment is done and a third set of diagnoses is made. These may include impaired physical mobility, impaired verbal communication, activity intolerance, sleep pattern disturbance, body image disturbance, self-esteem disturbance, knowledge deficit, anxiety, and fear.

Nursing Interventions

Kim (1986) defined three types of nursing interventions: independent, collaborative/interdependent, and dependent. *Independent* nursing interventions can be administered without a physician's order and can treat the patient's problem without consulting or collaborating with physicians or other health team members. *Collaborative/interdependent* nursing interventions are initiated with a physician's order and collaboration with other health team members who are responsible for the patient's care. *Dependent* interventions are carried out with a physician's order without the nurse being consulted and without the nurse's judgment or decision-making skills. It is hoped that this type of intervention is no longer in use.

The history of nursing functions or "who does what" has been discussed as much as nursing diagnosis. Nursing functions depended mostly on physician(s') orders in the 1960s and increasingly became more collaborative during the 1970s. With the increase in nursing research, particularly in the realm of interventions, it appears that the number of independent nursing interventions

Diagnosis	Characteristics/Cues
Ineffective breathing pattern	Altered chest expansion Rib fractures Pain Anxiety Decreased oxygen content in blood
Decreased cardiac output	Cardiac contusion Elevation of cardiac isoenzymes Ventricular ectopy ST depression Vital sign changes
High risk for decreased cerebral tissue perfusion	Concussion Inability to remember accident Possible loss of consciousness Retrograde amnesia
Pain	Verbal complaints Rib fractures Contusions/lacerations
Anxiety	Nervousness Inability to talk
Fear	Emergency setting Acknowledged fear of dying

(performed without physician involvement) will increase.

Recent discussion involving nursing intervention revolves around Gordon's (1976) definition of nursing diagnosis. She concludes that nurses can intervene in problems that they have experience in and are capable of treating, if they are licensed and educated for such. As a discipline, nursing is in the midst of deciding just what interventions nurses are licensed and educated for and experienced to do. The nursing scope of practice is difficult to define in the trauma setting because of the type of practice performed.

The line between independent and collaborative nursing interventions, particularly in the trauma setting, is sometimes very narrow. Because of the standards of practice and the increasing skills of the trauma nurse, he or she may practice more independently in the trauma setting than in the typical in-patient setting.

Application of Nursing Diagnosis

Nursing diagnosis provides an established mechanism for defining "what nurses do." Nursing diagnosis assists in (1) more clearly defining the domain of nursing; (2) influencing the quality of patient care by facilitating the use of the nursing process; (3) defining the scope of nursing accountability; (4) allowing nurses to speak the same language; and (5) costing out nursing interventions.

In the trauma setting, nursing diagnosis can assist in the identification of unique needs/human responses to injuries that identify the trauma patient. Nursing diagnosis provides a mechanism for documenting signs and symptoms that the nurse assesses.

Nursing diagnoses can become the organizing framework for quality assurance, patient teaching, staff development education, consultation, and research. Maibusch (1987) described six commonly occurring nursing diagnoses found in one emergency department setting. They were (1) ineffective airway clearance, (2) anxiety, (3) impaired skin integrity, (4) impaired physical mobility, (5) knowledge deficit, and (6) ineffective breathing pattern. These nursing diagnoses could be used to develop a patient classification system and framework for calculating charges based on the nursing process.

The potential usefulness of one of these diagnoses is to devise an assessment tool, to include the cues/characteristics from NANDA. In this way all of the staff can better diagnose the problem (e.g., anxiety) while communicating on the same level. A list of nursing interventions can then be written, which might include such actions as letting the patient express his feelings, listening, sitting quietly next to the patient, answering questions, or making a telephone call. This list may help less experienced nurses try different interventions. To complete the process, expected outcomes should be available to measure usefulness or efficacy of the interventions.

Nursing diagnosis can benefit quality assurance programs also. Using the nursing diagnosis *fluid volume deficit* as an example, the process can be developed as described in the box below.

Nursing diagnosis as an organizing framework

Fluid volume deficit

Etiology/risk factors

Trauma, blunt trauma, actual loss (hemorrhage, burns).

Process criteria

Assess for decreased urine output, site of loss, hypotension, tachycardia, dysrhythmias, change in mental status, thirst, anxiety, fear, decreased pulse pressure, concentrated urine, output greater than intake, dry mucous membranes, dry skin.

Intervention

Titrate fluids as appropriate, titrate medications as appropriate to maintain adequate blood pressure, apply pressure to external bleeding sites, administer oxygen, notify physician of changes in status.

Outcome criteria (projected goals)

Patient will demonstrate a systolic blood pressure of 90, pulse of 60 to 100, respiratory rate of 12 to 16, sinus rhythm, "normal" urinary output (30 ml/hr), awake and alert mental status, normal skin turgor.

Much controversy exists regarding the usefulness of NANDA's listing of nursing diagnoses because of the lack of diagnoses for all patient areas. Not all the diagnoses are appropriate for the trauma patient and not all of the nursing diagnoses the trauma nurse formulates are listed in the taxonomy.

The development of a listing of appropriate diagnoses is in an early stage. Many individuals incorrectly assume that the NANDA list is complete and accurate. When a diagnosis is accepted by NANDA, it is accepted for testing and validation. The current list is a compilation of work completed over 15 years by clinicians, educators, and theorists. It is just the beginning, and like all innovations in their early stages, nursing diagnoses are undergoing change and development.

Nursing diagnoses will assist the trauma nurse to demonstrate and document accountability, to provide continuity of care, and to have available a standardized language. Trauma nurses should identify those already-defined nursing diagnoses that are useful and identify new nursing diagnoses that are appropriate for the trauma patient. Testing of the cues/characteristics is important also. Nursing should know which of the cues are found and their frequency of occurrence in relation to a particular nursing diagnosis. Also of importance is the occurrence of the cues with such variables as age, sex, marital status, presence of significant others, or religion.

There is a definite need for collaborative and physiologic-oriented nursing diagnoses. The trauma nurse, although not diagnosing medical disorders, does assess, intervene, and evaluate the physiologic and behavioral or psychosocial responses to the medical disorder. The nurse should be able to consistently identify those responses in a standard format to clarify nursing's collaborative role with the physician in assisting the patient to receive the best care possible and to justify charging for nursing services. Roberts (1988) in discussing nursing diagnosis in the critical care area stated that the current list of nursing diagnoses may not be appropriate to all nursing settings. The same thought applies to the trauma setting.

A trauma nurse has the opportunity to define and describe his or her practice. Nursing diagnosis pertinent to trauma nursing provides information that can be used by educators to rewrite programs of study that more realistically represent what occurs in the practice setting.

Validation of the cues/characteristics that are actually seen in trauma patients is also important. These cues may be very different in the trauma setting from those seen in a less critical environment. For example, the patient with a fractured femur at the trauma scene might be screaming that he is in pain, whereas the same patient in pain in the critical care setting may exhibit the pain by signs of depression or withdrawal or by rubbing the area.

Many of these ideas and statements may seem obvious to the expert clinician, but less experienced nurses could benefit from written information. Nurses should assess, document, and share what they know, using a common language—nursing diagnosis.

NEW DIAGNOSES

Nurses often complain about a lack of nursing diagnoses for a particular patient situation. Nursing diagnoses can be submitted by any nurse. The purpose of NANDA, as described, is to develop, refine, and promote a taxonomy of nursing. The nurses *best* able to describe what nursing diagnoses are "needed" in the trauma setting are those working in that environment. Guidelines for submitting new nursing diagnoses are included in the box on pp. 47-49.

VALIDATION IN TRAUMA NURSING

One of the most important and immediate needs for using nursing diagnosis in the trauma setting is the validation of the currently available diagnoses. Nursing research must be conducted to validate the usefulness of the diagnoses, to identify what nursing diagnoses are seen with various medical diagnoses, to validate the cues/defining characteristics for the diagnoses, to identify how many cues are essential to validate a diagnosis, and to identify what cues, if any, are always found. Only then can nurses use the nursing diagnoses in the taxonomy with confidence.

NANDA guidelines for submission of nursing diagnoses

I. Newly proposed diagnosis

The North American Nursing Diagnosis Association (NANDA) solicits newly proposed nursing diagnoses for review by the Association. Such proposed diagnoses undergo a systematic review process for inclusion in NANDA's approved list of diagnoses. Approval indicates that NANDA endorses the diagnosis for clinical testing and continuing development by the discipline.

To assist with submission of proposed diagnoses, the NANDA Diagnosis Review Committee has prepared a set of guidelines. These guidelines are designed to promote the consistency, clarity, and quality of submissions. Diagnoses that are submitted but do not meet the guidelines will be returned to the submitter for appropriate revision. Questions regarding the submission process may be forwarded to the NANDA office.

Nursing diagnosis defined (approved at Ninth Conference)

A nursing diagnosis is a clinical judgment about individual, family, or community responses to actual or potential health problems/life processes. Nursing diagnoses provide the basis for selection of nursing interventions to achieve outcomes for which the nurse is accountable.

Actual nursing diagnosis

1. **Label** The label provides a name for the diagnosis, a concise phrase or term that represents a pattern of related cues. Diagnostic labels may include but *are not limited* to the following qualifiers:
   Altered A change from baseline
   Impaired Made worse, weakened; damaged, reduced; deteriorated
   Depleted Emptied wholly or partially; exhausted of
   Deficient Inadequate in amount, quality, or degree; defective; not sufficient; incomplete
   Excessive Characterized by an amount or quantity that is greater than is necessary, desirable, or useful
   Dysfunctional Abnormal; incomplete functioning
   Disturbed Agitated; interrupted, interfered with
   Ineffective Not producing the desired effect
   Decreased Lessened; lesser in size, amount, or degree
   Increased Greater in size, amount, or degree
   Acute Severe, but of short duration
   Chronic Lasting a long time; recurring; habitual; constant
   Intermittent Stopping and starting again at intervals; periodic; cyclic
2. **Definition** The definition of the diagnosis provides a clear, precise description. The definition delineates its meaning and helps differentiate this diagnosis from similar diagnoses.
3. **Defining Characteristics** Defining characteristics are clinical cues that cluster as manifestations of a nursing diagnosis. Diagnostic cues are clinical evidence that describes a cluster of behaviors or signs and symptoms that represent a diagnostic label. Diagnostic cues are concrete and measurable through observation or patient/group reports. Diagnostic cues are separated into major and minor.
   Major diagnostic cues are critical indicators of the diagnosis. Minor diagnostic cues are supporting indicators that are not always present but they complete the clinical picture and increase the diagnostician's confidence in making the diagnosis.* Differentiation of major from minor characteristics should be logically defended. If appropriate, the submitter may designate major as occurring 80% to 100% of the time and minor as occurring 50% to 79% of the time.
4. **Related Factors** Related factors are conditions or circumstances that can cause or contribute to the development of a diagnosis. Related factors that are associated with the proposed diagnosis must be listed and supported by an accompanying literature review.

Note. From North American Nursing Diagnosis Association, 1990, *Taxonomy I Revised 1990.* Copyright 1990 by North American Nursing Diagnosis Association.
*Gordon, M. *Nursing Diagnosis: Process and Application.* New York: McGraw-Hill Company, 1982.

Continued.

5. **Literature/Clinical Validation** A narrative review of the relevant literature is required to support the rationale for the diagnosis, the defining characteristics, and the related factors. If the diagnosis is similar to an approved NANDA diagnosis, the reason for its usefulness must be addressed. Literature citations for defining characteristics are required and should be cited for each cue. If defining characteristics are not supported by the literature, an explanation for their inclusion is required. In addition, the designation of major versus minor defining characteristics must be supported by clinical data. These data can be derived from case studies, nurse consensus, retrospective chart reviews, and/or other appropriate validation methods. A sample three-part (label, related factors, and signs and symptoms) nursing diagnostic statement with the associated outcome criteria and nurse-prescribed interventions must accompany the submission.

Sample

Activity Intolerance: Related to deconditioned status as evidenced by inability to wash body or body parts without tachycardia, dyspnea, and fatigue.

Outcome Criteria: Bathes independently without tachycardia or dyspnea

Interventions: Position to minimize energy requirements; assist to recondition; teach energy conservation techniques and pacing techniques; provide assistance as indicated

II. High-risk nursing diagnosis
(NANDA-approved diagnoses previously designated as "Potential" are labeled "High Risk for" after 1992)

A high-risk nursing diagnosis is a clinical judgment that an individual, family, or community is more vulnerable to develop the problem than others in the same or similar situation. High-risk nursing diagnoses are supported by risk factors that guide nursing interventions to reduce or prevent the occurrence of the problem.

1. **Label** The label provides a name for the diagnosis, a concise phrase or term that represents a pattern of related cues. Diagnostic labels may include but *are not limited* to the following qualifiers:

   Altered A change from baseline

   Impaired Made worse, weakened; damaged, reduced; deteriorated

   Depleted Emptied wholly or partially; exhausted of

   Deficient Inadequate in amount, quality, or degree; defective; not sufficient; incomplete

   Excessive Characterized by an amount or quantity that is greater than is necessary, desirable, or useful

   Dysfunctional Abnormal; incomplete functioning

   Disturbed Agitated; interrupted, interfered with

   Ineffective Not producing the desired effect

   Decreased Lessened; lesser in size, amount, or degree

   Increased Greater in size, amount, or degree

   Acute Severe, but of short duration

   Chronic Lasting a long time; recurring; habitual; constant

   Intermittent Stopping and starting again at intervals; periodic; cyclic

2. **Definition** The definition of the diagnosis provides a clear, precise description. The definition delineates its meaning and helps differentiate this diagnosis from similar diagnoses.

3. **Risk Factors** Risk factors identify behaviors, conditions, or circumstances that render an individual, family, or community more vulnerable to a particular problem than others in the same or similar situation. There are not signs and symptoms for high-risk diagnoses.

4. **Literature/Clinical Validation** A narrative review of the relevant literature is required to support the rationale for the diagnosis and the risk factors. If the diagnosis is similar to an approved NANDA diagnosis, the reason for its usefulness must be addressed. The submission must include a sample two-part (including label and risk factors) high-risk nursing diagnostic statement with related outcome criteria and nurse-prescribed interventions.

   Sample

   High Risk for Injury: Fall related to fatigue and altered gait.

   Outcome Criteria: Describes or demonstrates necessary safety measures

   Interventions: Teach measures to prevent falls; instruct to request assistance when needed.

Note. From North American Nursing Diagnosis Association, 1990, *Taxonomy I Revised 1990.* Copyright 1990 by North American Nursing Diagnosis Association.

*Gordon, M. *Nursing Diagnosis: Process and Application.* New York: McGraw-Hill Company, 1982.

NANDA guidelines for submission of nursing diagnoses—cont'd

III. Wellness nursing diagnosis

A wellness nursing diagnosis is a clinical judgment about an individual, family, or community in transition from a specific level of wellness to a higher level of wellness.

1. **Label** The label "Potential for Enhanced" will be the designated qualifier. *Enhanced* is defined as made greater, to increase in quality, or more desired. Wellness diagnoses will be one-part statements.
2. **Definition** The definition of the label provides a clear, precise description. The definition delineates its meaning and helps differentiate this diagnosis from all others.
3. **Literature/Clinical Validation** A narrative review of the relevant literature is required to support the rationale for the diagnosis and the risk factors. A sample one-part wellness nursing diagnostic statement with related outcome criteria and nurse-prescribed interventions must accompany the submission.

   Sample

   Potential for Enhanced Parenting

   Outcome Criteria: Will practice listening without advice-giving with children

   Interventions: Describe active listening; differentiate between listening and advice-giving

IV. Revision of NANDA-approved nursing diagnoses

Changes can be proposed for the label, the definition, and/or the defining characteristics. In order for any NANDA-approved nursing diagnosis to be refined or revised, the proposal must contain the following:

1. A narrative describing the rationale for the proposed change.
2. Research findings to support the proposed changes. These findings can be the results of research by the submitter or from research reported in the literature.

V. Deletion of NANDA-approved nursing diagnoses

Proposals can be submitted to delete a NANDA-approved nursing diagnosis. The proposal must contain a narrative describing the rationale for the proposed deletion. The rationale must be supported by the following:

1. Logical justification.
2. Research findings and/or relevant literature review.

VI. Diagnosis review committee review cycle

1. Submission Deadline: March 1 (year prior to conference, e.g., 1991, 1993, 1995).
2. Initial review by Diagnosis Review Committee (DRC) chairperson for inclusion of required components.
3. Incomplete submissions returned with a resubmission deadline date of July 1.
4. Submissions with all the required components will be reviewed by the DRC. One of the following decisions will be made for each submission:
   a. Not Accepted—The proposed diagnosis has not been accepted for review by the Expert Advisory Panel. Reasons for "not accepted" are:
      - Represents a medical diagnosis
      - Represents a treatment or procedure
      - Did not represent a human response
      - Defining characteristics for actual nursing diagnosis are not cues or signs or symptoms
      - Defining characteristics for high-risk diagnosis are not risk factors
   b. Hold for Revisions—This proposed diagnosis will be returned to the submitter for revisions. Examples of needed revisions are the following:
      - Research population was not representative for conclusions drawn
      - Inadequate literature support for proposed diagnosis
   c. Accepted for Expert Advisory Panel Review
5. After the Expert Advisory Panel and the DRC review, each proposed diagnosis or proposal (revisions or deletions) will receive one of the following designations:
   a. Returned to Be Developed (TBD)—This decision delineates submitted work as promising but requires substantive development. This work will require resubmission in its entirety to the DRC. This category acknowledges promising work in need of substantive revisions.
   b. Conditional Accept—This category indicates a provisional acceptance of the submitted work pending receipt of revisions agreed on by the committee and the submitter.
   c. Accepted—This category indicates the submitted work is accepted.
6. Accepted diagnoses or proposals for revisions/deletions will be forwarded to the Board of Directors for approval.
7. Board-approved proposed diagnoses or proposals for revisions/deletions will be presented at the NANDA conference and will be subject to membership mail vote.

SUMMARY Nursing diagnosis has the potential to address many of nursing's current limitations. Although the movement is less than 20 years old, it is widely accepted. Specialty groups now have the potential to define their specific areas of practice and to build on the foundation of nursing diagnosis. Likewise, trauma nurses have the unique opportunity to define and describe those nursing diagnoses that are particular to trauma care and to thereby enhance the practice of trauma nursing.

RESEARCH QUESTIONS

- What are the most commonly found nursing diagnoses in the various trauma settings (prehospital, transport, emergency and critical care)?
- What is the relationship between these nursing diagnoses and medical diagnoses?
- Are NANDA's cues/characteristics appropriate for a given diagnosis?
- What nursing diagnoses are not identified that occur in the trauma patient?
- Are there specific cues that are found in the trauma setting that are not found in other settings?
- Are there cues and nursing diagnoses that are pertinent for particular patient groups, e.g., age, sex, ethnic, religious, or socioeconomic group, presence of support group or significant other, or mechanism of injury?

RESOURCES

North American Nursing Diagnosis Association (NANDA)
Debi Folkerts, Executive Director
St. Louis University School of Nursing
3525 Caroline Street
St. Louis, MO 63104
(314) 577-8954

ANNOTATED BIBLIOGRAPHY

North American Nursing Diagnosis Association. (1990). *Taxonomy I Revised 1990.* St. Louis: Author.
  Contains official diagnostic categories, definitions, defining characteristics, related factors, critical factors, date accepted, development/submission guidelines, review cycle, and introduction to ICD-10.
Nursing Diagnosis. (1990-present). The official journal of the North American Nursing Diagnosis Association. Philadelphia: J.B. Lippincott.
  Contains original articles related to nursing diagnosis, book reviews, and NANDA news.
Wake, M. (Ed.). (1987). Symposium: Nursing diagnosis in critical care. *Heart and Lung,* 16(1), 593-635.
  Includes six papers presented at the 1987 National Conference on Nursing Diagnosis in Critical Care. It was intended to encourage discussion by nurses about issues related to nursing diagnosis pertinent to their clinical realm. Topics include nursing practice, administration, research, and education.

REFERENCES

Abdellah, F.B. (1957). Methods of identifying covert aspects of nursing problems. *Nursing Research,* 6, 4-23.
American Nurses Association. (1980). *Nursing: A social policy statement.* Kansas City: American Nurses Association.
American Nurses Association. (1973). *Standards of nursing practice.* Kansas City: American Nurses Association.
Chambers, W. (1962). Nursing diagnosis. *American Journal of Nursing,* 62, 102-104.
Durand, M., & Price, R. (1966). Nursing diagnosis: Process and decision. *Nursing Forum,* 5, 50-64.
Emergency Nurses Association. (1991). *Standards of emergency nursing practice.* St. Louis: Mosby–Year Book, Inc.
Gordon, M. (1976). Nursing diagnosis and the diagnostic process. *American Journal of Nursing,* 76, 1298-1300.
Kim, M.J. (1986). Nursing diagnosis: A Janus view. In M.E. Hurley (Ed.), *Classification of nursing diagnoses: Proceedings of the Sixth Conference* (pp. 1-4). St. Louis: Mosby–Year Book, Inc.
Maibusch, R.M. (1987). Implementing nursing diagnosis. *Nursing Clinics of North America,* 22, 955-969.
McCain, R.F. (1965). Nursing by assessment—not intuition. *American Journal of Nursing,* 65(4), 82-84.
McManus, L. (1950). Assumption of functions of nursing. In Teachers College, Division of Nursing Education, *Regional planning for nursing and nursing education.* New York: Teachers College Press.
McLane, A.M. (Ed.). (1987). *Classification of nursing diagnoses: Proceedings of the Seventh Conference* (pp. 464-465). St. Louis: Mosby–Year Book, Inc.
NANDA-approved nursing diagnostic categories. (1988). *Nursing Diagnosis Newsletter,* 15, 1.
Roberts, S.L. (1988). Physiologic nursing diagnoses are necessary and appropriate for critical care. *Focus on Critical Care,* 15(2), 42-49.
Webster's Ninth New Collegiate Dictionary. (1987). Springfield, MA: Merriam-Webster.

4 *Legal Issues*

■■■

Sarah D. Cohn

OBJECTIVES
- ❏ Describe the principles of law governing consent to treatment, autopsy, and organ donation in trauma.
- ❏ List selected professional liability risks in trauma and selected steps to minimize risk.
- ❏ Outline the legal aspects of risk of employee infection.

INTRODUCTION   At least as many legal questions arise in the delivery of trauma care as arise in the rest of health care, but those caring for trauma cases have far less time to consider questions and obtain answers. This chapter discusses some of the most important and frequently occurring legal issues for the trauma staff, including questions of consent for medical care and for autopsy, relationships with police and other nonhospital personnel, and professional liability concerns. The information provided should not be construed as legal advice; when a difficult situation arises, the trauma staff should refer to hospital policy or consult with appropriate hospital personnel.

PATIENT CONSENT ISSUES

Many consent issues are involved in trauma nursing. Discussed in this chapter are general consent for medical care, living wills and powers of attorney, consent for autopsy and consent for organ donation.

Consent for Medical Care

Case law since the early 1900s confirms that a patient must consent to his or her treatment. This principle remains true even for trauma patients, as long as they are able to consider the treatment and give consent. For example, an adult patient who has sustained a traumatic amputation of a digit without other injuries probably can consider

the alternatives for treatment. Unless he or she has psychiatric problems that impair judgment, the law permits the patient to refuse reattachment of the digit even if health care providers disagree with the decision. In the same situation, if the patient refuses surgery to stop life-threatening arterial bleeding, he or she might be considered suicidal and psychiatrically impaired. In these cases, it may be wise to document the patient's impairment and obtain substitute consent from a family member (Borak & Veilleux, 1984) or to consider an emergency court action.

Both early and modern cases confirm that a health care provider may provide treatment in an emergency without consent. Practical questions arise over the definition of an emergency. Generally, the definition involves two aspects. First, the patient must be incapacitated and unable to exercise his or her judgment and make an informed choice. A patient may be unconscious, delirious, or hallucinating, for example. Second, the patient must suffer from a life-threatening condition that requires immediate treatment. Hemorrhage from a ruptured spleen is an example. If these two conditions are met, it is presumed that a reasonable person would consent to the "preservation of his life or limb" and consent will be implied (*Mohr v. Williams*, 1905).

It is preferable to obtain consent before the patient receives medications such as analgesia, which may impair judgment. However, a patient is not necessarily disqualified from giving consent if he or she has received a narcotic; ability to consent may actually be improved, if pain had caused the patient to be out of control. The type of medication, dose, timing, route of administration, and effect must all be considered when a claim is made that consent was ineffective as a result of medication. When a patient has been medicated before giving consent, the patient's need for the medication and his or her mental status when the treatment was discussed should be documented in the medical record.

Many trauma situations involve true emergencies when the patient cannot consent. Adequate documentation of the patient's condition, preferably by the physician, will demonstrate the need for immediate evaluation and treatment and will show why an adequate discussion with the patient was not possible. When family members are available, substitute consent can be obtained in an emergency. Hospital policies should contain a procedure to be used when substituted consent or telephone consent is to be obtained. When a patient is physically unable to sign his or her name, a witnessed mark is acceptable. If the patient cannot make a mark, verbal consent may be obtained and documented by the physician in the medical record. If verbal consent to surgery is accepted or emergency trauma surgery has taken place without consent, the patient need not sign a consent form later. The patient remains responsible for payment for these emergency services even though he or she could not consent to them at the time.

Although many health care providers permit a family member to assent to planned emergency surgery, most do not permit that same family member to refuse life-saving treatment for the patient, particularly if the patient is admitted unconscious and the staff could not discuss the patient's wishes. For example, an unconscious adult patient who requires immediate blood transfusion for survival should be transfused despite relatives who refuse because of their own religious convictions. The general view is that because death from lack of blood or any other cause is irrevocable, when death may be preventable, the adult patient must make his own decision. When the patient regains consciousness, discussions may ensue and the patient may then be permitted to refuse further blood transfusions.

If the injured patient is a minor, many of the same principles apply. That is, the hospital should try to locate a parent from whom consent may be obtained, but indicated life-saving evaluation and treatment should proceed (Holder, 1985).

These principles remain part of the common law in many states. In others, state legislatures have enacted statutes that attempt to provide some guidance to health care providers. For example, current New York law states that (New York Public Health Law, 1988):

> (m)edical, dental, health and hospital services may be rendered to persons of any age without the consent of a parent or legal guardian when, in the physician's judgment, an emergency exists and the person is in immediate need of medical attention and an attempt to secure consent would result in delay of treatment which would increase the risk to the person's life or health.

When the emergency exception has been used to presume consent, the scope of the consent is limited to what must be done. No consent is presumed for elective treatment or surgery.

Living Wills and Powers of Attorney

By March, 1991, 42 states and the District of Columbia had enacted so-called living will or natural death acts. The provisions vary considerably, but in general these laws protect the right of a terminally ill person who has become incapable of expressing his or her wishes to refuse life-prolonging treatment when the treatment would be of no value. Twelve of these statutes also authorize the appointment of a health care agent or proxy. The powers of this agent may vary but may be limited to authorizing termination of treatment in accordance with the provisions of the living will (Society for the Right to Die, 1991).

By its terms, a living will should not usually be applicable to treatment decisions in a trauma setting, since it is not clear upon the patient's arrival that he or she is in a terminal condition. Instead, a patient's condition should be evaluated and stabilized in the emergency or trauma service. Only then can a decision about prognosis be made and treatment alternatives discussed with patient or family.

Widespread misunderstanding exists among the public about the applicability of a living will.

A living will should not be used to justify family refusal of treatment for a condition in an elderly person that could be treated and from which the patient is expected to recover. These patients are not in a "terminal" condition. In most states, a living will is not binding upon the health care provider, but is advisory only and is used to help determine what the patient would have wanted under the circumstances. The provisions of a living will statute are intended to supplement the common law rights of a patient to decline treatment, not replace them.

A durable power of attorney can be executed in addition to or in lieu of a living will. It is signed by a competent patient and used to designate a person (or institution, such as a bank) who will be responsible for managing that patient's affairs when he or she becomes unable to do so for self (an ordinary power of attorney is inapplicable when the patient becomes incompetent). In 24 states and the District of Columbia, a statute explicitly provides for a durable power of attorney for health care decisions. Under these statutes, a patient can explicitly designate who will make treatment decisions. In some of these states, statutes limit the power to certain types of decisions. In at least 7 other states, an ordinary durable power of attorney can be used to designate a treatment decision maker if the patient so desires.

If a living will or an applicable durable power of attorney exists, a copy should be placed in the patient's medical record. If the patient is competent, every effort should be made to clarify with the patient his or her desires, since the language of a living will is quite broad in most cases and patients differ about what types of treatment they wish to avoid (Eisendrath & Jonson, 1983).

Consent for Autopsy

A general rule of law is that autopsies are done only with patient or family consent unless there is statutory authority given a third party, such as a coroner or medical examiner. Most states have statutes that require the notification of a coroner or medical examiner when death occurs under certain circumstances. For example, statutes may require medical examiner notification when a death occurs at home, when death appears to be caused by a homocide or child abuse, when death occurs within 24 hours of arrival at a hospital, or

when the cause of death is unexplained (Connecticut General Statutes, 1988) Once the medical examiner or coroner is notified of the death and the known facts (this may be done by the police from the scene of a crime or by hospital personnel later), the medical examiner may choose to perform an autopsy or may decline. If an autopsy is to be done by the medical examiner, family consent is not required. Several cases have challenged the coroner's statutory authority to perform an autopsy without family consent; in most cases, this authority has been upheld as long as the case satisfies the statutory requirements.

When the medical examiner declines to do an autopsy or the circumstances of the death do not involve the medical examiner, the statutes may list those family members (in order of preference) who may give consent, or may simply state that the next of kin who takes responsibility for the burial of the body may consent. Some statutes explicitly authorize the patient to give permission for his or her own autopsy. When a family member consents to an autopsy, the autopsy may be limited to a particular body part or system, such as the head or heart. Any restrictions on the autopsy should be clearly noted on the autopsy consent form.

Consent for Organ Donation

All 50 states and the District of Columbia have enacted some form of the Uniform Anatomical Gift Act. These statutes are meant to encourage anatomical donation and to provide procedures to be followed for donation. Generally, any person who is at least 18 years of age and of sound mind may donate all or part of his or her body. Some laws permit donation by minors with parental consent. The states have provided methods by which persons may indicate their intent to donate organs upon death. For example, the gift of an organ may be made by will or by card; in some states a portion of the driver's license is marked if the driver is willing to be an organ donor.

Designation of an organ gift may be legal but may be opposed by family members. Many hospitals are reluctant to accept an otherwise legal organ gift if the family is hostile, because it is the family that will survive and may sue, whereas the organ donor will not be able to defend the hospital's decision. Adequate premortem documentation of the intent of the gift by the donor can encourage a hospital to act upon the gift.

When there is no organ gift by a designated method and the patient is a suitable donor, the statutes specify family members who may give permission. In order of preference, the statutes usually name the spouse, an adult child, either parent, an adult sibling, a guardian, or any person who is authorized to accept the body for burial. Although the statutes may specify that only one member of the consenting class may consent, the statutes often do not provide assistance when there are several family members who are in conflict about organ donation (when, for example, there are several siblings, some of whom approve of organ donation and some of whom disapprove). Some statutes indicate that a member of the same or higher class in terms of statutory preference may object, usually in writing.

Since 1986 many states have passed "organ request laws," which require that hospital personnel determine from the patient or family if organ donation is desired upon the patient's death. These laws do not require the patient or family to consent to donation. In fact, usually the staff need not even make the inquiry if the patient's medical condition renders him or her an unsuitable organ donor.

Because laws in the various states differ, each trauma center should have developed procedures or guidelines that govern consent to organ donation. Many large centers have organ donation or transplant coordinators who are familiar with state law and with hospital policy and can assist staff with family members.

PATIENT MEDICAL INFORMATION

It is a long-standing rule, by common law in some states and by statute in others, that although the institution makes and owns the medical record, the patient or guardian retains rights to the release of the record information. In general, trauma and other personnel should not discuss a patient's medical condition with anyone without the patient's permission (preferably in writing) or other legal authority. For example, many facilities perform a blood alcohol level on all trauma patients for medical treatment purposes. This is permissible but the results should not be released to the police without patient or family consent (if the patient is a minor), or without a court order

or search warrant. Because the law does not require a hospital to maintain chain of custody (a signed list of all those in the chain of possession of the specimen) documentation on tests done for medical reasons, police who obtain these test results via legal authority should be told whether the hospital maintains chain of custody documentation.

Some hospitals agree to take blood or tissue samples from certain patients for legal reasons. In these cases, there should be some legal authority to draw the blood, unless there is patient consent. A tube of blood should not be drawn and presented to the police without patient knowledge (unless there is an authorizing state statute). If the sample and its result are to be used in legal proceedings later, the chain of custody should be maintained in the processing of the sample or in its delivery to the appropriate law enforcement officer.

No patient consent is needed for certain statutory reporting. For example, a death that is probably a homocide is reportable to the medical examiner and, depending on state law, to the police if they do not already know about the death. In some states, a gunshot or stab wound that does not result in death is reportable to local police by statute, since it is presumed that a crime has been committed (although hospital personnel may not know by whom). Where there is no statute authorizing this type of reporting, it may be the local custom to report. A recent case involving a human bite has upheld the right of a health care provider to notify police of certain information when the health care provider believes that a crime may have been committed (*Bryson v. Tillinghast*, 1988). Information that is released about a possible crime should be limited to the fact of the wound and the identity of the patient. Thereafter, the police will obtain legal authority to obtain medical records and other information.

Emergency department personnel may examine the belongings of a trauma patient to determine identity and next of kin and to identify and store any valuables. If a weapon or an illegal or unidentified substance is found among the patient's belongings, the staff should consult with the hospital security force to determine how the items are to be treated under relevant state law.

A hospital emergency department often receives telephone calls from persons inquiring about a patient. Hospital personnel may confirm a patient's presence and may, but need not, give a general description of the injuries (e.g., head or abdominal). No further specific information should be given without further information about the caller and patient consent if the caller is not a family member. These rules apply to information released to the press as well. Hospital personnel should not discuss a patient's condition with non–hospital personnel without the patient's consent. The press may be able to videotape the trauma scene but should not be permitted into the treatment area without patient consent (or a hospital may refuse to permit the press into the treatment area under most or any circumstances).

PROFESSIONAL RELATIONSHIPS

Trauma personnel frequently deal with police, investigators, attorneys in personal injury cases, medical examiners, and others. So that the work proceeds with as little disruption as possible, the staff should maintain collegial relationships with everyone who may have a legal interest. However, this relationship should not be maintained at the expense of the patient. The police, for example, should not attempt to obtain medical information to which they are not entitled by misusing their authority or by presuming on a friendship with trauma personnel. In the same way, trauma personnel should not presume on their relationship with local police to influence legal proceedings for family or friends (e.g., trying to get a traffic ticket "fixed"). When these improprieties take place and are revealed, the integrity of the trauma service and of the police is damaged.

EMERGENCY DEPARTMENT TRANSFERS

Federal law (the Social Security Act) requires that a hospital that has an emergency department provide an "appropriate medical screening examination within the capability of the hospital's emergency department" to any individual who presents himself, regardless of the patient's ability to pay. The examination must determine if an "emergency medical condition" exists or if the person is in active labor. An emergency medical condition is defined in the statute as a (Social Security Act Section 1867):

> medical condition manifesting itself by acute symptoms of sufficient severity (including severe pain) such that the absence of immediate medical attention could reasonably be expected to result in:

- placing the patient's health in serious jeopardy;
- serious impairment to bodily functions; or
- serious dysfunction of any bodily organ or part.

Active labor is defined also.

The hospital is required (1) to provide examination and treatment within the staff and hospital capabilities to stabilize the patient or (2) to transfer the patient to another facility. Stabilization is said to have occurred when, within reasonable medical probability, no "material" deterioration is likely to result from the transfer or occur during the transfer. Patients may not be asked about payment before they are examined and provided with stabilizing treatment.

When transfer is to occur from one hospital to another and the patient has an emergency medical condition that is not stabilized (as is often the case in a trauma transfer), there are specific rules to follow to show that the transfer was appropriate. In general the following are required:

- The transferring hospital must provide medical treatment within its capacity to minimize risks to the individual being transferred.
- The receiving facility must be contacted and have available space and personnel to receive the transfer.
- The receiving facility must agree to accept the transfer.
- The transferring hospital must send copies of all available medical records related to the medical problem for which the patient is being transferred.
- The individual or family, after being informed of the risks, must request a transfer, or a physician must sign a certification that the benefits of the transfer outweigh the risks. A nonphysician can sign the certification after consultation with the physician, and the physician may countersign the document later.
- The transfer must be effected using qualified personnel and transportation equipment.

The transferring hospital must maintain thorough documentation that all these conditions have been met before any unstable patient is transferred. Individuals refusing treatment or transfer must be informed of the consequences of their refusal; this refusal and discussion should be documented and include a patient signature if possible. Other rules, e.g., posting signs to inform patients of their rights, are beyond the scope of this chapter.

The Health Care Financing Authority (HCFA) investigates instances of alleged violations of these requirements, called "anti-dumping" measures. Hospitals and individual physicians can be fined; as of March, 1990, two hospitals were barred from participation in federal health programs because of these investigations and three others were suspended from participation. One physician who was found to have transferred a patient in active labor was fined $20,000 ("Stricter Patient," 1990). Civil suits by patients can be and have been brought for violations of these federal requirements.

Hospitals with trauma services are more likely to receive than to transfer patients. However, the trauma staff must understand these rules so that they can assist the transferring hospital in complying and for those occasions when the trauma hospital itself transfers a patient out to another facility.

PROFESSIONAL LIABILITY IN TRAUMA CARE

The principles of professional liability are the same for trauma providers as they are for nursing and medical providers working in other specialties and will not be reviewed here. Many cases in the legal literature involve allegations of malpractice in the care of trauma patients, although no "trauma service" was identifiable when the incidents took place.

In some of these cases, physicians and hospitals have claimed that they are or should be immune from liability for ordinary negligence under the relevant state's Good Samaritan statute. Although there have been cases to the contrary, the majority opinion can be found in the court's ruling in *Colby v. Schwartz* (1978). In this case, a patient who was injured in an automobile accident was admitted through the emergency department to an intensive care unit. The on-call emergency physician arrived at about 1 PM, and the patient was taken to surgery at 3 PM. He died on the operating table at about 4:30 PM. The cause of death was hemorrhage as a result of multiple intraabdominal lacerations caused by blunt trauma during the accident. The estate of the patient sued the surgeon for negligent care. The surgeon, in an attempt to have the case dismissed, argued that he should be immune from suit under the

Good Samaritan statute. The court ruled that the statute was meant to protect those health care providers who, by chance and irregularly, were called upon to render emergency care. The surgeon in this case, who was part of the emergency call system, did not render the type of "emergency care," that would make him eligible for the statutory protection.

In other cases the allegations concern the adequate evaluation and treatment of an injured patient. An example is *Thomas v. Corso* (1972). In that case, Mr. Corso had been hit by a passing car while he was scraping ice off his own automobile. He was found by a friend who witnessed the accident. Mr. Corso was unconscious with blood coming from his mouth, but promptly regained consciousness. He was brought to the emergency service of a nearby hospital at 11:10 PM. On admission, his pulse was 84, respirations were 26, and blood pressure was 80/60. He was given meperidine, and a laceration on his head was cleaned. Although he complained of hip pain while at the site of the accident and numbness in the right anterior thigh at the hospital, the nurse observed that the right leg was not deformed and that the patient could move it. The on-call physician was called at 11:25 PM but did not come in. The patient was admitted, but since there was an influenza epidemic and there were no beds available, he remained in a hallway in the emergency department. The patient's blood pressure continued to be in the 70/50 range, and the nurses continued to take vital signs periodically. At 1 AM the blood pressure was 94/70 with a pulse of 100. The patient experienced a cardiopulmonary arrest at about 2 AM and was pronounced dead at 2:30 AM when Dr. Thomas arrived at the hospital. When Dr. Thomas arrived, he noted deformity of the patient's right leg. Autopsy showed a lacerated liver, comminuted fractures of the femoral neck and portions of the pelvis, and extensive hemorrhage associated with the fractures.

In the malpractice case that followed, disputes arose among the nurses and Dr. Thomas. The nursing staff attributed the patient's thirst to his intoxication, and his hypotension to the meperidine administration. Dr. Thomas claimed that it was the duty of the nursing staff to keep him informed of the patient's condition and that he had relied on them. The jury found against the physician and hospital and awarded damages of $99,609.24. On appeal, the court affirmed the jury award. It found that the physician had enough information about the patient from the nursing staff to determine that his presence at the hospital was needed, and it found that the nursing staff had misinterpreted the severity of the patient's symptoms.

This case and others like it hold that the trauma and emergency department staffs must use reasonable judgment in the care of their patients. These standards of care, which are judged as of the time of the incident, not as of a later date, are set in part by professional organizations in their publications and standards. In trauma care, relevant information may be found in the American College of Surgeons' Committee on Trauma Guidelines, and in American Association of Critical Care Nurses' and Emergency Nurses' Association Standards. These are supplemented by the professional literature and by protocols and procedures written by trauma staffs. Although the trend is to develop written standards, the standards cannot cover every aspect of care. Therefore a standard of care can be set also by reasonable practice patterns.

Trauma Service Protocols and Procedures

Many trauma services have found it useful to design action plans, protocols, or procedures for various types of injuries commonly seen by the service. These documents should be carefully designed. Although they can be quite useful for nursing, housestaff, and attending physicians, they should be broad enough to comport with legitimate individual and medical practice variations.

Because protocols, if relevant, are sure to be used in any professional liability action against hospital or trauma personnel, they should reflect current acceptable practice rather than aspirations for improvement in the future. To illustrate, it may be the standard of care within the profession that an aortogram team be available to the trauma service within 1 hour. If so, any protocol should reflect that (if any time limit is necessary in a protocol) rather than a shorter time, which some might prefer but which is currently unrealistic.

Unless the provisions are meant to be binding on everyone and under all circumstances, the protocols might better be called *guidelines*, because that term implies room for more staff flexibility and judgment. In a professional liability action, protocols and guidelines often are used to set

the standard of care to which the trauma personnel should have adhered. If the staff has not complied with its own rules, it will have the burden of explaining why the rule was not applicable under the circumstances of the case.

Professional Liability Insurance

Hospitals customarily provide professional liability insurance for employees in an amount considered adequate in that state or region. Employer-provided professional liability insurance is applicable only within the employee's scope of employment. Nurses who view the employer-provided insurance as inadequate or who sometimes practice elsewhere should carry their own professional liability insurance. When a nurse carries personal professional liability insurance, it usually is not primary in those cases when other (employer) insurance is applicable.

DOCUMENTATION IN TRAUMA CARE

Many cases in the legal literature demonstrate the effect of documentation of care on a professional liability case. If documentation of care is thorough, the case may not be brought at all, since the patient and his attorney may be satisfied with the contemporaneous written explanation. If a claim is made, thorough documentation makes it much easier to defend. By contrast, even a defensible professional liability case may be difficult to defend when the documentation is inadequate, and settlement may be necessary.

The trauma team members must document care. For example, if a patient experiences anterior tibial compartment syndrome, a claim may be made that the patient was not moved to the operating room in a timely manner. Gaps in medical record documentation could make it appear that the staff did not attend to the patient during those periods.

When the patient is in critical condition and events occur rapidly, the staff still must document care, although the documentation may be done after the crisis. Critical information can be jotted on a piece of paper and transferred to the trauma form later. If this is done, most experts see no need to include the scrap paper in the record along with the transcription. Notes should be dated and timed, and late entries should be recorded as such—not written between previously recorded lines. All charting, current *and* after-the-fact, should be recorded on-line—not squeezed between lines. Personal notes may be retained for those cases that may prove to be troublesome. However, although many nurses are not aware of it, if a malpractice action is brought, these notes must be released if the staff member's testimony is requested.

Finally, if a patient is uncooperative for any reason (intoxication, personality, or anger) and attempts to refuse care, the trauma staff must document the circumstances. At least enough evaluation must be done to ensure that the patient's uncooperative or aggressive behavior is not caused by physiologic conditions such as blood loss or a head injury. A patient who refuses evaluation must be informed of the potential consequences of the refusal; a clear note should reflect this discussion. If a patient's competence is at least questionable and the treatment is urgent but not a true emergency, the staff may consider the appointment of a temporary conservator or guardian to consider medical care. The speed with which this can be done varies by jurisdiction, but it often can be accomplished within 1 to 2 hours.

CLINICAL RISKS IN TRAUMA NURSING

The Centers for Disease Control (CDC) estimated that in a hypothetical hospital with 10,000 admissions per year and an HIV infection prevalence rate of 1%, there will be approximately 105 HIV-infected patients and at least 2 or 3 who are infectious but who are not yet HIV-positive (Centers for Disease Control [CDC], August 1987).

Although the actual number is not known (since HIV-positivity alone is not reportable to state health authorities in all states), it has been estimated that from 1 to 4 million persons are currently infected with HIV (Schurgin, 1988). As of August, 1991, more than 180,000 cases of AIDS have been reported.

The CDC has estimated also that there are 300,000 cases of hepatitis B in this country every year. Of health care workers whose work entails blood exposure, 500 to 600 are hospitalized annually, with more than 200 deaths annually (U.S. Department of Labor, 1987).

In May, 1987, the CDC reported that it knew of nine health care workers without other known risk factors who had acquired the human immunodeficiency virus through patient contact. The circumstances of three of those seroconversions were reported that month. In one, a female health care provider assisted with an unsuccessful attempt to insert an arterial catheter in a patient suffering from cardiac arrest in the emergency service. She then applied pressure to the insertion site to stop the bleeding and probably had blood on her index finger for about 20 minutes before she washed her hands. The worker was not wearing gloves during her blood exposure and had chapped hands. The patient was not known to the emergency service staff and was not suspected of carrying HIV. His resuscitation was not successful, and autopsy revealed that he had *Pneumocystis carinii* pneumonia and that he was HIV positive.

The health care worker was HIV positive 16 weeks after the incident and is presumed to have an occupationally related seroconversion (CDC, May 1987). In May, 1988, the CDC noted that at least 15 health care worker presumptive seroconversions (without other risk factors) had been reported in the literature (CDC, April 1988). Rare seroconversions have occurred when universal precautions were in use but when a needle stick or other blood exposures occurred despite the precautions.

Employers, including hospitals, are required by the Occupational Safety and Health Administration (OSHA) to provide a safe working environment for their employees. OSHA has published its final bloodborne pathogens rule (Dept. of Labor, 1991). As a result, hospitals must require the appropriate use of universal precautions by all employees, regardless of the employee's personal preference. This includes trauma service personnel who may have little time to put on protective equipment. The failure to enforce the universal precautions requirement can subject an employer to fines of more than $10,000 per violation.

With this background, hospitals must now educate employees in the proper use of universal precautions, (CDC, June 1988) and are beginning to implement discipline criteria for those employees who refuse to comply. Hospitals are also requiring that physicians and other staff not employed by the hospital adhere to required universal precautions or be denied hospital privileges, particularly if their careless practices endanger employees.

The hospital-employer also is responsible for providing necessary protective equipment in sufficient quantities and of sufficient quality to provide the required protection. Every trauma service employee should report blood exposures to the personnel health department at the time of the incident. Whether the patient's hepatitis or HIV status is known or unknown, the hospital should have a follow-up protocol that it offers to exposed employees.

Exposure to bloodborne infection is probably the most serious work-related risk for trauma service personnel. Regardless of the fact that the employer requires universal precaution protection, each employee must take steps with every patient to protect himself or herself from possible infection, since patients may be infectious even when tests are negative. Any slight delay in treating the patient while the staff dons protective equipment will be insignificant in the outcome of most patients, and in any case, the wearing of protective equipment is now the standard of care in the United States. Because by definition, trauma service patients sustain sudden injuries, the chance that the staff will know much about the patient and risk factors is slim; universal precautions are the only protections that have a chance of protecting staff.

Occupationally related employee seroconversions are treated as Worker's Compensation injuries for compensation purposes. The Worker's Compensation system is an administrative, no-fault system established by state statute. In most states, where the Worker's Compensation statute is applicable, suit against an employer is not permitted unless employer conduct is egregious.

SUMMARY Trauma personnel should be able to identify the most frequent legal questions that arise in trauma care. Because statutes and case law vary somewhat among the states, the trauma service must consult with the hospital attorney or risk manager about a specific situation and determine how state law may dictate the answer. Hospital risk managers can also be useful sources for information about any relevant changes in state law. Many hospitals have a risk manager or legal counsel available at all times for emergencies, so the nursing staff should know whom to contact and how. However, no amount of education about the legal background for practice can substitute for trauma care provided in accordance with a professional standard of care. Patients and families who are sensitively and well cared for are less likely to bring any legal action (Press, 1984).

CASE STUDY A 45-year-old single man is brought to the emergency department by ambulance accompanied by the police. He had been found wandering near his place of employment with blood on his trousers. He was carrying a plastic bag containing his penis, which he had amputated with a sharp instrument.

Upon arrival in the emergency department, he was lucid and oriented to person, place, and time. Although he had a history of psychiatric treatment some years before, he was not taking medications. A blood alcohol level and a toxicology screen were negative. He was not paranoid, hallucinating, or delusional. He could not state clearly why he had amputated his penis or why he then carried the penis with him after it had been amputated.

Urologic evaluation of the amputation site indicated that reimplantation was a surgical possibility, but in any case, the patient needed surgery to control arterial bleeding and to divert his urinary tract at least temporarily. The patient was informed of these findings. He agreed to the surgery to correct the bleeding and divert the urinary tract but refused reimplantation. The attending urologist thought that the patient was competent and declined to reimplant the penis without further authority.

The attending psychiatrist was called to the emergency department and examined the patient, whose vital signs had remained stable. He concluded that the patient showed no signs of psychosis but that his judgment was impaired. The psychiatrist feared that if the patient were permitted to refuse reimplantation of the penis, he might greatly regret his decision after psychiatric therapy.

By this time, 3 hours had passed since the patient's arrival in the emergency department. The urologist informed the staff that the likelihood of implantation success decreased as time passed.

What action should the emergency department staff take?

Should family be permitted to make the reimplantation decision?

Should the patient be permitted to refuse that portion of the surgery?

If the staff would accept his consent for the life-saving portion of the surgery, why not accept his refusal for the elective portion?

If the staff believes that reimplantation should be considered, they must contact the risk management department or the hospital legal counsel. The question in this case is one of competence. Had the patient been floridly psychotic, the staff may have been more comfortable permitting concerned family members to authorize the surgery. However, in this case, the urologist thought the patient was competent, and substitute family consent was not possible.

After discussion with the attending urologist and psychiatrist, the risk manager may call the appropriate judge and begin the process of having an emergency temporary guardian appointed for the patient. In all states, statutes provide for emergency appointments, and the judge may decide whether there is the time to come to the emergency department to interview the patient. If the judge decides that there is sufficient doubt about competence, a family member or third party may be appointed to consider the surgery. After this is done, the urologist may then proceed to inform the guardian about the risks, benefits, and alternatives to the surgery, including the reimplantation portion, and seek the guardian's informed consent. The urologist may also discuss aspects of the patient's care with the guardian, and in this case, may wish to inform the family that four-point restraints after surgery will be required (to prevent disruption of the surgical site by a patient who did not desire reimplantation).

ANNOTATED BIBLIOGRAPHY

American Hospital Association. (1989). *AIDS and the law: Responding to the special concerns of hospitals.* Chicago: AIDS Task Group of the American Academy of Hospital Attorneys.
This 83-page booklet contains text and questions and answers, along with an extensive bibliography on the topic.

American Hospital Association: Technical Advisory Bulletin. (1986). *Hospital responsibilities in requesting organ donations.* Chicago: Author.
Describes recent changes in the law.

Areen, J. (1987). The legal status of consent obtained from families of adult patients to withhold or withdraw treatment. *Journal of the American Medical Association, 258,* 229-235.
Describes statutory and case law on withholding and withdrawal of treatment.

Cotton, R.D., & Sandler, A.L. (1986). The regulation of organ procurement and transplantation in the United States. *Journal of Legal Medicine, 7,* 55-84.
Describes history and relevant law.

Ruark, J.E., & Raffin, T.A. (1988). Initiating and withdrawing life support. *New England Journal of Medicine, 318,* 25-30.
Describes practices and principles used in questions of life support.

Schmidt, S. (1983). Consent for autopsies. *Journal of the American Medical Association, 250,* 1161-1164.
A good background article on autopsy consent and liability for unauthorized autopsies.

REFERENCES

Borak, J., & Veilleux, S. (1984). Informed consent in emergency settings. *Connecticut Medicine, 48,* 235-239.

Bryson v. Tillinghast, 749 P. 2d 110 (Okla. 1988).

Centers for Disease Control (CDC). U.S. Public Health Service. (May 1987). Update: Human immunodeficiency virus infections in health care workers exposed to blood of infected patients. *Morbidity and Mortality Weekly Report, 36,* 285.

Centers for Disease Control (CDC). U.S. Public Health Service. (August 21, 1987). Recommendations for prevention of HIV transmission in health care settings. *Morbidity and Mortality Weekly Report, 36,* 135.

Centers for Disease Control (CDC). U.S. Public Health Service. (April 1988). Update: Acquired immunodeficiency syndrome and human immunodeficiency virus infection among health care workers. *Morbidity and Mortality Weekly Report, 37,* 232.

Centers for Disease Control (CDC). U.S. Public Health Service. (June 24, 1988). Update: Universal precautions for prevention of transmission of human immunodeficiency virus, hepatitis B virus, and other bloodborne pathogens in health care settings. *Morbidity and Mortality Weekly Report, 37,* 377.

Centers for Disease Control (CDC). U.S. Public Health Service. (October 1988). Quarterly report to the Domestic Policy Council on the prevalence and rate of spread of HIV and AIDS—United States. *Morbidity and Mortality Weekly Report, 37,* 551.

Colby v. Schwartz, 144 Cal. Rptr. 624 (1978).

Connecticut General Statutes Sections 19a-406-407 and Conn. Agencies Regs. Section 19a-401-9 (1988).

Department of Labor, Occupational Safety and Health Administration. *Occupational exposure to bloodborne pathogens.* 56 Federal Register 64004. Dec. 6, 1991.

Eisendrath, S.J., & Jonson, A. (1983). The living will: Help or hindrance? *Journal of the American Medical Association, 249,* 2054.

Holder, A. (1985). *Legal issues in pediatrics and adolescent medicine* (pp. 125-126). New Haven, Conn: Yale University Press.

Mohr v Williams, 104 N.W. 12 (1905).

New York Public Health Law, Section 2504 (4) (1988).

Press, I. (1984). The predisposition to file claims: The patient's perspective. *Law, Medicine & Health Care, 12,* 53-62.

Schurgin, W. (1988). The impact of AIDS upon health care employers. *Journal of Health and Hospital Law, 21,* 285-294.

Social Security Act Section 1867.

Society for the Right to Die. (1991) *Refusal of treatment legislation* (Handbook), Introduction, p. 1.

Stricter patient transfer rules effective July 1. (1990, June 29). *American Medical News,* pp. 1, 21.

Thomas v. Corso, 288 A. 2d 379 (Md. 1972).

U.S. Department of Labor (October 1987). Joint Advisory Notice: Department of Labor/Department of Health and Human Services; HBV/HIV. *Federal Register, 52.*

5 Forensic Aspects

▪▪▪▪▪▪▪▪▪▪▪▪▪▪▪▪▪▪▪▪▪▪▪▪▪▪▪▪▪▪▪▪▪▪▪▪▪▪▪

Lori D. Taylor

Allen Jones

OBJECTIVES

❑ Describe the value of the forensic autopsy to the improvement of trauma care.

❑ Discuss mechanism of injury relative to patterns of predictable injury.

❑ Identify types of forensic evidence encountered in trauma resuscitations.

❑ State the appropriate handling of each type of evidence.

❑ Perform appropriate postmortem care of medical examiner's cases, including reporting of deaths.

INTRODUCTION A majority of injury cases seen in trauma centers will come under medico-legal investigation, whether or not the victim dies. When death from trauma does result, it is even more likely that the case will be classified as a forensic case, because civil or criminal charges may be filed against the injuring person. One study of 100 consecutive admissions to a trauma service found that 62 of those cases involved the potential for criminal charges, which necessitated appropriate evidence gathering (Carmona & Prince-Johnson, 1988).

Trauma is also frequently encountered by forensic personnel, because violence in all of its forms and effects is observed daily by medical examiners or coroners. Based on the frequency with which these cases occur, it is crucial for trauma nurses to understand forensics and their role in evidence handling and preservation.

SCOPE OF FORENSIC MEDICINE

Forensics involves the study of violent, sudden, or unexpected death. In the United States, all county and state jurisdictions have laws governing how victims of violence and sudden death are handled. The duties and responsibilities of this are enormous—nearly 500,000 persons die each year under these circumstances. The system for death investigation varies from state to state, but generally falls into one of three types: (1) a medical examiner system, (2) a coroner system, or (3) a mixed medical examiner and coroner system. Trauma care providers should know the type of system that exists in their area.

A state medical examiner system consists of a physician-directed program that provides a uniform approach to death investigation throughout the state. The majority of medical examiners in metropolitan jurisdictions are specially trained in forensic pathology and are usually certified by the American Board of Pathology in forensic, anatomic, and clinical pathology. Forensic pathology is that subspecialty of pathology concerned with the interpretation of injuries, the determination of how those injuries were produced, and the investigation of the circumstances of the violent event.

Conversely, a coroner system consists of an elected person (often a lay person) who is assigned the task of death investigation for a particular region. The educational and training level of these individuals may vary greatly from county to county.

A mixed system within a state exists when some counties or regions have a medical examiner and others have a coroner.

Regardless of the type of system, the agencies responsible for death investigation have some

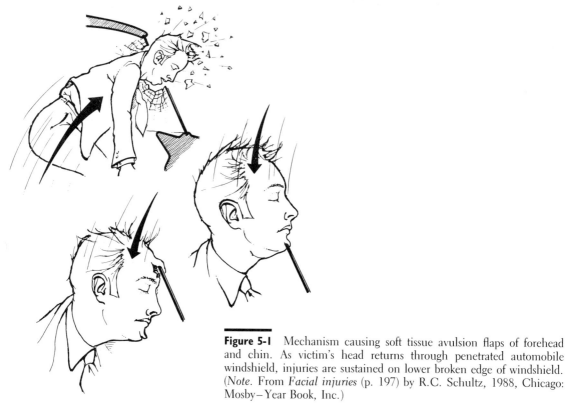

Figure 5-1 Mechanism causing soft tissue avulsion flaps of forehead and chin. As victim's head returns through penetrated automobile windshield, injuries are sustained on lower broken edge of windshield. (*Note.* From *Facial injuries* (p. 197) by R.C. Schultz, 1988, Chicago: Mosby–Year Book, Inc.)

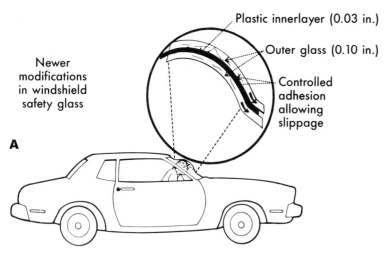

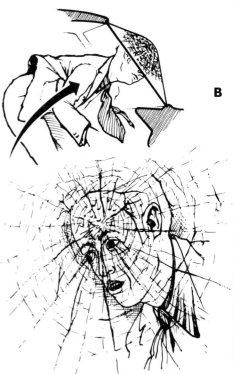

Figure 5-2 Windshields of automobiles manufactured after 1966 help to contain passenger within automobile. **A,** Thicker plastic innerlayer and looser bonding permit ballooning of windshield on impact; **B,** multiple small blunt glass particles can cause numerous small lacerations, small triangular avulsion flaps, and tiny avulsion injuries. (*Note.* From *Facial injuries* (p. 18) by R.C. Schultz, 1988, Chicago: Mosby–Year Book, Inc.)

common tasks. Any person or agency charged with death investigation has a duty to establish both the cause (e.g., motor vehicle collision, fall) and the manner (e.g., suicide, accident, natural, homicide) of death for all cases that fall under the particular jurisdiction. Death investigation necessitates working closely with law enforcement agencies; county, city, and state attorneys; physicians; nurses; dentists; and many other groups. Because the responsibility of death investigation is a government extension, the financial resources available vary enormously across the country. As mentioned, regional variations in the type of agencies create striking differences in the level and completeness of death investigation.

A major adjunct to establishment of circumstances of death is the forensic autopsy. Valuable information about injury can be obtained through postmortem analysis.

TRAUMA PREVENTION: AN OUTCOME OF FORENSIC INVOLVEMENT

The data collected at autopsy after injury are extremely useful, especially from an epidemiologic viewpoint. The autopsy findings, in addition to trauma data generated from emergency departments, operating rooms, and intensive care units, can be used to provide beneficial data to automotive design engineers and to develop trauma care systems and clinical practice standards.

The redesign of automobiles and their parts has been an area in which medical examiners have made great contributions. An example of such change is windshield design. Before 1966 windshields were made of a bonded, double layer of glass sandwiched over a very thin (.015 inch) plastic innerlayer. During that period, many persons sustained serious lacerations or were decapitated when they were ejected through the windshield (Figure 5-1). Therefore automotive engineers and private industry elected to redesign the windshield to prevent these catastrophic injuries. The new design sandwiched two layers of glass over a much thicker (.030 inch) layer of plastic (Spitz & Fisher, 1980). This thicker layer made tremendous differences in injury by absorbing the energy of the moving head and by preventing glass shards (Figure 5-2). Additionally, seat belt redesign, air bag development, roll bar design, and changes in steering wheel construction have resulted from a review of injuries sustained without proper protective devices.

In support of the value of the postmortem examination in discovering unrecognized injury, the American College of Surgeons (ACS) Committee on Trauma published a position paper calling for autopsy examination of all victims of fatal injury (Subcommittee on Emergency Services, 1986). Detection of unrecognized injury becomes crucial in trauma systems as a means of identifying those trauma deaths classified as "preventable." A comprehensive quality assessment program in a trauma system must look at preventable deaths to alter patient care and outcome.

A study comparing injury severity scores (ISS) based on clinical findings with those scores derived from autopsy findings supported the ACS recommendation for mandatory autopsies (Harviel et al., 1989). This study noted substantially higher ISS based on autopsy findings than ISS based on clinical findings in those patients dying 7 days or less after emergency department admission (Harviel et al., 1989). The higher ISS was the result of a greater number of injuries identified by autopsy findings. Stothert, Gbaanador, and Herndon (1990) noted similar "major discrepancies in clinical diagnoses versus the anatomic diagnosis at autopsy in approximately 30% of patients." Additionally, they noted an overall decline in the rate of autopsy in most hospitals, from 50% to less than 15% over the past 40 to 50 years. Factors cited as contributors to this decline include issues of cost and reimbursement, misconceptions regarding the amount of knowledge actually gained, and fear of litigation (Stothert et al., 1990).

AUTOPSY FINDINGS AND PREDICTABLE INJURIES

A primary contribution made by autopsy findings is the correlation of mechanism of injury (such as falls and motor vehicle crashes) with groups of common injuries. The development of anthropomorphic dummies fitted with elaborate, high-technology devices and photographed with high-speed, high-resolution cameras has also contributed to this body of knowledge (Figure 5-3). These test data, combined with the observations of trauma by surgeons and medical examiners, have led to a fundamental understanding of crash kinematics. For trauma care providers to effectively use this information in searching for occult injuries, details of the incident must be obtained from prehospital care providers. The following

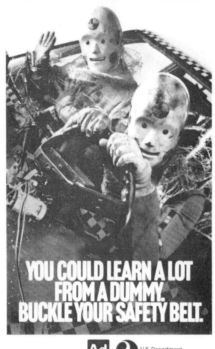

"I'LL JUST BRACE MYSELF WITH THE STEERING WHEEL."

YOU COULD LEARN A LOT FROM A DUMMY. BUCKLE YOUR SAFETY BELT.

A Public Service Message Ad Council U.S. Department of Transportation
© 1985 U.S. DOT

Figure 5-3 In addition to being used in sophisticated crash testing, these simulated, anthropomorphic dummies are used to heighten awareness and compliance with safety practices. (Courtesy U.S. Department of Transportation and the Advertising Council, Inc.)

discussion focuses on the predictability of injury based on mechanisms.

Pedestrians

Typically, adult pedestrians struck by the front of an automobile first contact the bumper of the vehicle, the most protruding portion. This can result in bony and soft tissue injury of the lower extremities, the severity of which is determined by such factors as speed of the vehicle and the amount of clothing in place at the time of impact. These injuries have been termed *bumper in-*

juries (Spitz & Fisher, 1980). If external signs of injury are lacking, the injuries may be identified on autopsy by incision into the calf area to examine soft tissue. When tibial fractures occur, they may be wedge shaped, with the apex of the wedge pointing in the direction of travel of the vehicle (Spitz & Fisher, 1980). Lack of bumper injuries suggests that the pedestrian was struck by the side of the vehicle (sideswiped).

Additionally, the distance of the injury above the heels is an important medicolegal observation that can be of evidentiary value. The interpretation of the height of the injury helps determine if the pedestrian was standing, walking, or running when struck and if the vehicle was braking at the time of impact. The front of a vehicle dips lower with braking.

Portions of paint, chrome, plastic, glass, or other materials may be found in the wounds created by impact. The trauma nurse should use care when cleaning or irrigating wounds, to prevent loss of these valuable pieces of evidence. Paint chips can be analyzed and become an important link regarding the vehicle involved in the crash, which is particularly crucial in hit-and-run incidents.

After initial impact with the bumper, the pedestrian may then suffer a secondary impact at the hood or fender level. This secondary impact may cause extensive pelvic fractures. With overstretching of the skin at this point, fresh stretch marks, or striae, are created. These striae are seen also when a victim is struck from behind or run over by a vehicle. Victims who are run over may also have tire mark impressions on their clothing and skin. Tire marks are specific for the vehicle that produced them and have high evidentiary value.

At speeds of less than 30 miles per hour, the adult victim struck below the center of gravity may then be thrown upward onto the hood of the vehicle. This creates elbow, shoulder, and head injuries (Spitz & Fisher, 1980). Then the victim rolls off the vehicle, usually striking the head on the roadway. These final injuries are frequently the most severe. At greater vehicular rates of speed, the victim may be thrown even higher into the air and may actually travel over the top of the vehicle, landing on the roadway behind. The victim then may be run over by other vehicles (Spitz & Fisher, 1980). This sequence of events is illustrated in Figure 5-4.

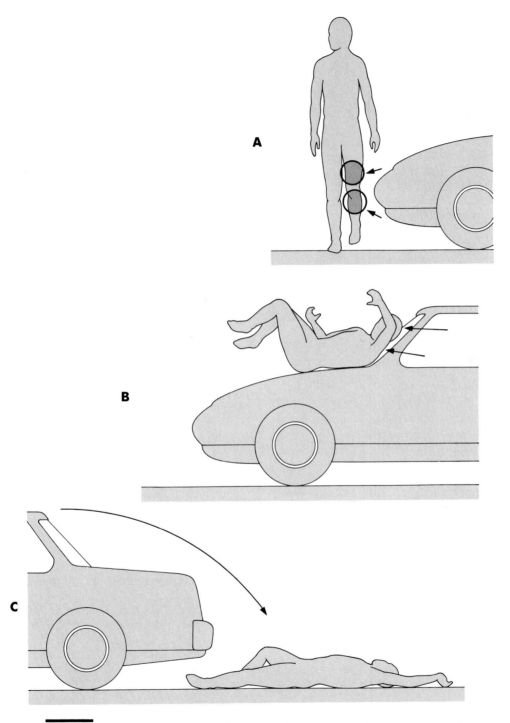

Figure 5-4 **A,** Adult victim struck below center of gravity sustains bumper injuries on legs and impact on hip by hood and front fender area. **B,** At normal city speed, adult victim is propelled upward after impact by front end of vehicle; he slides onto hood and sustains injuries of head and shoulders as they come in contact with windshield. When vehicle slows or stops, victim rolls from hood to ground. **C,** At greater speed, victim may be thrown higher and land on roof of automobile or on its trunk, or possibly on road behind automobile, risking being run over by oncoming vehicles.

Drivers and Passengers

Motor vehicle collisions occur in four basic modes: frontal impact, side impact, rear impact, and rollover (National Highway Traffic Safety Administration, 1981). The injuries sustained by drivers and passengers in such crashes vary, depending on the type of crash and use of appropriate safety restraints.

Currently, 34 states have laws regulating the use of safety restraints for all occupants, with an estimated 42% of all occupants using these devices nationally (National Highway Traffic Safety Administration, 1989). Appropriate safety restraints include the use of lap and shoulder restraints that are properly positioned. Repeat studies have documented instances of intraabdominal and spinal injuries associated with the use of safety restraints. A 1991 study, however, noted that belted and unbelted patients had an equal incidence of abdominal trauma, but a different spectrum of injuries—hollow viscus injuries were more common in belted crash victims (Rutledge et al, 1991). This group also found significantly fewer head injuries and deaths in belted occupants (Rutledge et al., 1991).

Mechanisms that are believed to cause injuries related to safety restraints include compression of the abdominal wall and viscera between the belt and the spine, sudden increases in intraluminal pressure, and shearing and deceleration forces against fixed intestinal points (Asbun, Irani, Roe, & Bloch, 1990). In addition to the hollow viscus injuries, rear-seat passengers belted only with a lap belt more commonly have Chance-type fractures of the lumbar spine than other types of spinal injuries (Anderson, Rivara, Maier, & Drake, 1991). However, injuries related to seat belt use generally occur in severe impact accidents and are considered an acceptable trade-off for more serious injuries that occur in unrestrained occupants (Gikas, 1983).

Patterned Injuries

Patterned injuries are those injuries seen when a fixed object imprints a pattern on the person striking the object. Patterned injuries are used by medical examiners to recreate the location of occupants within a vehicle. This is particularly useful when a question arises regarding which occupant was in control of the vehicle at the time of impact, since criminal or civil cases often follow motor vehicle crashes that result in serious injury or death. Contusions and abrasions across the chest, neck, and abdomen are examples of patterned injuries seen with shoulder restraint and lap belt use.

In frontal collisions (Figure 5-5), unrestrained drivers first hit the steering wheel and column. Serious chest injury often results, including multiple rib fractures, a flail chest, fractured sternum, myocardial contusions, aortic injuries, and pulmonary contusions and lacerations. However, since the advent of the energy-absorbing steering column, the frequency and severity of such driver injuries have declined considerably (Spitz & Fisher, 1980). These changes were incorporated in all General Motors, American Motors, and Chrysler Corporation automobiles in 1967 and in all Ford Motor Company vehicles in 1968 (Spitz & Fisher, 1980).

In addition to chest injuries, facial injuries (soft tissue and bony) are common in unrestrained drivers. These injuries occur from impact with either the upper portion of the steering wheel, the dashboard, or the windshield. The severity of facial injuries from windshield contact relates directly to the speed of the impact and the year of manufacture of the windshield. Regardless of the type of glass used in the windshield (pre- or post-1966), both will allow penetration by the head at high speeds. Both types also fracture in the typical "spider-web" pattern (Spitz & Fisher, 1980).

As the head of the unrestrained driver strikes one of these fixed objects, either flexion or extension injuries of the cervical spine may occur. The presence or absence of headrests is also a determining factor in the severity and type of spinal injury. Headrests prevent injury occurring from extension of the neck in rear-end collisions.

Side and rear windows are made of safety glass, which breaks into multiple, rectangular-shaped fragments when broken. These small cubes of glass become missiles, which may strike the face of the occupant. The incisions created can be extensive and quite disfiguring and are referred to as *dicing injuries* (Brady, 1982). This patterned injury also is useful in reconstructing occupant position. Typically, dicing injuries are found on the left side of the driver's face and the right side of the passenger's face. However, if seat belts are not worn and occupants move freely about the interior of the vehicle, this may not be a reliable

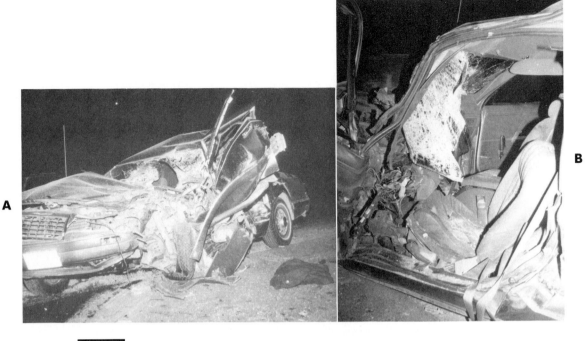

Figure 5-5 **A,** Frontal, high-speed collision demonstrating significant vehicular damage with resultant death of front seat driver and serious injury to three passengers. **B,** Interior view of driver's area of same vehicle. Collision of driver with steering wheel, column, dashboard, and windshield resulted in fatal chest and head injuries.

finding. When the wounds are debrided and sutured, cubes of glass found within facial wounds should be retrieved and saved as evidence.

Unrestrained drivers also may suffer lower extremity injury by contact with the dashboard and entaglement in the foot pedals. As the driver moves forward, the knees strike the dashboard, resulting in abrasions, contusions, lacerations, and fractures of the patella, distal portion of the femur, or tibial plateau. Dislocation of the femoral head, with or without fracture, may occur as force is transmitted up the femur. Acetabular fractures also may be produced. If the feet become entangled in the pedals, foot and ankle injuries may result (see Chapter 7, Figure 7-1). The sole of the driver's right shoe may show the imprint of the gas or brake pedal, indicating which of the two pedals was being applied at the time of the collision (Spitz & Fisher, 1980).

Unrestrained front seat passengers strike the windshield and dashboard as the first point of impact. This usually results in more serious head and facial injuries than those seen in drivers. Flexion injury to the cervical spine may occur. Lower extremity injuries occur by the same mechanism as with drivers, with the exception of absence of foot and ankle injuries. Knee, femur, hip, and pelvic injuries result from contact with the dashboard (see Chapter 7, Figure 7-2). The torso of the front-seat passenger also may strike the dashboard, with resultant thoracic and abdominal injuries (Daffner, Deeb, Lupetin, & Rothfus, 1988).

Rollovers and ejections from motor vehicles and motorcycles make interpretation of injuries and determination of seating arrangements more difficult, because injuries likely will be wide and varied. Ejection of occupants results in a much higher mortality because of the severe nature of the injuries sustained.

Natural Deaths and Motor Vehicle Collisions

Several studies have documented that a percentage of motor vehicle collisions are caused by the driver experiencing a sudden, catastrophic medical event. Peterson and Petty, in a 1962 review of this topic, found that death in 19% of all drivers in motor vehicle collisions was due to a natural cause. The majority of the deaths were caused by myocardial infarction and dysrhythmias. A similar study found a 15% death rate from natural causes in association with motor vehicle collisions (West, Nielsen, Gilmore, & Ryan, 1968). This may cause some confusion for the trauma care provider, because physical findings may be inconsistent with presenting signs and symptoms. The following case illustrates this discrepancy.

CASE STUDY A 32-year-old restrained female driver was traveling on a rural highway with three other family members in the vehicle. Her husband awakened to find her swerving across the center line. He thought she was asleep and tried unsuccessfully to bring the vehicle under control; the vehicle struck another car head-on. Prehospital personnel did note significant vehicular damage. As mentioned, the driver was fully restrained and lacked obvious external signs of injury. However, her Glasgow Coma Score was only 4, with the presence of fixed, dilated pupils. When the patient arrived at a definitive care facility, the physician also noted lack of signs of injury to explain the neurologic findings. An urgent CT scan of her head revealed a massive subarachnoid hemorrhage, and further studies revealed an internal carotid artery aneurysm. The patient eventually died from the hemorrhage.

Situations such as this emphasize the need for autopsy of victims of trauma. If the CT scan had not been done in this case, the determination of death may have been in error (accidental death instead of natural causes).

Suicide Attempts and Motor Vehicle Collisions

The use of the automobile as an instrument of self-destruction has been postulated repeatedly in recent years (Spitz & Fisher, 1980). It is difficult to obtain actual numbers of incidences, because investigation of this type of accident is difficult. Certain factors identified in the investigation (such as the lack of skid marks or the imprint of the gas pedal on the driver's right foot) may suggest that the crash was a suicide attempt. However, a driver falling asleep at the wheel may present in a similar manner. A careful investiga-

tion into the victim's psychiatric history becomes necessary, and only unequivocal cases should be ruled as suicides.

Gunshot Wounds

Trauma care providers are likely to encounter victims of violent crimes who have sustained gunshot wounds. Geography will influence the number of such cases seen: urban areas have a higher incidence than rural locales. With a basic understanding of wounding forces and ballistics, trauma nurses can anticipate the varying amounts of tissue damage that might be encountered. Once again, historical data regarding weapon type must be elicited from prehospital care providers.

Accurate investigation of gunshot wounds requires extensive training. These injuries are not ruled a suicide or homicide until a thorough investigation of the incident is completed, including interview of any witnesses, close examination of the wounds, inspection of clothing, and examination of the weapon and the hands of the victim. Consequently, victims of shootings presenting to emergency departments should always be viewed as potential medicolegal cases, which necessitates assisting in evidence preservation. Wounds should not be classified as self-inflicted until an investigation is completed. Usually, questions still exist at time of death as to wound appearance, and a forensic autopsy can establish such facts as range of fire, type of weapon, and type of bullet. Additionally, medical examiners in some areas examine gunshot wounds before a victim's death. This facilitates determination of characteristics of the wound before procedures are done that might alter the evidence found on the victim.

Types of weapons

Hundreds of different types of firearms and ammunition are available in the United States (DiMaio, 1985). Weapons can be divided into two general groups based on *muzzle velocity*, or the speed at which the bullet leaves the muzzle of the weapon. Low-velocity weapons have a muzzle velocity of 1400 feet/second or less and include all handguns (except for many of the "magnum" weapons) and .22 rimfire rifles. High-velocity weapons are those that have a muzzle velocity of 2400 to 4000 feet/second (DiMaio, 1985). Included in this category are centerfire rifles, such as those commonly used in hunting. Shotguns differ from rifles and handguns in a variety of ways and constitute a separate classification. Unlike rifles and handguns, which fire a single bullet at a time, shotguns fire multiple pellets. In close-range shootings, shotgun injuries may produce massive tissue destruction (DiMaio, 1985).

Kinetic energy

The severity of a gunshot wound is directly related to the transfer and loss of kinetic energy (KE) in the tissues. For bullets, this energy is determined by its weight and velocity, or by the following formula (French and Callender, 1962):

$$KE \;) \; \frac{WV}{2g}$$

W = weight of bullet; V = velocity; g = gravitational acceleration.

As can be shown by this formula, velocity (because it is squared) is the major determinant of tissue destruction, and wounds caused by high-velocity weapons are generally much more severe than those caused by low-velocity weapons.

As a bullet fired from a weapon strikes a victim, it imparts KE to the tissues and creates a path as it disrupts the tissue. This results in a *temporary cavity*—the dilation of the walls of the bullet hole as tissues surrounding the bullet path are stretched radially outward (Fackler, 1991). The tissues then recoil and contract, leaving the permanent wound track. The extent that the tissue returns to its former state and position depends on the elasticity of the tissue (Fackler, 1991). Low-velocity weapons impart little KE to the tissues, creating small temporary and permanent cavities. Conversely, high-velocity weapons may create temporary cavities up to 30 times the diameter of the bullet (DiMaio, 1985). This often results in damage to bone, tissue, and organs far removed from the suspected path of the bullet (Figure 5-6).

Deformation and erratic movements of bullets

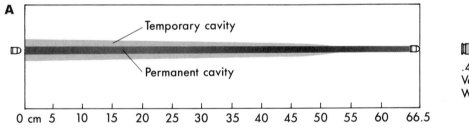

.45 automatic (11.4 mm)
Vel-869 ft/s (265 m/s)
Wt-230 gr (14.9 gm) FMC

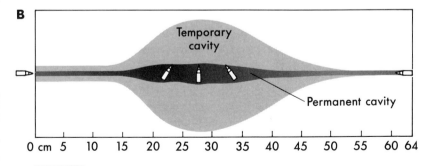

7.62 mm NATO
Vel-2830 ft/s (862 m/s)
Wt-150 gr (9.7 gm) FMC

Figure 5-6   **A,** Wound profile of 45 ACP pistol. Predominant wounding mechanism is tissue crush, typical of most low-velocity handgun wounds. **B,** Wound profile produced by 7.62 NATO rifle (high-velocity) with full-metal-jacketed military bullet. (*Note.* Redrawn from *Current Therapy of Trauma* (pp. 96, 97) by D.D. Trunkey and F.R. Lewis, 1986, Philadelphia: B.C. Decker.)

within the body also cause greater transfer of KE to tissue. Certain types of bullets, such as hollow points, are made to deform, or "mushroom", on impact. This increases the amount of tissue struck (cross-sectional area) by up to 6 times (Fackler, 1991). Bullets may also deviate from a straight path and tumble within tissues, which increases the amount of tissue damage by greater dissipation of KE.

Wound characteristics

The appearance of the wound depends on a variety of factors, including the type of weapon (high or low velocity) and the range of fire, or distance from the muzzle to the target. Range of fire is one of the most important factors used in ruling a death by gunfire as a suicide or homicide (Spitz & Fisher, 1980). In addition to the bullet, other materials leave the muzzle at time of firing, including particles of burning and unburned gunpowder, soot, and gases rich in carbon monoxide. All of these may create injury, depending on the range of fire.

Contact wounds are produced when the weapon is held in contact with the skin. The edges of the entrance wound may reveal deposits of grey-black soot, burned or seared skin edges, and particles of unburned gunpowder in the wound depths. On autopsy, powder and soot may be found deep in the tissues. Soot may even be found deposited on bone underlying a contact wound. The tissue immediately surrounding the wound also may have the typical cherry-red coloration from the binding with carbon monoxide (carboxymyoglobin) (Brady, 1982).

The area of the body involved affects the appearance of the wound. Contact wounds to the head often appear as large, irregular, stellate-type injuries. This occurs when the thin layer of the scalp overlying bone is torn by the compressive forces of the gases released into the tissue (Figure 5-7). Contact, high-velocity wounds to the head often result in a type of bursting injury because of the tremendous pressure created by expanding gases released inside the fixed cranial vault. The chest and abdominal areas consist of much more elastic tissues. The force of the gases released at the time of firing may be absorbed into the cavity

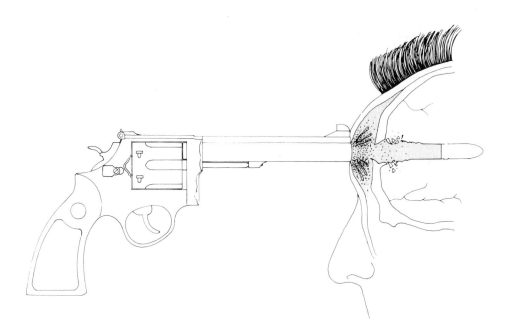

Figure 5-7   Contact wound of head showing dissection of gas between scalp and skull. (*Note.* From *Gunshot Wounds: Practical Aspects of Firearms, Ballistics, and Forensic Techniques* (p. 105) by V.J. DiMaio, 1985, New York: Elsevier Science Publishing.

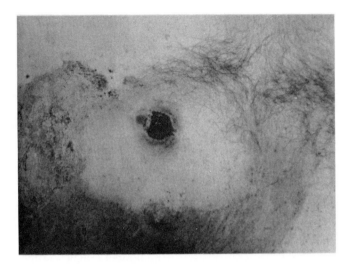

Figure 5-8   Contact gunshot wound to chest, resulting in blow-back of tissues and imprint of muzzle and sight of weapon around wound edges.

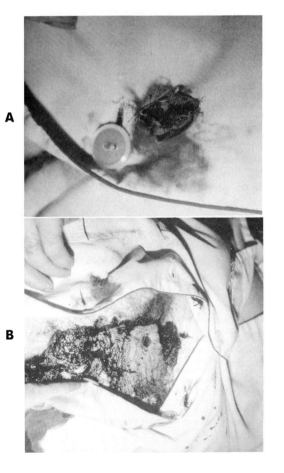

A

B

Figure 5-9   **A,** Soot and powder deposition on clothing around defect created by bullet in close-contact wound. **B,** Removal of clothing reveals entrance defect, which is nearly devoid of powder and soot deposition. Investigation of incident is hampered if clothing is removed and left at scene and/or discarded.

involved. However, the skin will usually blow-back around the muzzle, leaving an impression of the muzzle on the skin (Figure 5-8). Contact wounds are suggestive of self-inflicted wounds, but can be seen also in homicides (Brady, 1982).

Intermediate gunshot wounds are produced when the gun is further from the body, generally as far away as 2 to 3 feet. The wound edges may be slightly abraded and reveal gunpowder stippling or tattooing, produced by burning and unburned gunpowder striking and embedding in the tissues. If the gunpowder is loose on the skin, it can easily be cleaned away, making wound interpretation more difficult. Clothing in place at the time of the shooting may trap this powder (Figure 5-9). If the clothing is then removed and not turned over to the medical examiner or law enforcement personnel, the wound may be incorrectly classified as a distant wound.

Distant gunshot wounds are produced when the weapon is far enough away from the skin so as not to leave a deposit of gunpowder around the entrance wound. This usually occurs at distances of 2 to 3 feet or greater. These wounds reveal abrasions of the edges, but will lack any signs of powder tattooing or searing. Distant wounds are generally not consistent with a self-inflicted wound.

Entrance versus exit wounds

A myriad of factors can alter the appearance of gunshot wounds, and extensive training is required to accurately interpret such wounds. These interpretations are used by medical examiners and law enforcement personnel as a means of differentiating suicides from homicides. Unfortunately, prehospital and emergency department personnel often attempt to classify in the medical record entrance and exit wounds. This can create difficulties in legal proceedings, especially if the wounds have been incorrectly identified by trauma care providers. To document gunshot wounds, it is best to simply describe the appearance and location of the wounds and avoid further labeling or interpretation. For example, describing a wound as "small, round, located in the right temporal area, and surrounded by a black-colored ring" would likely support findings of an entrance wound without assuming further liability.

Another frequently made error occurs when attempts are made to classify the caliber of the bullet based on plain x-ray films of the injured area, because magnification of the bullet occurs. Plain x-ray films are helpful to trauma care providers as a means of assessing potential injury based on the bullet path. However, bullets may deflect and ricochet within the body, especially if they are small caliber and strike bone.

The bullet as a foreign object

The presence of an entrance and exit wound does not mean that a foreign object does not exist in the body. In the case of partially metal-jacketed bullets, the lead core may separate from the jacket and exit the body, leaving the jacket lodged internally. These jackets generally can be visualized on plain x-ray films. One exception is the Silvertip pistol ammunition manufactured by Winchester. Because the jacket is composed of aluminum, it is not radiopaque (DiMaio, 1985).

Bullet embolization can be associated with small-caliber, low-velocity weapons (DiMaio, 1985). If the missile loses velocity in a major vessel or the heart, it can be carried in the bloodstream to its final destination. This might be suspected when an entrance wound is seen without an exit wound, but plain x-ray films fail to show the bullet in the area of the wound. A common site for embolization is to the legs, with lodging in the popliteal artery. Multiple radiographs may be necessary to localize the bullet (Jones, Graham, & Looney, 1983).

ROLE OF THE TRAUMA NURSE IN EVIDENCE PRESERVATION

Victims of traumatic injury present at trauma facilities not only with injuries necessitating urgent evaluation and treatment, but with valuable pieces of evidence needed for successful medicolegal investigation. The role of the trauma team is to provide needed care; however, this can be done while assisting in evidence preservation. If the victim survives, this evidence likely will be turned over to law enforcement personnel. In the event of the death of the victim, the medical examiner also will be involved in the investigation. Items to be identified and preserved include physical evidence (bullets, bags of powder, weapons, pills, and other foreign objects); trace evidence (loose hair, paint chips, and fibers); biologic evidence (patient's blood, body fluids, and pulled head hair); and clothing and its contents (Baulch & Hall, 1991). The following discussion offers a general approach to actual care and appropriate handling and transfer of evidence, as well as chain-of-custody procedures. Because these procedures may vary from area to area, trauma care facilities must have written guidelines outlining procedures acceptable to local law enforcement and death investigation agencies.

Clothing

Articles of clothing are valuable pieces of evidence. Unfortunately, the victim's clothing often is removed and left at the scene of the accident or discarded in the emergency department. This impedes the investigation of the event. The types of evidence found in clothing vary, depending on the mechanism of injury.

In automobile crashes or auto-pedestrian collisions, minute pieces of paint or glass may be found in the victim's clothing. In hit-and-run incidents, paint chips may facilitate identification of not only the color of the vehicle, but also the year and model. An example of the importance of this piece of evidence is illustrated in the following case.

CASE STUDY An elderly couple were walking along a city sidewalk late one summer evening. Suddenly the woman, nearest the roadway, was struck from behind and killed by a motorist who left the roadway and ran onto the sidewalk with his vehicle. The victim was dead at the scene, and the driver of the vehicle left the scene. The woman's body was removed, and further examination was carried out, which revealed large flakes of an unusual shade of green paint throughout her clothing. The following morning, several members of the local law enforcement and death investigation agency were at the scene of the incident. During the processing of the scene, one of the investigators noticed a pickup truck with the same unusual shade of green paint moving slowly down a side street a few blocks away. The driver was stopped and subsequently arrested, because his vehicle contained significant front-end damage and fresh blood stains. The other person was knocked to the roadway at the time of the accident and was unable to provide a description of the vehicle. A suspect may never have been located without the link the paint chips provided.

Tire marks on clothing also may assist investigators in making a match with a particular vehicle. Because of imperfections in tires and variable wear in tread, tire marks are specific for the vehicle that produced them.

In the case of shootings and stabbings, direction of fibers around the defect in the clothing may help establish direction from which the shot or weapon originated. However, certain variables, such as fabric weave, movement of the body and clothing, and insect activity, may alter these findings. In contact and intermediate-range shootings, clothing may also contain gunpowder and soot. An incised defect in an article of clothing may help to identify the shape of the blade or object used in an assault. Certain materials such as leathers and synthetics will preserve the shape of the blade because of their low elasticity. Clothing is also useful in cases of unknown identity of the victim. Missing person reports include descriptions of clothing worn, and familiar articles of

clothing may be identified by a victim's relatives. Victims of sexual assault may have hairs and fibers on their clothing from the attacker and from the area in which the assault occurred.

Proper handling of clothing is essential if evidence is to be preserved intact. Whenever possible, defects in the clothing should not be cut through when the clothing is removed from the body. If heavy debris is noted on the clothing, removal of the clothing over a clean white sheet on the floor will aid in the collection of potential trace evidence. The sheet can then be folded up and turned over to law enforcement personnel. Clothing should always be placed in paper bags, not plastic—plastic bags accelerate mold and mildew growth by trapping moisture, which can destroy evidence. If the clothing is wet or damp, it should be air dried. If time does not allow this, the receiving agency should be informed of the condition of the clothing.

Chain of Custody

The chain of custody of clothing, as with all evidence, must be maintained at all times (Spitz & Fisher, 1980). Chain of custody establishes all parties who had contact with the items. Two ways in which chain of custody may be established in court are by demonstrating that (1) the piece of evidence has been in the continuous and secure possession of one or more identified persons at all times and (2) the evidence was in a marked, sealed, and tamper-proof container at all times. It is recommended that a preprinted form be used for this purpose, which facilitates items of evidence to be signed over to the receiving agency.

Hands

The hands of a victim of trauma may contain valuable evidence, especially in the cases of assaults and gunshot wounds. In assaults, the victim may scratch the assailant, which can be substantiated by scraping for tissue under the fingernail tips of the victim. Sexual assault examinations routinely include this procedure.

In cases of suspected suicidal gunshot wounds, hands may be examined for the presence of soot or gunpowder. A variety of tests for primer residues may be performed to establish whether the victim fired the weapon. This is often done even if no visible evidence of powder exists; therefore it should not be assumed that the lack of obvious

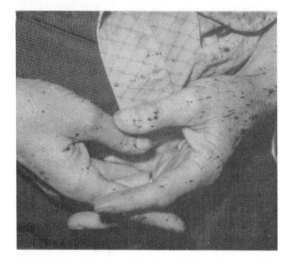

Figure 5-10 Characteristic blow-back blood spatters on hands of victim of low-velocity, self-inflicted gunshot wound. Examination of individual spatters allows calculation of direction and angle of source of origin of spatter.

powder means that no testing will be done. Additionally, this evidence is often found on both hands—the one used for firing the weapon and the one used to cradle the muzzle against the skin. This necessitates proper care of both hands. Blood spatters found on the hands may also take a characteristic appearance in self-inflicted gunshot wounds (Figure 5-10). This evidence can easily be lost or altered with improper care.

A relatively simple and expeditious way to preserve evidence on the hands of the victim involves the placement of a paper bag over each hand. The bags can then be secured at the wrist with a band of tape. Obviously this would not be feasible if the victim survives the injury. In the event of death or the unconscious critically ill patient, however, this procedure should be used. The victim's hands should not be washed unless absolutely necessary.

Bullets, Weapons, and Other Foreign Bodies

As with clothing, any bullets, weapons, or other foreign bodies (e.g., paint chips and pieces of windshield) should be signed over to the proper authorities on a chain-of-custody form. Bullets are an especially valuable piece of forensic evidence, because they are used to positively identify the weapon from which they were fired.

As a bullet moves down the barrel of a weapon, impressions are made in the soft lead by

riflings (grooves and elevations) in the barrel. These riflings are specific for the weapon used and may indicate the make and model of the gun. In addition to riflings, imperfections in the barrel can mark the bullet. These markings are even more specific for a particular weapon. Because most bullets are made of soft lead, handling of the bullets with metal instruments can alter these marks and this practice should be avoided.

Wounds

Vigorous cleansing of wounds and any incision into or around wounds should be avoided if possible. As discussed with gunshot wounds, valuable evidence can be found in and around the area. Alteration of the area may make determination of such factors as range and direction of fire more difficult. The wounds associated with stabbings may also contain fibers or trace evidence, which is lost with irrigation. If such care is necessary, any debris noted should be saved as evidence. The actual stab wound also may provide information about the inflicting weapon.

Laboratory Specimens

Blood alcohol levels and other drug concentrations are important to law enforcement personnel, attorneys, and the medical examiner in the investigation of motor vehicle crashes. Often the human factors of a crash center around the degree of intoxication of the persons involved. Local laws vary as to the consent needed for obtaining blood specimens, necessitating familiarity with various evidentiary laws in the area.

In many jurisdictions, all biologic specimens from the victim must be sent to the medical examiner with the body. The samples obtained on admission are usually the most valuable for toxicologic studies, particularly if massive fluid resuscitation has been carried out. Autopsy samples may reveal the dilutional effects of such fluid resuscitation. Therefore it is advantageous to have a designated area in the laboratory for the retention of initial specimens from trauma victims and other potential medicolegal cases. Urine is also used for drug testing and can be obtained premortem or postmortem. If a catheter for bladder drainage was used before death, the bladder will be empty at the time of the autopsy. Therefore it is important that a specimen be obtained before removal of the catheter.

Blood and urine samples cannot be identified in the same way as other pieces of evidence. With these types of specimens, chain of custody is demonstrated by establishing conclusively that the specimen in question is the same one that was taken from the patient and sent to the laboratory. This necessitates accurate labeling of the tube or container with the patient's identification, date, time, and initials of the person obtaining the specimen. It must be shown also that the sample has not been switched, altered, or tampered with from the time it is first taken until it is delivered to the appropriate investigating agency. Proper storage in a secure area of the laboratory will facilitate compliance with these criteria.

POSTMORTEM CARE AND ISSUES

Reporting laws vary from state to state, which makes it necessary for trauma facility personnel to be familiar with local regulations regarding deaths that are reportable to the medical examiner's office or to law enforcement agencies. Generally, when any person comes to a sudden, violent, or unexpected death or when the cause of death is unclear, a report must be made to the proper authorities. In most states, all deaths involving any type of trauma, accident, or violence fall within the medical examiner's jurisdiction. Additionally, deaths that occur within a certain period after admission (usually 24 hours or less) are generally reportable. If any question exists regarding the circumstances of a death, report should be made and the responsible agency can make a determination.

Once a death has been identified as falling under medical examiner jurisdiction, special handling of the body is necessary. The body should not be cleaned, and clothing in place at the time of death should be left in place. If clothing has already been removed, it should be packaged as previously described. Endotracheal tubes and nasogastric tubes, as well as intravenous lines, should be left in place so that placement of these devices can be assessed at time of autopsy. Improper intubation would obviously be of importance in the evaluation of a patient's clinical course. Venipuncture sites made before death by the prehospital or emergency department staff can be distinguished by encircling them in ink. Other clinically produced defects, such as needle thoracostomy or periocardiocentesis sites, should be similarly marked.

If biologic samples were obtained before death, either they should be sent with the body or the laboratory personnel should be notified that the particular case is being reported to the medical examiner. This will facilitate preservation of the admission specimens, which yield more accurate toxicologic results.

In some facilities, especially teaching institutions, postmortem procedures, such as intubation and venipuncture, are carried out. In addition to the ethical considerations and issues involving consent for such procedures, potential exists for the alteration of evidence in medical examiners' cases. Consequently, it is advisable for institutions to obtain appropriate consent from the medical examiner's office before these procedures are performed on potential medicolegal cases.

Organ Procurement

Frequently, trauma victims identified as suitable candidates for organ donation also will be reportable cases to the medical examiner. Therefore it is important to obtain appropriate consent from the medical examiner before proceeding with organ procurement. This may involve making contact before the patient's actual death (or at the time of pronouncement of brain death). Early notification of the medical examiner facilitates the completion of the investigation of the incident in a timely manner to facilitate successful organ retrieval.

Certain cases, such as homicides and motor vehicle crashes involving possible litigation, present potential conflict regarding the procurement of solid organs. When making a report of autopsy findings, the medical examiner is responsible for reporting on the condition of the entire body, including all organs. If the organs are removed before the autopsy, reporting may be incomplete. Additionally, removal of the ocular globes for corneal retrieval negates the possibility of completion of any studies on the vitreous fluid. Because diffusion into vitreous fluid occurs slowly, analysis of this fluid can be a reliable indicator of pre-death levels of such substances as drugs, alcohol, and various other plasma chemistries.

To facilitate organ retrieval in medicolegal cases, some areas have opted to have the medical examiner present at the time of retrieval of organs. An examination of the organs can be carried out at that time, and findings are then included in the final report. Facilitation of organ retrieval necessitates a close working relationship with death investigation personnel on potential or actual medicolegal cases.

Requests for Autopsy

Medical examiners and coroners are given authority by state law to carry out death investigation and establish manner and cause of death. If a question exists regarding the circumstances of the death, an autopsy may be ordered to assist in making such determinations. For this reason it should be stressed that permission for autopsy should never be requested by hospital staff for those patients who are medical examiner or coroner cases. If the family refuses permission, conflict results when the medical examiner or coroner must exert authority to perform an autopsy against the family's wishes (Smialek, 1983).

SUMMARY Trauma care providers are likely to encounter a number of patients in their day-to-day practice who have sustained injuries that may come under medicolegal investigation. Because the circumstances of the incident are not always known by the nurse on first contact with the trauma victim, it is difficult to readily identify those cases likely to proceed to an investigation. Based on this premise, hospital personnel should be familiar with types of evidence that can be found on these patients, as well as the appropriate procedure for evidence handling. Accurate and careful evidence preservation facilitates successful death investigation, as well as effective litigation of those guilty of criminal acts.

CASE STUDY A local ambulance company notifies the emergency department that they are en route with an approximately 45-year-old man who has sustained a gunshot wound to the right lower portion of his chest while cleaning his rifle. The victim has been hypotensive and tachycardic since the incident. Intravenous lines have been established, and the victim has been intubated and is being ventilated. The medics report that he is difficult to ventilate.

Shortly after the patient arrives in the emergency department, he suffers a cardiopulmonary arrest and resuscitation efforts are carried out. A right chest tube is immediately placed, and advanced cardiac life support protocols are followed. Efforts are unsuccessful and are discontinued after approximately 30 minutes. The wife of the patient arrives and confirms that she found her husband slumped over his rifle with the gun-cleaning materials around him.

What types of injuries and extent of tissue damage might be expected with this history?

With the history of a gunshot wound from a rifle, massive tissue destruction should be expected. Rifles are considered high-velocity weapons and can create a temporary cavity up to 30 times the diameter of the bullet. One exception to this is the .22 rifle (low velocity), so obtaining information about the specific weapon is helpful. Because the wound was in the right lower portion of the chest, injury within the chest and abdominal areas should be suspected, since diaphragm excursion ranges from the fourth to the twelfth intercostal spaces.

Is this a reportable death, and if so, what factors make it reportable?

This death is reportable to authorities for a variety of reasons. Deaths occurring in the emergency department (ED) are usually all reportable, since they occur within a short time after admission and, generally, deaths occurring within 24 hours of admission are reportable. This regulation may vary from area to area, so the trauma nurse should be familiar with local regulations. Additionally, this death occurred suddenly, violently, and certainly unexpectedly. Deaths in these circumstances are always reportable. Report must be made not only to the medical examiner or coroner's office, but also to law enforcement personnel.

What information regarding the history of this incident should be documented in the ED record?

Documentation regarding gunshot wound victims should be done carefully. The history in this case may initially appear to be a straightforward, accidental death. However, any information included in the documentation about the incident should be charted as quotes from witnesses when available (wife states "my husband was cleaning his gun, and I found him like this").

Does this incident seem to be an accidental death?

It is not uncommon for a victim of a self-inflicted gunshot wound to make the incident appear to be accidental. One of the most common ways is the "gun cleaning accident" (DiMaio, 1985). Whether a death is ruled suicidal or accidental may impact substantially on payments from life insurance policies. Some policies do not cover deaths ruled as suicides, but pay double indemnity for accidental death.

What items found on the patient would be considered evidence, and what would be the appropriate method for handling this evidence?

Evidence likely present on this patient would include any clothing in place, the wound, and the patient's hands. If a bullet were located, this also would be an important piece of evidence. Clothing still in place should be left on the patient. If clothing has already been removed, it should be placed in a paper bag and the bag then labeled with the patient's identifying data, date and time, and the initials of the person placing the items in the bag.

The nurse should remove the clothing carefully to avoid cutting through any defects. Because the patient died, paper bags can be placed over the hands and secured at the wrists with tape. When law enforcement personnel or the medical examiner arrives, the articles collected can be signed over on a chain-of-custody form to the receiving person.

RESEARCH QUESTIONS

- What impact does your current protocol for evidence preservation and chain of custody have on the outcome of cases?
- Does the height of headrests affect the injuries seen in front- and rear-end collisions?
- Are there any patterned injuries identifiable based on type of collision in motorcycle accidents (ejection over handlebars compared with ejection from a side collision)?
- What alternative restraint devices could be used to minimize the injuries associated with use of current restraint systems?

RESOURCES

Academy of Criminal Justice Sciences
    Focus: Study of the reaction to deviance in the areas of police, courts, correction, and commercial and industrial security.
Department of Police Studies
East Kentucky University
Richmond, KY 40475-3131
(606) 622-6173

American Association for Automotive Medicine
2350 East Devon Ave., Suite 205
Des Plaines, IL 60018
(708) 390-8927

American Academy of Forensic Sciences
    The first organization to accept Forensic Nursing as a discreet discipline in 1991.
PO Box 669
Colorado Springs, CO 80901-0669
(719) 636-1100

American Society of Criminology
    Focus: Theoretical issues of making and breaking of laws, and the reaction to breaking the laws; criminal theories.
1314 Kinnear Rd.
Columbus, OH 43212
(614) 292-9207

Association of Forensic Nursing
Route 2, PO Box 476
Lake Park, GA 31636
Contacts: Virginia A. (Lynch) Red Hawk, MSN,RN
            (912) 247-1160;
        Zug Standing Bear, PhD
            Director of Criminal Justice Program
            Valdosta State College, Valdosta, GA
            (912) 333-5943

Association of Police Surgeons
Contact: Derrick J. Pounder, Professor
Department of Forensic Medicine
The Royal Infirmary
Dundee, Scotland DD1 9ND
0382 22074

National Highway Traffic Safety Administration (NHTSA)
U.S. Department of Transportation Auto Safety Hotline
    NEF-11
400 7th St. SW
Washington, DC 20590
(202) 366-5972 or (800) 424-9393 **Hotline**

Occupational Safety and Health Administration (OSHA)
Department of Labor
Public Information
200 Constitution Ave. NW
Washington, DC 20210
(202) 523-8148

United Network for Organ Sharing (UNOS)
PO Box 28010
Richmond, VA 23228
(800) 446-2726 or (800) 24-DONOR (In VA)

U.S. Department of Transportation/Emergency Medical
Services Division
400 7th St. SW, Room 6124-A
Washington, DC 20590

ANNOTATED BIBLIOGRAPHY

DiMaio, V.J. (1985). *Gunshot wounds: Practical aspects of firearms, ballistics, and forensic techniques.* New York: Elsevier Science Publishing.
  A complete and current reference on a variety of aspects of gunshot wounds. Focus is on the forensic aspects, but does include valuable information about wounding forces.
Gikas, P.W. (1983). Forensic aspects of the highway crash. *Pathology Annual, 18,* 147-163.
  A detailed discussion of the pathogenesis of injury in specific crashes and a wide variety of case illustrations.
Hanzlick, R.L. (1985). Hanging in the balance: The scales of justice and forensic evidence. *Journal of the Medical Association of Georgia, 74,* 84-87.
  A concise but valuable reference presenting the guidelines for obtaining and preserving forensic evidence in the hospital setting. Also includes case reports.
Lynch, V.A. (1991). Forensic nursing in the emergency department: A new role for the 1990s. *Critical Care Nursing Quarterly, 14* (3), 69-86.
  An article written by the woman who spearheaded the concept of forensic nursing. The evolving role of the forensic clinical nurse specialist and its many facets and multidisciplinary input are described. Of most interest are the examples of a need for understanding of the protocols of the various disciplines to establish a functional medical-legal interface. Forensic medicine deals not only with death investigation, but with clinical forensics applied to the living, of which forensic nursing is a complementary clinical subspecialty. A model of the theoretic framework for forensic nursing and a sample job description are included.
Spitz, W.U., & Fisher, R.S. (1980). *Medicolegal investigation of death.* Springfield, IL: Charles C. Thomas, Publisher.
  A comprehensive book that includes detailed information about predictable and patterned injuries seen in motor vehicle crashes. Also includes valuable information about evidence preservation in a variety of circumstances.

REFERENCES

Anderson, P., Rivara, F., Maier, R., & Drake, C. (1991). The epidemiology of seat belt–associated injuries. *Journal of Trauma, 31*(1), 60-67.
Asbun, H., Irani, H., Roe, E., & Bloch, J. (1990). Intraabdominal seat belt injury. *Journal of Trauma, 30*(2), 189-193.
Baulch, S., & Hall, G. (1991). Evidence collection. In M. Mancini, & J. Klein (Eds.), *Decision making in trauma management: A multidisciplinary approach.* (pp 266-269). Philadelphia: B.C. Decker.
Brady, W.J. (1982). *Outline of death investigation* (3rd ed.). Portland, OR: Author.
Carmona, R., & Prince-Johnson, K. (1988). Trauma and forensic medicine. *Journal of Trauma, 28*(7), 1082. (48th Annual American Association for the Surgery of Trauma Abstracts.)
Daffner, R.H., Deeb, Z., Lupetin, A., & Rothfus, W. (1988). Patterns of high-speed impact injuries in motor vehicle occupants. *Journal of Trauma, 28*(4), 498-501.
DiMaio, V.J. (1985). *Gunshot wounds: Practical aspects of firearms, ballistics, and forensic techniques.* New York: Elsevier Science Publishing.
Fackler, M. (1991). Wound ballistics. In D. Trunkey, & F. Lewis (Eds.), *Current therapy of trauma* (3rd ed.) (pp. 40-43). Philadelphia: B.C. Decker.
French, R.W., & Callender, G.R. (1962). Ballistic characteristics of wounding agents. *Wound Ballistics.* Washington, DC: U.S. Government Printing Office.
Gikas, P.W. (1983). Forensic aspects of the highway crash. *Pathology Annual, 18,* 147-163.
Harviel, J.D., Landsman, I., Greenberg, A., Copes, W., Flanagan, M., & Champion, H. (1989). The effect of autopsy on injury severity and survival probability calculations. *Journal of Trauma, 29*(6), 766-772.
Jones, A.M., Graham, N.J., & Looney, J.R. (1983). Arterial embolism of a high-velocity rifle bullet after a hunting accident. *American Journal of Forensic Medicine and Pathology, 4*(3), 259-264.
National Highway Traffic Safety Administration. (1981). *An ounce of prevention.* Washington, DC: U.S. Department of Transportation.
National Highway Traffic Safety Administration. (1989). *Occupant Protection Facts.* Washington, DC: U.S. Department of Transportation.
Peterson, B.J., & Petty, C.S. (1962). Sudden natural death among automobile drivers. *Journal of Forensic Science, 7,* 274.
Rutledge, R., Thomason, M., Oller, D., Meredith, W., Moylan, J., Clancy, T., Cunningham, P., & Baker, C. (1991). The spectrum of abdominal injuries associated with the use of seat belts. *Journal of Trauma, 31*(6), 820-825.
Smialek, J.E. (1983). Forensic medicine in the emergency department. *Emergency Medicine Clinics of North America, 1*(3), 693-704.
Spitz, W.U., & Fisher, R.S. (1980). *Medicolegal investigation of death.* Springfield, IL: Charles C. Thomas, Publisher.
Stothert, J., Gbaanador, G., & Herndon, D. (1990). The role of autopsy in death resulting from trauma. *Journal of Trauma, 30*(8), 1021-1025.
Subcommittee on Emergency Services—Hospital of ACS Committee on Trauma. (1986). Position paper on trauma autopsies. *American College of Surgeons Bulletin, 71* (10), 37.
West, I., Nielsen, G.L., Gilmore, A.E., & Ryan, J.R. (1968). Natural death at the wheel. *Journal of the American Medical Association, 205,* 206.

6 *Trauma Quality Management*

■■■

Patricia A. Southard

Lynn E. Eastes

OBJECTIVES
❏ *Differentiate between quality management, quality improvement, and quality assurance.*

❏ *Describe three measures that should be used to assure confidentiality of regional quality management meetings.*

❏ *Identify and compare the features associated with case management and managed care.*

❏ *Discuss the problem associated with relying on injury severity scores as the only factor in determining probability of survival.*

❏ *Describe three organizational charts that can be used in the quality improvement process.*

INTRODUCTION Achieving quality care has been the aim of hospitals and all healthcare agencies for many years. Finding the perfect mechanism to assure quality patient care has been difficult. Numerous systems and plans for assuring quality care have been implemented, but only a few have resulted in measurably improved care. Few are outcome driven, and even fewer use a prospective approach to the problem.

Although those who deliver care to the trauma patient are no less committed in their desire to design a method of monitoring patient care and improving outcome, few references discuss quality management in patient populations that are exclusively trauma-related. This chapter provides an overview of trauma quality improvement and suggests various methodologies for monitoring and improving the care of the trauma patient.

HISTORICAL PERSPECTIVE

Avedis Donabedian's approach to quality assurance is one of the most frequently quoted (Donabedian, 1986). The Donabedian model emphasizes the elements of structure, process, and outcome in the overall approach to evaluating quality. It serves primarily as an organizational framework for designing a comprehensive evaluation process. It organizes areas of focus into (1) structural aspects of care (e.g., physical hardware, personnel, training of personnel, physical plant of the emergency department); (2) process aspects (e.g., activation of the trauma team, ordering and administration of blood products); and (3) outcome aspects (e.g., mortality and morbidity of trauma patients, length of stay). These categories are not mutually exclusive, and when patient care is evaluated, the categories overlap considerably. Although many quality improvement methodologies are moving away from the Donabedian model of structure, process, and outcome, understanding the concept is useful when considering a thorough approach to evaluating quality. In addition, the evaluation of processes of patient care and their outcomes of health care remain key concepts in current quality improvement approaches, as will be discussed later in this chapter.

The Joint Commission on Accreditation of Healthcare Organizations (JCAHO) is another influential body in the development of quality review systems. Since its inception in 1952 (at that time known as the Joint Commission on Accreditation of Hospitals [JCAH]), JCAHO has been at the forefront of developing standards for all aspects of patient care within hospitals. JCAHO's most recent impact on health care is its "Agenda for Change," which was first published in 1987. A part of the "Agenda for Change" included the now well-known "10-step process," which set a new direction and set of goals for quality assurance in health care. The box below describes the 10-step process. Future trends in JCAHO will be discussed later in this chapter.

A fundamental objective of the "Agenda for Change" was to encourage a systematic method of monitoring patient care by identifying important aspects of care and developing measurable performance standards, or indicators, for review. JCAHO first developed indicators for obstetrics and anesthesia, followed by ones for oncology, cardiovascular care, and trauma.

JCAHO 10-step process

1. Assign responsibility
2. Describe scope of service
3. Identify important aspects of care that are high risk, high volume, or problem prone
4. Develop indicators of quality
5. Establish thresholds for evaluation
6. Collect and organize data
7. Analyze data
8. Create action plan
9. Evaluate effectiveness of action plan
10. Communicate relevant information

Note. From *Accreditation Manual for Hospitals* by JCAHO, 1991, Chicago: Author.

In late 1991, JCAHO initiated beta testing of the trauma indicators (the final phase to establish reliability and validity); this process will be completed by 1993 (see box on p. 81).

The American College of Surgeons Committee on Trauma (ACSCOT) is the other influential body involved in developing performance standards and guidelines for trauma care. Similar to JCAHO's indicators, the American College of Surgeons (ACS) has put forth 22 audit filters to be used in evaluating the quality of trauma care. (American College of Surgeons, 1990). Some of these audit filters are similar to the JCAHO indicators.

FUTURE TRENDS IN JCAHO

The 1992 JCAHO requirements for quality improvement (QI) will differ significantly from previous standards. First, the term *quality assurance* (QA) will be dropped, and the term *quality assessment and improvement* will be adopted. The 1992 standards shift the emphasis from standards that inhibit the development of a continuous quality improvement approach to standards that assess and improve quality. These impediments to quality improvement include (1) exclusively focusing on clinical aspects of patient care, (2) compartmentalizing QA activities in accordance with hospital structure, (3) exclusively focusing on individual performance rather than on the processes involved in care, (4) initiating an action plan only when a problem is identified rather than identifying opportunities for improvement before an actual problem occurs, (5) separating appropriateness of care from the efficiency of care (JCAHO, 1992). Of importance also is JCAHO's new requirement for all hospital leaders, medical staff, and nursing leaders to receive education regarding quality improvement. In the past no specific education was required.

QUALITY IMPROVEMENT VERSUS TRADITIONAL QUALITY ASSURANCE

In the past 5 years, a revolution has been occurring in both industrial quality control and health-care QA. The entire impetus of this movement has been to deemphasize inspection of products and observation of the individual worker and instead focus on the processes of production or health care that could be performed better. W. Edwards Deming used much of this ideology to

---

JCAHO trauma indicators in beta testing

- Trauma patients with prehospital emergency medical services (EMS) scene times longer than 20 minutes
- Trauma patients with blood pressure, pulse, respiration, and Glasgow coma scale (GCS) score documented in the emergency department (ED) record on arrival and hourly until in-patient admission to operating room or intensive care unit, death, or transfer to another care facility (hourly GCS needed only if altered state of consciousness)
- Comatose patients discharged from the ED before the establishment of mechanical airway
- Trauma patients with diagnosis of intracranial injury and altered state of consciousness upon ED arrival receiving head computerized tomography (CT) scan longer than 2 hours after ED arrival
- Trauma patients with diagnosis of extradural or subdural brain hemorrhage undergoing craniotomy longer than 4 hours after ED arrival (excluding intracranial pressure monitoring), subcategorized by pediatric or adult patients
- Trauma patients with open fractures of the long bones as a result of blunt trauma receiving initial surgical treatment longer than 8 hours after ED arrival
- Trauma patients with diagnosis of laceration of the liver or spleen requiring surgery, undergoing laparotomy longer than 2 hours after ED arrival, subcategorized by pediatric or adult patients
- Trauma patients undergoing laparotomy for wounds penetrating the abdominal wall, subcategorized by gunshot and/or stab wounds
- Trauma patients transferred from initial receiving hospital to another acute care facility within 6 hours from ED arrival to ED departure
- Adult trauma patients with femoral diaphyseal fractures treated by a nonfixation technique
- Intrahospital mortality of trauma patients with one or more of the following conditions who did not undergo a procedure for the condition: tension pneumothorax, hemoperitoneum, hemothoraces, ruptured aorta, pericardial tamponade, and epidural or subdural hemorrhage
- Trauma patients who expired within 48 hours of ED arrival for whom an autopsy was performed

Note. Modified from *Accreditation Manual for Hospitals* by JCAHO, 1992, Oakbrook Terrace, IL.: Author.
The reader will notice that some of these indicators are worded positively, whereas others are worded "negatively." Trauma institutions can reword these indicators according to their particular needs and requirements.

---

help Japan's industry rebuild after World War II (Deming, 1986; Walton, 1986). The success of Japan's high-technology industries today is evidence that these methodologies work.

Though little empirical evidence exists to show that quality improvement (QI) will eliminate all of the healthcare quality shortfalls, many experts suggest that QI is far more likely to positively impact the quality of care than traditional QA methodologies.

Deming's approach to QI is based on 14 basic tenets (see box, p. 82), which lay the foundation for the entire approach to it (Deming, 1986).

QI's appeal to health care is that it focuses on the *processes* of patient care that cause problems and need improvement rather than the *people*. Health care providers, particularly physicians, often have viewed the traditional QA approach (looking for "bad apples") very negatively. Historically, physicians have been involved in mortality

and morbidity (M&M) conferences and have had to deal with the legal consequences of physician peer review. Because of these consequences, the QI approach is much more appealing.

Another significant aspect of QI's departure from traditional QA is its approach to problems. Traditional QA looks at processes (or people) involved in care and acts to change them only if a problem is identified. Contrary to this, QI examines key areas of care, whether specifically problematic or not, and determines how to improve performance. Thresholds for evaluation are a prime example of traditional QA methodologies that can artificially inhibit the identification of opportunities for improvement. When using thresholds, the QA coordinator does not act on a particular area of care unless the threshold is exceeded.

QI, unlike QA, also strives to avoid mediocrity. For example, performing merely up to "in-

---

Deming's 14 tenets of quality improvement

1. Create and publish to all employees a statement of the aims and purposes of the company or other organization. The management must demonstrate constantly their commitment to this statement.
2. Learn the new philosophy, top management and everybody.
3. Understand the purpose of inspection, for improvement of processes and reduction of cost.
4. End the practice of awarding business on the basis of price tag alone.
5. Improve constantly and forever the system of production and service.
6. Institute training.
7. Teach and institute leadership.
8. Drive out fear. Create trust. Create a climate for innovation.
9. Optimize toward the aims and purposes of the company the efforts of teams, groups, staff areas.
10. Eliminate exhortations for the work force.
11. a. Eliminate numerical quotas for production. Instead, learn and institute methods for improvement.
    b. Eliminate M.B.O. Instead, learn the capabilities of processes, and how to improve them.
12. Remove barriers that rob people of pride of workmanship.
13. Encourage education and self-improvement for everyone.
14. Take action to accomplish the transformation.

Note. From W. Edwards Deming, 1990.

---

dustry" standards or norms is no longer acceptable. QI programs avoid the "we're no worse" phenomenon (Bone & Griggs, 1989). For example, one might say "we're no worse than Trauma Center XYZ because our ICU readmission rate for respiratory failure is comparable to theirs." The QI approach to this problem is instead "our ICU readmission rate is comparable to Trauma Center XYZ's, but what is it about our ICU transfer policy that is contributing to these ICU readmissions that might be changed?" This QI approach pushes programs beyond the status quo.

Finally, key to the philosophy of QI is its integration into the very *culture* of the organization itself. For QI to be implemented successfully in any industrial or health care organization, it must be espoused and promulgated by those at the top. JCAHO's 1992 requirement for QI education of all top administrators, CEOs, and medical and nursing leaders is evidence that this organization recognizes that QI cannot be implemented without this step. Unlike QA, which can and often does begin and end with the QA Coordinator or small medical staff or nursing committee, QI takes the total burden off the QA department staff and places responsibility on those who have ultimate authority and power to act. Later in this chapter, the implementation of QI in a trauma program will be discussed.

DESIGNING A TRAUMA QUALITY MANAGEMENT (QM) PROCESS

Despite the tremendous shift in health care from traditional QA methodologies to QI philosophies, many fundamental processes remain the same. To design and implement a QI program in trauma, several key functions must be completed to lay the foundation for the overall program. First and most important, key players must decide who will be accountable for both the workload and results of the trauma QI program.

Typically, accountability is a shared responsibility between the trauma coordinator (TC) and the trauma medical director (TMD). The TC may assume full responsibility for working with other department directors and key individuals to resolve operational and nursing care quality issues. The trauma coordinator might even assume responsibility of QI education for the trauma staff in collaboration with the hospital-wide QI department. The TMD holds primary accountability for review of all medical (physician) care of the trauma patient. Although the TMD may choose to delegate data collection for various studies relating to physician medical care to the TC, the final evaluation of those results and determination of issues of appropriateness are completely within the purview of the TMD. The box on p. 83 further delineates the division of responsibilities between the TC and the TMD for trauma QI activities.

As responsibilities are delineated in the development of the trauma QI process, another key factor is the integration of trauma QI into the hospital-wide QI process. Trauma quality assessment and evaluation should not exist in a "vacuum." Trauma is a multidisciplinary disease process that crosses numerous professional disci-

---

Delineation of responsibilities for QI

Trauma coordinator

- Coordinates review of all operational issues relating to trauma, and implements action plans in collaboration with various hospital departments involved.
- Coordinates review of ACS, JCAHO, and other indicators.
- Compiles reports for hospital QI department and regional QI processes.
- Coordinates trauma nursing QI studies in collaboration with the nursing QI or hospital QI departments.
- Performs concurrent review of patient charts, evaluating for potential care issues, and refers these to the trauma medical director if physician related.

Trauma medical director

- Coordinates review of physician-related issues.
- Coordinates physician peer review of deaths, complications, and infections.
- Usually represents trauma program on hospital-wide committees and regional QI committees.
- May delegate some QI special study data collection to trauma coordinator or trauma registrar.
- Performs review of physician clinical pertinence.

---

plines. Therefore integration with other QI processes is imperative. At the beginning of the planning phase, the key QI department personnel should serve as consultants and expert advisors on how to best implement the QI plan without being duplicative or uninformed of processes already in place. JCAHO has recognized this problem, and the 1992 JCAHO standards (JCAHO, 1992) are specifically designed to shift the emphasis of QI activities away from an exclusively departmental and discipline-specific focus to a completely integrated approach that will encourage continual improvement. This will be accomplished by encouraging institutions to implement QI activities that cross multiple disciplines and solve problems with systems rather than individual practitioners. The TC and TMD should develop, in collaboration with the hospital QI department, a multidisciplinary QI committee for trauma. Membership on the committee includes medical and nursing directors for various departments (e.g., pediatrics, ED, radiology, blood bank, ICU). The TMD usually will be the chairperson of the trauma committee. The box at right shows a sample trauma committee membership roster.

The trauma committee is a policy-making body for all issues relating to trauma care. However, strong lines of communication must be established with other departmental QI committees to facilitate the exchange of problems and issues for review.

Trauma committee sample membership roster

Trauma medical director (chairperson)
Trauma coordinator
ICU nursing director
ICU physician director
Operating room nursing director
Department of anesthesia representative (physician)
Trauma ward nursing director
Pediatric intensive care nursing director
Pediatric intensive care medical director
Pediatric surgery representative
Transfusion services (blood bank) medical director
Radiology medical director
Emergency department nursing director
Emergency department medical director
Representatives from various medical subspecialties (e.g., plastic surgery, ophthalmology, rehabilitation, orthopedics, neurosurgery)

Note: Some trauma centers have a separate pediatric trauma QM committee. A core group may also be designated with subspecialty representation only for pertinent cases.

To be able to systematically design the trauma QI process, trauma program staff should develop a comprehensive written plan. This written plan (a requirement of JCAHO) allows the trauma program to delineate all of the reporting structures,

---

Components of the written QI plan

- Scope of services rendered to patients by the trauma program
- Organization and accountability of the trauma QI process
- Data analysis
- Action plans
- Planned reevaluation
- Mechanism for overseeing effectiveness of monitoring activities
- QI program evaluation
- Reporting

---

the areas of responsibility, and the scope of services rendered. The box above illustrates the components that should be thoroughly discussed in the written plan.

Developing Indicators

The next step in the design and implementation of a trauma QI plan is to identify the key activities involved in trauma care and develop indicators, or measurable, objective performance standards, to assess the care that is delivered. As mentioned, many such indicators are already provided by both ACS and JCAHO. Trauma programs, however, should develop their own program-specific indicators as well. Indicators are usually one of two types: sentinel events or rate-based events (JCAHO, 1989). Sentinel events are those incidents that are serious enough to warrant review with each occurrence. Such occurrences as patient deaths, serious complications, and failure of a surgeon or other required personnel to meet a trauma patient in the emergency department (ED), are examples of sentinel events. Rate-based events are generally less high-risk to the patient and may be viewed retrospectively as an aggregate of data or "rate." The trauma program may want to designate as rate-based events such indicators as "patients discharged home directly from the ED" and "trauma patients admitted to physician other than a general surgeon." Many other indicators may be either rate-based or sentinel events, depending on the specific problems and needs of the individual institution.

The determination of sentinel events versus rate-based events is trauma program specific. The

individual program and institution are responsible for choosing which categorization will help to best monitor care and identify opportunities for improvement. Additionally, these categorizations are not permanent and may be changed as needed. For example, if a particular trauma program is dissatisfied with physician response to trauma codes, the TC may choose to make this indicator a sentinel event (review and act on each occurrence) until the problem has been resolved to a manageable or acceptable level.

One caveat about sentinel events and rate-based events, however, should be given to the small trauma center. If the volume of trauma admissions is fewer than approximately 50 patients per month, viewing indicators as rate-based events may not be an effective tool. In this case, the trauma program should consider reviewing every indicator each time it occurs or fails to occur. With inadequate numbers for the denominator, rates can be misleading and meaningless. For example, if the trauma program examines the indicator "trauma surgeon present in ED on arrival of patient if 5-minute notification given" as a rate-based event and of 500 cases there were two occurrences in which the surgeon was not available, the rate is 2/500 or 0.4% (or a 99.6% compliance rate). If, however, the trauma program has a low volume of patients and has 3 occurrences of 10 cases, the rate will be 3/10 or 30% (only a 70% compliance rate) and would warrant review anyway.

The development of indicators is a serious process that requires deliberation and time. If the TC and the TMD carefully and appropriately develop the indicators, the results of data collection and analysis are much more likely to be valid and meaningful. JCAHO has led in the development of indicators by producing an indicator development tool (JCAHO, 1989), which is the same form they use in the alpha-testing phase of indicators for anesthesia, obstetrics, oncology, cardiovascular care, and trauma (Figure 6-1). The basic information required by this tool is (1) initial statement of the indicator, (2) definition of any ambiguous terms within the indicator statement, (3) classification of the indicator (i.e., sentinel event or rate-based event), (4) rationale for why the indicator is important to monitor, (5) description of the types of patients that the indicator will involve, (6) location of various data elements in

1

I.   INDICATOR:

II. DEFINITION OF TERMS: (define all terms within the indicator that might be ambiguous or in need of further explanation for data collection purposes).

III. TYPE OF INDICATOR:

    A.   Indicate whether this indicator is a:

        1. _____   Sentinel Event (all occurrences warrant investigation)

        2. _____   Rate Based indicator (further assessment occurs if the occurrence rate shows a significant trend, exceeds predetermined thresholds, or indicates significant differences when compared to other peer institutions).

    B.   Indicate whether this indicator primarily addresses:

        1. _____   a process of patient care

        or

        2. _____   a patient outcome

        or

        3. _____   both

IV. RATIONALE:

    A.   Explain the reason why this indicator is useful to assess and the specific process or outcome that will be monitored.

    B.   Supportive references (identify the sources of information used to develop the above rationale).

Figure 6-1 Example of clinical indicator development form. (*Note.* From JCAHO. (1989). Reprinted with permission from *Quality Review Bulletin*, 15(11), 1989.)

Continued.

2

C. Identify the practitioner and/or organizational processes assessed by this indicator, (e.g., judgement, capability of practitioner or staffing, systems, equipment/supplies).

V. DESCRIPTION OF INDICATOR POPULATION

A. Subcategories (identify patient subpopulations by which the indicator data will be separated for analysis, i.e., pediatric v. adult. If none, write "NONE."

B. Indicator Data Format (define the manner by which indicator data will be expressed).

1. Rate-based indicator format:

   a. Numerator(s):

   b. Denominator(s):

2. Sentinel event indicator format:

VI. INDICATOR LOGIC
List the specific data elements to be collected (e.g., ICD-9 CM codes) in the sequence of data element aggregation which will identify the patients assessed by the indicator. Also, enter the most likely sources of documentation where information will be found.

Data Elements   Data Sources

1.

2.

3.

Figure 6-1, cont'd Example of clinical indicator development form. (*Note.* From JCAHO. (1989). Reprinted with permission from *Quality Review Bulletin*, 15(11), 1989.)

3

VII. UNDERLYING FACTORS

List factors not included in the indicator that may account for significant indicator rates or indicator activity.

A. Patient-based factors (factors outside the healthcare organization's control contributing to patient outcomes).

1. Severity of illness (factors related to the degree or stage of disease prior to treatment).

2. Co-morbid conditions (disease factors, not intrinsic to the primary disease, which may have an impact on patient suitability for, or tolerance of, diagnostic or therapeutic care).

3. Other patient factors (non-disease factors which may have an impact on care, e.g., age, sex, refusal of consent).

B. Non-patient based factors (factors within the healthcare organization's control or problem areas causing indicator activity).

1. Practitioner based factors (factors related to specific health care practitioners).

2. Organization-based factors (factors related to healthcare organization which contribute either to specific aspects of patient care or to the general ability of direct care givers to provide services).

VII. FREQUENCY OF MONITORING AND EVALUATION (RATE-BASED EVENTS ONLY)

_____   Monthly

_____   Quarterly

_____   Semi-annually

_____   Annually

Figure 6-1, cont'd   For legend see opposite page.

the medical record or elsewhere that will be used by the data collector, and (7) delineation of underlying factors that may explain variations in indicator data (e.g., exclusions).

In the *rationale* portion of the indicator development tool, supportive references for the indicator are requested. This feature is particularly important because it forces TCs and TMDs to base their indicators on current scientific literature and research rather than on the opinions of the healthcare providers, increasing the likelihood of a positive impact on changing practice. However, some indicators will not have supporting literature.

The practice of using "generic" indicators, as prescribed by JCAHO and ACS, has been criticized. In a recent study, Rhodes, Sacco, Smith, and Boorse (1990) questioned the utility of generic screens in yielding significant problems. Rhodes found that modification of the indicators to be more specific improves their utility. The indicators development tool can assist in this refining process.

In a similar study the Health Care Financing Administration (HCFA) (HCFA, 1989) found that generic screens used by peer review organizations (PROs) to evaluate such areas as discharge planning, infections, unscheduled returns to surgery, and hospital injuries had high false-positive rates and thus identified cases in which no actual problem could be found on individual review.

Organizational Considerations

For organizational purposes, the TC and the TMD may want to consider designing a monitoring protocol to guide their QI activities. This can be an excellent tool to follow (1) the various indicators being monitored simultaneously, (2) the methodologies to be used, and (3) the frequency of evaluation, as well as whether the indicators are sentinel events or rate-based events. Table 6-1 illustrates an example of a monitoring protocol from a level I trauma program. Trauma programs can adopt monitoring protocols to meet their individual needs; they do not need to be as extensive as this example.

Trauma Nursing Quality Improvement

Trauma QI is by nature a multidisciplinary process, and nursing issues are usually integrated into the overall trauma QI plan. In some cases, however, TCs will want to collaborate with other nursing managers to address certain trauma issues specifically from a nursing perspective.

Most trauma nursing QI activities revolve around documentation. Specifically, nurses should review documentation of trauma resuscitation activities. Evaluation of the appropriateness of patient care during the initial resuscitation phase depends on complete, contemporaneous nursing documentation. The box below suggests some additional nursing issues that should be addressed in the trauma QI plan.

Although trauma physician standards are plentiful in the literature (e.g., ACS, JCAHO), available nursing standards for trauma care are limited. The Trauma Nursing Core Course (TNCC) (ENA, 1986), developed by the Emergency Nurses Association in 1986, provides a training curriculum for emergency nurses involved in the initial resuscitation of the trauma patient. Similar to the advanced trauma life support course offered to physicians by ACS, TNCC offers a systematic approach to the assessment and initial nursing management of the critically injured trauma patient. Emergency nurses may obtain 4-year verification through TNCC.

The Trauma Nursing Resource Document, a 1992 publication by a collaboration of nursing specialty organizations representing over 150,000 nurses, provides guidelines for nursing of the injured patient from injury through rehabilitation.

Nursing quality improvement indicators

- Review of emergency department documentation on resuscitation record
  Presence of hourly sequential vital signs
  ED admission and ED discharge Glasgow
  coma scale (GCS) score recorded
- Documentation of cervical spine clearance
  Neurovascular assessment documented after
  every patient move
  Collar removed only after physician order
- Skin integrity maintained in immobilized trauma patients
- Rigid cervical collar fitted properly
- Not more than 2 units of blood administered without the blood warmer

Table 6-1 Trauma quality management monitoring protocol

Important aspects	Indicators	Indicator type	Thresholds	Methodology*
Appropriate and timely care of trauma patients	**Operational**			
	Trauma team response times in accordance with:			
	1. Trauma surgeon (meet patient on arrival, assuming 5 minutes notification).	Sentinel event	100%	Review every occurrence until 100% compliance is reached.
	2. Anesthesia staff (meet patient on arrival, assuming 5 minutes notification).	Sentinel event	100%	Review every occurrence until 100% compliance is reached.
	3. Trauma nurses 1 and 2.	Rate-based event	99%	Monitor semiannually by registry report, 100% of trauma system patient charts.
	4. Neurosurgeon (consult on patient within 30 minutes of call requesting transfer).	Sentinel event	98%	Monitor semiannually by registry report, 100% of trauma system patient charts.
	Trauma system notification/activation			
	1. Notification to trauma communications center from prehospital setting.	Rate-based event	100%	Monitor annually by QA registry report, 100% of trauma system patient charts.
	2. Activation of trauma team by trauma communications center for all trauma system patients.	Sentinel event	100%	Review QA interdepartmental forms for any occurrences.
	Resource availability			
	1. Emergency department (ED) bed available for trauma patient arrival.	Sentinel event	100%	Review QA interdepartmental forms for any occurrences.
	2. CT scan available (assuming 30 minutes notification for trauma system patient arrival).	Sentinel event	100%	Review every occurrence. Refer to department manager for resolution.
	3. OR available for trauma system patient arrival.	Sentinel event	100%	Review every occurrence. Refer to department manager for resolution. Monitor annually by registry reports for any occurrences.
	4. Angiography suite available for trauma system patient arrival.	Rate-based event	100%	Review every occurrence. Refer to department manager for resolution.
	5. Critical care bed available for trauma system patient.	Sentinel event	100%	Monitor annually by registry reports for any occurrences. Review QA interdepartmental forms for any occurrences.

Continued.

*In addition to the methodology listed, all complaints and anecdotal reports will be evaluated.

Table 6-1 Trauma quality management monitoring protocol—cont'd

Important aspects	Indicators	Indicator type	Thresholds	Methodology*
Appropriate and timely care of trauma patients—cont'd	*Trauma admission procedures* 1. Trauma system patients are admitted to the general surgery service. 2. No trauma system patients will be discharged home directly from the ED.	Rate-based event Rate-based event	98% 100%	Previous evaluation yielded no significant problem. Evaluate annually. Previous evaluation yielded no significant problem. Evaluate annually. Analyze for increased incidence. Refer to systems assurance group (SAG) for review and action.
	Clinical			
	Delays in intervention 1. Trauma system patient disposition from the ED will be determined within 2 hours if systolic blood pressure is <90 or GCS score is 9 or less.	Rate-based event	90%	Retrospective review of registry report of all occurrences during the preceding 12 months. Evaluate annually. Previous evaluation yielded no significant problems.
	2. Trauma system patient will receive a CT scan or operative intervention in <2 hours if GCS score is <9.	Rate-based event	98%	Retrospective review of registry report of all occurrences during the preceding 12 months. Evaluate annually. Previous evaluation yielded no significant problems.
	3. Trauma patient with a diagnosis of a surgically correctable subdural or epidural hematoma will receive a craniotomy within 4 hours of ED arrival (excluding intracranial pressure monitoring device placement) and within 2 hours if systolic blood pressure is <90 or GCS score is 13 or less.	Rate-based event	100%	Retrospective review of registry report of all occurrences during the preceding 12 months. Evaluate annually. Previous evaluation yielded no significant problems.
	4. Trauma patients with open fractures or open joint injuries will receive operative intervention within 6 hours.	Rate-based event	95%	Retrospective review of registry report of all occurrences during the preceding 12 months. Evaluate annually. Previous evaluation yielded no significant problems.
	5. Trauma patients who have demonstrated hemoperitoneum by CT scan, diagnostic peritoneal lavage (DPL), or physical findings, and hemodynamic instability (BP of 90 or less and falling) will receive an exploratory celiotomy within 1 hour of diagnosis.	Sentinel event	95%	Every occurrence referred to trauma medical director for review.

Indicator	Type	Threshold	Methodology
6. Initial thoracic, abdominal, vascular, or cranial surgery will be performed within 24 hours of ED admission (excluding orthopedic, plastic, and hand surgery).	Sentinel event	95%	Every occurrence referred to trauma medical director for review.
7. All trauma patients with gunshot wounds or stab wounds to the abdomen with violation of peritoneum will receive an exploratory celiotomy.	Rate-based event	95%	Retrospective review of registry report of all occurrences during the preceding 12 months. Evaluate annually. Previous evaluation yielded no significant problems.
Delays in Intervention			
8. All trauma patients who have an injury severity score > 20 will have a nutrition consult within 48 hours of admission.	Rate-based event	95%	Evaluate data from QA registry report per monitoring calendar.
9. All trauma patients will receive occupational therapy and physical therapy consults within 48 hours of admission.	Rate-based event	80%	Evaluate data from QA registry report per monitoring calendar.
10. Trauma patients will receive social services consult within 48 hours of admission.	Rate-based event	80%	Evaluate data from QA registry report per monitoring calendar. Department of social work will also review on scheduled basis and report their findings to trauma program.
Documentation Contemporaneous accurate documentation of all care delivered to the trauma patient.			
1. Hourly, sequential vital signs will be documented for all trauma system patients from the time of ED arrival to OR or ICU admission or death (refer to policy and procedure for trauma documentation).	Rate-based event	95%	1) Perform focused reviews quarterly until performance to threshold.
2. All trauma system patients will have a progress note written by the trauma surgeon while the patient is in the ED.	Rate-based event	80%	2) Counsel individual nurses with poor compliance. Monitor annually by QA indicator report for any occurrences. Previous review yielded no significant problems.
3. Status of tetanus toxoid immunity will be documented.	Rate-based event	95%	Evaluate data annually on registry report.
4. All referring physicians for transferred trauma patients will receive a follow-up letter or telephone call from the medical director of trauma.	N/A	98%	1) Reminder sent by trauma registrar. 2) 100% review by trauma registrar. 3) Enter individual complaints by referring physicians or hospitals into QA data base.

Continued.

*In addition to the methodology listed, all complaints and anecdotal reports will be evaluated.

Table 6-1 Trauma quality management monitoring protocol—cont'd

Important aspects	Indicators	Indicator type	Thresholds	Methodology*
Clinically appropriate trauma care will be delivered to all trauma patients	*Procedures* 1. All trauma patients who have a GCS score of < 9 in the ED will have a mechanical airway placed before leaving the ED.	Rate-based event	100%	Review 20 randomly selected patient charts that meet criteria (GCS < 9) and report data annually. Previous evaluations yielded 100% compliance.
	Administration of Blood Products 1. All trauma patients who receive > 10 units of whole blood or packed red blood cells will receive either fresh frozen plasma or platelets as adjunctive therapy within 24 hours of blood administration.	Sentinel event	100%	Review semiannually all cases of massive transfusion (patient received > 10 units of whole blood or packed red blood cells within 24 hours). Cases obtained from trauma registry. Referred to transfusion services supervisor for verification. All cases not receiving adjunctive therapy referred to trauma medical director for review.
	Morbidity and Mortality 1. All patients who have an injury severity score of < 5 will survive their injuries.	Sentinel event and rate-based event	100%	1) Ongoing monthly review of all trauma deaths. 2) Monthly report of deaths to trauma audit group. 3) Review of registry report annually.
	2. Trauma patients who have been discharged from the ICU will not require unscheduled readmission to the SICU.	Sentinel event	100%	Trauma coordinators monitor patient's chart concurrently and report every occurrence to trauma medical director for review at M & M conference.
	3. Trauma patients who require CPR will be located in the ED, OR, or ICU. Cardiac arrests will not occur in areas outside of the ED, OR, or ICU.	Sentinel event	100%	1) Trauma coordinators monitor patient's chart concurrently and report every occurrence for review. 2) Monitor any anecdotal accounts of this problem.
	4. Trauma patients will recover from their injuries without complications/infections secondary to the injury.	Sentinel event and rate-based event	95%	1) Concurrent review by trauma coordinators, who report every occurrence for review in M & M conference. 2) Semiannual report of complications and infections to trauma audit group.

	Event type	Threshold	Methodology
			3) Semiannual tabulation of complications/infections to department of surgery. Monitor trauma death patient charts and review every occurrence.
Medical and nursing certification and continuing education			
5. Autopsy will be performed on all patients who die of trauma-related causes within 48 hours of admission.	Sentinel event	80%	
6. All trauma patients admitted to the ICU will be discharged from the unit within 6 days of admission.	Rate-based event	80%	Annual review by trauma registry report of all trauma patients remaining in the ICU for > 6 days from time of admission.
Physician credentialling			
Surgeons			
1. All trauma surgeons will have the following:			
a. Board certification/eligibility	Sentinel event	100%	Trauma director reviews individual surgeons' files annually for compliance.
b. ATLS verification or registration for next available course	Sentinel event	100%	
c. Credentialling documentation on file evidencing ability to perform trauma-related procedures	Sentinel event	100%	
d. Evidence of trauma continuing medical education (CME) activity on file	Sentinel event	100%	
Emergency Physicians			
1. All ED physicians caring for trauma patients will have the following:			
a. ATLS verification or registration for next available course	Sentinel event	100%	Chief of emergency medicine reviews individual ED physicians' files annually for compliance.
b. ACLS certification	Sentinel event	100%	
c. Evidence of trauma CME activity on file	Sentinel event	100%	

*In addition to the methodology listed, all complaints and anecdotal reports will be evaluated.

Continued.

Table 6-1 Trauma quality management monitoring protocol—cont'd

Important aspects	Indicators	Indicator type	Thresholds	Methodology*
Medical and nursing certification and continuing education—cont'd	*Anesthesiologists* 1. All anesthesiologists who respond to trauma will have the following:			
	a. ATLS verification or registration for next available course	Sentinel event	100%	Chairperson of anesthesiology reviews individual anesthesiologists' files annually for compliance.
	b. Evidence of trauma CME activity on file	Sentinel event	100%	Same as above.
	Nursing credentialing *Emergency Department* 1. All staff nurses who work in the ED will have the following:			
	a. ACLS certification	Sentinel event	100%	ED nursing director reviews individuals' records annually and reports results to trauma program.
	b. TNCC verification	Sentinel event	100%	
	c. Six hours of trauma education annually	Rate-based event	80%	Trauma coordinators review annually listing of trauma education for all nurses on trauma units.
	Surgical Intensive Care Unit 1. All staff nurses who work in the surgical intensive care unit will have the following:			
	a. ACLS certification		100%	Critical care nursing director reviews annually individuals' records and reports to trauma program.
	b. Six hours of trauma education annually		90%	
	Trauma Ward 1. All staff nurses who work on the trauma unit will have the following:			
	a. Six hours of trauma education annually		80%	Unit manager reviews annually individuals' records and reports to trauma program.
Patient, family, or referral agency satisfaction	Positive patient/referring agency satisfaction will be evidenced by positive responses on mailed surveys.		80%	Written survey given to all trauma patients on discharge, with an enclosed, stamped envelope for return.

Appropriate and timely care of the trauma patient	Patient with cervical spine injury will be diagnosed on admission or as soon as patient is alert enough to give subjective complaints of neck pain. (ACS-modified)	Sentinel event and rate-based event	100%	1) Focused review performed every 6 months of 1 month sampling of all patients admitted to ICU or ward in collars. 2) Referral of all missed cervical spine fractures to surgery M & M conference by trauma coordinators.
Appropriate and timely nursing care of the trauma patient	*Nursing indicators* Physician notification for > 3 liters of fluid infused in ICU or ward.	Sentinel event	100%	Focused study by individual unit-based QM committees
	If > 2 units of blood transfused, will use warmer.	Sentinel event	100%	Focused study by individual unit-based QM committees
	Notification of family members or significant others within 4 hours of patient arrival.	Sentinel event	100%	1) Focused review by ICU and unit-based QA committees on an ongoing basis until no problem occurrences. 2) Trauma coordinators track and review every occurrence.
	Trauma patients will not develop skin impairment caused by immobility.	Sentinel event and rate-based event	100%	1) Reviewed periodically by unit-based practice committee (UBPC). 2) Concurrent review by trauma coordinators—referral of any occurrences to UBPCs of individual unit.
Appropriate care of trauma patient	Central line insertions will be documented in patient chart. (QA department)	Rate-based event	100%	Study conducted periodically by hospital QA department in ICUs. Trauma subset extracted from these reports every time this study is completed.
Timely follow-up to referring physicians	Follow-up letters and/or calls to referring physicians by receiving physicians.	Rate-based event	100%	Study conducted periodically by hospital QA department in ICUs. Trauma subset extracted from these reports every time this study is completed.
Timely follow-up with patient's family	Family contact by physicians made at least once during hospitalization.	Rate-based event	100%	Study conducted periodically by hospital QA department in ICUs. Trauma subset extracted from these reports every time this study is completed.

*In addition to the methodology listed, all complaints and anecdotal reports will be evaluated.

Table 6-2 QI activity and corresponding data display technique

Quality improvement activities	Technique
1. To decide which areas should be addressed first for QI activity	Flow chart Pareto chart Brainstorming Nominal group technique
2. To describe the variations in systems/processes in terms of what it is specifically, where it occurs, when it happens, and its extent	Pareto chart Run chart Histogram Pie chart Stratification
3. To develop a complete picture of all the possible causes of the variation	Check sheet Cause-and-effect diagram Brainstorming
4. To agree on the basic cause(s) of the variations	Check sheet Pareto chart Scatter diagram Brainstorming Nominal group technique
5. To develop an effective and implementable solution	Brainstorming Force field analysis Pie chart Bar graph
6. To implement the solution and establish needed monitoring procedures action plan	Pareto chart Histogram Control chart Stratification PERT chart Gantt chart

Note. From *Health Care Quality: A Practical Guide to Continuous Improvement*. (p. 61). by P. Spath, 1991, Portland, OR: Brown-Spath & Assoc.

Graphic Tools for Quality Improvement

The TC and TMD may choose from a number of graphical tools to use in their QI data analysis. These are useful in translating information into a format that improves analysis, consolidating information into a "at a glance" format and effectively communicating data collected (Spath, 1991). Table 6-2 provides some examples of application of various graphical tools.

A histogram (Figure 6-2) is a graphic technique used to show the frequency of an event's occurrence. It is relatively easy to make (most computer graphics packages produce them), and it clearly depicts the data distribution over time (Spath, 1991).

A Pareto diagram (Fig. 6-3), similar to the histogram or bar graph, demonstrates the significant contributing factors to a particular problem and differentiates them from the less important contributing factors (Spath, 1991).

A run chart (Figure 6-4), or *line chart*, presents trends in data over time. Run charts are useful in assessing the stability of performance over time (Spath, 1991).

Stratification charts are similar to run charts, but they compare data on one chart. Control charts (Fig 6-5), or *statistical process control* are most commonly used in the industrial setting. However, they are useful for health care also. Control charts show statistically determined upper and lower limits on either side of the average or mean. The upper and lower control limits are calculated using data that has been collected over time and usually represent one or two standard deviations from the mean. Variations over time are plotted on this graph, and occurrences either above the upper control limits or below the lower control limits are easily identified.

Flow charts (Figure 6-6) are useful tools to graphically show the steps involved in a particular process. For example, if the problem is family notification of unidentified trauma patients, a flow chart depicts all of the steps involved in the notification process. Walking through the various steps facilitates pinpointing the areas in which a breakdown in the process can occur.

A cause-and-effect diagram (Figure 6-7) is a graphic display showing the relationship between an effect and all of the possible causes. The cause-and-effect diagram is useful in analyzing complex problems to better understand them.

A force field analysis (Figure 6-8) is a process that looks at the opposing forces relating to the solution of a problem. When the force field analysis is complete, the group using it can identify which factors they can influence and which they cannot. They can also determine if the effects of some of the impeding forces can be reduced and what forces might be developed to help carry out the strategy. The force field analysis is most useful in the development and implementation of action

Text continued on p. 101.

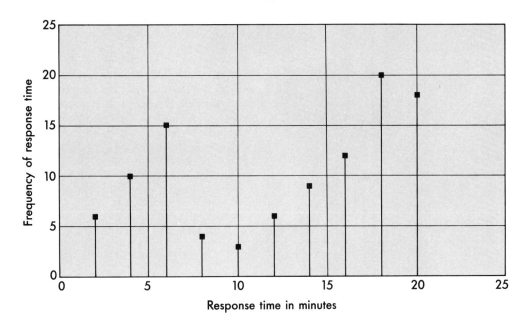

Figure 6-2 Example of histogram showing response times of radiology technicians to trauma resuscitations. (Observations made October, 1991.)

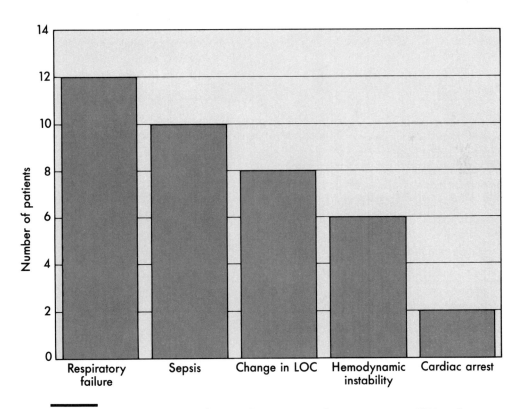

Figure 6-3 Example of Pareto diagram showing reason for trauma patient ICU readmissions. (January-June, 1991.)

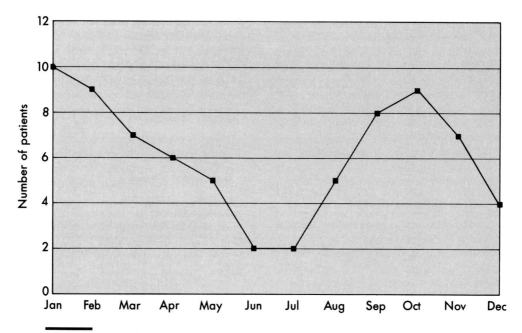

Figure 6-4   Example of run chart showing number of trauma patients with skin break-down. (Data from 1991.)

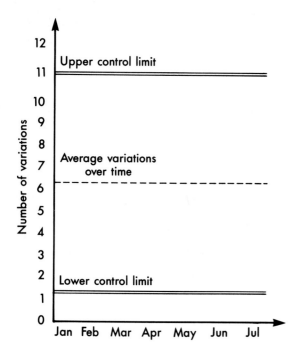

Figure 6-5   Example of control chart for use in plotting outliers. (*Note*. From *Health Care Quality: A Practical Guide to Continuous Improvement* (p. 67) by P. Spath, 1991, Portland, OR: Brown-Spath & Assoc.)

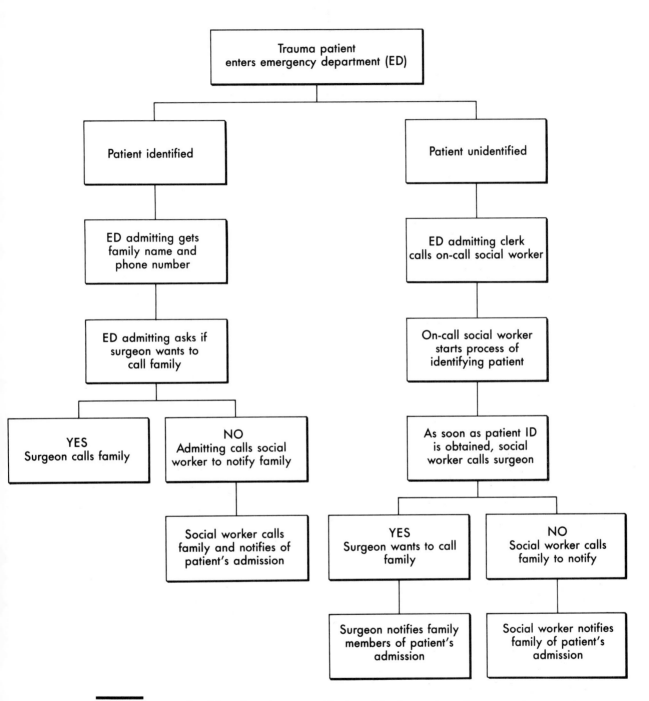

Figure 6-6   Example of flow chart showing notification of family members of trauma patients

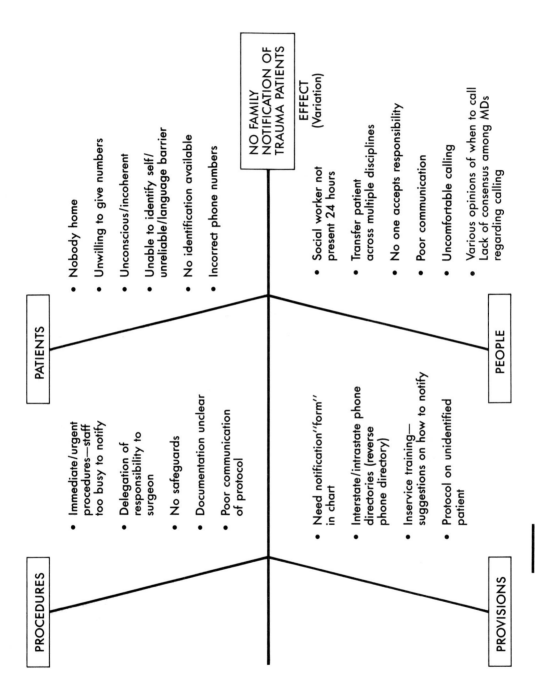

Figure 6-7 Example of cause-and-effect diagram showing the causes or factors associated with an effect—the lack of family notification.

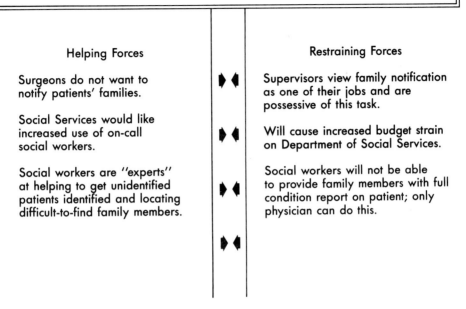

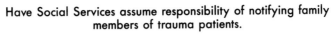

Figure 6-8 Example of force field analysis showing the identified helping and restraining forces that will impact decisions regarding an action plan. (*Note.* From *Health Care Quality: A Practical Guide to Continuous Improvement* (p. 67) by P. Spath, 1991, Portland, OR: Brown-Spath & Assoc.)

plans (Spath, 1991). Finally, a program evaluation and review technique (PERT) chart and Gantt chart are similar tools used to organize the steps required to implement an action plan. They are similar to timelines used for research and other projects. The PERT chart focuses on the various events that must occur to implement an action plan, with no regard for time, whereas the Gantt chart lists specific activities in relation to a specific schedule (Spath, 1991). Either tool is useful in tracking work on a particular quality improvement project and keeping it organized and manageable.

IMPLEMENTING QUALITY IMPROVEMENT

Moving from traditional QA into QI methodologies does not necessarily mean that all indicators and other means of systematically monitoring care are discarded. Instead, an integrated system of monitoring and QI is preferred, especially in environments where regulatory agencies (such as the state or county health division) still require documentation of certain monitoring activities. QI methodologies are excellent means of solving major issues within the trauma program that traditional QA techniques have been unable to resolve.

The first step in implementing QI involves education. As discussed earlier in this chapter, key administrative personnel, as well as those at the staff level, must become well versed in QI. Only through education can QI philosophies become ingrained in the organizational culture of an institution.

The next step is to set priorities for opportunities for improvement. This is best done in a governing committee, such as the trauma QI committee, through brainstorming. In this forum, key issues are identified and placed in order of significance. Next, QI teams are formed to address the problems identified, using various problem-solving techniques including nominal group process, brainstorming, and cause-and-effect diagrams.

As the QI teams discuss a given problem, they may begin with a flow chart to map out the process involved. Their goal is to identify the cause of the problem. They may use the cause-and-effect diagram to determine the relationship among potential causes of the variance and the variance itself. Once this is done, potential causes of the variance can be ranked as to their relative weight as contributing factors toward the problem (see Figure 6-7).

Problems are resolved only after the cause has been identified. This eliminates "quick fixing" a problem and later realizing that the solution is ineffective. Therefore the next step in identifying the cause of the problem is to collect data to verify that the possible causes of the identified problem are indeed the reasons for the variation. Extensive data collection may be needed to validate the QI group's "hunches."

Case Study: A QI Task Force on Problems with Notification of Family Members of Trauma Patients

Trauma Program XYZ experienced an ongoing problem of delayed notification of family members of trauma patients. Despite efforts, this problem remained unresolved. A QI task force met to address this problem. Using the cause-and-effect diagram (see Figure 6-7), they brainstormed for all of the possible reasons for this variation.

After the possible reasons were identified, the task force ranked the reasons according to their likelihood of contributing to the problem. Then they brainstormed for all of the possible means to verify these reasons. The trauma coordinator was then instructed to collect data about the various reasons to validate their contribution to the problem.

One month later the trauma coordinator reported the results of her data collection to the task force. The committee was surprised to learn that many of the possible "reasons" for the variation were not validated by the data collection. What became evident from the data collection was the following:

1. The majority of the problems were not taking place on night shift, as suspected.

2. The majority of the problems did not involve patients who were comatose and who could not identify themselves.
3. Family notification was done primarily by the social worker; however, no clear policy was in place to formalize this responsibility.
4. Nursing staff in the ED consistently failed to document attempts to notify family.

As a result of these findings, the task force developed a formal procedure to address this problem (see Figure 6-6), in which primary accountability for family notification was assigned to the on-call social worker. The nursing and physician staffs were eager to delegate this task to individuals who were well trained in family notification and counseling. Though the results of this QI task force's changes are yet to be measured, this example suggests a method that can be used when traditional QA methodologies have failed to rectify a problem.

It can be concluded, therefore, that QI techniques are complementary to some of the more traditional QA methodologies. Although it might seem more time consuming to the first-time observer, this methodical manner of studying long-standing issues is effective.

TRAUMA MANAGED CARE

Both the government and insurance companies (via health maintenance organizations [HMOs] and preferred provider organizations [PPOs]) are increasingly regulating health care. These regulations have stimulated hospitals to develop programs that are intended to continue to provide high quality care in spite of diminishing resources.

One of the most innovative programs, case management, was developed at Tufts University at the Center for Case Management. Case management is a proactive strategy that plots out expected hospital interventions for identified illnesses or injuries. The patient's hospital course is graphed on a CareMap™ (The Center for Case Management, Inc., Natick, Mass.). The purpose of the CareMap™ is to monitor and guide patient care delivery and to audit the cost and quality of the care provision (Zander, 1990).

Tracking Patient Progress

CareMaps™ are the most current instruments used in case management or managed care models. They serve a variety of functions, which include the following:

1. Replaces nursing care plans (Brider, 1991)
2. Provides data base for continuous quality improvement (CQI)
3. Provides schedule that sequentially integrates standards of care and standards of practice for a defined injury or multisystem injuries
4. Provides data base for acuity systems, financial systems, and research (Zander, 1991)

The CareMaps™ are developed with the input of all the disciplines that provide care for the injured patient. For example, if a CareMap™ is being developed for a patient with multiple extremity fractures, the following personnel should be included in the process: (1) trauma surgeon, (2) orthopedic surgeon, (3) intensive care unit nurse, (4) orthopedic nurse, (5) trauma coordinator, (6) physical therapist, (7) social worker, (8) discharge planner, and (9) nutritionist.

This group will meet and graph out in sequence the interventions and care expectations for each day the patient is hospitalized. Each patient who is subsequently admitted with this diagnosis will be placed on the prescribed CareMap™ course.

Some examples of interventions in such a CareMap™ include a physical therapy evaluation on the third hospital day, social work consult within 48 hours of admission, and internal fixation of fractures within 48 hours of admission. Every common intervention or expected care should be found in the daily sequences described in the CareMaps™.

If the intervention does not occur as scheduled, it becomes a variance that requires a review and explanation for the nonoccurrence. When CareMaps™ are first used, more variances may be found than will be expected after the CareMaps™ have been used for a period of time. The initial CareMaps™ may require adjustment if common variances are found. Some traumatic injuries are ideal for the managed care or case management model. Single-system injuries are the most adaptable to this model, whereas multiple-system injuries present a more complex problem for the Care Mapping™ approach. See Figure 6–9 for an example of a care pathway.

The consistent use of CareMaps™ will lead to (1) fewer variances and (2) highly predictable hospital courses for injuries (Zander, 1991). Ultimately, the length of stay by injury type can be predicted, which will result in the optimal use of scarce resources. Additionally, planned interventions coupled with predicted lengths of stay may help to decrease the costs associated with trauma care provision.

Staffing and Finances

Many hospitals are beginning to incorporate case management as part of both clinical and business practices. With case management, a designated hospital employee oversees the care delivery of a group of patients. This case manager assures that duplication is minimal, that interventions occur as scheduled, and that discharge is timely. Because trauma crosses so many disciplinary lines, it is ideal for the case management method.

An article by Songne and Holmquist (1991) describes a type of case management that has been in place for 10 years. A group of nurses in a hospital were designated as trauma nurse providers. They respond to all trauma team activations and coordinate all phases of care until the patient reaches the definitive care unit.

This hospital found that the presence of these trauma nurse providers results in an increase in continuity of care and improves documentation and rapid movement of the patient through the initial phases of hospital care. In a true case management approach, the trauma nurse provider follows the patient to discharge.

The case management model requires, the addition of full-time equivalent (FTE) personnel to function as case managers. However, the expense associated with hiring new personnel may be offset by the savings accomplished by case management oversight during the patient's hospitalization.

Trauma centers may choose to implement managed care rather than case management. Managed care follows the same planned care as case management. However, the responsibility for adhering to the scheduled care and interventions falls to all the caregivers rather than one case manager. Trauma coordinators can play an important role in managed care by assuring compliance with the CareMaps™ during rounds.

Case management or managed care provides

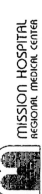

MISSION HOSPITAL REGIONAL MEDICAL CENTER

NAME _____
DX _____
SURGEON _____

MR# _____
ISS _____
PROJ. LOS _____

CRITICAL PATHWAY
NEUROLOGICAL SYSTEM: SEVERE HEAD INJURY
AIS 4-5, GCS 3-8, VENTILATED

	DAY 1: ICP IN DATE:	DAY 2	DAY 7	ICP OUT DATE:	DAY 1 P ICP
CONSULT	Trauma surgeon Neurosurgeon Consulting specialists prn		ENT prn		
ACTIVITY	ICU, HOB ↑ 30° control environment, ↓ stimulation, proper neck alignment		Graded stimulation prn	Progress as tolerated	
TESTS	CT, CBC, SMA-7, PT, PTT, UA, CXR ABGs, T & C (PRC's), nutrition labs, serial serum osmo, culture CSF qod, calorimetry, C & S prn	CT, CBC, SMA-7, CXR, ABGs Anticonvulsant levels	Anticonvulsant levels q week Nutrition labs q week, C & S prn Calorimetry q week	DC serum osmo	Weaning parameters
TREATMENT	Hemodynamic monitoring, CPP >50 Mech. vent. $ETCO_2$ 25 ±3 SaO_2 ≥ 95%, EKG monitor, ICP <20, Drain CSF prn, Foley, NG, SEQTEDs Normothermia, SBP ≥100 ≤150	EEG monitor prn Change NG to Dobbhoff prn	CONSIDER: trach, G-tube, J-tube removal ICP normalize $ETCO_2$		Wean ventilator
MEDICATION	BP control Sedation/analgesia per PCA/RN Antibiotics, anticonvulsants, H_2 blocker, Mannitol/Lasix prn	Pentobarb prn Bowel protocol		↓ sedation, DC diuretics	DC paralytics
FLUIDS/ NUTRITION	NPO, IV, strict I & O Restrict fluids Urine specific grav. q 12	Start TPN or tube feeding	Maintain target calories Consider liberalize fluids Meds by NG	↑ fluids	
REFERRALS	Social services, metabolic team	Nutrition assess, completed Rehab team assess, financial services, DC planning assess.	OT, PT treatment Rehab team conference q week	Active discharge planning	Develop rehab treatment sched.
TEACHING	Orient family to unit, short-term goals, assess family needs, impact of cultural background on support needs	Reinforce and reassure	Discuss changes in therapy	Reinforce pt. progress, offer community referrals, ↑ family involvement in patient care	Prepare for extubation
OTHER	Restrain patient Talk to the comatose patient				

PAGE TWO

	D/C VENTILATOR DATE:	DAY 2 P VENT	TO FLOOR DATE:	DAY PRIOR TO DISCHARGE	DAY OF DC:
CONSULTS	Continued as before			DC summaries dictated	Care to physiatrist
ACTIVITY	OOB as tol.	Progress as tol.			DC
TESTS	CXR, ABGs; Continue nutrition labs, Anticonvulsant levels q week	CXR	CBC, SMA-7	CBC, CXR, SMA-7, urine C & S; CT within 48° of DC	
TREATMENT	Cont. SaO_2, EKG monitor; Respiratory treatments; PT, OT treatments	Nasal cannula prn; Wean trach prn	O_2 prn; DC Foley	Trach out x24°; G-tube, J-tube clamped	
MEDICATION	Cont. sedation/analgesia prn; Cont. antibiotics, H_2 blockers; Bronchodilators; Cont BP control			All meds po or NG x24°	
FLUIDS/ NUTRITION	Cont. IV, tube feedings; Cont. strict I & O	Trial clear liquids per swallow eval.	Advance diet as tol, wean TF; Maintain target calories; Hep lock IV	Diet as tolerated; IV d'cd	
REFERRALS	Cognitive eval.; Cont. metabolic support team; Cont. rehab team	Swallow eval.	Rehab facility consult		Acute or sub-acute rehab
TEACHING	Discuss outcome & behavioral expectations R/T head trauma; Prepare for further changes in therapy	Pt. cognitive retraining; ADLs; Prepare for move from ICU	Begin prepare family for DC; Offer rehab options for family consideration	Max. self-care as tol.; Assess family p DC needs; Assure family has contact number for trauma/neuro case mgr	Follow-up appts. in DC orders
OTHER	Cont. close observation of confused patient		3:1 nursing	Meets rehab facility criteria	Copies of chart to receiving facility

* Copyright pending

Figure 6–9   Example of critical pathway for severe head injury. This proposed system of care-mapping demonstrates (1) event-driven rather than time-driven interventions to accommodate the unpredictable length of stay in severely injured patients; (2) systems-oriented rather than diagnosis-specific content, with one or more levels per system, depending on injury severity. It may consist of two or more interrelated pathways, directed at any one time by the most severely affected system. (*Note.* Developed by E Songne, RN, CCRN, and L Littlejohns, RN, BSN, in collaboration with physicians, nurses, and the Collaborative Care Committee at Mission Hospital Regional Medical Center, Mission Viejo, CA.)

hospitals with the most comprehensive information on the actual costs associated with providing care to injured patients. This may assist hospitals in arguing for enhanced DRG reimbursement for certain injury types. CareMaps™ are equally suited to use with both case management and managed care models.

Managed care and case management dovetail nicely with the principles of total quality management (TQM). The variances provide the data base for CQI activities. Additionally, the constant review of care for the injured patient also assists with the tracking of required indicators for the QA portion of TQM.

In addition to the usual hospital requirements for quality management, trauma centers have expectations from the designating authority, which include monitoring for the required state or county indicators, along with the ACS trauma indicators. These demands for quality monitoring place an additional burden on trauma centers, which can be mitigated with the implementation of case management or managed care.

Finally, trauma centers have another major advantage in data collection for quality review—the presence of an institutional registry, which is usually required in order to receive trauma designation. That registry generally contains a complete data base on every trauma patient who received care at that hospital and can be used to generate reports to assist in the TQM process.

TRAUMA REGISTRIES

In addition to the requirements for designated trauma centers to report to a state, county, or other jurisdictional registry, most trauma centers maintain an in-house registry. This registry can be used to provide data for research, to track financial information on trauma patients, to assign injury severity scale (ISS) scores, and to perform a myriad of other functions.

Before implementation of an institutional trauma registry, many issues must be addressed, including the type of person (e.g., nurse or medical records registrar) who should do the data abstraction, the type of registry that the institution will purchase, and the data points that will be collected. If the registry is to produce data for research, data cross-checks must be developed and implemented to assure the purity of the data.

Several factors should be considered when selecting a data abstractor: the person should be well versed in medical terminology, with some knowledge of ICD-9 coding, and should be skilled in reading and objectively interpreting medical records. Because the job is tedious, two part-time employees may be more effective to do the abstracting than one full-time employee.

Several commercial software trauma registries are available for purchase. Before investing in one of these registries, the institution should be assured that the registry will serve the needs of the trauma program. A key consideration is the availability of the vendor to provide support for registry problems and questions. Also, the reporting function must not require a computer expert to generate a requested report. The registry should be flexible to allow for periodic reviews of data that are not routinely collected. This function will allow the trauma program personnel to do focused reviews.

Several components should be considered for inclusion into the registry during the deliberations for determining the final data points for collection. Input for data points should be solicited from key personnel in the trauma program. Additionally, a decision must be made if the registry will be used for the storage of clinical data only or if financial data will be stored also. Suggestions for the components of the registry should be requested, but the final decision should be left to one or two people to avoid delay of the implementation of the registry.

One of the most important functions of the registry is reporting to the designating authority, which is usually accomplished by downloading information from the institutional registry. Therefore the institutional registry program must have the capability to accomplish this task.

In areas where regional trauma systems are in place, the designating authority will collect the data from each trauma center and pool the information to a central file. The information will then be used for purposes ranging from production of epidemiologic data to comparisons of trauma centers' effectiveness. One of the most important purposes for these data is to use it to generate reports on the required indicators for QA. The ability to generate indicator reports is especially helpful as trauma systems move to a regional QM process.

REGIONAL QUALITY MANAGEMENT

When a regional trauma system goes into effect, the designated trauma centers usually are expected to participate in some form of regional QM. The requirement for regional QM is set by the regulatory body responsible for the oversight of these centers. The San Diego trauma QA process is the most well-known for its multicenter trauma care review (Shackford, Hollingworth-Fridlund, Cooper, & Eastman, 1986). The committee that is charged with the responsibility of evaluating the trauma care provided at multiple institutions will function under the Total Quality Management (TQM) model rather than QA or QI. TQM will allow for the combination of both types of quality review, which is the most practical for a multicenter review process.

Obstacles can block successful implementation of a regional QM process. First and most important is the difficulty in finding physicians and nurses who are willing to dedicate a significant number of hours to prepare and participate in such a committee. Another potential obstacle is the confidentiality concerns associated with doing quality management outside the individual institutions. Also, anxiety is associated with presenting problem cases to medical and nursing colleagues from other healthcare institutions. Finally, it is laborious to determine which cases and or complications should be reviewed and whether indicators should be reviewed at the regional level.

The logistics for implementing the review process are not the only hurdles that must be cleared. Who will have the responsibility of reviewing prehospital trauma care must be decided also. The role of the medical examiner or coroner must be considered. Each of these potential impediments will be discussed with potential strategies for solutions presented. The following section will provide a guideline for the development of a system to perform trauma regional QM.

Authority for Regional Quality Management

The authority and requirement to perform regional QM generally comes from the body charged with the responsibility of regulating the trauma system. The obligations of this agency commonly include the power to designate trauma centers, to conduct site surveys to assure compliance with standards and to develop methodology to assure that care delivery is optimal.

The agencies that have the responsibility for all aspects of trauma centers generally have received that power via the legislative process, i.e., county or state law. This type of empowerment is necessary because the designation of trauma centers could be viewed as anticompetitive, which would put the process at risk for antitrust claims. Two actions have been described by the court that can provide protection from antitrust litigation (*Parker v. Brown*, 1943). The active participation of the government agency in the designation and regulation of trauma centers coupled with a clear recognition by the legislature that the effect of trauma center designation is anticompetitive will satisfy the legal requirements.

The designation process often dictates that an ambulance with a trauma patient bypass the closest hospital and instead transport that patient to the trauma center. It is incumbent on regulatory authority to assure that those hospitals that have been designated as trauma centers perform in compliance with all the required standards. It would be difficult to justify bypassing nondesignated hospitals if substantial noncompliance with defined standards existed in trauma-designated hospitals.

The presence of multiple trauma centers in a region requires the addition of a regional review process. This regional process accomplishes a variety of tasks including case review, education, policy revision, and system oversight.

Committee Review Parameters

One of the initial decisions that must be made is the parameters of the review responsibilities for the regional QM committee. The primary issue is whether one committee will be charged with reviewing both prehospital and hospital trauma care.

Including prehospital care in the hospital review process should be carefully considered, because the addition of prehospital care has the potential for creating an onerous workload for committee members. In regional trauma systems that have a significant trauma volume, reviewing prehospital and trauma care in one committee is impractical.

One other consideration in determining the parameters of review for the committee is that physicians may be disinclined to be candid in the presence of prehospital care personnel about problems that occurred with the care delivery. The question to be asked is whether prehospital personnel have the educational background to be involved in discussions relating to medical judgment and care delivery in the hospital setting. Paramedics may argue that the reverse is true and that physicians should not be allowed to review prehospital care. The fact is, however, that paramedics practice under the authority of a physician supervisor, who bears the ultimate responsibility for their care delivery. Therefore physicians have not only the right but the responsibility to participate in committees reviewing the quality of prehospital care.

In rural areas, it might be necessary to combine these two QM committees because of the low volume of trauma cases and the limited number of personnel available to serve on committees. If the committees are separated, some mechanism should be in place to allow the referral of cases between the committees.

Committee Membership

For the regional hospital, because of the importance of autopsies on trauma patients, the medical examiner or coroner must attend QM committee meetings. An autopsy provides the most accurate information for the ISS score assigned to a deceased trauma patient. The medical examiner or coroner can assist also by bringing for committee review trauma deaths that occurred at nondesignated trauma centers.

Committee representation should be from both designated and nondesignated hospitals because of the necessity of monitoring the undertriage rate and overtriage rate. All the hospitals in the trauma catchment area should agree that the overtriage rate will not be addressed until data are available to assure that undertriage is not occurring. These data can be obtained by the nondesignated hospitals providing information on injury patients who were transported to their hospitals.

In areas where the designation process is competitive, the inclusion of committee members from nondesignated hospitals helps to assure those hospitals that the community trauma care is kept at the highest standard. Also, an orthopedic surgeon may be selected as a member of the committee because of the number of patients who have some type of orthopedic injury or complication. Table 6-3 lists the essential members on the regional hospital QM committee.

Table 6-3 Essential members for regional hospital management committee

Trauma surgeons	Each designated trauma center
General surgeons	Representatives of nondesignated hospitals
Anesthesiologist	Appointed by state society
Neurosurgeon	Appointed by state society
Emergency physicians	One from a designated center and one from a nondesignated center
Medical examiner or coroner	County or state representative
Trauma coordinator	Each designated trauma center
Critical care nurse	Appointed by local AACN chapter
Emergency department nurse	Appointed by local ENA chapter

The prehospital care committee should have representation from all the fields that have a role in prehospital care. Physician representation should be primarily from the emergency department setting with the emphasis on physician advisors for the rescue and ambulance services. Table 6-4 lists the essential members for the regional prehospital QM committee.

Confidentiality Considerations

One of the most difficult impediments to overcome with a regional QM process is the reluctance of hospitals to share QM data outside of their own institution. The participating hospitals must get a firm commitment from the regulatory agency that all information discussed will be afforded protection from legal discovery. Generally, the commitment must be in the form of an ordinance or statute that grants specific protection to QM activities occurring outside the hospital confines.

The activities of the regional committees must follow standard practices for assuring confidentiality of proceedings. The methods used to protect the data will vary from state to state and institu-

Table 6-4 Essential members for regional prehospital management committee

Physician advisors	Representing ambulance and rescue services
Base hospital representative	From designated trauma center
Emergency department nurse	Appointed by the local ENA chapter
Emergency physician(s)	Representing designated trauma centers
9-1-1 representative	
County EMS representative	
Basic life support provider(s)	
Advanced life support provider(s) (ground and air)	

tion to institution. However, there are some standard actions that should be used.

These standards include having each committee member sign statements of confidentiality, which describe the applicable law for the proceedings and the penalties for violation of the law. Only one set of minutes and documents should be kept for records, and these sets should be locked in a secure place with access by only one or two people. When other copies of the minutes are brought to a meeting for committee approval, a designated staff person must collect and destroy all extra copies.

The single set of minutes and documents should be marked to reflect that they are QM documents. The applicable statute or county ordinance number that extends protection from legal discovery should be noted on the face of the documents. All patient identifiers should be removed from the documents, and trauma identifiers should be used in place of names or medical record numbers. No possibility should exist that the regional QM records could be traced to a patient medical record.

Each state and county has laws specific to that jurisdiction. Therefore the confidentiality procedures must comply with local statutes and/or applicable ordinances.

Standard for Review

Resources for Optimal Care of the Injured Patient (ACS, 1990) defines the categories that should be used when evaluating mortality and morbidity. The attributions for deaths and complications are (1) frankly preventable, (2) potentially preventable, and (3) nonpreventable. These standards are nationally recognized and should be used for the regional QM process. This adds consistency to the review process and allows for comparisons with other systems.

The *potentially preventable* designation often proves to be the most difficult for the committee to make because no clear-cut guidelines exist to determine what factors make a death or complication fit this category. These cases require intensive discussion, and the decision is made by majority rule. If the concerns of the case are purely a question of medical judgment, the voting probably should be limited to the physicians on the committee.

Probability of survival

The probability of survival scores help determine whether deaths were preventable. However, these scores cannot be relied on too heavily because often they do not represent the seriousness of the injuries that were sustained. For example, an 18-year-old patient with a single gunshot wound to the head arrives in the ED with BP, 140/90; P, 108; RR, 10; and a GCS Score of 5. A CT scan demonstrates that he has sustained an irreversible brain injury. He is declared dead 10 hours after admission. The injury to his brain is given an abbreviated injury scale (AIS) score of 5, which translates into an ISS score of 25. (Association of the Advancement of Automotive Medicine, 1990) Because the patient arrived in the emergency department with vital signs, a GCS score of 5, and an ISS of 25, his probability of survival prediction will probably be greater than 50%. However, the original injury was lethal and the patient could not have survived the insult to the brain. Probability of survival predictions must be used as only *one* of the factors when considering questions of preventability.

When the probability of survival prediction falls below 50%, it is reasonable for the committee to remove *frankly preventable* from possible choices. Since the patient was projected to have a less than 50% chance of survival, the death probably should not be counted as frankly preventable. This is not a hard and fast rule, but rather a consideration for the committee on a case-by-case basis.

When the committee decides that the death or complication was either *frankly* or *potentially preventable*, a further determination must be made as to the factors that contributed to the death or complication. Again following the guidelines set forth in *Resources for Optimal Care of the Injured Patient* (ACS, 1990) the committee must decide whether the death or complication occurred because of an error in diagnosis, judgment, interpretation, or technique or a delay in diagnosis. If the patient had comorbid factors of preexisting medical disease, that may be a mitigating factor in the cause of the death or complication.

It is beneficial to further delineate the error made by the phase of care in which the error or delay occurred. The phases are broken into the prehospital phase, resuscitation phase, operative phase, critical care phase, and postoperative phase. Listing the errors by where they happened will assist in determining where the primary education should be focused.

If a death or complication is deemed to be potentially or frankly preventable, a mechanism must be in place to give this information back to the trauma center or ambulance service and to the regulatory agency responsible for trauma center oversight. These reports to the regulatory agency should be used as triggers for medical record review during scheduled site survey visits. Furthermore, if an ongoing serious problem is identified with a particular trauma center, this information from regional review will alert the regulatory agency of the possibility that some action may be warranted to assure quality care is being delivered.

When the trauma center receives the information on regional QM review, the findings should be compared to assure that the institutional and regional QM reviews had the same result. If the trauma center consistently fails to identify its problem cases, education in the case review process may be needed.

Regional QM is an integral part of measuring the effectiveness of trauma systems. The process provides the method to assure nondesignated centers and the community that the trauma care in that particular system is of sufficient high quality to allow the anticompetitive effect of designating trauma centers.

SUMMARY   Trauma QM is a multifaceted approach to monitoring the varied aspects of trauma care delivery. The QI portion provides an innovative approach to problem solving with the focus on the *system* rather than the *individual* as the problem.

The QA portion retains the indicator review required by ACS and designating authorities. Case management or managed care methods provide data relevant to both QI and QA.

The presence of the trauma QM techniques coupled with regional oversight will assure the highest quality in trauma care delivery. Finally, the addition of case management or managed care will help to make trauma care more efficient and thus more economical.

RESEARCH QUESTIONS

- What could be done to increase the accuracy of probability of survival scores for single-system injuries?
- How effective are QI techniques for solving quality problems compared with traditional QA methods?
- What is the degree of disparity between ISS calculated using autopsy results and ISS calculated without using autopsy results?

- What is the utility of the beta test site trauma indicators from JCAHO in terms of providing meaningful information to trauma centers?
- Develop and evaluate trauma nursing indicators.

ANNOTATED BIBLIOGRAPHY

Berwick, D., Godfrey, A.B., & Roessner, J. (1991). *Curing health care: New strategies for quality improvement.* San Francisco: Jossey-Bass.

A description (using the reports of the National Demonstration Project), of how QA methodologies can be applied to health care. Includes case examples specific to health care QI, and offers practical examples of implementation.

Rhodes, M., Sacco, W., Smith, S., & Boorse, D. (1990). Cost effectiveness of trauma quality assurance audit filters. *Journal of Trauma,* 30(6), 724-727.

A study that examines the use of the American College of Surgeons Committee on Trauma (ACSCOT) generic audit filters in a trauma quality assurance program. Describes investigators' findings after assessing each indicator's yield of substantive problems in relation to the cost involved in monitoring it.

Shackford, S., Hollingworth-Fridlund, P., Cooper, G., & Eastman, A. (1986). The effect of regionalization upon the quality of trauma care as assessed by concurrent audit before and after institution of a trauma system: A preliminary report. *Journal of Trauma,* 26(9), 812-820.

A study that presents the model for implementation of a regional QA committee to study trauma care. Compares care for trauma patients before and after regionalization of trauma care. Describes the primary method to determine the effectiveness of the trauma system: evaluation of deaths as nonpreventable, potentially preventable, and preventable.

Spath, P. (1991). *Health care quality: A practical guide to continuous improvement.* Portland, OR: Brown-Spath & Assoc.

A practical book that provides an overview of the entire QI philosophy and its implementation into health care. Though examples are not written specific to trauma care, principles are easily adapted and applied to this setting. Many practical tools, check sheets, and other useful adjuncts may be used by readers for their own QI activities.

Zander, K. (1991). Differentiating managed care and case management. *Definitions* 5(2), 1-4.

A newsletter that provides a comprehensive description of the differences between case management and managed care. Presents a detailed chart that provides the differences in key elements of a variety of clinical systems, such as primary nursing and case management.

REFERENCES

American College of Surgeons (ACS), 1990. *Resources for optimal care of the injured patient.* Chicago: Author.

Association of the Advancement of Automotive Medicine. (1990). *The Abbreviated Injury Scale.* Des Plaines, IL: Author.

Bone, D., & Griggs, R. (1989). *Quality at work: A personal guide to professional standards,* Los Altos, CA: Crisp Publications.

Brider, P. (1991). Who killed the nursing care plan? *American Jounal of Nursing,* 91(5), 35-38.

Deming, W.E. (1986) *Out of Crisis* (pp 24-26). Cambridge, Mass: Massachusetts Institute of Technology Center for Advanced Engineering Study.

Donabedian, A. (1986). Quality assurance in health care system, *Quality Assurance and Utilization Review,* 1(1), 6-12.

Emergency Nurses Association (ENA) (1986). *Trauma nursing core course.* Chicago: Award Printing.

Health Care Financing Administration (HCFA) (1989). *Peer Review Organization data summary.* Baltimore: Office of Peer Review, Health Standards, and Quality Health Bureau, HCFA.

Joint Commission on the Accreditation of Healthcare Organizations (JCAHO) (1989). *Quality Review Bulletin,* 15(11), 330-339.

Joint Commission on the Accreditation of Healthcare Organizations (JCAHO) (1992). *Accreditation Manual for Hospitals,* Chicago: Author.

Parker v. Brown, 317 US 341, 87 L Ed 315 (1943).

Rhodes, M., Sacco, W., Smith, S., & Boorse, D. (1990). Cost effectiveness of trauma quality assurance audit filters. *Journal of Trauma,* 30(6), 724-727.

Shackford, S., Hollingworth-Fridlund, P., Cooper, G., & Eastman, A. (1986). The effect of regionalization upon the quality of trauma care as assessed by concurrent audit before and after institution of a trauma system: A preliminary report. *Journal of Trauma,* 26(9), 812-820.

Songne, E., & Holmquist, P. (1991). Comprehensive care by trauma nurse providers: Mission Hospital's 10-year experience. *Journal of Emergency Nursing,* 17(2):73-79.

Spath, P. (1991). *Health care quality: A practical guide to continuous improvement.* Portland, OR: Brown-Spath & Assoc.

Walton, M. (1986). *The Deming Management Method.* New York: Dodd, Mead.

Zander, K. (1990). Differentiating managed care and case management. *Definitions,* 5(2), 1.

Zander, K. (1991). CareMaps™: The core of cost/quality care. *Definitions,* 6(3), 1-4.

NURSING CARE OF THE TRAUMA PATIENT

7 Assessment of the Trauma Patient

Pamela Stinson Kidd

■■

OBJECTIVES

❏ Identify priorities in performing physical assessments of trauma patients.

❏ Recognize the differences in assessment techniques for pediatric, adult, and geriatric trauma patients.

❏ Analyze abnormal physical data, and anticipate appropriate nursing interventions.

❏ Recognize the legal and professional responsibilities in performing physical assessment.

INTRODUCTION In the acute care of trauma patients, nurses often observe and record the assessment of others', as well as their own actions, whereas in some trauma settings the nurse is expected to conduct and document a full nursing assessment. In either situation, the nurse must be aware of pertinent pathophysiology related to particular mechanisms of injuries and manifestations of abnormalities. To record other's actions the nurse must know what should be done. In a tense, busy environment, the nurse must be able to focus on and easily comprehend the significant findings to fully and accurately record the sequence of assessment and interventions, as well as patient responses. Knowledge of anatomy and physiology is prerequisite to understanding the pathophysiology of trauma. This chapter focuses on the epidemiology of trauma, particular patterns of injuries, important questions to elicit in the history, and the performance of the primary and secondary survey.

CASE STUDY A 25-year-old man is brought to the emergency department by friends after "hitting a tree with his motorcycle." The patient is alert and oriented and denies a loss of consciousness. He is limping and complains of pain in his right leg. Abrasions are visible on his upper torso, and a laceration of his right thigh is present.

How should the emergency nurse proceed in assessing this patient?

Regardless of the manner in which the trauma patient arrives (whether by ambulance or private vehicle), assessment should be conducted using the primary and secondary survey guidelines. One nurse should remove the patient's clothing and obtain vital signs to assess breathing and circulation while another health care provider checks airway patency and assesses breathing by a quick check of chest excursion and auscultation of breath sounds. Orientation of the patient can be evaluated simultaneously by asking the patient questions. Spinal immobilization should be initiated and maintained until radiographic evaluation is completed and spinal injuries have been ruled out.

What pertinent questions should the emergency nurse ask about the event to collect information related to care of this patient?

Several questions about the collision are important:

- Was the patient wearing a helmet?
- How fast was the patient traveling at time of impact?
- How far was the patient thrown and on what type of surface did the patient land?

Although a detailed history may not be possible, the trauma nurse can collect essential data in a short time using the mnemonic AMPLE. This includes questioning about allergies, present medications, past medical and surgical history, last meal and last tetanus immunization, and patient's recall of events.

MECHANISM OF INJURY

Typically, mechanism of injury is discussed from the perspective of forces and type of energy dissipated, e.g., whether the injury was the result of thermal energy (burn) or kinetic injury (motor vehicle crashes [MVC]). Kinetic energy is further classified as blunt or penetrating forces. In reality, the healthcare provider receives a report of the injury from a description of the agent or object that precipitated the event. Thus this section is organized around agents that produce injury, consistent with Haddon's matrix presented in Chapter 2, Prevention of Traumatic Injury. Anatomic and physiologic considerations are integrated.

According to 1982 statistics (most recent available), trauma accounted for an annual loss of approximately 4 million potential years of life (Committee on Trauma Research, 1985). The financial costs of health resources for the acute and chronic care of trauma patients is estimated at $133.2 billion annually (National Committee for Injury Prevention and Control, 1989). Injuries are the leading cause of death from birth to early 40s. This age span encompasses more than half of the average life span (Baker, 1987).

Clearly, trauma is a major national health problem. As with any disease or health problem, certain individuals have a higher risk of susceptibility. Half of all trauma deaths occur in the 13- to 34-year age range, with MVCs constituting the major cause of death (Baker, 1987). Fatal motorcycle crashes (MCCs) affect the early-20s age group. It appears that fatality risk is 25% greater for females than for similarly aged males in MVCs, from 15 to 45 years of age. Males younger than 15 years and older than 45 years have a higher risk of fatality (Evans, 1988). Falls are the leading cause of injury death in the el-

derly population (Baker, O'Neill, & Karpf, 1984).

Alcohol has been identified as a contributing factor in 40% of MVC-related traumatic deaths (Insurance Institute for Highway Safety, 1991). An elevated blood alcohol level (> 100 mg/dl) is a factor in approximately 20% of all MVCs (Soderstrom & Cowley, 1987). A descriptive survey completed by 154 trauma centers demonstrated an interesting pattern: 65.8% of the centers estimated that alcohol consumption contributed to the injury of more than half of their trauma patients (Soderstrom & Cowley, 1987).

When identifying mechanism of injury, the health care provider must maintain a high index of suspicion. The nurse should focus on what injuries can be predicted based on the type of force (penetrating or blunt) that produced the injury. Circumstances surrounding the injury, such as the age of the patient and agent of injury, may also suggest the probability of particular injuries. For example, when suspecting neurologic trauma, the nurse should remember that MVCs and falls are the leading causes of head injuries (McGuire, 1986). Young children and the elderly comprise the high-risk groups for sustaining neurologic trauma secondary to falls. MVCs account for the majority of cervical spine trauma until 80 years of age, when falls, regardless of the height involved, replace MVCs as the most prevalent precipitating cause (Bryson, Warren, Schwedhlem, Mumford, & Lenaghan, 1987). Sports and recreation injuries result in 10% of all brain injuries and 7% of spinal cord injuries (McGuire, 1986). Motorcyclists who do not wear helmets have twice the incidence of death from head injury and a 52% higher death rate overall than helmeted riders regardless of speed (Insurance Institute for Highway Safety, 1991; Lipe, 1985; Russo, 1978). Computed tomography screening of helmets may provide additional data about extent of the head injury. The data, in conjunction with the injury pattern and crash data, can improve understanding of head-helmet and helmet-environment interactions (Cooter, 1990).

Motor Vehicle–Related Crashes

The mechanical force involved in MVCs is usually kinetic energy. Kinetic energy is a function of the mass of an object and its speed. Velocity increases kinetic energy to a greater degree than the weight of an object. In blunt trauma, injuries oc-

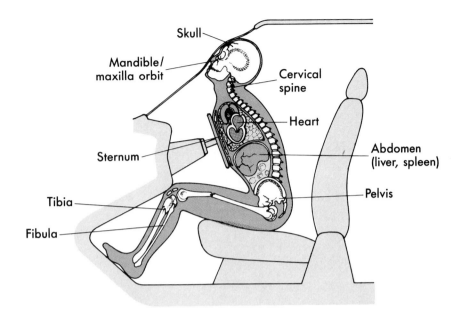

Figure 7-1   Potential injury sites of unrestrained driver.

cur as tissues are compressed. Three types of compressive forces are involved. The first force is produced when the motor vehicle collides with an object. The second force results when the occupant collides with the inside of the motor vehicle. The last force occurs when the internal organs of the occupant collide (Alexander, 1988). When assessing a patient involved in an MVC, the nurse should remember that the object hit, the traveling speed, the stopping time involved, and the proper use of protective devices will impact the resulting injuries. Figure 7-1 depicts potential injury sites of the unrestrained driver.

Because of the high incidence of traumatic injuries and deaths from MVCs, a review of predictable injuries that occur in a MVC is warranted. Table 7-1 summarizes common injuries as related to restraint status.

An unrestrained person has a greater chance of being ejected to the ground or another object. Ejected persons have a higher rate of spinal fractures and mortality (Demarest, 1986). Unrestrained front passengers are at risk for craniofacial injuries because the head and windshield often make contact, since the steering wheel is not a deterrent (Figure 7-2). Extremity injuries are similar to those of the unrestrained driver because of dashboard impact.

Table 7-1 | Predictable injuries in MVCs

Unrestrained driver	Restrained driver
Head injuries	**Caused by lap restraint**
Facial injuries	
Fractured larynx	Pelvic injuries
Fractured sternum	Spleen, liver, and pancreas injuries
Cardiac contusion	
Lacerated liver or spleen	**Caused by shoulder restraint**
Lacerated great vessels	
Fractured patella and femur	Cervical fractures
Fractured clavicle	Rupture of mitral valve or diaphragm

Injuries also depend on the site of impact. Rear-impact collisions result in hyperextension of the neck, predisposing the patient to cervical injury (Figure 7-3). Lateral impacts generally produce chest, pelvis, head, and neck injuries (Figure 7-4). Drivers are more susceptible to splenic injuries, whereas passengers have a higher rate of liver injury. Airbags, although designed for frontal crashes, provide greater protection in lateral crashes than lap belts alone. Spinal fractures occur more frequently with lateral collisions than with rear impact collisions. An unrestrained child

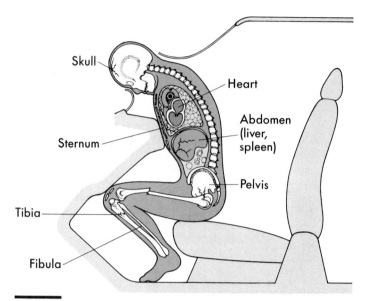

Figure 7-2   Potential injury sites of unrestrained passenger in front seat.

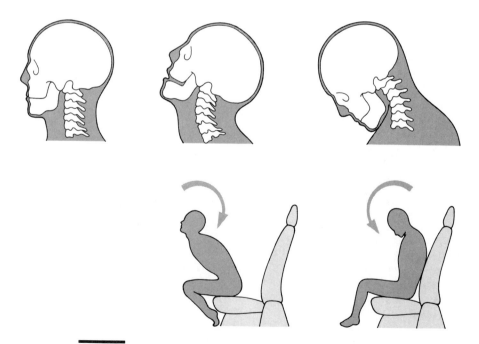

Figure 7-3   Rear-impact collision results in hyperextension of neck.

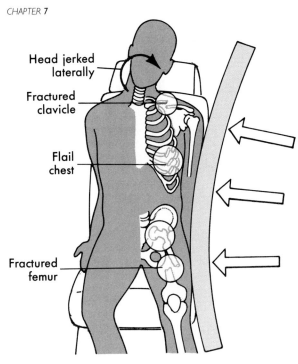

Head jerked laterally

Fractured clavicle

Flail chest

Fractured femur

Figure 7-4 Potential injury sites in lateral-impact collision. Note that injury is still possible in lateral crash, even with airbag inflation, because airbags were designed specifically for frontal crashes. However, injuries are usually fewer in lateral-impact crashes *with* airbag inflation than *without*.

experiences thorax and head injuries. This is especially true if the child is being held by an adult, since the combined weight in association with the speed of the vehicles involved can produce a force of approximately 2 tons (Lipe, 1985) (Figure 7-5).

Compression injuries to the spleen, liver, and pancreas can result when lap belts are not worn low across the pelvis and secured snugly. In one study of 42 individuals who were wearing lap belts and who died from injuries sustained from a MVC, liver injuries accounted for the greatest number of deaths. The injury mechanism was deceleration and gross crushing impact from a lateral-impact crash (Arajärvi, Santavirta, & Tolo-

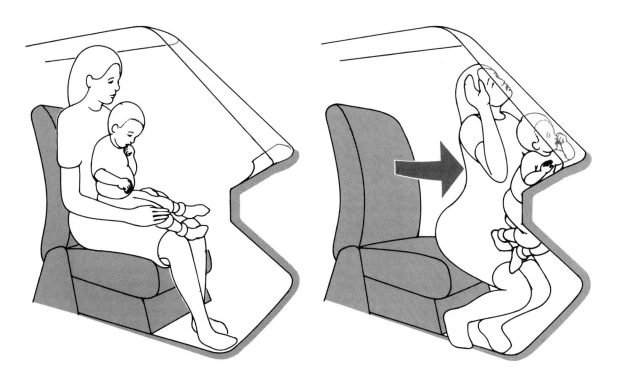

Figure 7-5   Potential injury sites of child held by adult.

nen, 1987). Diaphragmatic rupture can occur if the compressive force is great. If the diagonal strap is not worn, facial and head injuries can result even when the lap belt is correctly positioned and tightened. Neck injuries have occurred when the diagonal strap was in place but not the lap belt (Demarest, 1986). The ribs and sternum may be injured also (Schoenfeld, Ziv, Stein, Zaidel, & Ovadia, 1987). Pregnant women should wear

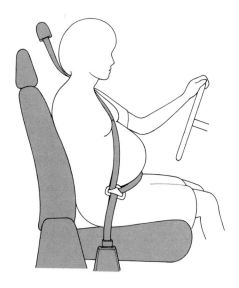

Figure 7-6 Proper positioning of lap-shoulder belt during pregnancy.

the lap belt low, across the bony pelvis. Wearing it presents no disadvantages, and it may prevent ejection from the vehicle (Schoenfeld, et al, 1987) (Figure 7-6). The trauma nurse should not assume the patient was protected from injury because he or she had been restrained. It is difficult to determine if the device was used properly. If the patient was wearing heavy, bulky clothing, is excessively overweight, or had unusual slack in the belt, the forward motion of the impact continues for a longer time. Additionally, the belt may have been used correctly but the headrest was improperly positioned, increasing the likelihood of cervical injuries (Alexander, 1988).

Restraints may give a false sense of security if they are used improperly. The anatomic characteristics of the child prevents adult seat belts from providing adequate protection. The child's iliac crests are immature and do not provide adequate anchoring of the belt. This allows for submarining: the belt rides up over the abdomen, and the child slides under the belt (Figure 7-7).

A study of children who were seat belted and received injuries in a MVC showed distinct injury patterns. Infants and toddlers sustained head injuries from going forward over and out of the belt and striking objects in the vehicle. Abdominal injuries were more common in the 4- to 9-year-old group from straining against the seat belt (Agran, Dunkle, & Winn, 1987). Therefore specially designed restraint devices should be used for children up to age 10.

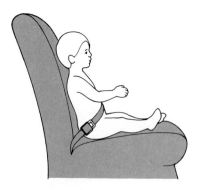
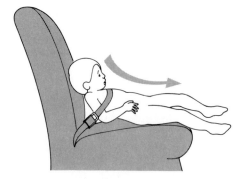

Figure 7-7 Potential movement of child restrained with adult lap belt during motor vehicle crash.

Pedestrian-vehicle injuries (PVI) occur less frequently but have a greater incidence of fatality than MVCs (Mueller, Rivara, & Bergman, 1987). Therefore healthcare providers must carefully assess patients involved in a pedestrian-vehicle collision. Children and adolescents are especially vulnerable to PVIs, and those younger than 5 years of age have the greatest risk of dying. Injury patterns for children involved in PVIs include fractures at the point of impact with the car bumper or hood. Usually the chest and upper leg are involved, as well as the head, constituting a series of injuries referred to as *Waddell's triad*. (Figure 7-8). Fractures also occur at point of secondary impact on the child or adult when the person is thrown as a result of force (Figure 7-9). Adult pedestrians commonly sustain similar fractures at the point of impact of the car hood and bumper, usually the upper and lower leg. Knee ligaments in the opposite knee from that which is struck by the car may be disrupted secondary to stress (Halpern, 1989) (Figure 7-10).

Cycles

The increased use of three-wheeled, all-terrain vehicles (ATVs) has resulted in a greater number of deaths and injuries. Recent statistics demonstrate an increase in injuries from 8600 in 1982 to 85,000 in 1985 (Sewell, Pine, & Hull, 1987). Children and adolescents appear to be at higher risk, since 46% of ATV injuries occur in users younger than 16 years. Injuries in ATV crashes are difficult to predict, since environmental factors, such as road surface consistency and its impact on ejected riders, influence injury. Head and spinal cord injuries are common. It is estimated that 60% of ATV fatalities may have been prevented if a helmet had been worn (Smith & Middaugh, 1985).

The popularity of the BMX off-the-road racing model bicycle has been cited as a reason for the increased number of bicycle injuries (Illingworth, 1984). Head injuries, fractured femurs, and supracondylar fractures of the humerus have been cited as major injuries resulting from BMX

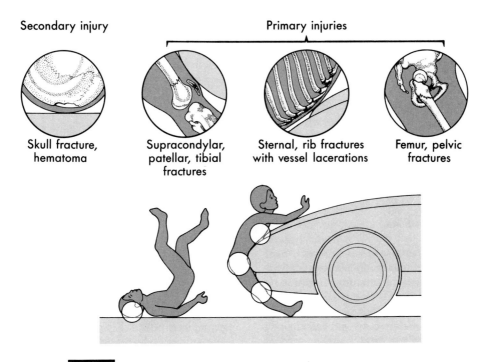

Secondary injury   **Primary injuries**

Skull fracture,   Supracondylar,   Sternal, rib fractures   Femur, pelvic
hematoma   patellar, tibial   with vessel lacerations   fractures
                   fractures

Figure 7-8   Potential initial injury site of child pedestrian (Waddell's triad).

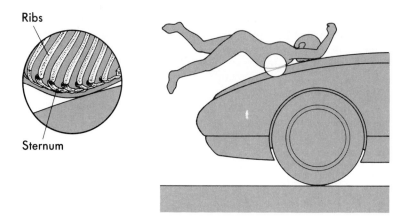

Figure 7-9 Potential secondary injury sites of child pedestrian.

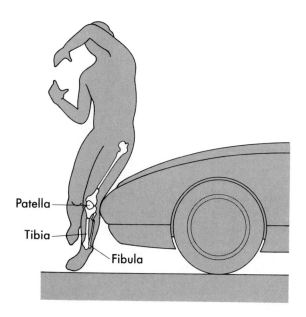

Figure 7-10 Potential primary injury sites of adult pedestrian.

crashes. Since the introduction of the BMX model, the severity of the resulting injuries has not increased (Park & Dickson, 1986). In fact, BMX bicycles may have had a positive effect because they are ridden "off the road" and the serious injuries usually occur as a result of road traffic collisions regardless of the type of bicycle involved (Park & Dickson, 1986). The use of bicycle safety helmets reduces the risk of head injury by 85% (Thompson, Rivara, & Thompson, 1989). Limited research is available that compares severity of injury with type of bicycle.

Falls

Falls are a common mechanism of injury, especially in the elderly population. The single greatest cause of accidental death in persons over 65 years of age is falls (Kidd & Murakami, 1987). Certain injury patterns may be present, depending on the circumstances of the fall. When a person lands on his or her heels when falling from a height, bilateral calcaneous fractures, Colles fractures of both wrists, and compression fractures of the vertebrae may occur (Halpern, 1989). Calcaneous fractures result from the extreme initial force of contact, whereas the wrists and vertebral injuries occur as the patient makes a secondary impact, absorbing additional energy through an outstretched hand or an extended leg. Renal injuries also are associated with a fall of this nature, secondary to deceleration forces (Kidd, 1987). If an anterior knee injury is suspected, the presence of an associated fracture dislocation of the hip should be considered. A fall that results in a hip fracture may also produce a dislocation of the opposite hip. Falls associated with a wrist injury may cause additional injuries to the elbow or shoulder (Barbarick, 1985).

Ballistics

Ballistic injuries vary in their severity based on (1) the amount of energy that the missile transmits to the tissue, (2) the velocity of the bullet, (3) the direction of the transmitted energy, and (4) the density of the tissue (Maloney, 1987). Gunpowder (chemical energy) is converted into a compressed gas that propels a projectile (kinetic energy) (Johnston, 1989). The kinetic energy of the missile depends primarily on its velocity and much less on its mass. Velocity can be modified by the barrel length of the gun used to discharge the missile (Barach, Tomlanovich, & Nowak, 1986). Within certain limits, the greater the barrel length, the higher the velocity. A missile with a lower kinetic energy can produce a greater degree of injury if it is designed to give up a greater amount of energy to the target. Missiles that tumble quickly (forward rotation around the center of mass) release more kinetic energy nearer the surface, producing a huge surface wound with little internal damage, whereas stable missiles produce small entrance wounds and greater internal organ destruction (Barach et al, 1986).

The degree of tissue damage depends on several additional factors, one of which is missile composition. Expanding bullets consist of a partially exposed bullet core that expands on impact. The expansion slows the bullet in the body, which increases the kinetic energy transmitted to organs and tissues, producing a greater wounded area. Small fragments break off, which can act as secondary missiles and result in multiple injuries. Fully jacketed bullets form a wound tract of a roughly cylindrical shape (Maloney, 1987). Shot shells filled with pellets instead of a solid projectile produce large surface wounds with major tissue destruction (Barach et al, 1986). Injuries produced by shotgun shells have an increased risk of infection because of severe vascular destruction and edema. These injuries can be further contaminated by shotgun shell wadding, especially if the weapon was fired at close range.

Shock waves can produce injury, since strong pressure changes within the tissue can easily rupture gas-filled organs. Temporary and permanent cavitation also damages tissue. Temporary cavitation is greater with high-velocity missiles since the greater the velocity, the greater the release of energy (Figure 7-11). The nose of the missile pushes forward and laterally, producing low-intensity pressure waves against tissue (Barach et al, 1986). The compression of the tissue forms a temporary cavity. The amount of damage associated with this cavity depends on the elasticity and density of the affected tissue. Lung and muscle tissues are the least damaged because of their expansion properties. On the other hand, the liver, spleen, and brain have no elastic properties and suffer the worst damage. Fluid-filled organs, such as the stomach, bowel, and distended bladder, can explode secondary to pressure waves. Pressure waves can also fracture bones and lacerate blood vessels. The negative pressure created inside the fluid-filled organ cavity can suck in foreign matter, since it communicates directly with the entrance and exit wounds (Maloney, 1987). The permanent cavity is smaller than the temporary cavity and is formed as tissue is excavated by the temporary cavity.

Generally, weapons are classified as rifles, shotguns, and handguns, with rifles being the most powerful of the three. The longer barrel of the rifle increases the velocity of the missile. Because of the cavity formation with rifle missiles, the severity of the wound cannot be estimated by the size of entrance and exit sites.

Shotguns can produce large wounds at close range, whereas at longer ranges the wounds may be minor (Barach et al, 1986). At close range the pellets act as one large mass and the wadding remains deep within the wound cavity. At longer distances the pellets start to disperse outward. Sawed-off shotguns allow maximum pellet spread because most of the barrel is removed.

Most handguns are considered low velocity; thus tissue damage is usually limited to tissue destroyed directly in the bullet path. Yet it is a misconception that low-velocity projectiles cause insignificant damage. Debridement in the operating room may be necessary (Fackler, 1988). A few handguns, such as the .44 magnum, can produce wounds with greater tissue damage. Handguns are the major type of weapon used in civilian shootings. The majority of handgun injuries in the urban emergency setting are from small-caliber, small-barreled guns (Barach et al, 1986).

Special Populations
Pediatric

Although the pediatric patient has been discussed briefly, additional epidemiologic factors require consideration. Age and injury patterns are closely correlated. Toddlers and preschoolers have a higher incidence of injuries associated with falls. School-aged children are more susceptible

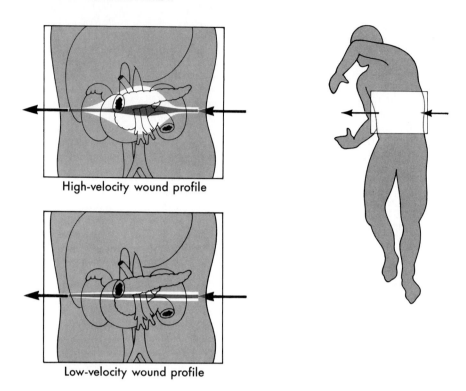

High-velocity wound profile

Low-velocity wound profile

Figure 7-11 Potential injury path of high- and low-velocity bullets.

to pedestrian-vehicle injuries and bicycling accidents. Adolescents are at greater risk for MVC and sports injuries (Schwaitzberg & Harris, 1987). Regardless of age, boys have a higher risk for fatal and nonfatal injuries in the pediatric population. Particular injury patterns in pediatric patients are discussed in Chapter 17.

Elderly

The discussion of the elderly patient has been limited and a more thorough discussion of elderly trauma injury is presented in Chapter 18. The statistics in this population must be evaluated cautiously. For example, elderly drivers have higher death rates from MVCs than younger people. However, death may be related to the higher susceptibility for complications and not to the kinetic forces involved in the crash. Less than 1% of elderly die from injuries sustained in MVCs. However, the elderly have the highest pedestrian death rates (Insurance Institute of Highway Safety, 1991).

GENERAL ASSESSMENT
Trauma Assessment Instruments

Several indexes have been developed for the classification of select patient characteristics to numerically quantify morbidity and mortality from traumatic injury. These indexes have the potential to (1) assist in the triage of patients, (2) provide data for clinical decisions, (3) support the evaluation of trauma care in prehospital and hospital settings, (4) provide information concerning epidemiologic patterns, and (5) allow for interfacility/system research, since common data are collected (Greenspan, McLellan, & Greig, 1985; Thompson & Dains, 1986; Trunkey, Siegel, & Baker, 1983). The indexes that are used most frequently will be discussed.

Abbreviated injury scale

The abbreviated injury scale (AIS) was first published in 1971 (Committee on Medical Aspects of Automotive Safety, 1971, 1972) and was revised in 1990 (Association for the Advancement

Table 7-2 Converting AIS score to ISS score

Region	Injury	AIS code	Highest AIS score	AIS²	ISS
Head/neck	Cerebrum: subdural hematoma, large (>50 ml in adult)	140656.5	5	25	3 highest AIS scores = 25 + 16 + 9 = 50
	Cerebral contusion	140602.3			
Face	Maxilla: *Le Fort III* fracture, with blood loss >20% by volume	250810.4	4	16	
Chest	Rib fracture: 2 to 3 ribs— any location, or multiple fractures of single rib with stable chest	450220.2	2	4	
Abdomen	Liver laceration: moderate (>3 cm deep with major duct involvement)	541824.3	3	9	
Extremities	Femur: fracture of shaft	851814.3	3	9	
External	Laceration: not further specified	710600.1	1	1	

of Automotive Medicine, 1990). The index is organized anatomically, with six body regions represented: head and neck, face, chest, abdomen or pelvic contents, extremities or pelvic girdle, and external. Each body region receives a score of *1* to *6*, with *1* representing minor injuries. Information for scoring is obtained from an AIS dictionary (Greenspan et al, 1985). The AIS requires a longer time to complete in comparison with other indexes. This makes it impractical for prehospital use, and generally it is calculated after stabilization and resuscitation. The AIS is used most often for research and quality assurance (QA) purposes.

The injury severity scale (ISS) was developed to incorporate severity of injury with the number and type of body regions involved (Baker, O'Neill, Haddon, & Long, 1974). It is based on the AIS, and each region is scored from 1 to 6, with 1 representing minor injury. The score is the sum of the squares of the highest AIS value in each of the three most severely injured parts of the body (Cayten, 1982). The ISS is a powerful predictor of mortality. Lethal doses have been calculated from the ISS according to age. A lethal dose is defined as a probability of survival less than 50%. Lethal dose is an ISS score of *40* for

ages 15-44, an ISS score of *29* for ages 45-64, and an ISS score of *20* for ages 65 and older. A drawback to the ISS is its retrospective use. Thus it is not helpful in the prehospital setting (Thompson & Dains, 1986). Table 7-2 illustrates a method of converting AIS scores to ISS scores.

Trauma score

The trauma score (TS) was developed from an earlier index, the triage score (Champion, Sacco, & Carnazzo, 1981). The TS uses physiologic criteria to assess patient severity. This index is used prospectively to assist in determining treatment needs and allocation of resources. Five variables were identified statistically as best predictors of mortality. These included respiratory rate, respiratory expansion, systolic blood pressure, capillary refill, and the Glasgow coma scale (CGS) (Teasdale & Jennett, 1974). The combination of the hemodynamic and respiratory score with the neurologic score may be referred to as the Champion-Sacco score (see box, p. 126) (Long, Bachulis, & Haynes, 1986). The TS value ranges from *1* to *16*, with *1* indicating major injury. Patients with a TS of *14* or less should be triaged to a trauma center. Presently the TS is not used alone

Champion-Sacco trauma score

Trauma score	Value	Points	Score
A. Respiratory rate			
Number of respirations in 15 seconds	10-24	4	
multiplied by 4	25-35	3	
	>35	2	
	<10	1	
	0	0	A._____
B. Respiratory effort	Normal	1	
Shallow: markedly decreased chest movement or air exchange			
Retractive: use of accessory muscles or intercostal retraction	Shallow or retractive	0	
			B._____
C. Systolic blood pressure			
Systolic cuff pressure (either arm): auscultate or palpate	>90	4	
	70-90	3	
	50-69	2	
	<50	1	
No carotid pulse	0	0	C._____
D. Capillary refill			
Normal: forehead, lip mucosa, or nail bed color refill in 2 seconds	Normal	2	
Delayed: more than 2 seconds for capillary refill	Delayed	1	
None: no capillary refill	None	0	D._____

E. Glasgow coma scale

	Value			
1. Eye opening				
Spontaneous	4	GCS 14-15	=	5
To voice	3	GCS 11-13	=	4
To pain	2	GCS 8-10	=	3
None	1	GCS 5-7	=	2
		GCS 3-4	=	1
2. Verbal response				
Oriented	5			
Confused	4			
Inappropriate words	3			
Incomprehensible words	2			
None	1			
3. Motor response				
Obeys commands	6			
Purposeful movement (pain)	5			
Withdraw (pain)	4			
Flexion (pain)	3			
Extension (pain)	2			
None	1			

E._____

Total GCS points = 1 + 2 + 3 _____   **Total trauma score = A+B+C+D+E** _____

Note. From "Trauma Score" by H.R. Champion, W. Saco, & A. Carnazzo, (1981). *Critical Care Medicine, 9,* p. 673.

to determine when to start or stop resuscitation procedures in most settings. However, because of the escalating costs of trauma care and restriction of resources, trauma assessment indexes may be used in the future for this purpose. Research exploring the use of the TS in predicting mortality suggests that of patients with a TS of 3 or less, 95% die and 77% were declared dead within 1 hour of hospital admission (Champion, Gainer, & Yackee, 1986). The study's results recommend reevaluating patients who have a TS of 1 or 2, 10 to 15 minutes after initiating life-saving interventions. A second TS of 1 or 2 at this time suggests that treatment can be discontinued (Fischer, Flynn, & Miller, 1985). The TS can be used to assess the quality of care the patient received. A survival curve has been developed that enables the comparison between expected number of survivors and actual number of survivors based on TS. Any deviation from the expected can be analyzed to determine areas of needed improvement or existing excellence (Hawkins, Treat, & Mansberger, 1988).

The TS has recently been modified and tested. Developers of the TS have tried to address the major criticisms of the instrument. These criticisms have focused on the difficulty in assessing capillary refill and respiratory expansion at night. Additionally, TS appears to underestimate the severity of head injury (Champion, Copes, Gann, Gennarelli, & Flanagan, 1989). The revised TS (RTS) still includes systolic blood pressure and respiratory rate but they have been categorized so that their associated survival probabilities parallel those of the nationally accepted GCS (Table 7-3). The scale ranges from 0 to 12. An RTS of 11 or less has been recommended as an indication for triage to a trauma center. The RTS more accurately classifies head injury. Preliminary research indicates that it is easier to apply at triage (Champion et al, 1989). It is too early to predict if the RTS will be accepted clinically and ultimately replace the original instrument.

The TRISS index combines the TS, ISS score, and the patient's age to quantify outcome. A probability of survival score is computed. The TRISS index has been criticized for underestimating head injury severity in adult patients who have sustained blunt trauma (Boyd, Tolson, & Copes, 1987). The R-TRISS was developed, which incorporates the RTS, ISS score, and patient age. As noted, the weight attached to the

Table 7-3 Revised trauma score

Glasgow coma scale	Systolic blood pressure	Respiratory rate		Coded value
13-15	>89	10-29	=	4
9-12	76-89	7-29	=	3
6-8	50-75	6-9	=	2
4-5	1-49	1-5	=	1
3	0	0	=	0
Range 12 to 0				

Note. "A Revision of the Trauma Score" by H.R. Champion, W.S. Copes, D.S. Gann, T.A. Gennarelli, and M.E. Flanagan, (1989). Journal of Trauma, 29(5), 624.

GCS score of the RTS has been increased in an attempt to correct the estimation of head injury. Both the TRISS and the R-TRISS have accurately predicted survival outcome in both adult and pediatric populations (Eichelberger et al., 1989; American College of Surgeons Committee on Trauma, 1990).

Pediatric trauma assessment instruments

The indexes mentioned up to this point were developed for the adult trauma patient. Mayer (1980) designed a pediatric index called the *modified injury severity scale* (MISS). The MISS incorporates the ISS, the GCS, pupillary response, presence of a surgical mass lesion, and oculocephalic reflexes. A score of 1 to 5 is possible for each variable, with 1 indicating a less severe injury. The MISS uses physiologic and anatomic factors to classify patients (Mayer, Walker & Clark, 1984). It requires information obtained through advanced assessment and use of sophisticated diagnostic equipment for completion.

The pediatric trauma score (PTS) was developed to provide rapid assessment of the injured child. The PTS is a prospective index that includes anatomic and physiologic data (see Chapter 17, Table 17-6). Scores may range from −6 to +12. The more severe the injury, the lower the score. Size is included as a criterion because of the body surface to volume ratio factor that affects physiologic reserve (Tepas, Mollitt, Talbert & Bryant, 1987). Cutaneous and skeletal injuries are included because of their frequency of occurrence with blunt pediatric trauma. Any child who presents with a penetrating injury regardless of location is graded as −1 in the open wound component. A prehospital score of 8 or less indicates the necessity for transport (possibly aeromedical evacuation) to a trauma center (Threadgill, 1987).

The need for a separate trauma assessment tool for the pediatric population has been debated. In one study the TS and PTS did not differ significantly in predicting severity of injury based on ISS scores calculated retrospectively (Eichelberger, Gotschall, Sacco, Bowman, Mangubat, & Lowenstein, 1989). The RTS performed as well as the TS and the PTS once it was adjusted for the rapid respirations of children until 3 years of age.

Prehospital assessment instrument

As discussed, the TS and RTS may be used in the prehospital setting. However, the CRAMS score was developed specifically for the prehospital setting to provide quick and easy data to help determine if the patient should be transported to a trauma center. It was a modification of the TS. The index consists of five variables: circulation; respirations; abdominal/thorax status; motor function; and speech, from which the tool got its name (CRAMS) (Table 7-4). Each variable may be scored from 0 to 2 for a total possible score of

10. A score of 8 or less indicates need for transport to a trauma center.

The committee on trauma of The American College of Surgeons has identified triage criteria that indicate when a person should be transported to a trauma center. The criteria include (1) GCS score 13 or less, (2) systolic blood pressure 90 or less, (3) respiratory rate of 10 or less or 29 or greater, (4) revised trauma score less than 11, (5) pediatric trauma score less than 9, (6) all penetrating injuries to head, neck, torso, (7) ejection from automobile, (8) death in same passenger compartment, (9) extrication time longer than 20 minutes, (10) falls greater than 20 feet, (11) auto-pedestrian injury with greater than 5 mph impact, and (12) motorcycle crash at greater than 20 mph (American College of Surgeons, 1990).

Few studies have compared trauma assessment instruments for their ability to predict the need for transport of a patient to a trauma center. These instruments may not be able to predict mortality based on initial presentation of the patient. Patients may appear physiologically normal when evaluated with existing trauma assessment instruments in the prehospital setting, but the ISS score at hospital evaluation may indicate major trauma

Table 7-4 CRAMS scale

CRAMS scale	Value	Points	Score
Circulation	Normal capillary refill and systolic BP >100 mm Hg	2	
	Delayed capillary refill or systolic BP of 85 to 100 mm Hg	1	
	No capillary refill	0	A._____
Respirations	Normal	2	
	Labored or shallow or > 35/min	1	
	Absent	0	B._____
Abdominal/thorax status	Nontender	2	
	Tender	1	
	Rigid abdomen, flail chest, or penetrating injury	0	C._____
Motor function	Normal	2	
	Responds only to pain (not decerebrate)	1	
	No response (decerebrate)	0	D._____
Speech	Normal	2	
	Confused	1	
	Unintelligible	0	E._____

Total CRAMS scale score = A+B+C+D+E_____

Note. Modified from "Comparison of Prehospital Trauma Triage Instruments" in a Semi-rural Population by J.R. Hedges, S. Feero, B. Moore, D.W. Haver, and B. Shultz, 1987, *Journal of Emergency Medicine, 5*(3), p. 207.

(Baxt, Berry, Epperson, & Scalzitti, 1989). No statistical differences exist between the sensitivity and specificity of the CRAMS, TS, and RTS in predicting need for transfer to a trauma center (Baxt et al, 1989). The CRAMS scale is a conservative instrument that has less specificity. Patients are triaged to a trauma center with this index who may not require this level of care. The use of mechanism of injury criteria alone is too liberal and may not predict the need for trauma center transport when it is actually necessary (Hedges, Feero, Moore, Haver, & Shultz, 1987). The combination of mechanism of injury, anatomic injury, and trauma score may have greater predictive power (Knopp, Yanagi, Kallsen, Geide, & Doehring, 1988).

The nurse working with trauma patients should be familiar with currently used trauma indexes, for the purposes of both data collection and interpretation. Knowledge of a particular score can provide valuable information that can be used in the immediate preparation period before arrival of the patient, to anticipate patient problems and plan future nursing care requirements.

Assessment and Intervention
Elicitation of the history: patient's perception of injury

Because of the acuity level of some trauma patients, eliciting a history from the patient is not always feasible. Family and friends, when available, as well as bystanders, can provide data on the patient's preexisting behavior and condition and immediate postinjury response. Information from prehospital personnel can greatly assist in "piecing together the injury," as well as tracking resuscitative measures, such as the volume and kind of intravenous fluids infused.

A trauma nurse functioning in the prehospital setting may have the first and last contact with a conscious patient and bystanders. Therefore any information the nurse may get from the patient and bystanders is vital.

When the trauma nurse must set priorities, information about the nature of the patient's pain can provide clues to underlying pathology. The PQRST mnemonic is a widely used tool to assist in pain data collection. It can be used by the trauma nurse in any setting:

P What produced your pain: e.g., was it the direct impact of the crash, or trying to open the door to get out of the automobile?

Q Quality of the pain: is it sharp, dull, pressure, or cramplike?

R Region and radiation: where is it, and where does it go?

S Severity: on a scale of 1 to 10, with 10 being the worst, how severe is your pain?

T Timing: is it intermittent or constant, and what associated factors influence the degree of pain experienced?

Assimilation of this information can assist in focusing the secondary survey. Other essential information includes preexisting medical history, allergies, and current medication use, both prescription and nonprescription. Determining the patient's compliance in taking medications can impact administration of medications in the trauma room. Determining the patient's immunization status and time of last meal is important also. Immunization status is always important; however, it is extremely important in the elderly population. Up to 66% of those over 65 years old lack a protective tetanus antitoxin level and have the potential of developing tetanus. Past military service and a definite history of three or more previous tetanus immunizations are good predictors of protection (Gareau, Eby, McLellan, & Williams, 1990). The mnemonic *AMPLE* may assist the provider to remember this information:

A Allergies

M Medications

P Past medical and surgical history

L Last meal and last tetanus immunization

E Events leading to injury

Information from the patient and/or family concerning consumption of alcohol and other mind-altering substances can assist in clarifying the patient's behavior in the emergent treatment phase. Recent behavior patterns and previous psychologic illness can also predispose a person to trauma. Silverman, Peed, Goldberg, Hamer, and Stockman (1985) studied the recognition of psychopathology in a nonrandom sample of 56 trauma patients. They found that 34% of 19 trauma patients demonstrated substantial treatable psychopathology, with alcohol abuse being the most common diagnosis. Of these 19 patients, 13 did not have documentation of a psychologic problem or treatment plan in their medical record. Many times trauma care providers do not recognize or initiate treatment of psychopathology, even by referring to specialists in this area.

An intoxicated person may have intentionally thrown himself or herself in front of a car in an attempt to commit suicide. The willingness of trauma patients to follow instructions and cooperate in their care can be influenced by these factors. In the intensive care setting the trauma patient may not be motivated to become involved in stabilization and rehabilitation. Physical limitations can affect emotional responses such as motivation. Participation in rather than resistance to the plan of care can assist recovery.

In some situations a patient may initially be declared a "trauma case" but actually, after assessment and diagnostic testing, only minor injuries are identified and the patient is discharged without hospital admission. Lack of psychologic data may expedite discharge of patients who should actually be hospitalized for psychologic treatment although their physical status is normal.

Additional complaints voiced by the patient may be indicative of underlying pathology. Organizing questions in a head-to-toe order can assist in eliciting these additional complaints. Starting with the head, the trauma nurse can ask about the patient's recall of the event and perception of any loss of consciousness. Patient complaints of shortness of breath, palpitations, nausea or vomiting, or incontinence of urine or bowels provide data concerning the presence of chest and abdominal trauma. Asking the patient about changes in sensation and motor capabilities of the extremities can provide valuable baseline data.

In this chapter, subjective data have been isolated and discussed as a separate entity. In reality, subjective and objective data are elicited almost simultaneously in the primary and secondary surveys. A partial history may be obtained from field personnel via radio communication before the patient's arrival, yet in some situations no subjective data are collected until initial interventions are executed in the primary survey to support oxygenation, ventilation, and perfusion. The reader should remember that the boundaries between history and assessment in this chapter are artificially drawn.

Objective data

The general overview is conducted simultaneously with the primary survey. It consists of collecting data about the trauma patient's behavior and physical state that may or may not be related to the traumatic event. Specifically, patient information is gathered concerning the following (Simoneau [1984]):
- Affect and cognition
- Quality of speech
- Appearance, including hygiene and nutritional aspects
- Spontaneous motor activity
- Odors
- Degree of distress

These data are assimilated with the objective data obtained in the primary survey.

Primary survey

A primary survey, which usually take 30 to 60 seconds to complete, is performed on every patient. Information that pertains to the elderly, pediatric, and pregnant patient will be integrated throughout discussion of the primary survey. The purposes of primary survey are to assess ABCs and to initiate appropriate measures in the presence of life- and limb-threatening injuries.

The patient's clothing can restrict accurate assessment. The caregiver should remove the clothing of patients who have experienced major trauma, GSW, or unconsciousness with unknown etiology (Bull, 1985). Figure 7-12 illustrates how clothes can be removed expeditiously from a supine- or prone-positioned patient. Hypothermia can occur quickly, and the nurse should ensure that the patient retains body heat. If a pneumatic antishock garment (PASG) is to be applied, clothing should be removed before this is done (Bull, 1985).

Airway   Assessment begins during the removal of clothing. Patency of the airway is assessed first. A noisy airway generally indicates obstruction, in which case the caregiver should reposition the patient's airway by using a jaw-thrust or chin-lift maneuver (Standards and Guidelines, 1986). Any debris should be removed by suctioning. Positioning should be reassessed continuously, since additional manual assistance may be necessary to prevent occlusion. An oropharyngeal airway may be inserted if the patient does not have a gag reflex (Sterner, 1987). This may be the preferred airway adjunct if the patient has a suspected cribriform plate fracture. Nasopharyngeal airways are preferred if the patient's teeth are loose or the tongue is swollen. If the patient is partially unresponsive, nasopharyngeal airway should be used, since insertion does not stimulate a gag reflex (Lynch & Bennett, 1986). Figure 7-13 demonstrates proper

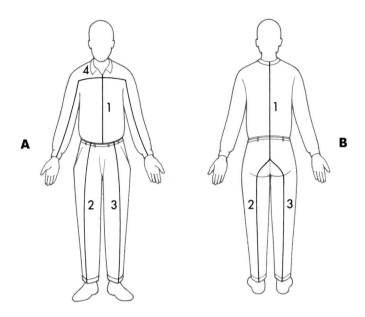

Figure 7-12   Technique for clothing removal in the supine and prone positions, also called "strip and flip." In the supine position: **A, 1.** Cut down midline of shirt, which exposes any emergent anterior chest injuries; **2 & 3.** Cut down legs of pants, which exposes any pelvic cavity, lower abdomen, thigh, or leg injuries. Cut through belt twice, keeping wide distance from genitals; **4.** Cut up arms, which will expose any peripheral injuries. Clothes will now fall away completely, allowing examination of back during logroll. In the prone position: **B, 1.** Cut down midline of shirt, which exposes any emergent posterior chest injuries; **2 & 3.** Starting at center, cut belt once; then continue down one leg. Finish by cutting down other leg by starting at midbuttocks. After patient is rolled onto backboard, clothes can be gently pulled away from front. (*Note.* Redrawn from "Strip and Flip" by G. Bull, 1985, *Emergency Medical Services, 14*[6], 14-16.)

placement of oropharyngeal and nasopharyngeal airways.

Which adjunct should be used in managing the airway depends on the patient's respiratory rate and injuries. Unconscious patients may need intubation to protect their airway from obstruction and to prevent aspiration. If severe facial trauma has occurred and the patient is acutely compromised (respiratory rate < 8/min), a cricothyrotomy may be preferred. Recent research suggests that complications after cricothyrotomy, such as tracheostomal stenosis, are not as prevalent as once thought (DeLaurier, Hawkins, Treat, & Mansberger, 1990). In some cases, orotracheal intubation under direct laryngoscopy may be possible (Gerold, 1988). In cases of blunt laryngeal trauma, tracheotomy is the preferred method of securing a patent airway. Hoarseness, intolerance of supine position, and subcutaneous emphysema

are symptoms of laryngeal injury (Fuhrman, Stieg, & Buerk, 1990).

Controversy exists over how to minimize cervical spine movement when the patient is being intubated orally. One study has demonstrated that less movement occurs with orotracheal intubation when in-line stabilization of the neck is provided by an assistant as compared with the use of a hard cervical collar and the use of curved or straight laryngoscope blades (Majernick, Bieniek, Houston, & Hughes, 1986). Axial (in-line) traction by means of an applied head halter (5 to 6.8 kg of weight) has been suggested as a stabilizing procedure during orotracheal intubation (Magnes, 1982). Recent research indicates that use of axial traction increases distraction of the spine, cord, and surrounding tissue (Bivins, Ford, Bezmalinovic, Price, & Williams, 1988). Blind nasotracheal intubation is preferred for the breathing pa-

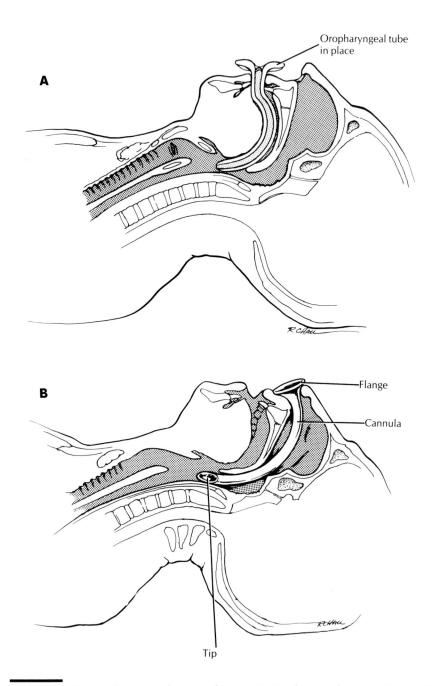

Figure 7-13   Proper placement of airway adjuncts. **A,** Oropharyngeal airway; **B,** nasopharyngeal airway. Airways are positioned to relieve upper airway obstruction. (*Note.* From Comprehensive Respiratory Care: A Learning System [2nd ed.] by D.H. Eubanks and R.C. Bone, 1990, St. Louis: Mosby–Year Book, Inc.)

tient. Insertion of the endotracheal (ET) tube nasally may require more time, but if proper technique is used, this intubation route has a 90% success rate (Sterner, 1987). When a cervical spine injury is suspected, nasotracheal intubation should be performed (Trunkey, 1984). Nasotracheal intubation results in less movement of the cervical spine than orotracheal intubation (Bivens et al, 1988).

Special populations

PEDIATRIC The most common cause of airway obstruction in pediatric patients is posterior displacement of the tongue, so early use of oral airways is recommended (Manley, 1987). If intubation is necessary, uncuffed tubes are used until age 8, since the pliable cricoid cartilage provides a natural cuff. Nasal endotracheal routes are preferred in children over 6 years of age, because the endotracheal tubes are easier to secure (Curley & Vaughan, 1987; Mayer, 1985). Orotracheal intubation, with axial traction to the head, is the first choice for obtaining a patent airway if head injuries are suspected (Ruddy & Fleisher, 1985).

PREGNANCY The patient who is in the third trimester of pregnancy is susceptible to airway compromise. Hormonal changes relax the cardiac sphincter of the esophagus, increasing the potential for regurgitation. The diaphragm is elevated, and intraabdominal pressure is increased, which can also contribute to vomiting with subsequent aspiration. Chapter 16, provides additional information.

Breathing When assessing breathing, chest excursion and symmetry of breathing pattern should be observed. Paradoxic chest wall motion may indicate the presence of a flail chest. The flail segment will move inward with inspiration and outward with expiration. The type of breathing pattern can provide clues about the presence of neurologic injury or metabolic disorders and help guide administration of oxygen. For example, no chest wall movement with abdominal breathing indicates a cervical cord lesion (Markovchick & Anderson, 1988). Generally breath sounds are briefly auscultated in the primary survey, since immediate stabilization is emphasized, not in-depth assessment. Breath sounds are assessed bilaterally. If they are absent on one side and the patient is intubated, the cuff should be released, the tube repositioned, the cuff reinflated, and breath sounds auscultated. If breath sounds do not exist after repositioning, a pneumothorax or hemothorax is suspected and chest tube insertion proceeds (Sterner, 1987). When ventilation is severely compromised (with unilaterally diminished breath sounds), a needle thoracostomy is performed with a 14-gauge intravenous catheter or needle inserted into the second intercostal space, midclavicular line, on the injured side. Subcutaneous emphysema is usually associated with a pneumothorax or a pneumomediastinum.

The choice of oxygen flow rate and delivery system depends on the ultimate percent of oxygen or FIO_2 that is to be delivered. Table 7-5 summarizes available systems and subsequent delivery ratios. Oxygen delivery is determined by the oxygen flow rate to the patient. If the patient normally retains carbon dioxide, 2 to 3 liters of oxygen is suggested (Wells-Mackie, 1981). Typically, delivery systems are referred to as high-flow or low-flow systems. A high-flow system has a gas flow suffi-

Table 7-5 Oxygen delivery systems

Device	Type	FIO_2	Flow rate (L/min)	Comments
Nasal cannula	Low flow	.24-.44	1-6	Valid for mouth or nose breathers; should humidify if the flow rate is greater than 4 L/min
Face mask	Low flow	.40-.60	6-8	Minimal rate of 6 L/min to ensure adequate release of exhaled air
Nonrebreathing mask	High flow	.60-.80	6-10	Prevents increase of CO_2 in patients needing high level O_2
Bag-Valve-Mask	High flow	.60-.80	6-10	For patients needing assisted ventilation

cient to meet all inspiratory requirements (e.g., bag, valve, mask with oxygen reservoir). A low-flow system supplements the patient's inspiratory requirements. A patient with a compromised respiratory pattern should receive oxygen from a high-flow system, since oxygen concentration can be measured and controlled in this system (Shapiro, Harrison, Kacimarek, & Cane, 1985). Generally, patients with symptoms of compromised respiratory function (gasping, stridor, wheezing, respiratory rate < 8/min or > 40/min, cyanosis, and restlessness), and/or thoracic injury should receive oxygen from a high-flow delivery system.

The chest should be scanned rapidly to identify any open chest wounds. An open chest wound should be covered immediately and the patient monitored for the development of a tension pneumothorax. A tension pneumothorax is suspected if the trachea is deviated and breath sounds are absent unilaterally. If a tension pneumothorax exists, it must be treated immediately by inserting a chest tube or performing a needle thoracostomy before further assessing the patient.

Special populations

PEDIATRIC   Certain facts should be considered when evaluating breathing in the pediatric trauma patient. Children normally have an abdominal breathing pattern. Retractions occur when lungs lose compliance. The child is unable to increase intrathoracic volume so the chest wall will move inward. Breath sounds are easily transmitted through the child's chest wall. A change in pitch, rather than intensity, may indicate diminished breath sounds (Curley & Vaughan, 1987). The midaxillary area should be auscultated, since if the endotracheal tube is incorrectly placed, breath sounds may be present in the anterior chest because they are referred from the abdominal area.

PREGNANCY   Oxygen should be administered to the pregnant trauma patient while the primary survey is conducted (Bremer & Cassata, 1986). This provides protection for the fetus until additional data are collected regarding the extent of injuries. Because of physiologic changes during pregnancy, the pregnant patient's tidal volume increases by 40%, and the carbon dioxide level in the blood decreases secondary to chronic hyperventilation in late pregnancy. The chronic hyperventilation is related to a diminished residual capacity. Initial blood gas analysis in the pregnant

trauma patient may reveal a functional respiratory alkalosis. This information can be important in the primary survey because the patient's ability to compensate for respiratory insults is limited. The ability of the blood to buffer is restricted, which can lead to metabolic imbalances.

ELDERLY   The elderly trauma patient may have preexisting disease that diminishes tidal volume and subsequent breath sounds. Also, carbon dioxide levels may be chronically elevated. Oxygen should be administered to these patients prophylactically during the assessment. Research has demonstrated that in elderly patients who experienced blunt trauma, the mortality was lower in those who had a higher initial hemoglobin level and diminished systemic vascular resistance and received increased oxygen delivery. The type of blunt trauma, history of preexisting disease, and presence of shock were not significantly related to survival (Horst, Obeid, Sorenson, & Bivins, 1986). The elderly patient's compensatory ability is limited also. Interventions to relieve respiratory compromise must be implemented swiftly.

Circulation   Assessing circulatory status is the next and final step in the primary survey. Vital signs are obtained as part of circulatory assessment. Capillary refill is assessed, and blood flow should return within 2 seconds for the pediatric and adult male patient. The adult female patient blood flow should return in approximately 2.9 seconds. The elderly patient's blood flow may take 4.5 seconds and still be considered normal (Schriger & Baraff, 1988). Skin temperature, color, and moisture is assessed also. Again, assessment and implementation occur simultaneously. External pressure is applied to obvious sites of bleeding. Two large-bore (16-gauge or larger) intravenous catheters are inserted peripherally. If hypotension is present, an initial fluid bolus of 2 liters of Ringer's lactate solution is infused and circulatory status is reassessed (Sterner, 1987). A pneumatic antishock garment may be applied and inflated if circulation is compromised (systolic blood pressure < 90 mm Hg in the adult). In some cases the hemodynamically compromised patient may have an acceptable blood pressure because of peripheral vasoconstriction, a compensatory attempt to improve core circulation. Generally, the presence of a carotid pulse indicates a systolic blood pressure of at least 60 mm Hg. Hypotension with bradycardia may indicate severe hypoxemia.

If severe hypotension is present, type 0-negative blood can be administered until the patient's blood is typed and crossmatched. Type-specific blood may be infused until crossmatched blood is available. All crystalloids and colloids should be warmed before administration. Central venous lines may be inserted to assist with fluid infusion or to help determine the source of hypotension if the patient does not respond to the initial fluid bolus. An elevated central venous pressure (CVP) reading may indicate cardiogenic shock related to cardiac tamponade, tension pneumothorax, or myocardial contusion. Distended neck veins may indicate cardiac tamponade or tension pneumothorax caused by an interference in venous return. Both of these conditions are life threatening and must be treated before the patient is further assessed.

Special populations

PEDIATRIC Children can become hypovolemic quickly without displaying an abnormal systolic blood pressure, because their catecholamine response functions efficiently. In the primary survey, the nurse should assess the pediatric trauma patient's capillary refill and skin color as parameters of circulation. Tachypnea and a decreasing pulse pressure may be present with hypovolemia in pediatric patients. Bradycardia may suggest inadequate ventilation. Hypovolemia is initially treated with a fluid bolus of 20 ml/kg of body weight infused quickly (Manley, 1987). Small tubes should be used for blood collection, since a child has only 80 ml of blood volume per kilogram of body weight (Manley, 1987). When a pneumatic antishock garment is used for the pediatric patient, the abdominal compartment should not be inflated because of impairment in diaphragmatic excursion.

PREGNANCY The pregnant trauma patient can compensate for a loss of 30% of circulating blood volume without symptoms (Bremer & Cassata, 1986). Because of hormonal influences, pregnant patients cannot vasoconstrict as well to compensate for blood loss. Therefore the skin may remain warm, pink, and dry in spite of advanced shock. Physiologic changes in pregnancy produce an increase in cardiac output, elevation in heart rate, and decrease in blood pressure as the pregnancy advances. Initial hematocrit levels may be decreased because of the increased plasma volume associated with pregnancy and may not be solely related to hypovolemia. As soon as it is determined that the cervical spine is not injured, the patient should be placed in left lateral position to avoid supine hypotensive syndrome (see Chapter 16). If the patient is well secured on a spine board, the board can be tilted to the left. Pneumatic antishock garments can be used with pregnant trauma patients but the abdominal section should not be inflated.

ELDERLY The elderly trauma patient may not present with tachycardia when experiencing hypotension secondary to physiologic changes associated with aging. As a general guideline, an elderly patient's heart can increase its rate by only one half a beat a minute for each 1 mm Hg drop in mean arterial pressure (Minaker & Weiss, 1986). Therefore a heart rate of 100 with a decreased blood pressure may signify severe hypovolemia.

Secondary survey

The secondary survey is a more thorough evaluation of the trauma patient's injuries. It is conducted after major injuries have been stabilized, oxygen administered, and intravenous therapy initiated. The secondary survey includes the conduction of diagnostic tests, reassessment, various tube insertions, and radiographic and laboratory analysis (Simoneau, 1984). An organized pattern of assessing the patient helps to ensure that injuries are not missed and also assists with documentation. Generally, the secondary survey begins at the head, neck, and face and proceeds throughout the rest of the body.

Head and face While the nurse assesses the head, he or she should also evaluate the patient's level of consciousness, verbal and motor response, and eye reaction. The Glasgow coma scale (GCS) is a frequently used neurologic assessment tool. The total score may range from 3 to 15, with *15* indicating the best response in all three categories (Teasdale & Jennett, 1974). Patients with a GCS score of less than 7 have a poorer prognosis. Further discussion is presented in Chapter 10.

As the nurse evaluates pupillary response, the eyes should be examined for foreign bodies and the conjunctival sac observed for discoloration. Visual acuity is assessed by asking the patient to state the number of fingers the examiner is displaying in the visual field. At this time contact lenses can be removed unless there is an obvious ocular injury. Cranial nerves can be assessed for intactness throughout examination of the head and neck. In conjunction with visual acuity, evaluating extraocular movements (assessing the patient's ability to follow the examiner's finger vertically, horizontally, and diagonally in the patient's visual field) reveals whether cranial nerves II, III, IV, and VI are intact.

The scalp should be palpated for lacerations, hematomas, and depressions; the facial bones should be palpated for deformity. If the patient is conscious, the nurse should ask the patient to smile and wrinkle the forehead. Symmetry is assessed, checking the intactness of cranial nerve VII. If the patient can clench the teeth and the strength of the muscle contractions is equal, cranial nerve V is not injured. This exercise also provides information about the stability of the mandible. The nose and ears are assessed for cerebrospinal fluid (CSF) drainage. If clear fluid is present, the nurse should test it with a dextrostick to determine if glucose is present, a positive finding for CSF. The orbital area and the mastoid area (behind the ears) are examined for bruising or an accumulation of blood. A positive finding for each of these areas, referred to as *raccoon eyes* and *Battle's sign* respectively, may indicate the presence of a basilar skull fracture. Further information is presented in Chapter 10.

The nurse should inspect the mouth for lacerations, broken teeth, vomitus, and any other material or condition that has the potential of compromising the airway. If the patient can stick out the tongue without the tongue vacillating and say 'ah' with the uvula rising symmetrically, cranial nerves IX, X, and XII are intact.

Neck The neck is stabilized until cervical spine films are read as normal. The cervical spine in children is very flexible. Spinal cord injury can occur without a fracture; therefore sole reliance on X-ray findings is not adequate (Manley, 1987). As mentioned, the GCS is the most frequently used neurologic assessment tool, yet it is difficult to use the GCS with the preverbal pediatric patient. A modified coma score (Hector, 1986) can be used or the mnemonic *AVPU* (alert, verbal, painful, unresponsive), to document assessment of the pediatric trauma patient's neurologic status. Chapter 16 provides additional information.

The elderly trauma patient is at greater risk of developing subdural hematomas with even minor injuries. The brain decreases in size with age, increasing the space between the dura and skull and diminishing the natural padding. Additionally, many elderly patients take oral anticoagulants, which compounds the physiologic effects of aging and increases the susceptibility of subdural hematoma formation (Kidd & Murakami, 1987).

The neck can be palpated for tenderness and crepitus and should be inspected for wounds. If the cervical spine is normal by X-ray studies, the patient should be asked to shrug the shoulders as the examiner places his or her hands on the shoulders to evaluate symmetry. The patient should be able to touch his or her chin to the chest. If both maneuvers are performed correctly, cranial nerve XI is intact. Cranial nerve VIII, acoustic (hearing), is evaluated throughout the assessment process. Generally, cranial nerve I, olfactory, is not assessed in the trauma setting.

The jugular veins are further assessed for degree of fullness. A 30-degree angle is preferred for inspection if the cervical spine is evaluated radiographically as normal. Full and bounding jugular veins are indicative of right heart failure, cardiac tamponade, or tension pneumothorax. Flat or difficult to see jugular veins at 30-degree elevation or when the patient is supine may indicate hypovolemia. The trachea is reassessed for its midline position. A tension pneumothorax, when severe enough, will displace the trachea to the opposite side of the tension pneumothorax.

Thorax The nurse assesses the thorax to a greater degree than it was in the primary survey. Breath sounds are reevaluated side to side, beginning at the apexes and moving toward the bases. Respiratory expansion is assessed for symmetry. Arterial blood gas studies may be initiated to evaluate oxygen delivery if they were not completed during the primary survey. Pulse oximetry and capnography (if the patient is intubated) may also be used to assess oxygenation. Heart sounds should be assessed. The presence of an extra heart sound, such as S_3 or S_4, suggests the possibility of ventricular failure. If these sounds occur, the nurse should evaluate the chest wall for abrasions, contusions, and open lacerations or impaled objects. Positive findings can assist the examiner in identifying the strength of the forces that produced the injury and anticipate such complica-

Inspiration   Expiration

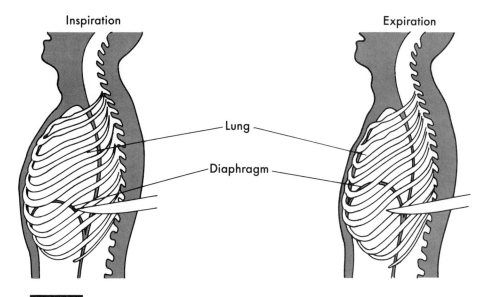

Lung

Diaphragm

Figure 7-14   Mechanism of diaphragmatic injury from penetrating trauma during inspiration.

tions as myocardial contusions. Any wound at or below the nipple line is considered an abdominal wound as well, since the diaphragm may be ruptured (Figure 7-14). The nurse should palpate the rib areas for crepitus and tenderness. A force strong enough to fracture the first or second rib can produce a laceration of the aorta. Lower rib fractures are frequently associated with renal injuries, because any force capable of fracturing a rib can compress the kidney (Kidd, 1987).

Blunt chest trauma in the elderly is generally associated with extrathoracic injury, such as fracture of the long bones (Allen & Schwab, 1985). The left side of the chest is injured more frequently than the right side. Pulmonary contusions, flail chest, and pneumothorax occurred with equal frequency in one study of elderly trauma patients (Allen & Schwab, 1985).

Abdomen   When the abdomen is assessed, the main concern is to determine if an acute abdominal emergency is present that requires surgical intervention. The nurse observes the abdomen for contusions, abrasions, and distention. Any wound above the umbilicus may have penetrated thoracic contents. Bowel sounds should be assessed in all four quadrants. Absent bowel sounds alone do not indicate a surgical emergency, but should

be considered in conjunction with other data. The presence of a bruit may suggest the possibility of injury to the great vessels, liver, or spleen. The nurse palpates the abdomen lightly for tenderness and notes any guarding or rigidity indicative of peritoneal irritation. Deep palpation can disrupt a tamponade and may be deferred with suspected organ and vascular injury. At this point in the assessment, it may be necessary to insert a gastric tube to decompress the stomach and prevent aspiration. A nasogastric tube should not be inserted if a basilar skull fracture is suspected secondary to discontinuity of the cribriform plate. A diagnostic peritoneal lavage may be performed to ascertain the need for laparotomy. Computerized axial tomography may be performed also. Kehr's sign, pain in the left scapula associated with abdominal palpation, suggests peritoneal irritation, usually from splenic rupture. The patient's abdomen is rigid, painful, and without bowel sounds, and he or she may also be hemodynamically unstable.

Femoral pulses are palpated bilaterally and assessed for equality simultaneously. The integrity of the pelvis can be evaluated by pushing on the wings of the iliac bones and determining if this action elicits pain. The urinary meatus is evaluated for the presence of blood, which may indicate a ruptured urethra. The nurse should inspect the vagina for the presence of blood and should evaluate rectal sphincter tone. In the male patient, the prostate is assessed during rectal examination to check for a free-floating condition, which may indicate a ruptured posterior urethra. The patient should be log rolled, with the head in alignment with the body, so that the posterior surface of the body can be assessed. Discoloration of the flanks may indicate retroperitoneal bleeding. The retroperitoneal space can accommodate a large amount of blood. The spine is examined for degree of symmetry and presence of tenderness. If the pelvis is intact, a urinary catheter may be inserted to monitor renal function and fluid infusion.

The pediatric trauma patient with abdominal injury may lie still and breathe shallowly to limit the pain. Children have a higher susceptibility to renal injuries because of their proportionately larger kidney size and lack of subcutaneous protection (Manley, 1987).

Abdominal assessment is slightly different for the pregnant trauma patient. As pregnancy increases, the uterus becomes a large, hollow organ filled with fluid and tissue, which predisposes it to injury. The bladder rises out of the pelvic region at approximately 4 months of pregnancy, becoming an abdominal organ with less protection. Intraabdominal organs are more susceptible to blunt trauma, since the uterus displaces the spleen and liver (Bremer & Cassata, 1986). A higher incidence of pelvic fractures occur in the last trimester because the symphysis pubis widens and the sacroiliac joints become less stable as the pelvic ligaments relax. Vaginal fluid can be tested with nitrazine pH tape to identify leaking amniotic fluid—the tape will turn blue if amniotic fluid is present. Fetal heart tones are assessed for at least one minute, and preferably a fetal monitor is applied to the patient. Fetal mortality increases whereas maternal mortality decreases in the last trimester (see Chapter 16).

Extremities The extremities are evaluated for quality and integrity of pulses. Diminished pulses in an extremity suggest entrapped or disrupted blood vessels. Traction applied to the affected extremity generally restores blood flow. The nurse notes and compares color, size, symmetry, and temperature of the extremities. In the conscious patient, sensation and motor ability are assessed. The nurse palpates the extremities for tenderness, crepitus, and deformity. Suspected fractures and dislocations are splinted for further radiographic and diagnostic evaluation and are reassessed after splinting. Hypovolemia can result from extremity fractures. A fractured femur or humerus can cause up to 2 liters of blood loss; a fractured ankle can cause up to 1.5 liters of blood loss (Kosmos, 1989).

The pediatric trauma patient with a fractured femur has a high possibility of associated solid-organ injury on the same side of the fracture (Simoneau, 1984). The elderly patient has a higher incidence of hip, Colles, and rib fractures from traumatic injury because of the osteoporotic changes associated with aging (Kidd & Murakami, 1987).

Vital signs Vital signs may be obtained during the primary survey if enough personnel are present. However, the focus during the primary survey is on whether the patient is breathing and has a pulse instead of the specific number of times a minute these processes are occurring. Vital signs usually are obtained during the secondary survey. A complete set of vital signs includes temperature assessment, which is especially important for the pediatric and elderly patient for whom hypothermia is a greater risk. Several devices are available for temperature assessment. Their use has not been examined in the trauma resuscitation phase of the patient's hospitalization. Research involving intensive care unit patients has demonstrated that axillary temperature measurement adequately reflects core body temperature in nonpostoperative patients (Giuffre, Heidenreich, Carney-Gersten, Dorsch, & Heidenreich, 1990). In the adult, the infrared tympanic thermometer has demonstrated a .98 correlation with core body temperature as measured by pulmonary artery catheter thermistor tip (Shinozaki, Deane, & Perkins, 1988). However, the tympanic thermometer has been less reliable in the pediatric population, probably because of the large size of the thermometer probe and improper user technique (Rhoads and Grandner, 1990). Until further research is conducted involving trauma patients, core body temperature should be obtained using the rectal route, esophageal probe, urinary catheter themistor tip, or pulmonary artery catheter thermistor tip.

SUMMARY   This chapter has addressed subjective and objective aspects when assessing the trauma patient. When appropriate, important subjective information is collected from field personnel concerning mechanism of injury. Questions valuable to ask in the history were discussed. The primary survey provides basic data essential to the patient's survival, and implementation occurs during this survey when life or limb is threatened. The secondary survey provides additional data that are integrated with the information obtained from the primary survey, the elicitation of history, and the epidemiology of the event. Throughout the chapter, particular assessment factors related to special populations have been included when appropriate.

As professionals, nurses working with trauma patients are responsible for conducting a systematic and pertinent assessment for each patient. Several professional organizations have identified standards relating to assessment. The *Standards of Emergency Nursing Practice* (ENA, 1990) delineates four areas of responsibility: practice, research, education, and professionalism. The second comprehensive practice standard addresses assessment:

> Emergency nurses shall initiate accurate and ongoing assessment of physical and psychosocial problems of patients within the emergency care system.

This assessment begins with triage and determining priorities of care and ends at discharge or transfer of the patient. The benefits to patient care as a result of nurses performing assessment are numerous; they include (1) setting priorities of care appropriately, (2) recognizing subtle changes, and (3) evaluating patients' response to therapy.

The basic principles of trauma assessment are the same whether the patient is being transported (1) from the field to a facility, (2) from one unit to another unit in the same facility, or (3) between facilities. A nurse working in any setting with trauma patients should be familiar with the information in this chapter.

CASE STUDY   A 22-year-old woman is brought to the emergency department by emergency medical services with a history of an MVC. She is 32 weeks pregnant and complains of abdominal and right leg pain. She was wearing a lap belt only. She had no loss of consciousness. She is wearing a hard cervical collar and is on a backboard. Vital signs in the field were: B/P, 90/70; AP, 120; R, 30.

What physiologic changes present during the third trimester of pregnancy could negatively impact the patency of the airway?
The physiologic changes are (1) elevation of the diaphragm, (2) hormonal changes resulting in relaxation of the cardiac sphincter of the esophagus, and (3) increase in intraabdominal pressure. All of these factors could produce regurgitation and subsequent aspiration and limited respiratory excursion.

Based on the complaint of abdominal pain, which organs have a higher incidence of injury in the third trimester and what signs and symptoms indicate that injury has occurred?
As pregnancy progresses, the uterus is predisposed to injury. Laceration or rupture of the uterus produces hypovolemic shock and fetal distress. The spleen and liver may be injured because they are displaced upward. If so, bowel sounds will be diminished or absent. The abdomen will be firm or rigid. Pain will be present on palpation. The bladder is less protected from injury; signs and symptoms of an intraperitoneal bladder tear can mimic an acute abdomen if the tear is large enough. An extraperitoneal tear will produce ecchymosis in the posterior flank area and suprapubic pain with possible radiation to the shoulder.

What initial interventions should be performed during the primary and secondary survey?

Initial interventions for the pregnant trauma patient should include administration of oxygen. Two large-bore intravenous lines should be initiated. Because blood pressure may be decreased in the last trimester, the nurse should assess circulation by checking capillary refill and skin temperature and color, as well as evaluating vital signs. If the cervical spine is evaluated as normal, a pillow can be placed under the left hip if the pelvis is not fractured, to facilitate venous circulation. If the patient is hypotensive, pneumatic antishock garments can be used with the abdominal section left uninflated. Because of the potential of vascular compromise, the fetus may already be in distress; the nurse should assess fetal heart tones. Measurement of the height of the fundus can provide a baseline from which to monitor blood loss. The height of the fundus will increase if intrauterine blood loss is occurring. Pulses must be evaluated in the extremities and traction splinting applied if the pulse is diminished or absent in the right leg. Last, a Foley catheter may be inserted if there is no evidence of pelvic fracture, to assist in monitoring hydration status. A nasogastric tube may be inserted to prevent aspiration and occlusion of the airway and prevent gastric distention, which would contribute to an even greater decrease in respiratory excursion.

RESEARCH QUESTIONS

- Would a trauma assessment instrument developed for the elderly patient that included scoring weighted for normal physiologic changes of aging better predict mortality than the revised trauma score?
- Does the infrared tympanic thermometer reliably measure core body temperature in the trauma patient?
- How accurate are emergency nurses' trauma assessment findings in identifying traumatic injury?

ANNOTATED BIBLIOGRAPHY

Baker, S. (1987). Injuries: The neglected epidemic. Stone lecture, 1985, America Trauma Society Meeting. *Journal of Trauma, 27*(4), 343-348.
An excellent synopsis of epidemiologic facts concerning trauma injuries. Longitudinal trends are discussed, as well as prevention strategies and their potential impact.

Halpern, J. (1989). Mechanisms and patterns of trauma. *Journal of Emergency Nursing, 15*, 380-388.

A discussion of traumatic injury patterns. Penetrating and blunt forces are addressed within the context of GSWs, falls, MVCs, and pedestrian-vehicle crashes.

Sterner, S. (1987). The multiply injured patient: Initial assessment and management. *Postgraduate Medicine, 81*(5), 119-127.
A brief and to-the-point review of the primary and secondary survey. Controversies in current interventions are included.

REFERENCES

Agran, P., Dunkle, D., & Winn, D. (1987). Injuries to a sample of seat-belted children evaluated and treated in a hospital emergency room. *Journal of Trauma, 27*, 58-64.

Alexander, M. (1988). Mechanism and pattern of injury associated with use of seat belts. *Journal of Emergency Nursing, 14*, 214-216.

Allen, J., & Schwab, C. (1985). Blunt chest trauma in the elderly. *American Surgeon, 51*, 697-700.

American College of Surgeons Committee on Trauma. Chicago: (1990). *Resources for Optional Care of the Injured Patient.* Author.

Arajärvi, E., Santavirta, S., & Tolonen, J. (1987). Abdominal injuries sustained in severe traffic accidents by seat belt wearers. *Journal of Trauma, 27*,(4) 393-397.

Association for the Advancement of Automotive Medicine. (1990). *The abbreviated injury scale: 1990 Revision.* Des Plains, IL. Author.

Baker, S. (1987). Injuries: The neglected epidemic. Stone lecture, 1985, American Trauma Society Meeting. *Journal of Trauma, 27*(4), 343-348.

Baker, S., O'Neill, B., Haddon, W., & Long, W. (1974). The injury severity score: A method for describing patients with multiple injuries and evaluating emergency care. *Journal of Trauma, 14*, 187-196.

Baker, S., O'Neill, B., & Karpf, R. (1984). *The injury fact book.* Lexington, MA: D.C. Heath.

Barach, E., Tomlanovich, M., & Nowak, R. (1986). Ballistics: A pathophysiologic examination of the wounding mechanisms of firearms: Part I and Part II. *Journal of Trauma, 26*, 225-235; 26, 374-383.

Barbarick, D. (1985). Initial assessment and triage of the multiple injured patient. *Orthopaedic Nursing, 4*, 19-22.

Baxt, W., Berry, C., Epperson, M., & Scalzitti, V. (1989). The failure of prehospital trauma prediction rules to classify trauma patients accurately. *Annals of Emergency Medicine, 18*, 21-28.

Bivins, H., Ford, S., Bezmalinovic, Z., Price, H., & Williams, J. (1988). The effect of axial traction during orotracheal intubation of the trauma victim with an unstable cervical spine. *Annals of Emergency Medicine, 17*, 25-29.

Boyd, C., Tolson, M., & Copes, W. (1987). Evaluating trauma care: The TRISS method. *Journal of Trauma, 27*, 370-378.

Bremer, C., & Cassata, L. (1986). Trauma in pregnancy. *Nursing Clinics of North America, 21*, 705-710.

Bryson, B., Warren, K., Schwedhlem, M., Mumford, B., & Lenaghan, P. (1987). Trauma to the aging cervical spine. *Journal of Emergency Nursing, 13*, 334-141.

Bull, G. (1985). Strip and flip. *Emergency Medical Services, 14*, 14-15.

Cayten, C. (1982). Trauma indices: A critical analysis. *Critical Care Quarterly*, 7, 79-89.

Champion, H.R., Copes, W.S., Gann, D.S., Gennarelli, T.A., & Flanagan, M.E. (1989). A revision of the trauma score. *Journal of Trauma*, 29(5), 623-629.

Champion, H.R., Gainer, P., & Yackee, E. (1986). A progress report on the trauma score in predicting a fatal outcome. *Journal of Trauma*, 26, 927-931.

Champion, H.R., Sacco, W., & Carnazzo, A., Copes, W., & Fouty, W. (1981). Trauma score. *Critical Care Medicine*, 9, 672-676.

Committee on Medical Aspects of Automotive Safety. (1971). Rating the severity of tissue damage I: The abbreviated scale. *Journal of American Medical Association*, 215, 277-280.

Committee on Medical Aspects of Automotive Safety (1972). Rating the severity of tissue damage: 2. The comprehensive scale. *Journal of American Medical Association*, 220, 717-720.

Committee on Trauma Research. (1985). *Injury in America: A continuing public health problem*. Washington, DC: National Academy Press.

Conference on Injury Severity Scoring and Triage. (1983). Sponsored by the U.S. Army Medical Research: Development Command Contract to DAMD 17-83-G-9259 and the American Trauma Society, Washington, DC: Author.

Cooter, R. (1990). Computed tomography in the assessment of protective helmet deformation. *Journal of Trauma*, 30, 55-68.

Curley, M. & Vaughn, J. (1987). Assessment and resuscitation of the pediatric patient. *Critical Care Nurse*, 7, 26-40.

DeLaurier, G., Hawkins, M., Treat, R., & Mansberger, A. (1990). Acute airway management. *American Surgeon*, 56, 12-15.

Demarest, J. (Ed.). (1986). *Pre-hospital trauma life support* (pp. 1-19). Akron: Educational Direction, Inc.

Eichelberger, M., Bowman, L., Sacco, W., Mangubat, E., Lowenstein, A., & Gotschall, C. (1989). Trauma score versus revised trauma score in TRISS to predict outcome in children with blunt trauma. *Annals of Emergency Medicine*, 18, 939-942.

Eichelberger, M., Gotschall, C., Sacco, W., Bowman, L., Mangubat, E., & Lowenstein, A. (1989). A comparison of the trauma score, the revised trauma score, and the pediatric trauma score. *Annals of Emergency Medicine*, 18, 1053-1058.

Emergency Nurses Association (ENA). (1990). *Standards of Emergency Nursing Practice* (2nd ed.). St. Louis: Mosby–Year Book, Inc.

Evans, L. (1988). Risk of fatality from physical trauma versus sex and age. *Journal of Trauma*, 28, 368-378.

Fackler, M. (1988). Wound ballistics: A review of common misconceptions. *Journal of American Medical Association*, 259, 2730-2736.

Fischer, R.P., Flynn, T.C., Miller, P.W., & Bowlands, B. (1985). The economics of fatal injury: Dollars and sense. *Journal of Trauma*, 25, 746-750.

Fuhrman, G., Stieg, F., & Buerk, C. (1990). Blunt laryngeal trauma: Classification and management protocol. *Journal of Trauma*, 30, 87-92.

Gareau, A., Eby, R., McLellan, B., & Williams, D. (1990). Tetanus immunization status and immunologic response to a booster in an emergency department geriatric population. *Annals of Emergency Medicine*, 19, 1377-1381.

Gerold, K. (1988). Special problems in post-trauma respiratory management: Maxillofacial, head, and chest injuries. *Critical Care Nursing Quarterly*, 11, 59-62.

Greenspan, L., McLellan, B., & Greig, H. (1985). Abbreviated injury scale and injury severity score: A scoring chart. *Journal of Trauma*, 25, 60-64.

Giuffre, M., Heidenreich, T., Carney-Gersten, P., Dorsch, J., & Heidenreich, E. (1990). The relationship between axillary and core body temperature measurements. *Applied Nursing Research*, 3, 52-55.

Halpern, J. (1989). Mechanisms and patterns of trauma. *Journal of Emergency Nursing*, 15, 380-388.

Hawkins, M., Treat, R., & Mansberger, A. (1988). The trauma score: A simple method to evaluate quality of care. *American Surgeon*, 54, 204-206.

Hector, J. (1986). Neurologic evaluation and support in the child with an acute brain insult. *Pediatric Annals*, 15, 17.

Hedges, J., Feero, S., Moore, B., Haver, D., & Shultz, B. (1987). Comparison of prehospital trauma-triage instruments in a semi-rural population. *Journal of Emergency Medicine*, 5, 197-208.

Horst, H., Obeid, F., Sorenson, V., & Bivins, B. (1986). Factors influencing survival of elderly trauma patients. *Critical Care Medicine*, 14, 681-684.

Illingworth, C. (1984). Injuries to children riding BMX bikes. *British Medical Journal*, 289, 956.

Insurance Institute of Highway Safety. (1991). Facts: 1991 edition. Arlington, VA: Author.

Johnston, J. (1989). Gunshot wounds: Initial assessment and treatment. *Emergency Nursing Reports*, 3, 1-8.

Kidd, P. (1987). Genitourinary trauma patients. *Topics in Emergency Medicine*, 9, 71-87.

Kidd, P., & Murakami, R. (1987). Common pathologic conditions in elderly persons: Nursing assessment and intervention. *Journal of Emergency Nursing*, 13, 27-32.

Knopp, R., Yanagi, A., Kallsen, G., Geide, A., & Doehring, L. (1988). Mechanism of injury and anatomic injury as criteria for prehospital trauma triage. *Annals of Emergency Medicine*, 17, 895-902.

Kosmos, C. (1989). Emergency nursing management of the multiple trauma patient. *Orthopaedic Nursing*, 8, 33-36.

Lipe, H. (1985). Prevention of neurosurgical trauma from travel in motor vehicles. *Journal of Neurosurgical Nursing*, 17, 77-82.

Long, W., Bachulis, B., & Haynes, G. (1986). Accuracy and relationship of mechanisms of injury, trauma score and injury severity score in identifying major trauma. *American Journal of Surgery*, 15, 581-585.

Lynch, J., & Bennett, B. (1986). A review of airway devices. *Emergency Care Quarterly*, 1, 51-61.

Magnes, B. (1982). Clinical recording of pressure on the spinal cord and cauda equina. *Journal of Neurosurgery*, 57, 64-66.

Majernick, T., Bieniek, R., Houston, J., & Hughes, H. (1986). Cervical spine movement during orotracheal intubation. *Annals of Emergency Medicine*, 15, 59-61.

Maloney, J. (1987). Principles of wound ballistics. *Emergency Care Quarterly*, 2, 8-17.

Manley, L. (1987). Pediatric trauma: Initial assessment and management. *Journal of Emergency Nursing, 13*, 77-87.

Mayer, T. (1980). The modified injury severity scale in pediatric multiple trauma patients. *Journal of Pediatric Surgery, 15*, 719-726.

Mayer, T. (1985). *Emergency management of pediatric trauma.* Philadelphia: WB Saunders.

Mayer, T., Walker, M., & Clark, P. (1984). Further experience with the Modified Abbreviated Injury Severity Scale. *Journal of Trauma, 24*(1), 31-35.

Markovchick, V., & Anderson, D. (1988). Initial assessment of chest injury. *Topics in Emergency Medicine, 10*, 11-18.

McGuire, A. (1986). Issues in the prevention of neurotrauma. *Nursing Clinics of North America, 21*, 549-554.

Minaker, K., & Weiss, M. (1986). The emergencies of old age: Homeostasis and surgery. *Emergency Medicine, 15*, 169-180.

Mueller, B., Rivara, F., & Bergman, A. (1987). Factors associated with pedestrian-vehicle collision injuries and fatalities. *Western Journal of Medicine, 146*, 243-245.

Munoz, E. (1984). Economic costs of trauma care: United States, 1982. *Journal of Trauma, 24*, 237-244.

National Committee for Injury Prevention and Control. (1989). *Injury prevention: Meeting the challenge.* DHHS. New York: Oxford University Press.

National Safety Council. (1985). Accident Facts. Chicago: Author.

Park, K., & Dickson, A. (1986). BMX bicycle injuries in children. *Injury, 17*, 34-36.

Rhoads, F., & Grandner, J. (1990). Assessment of an aural infrared sensor for body temperature measurement in children. *Clinical Pediatrics, 29*, 112-115.

Ruddy, R., & Fleisher, G. (1985). Pediatric trauma: An approach to the injured child. *Pediatric Emergency Care, 1*, 151-159.

Russo, P. (1978). Easy rider—hard facts: motorcycle helmet laws. *New England Journal of Medicine, 299*, 1074-1076.

Schoenfeld, A., Ziv, E., Stein, L., Zaidel, D., & Ovadia, J. (1987). Seat belts in pregnancy and the obstetrician. *Obstetrical and Gynecological Survey, 42*, 275-282.

Schriger, D., & Baraff, L. (1988). Defining normal capillary refill: Variation with age, sex, and temperature. *Annals of Emergency Medicine, 17*, 932-935.

Schwaitzberg, S., & Harris, B. (1987). The epidemiology of pediatric trauma. *Emergency Care Quarterly, 3*, 1-6.

Sewell, C., Pine, J., & Hull, H. (1987). Injuries and fatalities associated with off-road, three-wheeled, all-terrain vehicles. *Western Journal of Medicine, 146*, 497-498.

Shapiro, B., Harrison, R., Kacimarek, R., & Cane, R. (1985). *Clinical Application of Respiratory Care* (3rd ed.) (pp. 180-189). Chicago: Mosby–Year Book, Inc.

Shinozaki, T., Deane, R., & Perkins, F. (1988). Infrared tympanic thermometer: Evaluation of a new clinical thermometer. *Critical Care Medicine, 16*, 148-150.

Silverman, J., Peed, S., Goldberg, S., Hamer, R., & Stockman, S. (1985). Surgical staff recognition of psychopathology in trauma patients. *Journal of Trauma, 25*, 544-546.

Simoneau, J.K. (1984). Trauma assessment. *Topics in Emergency Medicine, 6*, 1-8.

Smith, S.M., & Middaugh, J.P. (1985). Injuries associated with three-wheeled, all-terrain vehicles: Alaska 1983 and 1984. *Journal of American Medical Association, 255*, 2454-2458.

Soderstrom, C., & Cowley, R. (1987). A national alcohol and trauma center survey: Missed opportunities, failures of responsibility. *Archives of Surgery, 122*, 1067-1071.

Standards and guidelines for cardiopulmonary resuscitation (CPR) and emergency cardiac care (ECC) (1986). *Journal of American Medical Association, 255*, 2905-2984.

Sterner, S. (1987). The multiply injured patient: Initial assessment and management. *Postgraduate Medicine, 81*, 119-127.

Teasdale, G., & Jennett, B. (1974). Assessment of coma and impaired consciousness: A practical scale. *Lancet, 2*, 81-84.

Tepas, J., Mollitt, D., Talbert, J., & Bryant, M. (1987). The pediatric trauma score as a predictor of injury severity in the injured child. *Journal of Pediatric Surgery, 22*, 14-18.

Thompson, J., & Dains, J. (1986). Indices of injury: Their development and status. *Nursing Clinics of North America, 21*(4), 655-672.

Thompson, R., Riveara, F., & Thompson, D. (1989). A case control study of the effectiveness of bicycle safety helmets. *The New England Journal of Medicine, 320*, 1361-1367.

Threadgill, D. (1987). An assessment and triage tool for the injured pediatric patient. *Trauma Nurse Network Newsletter, 1*, 2-5.

Trunkey, D. (1984). *Advanced trauma life support: Instructor's manual* (p. 159). (Chairman, FACS). Chicago: American College of Surgeons.

Trunkey, D., Siegel, J., & Baker, S. (1983). Current status of trauma severity indices. *Journal of Trauma, 23*, 185-201.

Wells-Mackie, J. (1981). Clinical assessment and priority setting. *Nursing Clinics of North America, 16*, 1-12.

8 Ventilation and Gas Transport

Pulmonary, thoracic, and facial injuries

Elizabeth A. Henneman

Philip L. Henneman

Kathleen S. Oman

OBJECTIVES
- ❏ Describe the four steps of the process of gas exchange.
- ❏ Describe the mechanism leading to altered ventilation and gas exchange in (1) pulmonary contusion and (2) tension pneumothorax.
- ❏ Describe at least two techniques for opening the airway in a trauma patient.
- ❏ Compare and contrast the cause and management of open, closed, and tension pneumothoraxes.
- ❏ Cite at least two nursing diagnoses appropriate for patients with maxillofacial, pulmonary, or thoracic trauma, and discuss three interventions for each.

INTRODUCTION A systematic approach to the assessment and management of the trauma patient with potential or actual respiratory failure is essential. Airway and breathing are among the first priorities in trauma resuscitation (Campbell, 1988). Normal respiratory function is critical to cellular metabolism. The buildup of carbon dioxide alters blood pH, resulting in acidosis and altered cellular function. Without oxygen, cellular processes stop, causing irreversible damage and eventual death. Care of the patient with acute respiratory failure (ARF) involves the expert skills of a multidisciplinary team. A collaborative approach is mandatory, and the nurse is an integral part of the team.

This chapter acquaints the reader with the multitude of processes that can result in ARF in the trauma patient. To facilitate the reader's understanding, a review of normal anatomy and physiology has been included. The importance of all four steps of the respiratory process (i.e., ventilation, diffusion, delivery of gases, oxygen utilization) in maintaining respiratory homeostasis is emphasized. Methods of monitoring these processes are included, as are formulas that are useful in evaluating respiratory function and the efficacy of therapy.

Pulmonary, thoracic, and maxillofacial injury all have the potential to cause ARF in the trauma patient. The specific injuries, clinical findings, and management approaches associated with each category are outlined in detail. Severe respiratory insufficiency usually does not present as an isolated entity; multiple injuries must always be considered in these patients. Associated injuries (e.g., neurologic and cardiovascular) are common in patients with ARF and are addressed in detail in Chapters 9 and 10.

Providing optimal treatment to patients with ARF depends on a continuum of care from the prehospital setting to the emergency department (ED), operating room (OR), and intensive care unit (ICU) as necessary. Although most of the information presented here is specific to emergency management, an effort has been made to provide a holistic approach to patient care, which includes information relative to secondary settings (e.g., OR, ICU, floor).

CASE STUDY A 25-year-old man sustained a single gunshot wound (GSW) to the right side of the chest. Paramedics found the patient awake and combative, with a palpable systolic blood pressure (BP) of 100 mm Hg, a pulse of 130/minute, and a respiratory rate of 30/minute. Approximately 500 ml of blood was observed at the scene. An occlusive dressing, taped on three sides, was placed over the single GSW in the fourth intercostal space, midaxillary line; the patient was placed into the ambulance, and oxygen therapy was initiated by a nonrebreathing mask at 15 L/minute (approximate FIo_2 of .85). An intravenous line was established via a 14-gauge needle, and 500 ml of normal saline was administered en route. On arrival in the emergency department (ED), the patient was promptly moved to a hospital guerney, his clothes cut away, the oxygen continued by face mask, and a cardiac monitor attached. The patient was lethargic, with a palpable blood pressure of 60 mm Hg, a sinus tachycardia of 140/minute, and a respiratory rate of 20/minute. He had tracheal deviation to the left, jugular venous distention, absent breath sounds, crepitus, and hyperresonance to percussion over the right side of the chest. A 14-gauge needle was placed in his right midaxillary line at the fifth intercostal space, with the sound of escaping air; then a 40-French chest tube was promptly inserted at the same site. The chest tube was connected to an autotransfusion and chest drainage device. A 7-French cordis introducer was placed in his right internal jugular vein. Repeat vital signs after chest tube placement revealed a BP of 130/80 mm Hg, a pulse of

100, and a respiratory rate of 24. The patient was awake, alert, and complaining of pain in the right side of his chest; no sensory or motor deficit was present. Breath sounds were equal and the abdomen nontender. He was log rolled, and no further injuries were noted. His central venous pressure (CVP) was 5 cm of H_2O. A portable chest x-ray film and an arterial blood gas specimen were obtained, as was venous blood for initial hematocrit, type and cross-matching, and basic chemistries. With the patient receiving O_2 at 15 L/minute, his Pao_2 was 220 mm Hg, the $Paco_2$ 25 mm Hg, and the pH 7.35. A pulse oximeter was placed on the patient. Chest x-ray studies confirmed proper chest tube and central line placement and revealed a normal heart and mediastinum, a fractured anterior fourth rib, multiple bullet fragments in the right side of the chest, and evidence of right pulmonary contusion. Lateral chest x-ray studies confirmed the presence of multiple bullet fragments lodged in the posterior chest above the tip of the scapula; abdominal x-ray films did not show any bullet fragments in the abdomen. The patient's initial hematocrit was 43% (hemoglobin 16 g/dl). Electrocardiogram was normal, and no blood was in his urine. Repeat vital signs, CVP, and physical examination were unchanged. A second hematocrit after a total of 2 L of normal saline was 36% (hemoglobin 11 g/dl). The patient was autotransfused the 450 ml of blood that had been collected from his chest tube. Morphine sulfate 5 mg was given slowly by intravenous push, and the patient was transferred to the intensive care unit.

What was the cause of this patient's hypotension?

The patient's hypotension resulted from his tension pneumothorax. The penetrating chest trauma allowed air to build up in the right pleural space, resulting in increased intrathoracic pressure. Increased intrathoracic pressure decreased blood flow to the right side of the heart by two mechanisms: (1) deviating the mediastinal structures (tracheal deviation) and causing mechanical obstruction of blood flow to the right side of the heart; and (2) elevating right atrial pressure (jugular venous distention), which decreased the pressure gradient of blood returning to the heart from the periphery. Decreased venous return to the heart resulted in decreased cardiac output and hypotension. The treatment of a tension pneumothorax is to promptly release the increased pressure by (1) tube thoracostomy or (2) needle thoracostomy followed by tube thoracostomy.

What are the mechanisms of this patient's hypoxemia?

This patient's expected Pao_2 on 85% oxygen (O_2 at 15 L/minute via nonrebreathing mask), assuming no injury, should have been between 400 and 500 mm Hg; instead, it was 220 mm Hg. His arterial-alveolar gradient was 356 mm Hg (A-a gradient = $.85 \times (760 - 47) - (1.2 \times 25) - 220$). His hypoxemia was caused by the pulmonary contusion that resulted from the multiple bullet fragments. These fragments disrupted the pulmonary architecture and caused bleeding within the alveoli and airways; this decreased oxygen exchange and caused ventilation/perfusion mismatching, which resulted in hypoxemia.

What are the respiratory risks of narcotic analgesia in this patient?

Narcotic analgesia can depress respiratory drive, resulting in hypoventilation, hypercapnea, and respiratory acidosis.

What respiratory complications is this patient at risk for from his GSW?

This patient is at risk for pulmonary contusion or hematoma, infection, hemorrhagic shock, and adult respiratory distress syndrome.

MECHANISM OF INJURY

Impaired ventilation and gas exchange can result from a variety of conditions, including damage to the airway, chest wall, pleura, pulmonary parenchyma, mediastinum, and diaphragm. The injuries can result from maxillofacial, thoracic, and abdominal trauma. Chest injuries account for 25% of all trauma deaths in this country (Ross & Cernaianu, 1990). Injuries typically are divided into those caused by blunt and those caused by penetrating trauma.

Blunt Trauma

Injuries sustained from blunt trauma typically result from acceleration/deceleration mechanisms, such as occur with motor vehicle accidents and falls (Creel, 1988). Motor vehicle accidents account for approximately one half of all accidental deaths (Jorden & Barkin, 1988). Blunt trauma can result in maxillofacial, neck, and thoracic injuries, including Le Fort and cervical spine fractures, tracheobronchial rupture, fractured ribs, flail chest, pulmonary contusion, pneumothorax, hemothorax, and ruptured diaphragm. Factors demonstrated to influence morbidity in blunt

chest trauma include severe associated thoracic injuries, the presence of shock, falls from height, combined pulmonary contusion and flail chest, and high injury severity scores (ISS) (Clark, Schecter, & Trunkey, 1988). Age plays a significant role in the extent of injury with blunt trauma. Children's bones have greater elasticity and therefore do not fracture as easily as those of the elderly, whose bones are more brittle. Elderly patients have a higher mortality than younger patients because they are less able to tolerate severe injury. Outcome for elderly patients sustaining blunt trauma is better if only conservative (nonventilator) therapy is required (Allen & Schwab 1985).

Penetrating Trauma

Penetrating trauma occurs when body structures are invaded by a foreign object, such as a knife, bullet, ice pick, or other impaling instrument. The extent of the injury is related to not only the location of the injury but, in the case of a bullet or missile, the amount of kinetic energy dissipated in the tissues. Kinetic energy is equal to one-half the mass of a missile times the square of its velocity. Therefore the amount of kinetic energy dissipated in the tissue with a bullet depends primarily on the change in velocity of that missile as it passes through the tissue. The damage that occurs from a penetrating injury results from the loss of structural and functional tissue. High-kinetic energy missiles, such as high-velocity bullets (assuming significant changes in velocity) and shotgun blasts, produce devastating tissue injury, whereas low-velocity objects (e.g., knives, bullets from short-barreled handguns) result in minimal tissue displacement (Barach, Tomlinovich, & Nowak, 1986). Lung tissue, which is elastic and of low density, has been shown to exhibit less damage after penetrating injury than more dense organs, such as liver and muscle (Amato, Billy, Lawsons, & Rich, 1974). Penetrating trauma results in such respiratory injuries as tracheobronchial disruption, pneumothorax, hemothorax, pulmonary contusion, and diaphragmatic laceration.

Associated Injuries

Injuries resulting in altered ventilation and gas exchange rarely occur as a singular entity. Concomitant neurologic and cardiovascular impairment should be suspected in any patient sustaining severe trauma. Damage to the respiratory control centers in the brainstem may result in severely compromised ventilation. Cardiovascular injuries that result in hypovolemia and impair perfusion will have a profound impact on the body's ability to deliver oxygen to the tissues. Management of the patient with hemorrhagic shock, cardiac shock, and altered neurologic status is discussed in detail in Chapters 9 and 10.

Inhalation of toxic gases during trauma, although uncommon, should be considered. Patients in automobile accidents or those who have sustained trauma during a fire (e.g., jumping out of the window to avoid the flames) or explosion should be considered at risk for carbon monoxide poisoning. Carbon monoxide is detrimental because it inhibits oxygen transport by binding to hemoglobin, thereby reducing the red blood cell's ability to carry oxygen. Additionally, carbon monoxide interferes with cellular metabolism and inhibits the utilization of oxygen (Martindale, 1989). The assessment and management of patients with inhalation injuries are discussed in Chapter 14.

ANATOMIC AND PHYSIOLOGIC CONSIDERATIONS
Normal Process of Respiration

The ultimate goal of respiratory function is oxygen utilization by the tissues and removal of carbon dioxide from the body so that normal cellular processes can occur. The four steps necessary to achieve this goal are ventilation, diffusion, gas transport, and oxygen utilization, as shown in Figure 8-1.

Step I: ventilation

Ventilation is the mechanical process of moving air into and out of the lungs. Normal ventilation depends on the structural integrity and patency of the conducting airways and the integrity of the respiratory muscles, chest wall, pleura, and pulmonary parenchyma. The process of ventilation requires an intact brainstem (medulla and pons). The respiratory center in the brainstem, which is affected by alterations in pH, P_{CO_2}, and P_{O_2}, regulates the depth and rate of respiration, adjusting ventilation to meet the metabolic demands of the body. An increases in CO_2 and a low pH (acidosis) stimulate the respiratory center to increase ventilation. Hypoxia also influences ventilation via chemoreceptors in the aortic and carotid arteries, which stimulate respiration via the glossopharyngeal and vagus nerves (Mullins & Garrison, 1987). During inspiration the diaphragm contracts, increasing the length and anteroposterior diameter of the thorax. As the chest expands, intrapulmonary pressure becomes more negative than atmospheric pressure, resulting in a pressure gradient that expedites air flow into the lungs. During expiration the diaphragm passively relaxes, decreasing thoracic size and increasing intrapulmonary pressures such that air flows out of the lungs. During full expiration the diaphragm ascends as high as the fourth intercostal space anteriorly (nipple line) and the tips of the scapulas posteriorly. Normal lung inflation depends on the negative pressure in the intrapleural space generated by thoracic expansion.

Normal, quiet breathing is performed almost exclusively by the diaphragm, which contracts during inspiration and passively relaxes during expiration. During stress states, such as exercise or acute respiratory failure, the intercostal and accessory muscles (e.g., sternocleidomastoid) take a more active role in ventilation. The diaphragm is innervated by the phrenic nerve, and the other respiratory muscles are innervated by nerves that exit the spinal column at various levels between the cervical and lumbar areas. As a result, patients with cervical and thoracic trauma are at high risk for injury to these nerves and possible impairments in ventilation.

The normal volume of air moved in and out with each breath is considered the tidal volume (V_T), which is equal to 5 to 7 ml/kg. Minute ventilation ($\dot{V}_E$) is a measure of the volume of air moved in and out of the lungs per minute; it is calculated by multiplying the tidal volume and the respiratory rate (RR). Minute ventilation is composed of both effective and dead space ventilation ($\dot{V}_D$). Effective, or alveolar, ventilation participates in gas exchange, whereas dead space ventilation does not. Normal anatomic dead space occurs between the mouth and bronchioles, where there is ventilation (i.e., gas flow) but no perfusion (i.e., blood flow) and therefore no gas exchange. It typically accounts for 25% of ventilation or approximately 2 ml/kg or 150 ml. Increases in the dead space to tidal volume ratio (V_D/V_T) occur in disorders that affect the pulmonary circulation. As dead space ventilation increases, less effective ventilation occurs and carbon dioxide removal is impaired.

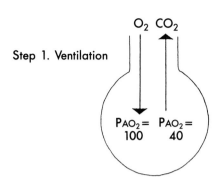

Step 1. Ventilation

O_2 CO_2

P_{AO_2} = 100 P_{AO_2} = 40

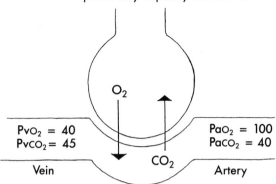

Step 2. Diffusion of gases across the pulmonary capillary membrane

O_2

PvO_2 = 40
$PvCO_2$ = 45

CO_2

PaO_2 = 100
$PaCO_2$ = 40

Vein   Artery

Step 3. Transport of gases

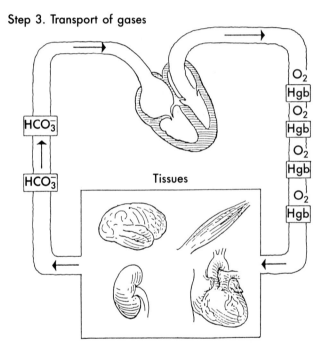

HCO_3^-

HCO_3^-

Tissues

O_2 Hgb
O_2 Hgb
O_2 Hgb
O_2 Hgb

Step 4. Oxygen utilization by the tissues

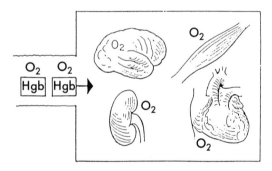

O_2

O_2 O_2
Hgb   Hgb →

O_2

O_2

O_2

O_2

Figure 8-1   Four steps in gas exchange process.

Alveolar ventilation ($\dot{V}_A$), also called *effective ventilation*, occurs when ventilated alveoli come in contact with well-perfused pulmonary capillaries. When the alveolar ventilation adequately meets the metabolic demands of the body, the partial pressure of arterial carbon dioxide (Pa_{CO_2}) will be normal. The relationship between Pa_{CO_2} and $\dot{V}_A$ is expressed in the following equation:

$$Pa_{CO_2} = \frac{V_{CO_2} \times P_B}{\dot{V}_A}$$

where P_B = barometric pressure and V_{CO_2} = CO_2 production. In the trauma patient, impaired ventilation can result from neurologic injury, obstructed airways, or structural damage to the chest wall, pleura, or lung parenchyma. These processes are described in Figure 8-2.

Step II: diffusion of gas between the alveoli and pulmonary capillaries

The transfer of oxygen into and carbon dioxide out of the pulmonary capillary depends on the diffusing capacity of the lung. Diffusion of gases

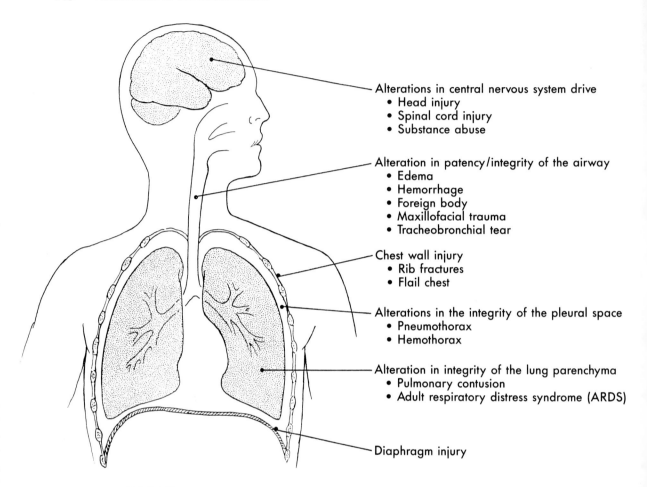

Figure 8-2 Causes of ventilatory failure and impaired gas exchange in trauma patient.

across the alveolar-capillary membrane depends on a number of factors, including (1) the surface area of the alveoli available for gas exchange, (2) the integrity of the alveolar capillary membrane, (3) the amount of hemoglobin in the blood, (4) the diffusion coefficient of the gases, and (5) the driving pressure between the alveoli and pulmonary capillary (Williams, 1985). Because CO_2 is 20 times more diffusable than O_2, problems with oxygenation are more common than problems with CO_2 elimination (Luce, Tyler, & Pierson, 1984). Alveolar and arterial partial pressure of carbon dioxide are almost always the same.

The efficiency of gas exchange is measured by evaluating how well alveolar oxygen equilibrates with the arterial circulation. Certain conditions alter the ability of oxygen to equilibrate across the alveolar-capillary membrane such that a significant difference can exist between the partial pressure of alveolar oxygen (PAO_2) and arterial oxygen (PaO_2). These conditions, which cause an increase in the PAO_2-PaO_2 difference (also called the A-a gradient), are responsible in most cases for the hypoxemia associated with traumatic injury. Conditions that impair equilibrium across the alveolar membrane include (1) ventilation/perfusion ($\dot{V}/\dot{Q}$) mismatching, (2) shunt, and (3) diffusion defects. Of these, $\dot{V}/\dot{Q}$ mismatch and shunt are the most common causes of hypoxemia (Figure 8-3).

Ventilation/Perfusion mismatch The normal ratio of ventilation to perfusion is 0.8, meaning that there is always slightly more flow past the alveoli via the pulmonary capillary than there is ventila-

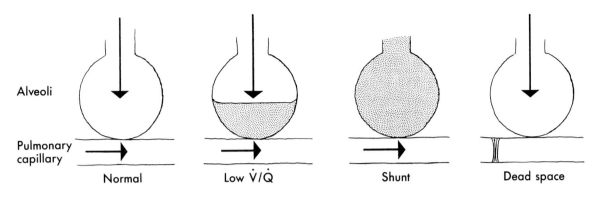

Figure 8-3 Normal and abnormal ventilation/perfusion units. In normal units, ventilation (to alveoli) and perfusion (in pulmonary capillary) are well matched. Areas of low ventilation relative to perfusion (low $\dot{V}/\dot{Q}$) and shunt units (no ventilation but normal perfusion) result in hypoxemia. Dead-space units receive normal ventilation but poor perfusion, resulting in impaired elimination of carbon dioxide.

tion into the alveoli. Under certain conditions this mismatching is exaggerated and an even greater amount of blood flow is wasted as it travels past underventilated alveoli. The result is under-oxygenated blood returning to the heart and mixing with oxygenated blood, lowering the Pao_2. A low $\dot{V}/\dot{Q}$ ratio is seen with such conditions as atelectasis and pulmonary contusion.

Shunt The most extreme form of low $\dot{V}/\dot{Q}$ mismatching is called *intrapulmonary shunting*. Shunting occurs when alveoli are completely collapsed or fluid filled, such that no gas exchange can occur between the alveoli and pulmonary capillary. The technique for differentiating shunt from $\dot{V}/\dot{Q}$ inequalities is to evaluate the effect of high FIo_2 (usually 100% O_2) on Pao_2. Hypoxemia secondary to low $\dot{V}/\dot{Q}$ will respond to high FIo_2, whereas hypoxemia secondary to shunting will not (Luce et al., 1984). This is because no gases are exchanged in shunting, and therefore no amount of oxygen can further facilitate the exchange of gases across the pulmonary capillary membrane. Shunting in the trauma patient can occur with severe pulmonary contusion, pulmonary edema, and the adult respiratory distress syndrome (ARDS).

External causes of hypoxemia Hypoxemia can result also from causes outside of the lung itself, such as hypoventilation or the administration of low FIo_2. These mechanisms rarely cause hypoxemia in trauma. Because both the alveolar and arterial Po_2 are affected by these conditions, the alveolar-arterial oxygen difference (A-a gradient) is normal.

Step III: transport of gases

Oxygen delivery Well-oxygenated blood is of little value unless it can be delivered to the tissues that need it. Adequate oxygen delivery (DO_2) requires two factors—a normal O_2 content of the arterial blood (Cao_2) and a normal cardiac output ($\dot{Q}T$).

$$DO_2 = Cao_2 \times \dot{Q}T$$

where $\dot{Q}T$ = blood flow over time. The arterial oxygen content (Cao_2) depends on three factors—hemoglobin (Hgb), oxygen saturation (Sao_2), and Pao_2—as evidenced in the following equation for a normal adult with a Pao_2 of 100 torr and a Hgb of 15 g/dl:

$$Cao_2 = Hgb \times 1.34 \times Sao_2 + (.0031 \times Pao_2)$$
$$Cao_2 = 15 \text{ g/dl} \times 1.34 \text{ ml } O_2/\text{g Hgb} \times .97 + (.0031 \times 100)$$
$$Cao_2 = 19.5 + 0.3 \text{ ml } O_2/\text{dl}$$
$$Cao_2 = 19.8 \text{ ml } O_2/\text{dl}$$

A normal Cao_2 therefore is approximately 20 ml O_2/dl blood. The constant 1.34 ml represents the carrying capacity of oxygen per gram of hemoglobin. The value derived by multiplying .0031 × Pao_2 is typically dropped from the equation, be-

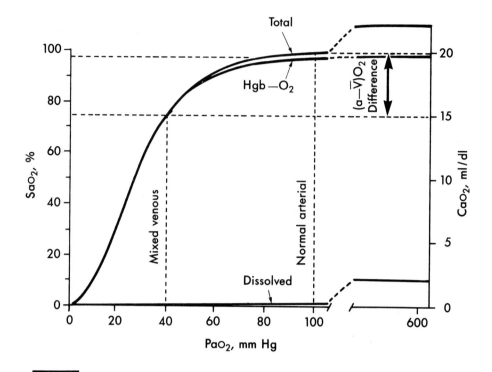

Figure 8-4 Oxyhemoglobin dissociation curve, relating partial pressure of oxygen in arterial blood (Pa_{O_2}), in millimeters of mercury (mm Hg), to arterial O_2 saturation (Sa_{O_2}) in percent and to O_2 content of arterial blood (Ca_{O_2}) and assuming normal hemoglobin concentration in millimeters per deciliter (ml/dl). Curve descends steeply below Pa_{O_2} values of 50 mm Hg, indicating severely reduced O_2-carrying capacity by hemoglobin below this Pa_{O_2}. Lower line represents O_2 in solution in blood; middle line depicts O_2 bound to hemoglobin plus O_2 dissolved. Note that dissolved O_2 contributes little to Ca_{O_2}, at Pa_{O_2} in normal range. (*Note.* From *Intensive Respiratory Care* [p. 26] by J.M. Luce, M.L. Tyler, and D.J. Pierson, 1984, Philadelphia: W.B. Saunders.)

cause it adds little to the final value.

As is evident from this formula, Ca_{O_2} is a function of Sa_{O_2} rather than Pa_{O_2}. It is important therefore to appreciate the relationship between the Pa_{O_2} and the Sa_{O_2}. The majority of oxygen (97%) is carried on hemoglobin; the remainder is dissolved in the plasma. The Pa_{O_2} measured via blood gas analysis is reflective of the amount of dissolved oxygen and does not depend on the presence of red blood cells.

The affinity of hemoglobin for oxygen is expressed by the oxyhemoglobin dissociation curve shown in Figure 8-4. The "S" shape of the curve reflects the nonlinear relationship that exists between the P_{O_2} and S_{O_2}. On the arterial side of the curve (upper right-hand portion), large

changes in Pa_{O_2} occur with very little change in Sa_{O_2}. On the venous side (lower left-hand portion), the reverse occurs, and even small changes in Pv_{O_2} are accompanied by large changes in Sv_{O_2}.

Certain conditions can influence the affinity of hemoglobin and oxygen, thereby shifting the curve from its normal position. A shift to the right occurs under the following conditions: acidosis, increased Pa_{CO_2}, increased temperature, and increased 2,3-diphosphoglycerate (DPG). A shift to the right indicates a decreased affinity of hemoglobin for oxygen; therefore at any given Pa_{O_2}, the saturation will be less than normal. A shift to the left occurs under the opposite conditions, reflecting an increased affinity of hemoglobin and oxygen. These shifts can be physiologically beneficial to the trauma patient. For example, a trauma patient who is acidotic as a result of lactate accumulation from hypoperfusion will have a rightward shift of the oxyhemoglobin curve, resulting in increased availability (i.e., unloading) of oxygen in the tissues. The relationship between SaO_2 and PaO_2 should emphasize the need for an evaluation of CaO_2 in trauma patients with respiratory insufficiency and anemia.

Adequate oxygen delivery (DO_2) depends on not only the content of arterial blood but also the cardiac output. Assuming a normal cardiac output of 5 L/minute, normal oxygen delivery is 1000 ml/minute. Example:

$$DO_2 = CaO_2 \times Q_T$$
$$DO_2 = 20 \text{ ml } O_2/100 \text{ ml} \times 5000$$
$$\text{ml/minute} \times 10$$
$$\text{(correction factor)}$$
$$DO_2 = 1000 \text{ ml/minute}$$

Impaired oxygen delivery in the trauma patient can result from poor oxygenation, low hemoglobin (e.g., hemorrhage), or diminished cardiac output (e.g., cardiac tamponade, hypovolemic shock). Studies suggest that cardiac output plays a major role in determining oxygen delivery (McCormick, Feustel, Newell, Stratton, & Fortune, 1988). Injuries impacting cardiac output and hemoglobin are discussed in more detail in Chapter 9. The variety of factors influencing oxygen delivery stress the importance of evaluating more than the PaO_2 or SaO_2 (i.e., CaO_2 and cardiac output) when evaluating the patient's oxygenation status.

Carbon dioxide transport   The carbon dioxide produced as waste in the cells diffuses out into the extracellular compartment where it reacts with water (H_2O) to form carbonic acid (H_2CO_3). The enzyme carbonic anhydrase (CA) catalyzes this hydration process, as well as the dissociation of carbonic acid into hydrogen and bicarbonate ions.

$$CO_2 + H_2O \overset{CA}{\rightleftharpoons} H_2CO_3 \overset{CA}{\rightleftharpoons} H + HCO_3^-$$

The hydrogen ions quickly bind to hemoglobin, whereas the bicarbonate diffuses back into the plasma. In the lungs, carbonic acid is converted back into CO_2 and H_2O, where the CO_2 is removed during ventilation (Mullins & Garrison, 1987).

The bicarbonate–carbonic acid system is the principal buffer of extracellular fluid. The relationship of the elements in this system is described by the Henderson-Hasselbalch equation:

$$pH = pK + \log (HCO_3/H_2CO_3)$$

where the pK of carbonic acid is 6.1. H_2CO_3 is calculated by multiplying a solubility factor (0.031 mM/liter/mm Hg) for carbon dioxide times the $PaCO_2$. For a normal $PaCO_2$ of 40 mm Hg, H_2CO_3 is calculated as $40 \times 0.031 = 1.2$ mM per liter. The normal concentration of carbon dioxide in body fluids is fixed at 1.2 mM per liter by the lungs; at this concentration pulmonary excretion equals metabolic production. Changes in blood pH result in almost instantaneous respiratory response; acidosis stimulates and alkalosis depresses ventilation. In this way the lung can maintain a balance in the acid-base status of the patient. The kidney functions in this system by retaining existing bicarbonate and generating new bicarbonate.

Carbon dioxide production in trauma patients may be increased by infection, seizures, or drugs (e.g., cocaine, phencyclidine) or decreased by hypothermia or drugs (e.g., barbiturates).

Step IV: tissue utilization of oxygen

The final step in the process of gas exchange is the uptake and utilization of oxygen by the tissues. In healthy persons, O_2 utilization matches the amount of O_2 required or demanded by the tissues. If, however, O_2 demand exceeds O_2 utilization (e.g., during stressed states such as trauma) lactic acidosis and ischemic injury may result. Typically, increases in O_2 demand result in increased O_2 delivery, primarily by enhanced cardiac output. In certain conditions, such as hemorrhagic or cardiogenic shock, cardiac output can not be increased even if demand is increased, and lactic acidosis develops as it did in the case study. In adult respiratory distress syndrome, O_2 demand is directly related to supply and not vice versa (Mohsenifar, Goldbach, Tashkin, & Campisi, 1983). Research has demonstrated a linear relationship between O_2 delivery and O_2 utilization when O_2 delivery is below a certain critical level (<21 ml/min/kg). These results suggest that O_2 utilization can be maximized in certain patients by optimizing oxygen delivery.

Impaired tissue O_2 utilization is rare in the

trauma patient but may result if the patient has carbon monoxide poisoning (such as in trauma involving inhalation injuries). Because carbon monoxide binds to hemoglobin, the arterial oxygen content and therefore oxygen delivery is reduced, leading to severe tissue hypoxia. In addition to binding to hemoglobin, carbon monoxide is toxic to the tissues. Carbon monoxide impairs cellular metabolism by binding to cytochrome oxidase a_3, resulting in tissue hypoxia (Martindale, 1989). Carbon monoxide poisoning is discussed in more detail in Chapter 14.

GENERAL ASSESSMENT
Primary Assessment and Intervention

Evaluation and management of the airway, breathing, circulation (ABCs), cervical spine, and level of consciousness are the initial priorities in the initial resuscitation of all trauma patients (Campbell, 1988). An extensive review of principles of the primary assessment is discussed in Chapter 7. This section highlights the initial assessment and management of the patient with maxillofacial, pulmonary, or thoracic trauma (and therefore potential alterations in gas exchange).

Cervical spine immobilization

The trauma patient's cervical spine should be promptly stabilized in a neutral position in the field. If this is not done, immobilization should be performed simultaneously with assessment of the airway in the ED. This immobilization should be maintained until cervical spine trauma is ruled out clinically or radiographically. Airway management (suctioning, intubation) should not compromise the cervical spine if at all possible. Patients should be assumed to have a cervical spine injury until proven otherwise, either clinically or radiographically. Cervical spine injuries can result in significant morbidity and mortality. Immobilizing the cervical spine with certain devices can result in decreased forced vital capacity (FVC) and forced expiratory volume in 1 second (FEV_1) when patients are strapped to the spinal board. (Bauer & Kowalski, 1988). Immobilization of the cervical spine may also increase the risk of aspiration if the patient vomits while he or she is unable to voluntarily turn the head to the side to clear vomitus. Patients who vomit during cervical spine immobilization should be promptly log

rolled onto their side while maintaining the cervical spine in a neutral position to prevent aspiration.

Airway

The evaluation of the patient's airway should be performed simultaneously with stabilization of the cervical spine. Loss of a patient's airway will quickly result in the death of the patient or significant neurologic injury if not promptly corrected. The airway must be assessed for patency, that is, the patient's ability to move air into and out of the lungs. Airway patency can be compromised in both awake and unresponsive patients. If the patient is awake, he or she may complain of progressive dyspnea or a feeling of tightness. Upper airway obstruction is associated with inspiratory crowing or stridor (wheezing) and the use of accessory muscles (retraction). Patients with severely compromised airways should be treated as if they had complete obstruction. Maintaining the integrity of the cervical spine must be a priority during all attempts at achieving airway patency.

Methods of relieving airway obstruction in the trauma patient differ for awake and unresponsive patients. An awake patient may be able to assist by pointing out the cause of the obstruction. If the patient is not responsive, a chin lift or jaw thrust may be the only intervention required for securing an airway (American Heart Association (AHA), 1986; Stewart, 1988). If this maneuver is not successful, the airway should be evaluated for the presence of foreign materials, such as vomitus, blood, or dislodged teeth. A variety of large-lumen, hard-plastic suction catheters (e.g., tonsil tip) are available to facilitate clearing the oral cavity. If the patient has suffered extensive facial injury, a soft, flexible suction catheter (e.g., red rubber) may cause less trauma. Care must be taken to avoid advancing foreign objects further down the oropharynx during suctioning attempts. If the oropharynx is clear of material, a nasopharyngeal or oropharyngeal airway can be inserted. These devices prevent the tongue and epiglottis from falling against the posterior pharyngeal wall and thereby help to maintain a patent airway. They also facilitate suctioning. Care must be taken not to provoke vomiting or gagging while inserting these devices. The nasopharyngeal airway is better tolerated than the oropharyngeal airway and can be used in the awake patient. The oropharyngeal airway should be used only in an unconscious patient. If a patient readily tolerates placement of an oropharyngeal airway (i.e; does not gag), he or she probably requires intubation to protect the airway (Stewart, 1988). Properly functioning suction equipment must be available to facilitate airway clearance. Portable devices used in prehospital settings may also be useful during in-hospital transport and in diagnostic areas.

If these conservative methods are not effective in clearing the airway, intubation, cricothyroidotomy, or tracheostomy should be performed. Endotracheal intubation (nasotracheal or orotracheal) by experienced clinicians is the preferred method of airway management. Some prehospital care personnel still use an esophageal obturator airway (EOA), but this should be converted to an endotracheal tube as soon as the patient arrives in the ED. When there are concerns about the cervical spine, in-line stabilization of the cervical spine must be maintained during intubation (Bivens, Ford, Bezmalinovic, Price, & Williams,

1988; Majernick, Bieniek, Houston, & Hughes, 1986; Stewart, 1988).

Endotracheal intubation can be accomplished either nasotracheally or orally; each approach requires a different technique (AHA, 1986; Stewart, 1988). Each method also has its own advantages, disadvantages, and complications, as listed in Table 8-1 (Kastendieck, 1988). Oral intubations require a lighted laryngoscope to visualize the vocal cords and facilitate proper placement. This method may result in neck flexion; therefore when a cervical spine injury is suspected, in-line cervical stabilization should be performed during intubation. In-line cervical stabilization with oral intubation may create the least cervical spine motion and therefore may be the preferred way to manage a patient's airway if the possibility of a cervical injury exists (Aprahamian, Thompson, Finger, & Darin, 1984; Majernick et al., 1986). Nasal intubations are performed blindly, and therefore only experienced personnel should perform this procedure. The advantage of nasal intubations is that neck flexion may not be required.

Table 8-1 Comparison of nasotracheal, orotracheal, and esophageal obturator airways

	Nasotracheal	**Orotracheal**	**Esophageal obturator**
Indications	Breathing patient Can be used with cervical spine injury if in-line stabilization is used	Apneic patient Decreased mental status/ lack of gag reflex Can be used with cervical spine injury if in-line stabilization is used	Prehospital setting— endotracheal intubation not available Can be used with cervical spine injury if in-line stabilization is used
Contraindications	Le Fort or basilar fractures	Oropharyngeal injury	Responsive patient with intact gag reflex
Advantages	Does not require neck extension (decreased risk of cervical spine injury) Can be used in an awake patient	Allows for direct visualization of vocal cords	Ease of insertion
Disadvantages	Technically more difficult Blind procedure	Requires obtunded/ sedated patient	Blind procedure Requires replacement with ET tube
Complications	Nasal bleeding Sinusitis Esophageal intubation Cord injury	Broken teeth Cord injury Esophageal intubation	Tracheal intubation Ruptured esophagus Aspiration Tracheal injury

Table 8-2 Equipment guidelines for intubation and chest drainage

Equipment	Age and weight				
	6 Months (7-8 kg)	1-2 Years (10-12 kg)	5 Years (16-18 kg)	8-10 Years (24-30 kg)	16 Years (adult) (60-70 kg)
Airway					
Oral	Small (1)	Small (2)	Medium (3)	Medium/Large (4)	Large (5, 6)
Nasal (F)	12	16-20	20-24	24-28	28-36
Breathing					
RR	22-32	20-30	16-24	12-20	12-16
HHR size	Child	Child	Child	Child/Adult	Adult
Mask size	Infant	Child	Child	Small adult	Adult
ET tube (mm)	3.5-4.0	4.0-4.5	5.0-5.5	5.5-6.5	7.0-9.0
Tracheostomy tube	0 or 1	1 or 2	3 or 4	4 or 5	5 or 6
Laryngoscope blade	1 (Straight)	1 or 2 (Straight)	2 (Straight or curved)	2 or 3 (Straight or curved)	4 or 5 (Straight or curved)
Suction catheter (F)	8-10	10	12	14	14
Chest tube (F)	14-20	14-24	20-32	28-38	36-40

Note. From *Pediatric Advanced Life Support* (p. 105) by L. Chameides (Ed.), 1988, Dallas: American Heart Association. *RR*, Respiratory rate; *HHR*, hand-held resuscitator (bag); *ET*, endotracheal tube; *F*, French.

Nasal intubation, however, results in significant movement of the cervical spine (Aprahamian et al, 1984). The digital or transluminal method can be used to assist with intubations and evaluation of proper placement. The digital method uses the middle and index fingers to guide the tip of the endotracheal tube into the trachea via the mouth. A variation of this may be used with nasotracheal intubation (Korber & Henneman, 1989). Digital methods cause significant cervical spine motion and should not be performed on patients with potential cervical spine injuries. Transluminal (lighted stylet) intubation is used in nasal intubations to guide the tube through the glottic opening without direct visualization of the cords (Stewart, 1988).

The nurse's role includes assisting with the intubation, evaluating proper tube position, and securing the tube. Equipment necessary for intubation includes various sizes of endotracheal tubes, functioning laryngoscope and blades, suction catheters and suction apparatus, and an appropriate size of hand-held resuscitator (Ambu bag). Proper tube size is essential, since a tube that is too small increases the work of breathing and may hamper the ability to wean off a ventilator (Table

8-2). The nurse should assist the physician and the respiratory therapist with the intubation when necessary, perhaps with in-line stabilization or assistance with evaluation of proper tube placement after intubation. Correct tube position is several centimeters above the carina. This position is ascertained by auscultating in the axillas for bilateral breath sounds, auscultating over the stomach for absent breath sounds, and obtaining a chest x-ray film. Breath condensation on the tube with each ventilation is suggestive of intratracheal placement, but not 100% reliable. End tidal CO_2 measurement can confirm intratracheal placement. If the patient can phonate, the tube may be in the esophagus or the cuff may be deflated. Unrelenting coughing after intubation suggests the tube is irritating the carina and should be withdrawn several centimeters. Maintenance of good oxygen saturation (as demonstrated by pulse oximetry) after intubation implies proper endotracheal tube position. Confirmation of proper tube placement should be performed whenever the tube is moved.

The endotracheal tube must be adequately secured to avoid such complications as inadvertent extubation, musosal damage, or tube migration.

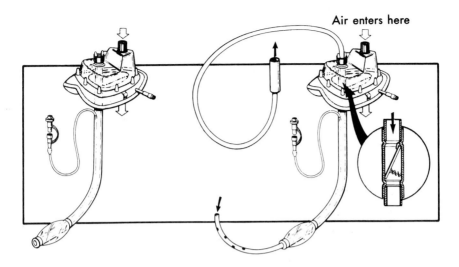

Figure 8-5   Esophageal gastric tube airway (EGTA). (*Note.* From *Basic Trauma Life Support* (p. 63) by J.F. Campbell [Ed.], 1988, New Jersey: Prentice Hall.)

Tubes can be secured with either adhesive tape or commercially available straps. Tape should not be wrapped around the necks of patients with head trauma to secure the tube, because the tape can impede venous outflow and increase intracranial pressure.

In the prehospital setting, an esophageal obturator airway (EOA) may be useful in securing the patient's airway. The EOA is a blind-ended tube that is inserted into the esophagus. Fenestrations in the proximal portion of the tube allow air to pass into the trachea during the administration of ventilations. The EOA was originally introduced to allow prehospital personnel to secure an airway without intubating the trachea. Since its inception in the early 1970s, the enthusiasm for its use has diminished, in part because of laws in many states permitting paramedics to perform tracheal intubations. Advantages and disadvantages of the EOA are discussed in Table 8-1. Of particular note is the difficulty ascertaining correct tube placement when EOA tubes are used. Despite this problem, studies suggest that the EOA provides gas exchanging capabilities comparable with those achieved with endotracheal intubation (Meislin, 1980). The latest models of these tubes have been refined to include a low-pressure, high-volume cuffed endotracheal tube, as well as a nasogastric tube. These esophagogastric airway

tubes have the advantage of being suitable for use as conventional endotracheal tubes if they are inadvertently inserted into the trachea (Figure 8-5).

Airway obstruction resulting from or accompanied by soft tissue swelling or mechanical disruption of facial structures necessitates cricothyroidotomy or tracheostomy. The preferred method of securing an airway when traditional methods are contraindicated is a cricothyroidotomy. A vertical incision is made in the skin and a horizontal incision made through the cricothyroid membrane; a small endotracheal tube (pediatric or tracheostomy) is then inserted (Figure 8-6). After the endotracheal tube is secured, it should be attached to oxygen via a T-piece or connected to a ventilator if the patient's ventilation is compromised.

As a temporary alternative, a large-bore (e.g., 14-gauge), over-the-needle catheter can be inserted into the cricothyroid membrane. A 10-ml syringe is attached to the catheter, which is advanced until air is aspirated, indicating placement in the trachea. The catheter is then directed caudally at a 30- to 45-degree angle and advanced over the needle. The needle is then withdrawn. The catheter must be adequately secured. Ventilation can be accomplished with one of a variety of commercially available jet ventilators (Figure 8-7). A makeshift ventilation system can be de-

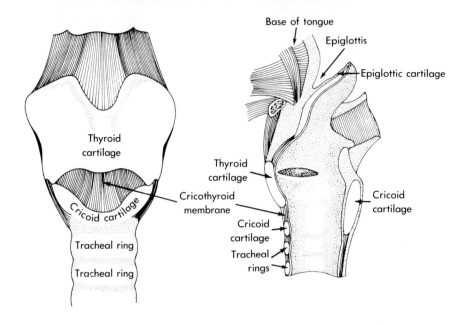

Figure 8-6 Important anatomic landmarks for performing surgical cricothyroidotomy. Assess for landmarks using inferior to superior approach. With fingers placed on thyroid and cricoid cartilages, make vertical skin incision and horizontal incision into trachea. (*Note*. From *Handbook of Medical Emergencies in the Dental Office* [3rd ed.] by S.F. Malamed, 1987, St Louis: Mosby–Year Book, Inc.)

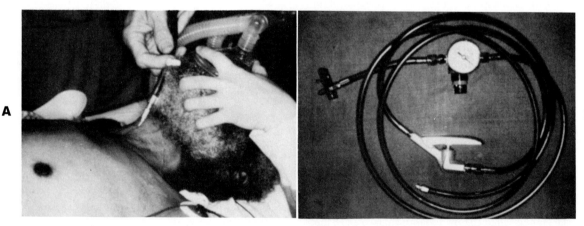

Figure 8-7 **A,** Needle cricothyroidotomy technique. After intravenous needle (14- or 16-gauge) insertion into cricothyroid membrane and aspiration of air, plastic cannula is slid over needle into trachea and luer fitting of high-pressure ventilating device is attached. This junction must be held and stabilized during ventilation. Gloves should be worn. **B,** Device for administering bursts of high-pressure oxygen for transtracheal ventilation by squeezing handle periodically (about 40 times/min). Luer fitting is at one end of high-pressure hose, and other contains adapter for high-pressure oxygen outlets. (*Note*. From *Early Care of the Injured Patient* [p. 93] by E.E. Moore (Ed.), 1990, Philadelphia: B.C. Decker.)

vised by attaching the port of a suction catheter to oxygen tubing that is attached to a flowmeter set at 15 L/minute or more. Intermittent ventilations (1-second inhalation, 2-second exhalations) are delivered by intermittently covering the thumb port (Barrett, 1986). Clearly, preparations for an emergent placement of a cricothyroid needle should be made *before* it is needed. Adaptors to connect O_2 tubing to the catheter may be difficult or impossible to locate. A commercial jet ventilation system or a system preassembled in-house should be available in every emergency department. Commercially available 13-gauge cannulas are available for jet ventilation, which are easily attached to a 50-PSI oxygen source. These cannulas also have attached straps, which make them simpler to secure. Complications reported with percutaneous jet ventilation include hemorrhage, perforation of the esophagus, subcutaneous emphysema, and arterial perforation (Smith, Schaer, & Pfaeffle, 1975). Because high pressures can build up in the chest with this type of system, it is contraindicated with complete upper airway obstruction, which impairs the escape of exhaled gases. In cases of complete airway obstruction, larger cannulas (3.5 mm internal diameter) can be inserted transtracheally, allowing for ventilation using hand-held resuscitators or oscillatory pressure devices (Goldman et al., 1988; Neff, Pfister, & Van Sonnenberg, 1983).

An emergency tracheostomy is rarely necessary except when laryngeal injury or fracture of the hyoid bone or thyroid or cricoid cartilage is evident. In children younger than 5 years, tracheostomy is the preferred surgical method of airway management, but is 4 times more risky than intubation (Kastendiek, 1988). The technique for performing a tracheostomy is described in detail in specialty texts (AHA, 1986). Identification of anatomic landmarks is essential to safe placement and is more difficult in obese patients and patients with short necks. Complications of tracheostomy include hemorrhage, thyroid laceration, pneumothorax, and inability to cannulate (Bayne, 1985). The tube must be secured to decrease the risk of dislodging. The nurse should dress the surgical wound carefully to avoid infection and control bleeding.

Breathing

Once the airway has been secured, the adequacy of breathing must be assessed. With the ex-

ception of apnea, it is often difficult to judge by the clinical examination alone whether ventilation is adequate. Any patient in whom ineffective breathing is suspected should have arterial blood gases (ABGs) drawn to evaluate the Pao_2 and $Paco_2$. If a patient's ventilations appear compromised, it is better to overtreat and provide ventilatory support than to wait for ABG results. All trauma patients should be given high-flow oxygen by mask, and any patient with a depressed level of consciousness should be hyperventilated. Patients who require artificial ventilatory support can be managed with a hand-held resuscitator bag and 100% O_2 until a ventilator is available. Clinicians should familiarize themselves with the features of the hand-held resuscitators used in their institution. The amount of air delivered by the "bagmask" or "bag-tube" depends on the type and size of the resuscitator and the technique used. An average adult can deliver 800 ml of gas using a one-handed technique (squeeze) and 1200 ml using two hands (Stewart, 1988). Significant volumes of air can be lost if the mask is not properly fitted or if the endotracheal tube cuff leaks. Special care must be taken during patient transport because proper bag-mask use is more difficult. Resuscitator bags can deliver from 21% to 100% oxygen if a reservoir is attached. Flow rates of at least 15 L/minute are necessary for delivering high FIo_2s. "Bagging" the patient every 3 to 4 seconds will provide a minute ventilation of 10 to 14 L/minute with most conventional units.

Patients requiring prolonged ventilatory assistance must be placed on a ventilator. Absolute indications for mechanical ventilation are CO_2 retention, acidemia, and hypoxemia (see box, p. 158). Initial ventilatory settings should include a tidal volume of 10 to 15 ml per kilogram of body weight, assist control or intermittent mandatory control, and an appropriate respiratory rate to provide an adequate minute ventilation (Table 8-3). All patients placed on a ventilator should have arterial blood gas studies to determine the effect of the ventilator settings.

Circulation

The assessment of a trauma patient's circulation begins before the patient's blood pressure (BP) is actually obtained. The patient's mental status, skin signs (including moisture, temperature, and capillary refill), and pulses can provide important clues in determining a patient's circula-

---

Indications for mechanical ventilation in the trauma patient

$Paco_2$ >45 mm Hg with pH <7.25
Sao_2 <90%
Respiratory rate <8 breaths/min or >30 breaths/min
Tidal volume <5 ml/kg
Vital capacity <15 ml/kg
Maximum inspiratory force (MIF) <−25 cm H_2O
Minute ventilation >10 L/min
A-a DO_2 >100 mm Hg on an Flo_2 of 100%
Pao_2/Flo_2 <350
Shunt fraction (Qs/Qt) >20%-30%
Acutely changing or depressed neurologic status after head trauma

Note: The decision to intubate in the ED usually is made on the basis of clinical factors (e.g., respiratory rate, mental status) and arterial blood gas results.

Table 8-3 Initial ventilator settings for the trauma patient

Setting	Comments

Ventilatory mode
  Assist control (AC)
  Intermittent mandatory
    ventilation (IMV)	

Respiratory rate 10-30	Variable: depends on patient's age and $Paco_2$ level; should be adjusted for patient comfort.
Tidal volume 10 ml/kg	Goal = $Paco_2$ within the normal range.
Flo_2 Variable	Goal = Sao_2 >90% Start at 100% and wean down, using Sao_2 as a guide.

Inspiratory : Expiratory
  (I : E) ratio
  1 : 2 or 1 : 3	

Positive end expiratory
  pressure (PEEP)
  3 to 5 cm H_2O
	Physiologic PEEP. Greater levels of PEEP should be guided by determinations of oxygen delivery (requires pulmonary artery catheter).

Sensitivity	Adjust to patient comfort.
Peak flow	Adjust to I : E ratio and peak pressures.

---

tory status. Patients with cold, clammy skin and prolonged capillary refill are in shock even if their blood pressure is normal. Determination of which pulses are present can give a clue as to a patient's approximate blood pressure. The presence of a dorsalis pedis pulse implies the patient's blood pressure is probably above 95 mm Hg; a radial pulse implies the patient's blood pressure is above 85 mm Hg; and a carotid pulse implies the patient's blood pressure is above 40 to 50 mm Hg. At least initially, tachycardia should always be assumed to be caused by hypovolemia. Determination of the patient's mental status, skin signs, and pulses is sufficient to initiate the resuscitation. Only after one's primary assessment and treatment of critical abnormalities (e.g., airway obstruction, tension pneumothorax, cardiac arrest), should the patient's actual blood pressure and pulse be determined. The appropriate interpretation of the patient's circulatory status depends on a complete assessment of the patient's mental status, skin signs, pulses, vital signs, and amount of fluid or blood already given to the patient.

If the patient with chest trauma has a cardiopulmonary arrest, chest compressions should be initiated and rapidly evaluated for their effectiveness. Should closed chest cardiopulmonary resuscitation (CPR) be ineffective, a thoracotomy should be considered. Although opening the chest and performing direct cardiac massage is not routinely recommended in blunt trauma arrest, it is indicated for penetrating chest trauma arrest (Cogbill, Moore, Millikan, & Cleveland, 1983).

Oxygen delivery depends on cardiac output and hemoglobin levels, as well as pulmonary factors. It is critical, therefore, to monitor closely the adequacy of O_2 transport during the initial phases of patient management. Methods of improving cardiac output and oxygen delivery in the trauma patient include (1) control of external hemorrhage, (2) use of pneumatic antishock garments (PASG) or military antishock trousers (MAST),

(3) administration of blood products and fluids, (4) delivery of adequate chest compressions during cardiac arrest, and (5) optimization of oxygenation and ventilation.

Use of PASG is controversial in the management of all trauma but especially in those cases with penetrating thoracic trauma; the use of PASG may increase mortality in patients with penetrating thoracic trauma (Ali, Vanderby, & Purcell, 1991; Henneman, 1987; Mattox, Bickell, Pepe, Burch, & Feliciano 1989; Mattox, Bickell, Pepe, & Mangelsdorf, 1986). The PASG is contraindicated in patients with pulmonary edema and should be used with caution in the patients with impaired respiratory function, since it decreases vital capacity when the abdominal section is inflated (McCabe, Seidel, & Jagger, 1983). Also, it should not be used in patients with a tension pneumothorax (Kaback, Saunders, & Meislin, 1984).

Initial level of consciousness

The nurse should assess the initial level of consciousness (LOC) early in the evaluation to determine (1) the need for hyperventilation and (2) the reliability of the rest of the examination. Patients with altered mental status often cannot confirm or deny pain from their injuries and therefore make physical examination less reliable. Patients with altered consciousness require more diagnostic testing to determine the extent of injury.

Secondary Assessment

Once basic and advanced life-support measures have been addressed, the nurse focuses on identification and management of specific injuries. The secondary assessment continues to rely heavily on the clinical examination, although obtaining an accurate health history and securing appropriate diagnostic tests are important also. The ability to perform a systematic evaluation and prioritize interventions is mandatory.

This section presents an overview of the secondary assessment and treatment of the patient with chest, pulmonary, and maxillofacial trauma. Assessment findings related to a specific condition (e.g., pneumothorax, fractured ribs) will be addressed in greater detail within that section. Secondary assessment of the abdomen, pelvis, and extremities and complete neurologic evaluation will not be discussed in this chapter.

History

An accurate history is valuable in determining diagnosis and guiding therapy. Historical data can be obtained from the patient, witnesses, and prehospital personnel. Important information to obtain includes the mechanism of injury and details of the event leading to the injury. For example, if a patient has sustained blunt trauma in an automobile accident, the nurse should ascertain details of the accident, such as the speed of the automobile before the event, time of the accident, degree and location of vehicle damage (e.g., steering wheel, windshield), patient's position in the vehicle, extrication, ejection, number of fatalities in the vehicle, and seat belt use. The use of seat belts is of particular importance, because it will influence the extent and type of injury (Green & Petrucelli, 1981; Stewart, 1988; Rutledge, et al., 1991). For example, the use of a lap belt only may result in maxillofacial trauma, whereas collisions involving no seat belts are likely to result in head, neck, and chest injuries. The driver of the vehicle is at additional risk for steering wheel injuries, particularly if he or she is unrestrained. These patients are at high risk for face, neck, thoracic, and abdominal injury. The nurse should investigate the type of instrument involved with penetrating trauma. If firearms have been involved, the type of weapon, caliber of the bullet, and distance it was fired from should be noted. High-velocity, large-caliber weapons result in higher kinetic energy missiles that have a greater potential for tissue destruction than shorter-barreled, low-caliber hand guns. In all accidents the nurse should determine the time of injury, the approximate amount of blood at scene, initial vital signs and physical examination, interventions performed by the prehospital care personnel, and fluids given en route.

Basic medical data obtained on all patients should include past medical history (particularly the preexistence of pulmonary or cardiovascular problems), allergies, medications, tetanus immunization status, and drug or alcohol history, last meal, areas of pain, and whether they are having difficulty breathing.

Physical assessment

The essentials of the physical assessment are inspection, palpation, percussion, and auscultation. Of these, inspection is probably used the most and percussion the least. Inspection entails evaluating skin color, respiratory rate and depth, evidence of external hemorrhage, penetrations, contusions, paradoxical motion, and deformities. Severe respiratory failure is usually easy to appreciate simply by observing the patient, noting facial expression, skin color, respiratory pattern or rate, and chest movements. Palpation is a valuable tool for evaluating tenderness, instability, crepitus (subcutaneous air), and chest excursion and identifying abnormal or deviated structures. Auscultation reveals information about airway patency (e.g., wheezing) and intraalveolar or intrapleural fluid (e.g., crackles, decreased breath sounds). Decreased breath sounds suggest lung collapse, atelectasis, and contusion or pleural fluid, and abnormal sounds (e.g., bowel) may indicate diaphragmatic rupture. Percussion is a useful technique in ascertaining the density of underlying structures. It can quickly differentiate a pneumothorax (hyperressonance) from a hemothorax (dullness). Although this technique is a valuable tool, unfortunately, it has been abandoned, largely because of the ease of rapidly obtaining chest x-ray results.

A variety of methods can be used in performing an organized physical assessment (e.g., systems, head to toe). The method presented here is a modified systems approach. Clinicians should use the method they feel most comfortable with. Access to the patient may be difficult because of the multitude of personnel involved in the patient's care and diagnostic procedures. Nonetheless, the nurse must collect his or her own set of assessment data to have a baseline with which to make subsequent comparisons. During this secondary assessment, the patient's airway, breathing, and circulation should be reevaluated.

Mental status Evaluating the patient's mental status begins in the primary assessment of level of consciousness (LOC) and continues with obtaining the history. Mental status is an important indicator of respiratory function. Confusion, agitation, and restlessness may be the earliest indicators of impaired gas exchange (Petty, 1974). Patients with depressed levels of consciousness should be suspect for brainstem injury and ventilatory impairment. If the patient is apneic, severe brainstem injury is likely. A standardized tool, such as the Glasgow coma scale, is useful for

evaluating trends in the patient's neurologic status.

The nurse should obtain information from prehospital care providers about the patient's LOC at the scene. A neurologic assessment should be obtained on admission to the ED and then at frequent intervals (i.e., every 15 to 60 minutes). The frequency of neurologic checks depends on the patient's risk of neurologic impairment. Emergency management of patients with neurologic injury includes providing ventilatory support and close monitoring of arterial blood gases, because Pao_2 and $Paco_2$ levels will impact cerebral blood flow and intracranial pressure. (See Chapter 10 for more information on patients with altered neurologic status.)

Head and neck The nurse should inspect the head for external signs of trauma, such as abrasions, contusions, penetrating wounds, or swelling. Areas of ecchymosis should be noted because they may indicate an underlying fracture. For example, ecchymosis in the periorbital area (raccoon eyes) and over the mastoid area (Battle's sign) is associated with a basilar skull fracture (Barrett, 1986). The ears and nose also should be inspected for bleeding or drainage. Serosanguineous fluid should be tested for the presence of cerebrospinal fluid (CSF) by placing a few drops on filter paper. If the fluid is CSF, a halo-like or bull's-eye configuration will appear. Patients with CSF leak or midface fractures should not be intubated nasally because the tube may inadvertently be passed into the brain (Jorden & Barkin, 1988). The nurse should examine the mouth, including the teeth, lips, gums, and palates, necessitating opening the patient's mouth and using a bright examination light. The nurse should note if any teeth are broken, loose, or missing, because they may have been aspirated and will contribute to airway obstruction. Any necessary airway suctioning or clearing should be performed as soon as the need is identified. The color of the mucous membrane can signify central cyanosis, a late sign of hypoxemia. The neck should be inspected for lacerations, hematomas, or ecchymosis. Both the head and neck should be gently palpated for tenderness, swelling, crepitus, and deformities. The nurse should carefully measure and describe hematomas and swelling so that any changes can be quickly appreciated. Abnormalities such as tracheal deviation are identified by palpation, although severe deviations may be apparent on inspection. The nurse should examine the head and neck carefully to maintain immobilization of the cervical spine until bony or spinal cord injury has been ruled out. The neck should be auscultated for abnormal sounds, such as wheezing or stridor, which accompany an obstructed airway. If the patient is intubated, the adequacy of cuff inflation should be assessed. Large leaks are evident by air escaping from the mouth and the patient being able to phonate. Less obvious leaks can be ascertained by auscultating the lateral neck. Air is injected into the pilot balloon cuff until the leak disappears. A small amount of air is then removed from the cuff until a slight leak is appreciated (i.e., minimal leak technique). This technique assures airway protection should further bleeding or emesis occur and minimizes tracheal injury from excessive cuff pressure.

In the management of head and neck injuries, the nurse should give priority to those conditions that result in airway obstruction, such as hematoma formation, edema, and bleeding. Trauma to the face can be potentially life threatening and is discussed in detail in the section on maxillofacial injuries.

Chest The secondary assessment of the chest should begin with a more in-depth assessment of respiratory rate, depth, and pattern. Gross abnormalities in ventilation (e.g., apnea) should have already been identified and managed. More subtle variations should be ascertained during this phase. For example, an increased respiratory rate may be a normal respiratory rate for that age (see Table 8-2); it may be a response to pain and anxiety; it may be a compensatory mechanism for metabolic acidosis; or it may represent respiratory decompensation. An increased respiratory rate, in combination with the use of accessory muscles, is suggestive of respiratory insufficiency. If the patient is awake, the nurse should ask about sensations of dyspnea or pain with respirations (pleuritic pain).

The nurse should then examine the patient for evidence of penetration, contusions, paradoxical motion, and deformities. Asymmetric chest movements such as occur with flail chest, ruptured diaphragm, or pneumothorax should be noted. Large flail segments can be stabilized by gentle but firm pressure, followed by application of a bulky dressing. Paradoxical breathing also may be

seen with respiratory failure. In this situation, the abdomen and respiratory muscles move out of synchronization with one another, resulting in ineffective ventilation. Palpation of the chest is useful in identifying areas of tenderness, instability (flail segments), embedded foreign objects, and crepitus. Crepitus occurs as air escapes from the lung and migrates into the soft tissues of the neck and upper torso.

Chest percussion may reveal air-filled spaces (hyperresonance) or consolidation (dullness), such as occur with pneumothorax and hemothorax, respectively. Percussion may be technically difficult in patients with massive chest injury or severe pain. Auscultation of the chest may reveal absent or abnormal (adventitious) breath sounds. Auscultation of the lower lung fields requires that the patient be log rolled to access the back. This is also the time to inspect and palpate the back. If it is impossible to move the patient, a reasonable alternative is to listen to the lateral chest in the midaxillary line at the fifth or sixth intercostal space. Until the cervical spine has been cleared for injury, the neck and upper torso should be handled as if an injury exists. Suspicion or even documentation of a cervical spine injury should not preclude examining the back.

Wheezing, stridor, or rhonchi are indicative of narrowed airways. When severe, these conditions are apparent without the aid of a stethoscope. Inspiratory wheezes are suggestive of upper airway obstruction; expiratory wheezing, lower airway obstruction. Crackles, formerly called *rales*, occur when air flows through fluid-filled passages, such as with pulmonary edema or hemorrhage. The absence of breath sounds indicate a lack of air flow, such as occurs with a pneumothorax. Some patients, such as those with emphysema, have chronically diminished breath sounds, making it difficult to recognize an acute process. Other patients may appear to have breath sounds, but actually have only referred sounds from the opposite lung (e.g., with pneumothorax or after pneumonectomy). Trauma patients with abnormal pulmonary sounds should undergo diagnostic studies.

DIAGNOSTIC AND MONITORING PROCEDURES

Routine diagnostic studies in the trauma patient with suspected alterations in gas exchange include

---

Normal blood gas values on room air at sea level

Arterial	Mixed venous
pH = 7.35 − 7.45	pH = 7.32 − 7.42
$Paco_2$ = 35 − 45 mm Hg	$Pvco_2$ = 41 − 51 mm Hg
HCO_3^- = 20 − 28 mEq	HCO_3^- = 20 − 28 mEq
Pao_2 80 − 100 mm Hg	Pvo_2 = 35 − 45 mm Hg
Sao_2 = 95%	Svo_2 = 75%

---

arterial blood gases and x-ray (cervical and chest) examinations. In addition to routine monitoring of vital signs, the patient with actual or suspected alterations in breathing patterns or gas exchange may require continuous or intermittent monitoring of oxygenation and carbon dioxide elimination. More definitive assessment may be required to manage unstable or critical patients (determination of pulmonary artery pressures, cardiac output, and mixed venous blood gas values).

Arterial Blood Gases

ABG analysis is considered the most accurate and reliable method of evaluating arterial oxygenation, carbon dioxide elimination, and acid-base status. Normal ABG values on room air (see box above) indicate that ventilation and alveolar pulmonary gas exchange are normal.

Oxygenation

Hypoxemia is the term to describe a partial pressure of oxygen (Pao_2) of less than 80 mm Hg (at sea level). Trauma patients may experience hypoxemia secondary to ventilation/perfusion ($\dot{V}/\dot{Q}$) mismatching (e.g., atelectasis, pulmonary contusion) or shunt, or impaired ventilation (e.g., secondary to head injury).

Many formulas are available to assist the clinician in identifying the cause and extent of hypoxemia (Table 8-4). The alveolar-arterial oxygen difference (A-a gradient) and shunt fraction (Qs/QT) are among the most common. Many of these equations are too cumbersome to be practical in the ED setting. To determine shunt, for example, requires placement of a pulmonary artery catheter. The A-a gradient on the other hand requires only results from an ABG study and knowledge of

the FIo_2. The A-a gradient is calculated by the following equation:

$$FIo_2 \ (760 \ mm \ Hg - 47 \ mm \ Hg) - 1.2 \ (Paco_2) - Pao_2$$

where FIo_2 equals the percent of oxygen in the inspired air, 760 mm Hg equals atmospheric pressure at sea level, and 47 mm Hg equals water vaper pressure. If the patient is breathing room air at sea level, this equation can be simplified to the following:

$$A\text{-}a \ gradient = 150 - 1.2 \ (Paco_2) - Pao_2$$

Normal, healthy adults have an A-a gradient of 10 mm Hg on room air. The A-a gradient increases with age and FIo_2, but should not be greater than 100 on an FIo_2 of 100%. An A-a gradient of greater than 350 on 100% oxygen suggests severe gas exchange abnormalities (Sahn, Lakshminarayan, & Petty, 1967). If an A-a gradient is widened, the hypoxemia is likely to be the result of pulmonary dysfunction rather than hypoventilation. Recently the Pao_2/FIo_2 ratio has been suggested as a means of evaluating gas exchange in the lung at varying levels of supplemental oxygen. A normal Pao_2/FIo_2 ratio is greater than 350 (Tashkin, Flick, Bellamy, & Mecurio, 1987).

CO_2 elimination

The $Paco_2$ is directly related to the alveolar ventilation. A low $Paco_2$ (i.e., hypocapnia) may suggest that the patient is ventilating more than the metabolic needs of the body (i.e., hyperventilation). This may be a normal response to pain or anxiety or a compensatory response to a metabolic acidosis. Patients compensate for a metabolic acidosis by hyperventilating, which creates a respiratory alkalosis.

To determine if a patient is adequately responding to a metabolic acidosis by hyperventilation, the following equation is used:

$$Paco_2 = 1.5 \ (HCO_3^-) + 8 \pm 2$$

where $Paco_2$ is the expected $Paco_2$ and HCO_3^- is the measured plasma bicarbonate. This equation predicts how much a normal individual should be hyperventilating in response to the degree of metabolic acidosis (Gardner, 1986). If a patient's measured $Paco_2$ is higher than the predicted $Paco_2$, he or she is hypoventilating in response to

Table 8-4 Formulas for evaluating oxygenation

Term	Formula	Use	Normal value	Comments
A-a gradient	$PAO_2 - PaO_2$ $PAO_2 = FIO_2 (P_B - 47) -$ 1.2 $PaCO_2$ P_B = barometric pressure	Measures the difference between the oxygen tension in the alveoli and in the artery. The A-a gradient is widened when the problem with oxygenation lies in the lung itself, and is normal when extrapulmonary factors are responsible for the hypoxemia.	<10 on room air <100 on FIO_2 of 1.0	Also called A-a DO_2 (Alveolar-arterial O_2 difference)
Shunt fraction	$\dfrac{Q_S}{Q_T} = \dfrac{CcO_2 - CaO_2}{CcO_2 - CvO_2}$ $CcO_2 = O_2$ content of end capillary blood $CaO_2 = O_2$ content of arterial blood $CvO_2 = O_2$ content of venous blood	Used to determine how much blood is being shunted past unoxygenated alveoli.	5%	Requires a pulmonary artery catheter to calculate. Can be estimated as follows (on 100% FIO_2): For each 20 mm Hg reduction in PaO_2 below 700, there is a 1% shunt. So, if the PaO_2 is 600, there is a 5% shunt.
P/F ratio	$\dfrac{PaO_2}{FIO_2}$	Used to roughly approximate the A-a gradient with patients receiving from 4%-70% FIO_2.	>350	Is useful in following trends at varying levels of FIO_2.

A, alveolar; *a*, arterial; *Q*s, shunt flow; *Q*T, cardiac output or total flow.

acidosis. This implies that the patient may be in respiratory failure even if he or she still has a respiratory alkalosis. This may occur in a hypotensive patient with a metabolic acidosis from lactate accumulation who is not adequately hyperventilating because of a head injury.

Hypocapnia may also be iatrogenically induced via dialed-in ventilator settings that overshoot the patient's minute ventilation needs. Patients may be admitted with a normal or low $PaCO_2$, which gradually or acutely increases as they tire or respiratory failure worsens.

Increases in the $PaCO_2$ (i.e., hypercapnia) indicate the minute ventilation is inadequate in meeting the metabolic needs of the body (i.e., hypoventilation). Hypoventilation results in respiratory acidosis and is best treated by increasing minute ventilation (e.g., naloxone to reverse narcotic-

induced respiratory depression, intubation and hyperventilation for the head-injured patient). Bicarbonate is not appropriate for the treatment of respiratory acidosis.

Interpreting acid-base status

The acid-base status is evaluated by measurement of pH and $PaCO_2$ in arterial blood gases, and bicarbonate (i.e., carbonic acid) concentration. The bicarbonate concentration reported with most blood gas results is a calculated value rather than an actual measurement. Measured serum CO_2 concentration (carbonic acid, which reflects the bicarbonate level) is most often obtained with venous electrolyte determinations.

To determine the acid-base status of the patient, one first determines the respiratory component for the patient's pH. Changes in $PaCO_2$ result in immediate changes in pH. Hyperventilation ($Paco_2$ <35 torr) results in a respiratory alkalosis, and hypoventilation ($Paco_2$ >45 torr) results in a respiratory acidosis. One can estimate the change in pH caused by alterations in $Paco_2$ in that for every change of 10 mm Hg $Paco_2$, pH changes in the reverse direction approximately 0.08 units (AHA, 1986).

After correcting for the respiratory component, one can determine if the patient has a metabolic acidosis (pH <7.35) or metabolic alkalosis (pH >7.45). Patients often have a mixed acid-base disorder, in which the primary disorder (e.g., metabolic acidosis caused by lactate accumulation in a hypotensive patient) is partially compensated for with an opposing disorder (respiratory alkalosis from hyperventilation).

Chest X-ray Examination

Chest x-ray (CXR) examinations are useful in identifying injuries and assessing placement of invasive devices (e.g., endotracheal tubes, central venous lines). Initial evaluation is usually performed with a portable anteroposterior film; in patients who have sustained blunt trauma and those in whom cervical spine injury has not been ruled out, this film is obtained with the patient supine. Supine chest films may make it more difficult to diagnose a hemothorax (diffuse opacification as blood layers out evenly along the back of the lung) or widened mediastinum. Once the patient has been stabilized and the cervical spine cleared, a posterioanterior film should be taken with the patient sitting upright. With the patient upright, it is easier (1) to detect hemothorax (opacification of the costophrenic angle), pneumoperitoneum (air under the diaphragm), and pulmonary contusions (area of increased opacification), and (2) to determine heart size and width of mediastinum. Small hemothoraxes (< 300 ml) require lateral views to detect. Pneumothorax is best detected by expiratory chest x-ray films, but an inspiratory film should always be obtained first to detect a widened mediastinum (suggestive of aortic disruption), an enlarged cardiac silhouette (suggestive of hemopericardium), a pulmonary contusion, or a significant pneumothorax. Chest x-ray examinations can sometimes detect rib fractures, spinal fractures, and, rarely, a ruptured diaphragm. A CXR film should be obtained promptly after placement of central lines, endotracheal tubes, and chest tubes to ensure correct position, infla-

tion of collapsed lung, or drainage of a hemothorax, and to rule out iatrogenic complications (e.g., pneumothorax).

Monitoring Gas Exchange
Po_2 and oxygen saturation

A variety of methods is available to monitor Sao_2 or Po_2 in the ED. These include pulse and ear oximetry and transcutaneous and transconjunctival Po_2 monitoring. Pulse and ear oximetry are widely used in critical care areas to noninvasively monitor Sao_2, either continuously or intermittently. This technique uses fiberoptics to determine the saturation of hemoglobin with oxygen. Studies indicate that a close correlation exists between measured arterial saturations and saturations detected by pulse oximetry and that pulse oximetry is a reliable indicator of hypoxemia (Niehoff et al., 1988; Yelderman & New, 1983). Oximetry has been demonstrated to be unreliable in patients with carbon monoxide poisoning and in patients who are jaundiced (Chaudhary & Burki, 1978; Douglas et al., 1979). Two common clinical problems with pulse and ear oximetry are the difficulty securing the sensors in agitated patients and the inability to detect a pulse signal during low-flow states. Despite its limitations, this method of noninvasive monitoring can be valuable in the detection of life-threatening hypoxemia and provides a simple means of evaluating the effectiveness of therapy (e.g., titrating the FIo_2, placement of a chest tube). Normal Sao_2 is 95%-97%; however, saturations greater than 90% (i.e., Pao_2 >60 mm Hg) are generally considered acceptable.

Newer but less widely used techniques of monitoring oxygenation are transcutaneous and transconjunctival Po_2 monitoring ($TcjO_2$). Transcutaneous Po_2 monitoring is used primarily in neonates and infants, whose thin skin allows properly placed electrodes to monitor capillary blood gas tension. Warming the skin underneath the electrode increases flow to the skin where Po_2 is measured. This technique has been demonstrated to be a reliable method of monitoring Po_2 in infants (Peabody, Willis, Gregory, Tooley, & Lucey, 1978). Disadvantages of this technique include the potential for burns, requiring repositioning of the electrode every 2 to 3 hours. Conjunctival oxygen tension monitoring uses miniaturized polarographic oxygen electrodes placed on the palpebral conjunctiva to continuously measure tissue oxygenation. In patients with normal cardiac output and tissue perfusion, the $TcjO_2$ correlates well with the PaO_2. However, because the $TcjO_2$ is flow dependent, it becomes disassociated from the PaO_2 in patients with impaired perfusion. In multiple trauma patients, a $PaO_2/TcjO_2$ index below 0.5 may identify patients with blood loss in excess of 1000 ml before any alteration in blood pressure has occurred (Abraham, Lee, & Morgan, 1986). Studies also suggest that the conjunctival oxygen tension index (the ratio of PaO_2 to $TcjO_2$) can be used to differentiate hypoxemia alone from hypoxemia associated with poor cardiac output (Abraham & Fink, 1988). Conjunctival monitoring may therefore be useful in monitoring patients with perfusion and ventilation problems, such as occurs with tension pneumothorax and hemothorax.

Carbon dioxide (capnography)

Bedside capnography allows for intermittent or continuous evaluation of CO_2 elimination. A capnogram is a displayed waveform of CO_2 content in the exhaled gas (Figure 8-8). Although primarily used in intubated patients, it can also be adapted for spontaneously breathing patients. Immediately after intubation it can be used to detect inadvertent esophageal placement (absence of CO_2). Capnography can also be useful in detecting altered ventilatory patterns not apparent by the clinical examination. The reliability of these devices continues to come under scrutiny. Some investigators have suggested that although measurement of end tidal CO_2 is helpful in evaluating trends, it is not a reliable indicator of hypercapnia (Niehoff et al., 1988).

Pulmonary artery catheters

Although most trauma patients do not require invasive monitoring to determine cardiopulmonary and fluid status, some critically ill patients may ultimately require it. Pulmonary artery (PA) catheters allow for the measurement of cardiac output, preload (pulmonary capillary wedge pressure) and afterload (systemic vascular resistance). Mixed venous blood gases obtained via the distal port of the PA catheter allow for the evaluation of the amount of oxygen utilized at the tissue level.

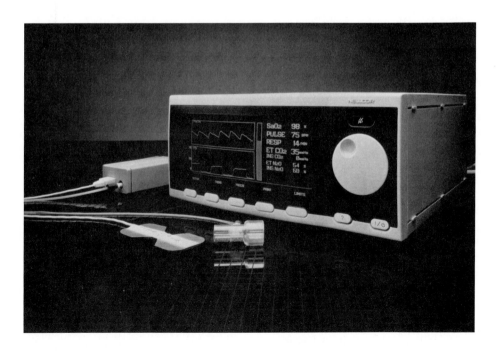

Figure 8-8 Nellcor® N-1000 bedside capnographer. New technology allows for both oxygen saturation (SaO_2) and end tidal carbon dioxide ($ETcO_2$) monitoring. (Courtesy Nellcor Inc. Hayward, Calif.)

Normally, 25% of the oxygen delivery to the tissues is utilized, and therefore the blood returning to the heart (mixed venous) is 75% saturated ($SvO_2 = 75\%$). Recently a PA catheter has been introduced that allows for the continuous monitoring of SvO_2. Low levels of SvO_2 ($< 60\%$) suggest decreased O_2 delivery or increased O_2 demand. When the SvO_2 decreases to 40%, lactic acid is produced and outcome is adversely affected. Higher than normal SvO_2 ($> 80\%$) indicates increased O_2 delivery or decreased O_2 utilization at the tissue level. Abnormally high SvO_2 is seen in patients with sepsis secondary to peripheral shunting and with cyanide or carbon monoxide poisoning, where tissue uptake of O_2 is impaired. SvO_2 has been reported to be a predictor of outcome in trauma patients with hemorrhagic shock and was considered to be a helpful parameter during the resuscitative, operative, and postoperative period (Kazarian & DelGuercio, 1980). The continuous evaluation of SvO_2 in the ED currently is not a standard of care. However, central venous O_2 saturation can be used to approximate SvO_2 and may be useful in managing patients. Further studies investigating the usefulness of SvO_2 monitoring in trauma patients are needed.

Data obtained with the PA catheter (specifically, cardiac output) together with arterial and venous blood gas results can be used in the determination of oxygen delivery and utilization. PA catheters in the trauma patient may be used to optimize PEEP therapy in patients with pulmonary contusions or the adult respiratory distress syndrome (ARDS).

ASSESSMENT AND INTERVENTIONS RELATED TO SPECIFIC INJURIES

This section discusses the most common injuries leading to impaired gas exchange secondary to thoracic, pulmonary, and maxillofacial trauma. These injuries include soft tissue injuries, maxillofacial trauma, sternal fractures, fractured ribs, flail chest, pulmonary contusion, pneumothorax, tension pneumothorax, hemothorax, ruptured diaphragm, and tracheobronchial injuries.

Soft Tissue Trauma

Soft tissue injuries   Ineffective airway clearance
High risk for infection
High risk for body image
    disturbance
Pain

Trauma to the soft tissue includes lacerations, abrasions, contusions, burns, and avulsions. Soft tissue injury may occur alone or in combination with facial fractures. Effective management of soft tissue injury includes pain control, cleaning, debridement, and closure when necessary. Pain management may necessitate local or regional anesthetics or parenteral medications. Parenteral narcotics should be administered judiciously if neurologic involvement is suspected.

Conservative debridement of the face is recommended. The face is vascular, and therefore tissue that might otherwise seem devitalized may survive on the face. All wounds should be thoroughly cleaned; irrigation is ideal. Superficial wounds need only be cleaned and dressed. Lacerations should be repaired promptly, often with a layered closure. If wounds are superficial but closure is desirable, Steri-Strips should be considered. Repair of complicated wounds may require the skills of an experienced plastic surgeon.

Skeletal Injuries

The diagnosis and management of facial fractures depends on the type of injury involved. A brief review of several types of facial fractures is presented here. The reader is referred to other writings for more detail on this subject (Barrett, 1986; Manson, 1984).

Maxillofacial injuries   Ineffective airway
    clearance
High risk for aspiration
High risk for fluid volume
    deficit
High risk for body image
    disturbance
Pain

The face has many prominent areas and is, therefore, highly susceptible to different types of deceleration injuries. Maxillofacial injuries are frequently dramatic and may be disfiguring. Penetrating trauma may cause severe structural damage, which is not as readily apparent. Nasal, zygomal, orbital, and mandibular fractures are common. In addition to the fractures and soft tissue injury associated with maxillofacial injury, these patients are at high risk for life-threatening airway obstruction. Optimal management of maxillofacial trauma demands the combined efforts of a skilled ED and head and neck or plastic surgery team. The psychosocial as well as the physical trauma associated with these injuries challenge the nurse.

In the management of patients with maxillofacial trauma, priority must be given to ensuring a patent airway. Obstruction may occur instantaneously or slowly, as edema and bleeding progressively occlude the airway. Initial airway management involves clearing the mouth and throat of foreign material, including blood, vomitus, fractured teeth, and bridgework. A firm, plastic catheter (e.g., tonsil tip) may be helpful in clearing secretions from the mouth. The nurse must not aggravate existing injuries with overzealous suctioning techniques. Injury to the cervical spine should be ruled out quickly, either clinically or radiographically, in case intubation is required later. If the patient is unresponsive, airway management includes (1) radiographic clearance of a stabilized cervical spine and (2) either placement of an oral airway to move the tongue away from the pharynx or intubation. The nurse must be careful to avoid aggravating cervical spine injuries, which are frequently associated with facial trauma (Manson, 1984). Intubation may be technically difficult with significant maxillofacial trauma, making a cricothyroidotomy the method of choice in securing an emergency airway. The clinician must be alert for signs and symptoms of airway obstruction, including agitation, intercostal retractions, dyspnea, cyanosis, gurgling, stridor, wheezing, and a SaO_2 less than 90% (PaO_2 ~ 60 mm Hg).

In the secondary survey, careful, systematic assessment of the head and face is mandatory. The nurse should carefully observe for evidence of bleeding and swelling. Open fractures will be obvious; underlying fractures should be suspected under areas of ecchymosis or contusion. The face should be inspected for symmetry and the presence of any obvious deformity. A wallet photograph, such as the one on the driver's license, may be used as a reference to the patient's premorbid appearance. The head and face should be palpated for crepitus bony irregularity, tenderness, and swelling. The upper jaw and face should be checked for mobility to determine the presence of a Le Fort fracture. Sensory and motor nerve function should be evaluated. Patients who are able should be asked to bite down while the examiner palpates the temporomandibular joint. If the patient admits malocclusion, a fracture should be suspected. Pain on palpation is also

suggestive of a fracture. Visual disturbances, such as diplopia or diminished vision, may indicate ocular injury, muscle entrapment, or globe rupture.

Life-threatening complications and injuries associated with maxillofacial trauma include aspiration, cervical spine injuries, intracranial injury, and hemorrhage. These conditions must be treated before definitive therapy can be initiated. Aspiration of gastric contents, blood, or secretions is always a potential problem in patients with maxillofacial trauma. Suctioning is the primary method of clearing secretions. The patient should be positioned appropriately (i.e., upright or on the side) as soon as cervical spine injury has been ruled out, to avoid aspiration. Patients with decreased level of consciousness (LOC) or who are sedated are at increased risk for aspiration. Blood in the stomach also increases nausea and vomiting, increasing the risk of aspiration.

Airway patency is of critical importance in patients with maxillofacial trauma. The nurse must be careful when positioning these patients to avoid iatrogenic spinal injury. If airway management is immediately necessary before cervical spine injury can be ruled out, in-line stabilization of the neck should be performed during intubation (Majernick et al., 1986). Patients with maxillofacial trauma may also present with associated intracranial injury, particularly with severe nasal, nasoorbital, frontal, and Le Fort fractures. The patient's neurologic status, including LOC and motor function, should be assessed frequently.

Hemorrhage can result from facial lacerations, as well as from lacerations of arteries and veins in fractured sinuses of the face. Bleeding from facial wounds can be significant and should be controlled by direct pressure or quick suturing. Hemorrhage from facial fractures often manifests as nasal bleeding. Controlling this type of bleeding is accomplished with manual reduction of the fracture, nasal packing, and external compression dressings (Manson, 1984).

Radiographic evaluation can be used to confirm clinical suspicions of facial fractures. Emergent computerized tomographic scanning should be considered on patients with frontal, orbital, nasoethmoid, sinus, supraorbital, and Le Fort II and III fractures. Definitive management of maxillofacial trauma includes treatment of soft tissue wounds and facial fractures but should be performed after treating more life-threatening injuries. Fractures of facial bones having high resis-

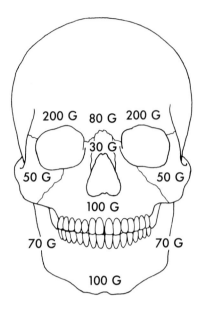

Figure 8-9   Resistance of various parts of facial skeleton to fracture-producing forces. Medial orbital walls, ethmoid sinuses, and cribriform area are fragile, whereas substantial force is required to fracture supraorbital ridge. G, gravitational forces. (*Note*. Redrawn from "Review of 1000 Major Facial Fractures and Associated Injuries" by E.A. Luce, T.D. Tubb, and A.M. Moore, 1979, *Plastic and Reconstructive Surgery*, 63, [1], p. 29.)

tance to impact (high gravitational [G]-force required to break bone) are more often associated with other major injuries. Figure 8-9 illustrates the G-forces required to produce fractures of the facial skeleton (Luce, Tubb, & Moore, 1979).

| **Nasal fractures** | High risk for infection
High risk for body image
disturbance
Pain |

Nasal fractures are common with blunt trauma because of the prominence of the nose and lack of supportive structures. Clinical findings with nasal fractures included pain, swelling, bruising, lateral deviation, flattening of the nasal pyramid, crepitus, and tenderness. When there is nasal trauma, a septal hematoma should be ruled out. Nasal x-ray films generally are not helpful in the acute treatment of nasal fractures. Definitive treatment may require manipulation of displaced fragments and open reduction with internal wiring.

| **Nasoorbital fractures** | High risk for infection
High risk for body image
disturbance
Pain |

A direct, intense blow to the bridge of the nose may result in a fracture of the nasoorbital area. Clinical findings of these fractures include tenderness, epistaxis, hematoma, and rhinorrhea. Altered neurologic findings in conjunction with a nasoorbital fracture are suggestive of bone infringing on brain tissue. Treatment of these fractures includes surgical repair and prophylactic antibiotic therapy (e.g., penicillin), to lessen the risk of meningitis.

| **Mandibular fractures** | Ineffective airway
clearance
High risk for body image
disturbance
High risk for altered
nutrition: less than
body requirements
Pain |

The mandible may be fractured or displaced secondary to blunt trauma. The severity of the fracture depends on the mechanism of injury and the dentition of the jaw (the more teeth, the less severe the fracture). Clinical findings depend on the area of the mandible affected, but typically include tenderness, edema, crepitus, ecchymosis, and malocclusion. Panoramic views of the mandible are the best way to diagnose mandibular fractures, but regular mandibular films will detect most of the fractures. Treatment of mandibular fractures requires surgical intervention, which is usually delayed until the patient has stabilized.

| **Le Fort fractures** | Ineffective airway clearance
High risk for aspiration
High risk for body image
disturbance
High risk for infection
Pain |

Maxillary fractures (Le Fort I, II, and III) are classified according to the level at which the maxillary dentition is separated from the upper facial or cranial skeleton (Figure 8-10). Le Fort I fractures result in a horizontal fracture through the body of the maxilla and separate the maxillary alveolus from the upper facial skeleton. Le Fort II

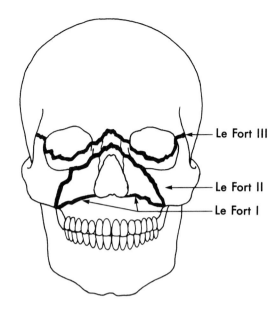

Le Fort III

Le Fort II

Le Fort I

Figure 8-10 Le Fort's classification of maxillary fractures.

fractures separate the central pyramid-shaped nasomaxillary segment from the zygomatic and orbital portion of the facial skeleton. Le Fort III fractures, also called *craniofacial fractures,* separate the facial bones from the cranial skeleton through the orbits.

Clinical findings associated with Le Fort fractures include pain, swelling, nasopharyngeal bleeding, tenderness, mobile maxilla, and malocclusion. A cerebrospinal fluid (CSF) leak may occur in 25% to 50% of Le Fort II and III fractures (Manson, 1984). Management of Le Fort fractures initially is directed at maintaining the airway, which may be compromised secondary to edema or bleeding. If a CSF leak is present, a cricothyroidotomy is typically the airway of choice. Definitive treatment of Le Fort fractures is typically delayed for several days until the edema subsides. If CSF leakage is present, proper antibiotic therapy should be instituted.

Sternal fractures   Ineffective breathing pattern
Pain

Sternal fractures result from significant force to the chest such as occurs with blunt trauma (e.g., steering wheel injury). The major concern with sternal fractures is the potential for associated in-

jury, such as myocardial or pulmonary contusion and cardiac tamponade. Clinical findings of sternal fractures include point tenderness and sternal pain. A lateral chest x-ray study will confirm the presence of a sternal fracture. Management of sternal fractures includes analgesics and observation for respiratory difficulty. Seriously displaced fractures may produce a flail chest and in some cases will require internal stabilization with mechanical ventilation (Vukich & Markovchick, 1988).

Fractured ribs   Ineffective breathing pattern
High risk for infection
Pain

Simple rib fractures are the most common form of significant chest injury seen with blunt trauma (Dougall, Paul, & Finely, 1977). Patients who are young and otherwise healthy do not typically experience any pulmonary complications with rib fractures. Children's ribs in particular have resilient cartilage, which can deform without fracturing. On the other hand, elderly patients or those with underlying lung disease have the potential to develop life-threatening complications, such as pneumonia. When assessing rib fractures, the nurse must be alert to the potential for associated injuries, such as damage to the mediastinum, pleura, lung, liver, kidney, or spleen. Fractures of the first and second ribs are associated with a high incidence (60%) of vascular injury (Phillips, Rogers, & Gasper, 1981). Lower rib fractures (ninth through eleventh) are more commonly associated with abdominal injury (Kattan, 1978). Rib fractures are diagnosed frequently on the basis of clinical findings (e.g., pain, ecchymoses, crepitus) and may be verified by x-ray examination. The pain associated with fractures may be elicited or aggravated by palpation (point tenderness), movement, or breathing. The patient's respiratory rate may be normal or increased secondary to pain, but is typically shallow as the patient attempts to splint. Management of the patient with rib fractures entails providing adequate pain control without impairing ventilation. In most cases this goal is achieved by the administration of oral analgesics, such as codeine (30 to 120 mg every 4 hours). Patients with a tenuous pulmonary status require close monitoring of ventilatory status and signs of oversedation (e.g., drowsiness, confusion). Optimal pain control in some patients will require the use of intercostal block with long-acting anesthetics, such as bupivacaine (Marcaine), which may provide relief from pain for up to 48 hours. The use of binders or belts to stabilize the chest are not recommended because they promote hypoventilation (Barrett, 1987; Vukich & Markovchick, 1988).

Patients with two or more rib fractures who are at high risk of developing complications (e.g., the elderly) should be considered for hospitalization. These patients require monitoring and encouragement of mobility, coughing, and deep breathing to prevent atelectasis and pneumonia. Appropriate pain management is critical to ensure that patients can tolerate these important activities. Seven or more rib fractures are associated with a high incidence of concomitant intrathoracic injury, such as pneumothorax, hemothorax, and pulmonary contusion. Patients with rib fractures who require positive pressure ventilation are at increased risk of developing a pneumothorax and should be monitored closely for this complication.

Flail chest   Ineffective breathing pattern
Impaired gas exchange
High risk for infection
Pain

A flail chest is present when three or more adjacent ribs are fractured at two points. The result is a loose, or flailing, segment that alters normal ventilation. The flailing segment moves opposite to normal; that is, it moves inward on inspiration and outward on expiration. This paradoxical breathing, known as *pendelluft*, is the hallmark of a flail chest (Figure 8-11). Impaired ventilation secondary to this pendelluft was once believed to be solely responsible for the derangement in gas exchange seen in these patients. It is now believed that a variety of factors influence the ventilation and gas exchange process, including underlying pulmonary injury, atelectasis, and pain secondary to splinting (Shackford, Virgilio, & Peters, 1981; Treasure, 1979).

The diagnosis of flail chest requires careful inspection of the patient's respiratory movements. This is particularly challenging in patients with posterior flails. Not only is the back of the patient difficult to observe, but the muscles of the scapula and sacrospinals support the chest wall and reduce paradoxical motion. Muscle spasm can also

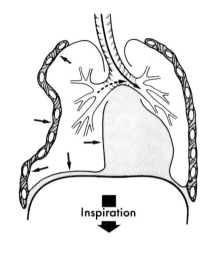

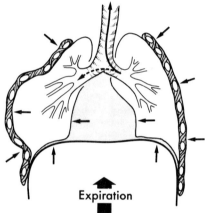

Figure 8-11   Flail chest. (*Note.* From *Trauma: The First Hour* [p. 108] by W.G. Baxt (Ed.), 1985, Norwalk, CT: Appleton & Lange.)

splint the flail segment and hinder important findings. A flail may become more obvious as the patient fatigues or the level of consciousness diminishes and splinting becomes less effective. The examiner must retain a high degree of suspicion when examining a patient with a potential for flail chest. If ventilation is impaired, the patient will exhibit signs and symptoms of acute respiratory failure, including altered mental status, decreased Sao_2, increased A-a gradient, and increased $Paco_2$.

Management of the patient with a flail chest in the field begins by ensuring an airway, administering oxygen, assisting ventilation as needed, and stabilizing the flail segment with manual pressure followed by a bulky dressing taped to the chest wall (Peitzman & Paris, 1988). When the patient arrives in the ED, the nurse should assess and maximize gas exchange, identify associated injuries, avoid fluid overload, and provide adequate pain control. Hemothoraxes and pneumothoraxes are commonly associated with flail chests and should be rapidly diagnosed and treated. Controversy exists over the value of stabilizing the chest to improve ventilation. Both internal and external methods have been recommended. Simple maneuvers are recommended to externally provide support to the chest wall; these include manual pressure, bulky dressings, sandbags, and positioning the patient on the flailing side. The effect of these maneuvers on gas exchange has not been well documented. Studies on the use of internal stabilization suggest that mechanical ventilation should be reserved for high-risk patients (i.e., those in respiratory failure or shock and older patients) (Adams, & Flint, 1982; Miller et al., 1983; Richardson, Shackford et al., 1981). Experts agree that a conservative approach using pain management and pulmonary hygiene is appropriate in most cases.

Patients with a flail chest who are placed on positive-pressure ventilation (e.g., in the operating room) are at increased risk of developing a pneumothorax and should be monitored closely for this complication or have a prophylactic chest tube placed. Surgical repair of the patient with a flail chest using open reduction and internal fixation has been recommended also. Regardless of the technique used, oxygenation and carbon dioxide elimination must be carefully monitored with all procedures. For example, repositioning the patient on the side of the flail may result in altered $\dot{V}/\dot{Q}$, resulting in alterations in gas exchange. Studies suggest that placing patients with pneumonia with the "good lung down" improves $\dot{V}/\dot{Q}$ matching and results in increased oxygenation (Dhainaut, Bons, Bricard, & Monsallier, 1980). Therefore placing the flail side down may be detrimental to the patient, in that the "bad lung" may be down, such as when the patient has a pulmonary contusion or pneumothorax. All patients need good pulmonary toilet, adequate pain control, supplemental oxygen, avoidance of excessive fluids, and judicious use of diuretics.

The morbidity and mortality of flail chest is related to the extent of underlying injuries (e.g., pulmonary contusion). Increased age, depressed level of consciousness, decreased preinjury pulmonary reserve, and shock are associated with poor prognosis (Miller et al., 1983; Shackford et al., 1981; Treasure, 1979).

Other Injuries

Pulmonary contusion   Impaired gas exchange
High risk for infection
Pain

A pulmonary contusion is a traumatic parenchymal injury associated with edema and hemorrhage without an actual laceration of lung tissue. A large percent of patients with blunt chest trauma suffer pulmonary contusions—most commonly those who experienced rapid deceleration in automobile collisions. Pulmonary contusion is considered the most common, potentially lethal, traumatic chest injury seen in the United States (Granovetter, 1985). The lung damage associated with pulmonary contusion develops gradually, requiring prolonged, close monitoring. A high degree of suspicion for pulmonary contusion should be maintained whenever a patient experiences a high-speed automobile collision, a significant fall, or other injury related to an intense force. It should also be suspected in patients with chest wall tenderness, ecchymoses, rib fractures, and hypoxemia. Pathologic changes associated with pulmonary contusion include extravasation of blood into the intraalveolar and interstitial spaces, increased capillary membrane permeability, and pulmonary edema. The result of these events are $\dot{V}/\dot{Q}$ mismatching, shunt, and poor lung distensibility (i.e., decreased compliance).

Clinical manifestations of pulmonary contusion can vary markedly, depending on the extent of the injury. Patients may be asymptomatic, or they may be dyspneic, tachypneic, hypoxemic, and hypotensive. Hemoptysis associated with a constant, loose cough may be present. Crackles and diminished breath sounds on the affected side may be noted also. Fractured ribs or a flail chest is commonly associated with pulmonary contusions. The chest x-ray film is characterized by a hazy lobar or segmental opacity, which typically occurs within minutes of the injury (Figure 8-12).

Treatment of pulmonary contusion is supportive and aimed at improving gas exchange. Hy-

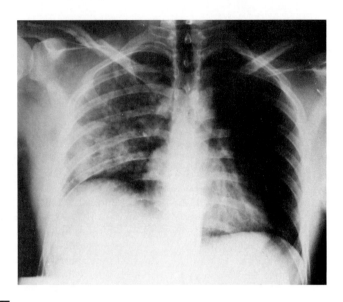

Figure 8-12 Pulmonary contusion. Chest x-ray film of 28-year-old man involved in motor vehicle accident. Note diffuse alveolar pattern in right chest from pulmonary contusion. (Courtesy Harbor-UCLA Medical Center.)

poxic patients should be treated with high-flow supplemental oxygen. Nonrebreathing face masks (oxygen at 15 L/min) usually deliver a maximum FIO_2 of approximately 85%. If conventional therapy does not improve the patient's oxygenation, a CPAP (continuous positive airway pressure) mask should be tried. This therapy may eliminate the need for more invasive management for patients who are hypoxemic but not in ventilatory failure. If the patient's condition deteriorates despite CPAP therapy, an endotracheal tube should be placed and 100% oxygen delivered. Patients who are awake may require sedation and possibly paralysis to facilitate intubation. Patients with large pulmonary contusions and significant shunts (greater than 20%) may benefit from the use of positive end expiratory pressure (PEEP). When PEEP is used, its potential effect on cardiac output must be considered. Studies suggest that PEEP therapy decreases cardiac output for a variety of reasons, including diminished venous return and decreased cardiac distensibility. Ultimately, the clinician is interested in evaluating the impact of PEEP on oxygen delivery (cardiac output $\times$ 1.38 $\times$ Hgb $\times$ Sao_2) and not just on oxygenation (Pao_2 or Sao_2). Additional supportive

care includes fluid administration, bronchial hygiene, and pain management.

The definitive treatment of significant pulmonary contusions occurs in an ICU setting where continuous monitoring of oxygenation, ventilation, and hemodynamic status is feasible. Patients benefit from a variety of monitoring modalities, including pulse oximetry, pulmonary artery, and Svo_2 monitoring. Formulas such as the A-a gradient, Pao_2/FIO_2 and shunt equation can be used to help follow trends in the patient's progress. Additional supportive care includes appropriate fluid administration, optimization of hematocrit, bronchial hygiene, and pain management. Mortality in patients with pulmonary contusions is increased when the injury severity score is equal to or greater than 25, initial Glasgow coma scale score is equal to or less than 7, transfusions of more than three units of blood are required, and Pao_2/FIO_2 is less than 300 (Johnson, Cogbill, & Winga, 1986).

Pneumothorax Impaired gas exchange
High risk for decreased cardiac
  output
High risk for infection
Pain

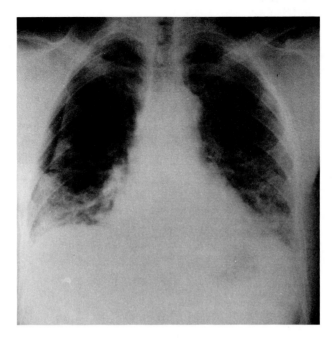

Figure 8-13   Pneumothorax. Expiratory chest x-ray film of 65-year-old man with right-sided pneumothorax. (Courtesy Harbor-UCLA Medical Center.)

Normal ventilation requires an intact chest wall and pleura. The accumulation of air in the pleural space alters the normal pressure gradient between the intrapleural and intraalveolar spaces, resulting in impaired ventilation and gas exchange. Pneumothoraxes are divided into three classes: simple (closed), communicating (open), and tension.

Simple pneumothorax   Simple (noncommunicating, or closed) pneumothorax is generally seen with blunt chest trauma. In this injury no communication exists between the pleural space and the atmosphere. These pneumothoraxes may be large or small, but usually do not cause severe complications, such as cardiovascular collapse, unless they are associated with more serious injuries. Simple pneumothoraxes in trauma patients are typically the result of a fractured rib lacerating the parietal pleura. Blunt trauma in children may produce a pneumothorax without rib fractures because of the resiliency of their chest walls. The pneumothorax results instead from the sudden increase in intrathoracic pressure generated when the chest wall is compressed against a closed glottis. The result is an increase in airway pressure and ruptured alveoli, which lead to a pneumothorax. Penetrating trauma may also cause a simple pneumothorax if a tear occurs that does not allow communication with the atmosphere. A simple pneumothorax may also be iatrogenically produced, such as during the placement of a central venous line (e.g., subclavian), particularly if the patient is receiving positive-pressure ventilation.

The clinical findings associated with a simple pneumothorax may be variable, ranging from essentially no symptoms to severe respiratory distress (e.g., cyanosis, tachypnea, hypoxemia). Crepitus may be present; breath sounds are typically decreased or absent on the affected side, and the affected lung may be hyperresonant to percussion. A chest x-ray film should be obtained to confirm a suspected diagnosis of a simple pneumothorax (Figure 8-13). Small pneumothoraxes can best be diagnosed with upright, expiratory chest x-ray films. Any patient in severe distress and exhibiting clinical evidence of a pneumothorax should receive tube thoracostomy before radiographic confirmation of the pneumothorax. Patients with small pneumothoraxes can often be treated conservatively (no chest tube) if they are monitored carefully. However, many clinicians will insert a chest tube into all patients with a traumatic pneumothorax, even if only as a prophylactic measure (Vukich & Markovchick, 1988).

Open pneumothorax   An open pneumothorax occurs when there is communication between the atmosphere and the pleural space. This wound occurs primarily with penetrating trauma, particularly gunshot wounds. The clinical findings of an open pneumothorax are usually more dramatic than with a closed pneumothorax in that the wound is visible and air can be heard flowing in and out of the chest (hence the term *sucking chest wound*). The lung expands paradoxically, increasing in size on expiration as air is pushed out of the wound.

Immediate treatment of a sucking chest wound is to cover it with a clean dressing until the chest tube is placed. Covering the wound converts it from an *open* to a *closed* pneumothorax. Wounds should not be packed tightly, because the sucking action may pull the dressing into the chest. Dressings should allow the escape of air but not the inflow. One method of closing a sucking chest wound is to tape a surgical glove with the fingers cut off over the defect. The glove acts as a one-way valve, allowing air to escape but not enter the chest. Contaminated wounds should be debrided and, if gaping, closed. It is preferable not to suture gunshot or stab wounds, to minimize the risk of infection (Henneman, 1989).

Tension pneumothorax   If air is allowed to accumulate unchecked in the pleural cavity, pressure will build up, affecting not only the lungs and gas exchange, but ultimately the heart and great vessels, resulting in complete cardiopulmonary collapse. Initially, as air accumulates in the pleural space, the affected lung collapses. Further buildup of air eventually results in enough pressure to compromise ventilation in the contralateral lung. Right atrial pressure also increases (as evidenced by jugular venous distention), decreasing the pressure gradient from the periphery to the right heart and thereby decreasing the amount of blood returning to the heart. At the same time, the mediastinum is compressed, distorting the vena caval arterial junction, which causes a mechanical obstruction that decreases the flow of blood into the heart. These effects result in de-

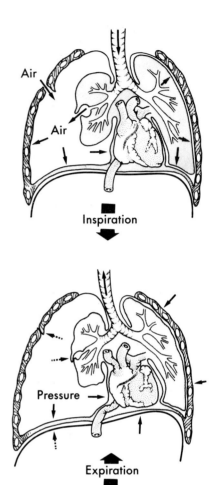

Figure 8-14   Tension pneumothorax. (*Note.* From *Trauma: The First Hour* by W.G. Baxt [Ed.], 1985, Norwalk, CT: Appleton & Lange.)

creased venous return to the heart and decreased cardiac output (Oparah & Mandal, 1976) (Figure 8-14). A tension pneumothorax may occur with either penetrating or blunt trauma. One phenomenon that leads to a tension pneumothorax in trauma patients is a "ball-valve" wound, usually created by a stab injury. In this situation, air can enter the chest, but during expiration the flap closes and air cannot escape.

The clinical presentation of a tension pneumothorax is dramatic. Findings typically include an acute onset of severe respiratory distress, hypoxemia, hypotension, tachycardia, dyspnea, chest pain, and altered levels of consciousness. Breath

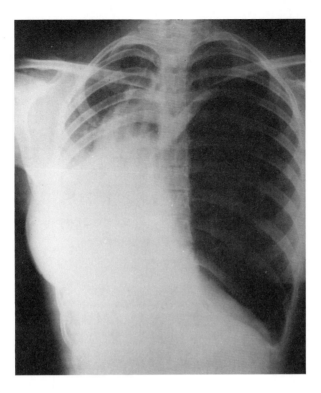

Figure 8-15   Tension pneumothorax. Chest x-ray film of right-sided tension pneumothorax in 25-year-old man who was in a fight. (Courtesy Harbor-UCLA Medical Center.)

sounds are absent, and hyperresonance is noted on the affected side. The chest expands asymmetrically, and the trachea deviates away from the side with the pneumothorax. Elevation of the central venous pressure may be noted by increased jugular venous distention unless the patient is significantly hypovolemic. Chest x-ray findings verify the presence of a collapsed lung and demonstrate a mediastinal shift toward the unaffected lung (Figure 8-15). If the patient has severe cardiopulmonary instability and a high suspicion of tension pneumothorax exists, immediate treatment should be instituted without obtaining a chest x-ray film.

Treatment of a tension pneumothorax involves immediate decompression of the pleural space. If a chest tube cannot be rapidly inserted, a large-bore (14- or 16-gauge) needle should be inserted over a rib (fifth intercostal space, midaxillary line) to temporarily relieve pressure. Other temporary devices are available commercially that were de-

signed primarily for use in the field (e.g., flutter [Heimlich] valves). Needle thoracostomy should always be followed by chest tube placement (Figure 8-16).

Hemothorax   Hemothorax, the presence of blood in the pleural space, is one of the more common complications of chest trauma. Impaired ventilation and gas exchange result from a reduction in vital capacity and associated pneumothoraxes (Vukich & Markovchick, 1988). Pressure within the chest from large amounts of blood can compress the mediastinal structures, impeding cardiac filling similarly to a tension pneumothorax. Decreased cardiac output and altered tissue perfusion (shock) also occur secondary to hypovolemia, which results from bleeding of the pulmonary, intercostal, or internal mammary vessels. Blood loss in the patient with chest trauma may occur also from other injuries, such as pelvic fractures and intrathoracic and intraabdominal injuries (Naclerio, 1970). Intraabdominal injury

Parietal pleura
Pleural space
Visceral pleura

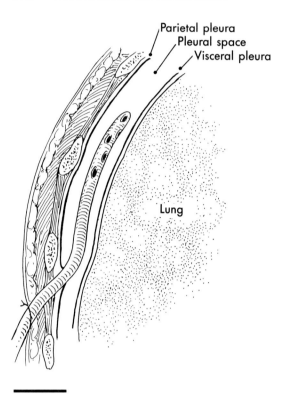

Lung

Figure 8-16 Chest tube insertion. Chest tube is tunneled over rib into pleural space.

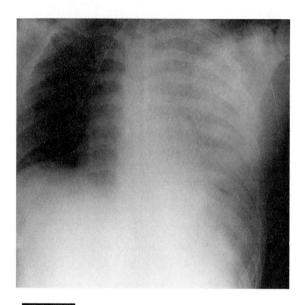

Figure 8-17 Hemothorax. Supine chest x-ray film of 30-year-old man who was stabbed in left anterior chest. Note opacification of left chest caused by layering of blood. Upright chest x-ray film would reveal pleural fluid (i.e., blood) obscuring left hemidiaphragm with otherwise clear lung fields. (Courtesy Harbor-UCLA Medical Center.)

can occur from penetrating trauma to the lower chest (i.e., below the nipple line anteriorly [fourth intercostal space] and below the inferior tips of the scapulas posteriorly) (Henneman, 1989).

The clinical presentation of the patient with a hemothorax will vary, depending on the extent of the injury. If bleeding is profuse, the patient will exhibit signs and symptoms of hypovolemic shock (restlessness, anxiety, tachycardia, hypotension, pallor), as well as respiratory insufficiency. Signs of hemothorax include diminished or absent breath sounds and dullness to percussion over the affected side. The upright chest x-ray film will exhibit blunting of the costophrenic angle if a significant amount of blood (>300 ml) is present in the thoracic cavity. Supine films will show opacification of the affected side (Figure 8-17). Unfortunately, the critical nature of the patient often demands that a supine x-ray film be obtained.

Therapy consists of replacing vascular volume with blood and crystalloid fluid, removing accumulated blood from the pleural space by means

of tube thoracostomy, and assisting with ventilation if necessary. A large chest tube (36 to 40 French in adults) should be used to remove blood from the pleural space; smaller tubes easily obstruct. Reexpansion of the lung after chest tube insertion has the additional potential benefit of tamponading bleeding from the lung parenchyma. The nurse should accurately record the amount of blood collected in the chest drainage system. Significant blood loss (600 ml over 3 hours) should be reported to the physician because it may indicate severe vascular injury and the need for a thoracotomy. Autotransfusion chest drainage systems (e.g., Pleur-Evac) allow blood that is removed from the pleural cavity to be collected and returned intravenously to the patient. These systems have the advantage of allowing for rapid transfusion of blood without the delay inherent in typing and crossmatching and the risk of disease transmission (e.g., hepatitis, acquired immunodeficiency syndrome [AIDS]). When available, these devices should be used in all patients with large hemothoraxes.

Ruptured diaphragm   Ineffective breathing
pattern
Impaired gas exchange
Pain

Traumatic rupture or injury of the diaphragm can result from penetrating and blunt trauma. Penetrating trauma commonly results from instruments such as knives, which impart little damage to tissues not directly in the path of the instrument. In blunt trauma, diaphragmatic injury occurs when intense blunt force to the lower chest or abdomen generates high intraabdominal pressures, rupturing the diaphragm (Ramponi, 1986). Penetrating trauma may cause minimal injury, whereas blunt trauma tends to result in larger diaphragmatic tears that are more likely to herniate. The majority of diaphragmatic ruptures or injuries occur on the left side; in blunt trauma this is believed to be the result of the protection of the right diaphragm provided by the liver. Injury to the diaphragm from knives more commonly affects the left side, probably because most assailants are right-handed.

The clinical picture associated with diaphragm injury depends on the size and site of the injury, the presence of the herniation, and associated injuries. Most diaphragmatic injuries are difficult to diagnose acutely because they bleed minimally and often are asymptomatic. Physical examination does not reveal diaphragmatic lacerations unless associated injuries exist (Miller, Bennett, Root, Trinkle, & Grover, 1984). If herniation has occurred, bowel sounds may be auscultated in the chest. Chest x-ray studies are usually normal or nonspecific, and they rarely diagnose acute diaphragmatic injury (Fataar & Schulman, 1979; Troop, Myers, & Agarwal, 1985). Nonspecific radiographic findings include elevated hemidiaphragm, opacification of the lower lung field, and hemothorax. When frank herniation occurs, abdominal contents will be visualized in the thorax. Unfortunately, many diaphragmatic injuries are not diagnosed acutely and patients present later (months to years) with significant complications (e.g., strangulation of herniated bowel). In the most severe situations, herniated abdominal contents compress large blood vessels and impair ventilation, resulting in cardiopulmonary collapse. The clinical findings of a ruptured diaphragm with this degree of herniation (decreased breath sounds with dullness to percussion) may be misinterpreted as a large hemothorax requiring emergent thoracostomy and replacement of presumed lost blood. Placement of a chest tube in this situation may result in damage to the herniated bowel. If time allows, chest x-ray examination will often prevent this clinical error.

Specific diagnostic tools, such as diagnostic peritoneal lavage (DPL) and barium swallow, may help in diagnosing diaphragmatic injury. Acutely, DPL is the most sensitive test for detecting diaphragmatic injury in penetrating lower thoracic trauma when a red blood cell (RBC) threshold of 5000 or 10,000 RBC/mm^3 is used (Henneman, 1989; Henneman, Marx, Moore, Cantrill, & Ammons, 1990; Merlotti, Marcet, Sheaff, Dunn, & Barrett, 1985). In blunt trauma the standard RBC threshold is 100,000 RBC/mm^3; at this threshold DPL is insensitive to diaphragmatic injury (Freeman & Fischer, 1976). Upper gastrointestinal series have proven to be useful in identifying abdominal contents above the diaphragm and in diagnosing a strangulated bowel (Drews, 1973). Management of diaphragmatic injury requires stabilizing and supporting the patient until surgical intervention is possible.

Tracheobronchial injuries   Impaired gas
exchange
High risk for
ineffective airway
clearance
High risk for
decreased cardiac
output
Pain

Injuries to the tracheobronchial tree are rare, occurring more in blunt than penetrating trauma. The mechanism of injury in blunt trauma is related to the traction produced during a decelerating automobile accident, which results in the lung being pulled away from the mediastinum. When the amount of the traction overcomes the elasticity of the trachea, the trachea ruptures. Most tracheobronchial injuries occur close to the carina.

Clinical findings depend on the type and extent of the injury. Penetrating wounds to the neck or chest are generally obvious, especially when associated with an air leak (e.g., subcutaneous emphysema) or bleeding (e.g., hemoptysis). Patients with severe blunt trauma must be examined with a high index of suspicion for tracheobronchial injury, especially when the first three ribs are involved. Signs and symptoms of acute respiratory failure (ARF), hemoptysis, and a crunching sound with each heart beat created by air surrounding the pericardial sac (Hamman's sign) may be present. Radiologic findings may include subcutaneous or mediastinal emphysema, and pneumothorax. Intense, continuous bubbling from the water-seal chamber of a chest tube, which may have been inserted for a pneumothorax, may signify an air leak from the tracheobronchial tree. Fiberoptic bronchoscopy may also be useful in diagnosing tracheobronchial injury, as well as in facilitating airway placement.

The priority in management of these patients is stabilization of the airway, which may be challenging. If the airway is obstructed secondary to a ruptured cervical trachea, an emergency tracheostomy must be performed. More distal injuries necessitate selective intubation, accomplished by visualization of the bronchi with a flexible bronchoscope and then passing an endotracheal tube over the scope.

Insertion of a chest tube may be necessary if a pneumothorax is present. Large air leaks from the trachea or bronchi typically require that suction (20 to 30 cm H_2O) be added to the water-seal system to retain negativity in the pleural space. Surgical intervention to repair the airway should be undertaken as soon as possible.

GENERAL INTERVENTIONS
Chest Tubes

The nurse is responsible for assisting with the thoracostomy, as well as setting up and monitoring the chest drainage system. Clinicians have debated the optimal site to place a chest tube. The best site allows for the removal of air and the drainage of fluid and is cosmetically acceptable. To achieve this end, it has been recommended that the tube be directed posteriorly and toward the apex of the lung. A study comparing the use of anterior (midclavicular, second intercostal space) with lateral (midaxillary, fifth intercostal space) chest tube positions demonstrated no difference in outcome (Hegarty, 1976). Most authorities recommend the midaxillary approach to decrease the risk of vascular injury and because it is more cosmetically acceptable. The caliber of chest tube will depend on the size of the patient and whether the patient also has a hemothorax, in which case a large-bore (36 to 40 French) tube should be used (see Table 8-2).

The chest tube must be connected to a device that allows the removal of air and fluid but does not permit reentry of air into the pleural space. A variety of techniques can accomplish this, including a bottle drainage system or disposable device (Figure 8-18). In certain situations the addition of suction may be required to enhance the removal of air or fluid. In these cases, an additional bottle can be added to the system or the disposable device attached to suction. Typically, 20 to 30 cm (H_2O) of suction is required for significant air leaks and will create constant bubbling in the suction chamber. The actual techniques for set up and monitoring differs slightly, depending on the system used. For example, addition of fluid to establish a "water seal" is required by some systems, whereas others are "dry" units. All systems have the capability of assessing for air leaks and monitoring tube placement. The water-seal chamber directly reflects changes in pressure occurring in the intrapleural space. Consequently, fluid in the water-seal chamber will fluctuate with respirations. If there is no fluctuation, the nurse should suspect that the tube is improperly placed or is clotted or kinked. Initially after placement, there will be bubbling in the water-seal chamber, indicating that air is being removed from the pleural space. Once the bulk of air has been removed from the pleural space, bubbling will be seen only on expiration or when the patient coughs. If bubbling continues, the physician should be notified, because this may represent a worsening tear. Very large leaks (i.e., vigorous bubbling) that do not respond to suction suggest a tracheal or bronchial tear. Drainage from the chest tube must be monitored also and significant blood loss reported to the physician.

Chest tubes, especially those with an air leak, should never be clamped for more than 2 to 3 minutes without a physician's order. Occluding the tubing with clamps restricts the release of air and may result in an accumulation of air within the chest and the development of a tension pneumothorax, which is potentially life threatening. If a break or leak in the system occurs, it is better to wait and replace the system than to risk the development of a tension pneumothorax by clamping the tube. When clamping is desired for 1 to 2 minutes, as when changing the drainage system or auscultating the lungs, it is best accomplished by pinching the tube between the fingers. If the chest tube should fall out, the wound can be covered with a clean but not tightly sealed dressing

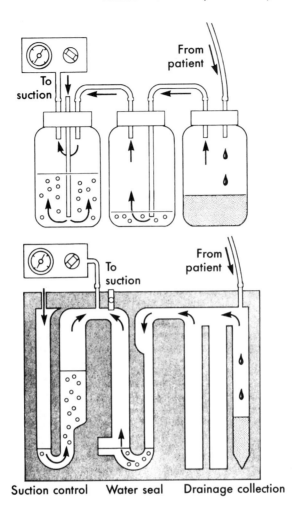

Figure 8-18   Comparison of three-bottle and Pleur-Evac® drainage systems. The Pleur-Evac can be used with or without suction. (*Note.* From *Intensive Respiratory Care* [p. 166] by J.M. Luce, M.L. Tyler, and D.J. Pierson, 1984, Philadelphia: W.B. Saunders.)

until the chest tube can be replaced. If the drainage system breaks, it should be replaced as quickly as possible. If a new system is not readily available, the end of the chest tube can be placed temporarily in a bottle or cup of water. This creates a makeshift water-seal system, which prohibits air from entering the chest.

Mechanical Ventilation

Mechanical ventilation is necessary when patients cannot independently meet their metabolic needs. Indications for mechanical ventilation in the trauma patient are ventilatory failure second-

ary to head injury or trauma to the chest wall, pleura, or lung parenchyma. Assisted ventilation is useful also in patients with altered gas exchange at the pulmonary capillary level (e.g., pulmonary contusion, ARDS), because it allows the administration of high concentrations of oxygen and PEEP therapy.

A variety of ventilators are available for use. Newer models (e.g., Siemens Servo 900C, BEAR 5) have the advantages of computerized functions and sophisticated monitoring systems, but require skilled respiratory personnel to operate. The optimal ventilator in the ED is one that provides appropriate therapy, has adequate alarm functions, is user-friendly, and is easy to transport. Both pressure and volume ventilators are currently used, but the volume cycled types are more common. Volume ventilators deliver a preset tidal volume at a predetermined rate per minute. The modes of ventilation that are most commonly used with volume ventilators are the assist-control (AC) and intermittent mandatory ventilation (IMV) mode. Guidelines for instituting mechanical ventilation with a volume ventilator are presented in Table 8-3. Adjustments in ventilator settings should be guided by arterial blood gas measurements, hemodynamic responses, and patient comfort.

New methods of mechanical ventilation include high-frequency, pressure support, and inverse ratio ventilation.

High-frequency ventilation

High-frequency ventilation (HFV) uses a variety of techniques to deliver small volumes of air at rapid rates. Three types of HFV are currently used: high-frequency, positive-pressure ventilation (60 to 100 breaths/min), high-frequency, jet ventilation (100 to 600 cycles/min), and high-frequency oscillation (90 to 3000 cycles/min). The actual method used depends on clinician preference and experience. Use of HFV is still considered experimental and is commonly employed as a last resort when other modes of ventilation have failed.

HFV has been tried with varying degrees of success in a variety of clinical situations. Some suggest that HFV may be useful in patients with tracheobronchial injuries that would benefit from low airway pressures (Frantz, Werthammer, & Stark, 1983). Another purported benefit of HFV is the lack of circulatory compromise often seen with conventional ventilatory methods (Carlon, Kahn, Howland, Rey, & Turnbull, 1981).

Inverse ratio ventilation

Inverse ratio ventilation is typically used to treat hypoxemia refractory to more conventional methods. By prolonging the inspiratory time relative to the expiratory time, a higher than normal residual volume remains in the lungs. This effect is referred to as "auto" PEEP. Like PEEP, inverse ratio ventilation increases the functional residual capacity of the lungs and allows for greater gas diffusion. (Gurevitch, Van Dyke, Young, & Jackson, 1986) Inverse ratio ventilation has been sug-

gested for patients with severe hypoxemia and noncompliant lungs, such as is seen with ARDS (Gurevitch et al., 1986; Lain et al., 1989; Rivizza et al., 1983).

Pressure support ventilation

Pressure support ventilation (PSV) is gaining popularity as a means of providing mechanical ventilatory assistance to patients with stable ventilatory drives who require an inspiratory assist. Some suggest that PSV decreases the work of breathing (WOB), increases patient comfort, and conditions respiratory muscles (Kanak, Fahen, & Vanderwarf, 1985; MacIntyre, 1986; Prakash & Meij, 1985).

PSV typically is used as a form of weaning patients from the ventilator. When the patient initiates a breath, the ventilator can sense the patient's effort and provides a rapid flow of gas. Patient comfort is enhanced because the patient can determine the length of inspiration, the inspiratory flow, and the respiratory rate. PSV is useful in overcoming the work of breathing associated with breathing through small-diameter endotracheal tubes and demand flow circuitry (Fiastro, Habib, & Quan, 1988; Viale et al., 1988). Because PSV requires an intact ventilatory drive, it must be used with caution in trauma patients with suspected or actual head injury.

Regardless of the type of ventilation provided, patient discomfort or agitation may result in "bucking" or breathing out of synchronization with the ventilator. This is of particular concern when alternative methods of ventilation, such as HFV or inverse ratio, ventilation, are used, because they do not mimic normal breathing patterns. Pain management and sedation frequently are required to relax the patient and allow the ventilator to assume some of the work of breathing. In extreme cases of agitation when it is important to control the patient's ventilation (e.g., severe flail chest), it may be necessary to use paralyzing agents (e.g., pancuronium). Paralyzing agents should not be used unless the patient is adequately sedated or already unconscious.

Positive end expiratory pressure

When positive pressure is maintained at end expiration, the alveoli remain open and gas exchange is enhanced. Positive end expiratory pressure (PEEP) is commonly employed in the clinical setting to treat hypoxemia refractory to high FIO_2 levels, such as occurs with shunting. The clinician also may add PEEP to the ventilatory regimen in the hopes of lowering the FIo_2 to a less toxic level.

Although PEEP may be useful in improving arterial oxygenation, it may have a detrimental effect by decreasing cardiac output and hence oxygen delivery. The mechanism by which PEEP decreases cardiac output includes decreasing ventricular filling and reducing coronary blood flow (Tittley, Fremes, & Weisel, 1985). Any attempt to adjust PEEP levels must be accompanied by appropriate monitoring of oxygen delivery variables, including oxygen saturation and cardiac output.

COMPLICATIONS
Psychologic Aspects of Maxillofacial Injury

Maxillofacial injuries can be psychologically, as well as physically, devastating. The nurse plays a critical role in supporting the patient during the early hours after injury. Providing explanations and reassurance, allowing the patient some control over the treatment, and ensuring privacy and dignity can all help the patient to cope psychologically. Patients are frequently awake after facial trauma and may be extremely anxious and uncomfortable. Simple explanations regarding procedures may decrease anxiety, as may allowing family members to stay with the patient. If patients can cooperate, they may be able to assist with suctioning to gain a sense of control over their environment. The nurse should provide the patient with privacy by pulling the curtain around the patient's guerney and minimizing the number of personnel attending to the patient. The reactions and support of staff may be crucial to successful patient adaptation after a disfiguring injury.

Adult Respiratory Distress Syndrome

Posttraumatic respiratory failure, or the adult respiratory distress syndrome (ARDS) may occur after a variety of traumatic events, such as fractures, pulmonary contusions, and shock. The exact mechanisms leading to the pathologic changes associated with ARDS remain unclear. The alveolar capillary membrane is damaged, allowing fluid to leak into the alveoli and interstitial spaces. Decreased functional surfactant results in alveolar collapse, adding to the injury. Pulmonary hypertension may occur also, secondary to hypoxemia and vasoconstriction.

The result of these changes is severe $\dot{V}/\dot{Q}$ mismatching, shunt, hypoxemia, and hypercapnia. Symptoms of ARDS typically appear 12 to 24 hours after the traumatic event. Clinical findings include anxiety, restlessness, cough, dyspnea, tachypnea, crackles, and low Sao_2. The chest x-ray film shows a characteristic "white out" pattern of diffuse bilateral infiltrates (Figure 8-19).

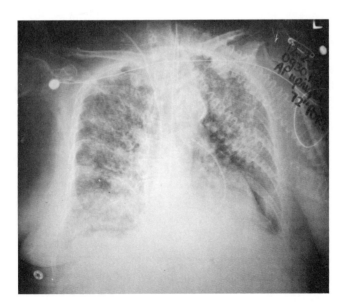

Figure 8-19   Chest x-ray film of patient with adult respiratory distress syndrome. (Courtesy Harbor-UCLA Medical Center.

The A-a gradient is typically widened, and significant shunts of greater than 50% are not unusual. The Pa_{CO_2} may be low initially as the patient hyperventilates, but will rise as the disease progresses. The terminal stages of ARDS are characterized by severe hypoxemia refractory to high FI_{O_2} and hypercapnia (Bone, George, & Hudson, 1987).

Management of ARDS is primarily supportive, with therapy directed at intervening in the underlying event and maximizing gas exchange. Major efforts are directed at optimizing oxygen delivery via PEEP therapy (to increase Sa_{O_2}), hemodynamic monitoring (to optimize cardiac output), and transfusion therapy (to optimize hemoglobin). High levels of PEEP (10 to 15 cm H_2O) typically are needed to maintain Sa_{O_2} greater than 90%. Hemodynamic monitoring is necessary not only for the determination of cardiac output, but for proper evaluation of fluid and PEEP therapy.

WEANING THE TRAUMA PATIENT

The critical care nurse plays a pivotal role in assisting the patient to wean from the ventilator. Responsibilities of the nurse include (1) assessing the patient's readiness to wean, (2) preparing the patient physically and psychologically for weaning, and (3) monitoring and supporting the patient through the weaning process.

Assessing Weaning Readiness

Many factors, both respiratory and nonrespiratory, influence the patient's ability to wean (see box at right). Most important, the underlying condition that necessitated mechanical ventilation must be resolved or significantly improved.

An evaluation of ventilatory capacity is usually performed before weaning is attempted. Although a number of sophisticated tests are available, a simple assessment of basic parameters is often sufficient. In fact, research suggests that the ratio of respiratory rate to tidal volume (f/V_T) is the most accurate predictor of weaning failure (Yang & Tobin, 1991).

Patient Preparation

A patient who has been ventilated for short periods (e.g., postanesthesia) generally has little difficulty making the transition from assisted to spontaneous breathing. This is in contrast to the patient who has been on the ventilator for prolonged periods and has come to rely on its support. In

Respiratory and nonrespiratory factors to consider before weaning	
Respiratory	**Nonrespiratory**
Arterial blood gases	Nutrition
Tidal volume	Hemoglobin
Respiratory rate	Electrolytes
Inspiratory force	Neurologic status
Shunt fraction	Pain, fear, anxiety
Dead space/ tidal volume	Sleep
Vital capacity	Fever
Work of breathing	Hemodynamic status

these instances, a significant amount of time may be spent preparing patients to breathe on their own. Physical preparation includes ensuring adequate rest, providing a quiet, relaxed environment, controlling pain, and positioning the patient comfortably. Gas exchanged should be optimized with bronchial hygiene measures and suctioning as needed. Psychologic preparation is a more complex process and one that is often overlooked when preparing the patient to wean. Patients often have concerns and fears about being able to breathe on their own, especially if they have "failed" weaning in the past. The nurse must discuss these concerns with the patients and provide reassurance by explaining to them that they will be closely monitored at all times while they wean.

The Weaning Process: the Nurse's Role

Once weaning has begun, the nurse assumes primary responsibility for monitoring the patient's neurologic, respiratory, and cardiovascular function. A patient must **never** be weaned unless a nurse, physician, or respiratory therapist is in constant attendance. A flow sheet should be used to record the events of the weaning process, such as the type of weaning employed and problems encountered. In particular, notes should be made as to why a weaning trial was discontinued.

The patient's response to weaning is evaluated by clinical findings and blood gas results. Pulse oximetry and capnography can be useful in monitoring trends in the patient's condition and limiting the number of ABGs drawn (Niehoff et al., 1988). Respiratory distress, arrhythmias, and agitation are generally considered indications for discontinuing the weaning trial. Care must be taken to differentiate the feeling of increased effort, which accompanies the change to spontaneous ventilation, from the dyspnea of respiratory failure. This is usually avoided if the patient is told before weaning of the potential for a feeling of increased "work" associated with being off the ventilator.

Methods of Weaning

Three methods are currently used to wean patients: (1) intermittent mandatory ventilation (IMV); (2) traditional, or T-piece; and (3) pressure support. To date, no data indicate that any method is superior to another in terms of efficacy. Efforts are underway to develop a more rigorous and scientific approach to weaning, but a successful weaning plan will always require a creative and individualized approach.

IMV

Patients on IMV receive a preset number of breaths per minute and can breathe spontaneously between the delivered breaths. When IMV weaning is used, the number of breaths delivered by the machine is progressively decreased. A blood sample for ABGs generally is drawn 20 to 30 minutes after each rate change.

Even though patients are still connected to the ventilator, they require as much attention as patients weaning with T-piece. Patients weaning by IMV may still develop respiratory failure if they cannot meet their ventilatory needs with the preset IMV rate. Disastrous consequences can be predicted in any situation where a weaning patient is not closely monitored.

T-Piece

When T-piece ventilation is used, the patient is removed from the ventilator and placed on a T-piece assembly that delivers humidified, heated oxygen. The time the patient is left off the ventilator is progressively increased, while allowing for rest periods on the ventilator in between. The actual routine of T-piece weaning varies, depending on the clinician's preference and the patient's condition. For example, a short-term ventilator patient may be allowed to stay on the T-piece indefinitely, whereas the long-term ventilator patient with chronic obstructive pulmonary disease (COPD) may tolerate being off the ventilator for only 5 minutes initially.

Pressure support

Pressure support is the newest mode of weaning from mechanical ventilation. Its popularity has resulted in many manufacturers adding this feature to their newer models of ventilators. Pressure support weaning can be accomplished in a variety of ways. One is to gradually decrease the amount of pressure given to the patient in a stepwise fashion. The other is to use it to augment IMV weaning. As the IMV rate is decreased, pressure support is used to assist the patient's spontaneous breaths.

SUMMARY Impaired ventilation and gas exchange can occur after a variety of pulmonary, thoracic, and facial injuries. The potentially life-threatening nature of these injuries mandates an organized approach to patient care by an experienced team of skilled, knowledgeable clinicians. Appropriate monitoring and intervention demand an appreciation of the normal physiology of ventilation and gas exchange, as well as the possible derangements associated with trauma that may lead to respiratory failure.

Monitoring of trauma patients is increasingly being assisted by sophisticated techniques (e.g., transconjunctival O_2 sensors). Despite this technology, the majority of life-threatening problems are diagnosed solely on the basis of the clinical examination, necessitating expert physical assessment skills. Management of the patient with impaired gas exchange may be fairly straightforward (e.g., chest tube for a tension pneumothorax) or complex (e.g., ARDS). In all cases, optimal treatment demands a coordinated effort that begins in the prehospital setting and continues into the ED, OR, ICU, acute care, and, at times, rehabilitation.

The nurse plays a vital role in the monitoring and treatment of these patients. A holistic approach mandates an appreciation of both the physical and psychosocial imbalances inherent in pulmonary, thoracic, and facial trauma. The patient will benefit from an organized, problem-oriented approach to nursing care. This may be accomplished in a variety of ways, such as via nursing diagnoses. Examples of potential nursing diagnoses for patients with impaired ventilation and gas exchange are presented in the table on pp. 184-189. These diagnoses include ineffective airway clearance, high risk for aspiration, ineffective breathing pattern, impaired gas exchange, decreased cardiac output, high risk for infection, pain, anxiety, body image disturbance, impaired verbal communication, and altered nutrition. The use of a comprehensive yet practical plan of care is critical to the successful nursing management of the trauma patient.

The trauma patient with impaired ventilation and gas exchange

Nursing diagnosis	Nursing intervention	Evaluative criteria
Ineffective airway clearance Related to foreign body, hemorrhage, edema, altered level of consciousness (LOC) As evidenced by noisy or absent respirations	**Ensure airways are clear** Secure airway by: • suctioning foreign material from mouth (e.g., blood, vomitus) using tonsil-tip catheter; • opening airway using chin-lift or jaw-thrust method to maintain cervical spine alignment; • inserting oropharyngeal or nasopharyngeal airway to relieve obstruction and facilitate suctioning; • preparing for endotracheal intubation or cricothryroidotomy; • anticipating need for sedation and paralytic agents during intubation; • evaluating endotracheal tube placement (i.e., auscultating lungs, obtaining CXR); • securing artificial airway (particularly important during transport). Control hemorrhage (with maxillofacial injury) by: • applying pressure over injured area; • avoiding blind clamping of vessels with maxillofacial trauma; • having wire cutters available in case of vomiting or hemorrhage; • anticipating surgical ligation of bleeding vessel. Monitor respiratory rate, depth, pattern, use of accessory muscles. Monitor LOC; heart rate and rhythm; skin temperature and color. Evaluate breath sounds, symmetry of chest movements, quality of secretions. Maintain patency of airway via suctioning, positioning, humidification. Evaluate oxygenation (Sao_2, Pao_2). Evaluate ventilation ($Paco_2$, pH, $ETco_2$).	Patient will have the following: • bilateral breath sounds; • respiratory rate, depth, and pattern within normal limits (WNL); • Pao_2 >60 mm Hg; Sao_2 >90%; • $Paco_2$ 35-45 mm Hg; • normal LOC; • Vital signs (VS) WNL for the patient; • Skin pink, warm, and dry.

The trauma patient with impaired ventilation and gas exchange—cont'd

Nursing diagnosis	Nursing intervention	Evaluative criteria
High risk for aspiration Related to altered LOC, hemorrhage, vomiting	**Ensure aspiration does not occur** Insert nasogastric (NG) tube into patients with compromised or artificial airway. (CAUTION: patients with maxillofacial fractures (e.g., Le Fort III) should have gastric tubes inserted orally. Facilitate obtaining serial CXRs if aspiration is suspected. Maintain high index of suspicion for aspiration in patients with head injury or those receiving sedation/analgesics. Maintain patent airway by positioning patient in high Fowler's or lateral position (after confirmation that no cervical spine injury exists). Evaluate breath sounds (crackles, rhonchi may indicate the patient has aspirated). Evaluate ABGs, Sao_2, VS, LOC. Suction patient as necessary. Maintain patent NG tube by: • maintaining low suction; • irrigating as necessary. Anticipate use of mechanical ventilation if aspiration occurs.	Patient will have the following: • patent airway (see criteria for *ineffective airway clearance*); • clear CXR without evidence of infiltrates.
Ineffective breathing pattern Related to altered LOC, obstructed airway, loss of integrity of thoracic cage (e.g., flail chest, sternal fractures) As evidenced by retractions, paradoxical movement of chest, labored respirations, asymmetry, abnormal respiratory rate	**Ensure breathing pattern is normal or improving** Secure airway (see *Ineffective Airway Clearance*). Anticipate artificial ventilation to provide internal stabilization for patients with flail chest or sternal fractures by: • monitoring respiratory rate, depth, pattern, use of accessory muscles; • evaluating for paradoxical movement; • monitoring LOC, heart rate and rhythm, skin temperature, and color; • evaluating oxygenation (Sao_2, Pao_2); • evaluating ventilation ($Paco_2$, pH, $ETco_2$).	Patient will have the following: • patent airway (see criteria for *ineffective airway clearance*); • respiratory rate, depth, and pattern WNL; • ABGs, Sao_2 WNL for the patient; • VS WNL for the patient; • Normal LOC.

Continued.

Nursing diagnosis	Nursing intervention	Evaluative criteria
Impaired gas exchange Related to obstructed airway, impaired ventilation, ventilation/perfusion mismatching (e.g., secondary to pulmonary contusion, pneumothorax, hemothorax), shunt (e.g., secondary to ARDS), decreased O_2 delivery/utilization (e.g., secondary to CO poisoning) As evidenced by abnormal ABG, increased A-a gradient, decreased Pao_2/Flo_2 ratio	**Ensure gas exchange is normal or improving** Secure airway (see *Ineffective Airway Clearance*). Evaluate patient's oxygenation status (Pao_2, Sao_2, A-a gradient, Pao_2/Flo_2). Administer O_2 therapy. Evaluate patient's ventilation status ($Paco_2$, pH, $ETco_2$). Anticipate need for mechanical ventilation, particularly in patients with flail chest, pulmonary contusion. Improve ventilation/perfusion mismatch, shunt by: • administering high Flo_2; • suctioning; • PEEP therapy. Reestablish negative pressure in pleural space with needle thoracostomy or chest tube when pneumothorax or hemothorax is present; obtain CXR after tube is placed. Provide chest tube care by: • evaluating for proper position; • assessing for presence of air leaks; • maintaining patency; • monitoring; • recording drainage. Optimize O_2 delivery (i.e., Sao_2, Hgb, cardiac output); consider use of autotransfusion device for large hemothorax. Evaluate O_2 utilization (Svo_2, carbon monoxide level). Monitor respiratory rate, depth, pattern, use of accessory muscles. Monitor LOC, heart rate (HR) and rhythm, skin temperature, and color. Evaluate breath sounds, symmetry of chest movements, quality of secretions. Maintain patency of the airway via suctioning, positioning, humidification	Patient will have the following: • normal Sao_2, Pao_2, $Paco_2$, pH, A-a gradient, shunt fraction, O_2 delivery, O_2 utilization, Svo_2; • Respiratory rate, depth, and pattern WNL; • normal LOC; • skin pink, warm, and dry.
High risk for decreased cardiac output Related to decreased venous return and impaired cardiac filling Secondary to hemorrhage (maxillofacial trauma, hemothorax), tension pneumothorax	**Ensure cardiac output is normal or improving** Secure airway; provide O_2. Consider Trendelenburg position if signs of shock. Control external bleeding (pressure).	Patient will have the following: • normal LOC; • stable VS with systolic BP >90 mm Hg; • ABGs WNL for the patient; • Amount of chest drainage gradually decreased;

Nursing diagnosis	Nursing intervention	Evaluative criteria
	Anticipate needle thoracostomy. Place two large-bore (14- or 16-gauge) intravenous (IV) lines; use blood tubing and normal saline or lactated Ringer's solutions. Obtain vital signs and ECG. Obtain blood specimen for type and crossmatch and hematocrit. Maintain IV rate to maintain systolic blood pressure >90 mm Hg, warm fluid, use pressure bags as needed. Anticipate placement of chest tube (> 36 French) and connect to 20 cm H_2O suction. Anticipate autotransfusion for large hemothorax. Anticipate blood replacement. Anticipate surgical intervention (i.e., thoracotomy). Anticipate central line placement. Obtain CXR after chest tube or central line placement. Place indwelling urinary catheter; assess for presence of hematuria. Monitor VS, LOC, ECG, skin color, temperature, fluid and blood input, and urine output. Monitor pulse oximeter, ABGs, Sao_2. Maintain patency of chest drainage system by: • ensuring there are no dependent loops; • not clamping; • gently stripping only if clots are present; • inspecting for proper fluctuation/bubbling; • maintaining system lower than patient's chest.	• Urine output >30 ml/hr; • Skin pink, warm, and dry.
High risk for infection Secondary to maxillofacial trauma, pneumonia/empyema	**Ensure infection is absent** Obtain baseline white blood cell (WBC) count with differential. Culture wounds and sputum before administration of antibiotics. Administer IV antibiotics as ordered. Administer diphtheria tetanus toxoid vaccine as ordered with open wounds. Monitor patient's temperature Q 4 hours. Use sterile technique during invasive procedures.	Patient will have the following: • WBC WNL; • wound site without redness, swelling, or purulent drainage; • temperature WNL; • breath sounds equal and clear bilaterally; • ABGs WNL for the patient; • clear CXR; • absent pleuritic pain

Nursing diagnosis	Nursing intervention	Evaluative criteria
High risk for infection—cont'd	**Ensure infection is absent**—cont'd Cover facial wounds with saline-soaked sterile dressings until closure is accomplished. Provide wound care by cleaning lacerations; applying antibacterial ointment. Monitor wound for evidence of infection: redness, swelling, purulent drainage. Monitor CXR studies, ABGs. Monitor breath sounds; sputum color, consistency, amount, odor (pneumonia). Monitor chest tube drainage (empyema). Turn patient Q2 hours; anticipate use of kinetic beds in immobilized or unconscious patients. Provide bronchial hygiene (postural drainage, percussion, suctioning) Q 2-4 hours as necessary.	
Pain Related to soft tissue injuries, fractures, pleural irritation, stimulation of nerve fibers As evidenced by verbal complaint of pain, moaning, grimacing, tachycardia, tachypnea, hypertension	**Ensure pain is absent** Avoid administration of pain medication until major injuries have been identified and evaluated and a treatment plan established; explain to patient reason for withholding pain medications until evaluation complete. Administer narcotics after above condition is met. (Small frequent IV doses may be more beneficial than larger intramuscular (IM) doses.) Anticipate use of regional nerve blocks for pain control with multiple rib fractures. Assess level of pain using an analog scale (e.g., "Rate the pain on a level from 0 to 10 with 0 being no pain and 10 being the worst pain you've ever felt."). Assess patient for nonverbal signs of pain—tachycardia, tachypnea, grimacing. Investigate the use of alternative methods of pain control (e.g., positioning (splinting and elevation), cold packs, distraction (e.g., family visiting). Inform patient and medicate before uncomfortable procedures, such as wound care and dressing changes.	Patient will: • report a decreased level of pain; • not exhibit signs of pain (i.e., tachycardia, tachypnea, grimacing).

Nursing diagnosis	Nursing intervention	Evaluative criteria
Anxiety Related to emergent nature of illness, lack of knowledge, fear As evidenced by nonverbal gestures, tachycardia, verbal statements of anxiety	**Ensure anxiety is absent or decreasing** Allow patient to express concerns regarding nature of illness and fears. Acknowledge patient's concerns (e.g., about "so much happening at once"). Provide simple but clear explanations regarding procedures.	Patient will do the following: • verbalize concerns and fears; • state that he or she is less anxious.
Body image disturbance Related to disfiguring injury As evidenced by verbal comments, avoidance of interpersonal contact	**Foster positive body image** Allow patient to express concerns regarding body changes. Inform patient that his or her feelings/concerns are normal. Demonstrate acceptance of the patient's body changes (e.g., maintain eye contact). Provide the patient with realistic information regarding the extent of damage and potential for recovery/reconstruction. Assist family members in accepting the patient's body changes. Involve patient in self-care activities as appropriate (e.g., suctioning, positioning).	Patient will do the following: • verbalize concerns regarding body changes; • verbalize feelings of sadness/loss; • share feelings with family; • verbalize an acceptance of body changes by time of discharge.
Impaired verbal communication Related to intubation, neuromuscular blockade, fixation devices, maxillofacial trauma As evidenced by incoherent speech, inability to move air past vocal cords	**Encourage patient's ability to communicate** Reassure intubated patients that they are unable to talk because of the temporary endotracheal tube. Acknowledge the patient's frustrations with being unable to communicate. Encourage the patient to communicate with alternative methods, such as pen/paper, alphabet boards). Ask *yes/no* questions as much as possible. Advance to fenestrated tracheotomy tube as soon as possible. Encourage family to talk and touch patient.	Communication will be apparent as follows: • patient will communicate at some level; • patient will be able to communicate needs to staff; • family will communicate with patient.
High risk for altered nutrition: less than body requirements Related to inability to chew or swallow Secondary to intubation, maxillofacial trauma As evidenced by weight loss, decreased albumin/globulin ratio, decreased total protein level	**Ensure nutritional intake meets patient's metabolic requirements** Assess patient's caloric requirements (consult dietician). Initiate and maintain enteral (preferable) or parenteral feedings. Monitor caloric intake. Monitor percent of calories delivered as carbohydrate.	Patient will receive 30-40 kcal/day. P_{CO_2} will remain stable.

COMPETENCIES
The following clinical competencies pertain to **caring for the patient with ventilation and gas exchange problems.**

☑ Perform initial assessment and subsequent assessments appropriately and in a timely fashion to auscultate breath sounds, detect evidence of impending respiratory failure, and evaluate weaning parameters.

☑ Accurately interpret ABG results.

☑ Maintain a patent airway.

☑ Set up and maintain a chest drainage system.

☑ Evaluate and dress facial wounds appropriately.

☑ Employ techniques to maximize ventilation for immobilized patients or patients in pain.

CASE STUDY A 25-year-old man who sustained a gunshot wound to the right side of the chest that resulted in a hemopneumothorax and pulmonary contusion was transferred from the emergency department to the ICU for continued observation. Twenty-four hours after admission he became restless, complaining of dyspnea and increased pain at the wound site. His respiratory rate was 36, rapid and shallow; diffuse crackles were auscultated bilaterally. The SaO_2 by pulse oximetry was 85% on 15 L O_2 nonrebreathing mask. ABGs were drawn and a chest x-ray film obtained. Arterial blood gases revealed a PaO_2 of 90 mm Hg, $PaCO_2$ of 30 mm Hg, and pH of 7.48. The chest x-ray showed no evidence of a pneumothorax, but diffuse bilateral infiltrates were present. A CPAP mask was tried in an attempt to improve oxygenation. The patient became increasingly restless and agitated on the CPAP mask despite pain medication (morphine sulfate 5 mg IV push every 1 to 2 hours). His saturations continued to decline, and his breathing became more labored. An orotracheal tube was placed and mechanical ventilation initiated (assist control at rate of 30/minute, FIO_2 100%, tidal volume 800 ml, PEEP 5 cm H_2O). The patient was extremely restless and "bucking" the ventilator, inhibiting adequate ventilations. A paralytic agent (pancuronium) was initiated after the patient was well sedated. A continuous morphine drip was added for pain management while the patient was paralyzed.

Despite these interventions the patient could not be well oxygenated and saturations remained in the 80th percentile. An SvO_2 pulmonary artery catheter was inserted to assist in the evaluation of the patient's cardiopulmonary status. PEEP was added to the patient's regimen at 2 to 5 cm increments. Even-

tually, on 10 cm of PEEP, the SaO_2 was 92%, the SvO_2 60%, and the cardiac output 5.5 L/min. The PEEP was then raised to 15 cm H_2O, resulting in an SaO_2 of 97%, SvO_2 of 50%, and cardiac output of 4 L/min. The fall in SvO_2 and cardiac output on 15 cm of PEEP indicated that although oxygenation had improved, the oxygen delivery had diminished, indicating an overshoot in the amount of PEEP. The patient was returned to 10 cm of PEEP to allow for maximal oxygen delivery (optimal PEEP).

Three days after admission, the patient's lungs began to clear and his oxygenation improved. He was extubated and discharged from the unit 14 days later.

What are the signs and symptoms of ARDS?
Restlessness, tachypnea, rapid shallow breathing, refractory hypoxemia, cyanosis, crackles, diffuse pulmonary infiltrates on x-ray film, and decreased lung compliance.

Why is the hypoxemia associated with ARDS refractory to high FIO_2 levels?
The primary mechanism of hypoxemia in ARDS is shunt. Shunt occurs when alveoli are completely filled with fluid or pus such that no oxygen can pass from the alveoli into the pulmonary capillary. In fact, this is the hallmark of shunting—hypoxemia that cannot be improved with the administration of 100% O_2.

Why was the PEEP reduced to 10 cm even though the SaO_2 had improved on 15 cm?
The ultimate goal of PEEP therapy is to improve oxygen delivery. Although the SaO_2 increased on 15 cm of PEEP, the cardiac output, O_2 delivery, and SvO_2 decreased. These changes indicated that 10 cm was the more effective level of PEEP.

RESEARCH QUESTIONS

- What is the effect of positioning a patient with a flail chest on the "good side" down (i.e., lying on the side opposite the flail) on oxygenation (SaO_2) and level of pain?
- What is the effect of positioning a patient with a pulmonary contusion on the "good side" (side opposite the contusion) on oxygenation?
- What is the effect of external stabilization of rib fractures/flail chest (e.g., taping) on oxygenation and carbon dioxide elimination?
- Is end tidal CO_2 measurement an accurate predictor of ventilatory failure in the trauma patient?
- Can conjunctival PO_2 monitoring be used to predict blood loss and impaired gas exchange in patients with massive hemothorax?

ANNOTATED BIBLIOGRAPHY

Barrett, A.S. (1986). Maxillofacial trauma. In M.K. Finke & N.E. Lanroe (Eds.). *Emergency nursing: A comprehensive approach* (pp. 196-219). Rockville, MD: Aspen.
A review of the emergency management of maxillofacial trauma including principles of assessment and nursing care.

Baxt, W.G. (Ed.) (1985). *Trauma: The first hour* (Chapters 2 and 5). Norwalk, CT: Appleton-Century-Crofts.
A comprehensive yet concise approach to the early management of airway and chest injuries in the trauma patient.

Campbell, J.E. (Ed.). (1988). *Basic trauma life support.* Englewood Cliffs, NJ: Prentice-Hall.
A text developed by the American College of Emergency Physicians to guide prehospital personnel in the care of trauma patients. The generous use of illustrations is helpful in understanding the basic techniques of airway and ventilatory management.

Manson, P.N. (1984). Maxillofacial injuries. *Emergency Medicine Clinics of North America, 2,* 761-798.
An extensive review of the emergency treatment and management of a variety of maxillofacial injuries, including soft tissue and bony injury. Also covered are such topics as the emergency management of airway obstruction, hemorrhage, aspiration, and cervical spine injuries.

Richardson, J.D., Polk, H.C., & Flink, L.M. (1987). *Trauma: Clinical care and pathophysiology.* St. Louis: Mosby–Year Book, Inc.
A text that contains several chapters useful in managing the trauma patient with impaired gas exchange. Chapter 8 provides a comprehensive review of respiratory pathophysiology and emphasizes the posttraumatic sequalae of multiple system failure and the adult respiratory distress syndrome. Chapters 10 and 11 describe in detail the mechanism of injury and management of facial and thoracic injury.

Rosen, P., Baker, F.J. II, Barkin, R.M., Braen, G.R., Dailey, R.H., & Levy, R.C. (Eds.). (1988). *Emergency medicine: Concepts and clinical practice* (2nd Ed.). St. Louis: Mosby–Year Book, Inc.
A discussion of thoracic trauma, including pulmonary chest wall, pleural, and diaphragmatic injuries (Chapters 23-26). The material includes extensive diagrams and examples of abnormal CXRs, which facilitate an understanding of both pathophysiology and diagnostic findings.

Waxman, K. (1986). Oxygen delivery and resuscitation. *Annals of Emergency Medicine, 15,* 1420-1422.
A review of the important concepts of oxygen delivery and oxygen consumption as they relate to resuscitative therapy. Determinants of oxygen delivery and factors that impair oxygen consumption are highlighted, as is the relationship between oxygen delivery and consumption in normal and stressed states.

REFERENCES

Abraham, E., & Fink, S. (1988). Conjunctival oxygen tension monitoring in emergency department patients. *American Journal of Emergency Medicine, 6,* 549-554.

Abraham, E., Lee, G., & Morgan, M.T. (1986). Conjunctival oxygen tension monitoring during helicopter transport of critically ill patients. *Annals of Emergency Medicine, 15,* 782-786.

Ali, J., Vanderby, B., & Purcell, C. (1991) The effect of the pneumatic antishock garment (PASG) on the hemodynamics, hemorrhage, and survival in penetrating thoracic aortic injury. *Journal of Trauma, 31,* 846-851.

Allen, J.E., & Schwab, C.W. (1985). Blunt chest trauma in the elderly. *American Surgeon, 51,* 697-700.

Amato, J.J., Billy, L.J., Lawsons, N.S., & Rich, N.M. (1974). High velocity missile injury. *American Journal of Surgery, 127,* 454-459.

American Heart Association (AHA). *Advanced Cardiac Life Support.* (1986).

Aprahamian, C., Thompson, B.M., Finger, W.A., & Darin, J.C. (1984). Experimental cervical spine injury model: Evaluation of airway management and splinting techniques. *Annals of Emergency Medicine, 13,* 584-587.

Barach, E., Tomlinovich, M., & Nowak, R. (1986). A pathophysiologic examination of wounding mechanisms of firearms. *Journal of Trauma, 26,* 225-235; 374-383.

Barrett, A.S. (1986). Maxillofacial trauma. In M.K. Finke & N.E. Lanroe (Eds.), *Emergency nursing: A comprehensive approach* (pp. 196-213). Rockville, MD: Aspen.

Barrett J. (1987). Chest trauma. In T.C. Kravis & C.G. Warner (Eds.), *Emergency medicine: A comprehensive approach* (pp. 1123-1135). Rockville, MD: Aspen.

Bauer, D., & Kowalski, R. (1988). Effect of spinal immobilization devices on pulmonary function in healthy, non-smoking man. *Annals of Emergency Medicine, 17,* 915-918.

Bayne, C.G. (1985). Management of the airway. In W.G. Baxt (Ed.), *Trauma: The first hour* (pp. 39-60), Norwalk, CT: Appleton-Century-Crofts.

Bivens, H.G., Ford, S., Bezmalinovic, Z., Price, H.M., & Williams, J. (1988). The effect of axial traction during orotracheal intubation of the trauma victim with an unstable cervical spine. *Annals of Emergency Medicine, 17,* 25-29.

Blaisdell, F.W., & Schlobohn, R.M. (1973). The respiratory distress syndrome: A review. *Surgery, 74,* 251-262.

Bone, R.C., George, R.B., & Hudson, L.D. (1987). Adult respiratory distress syndrome. In R.C. Bone, R.B. George, & L.D. Hudson (Eds.), *Acute respiratory failure* (pp. 173-196). New York: Churchill Livingstone.

Campbell, J.E. (1988). Field evaluation and management of the trauma patient. In J.E. Campbell (Ed.), *Basic trauma life support* (pp. 21-41). Englewood Cliffs, NJ: Prentice Hall.

Carlon, G., Kahn, R., Howland, W., Rey, C., & Turnbull, A. (1981). Clinical experience with high-frequency ventilation. *Critical Care Medicine*, 9, 1-6.

Chaudhary, B.A., & Burki, N.K. (1978). Ear oximetry in clinical practice. *American Review of Respiratory Disease*, 117, 173-175.

Clark, G.C., Schecter, W.P., & Trunkey, D.D. (1988). Variables affecting outcome in blunt chest trauma: Flail chest versus pulmonary contusion. *Journal of Trauma*, 28, 298-303.

Cogbill, T.H., Moore, E.E., Millikan, J.S., & Cleveland, H.C. (1983). Rationale for selective application of emergency department thoracotomy in trauma. *Journal of Trauma*, 23, 453-458.

Creel, J.H. (1988). Mechanisms of injuries due to motion. In J.E. Campbell (Ed.), *Basic trauma life support* (pp. 1-20). Englewood Cliffs, NJ: Prentice Hall.

Dhainaut, J.F., Bons, J., Bricard, C., & Monsallier, J.F. (1980). Improved oxygenation in patients with extensive unilateral pneumonia using the lateral decubitus position. *Thorax*, 35, 792-793.

Dougall, A.M., Paul, M.E., & Finely, R.J. (1977). Chest trauma: current morbidity and mortality. *Journal of Trauma*, 17, 547-553.

Douglas, N.J., Brash, H.M., Wraith, P.K., Calverley, P.M., Leggett, R.J., McElderry, L., & Fenley, D.C. (1979). Accuracy, sensitivity to carboxyhemoglobin and speed of response of the Hewlett-Packard 47201A ear oximeter. *American Review of Respiratory Disease*, 119, 311-313.

Drews, J.A. (1973). Acute diaphragmatic injury. *Annals of Thoracic Surgery*, 16, 67-70.

Fataar, S., & Schulman, A. (1979). Diagnosis of diaphragmatic tears. *British Journal of Radiology*, 52, 375-381.

Fiastro, J.F., Habib, M.P., & Quan, S.F. (1988). Pressure support compensation for inspiratory work due to endotracheal tubes and demand continuous positive airway pressure. *Chest*, 93, 499-505.

Frantz, I.D., Werthammer, J., & Stark, A.R. (1983). High frequency ventilation in premature infants with lung disease: Adequate gas exchange at low tracheal pressures. *Pediatrics*, 71, 483-488.

Freeman, T., & Fischer, R.P. (1976). The inadequacy of peritoneal lavage in diagnosing diaphragmatic rupture. *Journal of Trauma*, 16, 538-541.

Gardner, L.B. (1986). Severe acid-base abnormalities. In L.B. Gardner (Ed.), *Acute internal medicine* (p. 499). New York: Medical Examination Publishing.

Goldman, E., McDonald, J.S., Peterson, S.S., Stock, M.C., Betts, R., & Frolicher, D. (1988). Transtracheal ventilation with oscillation pressure for complete upper airway obstruction. *Journal of Trauma*, 28, 611-614.

Granovetter, B. (1985). Blunt chest trauma. In B.E. Brenner (Ed.), *Comprehensive management of respiratory emergencies* (pp. 57-77). Rockville, MD: Aspen.

Green, N., & Petrucelli, E. (Eds.). (1981). *Proceedings: International symposium on occupant restraint*. American Association for Automotive Medicine. Morton Grove, Toronto.

Griffith, L.D. (1985). Chest trauma. In W.G. Baxt (Ed.). *Trauma: The first hour* (pp. 103-139). Norwalk, CT: Appleton-Century-Crofts.

Gurevitch, M.J., Van Dyke, J., Young, E.S., & Jackson, K. (1986). Improved oxygenation and lower peak airway pressures in severe adult respiratory distress syndrome: Treatment with inverse ratio ventilation. *Chest*, 89, 211-213.

Hegarty, M.M. (1976). A conservative approach to penetrating injuries of the chest: Experience with 131 successive cases. *Injury*, 8, 53-59.

Henneman, P.L. (1987). MAST (letter). *Journal of Trauma*, 27, 1095.

Henneman, P.L. (1989). Penetrating abdominal trauma. *Emergency Medicine Clinics of North America*, 7, 647-666.

Henneman, P.L., Marx, J.A., Moore, E.E., Cantrill, S.V., & Ammons, L.A. (1990). Diagnostic peritoneal lavage: Accuracy in predicting necessary laparotomy following blunt and penetrating trauma. *Journal of Trauma*, 30, 1345-1355.

Johnson, J.A., Cogbill, T.H., & Winga, E.R. (1986). Determinants of outcome after pulmonary contusion. *Journal of Trauma*, 26, 695-697.

Jorden, R.C., & Barkin, R.M. (1988). Multiple trauma. In P. Rosen, F.J. Baker II, R.M. Barkin, G.R. Braen, R.H. Dailey, & R.C. Leuy (Eds.), *Emergency medicine: Concepts and clinical practice* (pp. 159-177). St. Louis: Mosby-Year Book, Inc.

Kaback, K.R., Saunders, A.B., & Meislin, H.W. (1984). MAST suit update. *Journal of the American Medical Association*, 252, 2598-2603.

Kanak, R., Fahey, P., & Vanderwarf, C. (1985). Oxygen cost of breathing: Changes dependent upon mode of mechanical ventilation. *Chest*, 87, 126-127.

Kastendieck, J.G. (1988). Airway management. In P. Rosen, F.J. Baker II, R.M. Barkin, G.R. Braen, R.H. Dailey, & R.G. Levy (Eds.), *Emergency medicine: Concepts and clinical practice* (pp. 41-68). St. Louis: Mosby-Year Book, Inc.

Kattan, K.R. (1978). Trauma of the bony thorax. *Seminars in Roentgenology*, 13, 69-77.

Kazarian, K.K., & DelGuercio, L.R.M. (1980). The use of mixed venous blood gas determinations in traumatic shock. *Annals of Emergency Medicine*, 9, 179-182.

Korber, T.E., & Henneman, P.L. (1989). Digital nasotracheal intubation. *Journal of Emergency Medicine*, 7, 275-277.

Lain, D.C., Dibenedetto, R., Morris, S.L. Van Nguyen, A., Saulters, R., & Causey, D. (1989). Pressure control versus inverse ratio ventilation as a method to reduce peak inspiratory pressure and provide adequate ventilation and oxygenation. *Chest*, 95, 1081-1088.

Luce, E.A., Tubb, T.D., & Moore, A.M. (1979). Review of 1,000 major facial fractures and associated injuries. *Plastic and Reconstructive Surgery*, 63(1), 26-30.

Luce, J.M., Tyler, M.T., & Pierson, D.J. (1984). *Intensive respiratory care* (pp. 1-32). Philadelphia: W.B. Saunders.

MacIntyre, N. (1986). Respiratory function during pressure support ventilation. *Chest*, 89, 677-683.

Majernick, T.G., Bieniek, R., Houston, J.B., & Hughes, H.G. (1986). Cervical spine motion during orotracheal intubation. *Annals of Emergency Medicine*, 14, 417-420.

Manson, P.N. (1984). Maxillofacial injuries. *Emergency Medicine Clinics of North America*, 2, 761-798.

Martindale, L.G. (1989). Carbon monoxide poisoning: The rest of the story. *Journal of Emergency Nursing*, 15, 101-111.

Mattox, K.L., Bickell, W.H., Pepe, P.E., & Mangelsdorf, A.D. (1986). Prospective randomized evaluation of antishock MAST in post-traumatic hypotension. *Journal of Trauma*, 26, 779-786.

Mattox, K.L., Bickell, W., Pepe, P.E., Burch J., & Feliciano, D. (1989). Prospective MAST study of 911 patients. *Journal of Trauma*, 29, 1104-1111.

McCabe, J.B., Seidel, D.R., & Jagger, J.A. (1983). Antishock trouser inflation and pulmonary vital capacity. *Annals of Emergency Medicine*, 12, 290-293.

McCormick, M., Feustel, P.J., Newell, J.C., Stratton, H.H., & Fortune, J.B. (1988). Effect of cardiac index and hematocrit changes on oxygen consumption in resuscitated patients. *Journal of Surgical Research*, 44, 499-505.

Meislin, H.W. (1980). The esophageal obturator airway: A study of respiratory effectiveness. *Annals of Emergency Medicine*, 9, 54-59.

Merlotti, G.J., Marcet, E., Sheaff, C.M., Dunn, R., & Barrett, J.A. (1985). Use of peritoneal lavage to evaluate abdominal penetration. *Journal of Trauma*, 25, 228-231.

Miller, H.A.B., Taylor, G.A., Harrison, A.W., Maggisano, R., Hanna, S., DeLacy, J.L., & Shulman, H. (1983). *Canadian Medical Association Journal*, 129, 1104-1107.

Miller, L.W., Bennett, E.V., Root, D., Trinkle, J.K., & Grover F.L. (1984). Management of penetrating and blunt diaphragmatic injury. *Journal of Trauma*, 24, 403-408.

Mohsenifar, Z., Goldbach, P., Tashkin, D.P., & Campisi, D.J. (1983). Relationship between oxygen delivery and oxygen consumption in the adult respiratory distress syndrome. *Chest*, 84, 267-271.

Mullins, R.J., & Garrison, R.N. (1987). In J.D. Richardson, H.C. Polk, & L.M. Flint (Eds.), *Trauma: Clinical care and pathophysiology* (pp. 167-212). Chicago: Mosby–Year Book, Inc.

Naclerio, E.A. (1970). Chest trauma. *Clinical Symposia*, 22, 75-109.

Neff, C.C., Pfister, R.C., & Van Sonnenberg, E. (1983). Percutaneous transtracheal ventilation: Experimental and practical aspects. *Journal of Trauma*, 23, 84-90.

Niehoff, J., DelGuercio, C., LaMorte W., Hughes-Grasberger, L.H., Heard, S., & Dennis, R. (1988). Efficacy of pulse oximetry and capnography in postoperative ventilator weaning. *Critical Care Medicine*, 16, 701-705.

Oparah, S.S., & Mandal, A.K. (1976). Penetrating stab wounds of the chest: Experience with 200 cases. *Journal of Trauma*, 16, 868-872.

Peabody, J.L., Willis, M.M., Gregory, G.A., Tooley, W.H., & Lucey, J.F. (1978). Clinical limitations and advantages of transcutaneous oxygen electrodes. *Acta Anaesthesiologica Scandinavica (Supplementum)*, 68, 88-90.

Peitzman, A.B., & Paris, P. (1988). Thoracic trauma. In J.E. Campbell (Ed.), *Basic trauma life support* (pp. 91-96). Englewood Cliffs, NJ: Prentice-Hall.

Petty, T.L. (1974). Acute respiratory failure In T.L. Petty (Ed.), *Intensive and rehabilitative respiratory care* (pp. 3-13). Philadelphia: Lea & Febiger.

Phillips, E.H., Rogers, W.F., & Gasper, M.R. (1981). First rib fractures: Incidence of vascular injury and indications for angiography. *Surgery*, 89, 42-47.

Prakash, O., & Meij, S. (1985). Cardiopulmonary response to inspiratory pressure support during spontaneous ventilation vs. conventional ventilation. *Chest*, 88, 403-408.

Ramponi, D.R. (1986). Chest trauma. In M.K. Finke & N.E. Lanros (Eds.), *Emergency nursing: A comprehensive review* (pp. 215-239). Rockville, MD: Aspen.

Richardson, J.D., Adams, L., & Flint, L.M. (1982). Selective management of flail chest and pulmonary contusion. *Annals of Surgery*, 196, 481-487.

Rivizza, A., Carugo, M., Cerchiari, E., Ferrante, M., Della Puppa, T., & Villa, L. (1983). Inversed ratio and conventional ventilation: Comparison of the respiratory effects. *Anesthesiology*, 59, 523.

Ross, S.E., & Cernaianu, A.C. (1990). Epidemiology of thoracic injuries: Mechanisms of injury and pathophysiology. In A.J. DelRossi (Ed.), Thoracic trauma. *Topics in Emergency Medicine* (pp. 1-6). Frederick, MD: Aspen.

Rutledge, R., Thomason, M., Oller, D., Meredith, W., Moylan, J., Clancy, T., Cunningham, P., & Baker, C. (1991). The spectrum of abdominal injuries associated with the use of seat belts. *Journal of Trauma*, 31, 820-825.

Sahn, S.A., Lakshminarayan S., & Petty, T.L. (1967). Weaning from mechanical ventilation. *Journal of the American Medical Association*, 235, 2208-2212.

Shackford, S.R., Virgilio, R.W., & Peters, R.M. (1981). Selective use of ventilator therapy in flail chest injury. *Journal of Thoracic and Cardiovascular Surgery*, 81, 194-201.

Smith, R.B., Schaer, W.B., & Pfaeffle, H. (1975). Percutaneous transtracheal ventilation for anaesthesia and resuscitation: A review of complications. *Canadian Anesthetists Society Journal*, 22, 607-612.

Stewart, R.D. (1988). Field airway control for the trauma patient. In J.E. Campbell (Ed.), *Basic trauma life support* (pp. 42-90). Englewood Cliffs, NJ: Prentice-Hall.

Tashkin, D.P., Flick G., Bellamy, P., & Mecurio, P. (1987). Pulmonary function. In W.C. Shoemaker & E. Abraham (Eds.), *Diagnostic methods in critical care*. New York: Marcel Dekker.

Tittley, J.G., Fremes, S.E., Weisel, R.D., Christakis, G.T., Evans, P.J., Madonik, M.M., Ivanov, J., & McLaughlin, P.R. (1985). Hemodynamic and myocardial metabolic consequences of PEEP. *Chest*, 88, 496-502.

Treasure, R.L. (1979). Management of flail chest. *Military Medicine*, 144, 588-589.

Troop, B., Meyers, R.M., & Agarwal, N. (1985). Early recognition of diaphragmatic injuries from blunt trauma. *Annals of Emergency Medicine*, 14, 97-101.

Versmaol, H.T., Linderkamp, O., Holzmann, M., Strohhacker, I., & Riegel, K.P. (1978). Limits of $tcPo_2$ monitoring in sick neonates: Relation to blood pressure, blood volume, peripheral blood flow, and acid-base status. *Acta Anaesthesiologica Scandinavica (Supplementum)*, 68, 88-90.

Viale, J.P., Annat, G.J., Bouffard, Y.M., Delafosse, B.X., Bertrand, O.M., & Motin, J.P. (1988). Oxygen cost of breathing in postoperative patients:Pressure support ventilation vs. continuous positive airway pressure. *Chest*, 93, 499-505.

Vukich, D.J., & Markovchick, V.J. (1988). Pulmonary and chest wall injuries. In P. Rosen, F.J. Baker, R.M. Barkin, G.R. Braen, R.H. Dailey, & R.G. Levy (Eds.), *Emergency medicine: Concepts and clinical practice* (pp. 473-518). St. Louis: Mosby–Year Book, Inc.

Williams, S.M. (1985). The Pulmonary system. In J.G. Alspach & S.M. Williams (Eds.), *Core curriculum for critical care nursing* (pp. 1-100). Philadelphia: W.B. Saunders.

Yang, K.L., & Tobin, M.J. (1991). A prospective study of indexes predicting the outcome of trials of weaning from mechanical ventilation. *New England Journal of Medicine*, 324, 1446-1495.

Yelderman, N., & New, W. (1983). Evaluation of pulse oximetry. *Anesthesiology*, 59, 349-352.

9 Perfusion
Cardiac and vascular injuries
■■■

Janet A. Neff

OBJECTIVES

❏ Identify the relationship between mechanism, site of injury, and potential perfusion abnormality.

❏ Describe the anatomic and pathophysiologic basis for vascular changes in shock.

❏ Recognize the clinical manifestations associated with altered tissue perfusion.

❏ Recognize the impact of fluid resuscitation on perfusion and gas transport.

❏ Anticipate the complications associated with inadequate perfusion.

❏ Explain the rationale for altered cardiovascular responses in pediatric, pregnant, and elderly patients.

❏ Describe the signs and symptoms, clinical significance, and nursing management of patients with specific perfusion disorders.

❏ Recognize the current and ongoing controversies in treatment modalities related to perfusion deficits.

INTRODUCTION Adequate perfusion of life-sustaining organs, such as the brain, heart, and lung, is of utmost importance. The importance of maintaining circulation (**C**) after assessing and supporting the airway (**A**) and breathing (**B**) is repeatedly emphasized to trauma care providers for good reason. This chapter focuses on maximizing the transport of needed gases, nutrients, and chemicals. Adequate perfusion means the maintenance of vascular flow, pressure, and volume to meet the demands of the tissues. Hemorrhage associated with facial injuries or within the bronchopulmonary tree or pleura may directly impact airway clearance and the capacity for gas exchange, but perfusion deficits without direct pulmonary involvement will also hinder tissue oxygenation and acid-base status.

The nursing role in maintaining adequate perfusion involves (1) awareness of the principles of oxygen transport, vascular flow, and indicators of hidden hemorrhage; and (2) astute anticipation and assessment of inadequate perfusion. These topics plus general treatment modalities and specific vascular injury assessment and intervention will be reviewed after a discussion of pertinent anatomy, physiology, and principles of physics.

CASE STUDY The following paramedic radio report is received: "We have an 18-year-old male warehouse worker with a chief complaint of pain and shortness of breath. He was hit by a carton of pipe clamps that fell from a shelf 10 feet off the ground. The object struck his right posterior thorax, and the patient fell onto another carton, striking the left side of his chest and abdomen. He is receiving oxygen at 4 L/min by nasal prongs and has one large-bore IV catheter in place with lactated Ringer's solution 'running wide open.'"

In planning for patient arrival at the facility, what additional history and assessment data are helpful?

Information regarding vital signs, especially respiratory rate (RR), effort, depth of excursion, and equality of breath sounds; heart rate (HR); blood pressure (BP); and level of consciousness is necessary. Also, location and description of pain may help in assessing degree of injury.

Radio update: "RR is 30/min, slightly labored, equal excursion, moderate depth, and decreased breath sounds bilaterally at bases; HR is 126; and BP is 90 palpated. Glasgow coma scale score is 15 with no loss of consciousness after injury. No flail segment noted. Patient complains of dull left upper quadrant pain and bilateral chest pain, which is accentuated by respiration."

What interventions have not been reported yet that should be done?

The prehospital crew should initiate spinal precautions and high-flow oxygen delivery and should attempt to place a second IV catheter en route.

What is the goal for prehospital fluid replacement?

The first goal is to establish an IV access before vascular collapse. Fluid replacement in the field begins to restore blood loss and maintains perfusion by improving intravascular volume. With short transport times, significant volume is usually not delivered, but with use of new solutions and equipment, vascular volume can be impacted.

Based on the available information, what injuries are suspected?

Injuries are listed according to physiologic process that is impacted:

- Ventilation: Flail chest (when awake and in pain, flail segment may not be noticeable)
  Pneumothorax/hemothorax
- Perfusion: Hemothorax
  Chest wall or cardiac contusion
  Cardiac tamponade
  Splenic/Hepatic injury
- Mobility: Vertebral and/or spinal cord injury

MECHANISM OF INJURY

The source of impact (e.g., motor vehicle collision, fist, bullet, horse's hoof), direction and rate of impact, and body composition and position all influence the potential for vascular injury and altered perfusion. Some organs, such as the brain and kidney, can autoregulate blood flow, whereas other organs and tissues depend on cardiac output and systemic changes in vascular tone for their blood supply.

The very structures that serve to protect the thorax may cause additional injury when the force applied is great enough, such as a fractured rib lacerating an intercostal artery. The pericardial tissue surrounding the heart allows the development of cardiac tamponade, a life-threatening condition, but also may contribute to saving a patient's life by literally tamponading a critical cardiac hemorrhage until definitive repair by emergent thoracotomy. Both blunt and penetrating injuries can lead to perfusion deficits.

Penetrating Injury

Penetrating injuries may appear confined. They usually traverse a well-defined area. However, multiple stabbings, shotgun injuries, proximity of other organs, blast effects, and the emboli cavitation and ricochet effects associated with missile injuries increase their scope of injury.

Degree of penetration depends on the size and shape of the object, the force applied, and tissue resistance. Objects with tapered ends facilitate penetration, since the contact area is initially small. Resistance is successively reduced the further the object advances. Intravenous catheter manufacturers use these principles in their design to ease insertion, for example, tapered tips, beveled needles, and low-"drag" materials. External force must overcome tissue tolerance to disrupt structure or function. If a force is applied but does not penetrate, structures (including vessels) can be contused beneath *intact* skin (Halpern, 1989). In thoracic trauma, skin, muscles, and bones serve to deflect or to reduce penetration, but the magnitude of forces involved in motor vehicle crashes (MVCs), falls, and intentional assault often exceed their protective capacity. Although the mass of a penetrating object is important, the velocity has the greatest wounding effect, since kinetic energy transmitted (KE) is proportional to the mass (m) and to the *square* of the velocity (v) (i.e., $KE = \frac{1}{2} mv^2$).

Blunt Injury

Blunt trauma is less apparent and is diffuse in nature, creating a more complex diagnostic challenge and potential for occult shock. The collision of organs after the body's collision with an object results in rupture, contusion, and tears. The two main blunt forces are *deceleration* and *compression* (refer to Chapter 7). Factors affecting deceleration force are velocity and stopping distance. Gravitational (g) force is a term used to convey the force experienced in acceleration or deceleration.

$$G \text{ force } = \frac{(\text{change in velocity})^2}{30} \times \text{stopping distance (SD)}$$

where 30 is a constant and SD is the distance over which the velocity changed (Martinez, 1989).

Human tolerance to deceleration is 30 g's, with injury predictable at greater than 45 g's. Velocity is a major factor, since it is squared in the g force equation. If speed is reduced by one half, the g force decreases by a factor of 4. During a fall, the body accelerates and then abruptly halts on impact with a noncompressible substance, such as concrete. The deceleration force from a fall of about 53 feet is equivalent to a 40 mph crash. By extending the stopping distance after impact (brakes, compressible barriers, and internal vehicle cushioning), the g forces are also reduced, thereby reducing injury. In the case of an MVC in which a driver's chest collides with the steering column of an older model vehicle without a collapsible steering wheel, the g forces are greater than in a more recently designed car in which the stopping distance is prolonged because of compressible materials.

Compressive forces

Injury occurring from lateral collisions may result in hemodynamic instability (hemothorax and pelvic hemorrhage), since the force is exerted against the thorax and against the pelvis (McSwain, 1984). When compressive forces trap the abdominal contents between the vertebral column and the object of impact, the liver and spleen can rupture. In the thorax, compression between the vertebral column and the sternum may lead to cardiac contusion. It should be remembered that 40 to 50 pounds of pressure exerted on the thorax for external cardiac compressions depresses the sternum 1½ to 2 inches and increases intrathoracic pressure. The pressure from an MVC or pedestrian collision is much greater. A simple method of calculating the force

involved and the strength required to prevent forward motion is to multiply the speed of the motor vehicle (in mph) by the patient's weight (in pounds)—a 10-pound infant "held" by a restrained adult in a 30-mph crash requires the strength equivalent to lifting 300 pounds 1 foot. (McSwain, 1984; Robertson, 1985). Sternal fractures are relatively rare but may be more common in the elderly and in osteoporetic patients. Children, in contrast, have a very compliant, elastic chest and may evidence less chest wall damage but may sustain internal injury (Eichelberger & Anderson, 1988).

During horizontal or vertical deceleration, the tissues make direct contact at different times, creating the potential for shearing, bending, and torsion stress. The aorta, for example, has a fairly mobile ascending portion and a relatively immobile descending portion held by the ligamentum arteriosum, intercostal arteries, and parietal pleura. Shearing stress (the movement of tissues in opposite directions along the same plane) and bending stress (the creation of tension as a tissue is compressed and forced to bend) occur in the descending aorta. In the ascending aorta the damage occurs during compression as the heart is displaced and the aorta rotates, resulting in torsion or twisting (Cammack, Rapport, Paul, & Baird, 1959). The liver is also impacted by bending stresses as it collides with the ligamentum teres hepatis, and the spleen may be torn from its mesenteric attachment, resulting in serious blood volume loss (McSwain, 1984).

Associated Injuries

The heart and the great vessels (inferior and superior vena cava, brachiocephalic and subclavian vessels, carotid arteries, and pulmonary arteries) are thoracic structures responsible for perfusion. Thoracic injuries are often combined with abdominal injury (Andrews, 1989) (Figure 9-1). Liver and spleen lacerations are usually the result of direct impact or contrecoup forces. However, it has been demonstrated in animals that nonpenetrating cardiac trauma can result in hepatic and splenic injury, related to a sudden, high elevation of venous pressure (Stein et al., 1983). Fluid loss from chemically induced inflammation, the need for additional surgery, and the potential for sepsis in abdominal injuries complicate hemodynamic maintenance.

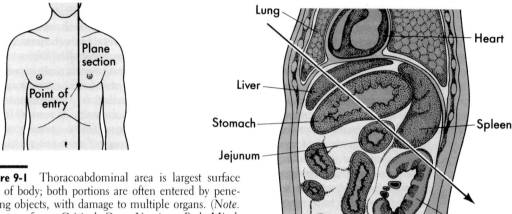

Figure 9-1 Thoracoabdominal area is largest surface area of body; both portions are often entered by penetrating objects, with damage to multiple organs. (*Note.* Redrawn from *Critical Care Nursing: Body-Mind-Spirit* [p. 1044] by C.V. Kenner, C.E. Guzzetta, and B.M. Dossey [Eds.], 1985, Boston: Little, Brown.)

ANATOMIC AND PHYSIOLOGIC CONSIDERATIONS
Principles of Blood Loss

The severity of the perfusion defect is related to the vascularity of the injured tissue and the ease of hemostasis. Blood loss will be proportional to the size of the vascular defect and the rate and pressure of flow (Table 9-1). Therefore the heart and its major outflow tracts, the aorta (high pressure) and the pulmonary artery (low pressure), have the greatest potential for immediate exsanguination from significant injury because of their flow rates of 5 liters of blood/min. However, these are not the most commonly injured sites. The liver is a particularly vascular organ that requires great skill to achieve hemostasis (Figure 9-2). The large, short, tortuous hepatic veins drain posteriorly into the inferior vena cava, making surgical access and repair difficult (Brown, 1988). In-depth analysis of 185 patients with blunt traumatic liver injury linked exsanguination to early mortality as a result of the associated damage from hypovolemic cardiac arrest and hypoxic progression of brain injury (Rivkind, Siegel, & Dunham, 1989). As the severity of liver injury increases, tremendous blood loss and a high mortality occur, especially with hepatic venous and vena caval injuries. Suggested management includes immediate intravascular fluid replacement and institution of rapid operative repair with packing.

Table 9-1 Relative flow rates of organs and vessels

Organ/vessel	Flow rate (ml/min)*
Heart	6000
Lungs	6000
Abdominal aorta	4000
Hepatic vein	1800
Kidneys	1500
Portal vein	1300
Brain	750
Superior mesenteric artery	700
Hepatic artery	500
Coronary circulation	250

*Approximations based on percent of blood flow in 70-kg person with a cardiac output of 6L/min.

Splenic and hepatic injuries are rated according to various classification schemes, e.g., from a minor hepatic nonexpanding hematoma <10% surface area to retrohepatic vena cava injury or hepatic avulsion (Moore et al., 1989).

The retroperitoneal and peritoneal spaces can hold tremendous amounts of blood without an obvious external change in appearance or girth. Whereas peritoneal bleeding may be detected by peritoneal lavage, retroperitoneal bleeding is evident only by general signs of shock and more advanced diagnostic techniques, such as CT scanning. Retroperitoneal structures of concern are

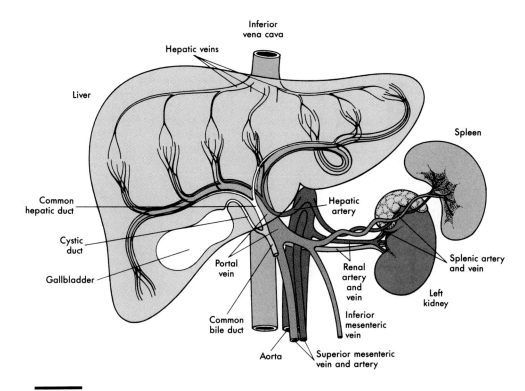

Figure 9-2   Hepatic arterial and venous flow is significant, creating great difficulty in obtaining hemostasis.

the abdominal aorta, the inferior vena cava, kidneys, pancreas, and iliac vessels.

Pelvic cavity hematomas may cause the traditional peritoneal tap to be positive, necessitating a supraumbilical approach in the presence of known pelvic fractures (Sherman et al., 1989). Vascular blood loss may be expected to be greatest from arterial sources, but this is not necessarily the case. Veins seal less efficiently than arteries when injured (Sedlak & Mace, 1989). A dramatic example is iliac venous bleeding, which may be more difficult to control than arterial bleeding, leading to high mortality (Duncan et al., 1989). Scalp lacerations may be misleading in estimation of blood volume lost, but the scalp has a very rich blood supply. Lemos and Clark (1988) report eight cases of adults sustaining hemorrhagic shock from inadequate control of scalp lacerations as suggested by clinical and laboratory findings. In the infant, intracranial bleeding can result in hemorrhagic shock because of an expandable cranium (Moylan, 1988) and cephalohematomas can be significant. In contrast, blunt head injury

when combined with hypotension indicates that another source of bleeding exists (other than the head) that must be evaluated.

Blood loss from arterial lacerations is affected by the type of vascular damage; that is, in arteries of similar size, flow, and pressure a partial laceration with or without associated crush will generally bleed more than a cleanly transected vessel (Richardson, Polk, & Flint, 1987) (Figure 9-3).

Bone is another potential source of blood loss. Bone is well supplied with blood in the outer layer of the periosteum and in the medullary cavity and haversian system (the unit of bone structure) via the nutrient artery and its tributaries (Gosling, Harris, Humpherson, Whitmore, & Willan, 1985). When a fracture occurs, these vessels are disrupted and profuse bleeding ensues. Additional hemorrhage may occur because of injury to vessels in approximation to bone. This is especially significant when major arteries and veins are damaged or when small vessel hemorrhage is unimpeded, exemplified by blood loss associated with posterior pelvic fractures (Richard-

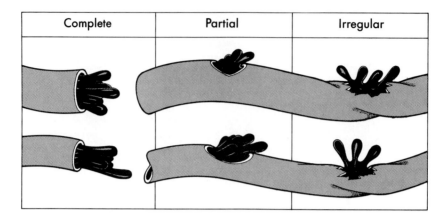

Figure 9-3 Vessel injury. Complete transection results in longitudinal and circumferential contraction of vein, which reduces diameter of vessel lumen and flow through it. Partial tear of vessel, resulting in same compensatory measures, which in this instance create larger defect, leading to greater blood loss. Irregular lacerations with or without crush and torsion cannot compensate as fully as complete injuries. In general, veins contract more effectively than arteries.

son et al., 1987). It is of particular importance in infants to recognize the possibility of significant blood loss into soft tissues after fracture of an extremity. Further discussion of orthopedic blood loss is found in Chapter 11.

It is obvious that the trauma patient suffering blunt or penetrating trauma has the potential for catastrophic hemorrhage and altered perfusion. The next section explains the significance of vascular anatomy, the physics of flow and pressure, and oxygen-carrying capacity.

Circulatory Processes

Arteriolar contraction and dilation can vastly change capillary flow and therefore tissue perfusion at the cellular level. These vascular changes occur because of sympathetic innervation in the muscular walls and the effect of local tissue factors, such as *oxygen*, carbon dioxide, and hydrogen ion concentration. Therefore flow should generally reflect the need of tissues. Preferential flow can be controlled by precapillary sphincters (rings of smooth muscle surrounding the entrance to capillaries).

The capillaries constitute the exchange system for diffusion of fluid, nutrients, gases, and electrolytes between the blood and alveoli and between the blood and interstitial spaces, allowing cellular exchange. The capillaries are explicitly designed for this function by way of their thin walls and extensive branching, contributing to a tremendous surface area for exchange (500 to 600 ml). Capillary walls consist of only one layer, the tunica intima, which comprises the endothelium and its basement membrane. This single, thin layer facilitates diffusion. In contrast, other vessels have three layers: intima, media, and externa (adventitia).

Capillary Exchange

Solvents and solutes are transported across the capillary, creating continual mixing of the capillary and interstitial contents. Although the permeability of capillaries in different tissues is varied, it is always greatest at the venous end (Berne & Levy, 1986). Lipid-soluble molecules, such as O_2 and CO_2, easily diffuse through the lipid membranes of the endothelial cells. The concentration of oxygen is the most important factor in the autoregulation of the terminal arterioles and precapillary sphincters (Guyton, 1987). Small, non-lipid-soluble molecules, such as Na^+, Cl^-, glucose, and water, are flow limited; there is little restriction to their passage via capillary pores. Therefore as blood flow increases, the capillary diffusion capacity increases. In a low-flow state, these molecules are less available for exchange to meet the cellular demands. Another inhibiting factor to diffusion is interstitial edema.

As the size of the molecular solute increases,

its diffusion is progressively restricted. A molecule the size of albumin is almost totally impermeable, creating a concentration difference between the capillary plasma and the interstitial fluid. Albumin is the main protein of significance in capillary dynamics and contributes to the oncotic pressure of about 28 mm Hg. Though this is a small pressure in relation to the total osmotic pressure of the plasma (600 mm Hg), it is significant because of the much lower protein concentration in the interstitium. This osmotic force is crucial to maintaining fluid within the capillary. In severe shock a permeability state develops that even allows leakage of albumin.

Fluid exchange through the capillary depends not only on the ease of water diffusion and the oncotic pressure, but also on the capillary hydrostatic pressure (blood pressure) and its impact on filtration and absorption. Capillary hydrostatic pressure is increased by elevated arterial or venous pressure and by increased postcapillary venous resistance but is decreased by closure of precapillary sphincters (Berne & Levy, 1986). When hydrostatic pressure exceeds oncotic pressure, filtration of fluid into the interstitium occurs. As vasoconstriction occurs in response to shock, capillary hydrostatic pressure is lowered, promoting fluid transfer from the tissues to the plasma. Also, if the oncotic pressure is decreased too much by hemodilution with crystalloids or by interstitial fluid reabsorption, retention of capillary fluid volume will be less certain.

The venous system has 2 to 3 times the volume and 5 to 6 times the distensibility of the arterial system, accounting for a 12 to 18 times larger capacity for blood storage (Smith & Kampine, 1980). Flow is impacted by this such that during fluid resuscitation, the volume will seek pressure equilibrium and will therefore distribute mainly in the venous system.

Pressure and flow dynamics

Pressure and flow within the vascular system depend on the characteristics of the fluid, vessel size, flow, and pressure. According to Poiseuille's law

$$Q = (\text{change in P})r^4 Pi/nL8$$

where Q = flow; (change in P) = the difference in pressure between two ends of the tube (vessel); r = radius; n = viscosity of the fluid; L = length of the tube (vessel); and Pi and 8 are constants. Of

these factors, the radius is predominant because of the fourth power effect. The aorta has the least fall in pressure and therefore the least resistance, whereas the arterioles have the greatest pressure fall and thus the greatest resistance to flow.

Viscosity   Viscosity is inversely proportional to flow, so a low hematocrit (decreasing viscosity) creates less resistance, and flow increases. When blood loss and hemodilution occur during resuscitation, the higher flow rate from the lowered hematocrit assists in distributing oxygen to tissues in the context of limited hemoglobin.

Fluid viscosity will increase about 2% for every 1°C drop in temperature. Allowing the infusion of cold fluids, therefore, decreases flow and the effectiveness of volume replacement. Higher hematocrit, as in polycythemia, is rarely seen in trauma, but the concept can be applied to transfusion principles. Whole blood has a hematocrit about equal to 45%, whereas packed red blood cells have a hematocrit between 60% to 65% and 75% to 80%, depending on the type of anticoagulant added. This higher hematocrit will increase resistance to flow unless dilution precedes administration.

In thoracic injuries the development of a partial tear of the aorta through the intima and media decreases the wall thickness and the radius increases as a pseudoaneurysm develops. If pressure remains the same, the wall stress increases as a result of the increased radius and sets the stage for aortic rupture.

Pulse pressure   The difference between systolic and diastolic pressures is the pulse pressure (normally 50 mm Hg), which corresponds to an increment of volume. The mean arterial pressure (MAP) exerted can be estimated as the diastolic pressure plus one third of the pulse pressure. For example, if the blood pressure = 90/70, the MAP = 70 + ⅓ (20) = 77. The MAP is the best single measure of driving pressure and is the prime variable regulated by hemodynamic mechanisms in defense of circulatory function. The level of the MAP depends on cardiac output (CO) (heart rate × stroke volume) and on total peripheral resistance (TPR), so MAP = CO × TPR. An increase in heart rate (HR), which occurs in response to pain, fear, and the volume loss of trauma, will be reflected in the pulse pressure and impacts cardiac output. The more rapid HR interrupts the diastolic decline, thereby raising diastolic pressure. If a temporary rise in CO does result, the systolic pressure increase usually will not match the diastolic, so the pulse pressure decreases, and a rapid, thready pulse is palpated (Smith & Kampine, 1980). A rapid HR also reduces the length of the cardiac cycle, mainly the diastolic portion, resulting in restricted ventricular filling (decreasing stroke volume) and eventually decreased CO.

Oxygen delivery

Oxygen delivery depends on blood flow to tissues, on the oxygen content, and on the ease of releasing oxygen to the tissues. Oxygen content comprises dissolved plasma oxygen (dependent on the Pao_2) and oxyhemoglobin, the primary oxygen carrier. Each gram of hemoglobin can combine with 1.34 ml of oxygen when exposed to high enough O_2 pressures. This creates an oxygen capacity of about 20 ml/dl for a normal (male) hemoglobin of 15 g/dl. The tissues continuously use O_2, thereby lowering the PO_2 in nearby interstitial fluid and in the capillary blood. In optimal circumstances, the arterial blood flows into the tissue capillaries with high O_2 saturation and tension. The oxygen, a lipid-soluble molecule with a high pressure gradient, diffuses across the capillary into the extracellular fluid and the cells. By doing so, the plasma PO_2 decreases, causing HbO_2 to dissociate and release more O_2 to the tissues (Comroe, 1965).

Oxyhemoglobin curve The shape of the curve offers physiologic advantages. The flat "lung" portion of the curve facilitates O_2 loading. As the hemoglobin (Hgb) loads O_2, it needs only a sufficient PO_2 level, usually about 80 mm Hg, to fully saturate. Therefore even if alveolar PO_2 is altered ± 20 mm Hg from its normal level of 100 mm Hg, the same amount of O_2 will be associated with the hemoglobin (Mines, 1986). The steeper "tissue" portion of the curve allows peripheral tissue withdrawal of large amounts of O_2 with only a small drop in capillary PO_2, thereby maintaining the partial pressure necessary to drive O_2 from the capillaries into the cells, specifically the mitochondria (West, 1979).

It is especially pertinent in trauma patients to note the effect of anemia on the oxyhemoglobin dissociation curve (Figure 9-4). Although Hgb is fully saturated, the limited Hgb available in anemia reduces the total O_2 content available to the tissues. In the presence of anemia, a lower percent of HbO_2 exists for any given oxygen tension.

This also occurs with a drop in pH, such as with metabolic acidosis in shock. This "right shift" aids the release of O_2 from Hgb to the tissues, but the amount available is limited. On the other hand, a "left shift" occurs with hypothermia (caused by exposure or by cold fluids) and with decreased 2,3-diphosphoglycerate (2,3 DPG), which is associated with storage of blood and is of concern in massive transfusion. A "left shift" increases O_2 affinity, which does increase O_2 content, but the effective release of O_2 to tissues is decreased.

Shock-Altered Circulation*

Shock refers to tissue perfusion that is inadequate to meet the metabolic needs of the cells and tissues. This may be the result of an increase in metabolic activity, a decrease in flow to the tissues, or a decrease in blood oxygenation. Regardless of the cause, a host of compensatory mechanisms is put into place in an attempt to prevent end organ damage.

Categories of shock

Shock may be classified into the following categories: cardiogenic, obstructive, distributive, and hypovolemic (Table 9-2). Cardiogenic shock may be the result of an arrhythmia caused by cardiac contusion, an electrolyte imbalance, direct cardiac or coronary trauma, or hypoxia. Obstructive shock may occur in response to pericardial tamponade, tension pneumothorax, or obstruction of venous return by soft tissue edema after a crush injury. Distributive shock may present as (1) anaphylactic shock caused by a reaction to contrast dye or a transfusion, (2) neurogenic shock with transection of the cord and loss of neural input, or (3) septic shock. Hypovolemia is perhaps the most common type of shock seen in the trauma patient. Internal volume losses include third spacing of fluid or blood into the interstitium, peritoneum, or tissues surrounding fracture sites. External losses primarily refer to hemorrhage and evaporative fluid loss and protein weeping secondary to burns. Finally, renal losses may be seen with excessive use of diuretics or with the syndrome of inappropriate antidiuretic hormone (SIADH) associated with head injury.

Any factor that decreases venous return (preload), such as hemorrhage, venous pooling, or a

---

*This section contributed by Margaret J. Neff, B.S.

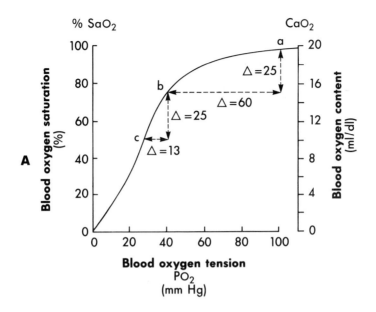

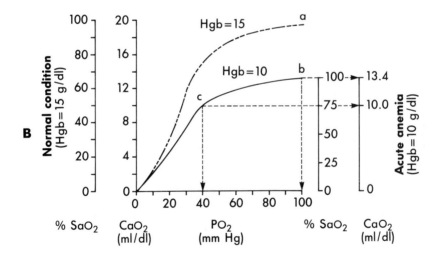

Figure 9-4 **A,** Normal oxyhemoglobin dissociation curve. Conditions: Hgb = 15 g/dl; pH = 7.40; temperature = 37.0° C; Pco_2 = 40 mm Hg. Note that reduction in Po_2 from 100 to 40 mm Hg produces only 25% reduction in Sao_2, but on the steep portion of curve, a mere 13 mm Hg reduction in PO_2, from 40 to 27 mm Hg, also produces a 25% decrease in Sao_2. **B,** Greatest effect on arterial oxygen content is by change in hemoglobin (*point a to b*), not change in arterial partial pressure of oxygen (*point b to c*). Therefore anemia is of greater concern than moderate hypoxemia. (*Note.* Modified from *Trauma Anesthesia and Intensive Care* [p. 117-118] by L.M. Capan, S.M. Miller, and H. Turndorf, 1991, Philadelphia: J.B. Lippincott; [**B** modified]).

Table 9-2 Categories of shock

Type	Cause	Mechanism	Outcome
Hypovolemic	Hemothorax Vessel injury Cardiac injury Bone injury	Hemorrhage, intravascular volume loss	Fluid volume deficit
Cardiogenic	Cardiac contusion Heart failure Myocardial depressant factor, e.g., burns, sepsis	Cardiac ischemia, contusion resulting in altered contractility	Altered cardiac output
Distributive	Spinal shock Sepsis Anaphylaxis	Altered vascular tone (vasodilation)	Relative fluid deficit
Obstructive	Cardiac tamponade Tension pneumothorax Embolism	Increased afterload and restricted ventricular filling	Decreased stroke volume and cardiac output

high central venous pressure, will cause a decrease in MAP because of the decreased cardiac output. An overall decrease in systemic vascular resistance (SVR), as seen in sepsis, anaphylaxis, cord transection, and any autonomic dysfunction (as in diabetes), decreases MAP. An increase in afterload has dual effects on MAP. The increase in SVR serves to directly increase MAP, but it also acts negatively on cardiac output because of increased resistance against which the left ventricle must eject.

Stages of shock

Shock may be described as progressing through three different stages: nonprogressive (compensated), progressive, and irreversible (refractory). A healthy person can compensate for a 10% to 15% loss in intravascular volume, but 20% to 25% loss will generally ovewhelm the body's ability to compensate and the shock will progress (Parrillo, 1991). In the progressive stage, the decrease in tissue perfusion worsens. At this point, the compensatory mechanisms begin to cause end organ damage because of prolonged vasoconstriction. Finally, in the irreversible phase, even if the underlying cause is corrected, too much tissue and cellular damage has occurred and death ensues.

The classic symptoms of hypovolemic shock are sinus tachycardia and oliguria. Blood pressure is reduced, decreased responsiveness is present, extremities are cool and mottled, and the body exhibits signs of sympathetic nervous system stimulation, including diaphoresis and pupillary dilation. In obstructive shock, jugular venous distention and possibly tracheal deviation are present. Early distributive shock will manifest with warm, pink extremities and an increase in cardiac output with bounding pulses. Bradycardia is evident in neurogenic shock when cord transection is above T10. Key components of shock assessment include cutaneous capillary perfusion, heart rate, pulse pressure, and renal output. Blood pressure is used as an indicator of shock but does not provide a direct assessment of *tissue* perfusion. In addition, the blood pressure may be well compensated for and may not drop significantly until later in the course of shock. Table 9-3 shows the American College of Surgeons' (ACS) classifications of hypovolemic shock and their accompanying clinical presentations.

A variety of atypical presentations can make the signs and symptoms presented in Table 9-3 less reliable. For instance, someone who is usually hypertensive may appear to have a "normal" blood pressure but in reality is in shock, because this "normal" pressure is too low to perfuse the person's tissues. Similarly, someone on a beta blocker may not be able to mount a tachycardia in response to a decreased circulating blood volume. Also, patients with a cord transection above T10 may not be able to elevate the heart rate. It is not uncommon for trauma patients to experience

Table 9-3 Classifications of hypovolemic shock and estimated fluid and blood requirements

	Class			
	I	**II**	**III**	**IV**
Blood loss (ml)	Up to 750	750-1500	1500-2000	2000 or more
Blood loss (%BV)	Up to 15%	15%-30%	30%-40%	40% or more
Pulse rate	<100	>100	>120	140 or higher
Blood pressure	Normal	Normal	Decreased	Decreased
Pulse pressure (mm Hg)	Normal or increased	Decreased	Decreased	Decreased
Capillary refill test	Normal	Positive	Positive	Positive
Respiratory rate	14-20	20-30	30-40	>35
Urine output (ml/hr)	30 or more	20-30	5-15	Negligible
CNS—mental status	Slightly anxious	Mildly anxious	Anxious and confused	Confused, lethargic
Fluid replacement (3:1 rule)	Crystalloid	Crystalloid	Crystalloid + blood	Crystalloid + blood

Note. Adapted from *Advanced Trauma Life Support Course* (p. 72) by American College of Surgeons, 1989, Chicago: Author.
Note. For 70-kg male, fluid needs for class I are 2250 ml; for class II, 2250-4500 ml; for class III, up to 6000 ml; for class IV, >6000 ml.

more than one type of shock concurrently (e.g., combined hypovolemic and spinal shock, or combined cardiogenic and anaphylactic shock from intravenous dye used during aortography).

Compensatory responses

A decrease in MAP and tissue perfusion results in stimulation of baroreceptors and chemoreceptors and activation of the sympathetic nervous system, resulting in a rapid increase in sympathetic tone and decrease in vagal tone. The effect of such stimulation is tachycardia, a positive inotropic response with increased stroke volume, and systemic vasoconstriction. This rapid response to a decrease in circulating pressure and volume occurs within seconds to minutes. However, this neural response will adapt rapidly (1 to 2 days) and will not provide the long-term compensation required to bring the MAP completely back to normal (Guyton, 1987).

Additional rapid-acting compensatory mechanisms include the release of antidiuretic hormone (ADH) from the posterior pituitary in response to a decrease in MAP or an increase in serum osmolality. In high concentration, ADH acts as a very potent vasoconstrictor (Guyton, 1987). Furthermore, a decrease in the MAP will be sensed by the juxtaglomerular cells in the afferent arterioles of the glomeruli. Also, a drop in the glomerular

filtration rate will result in a decrease in sodium, which will be noted by the macula densa cells of the glomerulus. Both mechanisms trigger the release of renin from the juxtaglomerular cells, as can direct sympathetic nervous system stimulation. Renin then initiates a cascade: it stimulates the activation of angiotensinogen (made by the liver) to angiotensin I. Angiotensin I is then converted to the active form (angiotensin II) by angiotensin converting enzyme, which is found primarily in the lung. Angiotensin II is a very potent, rapidly acting vasoconstrictor. As with the neural response, these effects of ADH and angiotensin II are short-lived.

Compensatory mechanisms, which are slower to respond but which are longer-acting, include the following. ADH, in addition to being a vasoconstrictor, also acts on the collecting tubules of the glomerulus to increase water permeability, thus allowing water reabsorption. Angiotensin II not only is a potent vasoconstrictor but also simulates release of aldosterone from the adrenal cortex. Aldosterone acts on the distal tubule to retain sodium, and thus water. Another mechanism by which the intravascular volume is increased is the following. In hemorrhage, the decrease in systemic pressure serves to decrease intracapillary hydrostatic pressure. As a result, fluid leaks or shifts into the capillaries from the interstitium. This has the effect of providing a transient increase in plasma volume and also contributes to the drop in hematocrit noted during hypovolemic shock caused by the fluid shift and resulting dilutional effect (Berne & Levy, 1986; Marino, 1991). Also, the bone marrow is stimulated to produce erythrocytes within a few hours of hemorrhage; however, complete replacement can take several months (Marino, 1991).

As shock worsens with progressively less perfusion to the tissues, vasodilating agents are released locally by the damaged tissues and override the systemic vasoconstriction. These agents include serotonin, bacterial endotoxins, prostaglandins, histamine, and lactate (Guyton, 1987). In addition to vasodilation, histamine and lactate also increase vascular permeability, resulting in fluid extravasation into tissue and a subsequent decrease in effective intravascular volume (Perlroth, 1989).

End organ effects

Unfortunately, the very compensatory mechanisms used to respond to shock can result in significant end organ damage. Vasoconstriction of the kidneys, intestines, and extremities is vital to provide elevated peripheral resistance and thus flow to the brain and heart. However, these organs will ultimately fail if not perfused. The result can include acute tubular necrosis of the kidneys and thus acute renal failure, as well as ischemia of the intestines and peripheral digits, resulting in necrosis and predisposing the body to sepsis. The lung responds to a decrease in oxygen and an increase in carbon dioxide by vasoconstricting, in contrast to the more common systemic response of vasodilation. This vasoconstriction can compromise lung perfusion and lead to tissue damage and subsequent development of adult respiratory distress syndrome (ARDS). The liver is particularly affected by prolonged hypoperfusion. With its high metabolic needs, it is less able to sustain a decrease in perfusion for an extended period. Its additional role in detoxification and in protein synthesis means that a decrease in its function can result in the systemic release of toxins and a decrease in serum proteins and coagulation factors. The body's overall response to shock may result in survival through the initial insult, only to succumb later to acute renal failure, sepsis, or respiratory distress.

Mechanism of cellular injury Decreased perfusion and the resultant acidosis can cause direct cellular damage. Further damage can occur during reperfusion. During prolonged ischemia, xanthine oxidase, a normal enzyme in the pathway of purine metabolism, accumulates. With the reintroduction of oxygen, the xanthine oxidase and oxygen can combine to produce uric acid, hydrogen peroxide, and superoxide. These local oxidants damage the cell membrane. Further damage can be caused by mediators released during tissue injury. For instance, thromboxane is released by injured tissue but then serves to impede microvascular blood flow to this very tissue by causing an increase in arteriolar constriction. Endotoxins released by bacteria in ischemic tissue (especially the GI tract) can evoke release of tumor necrosis factor (cachectin), which is toxic to the vascular endothelium and can result in increased cellular permeability. Myocardial depressant factor, also released by ischemic tissue (especially the pancreas and small intestine), is known to affect cardiac function, although the exact mechanism is as yet unknown (Haglund, 1989). Finally, study has revealed that shock can induce the release of not only ACTH but also beta endorphins from the anterior pituitary. Given the similarity of the β-endorphin receptors to opiate receptors, it is believed that the β-endorphin release may contribute to the hypotension seen in shock (Perlroth, 1989).

Treatment modalities

Table 9-3 provides guidelines for resuscitation based on estimated blood loss in hypovolemic shock, as well as physical and clinical parameters. Additional treatment is aimed at correcting imbalances. For instance, acidosis can be compensated by giving bicarbonate (especially if serum HCO_3 is <10 mEq/L) or by hyperventilating the patient. The lysosomal release seen as a result of local acidosis has been averted in one research setting with the administration of corticosteroids and has shown some efficacy in clinical trials of distributive shock. Because corticosteroids also block the release of ACTH (associated with β-endorphin release), another role for the use of steroids seems likely. Trials using naloxone to block the β-endorphin receptors have proven to increase MAP, pulse pressure, and survival (Perlroth, 1989), Also, experimentally, the production of superoxide may be blocked by inhibiting xanthine oxidase with allopurinol (Demling, 1989) or the enzyme superoxide dismutase (SOD) (Grisham & Granger,

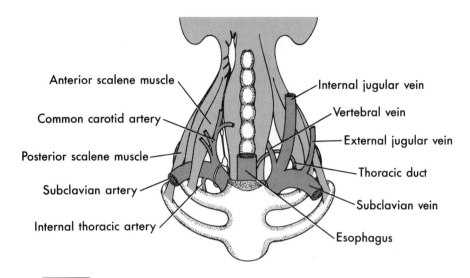

Figure 9-5   Vascular supply of the neck and main branches of the thoracic aorta.

1989) The optimal treatment is · still elusive, but the overall treatment goal is to improve tissue perfusion by trying to increase cardiac output via fluid resuscitation and maintenance of adequate oxygen-carrying and diffusing capacity.

GENERAL ASSESSMENT
Anatomic Considerations

The thorax contains essential and highly vascular structures. Their anatomic relations help to clarify the level of risk from particular mechanisms of injury. Figure 9-5 shows the structures and vasculature of the neck. Figure 9-6 outlines the thoracic structures seen on posteroanterior and lateral chest x-ray films.

Primary Survey

A system of approach for the primary and secondary survey can be remembered by linking systems for review to the alphabet. An instructor for the Trauma Nurse Core Curriculum Instructor Course used this technique, and it has been used successfully by numerous other instructors. The steps are covered from A to I (see the box on the right).

Airway

Airway is always the first priority and has been fully reviewed in Chapter 8. Hypoxia obviously is detrimental to the patient with poor perfusion because the low flow carries less available oxygen. A

Mnemonic system for primary and secondary assessment	
A	Airway
B	Breathing
C	Circulation
D	Disability/level of consciousness
E	Exposure
F	Fahrenheit
G	Get full set of vital signs
H	Head-to-toe assessment
I	Inspect the back

concern for the airway related to perfusion is the development of edema (e.g., from direct trauma, or burn edema after 24 hours) and hematoma formation. Figure 9-5 shows the numerous vessels in the upper thoracic and neck area. If bleeding occurs, pressure on the trachea can result from an expanding hematoma.

CASE STUDY   A young construction worker fell through flooring and impaled himself on a 1-inch reinforced steel bar (rebar), which entered below the jaw and exited through the right orbit. The path of the rebar led to concern for possible development of a hema-

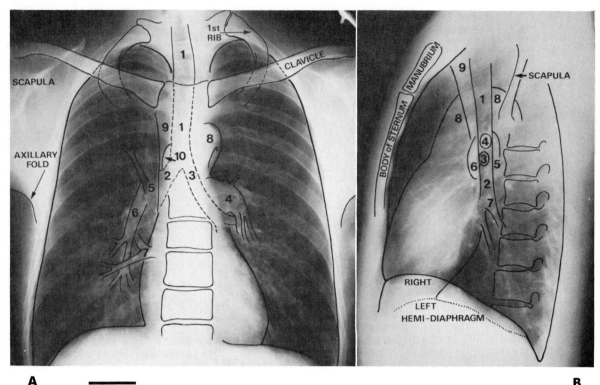

A   **B**

Figure 9-6   Anatomy of chest as shown by posteroanterior and lateral chest x-rays. **A**, Posteroanterior view: numbers refer to anatomic structures as follows: *1*, trachea; *2*, right main bronchus; *3*, left main bronchus; *4*, left pulmonary artery; *4*, right upper lobe pulmonary vein; *7*, right interlobar artery; *7*, right lower and middle lobe vein; *8*, aortic knob; *9*, superior vena cava; *10*, aortic arch. **B**, Lateral view: structures identified are as follows: *1*, tracheal air column; *2*, right intermediate bronchus; *3*, left upper lobe bronchus; *4*, right upper lobe bronchus; *5*, left interlobar artery; *6*, right interlobar artery; *7*, confluence of pulmonary veins; *8*, aortic arch; *9*, brachiocephalic vessels. (*Note.* From *Diagnosis of Diseases of the Chest* [2nd ed.] [Vol. 1] by R.G. Fraser and J.A.P. Pare, 1977. Philadelphia: W.B. Saunders.)

toma (Figure 9-7). As a precaution, he was successfully intubated by fiberoptic laryngoscopy; his angiogram was negative. His C-spine was maintained immobile by the rebar itself until it was removed intraoperatively; full radiographic studies followed. Further discussion of this case is found in Chapter 11.

Breathing

In terms of perfusion, loss of hemoglobin (Hgb) will result in lower oxygen content and shock will reduce the oxygen delivery to tissues. Development of a significant hemothorax will impede gas exchange, and a tension pneumothorax/hemothorax not only will alter gas exchange, but the mediastinal shift can compromise cardiac out-put. Use of auscultation to detect areas of decreased air movement, percussion to detect hyperresonance for pneumothorax or dullness for hemothorax, and inspection and palpation to detect an open, sucking wound, multiple rib fractures, or flail chest will facilitate detection of life-threatening conditions that can impact perfusion.

Circulation

Circulation is assessed in the primary survey by inspection for signs of uncontrolled hemorrhage and general assessment of perfusion by palpation of the strength of the pulse, skin temperature and moisture, and/or assessment of the rapidity of capillary refill. These steps allow rapid assessment of

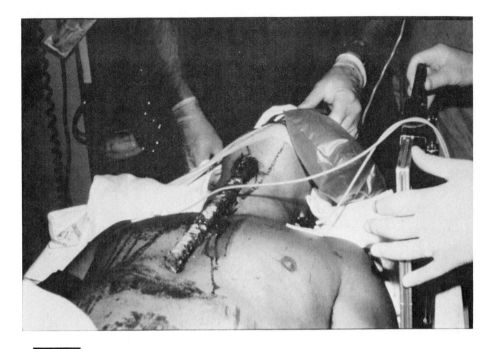

Figure 9-7 Impalement by reinforced steel bar (rebar) through neck and orbit. Elective fiberoptic laryngoscopy procedure followed to ensure airway patency because of potential for hematoma formation that could compromise airway. Angiography was negative. (*Note.* Courtesy Stanford University Trauma Service, Stanford, CA.)

gross perfusion and require minimal technologic aids. In most trauma centers, concurrent assessment and intervention occur, allowing a more rapid progression through the primary and secondary survey. For example, vital signs are routinely measured early in trauma centers by one of the many personnel, but the specific values are not required early to determine whether the person has a perfusion deficit. Therefore in instances where the number of personnel is limited, the steps of primary and secondary survey as typically prescribed allow safe, prioritized assessment and intervention.

Disability/level of consciousness

The level of consciousness is used as another indicator of perfusion. Once the higher level centers in the brain are affected by decreased perfusion, the brain uses autoregulation to maximize oxygen delivery. When this is insufficient, altered consciousness ensues. Other associated factors must be concurrently evaluated, such as direct head injury and the presence of ethanol or de-

pressant drugs. Bedside alcohol sensors are useful in rapidly determining whether alcohol is contributing to altered consciousness.

Secondary Survey
Exposure

Exposing the patient is necessary to maximize assessment. Early awareness of signs such as subtle contusions and seat belt marks can help predict underlying perfusion injury (Figure 9-8).

CASE STUDY A 36-year-old woman was walking with her husband after attending the theatre. They heard a "shot," and she felt considerable pain in her abdomen and saw blood stains on her clothes. A nearby police officer rushed her to the local trauma center. On arrival, she complained of abdominal pain and was quite anxious. She was rushed into the trauma room, and her clothes were cut off. It was then found that the injury resulted from a red dye gun, and except for some bruising from the impact, she was uninjured. However, she had no clothes to wear. This patient was very grateful for her care, but others may

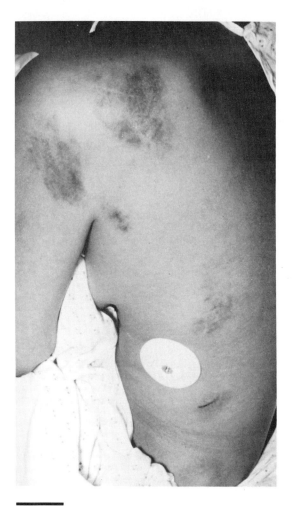

Figure 9-8 Injury to a restrained driver from a roll-over. Bruising and abrasions to left lateral chest and flank from contact with interior of car are obvious.

be furious when expensive jackets or favorite clothes are cut through only to find they have minor injuries and are discharged from the emergency room. Nevertheless, the principle of early and complete exposure is essential and starts in the field. It may be helpful to expose the obvious site of injury first to apply pressure or to evaluate the extent of injury.

Fahrenheit

After exposure, every attempt to maintain the patient's temperature should be made. Low body temperature (1) affects skin signs and the ability to properly palpate vital signs, (2) results in shivering, which can interfere with SpO2 and invali-

date oscillometric, noninvasive blood pressure monitoring, and (3) contributes to coagulopathy. The effects of body temperature are shown in Table 9-4. Most sources define hypothermia as ≤35° C (95° F). Knowledge of the patient's current temperature is also required for accurate interpretation of arterial blood gas values. As temperature drops, the sample measurements of oxygen and carbon dioxide tension are lower, and pH values are higher than actually exist in the patient (Shapiro, Harrison, Cane, & Templin, 1989). To detect hypothermia, the core body temperature must be measured and recorded. Core temperature can be obtained from the esophagus, bladder, pulmonary artery, and tympanic membrane. Mize, Koziol-McLain, and Lowenstein (1991) retrospectively found that 23% of trauma patients brought to a level I trauma center did not have body temperature recorded in the emergency department and that temperature correlated negatively with injury severity scale score. In a prospective pilot study, Neff and Shaver (1987) measured core body temperature in trauma patients and found that 60% had hypothermia (<35° C) on admission to the emergency trauma center. Temperature was monitored throughout the resuscitation phase, and trajectories varied, but showed drops in temperature during thoracotomy and on transfer to other departments for diagnostic studies. During transfer the patients were hand-ventilated with room temperature air and were influenced by convection and arrival in a cool room. In another study, body temperature <36° C in trauma patients transferred from the ED to the OR was linked to fluid infusion and severity of injury, but not to length of time in transport, ED, or OR, patient age, or time of year (Gregory, Flancbaum, Townsend, Cloutier, & Jonasson, 1991). They found a greater mean temperature decline (heat loss) in the ED than in the OR.

Get full set of vital signs

A full set of vital signs should be obtained by this stage of the secondary survey. Blood pressure on ED arrival is one of the required components to determine the revised trauma score. Without it, the trauma score cannot be calculated and therefore the probability of survival (Ps) for the patient will be unavailable. Some advise obtaining a manual auscultatory BP to determine correlation with invasive or noninvasive readings. The

Table 9-4 Signs and symptoms associated with hypothermia

| Temperature | | Characteristics |
Fahrenheit (F)	Centigrade (C)	
98.6°	37.0°	Core body temperature "normal"
95.0°	35.0°	Level of consciousness normal HR, RR, BP, CO, metabolic rate, and renal function increase Shivering to maintain body heat; vessel constriction Ileus and depressed liver detoxification below 34° C Definition of hypothermia is <35° C
89.6°-86.0°	32°-30°	Reactions delayed, stuperous; motor response slow HR decreased; systole prolonged; CO decreased at least 30% RR and metabolic rate decreased Characteristic Osborn, or J, wave appears on ECG after QRS
84.2°-80.6°	29°-27°	Answers simple questions or grunts only Renal blood flow decreased by 50%, but depression of distal tubule enzyme activity may result in cold diuresis Dysrhythmias appear; atrial initially followed by ventricular excitability Shivering has ceased Little voluntary motion; limbs move to noxious stimuli Pupillary response to light is minimal Basal metabolic rate falls 50%; apnea
80.6°-78.8°	27°-26°	Does not speak; rigor only Loss of gag, deep tendon, and pupillary light reflexes BP drops severely; CO decreased Ventricular fibrillation or standstill
78.8°-75.2°	26°-24°	Unconscious; no motor movement; corneal reflex absent
68.8°	20°	Cardiac standstill (although a bradycardia may be present at lower temperatures)
62.6°	17°	Isoelectric electroencephalogram (EEG)

Note. Modified from "Hypothermia: The Chill that Need Not Kill" by R.S. Pratt, 1980, *Bulletin of the American College of Surgeons,* 65(10),pp. 30-31; and from *Accident Analysis and Prevention, 14* (2), 1982, p. 148.

main value in this is the hands-on requirement with subsequent assessment of pulse strength and equality and skin signs. Because BP may be hard to auscultate during vasoconstriction, other techniques, such as Doppler scan or continuous, direct monitoring, may be more accurate. Nevertheless, if the assessments raise questions about the accuracy of a result, a manual check should be done. The mode of BP measurement should be clearly recorded on the trauma data base/flowsheet. For all major trauma patients, the BP should be measured in both arms and recorded to determine any variance that might reflect a preexisting vascular defect or an aortic hematoma or dissection, especially when mechanism of injury points to deceleration injury or significant blunt chest trauma. When the number of personnel is limited, assessment of equality of upper and lower extremity pulses may be sufficient.

Trends in HR and BP, as well as narrowing of the pulse pressure, should be monitored and evaluated in terms of the ACS levels of shock (Table 9-3). The stability of findings in relation to ongoing fluid requirements and known injuries will help to determine whether the patient should have continued monitoring, would be considered safe for transfer to CT department, or should proceed directly to the OR.

Head-to-toe assessment

In the process of completing this whole body assessment, distal vascular compromise should be found and intervention begun. Some minor injuries such as a nondisplaced ankle fracture may be missed in very unstable patients requiring rapid resuscitation and even with a careful assessment in patients with less severe conditions. This oversight may be the result of limited swelling, other distracting pain, or unconsciousness. This places great importance on the continued nursing assessment on admission to an in-patient unit. Some injuries are detected at the time of first attempts at increased mobility.

Inspect the back

The evidence of major damage from an exit wound of a benign-appearing anterior gunshot, a tender or unstable spine, or other previously undetected injury may be found on the posterior surface of the body. This inspection should be done with proper alignment until spinal integrity is known.

CASE STUDY A 22-year-old man was brought to a trauma center with no vital signs or signs of life and a somewhat extended downtime. He had been found "down" in his car. The patient was pronounced dead after a short resuscitation attempt. On review of the coroner's autopsy report, it was found that the victim had a bullet entrance wound behind the left shoulder, which was not documented by the trauma team. In this case, the cause of death was still nonpreventable because of the downtime without vital signs. However, it certainly brought attention to the trauma center's initial patient assessment process.

Special Considerations
Pregnancy

The physiologic changes in pregnancy are significant in an effort to provide the optimal environment for the developing fetus. Changes related to perfusion include blood volume, positional aortocaval flow, and the heart itself. The blood volume increases substantially by increasing plasma volume, as well as the number of red and white blood cells. The increase in plasma volume predominates, leading to a 12% decrease in viscosity (Bonica, 1981; Ramanathan & Porges, 1991). The majority of fluid gain in pregnancy is within the fetus, uterus, plasma volume, and interstitial fluid, for an approximate total of 7.5 liters (Ramanathan & Porges, 1991). Such significant volume increases might be expected to raise the central venous pressure (CVP), but a reduction in peripheral vascular resistance maintains a normal CVP.

The aorta and inferior vena cava may be compressed by the weight of the uterus after 24 to 28 weeks of gestation (Ramanathan & Porges, 1991). The vena caval compression may reduce venous return sufficiently to reduce maternal cardiac output, whereas the aortic compression can result in placental insufficiency, as well as reduced renal blood flow. Therefore women in their third trimester of pregnancy should avoid the supine position. The inferior vena cava is to the right of the aorta, so during transport, resuscitation, or operation, proper positioning can be accomplished by propping up the right hip to displace the uterus. When the presence of spinal injuries is uncertain, careful logrolling to the left lateral position is an alternative (Figure 9-9). The heart itself is displaced anterolaterally, and ECG changes that typically reflect ischemia can be normal in pregnancy, complicating evaluation of cardiac injury. Fetal heart tones must be checked during care of

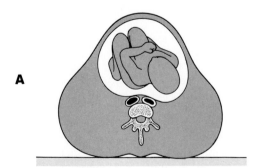 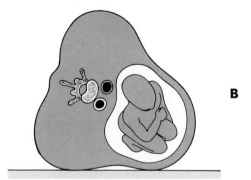

Figure 9-9 **A,** Location of vena cava and aorta in relation to pregnant uterus. **B,** Effect of lateral positioning on reduction of vascular compression.

the pregnant trauma patient. Extensive discussion of the pregnant trauma patient is found in Chapter 16.

Pediatrics

Differences in compensatory mechanisms, blood volume, Hgb levels, vascular access potential, and heart rate response to ventilation exist in children younger than 14 years. Their ability to compensate for shock to a greater extent can lead to delayed diagnosis of the severity of their injuries. In the child, 7% to 8% of body weight is blood, compared with 5% to 6% in adults. Therefore their blood volume is comparatively larger than that of adults, but when hemorrhage occurs, small amounts still account for a significant portion of their total blood volume. For example, a loss of 180 ml of blood (equivalent to a 6-ounce can of juice) is almost 20% of the blood volume in a 12-kg 1-year-old. Estimation of blood volume is always difficult, so great care must be taken to halt external hemorrhage and to measure or weigh blood loss (1 ml = 1 mg) in an attempt to quantify the volume.

Cautious calculation of fluid volume through the use of automated pumps, 250- to 500-ml IV bags, syringe bolus technique and in-line volume burettes will help prevent rapid, uncontrolled, "runaway" IV rates, which could be disastrous in children. It is especially important to quickly determine prehospital fluid intake, since many ambulance systems may hang microdrip tubing for children but still use 1000-ml bags. Table 9-5 shows the volume estimates for replacement by age and weight and a list of expected maintenance fluid rates. Although these serve as guidelines, it is also suggested that fluid replacement volumes be based on total body surface area because of the large surface area-to-weight ratio of children relative to that of adults.

Vascular access is more difficult in children and requires expert clinicians and special techniques. The saphenous vein cutdown is commonly used for rapid access when percutanous access in the upper extremity is difficult. The resurrection of intraosseous infusion has greatly assisted in rapid access for fluid and blood components in emergency situations. Detailed discussion of pediatric trauma is found in Chapter 17.

Elderly

Knowledge of the elderly person's medical history is very important because of the higher fre-

Table 9-5 Pediatric volume estimates for age, weight, and blood product doses; guidelines for calculation of maintenance fluids

Volume estimates by age and weight

Age	Weight (kg)	Volume at 20 ml/kg
Newborn	3.5	70 ml
6 Months	6.0	120 ml
1 Year	12	240 ml
4 Years	16 (¼ adult)	320 ml
10 Years	35 (½ adult)	700 ml

Blood products (IV administration)

Constituent	Volume (ml/kg)
Whole blood	20
Plasma	20
5% Albumin	20
Packed red blood cells	10
25% Albumin	4

Maintenance fluids (5% dextrose, 0.25 normal saline)*

Weight (kg)	Volume
1st 10 kg	100 ml/kg/24 hours
2nd 10 kg	50 ml/kg/24 hours
Each additional kg	20 ml/kg/24 hours
More than 40 kg	2500 ml/24 hours (adult requirement)

Note. Modified from *Pediatric Trauma Care* (p. 76) by M.R. Eichelberger and G.L. Pratsch (Eds.), 1988, Rockville, MD: Aspen Publishers.
*10% Dextrose for the newborn.

quency of medication usage and cardiopulmonary disease in this group. Awareness of the elderly person's usual blood pressure could alert the clinician to inadequate perfusion; e.g., the patient's present BP is 110/74 and his or her norm is 180/90. The ability to increase cardiac output is limited by ventricular compliance changes that hinder increases in stroke volume; therefore increasing preload may not be effective. Thus the elderly may respond differently to fluid resuscitation. Compensatory increases in heart rate may also be restricted by the prescribed use of beta blocking agents and a decreased responsiveness to catecholamines. Detailed discussion of trauma in the elderly is found in Chapter 18.

DIAGNOSTIC AND MONITORING PROCEDURES
Estimated Blood Loss

Accurately estimating blood loss can be difficult. Visual determination of external bleeding is often inaccurate and especially so when bleeding occurs at the scene of injury and the patient is transported. Some bleeding can be directly measured in calibrated containers, such as chest tube output. Intraoperative blood loss is also estimated by weighing blood-soaked gauze packs in conjunction with the nursing responsibility of "counting" the gauze. Skeletal blood loss may be grossly calculated by reference to ranges of blood loss associated with varied fractures (see Chapter 11). Computed tomography can be used to estimate minor versus major intraperitoneal or retroperitoneal hemorrhage.

Orthostatic hypotension

One method of detecting a deficit in vascular volume or vasomotor tone is the measurement of orthostatic vital signs. The pulse and blood pressure are obtained when the patient is supine and then when standing. Obviously, major trauma patients or those with potential spinal cord injuries or fractures inhibiting the upright position are not candidates for this test. Orthostatic vital signs are often obtained for minor and moderate trauma patients and those being evaluated for inpatient observation versus discharge home. It has been used in EDs for such patient complaints as dizziness or syncope, abdominal pain, gastrointestinal and vaginal bleeding, influenza symptoms, and heat exposure, to assist in determining the need for intravenous access and volume replacement. Generally the literature has described inconsistency in technique and a wide range of published "normal" and "abnormal" values (Halpern, 1987; Knopp, Claypool, & Leonardi, 1980; Koziol-Mc-Lain, Lowenstein, & Fuller 1991; Moore & Newton, 1986; Schulte, 1986).

Levitt, Lieberman, and Lopez (1989) evaluated orthostatic vital signs (VS) in emergency department patients in relation to degree of dehydration as calculated from serum osmolality and body weight. Although a significant statistical difference was found, the results were not clinically useful. The great individual variation in orthostatic VS changes led them to conclude that vital signs could not be used to determine the degree of dehydration or blood loss. Koziol-McLain et al. (1991) evaluated a sample of 132 ED patients with no history of acute, overt fluid or blood loss for the normal range of orthostatic changes and how relationships identified related to current critical values of orthostatic VS. Heart rate and BP were measured by an automated device. The fluid or blood loss was a subjective measurement based on patient report of external losses within 24 hours of ED arrival. Therefore any possible internal blood loss or fluid shifts could not be accounted for. The criteria considered currently accepted as indicators of "positive" orthostatic VS were a HR increase of ≥ 20 beats/minute and a systolic BP (SBP) or diastolic BP (DBP) decrease of ≥ 10 mm Hg. No statistically significant differences existed between those who experienced thirst and those who did not or those who did or did not feel dizzy upon standing. Koziol-McLain concluded that the variation in orthostatic VS was so large that discrimination between normal-volume and volume-deficient patients was not possible.

Elderly

There is no developmental chart for VS changes in aging as there is for childhood. Aging is an individualized phenomenon impacted by life-style, physical and mental health, medications, heredity, and functional ability, which affect musculoskeletal, neurologic, and vascular responses. Schulte (1986) evaluated differences in orthostatic changes in HR, SBP, and DBP between elderly (≥ 60 years) and nonelderly healthy subjects immediately upon standing and at 30 seconds and 1, 2, 3, 4, and 5 minutes. The only statistically significant difference was in HR, where change scores were greater in the *non*elderly. Norris, Shock, & Yiengst (1953) also found smaller HR increases upon standing in elderly as compared with younger subjects. In patients without a history of acute overt fluid or blood loss, Koziol-McLain et al. (1991) found a negative correlation between age and orthostatic HR. Thus the change in HR may not be as pronounced in the elderly patient, and orthostatic VS may be less reliable.

Practice implications

It appears that HR, SBP, and DBP of healthy people will generally adjust to standing within 30 seconds (Borst et al., 1982; Borst & Karemaker, 1983; Wieling & Dambrent, 1984). When trauma patients exhibit dramatic changes in HR or BP after standing 1 minute compared with their supine VS, volume loss, neurogenic alteration, or the sequelae of pain should be considered on an individual basis. It should also be realized that in a trauma patient who has been maintained supine and relatively immobilized for 30 minutes to a few hours, a change in vital signs may be a response to the immobility and not necessarily reflect acute blood loss. Borst, van Brederode, Wieling, Von Montfrans, & Dunning (1984) found that although the time frame of HR and BP response to standing was not different, the magnitude of change was significantly less after short-term supine rest as compared with 20-minute supine rest.

Indirect (Noninvasive) Blood Pressure Measurement

Environmental noise levels, peripheral vasoconstriction secondary to cold, fear, pain, or shock, and reduced cardiac output make BP measurement difficult. To facilitate auscultation of the BP, a change of ear pieces, use of the bell versus diaphragm, or switching to ear phones and a Doppler device might be tried. Kirkendall, Feinleib, Fries, and Mark (1980) and Mauro (1988) recommend the use of the bell versus the diaphragm of the stethoscope for accurate systolic readings. Palpation and Doppler technology (ultrasound) are more reliable alternatives for systolic pressure measurement during hypovolemic states, but the diastolic pressure is not measured (Poppers, Epstein, & Donham, 1971). This eliminates the ability to monitor pulse pressure, a noninvasive indicator of the patient's ability to maintain cardiac output (Underhill, 1986). Normal pulse pressure is 50 mm Hg, and a value less than 30 is of concern. Kelley (1988) reports that auscultation of systolic and diastolic pressures is difficult in infants and toddlers so the Doppler or palpation method may be the viable solution. The elderly frequently have some component of arteriosclerosis or atherosclerosis with decreased aortic distensibility leading to higher systolic pressures (Guyton, 1987). Therefore a systolic BP of 90 mm Hg may be much lower than the elderly person's norm. The elderly patient with vascular disease is at particular risk for heart, brain, and bowel hypo-

perfusion in the presence of hypotension (Bryan-Brown, 1988). Systemic vascular resistance also affects cuff versus direct BP measurements. When SVR was less than 1500 dynes/sec/cm^5, a mean discrepancy between brachial cuff and radial direct was only 6 mm Hg, whereas at an SVR greater than 1500, the cuff underestimated direct by an average of 64 mm Hg (Quaal, 1988).

Other sources of inaccuracy are inappropriate cuff size and mercury or gravity sphygmomanometer defects. A cuff that is too wide generally causes less error than a cuff that is too narrow (American Heart Association, 1987). Small cuffs generally result in overestimation of BP, which could negatively alter fluid resuscitation. Sphygmomanometers should be routinely calibrated, especially in the environment of trauma where equipment is often roughly handled and fluid exposure is common. The use of disposable cuffs helps in serial monitoring trends, since the same cuff can be used from the prehospital setting to the ED, ICU, and floor for patients without arterial lines. Another useful device for rapid, indirect measurement is the oversized inflation bulb, which is normally supplied with a thigh cuff. The bulb volume is 75 ml, about double the normal capacity of standard bulbs, which increases the rate of inflation to about two or three puffs (Dick, 1988).

The use of indirect measurements that use technology such as oscillometric digital sphygmomanometry will be discussed in comparison with direct measurement in the next section. The Dinamap (an acronym for device for indirect noninvasive mean arterial pressure) is one type of indirect, or noninvasive, BP (NIBP) measuring device. Another form of indirect pressure monitoring, the Ohmeda Finapres 2300, can provide continuous measurements allowing for detection of transient or sudden changes (Dorlas et al., 1985; Gorback, Quill, & Lavine, 1991). It is applied to the finger, reducing the incidence of upper arm pain and petechiae associated with frequent oscillometric readings; it functions by photoelectric and plethysmography evaluation. Of interest, a comparison of arterial BP to NIBP in the same patients showed no "alerting reaction" to automatic and semiautomatic BP measurement. No emotionally induced pressor effect or change in HR occurred 1 minute before, during, or after inflation (Parati, Pomidossi, Casadei, & Mancia, 1985; Parati et al., 1990).

Direct (Invasive) Blood Pressure Measurement

Critically ill trauma patients are often monitored by direct arterial measurement of blood pressure. This not only allows a continuous read-out, which is helpful during periods of rapid change and intraoperative and postoperative management, but also provides access to blood specimens without the need for arterial or venous puncture. Because it is a direct measurement, it is often considered to be the most accurate, although it still will be affected to some extent by peripheral vasoconstriction. Chyun (1985) compared palpated, auscultated, and intraarterial blood pressure readings in 14 patients in intensive care after open heart surgery. Palpatory readings were found to correlate better with intraarterial than auscultatory readings, although in some patients palpatory pressures could not be obtained. Venus, Mathru, Smith, and Pham (1985) report that automatic indirect measurements accurately measured MAP but underestimated SBP by a mean of 9.2 mm Hg and overestimated DBP by a mean of 8.7 mm Hg in 43 hemodynamically unstable patients. A thorough review of the physical components of blood pressure monitoring, both direct and indirect, describes the rationale for the variance seen between these methods (Henneman & Henneman, 1989). The creation and propagation of the pressure pulse reflects that the radial pulse is not actually related to the flow of blood but to the pressure pulse preceding it. Also, because resistance does not remain constant secondary to varying peripheral resistance according to body needs, BP and blood flow are not necessarily directly correlated. Therefore direct and indirect monitoring will not necessarily correlate. When indirect, flow-dependent methods are used in low-flow shock states, they may be unreliable. Oscillation amplitudes become very small in the presence of hypotension and severe vasoconstriction, without which only the mean arterial pressure (MAP) and heart rate can be determined (Gorback, Quill, & Lavine, 1991). The reason the Dinamap can measure MAP is because the MAP is determined at the maximum oscillation amplitude. If oscillometric units stop reading, patient status should be checked and the cuff deflated, all air removed, and the cuff reapplied snugly. Empiric observations have shown that more than one inflation may be necessary to once again measure MAP,

usually followed by return of SBP and DBP readings. When cardiac output is decreased or peripheral resistance is increased, direct arterial monitoring is optimal and generally indicated.

Age factors

Blood pressure, although difficult to measure in the young child, should nevertheless be obtained in the patient with traumatic injury. For the infant, the flush method is easy to use. The BP cuff is first properly fitted, and then, with the arm elevated, an elastic bandage is wrapped from the fingers to the antecubital fossa to essentially empty the capillary and venous network. The cuff is then inflated to a level over the estimated systolic pressure, the arm is placed at the infant's side, and the cuff is then slowly deflated. The point at which a rapid flushing of the forearm and hand is seen marks the systolic pressure (Bates, 1987). It may seem surprising to use the same SBP (90 mm Hg) for the top value in both the revised trauma score and pediatric trauma score, but the SBP of 95% of children between the ages of 1 and 14 years is greater than 80 mm Hg (Blumenthal et al., 1977; Mangubat & Eichelberger, 1988).

Heart Rate

In the absence of more elaborate monitoring, such as pulmonary artery pressures, knowledge of the heart rate in conjunction with the BP can help evaluate response to fluid administration. If the BP is at least 90 mm Hg but the HR is more than 120, fluid challenge can help to determine whether the tachycardia is the result of low volume, which is compensated by vasoconstriction and tachycardia, or if it is induced by pain and fear. If the pulse does gradually drop with fluid administration, it may reflect improved vascular volume and less need for a chronotropic cardiac effect. Yet, bradycardia also serves as a protective reflex by increasing diastolic filling time and therefore stroke volume. In a study of 43 trauma patients with isolated penetrating abdominal injury, Snyder and Dresnick (1989) evaluated the lack of tachycardic response to hypotension. These patients were not taking beta blockers or analgesics, yet a number had no tachycardia (HR > 100) in association with SBP less than 90. In fact, a wide variation in HR existed for both normotensive and hypotensive patients and no significant dif-

Table 9-6 Expected heart rate and blood pressure by age

Age	Heart rate*	Systolic blood pressure†
6 Wk-6 mo	130	$\frac{70}{40}$
6 Mo-12 mo	115	$\frac{80}{50}$
1 Yr-3 yr	110	$\frac{90}{60}$
4 Yr-7 yr	104	$\frac{100}{60}$
8 Yr-12 yr	95	$\frac{110}{60}$
13 Yr-16 yr	85	$\frac{120}{70}$
>16 Yr	80	$\frac{90\text{-}140}{60\text{-}90}$
Elderly	80	$\frac{130\text{-}140}{90\text{-}95}$

*Children's heart rates are more labile than those of adults and are very sensitive to emotion and illness.
Elderly patients on beta blockers or set pacemaker rates will have limited chronotropic response.
A HR of 30 to 50 bpm is not uncommon in well-conditioned athletes.
†Pediatric systolic blood pressure can also be estimated by adding 80 + (2 × age in years).

ference in mean HR was found between the groups. They concluded that minor bleeding and intraperitoneal fluid leakage in the context of mechanical trauma may trigger a parasympathetic reflex via peritoneal irritation, accounting for the bradycardic hypotension. Although this study could not evaluate HR with parameters other than BP, such as mentation or skin signs, it does challenge the long-held concept that tachycardia is a reliable sign of early hypovolemic shock. There is not a clear relationship between volume of blood lost and heart rate (Little, 1989).

The expected HR and BP values for all ages are shown in Table 9-6.

Skin Signs

Signs of peripheral perfusion reflect cardiovascular status but are qualitative measures that are subject to error. However, determination of skin temperature and the strength of peripheral pulses has been shown to accurately predict postoperative mortality and to correlate with cardiac output in children (Kirklin et al., 1981; Moodie, 1980). Fagan (1988) examined the relationship between methods of evaluating peripheral perfusion and toe temperature. She found that classifying peripheral pulse as absent, barely palpable, and normal was the most specific scale. Schriger and Baraff in a series of studies (1988, 1990, 1991) demonstrated that capillary refill varies with age, temperature, and sex. For patients older than 65 years, the upper limit of normal should be 4.5 seconds to maintain a specificity of 95%. Even after a 10-minute phlebotomy of 10% of their blood volume, 47 volunteers had capillary refill times (CRT) less than 2 seconds, and in patients who were not initially hypotensive but became orthostatic, capillary refill had a sensitivity of only 47% (Schriger & Baraff, 1991). In order for the CRT to be reliable, it must be performed using a specific technique (5 sec squeeze of middle or index phalanx tip), careful timing, and good lighting.

Jugular Venous Filling

In traumatic shock, lack of jugular venous distention (JVD) in a supine position is an important finding, since it is normal to find as much as 2 cm distention above the sternal angle with the head elevated 30 to 45 degrees. The best estimate of right atrial pressure is from the internal jugular veins, since they have the most direct access to the right atrium. Although the external jugular veins are less reliable, they may be used if the internal veins cannot be seen. If JVD is present with the patient supine, such as in obstructive cardiac flow secondary to tamponade or tension pneumothorax, the veins may distend up to the earlobe, and accurate measurement will not be possible unless the head of the bed can be safely elevated (C-spine cleared). This, nevertheless, likely indicates either thoracic injury, requiring immediate treatment, or fluid overload, especially in the elderly. Central venous pressure (CVP) or pulmonary artery (PA) monitoring may be indicated. A jugular venous distention of 2 cm is roughly equivalent to a CVP of 7 cm where the norm for CVP is 2 to 8 (Bates, 1987). Converting centimeter (cm) H_2O to millimeter mercury (mm Hg) is done by dividing cm by 1.36. In children younger than 12 years, it is very difficult to visualize the jugular veins.

Central Venous Pressure

Central venous pressure (CVP) may be monitored in the resuscitative phase of the trauma patient, but early access to a central vein would optimally be used for rapid fluid administration, and blood in the line would negate taking measurements. Subclavian and jugular central lines have a propensity for kinking and therefore giving false readings, although this can often be determined by watching for fluctuations with respiration and by checking for ease of blood return. CVP lines can be monitored with a fluid manometer (cm H_2O) or transduced (in mm Hg). As with all hemodynamic monitoring, readings should be taken at the level of the heart, or the phlebostatic axis. Patients needing close monitoring deserve a PA line, which will accurately reflect left heart function. The CVP reflects preload and right heart function and will be affected by pulmonary hypertension. Once a PA catheter is placed, a CVP reading can be taken from the port in the right atrium (RA) to compare left and right heart function.

Pulmonary Artery Catheter

The pulmonary artery or Swan-Ganz catheter is placed percutaneously or via cutdown through an introducer into a major vein and threaded into the pulmonary artery. The benefits of PA catheters include (1) monitoring CVP (proximal right atrium) and pulmonary wedge pressure (PWP)—sometimes referred to as pulmonary artery occlusion pressure (PAOP), (2) measuring cardiac output (CO) by thermodilution technique, and (3) having the capacity in specialized models to measure mixed venous blood oxygen saturation (Figure 9-10). Cardiac output can be converted to cardiac index (CI) based on body surface area (BSA). The normal values and equations to calculate units are listed in Table 9-7. Additional infusion ports are available, and some models contain atrial and ventricular pacing electrodes. The thermistor allows for continuous measurement of core body temperature.

Pulmonary wedge pressure reflects the left ventricular end-diastolic pressure (LVEDP), thereby

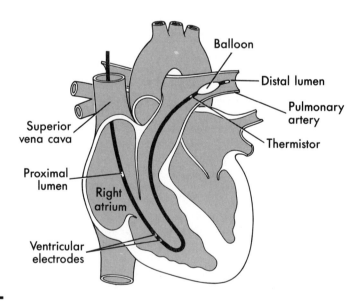

Figure 9-10 Pulmonary artery catheter in relation to cardiac anatomy. Ports for proximal and distal fluid infusion, thermistor for determination of cardiac output injectate temperature change and ongoing core body temperature measurement, balloon for PAOP measurement, and site for cardiac pacing electrode.

Table 9-7 Calculation, norms, and significance of physiologic parameters

Parameter	Calculation	Norms (value)	Significance
CVP	Direct transducer or fluid manometer (cm H_2O/ 1.36 = mm Hg)	3-10 mm Hg or 4-14 cm H_2O	Right heart preload indicator
CO	Thermodilution technique	4-8 L/min	Influenced by preload, afterload, and cardiac contractility
CI	CO/BSA	2.5-4 L/min/m²	Adjusted for individual size
PWP/PAOP	Transducer	6-12 mm Hg	Left heart preload indicator
PAP (systolic/diastolic)	Transducer	15-30/8-16 mm Hg	
SVR	$\dfrac{(MAP - CVP)}{CO} \times 80$	850-1400 dynes/sec/cm⁵	Left ventricular afterload or total peripheral resistance

CVP, central venous pressure; *CO*, Cardiac output; *BSA*, body surface area; *CI*, cardiac index; *PWP*, pulmonary wedge pressure; *PAOP*, pulmonary artery occlusion pressure; *PAP*, pulmonary artery pressure; *SVR*, systemic vascular resistance; *MAP*, mean arterial pressure.

serving as a barometer of blood volume and left ventricular function. In the presence of increased afterload (SVR), PWP will increase when the heart cannot adequately compensate. PWP is a valid indicator of preload or left ventricular end-diastolic volume (LVEDV) only when LVEDP is consistently equivalent to LVEDV. This will vary when the compliance or distensibility of the ventricle changes and when the intrathoracic pressure is changed by positive pressure ventilation. The effect of intrathoracic pressure depends on the degree of lung stiffness. Fink (1989) concludes that PWP is most useful for determining gross under-resuscitation in critically ill patients and recommends gauging treatment by incremental fluid increases while monitoring CI, not just PWP. In a prospective study of 385 high-risk surgical patients, the PWP was considered no more valuable than CVP unless the goal of therapy was to monitor PWP while augmenting CI and DO_2 (oxygen delivery) to supranormal values (Shoemaker, Appel, Kram, Waxman, & Lee, 1988).

Documentation of both PAD (PA diastolic pressure) and PWP creates a trend for comparison in the event that the PA catheter fails to wedge. In the presence of increased pulmonary vascular resistance, PWP should be directly measured.

Oxygen Consumption

Oxygen consumption (VO_2) is another indicator of cellular metabolism that can be monitored when advanced technology is available. This parameter can be calculated by the Fick equation or measured through inspiratory and expiratory gas sampling. The normal value range is 180 to 280 ml/min based on 3.5 ml/kg/min. A reduction in VO_2 may be caused by (1) a decrease in body temperature as a result of decreased metabolic need or (2) poor perfusion and inadequate tissue oxygenation (Shoemaker, 1982; Siegal, Linberg, & Wiles, 1987; Vary & Linberg, 1988).

Tissue Oxygen Indicators

The arteriovenous oxygen content difference ($AVDO_2$) is a critical variable to measure as an indicator of adequate perfusion. It is possible to calculate $AVDO_2$ when samples of arterial and mixed venous blood are available.

Mixed venous oxygen saturation

By comparing mixed venous oxygen saturation (SvO_2 or $SmvO_2$) from the pulmonary artery (venous blood) with arterial oxygen saturation (SaO_2) from an arterial line, the dynamics of oxygen delivery versus demand can be examined. Normally a ratio of oxygen consumption to oxygen delivery of 0.25 is expected. This means that the tissues extract 25% of the oxygen delivered. Because normal SaO_2 values are 95% to 100% and SvO_2 60% to 80%, there is usually a similar difference of 25% (Hardy, 1988). The body will attempt to increase cardiac output in the presence of decreased

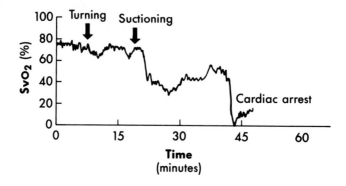

Figure 9-11 Mixed venous oxygen saturation (Svo_2) tracing during routine nursing care. Continuous Svo_2 monitoring can signal clinician when modifications in care are needed. A small and then a larger drop in Svo_2 accompanied turning and suctioning patient. Svo_2 remained depressed and preceded cardiac arrest by 15 to 20 minutes. (*Note.* From "Continuous Monitoring of Mixed Venous Oxygen Saturation by M.B. Divertie and J.C. McMichan, 1984, *Chest*, 86 (5), pp. 423-428.)

Hgb levels, decreased O_2 saturation, or increased O_2 consumption. If this is inadequate, oxygen extraction by the tissues increases, at least in supply-independent tissues such as the kidneys and the splanchnic area (Bryan-Brown, 1988). The result is a decrease in oxygen returned to the heart, which is detected by a decrease in Svo_2. With continuous monitoring of Svo_2, changes in patient pulmonary and circulatory parameters can be detected early. Use of Svo_2 in calculating VO_2 is a valuable maneuver (Figure 9-11). When oxygen delivery is increased and oxygen consumption also increases, a substantial oxygen debt is present and poor outcome is expected (Fink, 1989).

The value of oxygen saturation determinations and arteriovenous oxygen content difference is explained by the delineation of essentially two "compartments" during hypovolemic shock. The central compartment remains perfused secondary to compensatory mechanisms (if effective) while the peripheral compartment contains the tissues that constrict. The peripheral tissues have decreased flow, and their decreased venous oxygen content (less oxygen delivery and greater oxygen extraction) combines with the normal venous O_2 content of the perfused central organs, resulting in a lower mixed venous O_2 (without supplemental oxygen). The net result is a wider arterial-to-venous oxygen content difference. This is demonstrated further by measuring venous samples from the superior vena cava ($Ssvco_2$) and comparing them with the pulmonary artery mixed venous O_2

($Smvo_2$). When compared with normal volunteers, $Ssvco_2$ is higher in patients in shock than $Smvo_2$, since the superior vena cava does not include the venous blood shunted from peripheral sites (Johnson & Mellors, 1988; Kandel & Aberman, 1983).

Conjunctival, transcutaneous, and liver surface oxygen tension

Other devices are being investigated for their value in reflecting peripheral tissue perfusion, such as palpebral conjunctival oxygen tension ($Pcjo_2$), transcutaneous oxygen tension at the skin surface ($Ptco_2$), and liver surface oxygen tension (Plo_2). Because altered tissue perfusion often precedes deterioration in other commonly monitored variables, effective indicators of diminished peripheral tissue oxygenation should allow earlier intervention. Arterial oxygen tension (Pao_2) cannot be relied on to reflect oxygen transport or tissue oxygenation during hemodynamic instability.

Measured $Pcjo_2$ has been shown to reflect local oxygen transport at the tissue level (Kram & Shoemaker, 1985). In their canine experiments, $Pcjo_2$ and $Ptco_2$ correlated with Pao_2 during hyperoxia and hypoxia. However, during induced hemorrhagic shock, $Ptco_2$ and $Pcjo_2$ closely paralleled cardiac output and oxygen delivery but not Pao_2. Clinical studies demonstrated variation in the $Pcjo_2$/Pao_2 ratio in relation to the patient's circulatory status. This indicates a risk in reliance

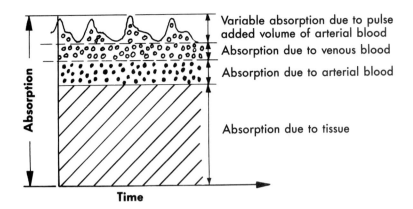

Figure 9-12   Ohmeda pulse oximeter wavelength signals through peripheral vascular bed are received by a photodiode. Variable absorption occurs from different tissue levels. Absorption from pulsating arterial bed is variable in comparison with other layers. (Courtesy BOC Health Care, Louisville, CO.)

on monitoring PaO_2 levels in hemorrhagic shock. Another clinical scenario that is hard to detect is normotensive shock. In this instance, there is low flow but a normal BP secondary to high systemic vascular resistance. Tremper, Barker, Hufstedler, and Weiss (1989) studied the response of $PtcO_2$ and PlO_2 during experimentally induced hemorrhagic shock and normotensive shock in the dog model. $PtcO_2$ followed the same trend as PlO_2 during canine hemorrhage and resuscitation. Values for $PtcO_2$ followed cardiac output and not BP in low-flow states; therefore this tissue oxygen indicator may prove more valuable to monitor than blood pressure.

Pulse oximetry

When technology such as a pulmonary artery catheter is not available, the oxygen status can be monitored continuously by pulse oximetry (SpO_2). Chapter 8 further discusses the use of pulse oximetry.

Pulse oximetry measures pulsatile *changes* in light transmission through tissue to calculate arterial saturation (Figure 9-12). A pulse oximeter relates the ratio of transmitted to absorbed light at wavelengths of reduced hemoglobin and oxyhemoglobin. There is an advantage to using a pulse oximeter with a waveform. The waveform represents pulsatile blood flow or, to some degree, perfusion. It is not quantifiable, but a pulse oximeter needs a minimum threshold of data points for a

quality reading. Ohmeda developed a signal strength indicator to reflect this (Figure 9-13). The practitioner can see the integrity of the signal and the digital number for the SpO_2 value. If the pulse becomes weak, a message is given that there is a low quality signal, and if perfusion worsens, the device will cease to give a reading.

Errors can occur in the presence of elevated carboxyhemoglobin. Smoke inhalation is the most likely cause of this, although a heavy smoker would also have a greater percentage of COHb. The end result is a seemingly normal SpO_2 and PaO_2 in the face of a drastically decreasing SaO_2 (arterial O_2 saturation). Monitoring of these patients with SpO_2 is inappropriate (Barker & Tremper, 1987; Szaflarski & Cohen, 1989). Although some oximeters have difficulty monitoring through nail polish or at certain body temperatures, the quality brightness of the light-emitting diodes and self-adjusting intensity capability can overcome some of these impedances. It is imperative that the device be applied correctly (photo light emitter against the nail; detector on the fleshy side of finger), although newer versions are less sensitive to position. A range of compatible probes should be available for various testing sites (finger, toe, nose) that are pertinent to all ages.

Benefits of pulse oximetry have been reported in prehospital, emergency, and postanesthesia units. Patient monitoring has improved, clinically unsuspected changes in arterial oxygenation are

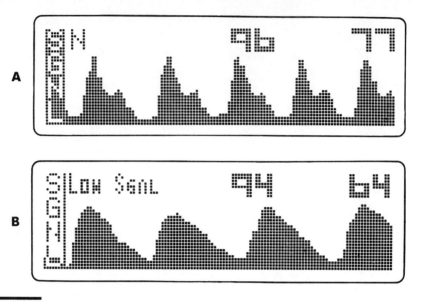

Figure 9-13 Ohmeda Biox 3700 pulse oximeter. Tracings demonstrate **A,** normal waveform and **B,** low quality signal. (Courtesy BOC Health Care, Louisville, CO.)

detected, and changes in therapy are instituted based on SpO_2 values. Of 202 patients in a pre-hospital setting, 32% needed a change in O_2 therapy based on abnormal SpO_2 values and 21% did not require supplemental O_2 based on normal SpO_2 values (Giard & Ross, 1989).

In flight, oximetry has been helpful in conjunction with clinical assessment to identify the need for intervention in critically ill patients (Melton, Heller, Kaplan, & Mohan-Klein, 1989). Absolute saturation levels (i.e., 90%) are set as alarm points, but the trend of SpO_2 aids in awareness of physiologic change and prediction of patient deterioration. Further research of oximetry findings in air transport may delineate which patients need oxygen support secondary to altitude effects in fixed-wing (primarily) and rotor craft. At present it appears to be a useful adjunct in the complex prehospital assessment process that is further impacted by the physics of flight.

Urine Output

Measurement of hourly urine output (UOP) is a time-honored method for assessing the adequacy of perfusion. It is generally expected to be 0.5 to 1.0 ml/kg/hr, although it is somewhat lower in the elderly and higher in children. The presence of neurologic disease, such as SIADH, and the use of osmotic diuretics to reduce intracranial pressure or to protect the kidneys in the presence of crush injury and urine myoglobin will obviously alter the validity of hourly urine output in relation to general perfusion. Care should be taken to adequately document the urine output from the time of initial placement of the urinary catheter by ED personnel. It is important to clearly report the total output that occurred in the ED or to drain the collection set before transfer to the OR so that UOP from the various phases of resuscitation and intervention can be accurately determined. Knowledge of the specific gravity of the urine can be helpful when evaluating patient response to fluid management. When blood volume and flow diminish, the specific gravity increases, as does the serum osmolality.

Radiography
Chest radiograph

Chest radiographs or x-rays are the most routine films ordered for the trauma patient. The chest x-ray is usually the first film requested to verify clinical impressions of endotracheal tube placement and evidence of the cause of altered breath sounds, such as a hemothorax or pneumothorax. The optimal view is posteroanterior (PA), since the x-ray beam passes from back to front with the film plate on the anterior surface. The heart is anteriorly situated, resulting in less magnification of the heart and mediastinum than in the typical portable anteroposterior (AP) view. Most initial x-rays are supine AP films, but an upright film should be attempted if the C-spine is cleared. The upright position maximizes lung size, and pleural fluid is easier to detect in the dependent position. Pleural fluid or blood accumulation of 500 ml or more may not be detected in the supine position. Lateral decubitus films can detect 25 to 50 ml and are an option when the patient can be logrolled but not placed upright (Matthay & Sostman, 1990). Rib fractures can be seen on plain films, but costal cartilage fractures are often missed unless grossly displaced (Lange, 1990). Some centers obtain oblique films to detect the full extent of rib fractures, but these studies are expensive and clinical examination and point tenderness will usually suffice. Suspicion of rib fractures with a pneumothorax is important in the operative patient, since a small pneumothorax may enlarge with positive-pressure ventilation and create a tension pneumothorax. Routine placement of chest tubes preoperatively in patients with rib fractures is often standard policy, but another option is to alert the anesthesiologist to the rib fractures and closely monitor peak inspiratory pressures and volume during the surgical procedure. Evidence of a widened mediastinum will trigger the need for further films or recommendation of aortography. The aorta and pulmonary arteries and veins are the main vascular structures identifiable on plain films (Matthay & Sostman, 1990). Diaphragmatic herniation from rupture may be detected and should arouse concern for associated splenic injury with hemorrhage.

CASE STUDY Frequently, patients who are rushed to surgery have recently had a chest x-ray film. It is very important that this film be read by the surgical team and/or radiologist. A 34-year-old man who was shot in the chest and abdomen was brought to the ED resuscitation room in extremis. He was rapidly intubated, initial venous access established, O-negative blood started, and a nasogastric tube (NGT) placed. A postintubation film was obtained just before transfer to the operating room. The anesthesiologist's report showed that when the NGT was placed to suction intraoperatively, a significant drop in pulmonary volume was noted. Therefore the NGT was removed. A cuff leak in the ETT had also been

appreciated. On review of this chart and the x-ray reports, the trauma coordinator found that the NGT was in the right lung. The anesthesiologist acted correctly by removing the NGT, but neither the surgical team nor the radiologist had viewed the film or informed the team of the incorrect NGT placement. When procedures are done under pressure, it is even more important to ensure that the normal steps of assessment are followed.

Angiography

Angiography is valuable for definitive diagnosis of vascular injury and affords interventional value as well when embolization of a vessel is required. Aortography is the most sensitive and most specific test currently available to diagnose traumatic aortic rupture (Armstrong, 1989). Digital subtraction angiography uses less of a contrast load, reduces artifacts, and can enhance difficult areas to image, such as vessels beneath bone (Harman & Floten, 1991). Penetrating extremity trauma in proximity to major vessels is a potential source of severe hemorrhage. Hartling et al. (1987) studied 61 stab wound cases retrospectively and found that arteriography was not warranted in stab wounds when the only indications were great vessel proximity or a nonexpanding hematoma (considered minor physical findings). Major physical findings included diminished or absent pulses, active bleeding or expanding hematoma, bruit or murmur, isolated neurologic deficit, or hypotension. These data are supported by Frykberg et al. (1989) in a prospective study of the value of routine arteriographic evaluation in 135 patients. Arteriographic evaluation was not justified when absent or only "soft" or minor signs of vascular injury were apparent except in the case of gunshot wounds.

CASE STUDY A 32-year-old man reported that the blade of a Sawsall, a power, narrow-bladed, rapid-oscillating saw, fell from a truck and became imbedded in his thigh. He had to climb out of a pit and was diaphoretic and pale with a trail of blood nearby when found by his co-workers. Paramedics documented approximately 2 liters of blood loss and initial vital signs of BP, 84/60; HR, 120; RR, 24 in the supine position; with a GCS of 15. A dressing was applied, and the patient was placed in shock position. Two large-bore IVs were placed. Upon ED arrival, his VS were stable, hematocrit was 36% and distal pulse and sensation were normal. The wound was dressed, and the

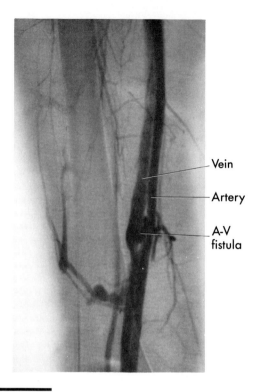

Vein

Artery

A-V
fistula

Figure 9-14 Angiographic evidence (*arrows*) of arteriovenous (A-V) fistula of superficial femoral artery and vein from penetrating injury to thigh. (Courtesy Valerij Selivanov, M.D., Stanford University Trauma Service, Stanford, CA.)

patient was admitted overnight. The following morning, his hematocrit was 31%, and a thorough predischarge assessment discovered a thrill and bruit over the site, and an angiogram showed an arteriovenous fistula of the right superficial femoral artery and vein (Figure 9-14). The vessels were reconstructed, but he developed infrapatellar paresthesia along the greater saphenous nerve distribution and some thigh swelling and claudication. A Doppler study revealed a thrombus in the superficial femoral vein. He was discharged 9 days after surgery. Coumadin (warfarin) was prescribed, and the patient was instructed to maintain a non-weight-bearing status for the involved leg.

Computed tomography

Abdominal CT scans show evidence of hematomas, free intraperitoneal fluid, and lacerations of vascular organs. The amount of free fluid must be differentiated from remaining lavage fluid, although it is rare to have the CT preceded by diag-

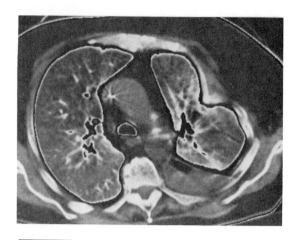

Figure 9-15 Flail chest with multiple rib fractures. Computed tomography shows inward displacement of rib fragments; clinical assessment revealed paradoxic respiratory movement. (*Note.* From *Radiology of Chest Diseases* (p. 165) by S. Lange, 1990, New York: Thieme Medical Publishers.)

nostic lavage. An estimation of blood loss can be grossly quantified by the surgeon or radiologist. In a study of 100 abdominal CT films in patients with blunt abdominal trauma, seven showed evidence of a collapsed infrahepatic inferior vena cava at multiple levels. Six of the seven had major blood loss that had not been clinically suspected. Although the CT films documented the sources of hemorrhage for five of the six, the source of hemorrhage for one case had been facial lacerations (Jeffrey & Federle, 1988). Thoracic injuries may be detected solely on abdominal CT scans in multiple trauma patients. In a retrospective 2-year study it was found that 55 of 109 chest injuries were detected only by abdominal CT scan initial portable chest films (Rhea, Novelline, Lawrason, Sacknoff, & Oser, 1989). These injuries included hemothoraxes, pneumothoraxes, and sternal and thoracic spine fractures. However, only 4% of the total population scanned had an alteration of clinical management as a result of the scan. It was suggested that in the unconscious patient or operative candidate, these findings would be more significant. A CT film confirmed the extent of thoracic injury in a patient with flail chest while scanning for other injuries (Figure 9-15). New spiral CT scanners allow creation of three-dimensional CT images, shorter scanning times, and use of less contrast media.

Magnetic resonance imaging

Newer versions of magnetic resonance imaging (MRI) units are becoming more rapid and more compatible with the supportive needs of acute injury. Blood has a characteristic appearance on MRI and can be differentiated as acute blood (1 to 6 days), subacute blood (1 to 4 weeks), and old blood (>4 weeks), depending on the presence of deoxyhemoglobin, methemoglobin, or hemosiderin respectively (Muhr, Teplick, & Wolferth, 1990). The contrast between signals for soft tissues and flowing blood allows delineation of the lumens of large vessels and chambers.

Laboratory Findings
Hemoglobin and hematocrit

Numbers tend to command attention, but what does the hemoglobin (Hgb) and hematocrit (Hct) reveal about the condition of trauma patients? It is known that the Hgb level impacts oxygen-carrying capacity and the Hct level alters viscosity and blood flow, but how is the desired range for critically ill patients determined, and what are the factors that alter them? First, the relationship of Hct to Hgb should be understood. The Hct is equivalent to the packed red cell volume (PCV), the percentage of red cells in a volume of whole blood expressed as a percentage. It is generally equivalent to 3 times the Hgb level, in agreement with the expected physiologic Hct/Hgb ratio of 2.9 to 3.1:1 (Savage, 1987; Simpson, 1989). The Hgb concentration is expressed as grams per deciliter (g/dl). Some red blood cells contain more Hgb than others. Both Hct and Hgb are highest within the first month of life and decline in the later years from (1) the male adult norms of Hct, 47 ± 7; Hgb, 16 ± 2 and (2) female adult norms of Hct, 42 ± 5; Hgb, 14 ± 2 (Finley, 1992). Values for Hct and Hgb may be normal after acute hemorrhage, since whole blood is lost, while the circulating Hgb and blood volume would be decreased. However, once fluid resuscitation is begun and the body begins its recovery process, the dilutional effects of crystalloids and fluid shifts will result in remarkable drops in Hct and Hgb (Fischbach, 1988; (Sutcliffe, 1987). In patients (n = 20) without hemorrhage, infusion of crystalloid at 20 ml/kg over 45 minutes resulted in a drop of Hct of 1.7 to 6.3

points. Half of the subjects' Hct levels dropped more than 5 points. When fluid was sequentially infused at 15 ml/kg over 1 hour and over 3 hours, the Hct began to increase, apparently as a result of equilibration of the infused fluid between intracellular, interstitial, and intravascular compartments (Stamler, 1989). When volunteers were phlebotomized 14.5% of total blood volume (equivalent to an expected Hct drop of 6.5 points), the investigators found that the reliability of the Hct value was optimized when drawn 10 minutes after bolus administration of crystalloid (Henneman, Greenfield, & Bessen, 1989).

The technique for drawing blood samples must be accurate to avoid contamination by distal IV fluids. Contamination from fluids infusing below the draw site has resulted in very erroneous values, which may or may not be obvious when reported, leading to unnecessary concern, treatment, or diagnostic studies. It could be helpful to have field blood samples for comparison of preresuscitation and postresuscitation values. This has been done in trauma systems, but research data to aid in interpretation have been scarce. A variety of portable devices are available for use in patient care areas to rapidly determine Hgb and/or Hct values from venous or fingerstick (microhematocrit) samples. Reliability, validity, and efficiency have been documented (Bridges, Parvin, & van Assendelft, 1987). Use of these devices outside of the laboratory has come under scrutiny by the Joint Commission on Accreditation of Healthcare Organizations and will require ongoing documentation of training and testing for competency. (Use of urine dipsticks and glucose and Hemoccult checks is being scrutinized also.) Arterial specimens may also be used, and in some pulmonary function labs, the Hgb is reported from arterial blood gas specimens.

Arterial blood gases

Arterial blood gas values facilitate determining oxygenation and detecting the degree of metabolic acidosis. The pH and bicarbonate levels are of most value to perfusion assessment, reflecting low-flow states in the presence of acidosis and low bicarbonate. It is presumed that ventilation will be supported in critical trauma patients, thereby avoiding any respiratory acidosis, but the level of Pco_2 in a spontaneously breathing patient without head injury can be of interest in determining the degree of respiratory compensation.

Lactate levels

Serum lactate levels indicate the presence of inadequate tissue perfusion and the cellular conversion to anaerobic metabolism. Normal venous values are 5 to 15 mg/dl. When cardiac output is decreased, arterial lactate may be normal but venous blood will reveal a lactic acidosis (Marino, 1991).

Serum osmolality

Serum osmolality can be measured in the laboratory, or an estimate can be calculated from the plasma concentrations of sodium (Na), glucose, and blood urea nitrogen (BUN). Plasma osmolality is calculated as follows:

$$(mOsm/kg\ H_2O) = 2 \times [Na] + [glucose]/18 + [BUN]/2.8.$$

The serum osmolality is often used to monitor effective fluid restriction in the trauma patient with head injury and to evaluate the degree of hydration in relation to other hemodynamic parameters. The normal value is 285 to 295 mOsm/kg; 270 to 290 for children. Serum osmolality is rather stable in comparison with urine osmolality, which has a large range. The usual ratio of urine to serum osmolality is 4:1. The urine and serum osmolalities will be elevated in the presence of shock, hemoconcentration, and acidosis (McFarland, Grant, & Schumacher, 1988).

GENERAL INTERVENTIONS
Hemostasis/Vascular Control

Bleeding cannot always be prevented, but the next goal is to halt the hemorrhage. A variety of techniques are available, and controversy abounds. Valuable methods range from the most simple, pressure, to definitive operative repair.

Pressure

First aid classes teach the basic principle of pressure to stop bleeding. This is effective and is relatively easy on exposed vascular and soft tissue injuries. Direct pressure with a double-gloved finger or fist, use of gauze rolls, or point pressure at sites where the vessels supplying the injured area are accessible to pressure is usually effective and requires only basic training. Once the clot has begun to form, pressure may be transferred to gauze packing and a tight elastic wrap, but this must be done carefully to ensure continued hemostasis, avoid hidden hemorrhage, and avoid nerve or vascular compromise. It is not always possible to maintain flow to distal tissues, and the priority focus must be given to halting the blood loss. Tourniquets are resorted to at times when a person must be moved for his or her safety and the number of personnel is limited, or when hemorrhage cannot be limited with direct pressure. Blind attempts to clamp bleeders can result in serious damage to adjacent structures.

CASE STUDY An angry, intoxicated 20-year-old man punched his dominant left arm through a plate glass window at home, creating a significant laceration and blood loss. Upon paramedic arrival, he was alert but lapsed in and out of consciousness during ambulance transport. Direct pressure with gauze was applied by the paramedics, and a large-bore IV line was placed in the opposite arm. Upon arrival at the local hospital, IV fluids were continued and the wound explored, whereupon an apparent pulsating stream of blood was noted along with a cool hand and delayed capillary refill on the injured side. The gauze and wrap were reapplied, and a call was placed to the regional trauma center for microsurgery referral. The patient was transported by helicopter, and during the flight the hand had limited motor function and remained cool. The flight nurse opted to try loosening the wrap in an attempt to provide better distal flow; however, the result was another bout of significant bleeding at the site of injury. The wound was rewrapped.

On the patient's arrival at the trauma center, the operating room and surgeons were ready, but the wound was reevaluated in the ED, causing continued bleeding and prompting application of a clamp within the wound. The operative note reported that this clamp was infringing on a nerve. Tendon, vascular, and nerve repairs were completed, and the patient was kept sedated to maximize alignment and repair potential. The patient had tenuous vascular supply the first postoperative day, but perfusion was successful. Full motor/neurologic capability did not return immediately, but neural regeneration is expected within the reanastomosed sheath and may ultimately provide improved function. The desire to "see for yourself" resulted in repeated potential impairment of blood volume and prompted a less than optimal application of a clamp. The patient's distal perfusion defect was present according to the paramedic report, as well as the motor deficit; therefore operative care was the only definitive treatment nec-

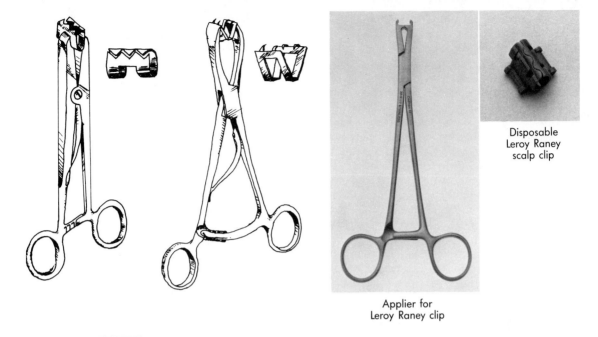

Disposable
Leroy Raney
scalp clip

Applier for
Leroy Raney clip

Figure 9-16 Scalp clip appliers and clips and disposable Leroy Raney scalp clip with applier. (*Note.* Courtesy Codman & Shurtleff, Inc., Randolph, MA. From *Alexander's Care of the Patient in Surgery* [9th ed.] [p. 720] by M.H. Meeker and J.C. Rothrock, 1991, St. Louis: Mosby–Year Book, Inc.)

essary besides basic pressure to halt the hemorrhage and replacement of intravascular volume.

Rapid mechanical hemostasis is invaluable in large, bleeding scalp lacerations. In multiply injured patients, a head laceration may be overlooked before a significant amount of blood is lost. One approach has been to place large sutures to grossly approximate the tissues and provide tamponade until definitive suturing can be done. Another helpful device to have available in the ED is a set of scalp clip appliers and disposable Leroy Raney scalp clips (Figure 9-16). These are used routinely in neurosurgery and are rapidly applied in resuscitation areas (Meeker & Rothrock, 1991). Disposable clips are recommended because they are made of plastic and therefore do not interfere with CT scanning; also, the metallic, reusable clips present a "sharps" hazard.

Pneumatic antishock garments

Pneumatic antishock garments (PASG) or military antishock trousers (MAST) began as a simple technique for prevention of orthostatic hypotension in neurosurgical patients and in aviation in the early 1900s. The trousers were modified and used during air evacuation in Vietnam to stabilize patients who were in hypovolemic shock. The trousers were converted to civilian use in the early 1970s (Cutler & Daggett, 1971; Schneider, Mitchell, & Allison, 1989). The MAST were deemed to increase external pressure, enhance venous return and thereby increase blood volume, increase BP, and splint fractures. However, considerable controversy has developed in terms of their efficacy, associated physiologic changes, and the impact on patient outcome. It has been shown that although MAST do increase BP, it is not by an autotransfusion effect but rather through elevation of systemic vascular resistance by as much as 48% (Bivins, Knopp, & Tiernan, 1982; Gaffney et al., 1981; Goldsmith, 1983). Although the intent was to promote direct hemostasis by tamponade through increased transmural pressure, the decreased bleeding time in some studies may be related to a generalized decrease in venous return (Schneider, Mitchell, & Allison, 1989). The benefits of MAST in splinting, especially related to pelvic injury, are still not certain, but in some systems it remains one of the few recommendations for field or hospital use. Stabilization of vital signs and apparent reduction in pelvic hemorrhage have been reported in children (Brunette, Fifield, & Ruiz, 1987).

The issue remains as to whether MAST is detrimental to patients and should be removed from the practice of trauma care. Greatest concerns are about pulmonary compromise from an elevated diaphragm (of even greater consequence in children with the pediatric MAST) and the potential for increased intracranial pressure. Studies do not prove that ventilation and brain function are adversely impacted by MAST (Schneider et al., 1989). Decreased survival and some degree of metabolic acidosis after deflation have been demonstrated when used in the presence of thoracic trauma and compartment syndrome. Central venous access (often desired in femoral vessels) and examination of the abdomen and extremities are hindered by the inflation of the abdominal compartment.

The prospective, randomized, 3½-year study of 784 patient outcomes after MAST or no-MAST usage revealed a statistically significant difference for length of ICU stay (increased) and survival (decreased) for the MAST group (Mattox, Bickell, Pepe, Burch, & Feliciano, 1989). In addition, the number of dead-on-arrival patients after cardiac injury was statistically higher in the MAST group. Mattox et al. related the use of MAST in patients with uncontrolled thoracic bleeding to the intraoperative scenario of vascular bleeding: the time-honored concept of never applying a vascular clamp **below** or distal to an area of arterial hemorrhage is disrupted by the use of MAST (a clamp effect) below the level of injury. The use of MAST in trauma care is not advocated by the authors. An obvious contraindication appears to be uncontrolled thoracic bleeding. Potential contraindications are diaphragmatic injury, significant lower extremity injury, and severe head injury. A possible benefit may be temporary pelvic stabilization.

Operative repair

The goal is rapid access to appropriate surgical intervention. To facilitate this, some trauma centers have designed protocols to identify patients who should be admitted immediately to the oper-

ative resuscitation suite upon arrival; others rely on rapid evaluation and transfer to the surgery suite or emergent thoracotomy while in the emergency department. Bypass of the ED and direct transport to a special operating room for resuscitation based on prehospital triage criteria showed a higher survival rate than predicted by TRISS for non-arrested, hypotensive, blunt trauma patients requiring laparotomy (Rhodes, Brader, Lucke, & Gillott, 1989).

Nonoperative management or repair of injured organs (e.g., splenorrhaphy) rather than removal (splenectomy) is generally practiced today except in instances of life-threatening, multiple-organ hemorrhage or when massive splenic destruction is present (Cogbill et al., 1989; Malangoni, 1990; Pickhardt, Moore, Moore, McCroskey, & Moore, 1989). In this instance, often the spleen is removed to focus attention and skill on the remaining viable and essential organs and tissues. One study of 67 blunt trauma patients with minor splenic injury showed similar transfusion requirements for those who had operative exploration and those who were managed nonoperatively (Flaherty & Jurkovich, 1991).

Fluid Therapy

Significant variation in approach exists related to fluids chosen for resuscitation. Aspects pertinent to vascular access, flow rates, timing of fluid delivery, and types of fluids in use will be reviewed.

Vascular access

In cases of severe vasoconstriction or poor vascular status, such as IV drug abuse, obesity, or tortuous or friable veins, the peripheral approach is not viable. In these instances, techniques for central vein access are necessary. Percutaneous thoracic central venous access may result in pneumothorax or hematoma formation and is often difficult to achieve in the severely injured patient in shock. The femoral and jugular veins are frequently used. Surgical cutdowns provide a rapid technique for access to a viable vein that can accept large volumes of fluid through a regular 14-gauge IV catheter or 5 French feeding tube. A cutdown can be accomplished with little disruption to resuscitation, since the surgeon is working at the foot of the bed. Saphenous cutdowns will support the circulation even in the presence of a proximal injury to vessels, such as the iliacs or vena cava, because of excellent collateral flow (Holcroft & Blaisdell, 1991).

Although the intraosseous (IO) route can be used on adults, it is generally reserved for use in children. Hematologic values, such as the differential WBC count and RBC morphology, may be altered shortly after IO infusion because of displacement of bone marrow contents into the peripheral circulation (Ros, McMannis, Kowal-Vern, Zeller, & Hurley, 1991). Intraosseous infusion is discussed in greater detail in Chapter 17.

Flow rates

As discussed in the review of circulatory processes, flow depends significantly on the radius of the vessel. When vascular access is obtained, the catheter and tubing can restrict the flow regardless of the size of the vessel. The shortest and largest internal diameter intravenous catheter should be used when fluid resuscitation is anticipated, to maximize fluid flow by gravity or with pressure.

Resistance   Resistance for an 18-gauge, 2-inch long, 1.3-mm inner diameter catheter is 7 times that of a 14-gauge, 2-inch, 2.1-mm catheter (Elboim, 1985). Many trauma centers use introducer sheaths as an IV access. These sheaths usually serve as conduits for a PA line or multilumen catheters, but they can be used as the catheter (Marino, 1991). Figure 9-17 illustrates the flow rates of crystalloid through different types of tubing and with varying degrees of catheter angulation (kinking) (Dutky, Stevens, & Maull, 1989). Trauma tubing does not limit the flow through an 8.5 French catheter; however, regular blood tubing, regular-bore extension tubings, and needles will reduce flow in varying degrees (Table 9-8). Special care must be taken to evaluate items attached to the main catheter, such as a T-piece that allows for use of a stopcock. When this is used, the fluid must infuse through the attached port, which is much smaller, thus defeating the purpose of a large-bore catheter. The side port

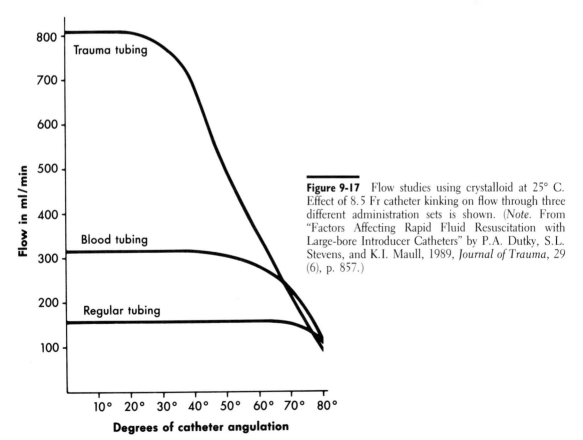

Figure 9-17   Flow studies using crystalloid at 25° C. Effect of 8.5 Fr catheter kinking on flow through three different administration sets is shown. (*Note.* From "Factors Affecting Rapid Fluid Resuscitation with Large-bore Introducer Catheters" by P.A. Dutky, S.L. Stevens, and K.I. Maull, 1989, *Journal of Trauma, 29* (6), p. 857.)

Table 9-8 Effect of tubing size on flow rates (ml/min) of crystalloids and blood products (25° C) using common intravenous cannulae

IV cannula size	Crystalloids			Dilute packed cells (Hct = 33%)	
	Regular IV tubing (2.54 mm I.D.)	Blood tubing (3.05 mm I.D.)	Trauma tubing (5.72 mm I.D.)	Blood tubing (3.05 mm I.D.)	Trauma tubing (5.72 mm I.D.)
18 gauge (0.97 mm I.D.)	87	108	117	72	87
16 gauge (1.37 mm I.D.)	125	193	247	120	188
14 gauge (1.70 mm I.D.)	147	268	417	162	328
8.5 French (2.85 mm I.D.)	160	316	805	193	642

Note. Modified from "Factors Affecting Rapid Fluid Resuscitation with Large-Bore Introducer Catheters" by P.A. Dutkey, S.L. Stevens, and K.I. Maull, 1989. *Journal of Trauma, 29* (6), p. 857.)
Note. I.D., Internal diameter; *dilute packed cells,* PRBC combined with equal volume of normal saline.

should be discarded and the IV tubing attached directly to the end of the introducer sheath. Reduction in flow can also occur when tapered catheters are used. Piggybacking of fluid through a needle should also be avoided for the same reason.

Pressure A variety of systems are available for increasing the pressure gradient for fluid infusion. The simplest form of pressure is gravity flow. This is often augmented by squeezing an in-line, positive-pressure chamber (or blood pump) to deliver 30 to 50 ml per "pump" (Elboim, 1985). This procedure is labor intensive, since someone must remain to pump the blood. A study designed to emulate the options available to prehospital personnel evaluated the effect of manual squeezing of the fluid container, kneeling on the container, inflating a BP cuff around the bag, and using commercial pressure infusors. Manual squeezing increased infusion by .5 times faster than gravity flow, and commercial pressure infusors were 2 to 5 times faster (White, Hamilton, & Veronesi, 1991). In place of manual pressure, EDs use manually inflated pressure bags (200 to 300 mm Hg), which are effective in doubling flow rates (Dutky et al., 1989). However, it is time-consuming to place the fluid bag inside the pressure bag and then inflate it to pressure. Manufacturers have now designed pressure infusors that use compressed air to rapidly inflate and deflate the device, requiring only placement of the bag on a hook and closure of a latched door. This is more expensive, but fully allows personnel to infuse fluid as fast as the tubing will allow. It is very important (1) that when infusing fluid under pres-

sure, any air in the fluid bag be expressed before infusion or (2) that a "fail-safe" set of air filter eliminators exists within the infusion system. Otherwise, air embolism could occur. Mechanical pumps (similar to IV rate controllers) are also available to infuse blood components at controlled rates, but each brand must be carefully evaluated in conjunction with the blood bank to assure that hemolysis will not result.

Viscosity Fluid viscosity will impact the rate of flow of the fluid. Blood products have greater viscosity than crystalloids because of the presence of cells, which results in more turbulent flow. In addition, most blood products are quite cold when delivered for patient administration; packed red blood cells (PRBCs) are stored at 4° C. The fact that PRBCs only partially fill the blood collection bag allows various approaches to changing its viscosity. The type and amount of anticoagulant used affects viscosity, since it impacts the hematocrit of the unit, which can vary from 60% to 85%. Dilution of the PRBCs with saline will thin the mixture, decreasing viscosity. Only normal saline is allowed by the American Association of Blood Banks (AABB) to be instilled into packed cells. (Holland, 1989). The AABB *Technical Manual* states that the entire unit of blood should not be warmed at one time, specifying that it should be warmed as it passes through the administration set (Walker, 1990). However, research has shown that PRBCs can be safely and effectively warmed by rapid admixture. No detrimental change in plasma hemoglobin levels and no RBC damage in vivo and in vitro occurred (Jud-

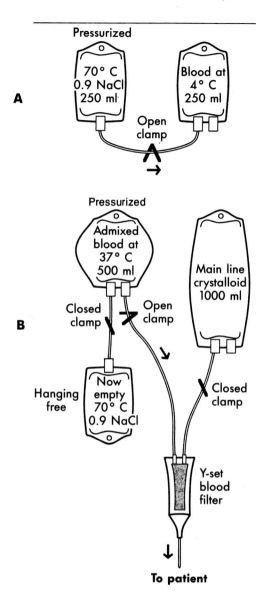

Figure 9-18   Technique for safe, rapid admixture blood warming. **A,** Use of transfer set to instill 250 ml of 70° C normal saline into cold packed red blood cells. **B,** Addition of admixture unit with blood administration set for infusion. (*Note.* From "Rapid Admixture Blood Warming" by D. Judkins and K.V. Iserson, 1991, *Journal of Emergency Nursing, 17* (3), p. 147.)

kins & Iverson, 1991). This involves mixing 250 ml of 70° C normal saline into the bag of PRBCs, which can warm 4° C blood to 37° C within less than 1 minute. The 250-ml aliquot of saline was accommodated in the standard PRBC bag for units weighing 220 to 420 g. The method requires use of a transfer set to transfer the hot saline into the PRBCs (Figure 9-18). The reason for this technique is to prevent inadvertent direct administration of the hot saline through the blood tubing into the patient, as might occur accidentally with a Y-set. A detailed protocol is listed in the article by Judkins and Iserson. A reminder is given that this procedure could be described as experimental, since it is not yet approved by the AABB. Advantages of this technique are the rapidity of warming, limited space requirements and cost of equipment, and the ability to use the system for multiple patients and for multiple vascular access lines in the same patient. The quality assurance and record-keeping steps listed in the protocol may require substantial staff time. Zorko and Polsky (1986) also showed a warming effect and increased delivery rate, without evidence of significant hemolysis with addition of 45° C normal saline to PRBCs.

Timing of fluid delivery

Considerable discussion continues regarding when IV fluid should be administered. Cannon, Fraser, and Cowell (1918) commented that "injection of a fluid that will increase blood pressure has dangers in itself." In a case of shock, hemorrhage may not have occurred to a marked degree because blood pressure was too low and the flow too scant to overcome the obstacle offered by a clot (Bickell, Shaftan, & Mattox, 1989). If the pressure is raised before the surgeon is ready to check any bleeding that may take place, bleeding may occur. Of note is that the Advanced Trauma Life Support Course (as well as most texts) recommends fluid infusion to maintain a normal blood pressure. These recommendations came in part from animal studies that used controlled hemorrhage from a cannula (rather than via bleeding vessels and organs) and did not develop a clot that could be disturbed. Determining whether practice should continue to elevate BP in the presence of traumatic hypovolemia and whether this practice is deleterious requires further study. A randomized, prospective study of IV access and infusion versus heparin lock insertion in the field is ongoing (K. Mattox [personal communication, January 1992]). This principle relates to the argument stated for reduction in use of the MAST when penetrating injuries are present because the pressure of the suit acts as a distal clamp, allowing increased proximal hemorrhage.

Prehospital issues The insertion of IVs is not the first priority in field treatment of trauma. IV insertion may be carried out while en route and is encouraged by the *Basic Trauma Life Support* manual for the "load and go" or "scoop and run" patient (Baldwin & Smit, 1988) and *Prehospital Trauma Life Support* training manual (Butman & Paturas, 1986). Generally, the only time an IV is started at the scene for a trauma patient is during prolonged extrication. Once intravenous access is established, a warm fluid supply is optimal and the capability to increase flow via a pressurized system generally is essential because of (1) the low interior height of the vehicle and (2) the limited number of personnel. Time required for field IV starts has been debated and is impacted by varied data collection methods and definition of the process. In one rural study, it was recommended that field manuevers be minimized in critically injured patients to decrease mortality (Smith, Bodai, Hill, & Frey, 1985), whereas in another rural study, prehospital ALS care was considered beneficial in 85% of multisystem injury cases (Reines, Bartlett, Chudy, Kiragu, & McKnew, 1988). Time required for field IV insertion has been reported to range from 2.3 to 13 minutes (Reines et al., 1988; Donovan, Cline, Whitley, Foster, & Outlaw, 1989; Feldman, 1986; Jones, Nesper, & Alcouloumre, 1989).

The field placement of an adequate-sized access line allows immediate use of a rapid infusor device in the ED and allows immediate access for paralytics or analgesics as indicated on arrival.

Types of fluid

Crystalloid Crystalloid refers to saline-based fluids that contain ions (electrolytes), all particles that can traverse between the intravascular, interstitial, and intracellular spaces when membranes are intact. Intravascular retention of crystalloid is only about 20% (Marino, 1991; Shippy & Appel, 1984). The relative efficiency of plasma volume filling decreases as more balanced salt solutions are administered; once the interstitial space is expanded, more distributes there. Examples of balanced salt solutions include 0.9% sodium chloride (normal saline), lactated Ringer's solution, and Plasma-Lyte A. Table 9-9 lists the osmolality, pH, and electrolyte contents of common solutions. Normal saline is often used in preparation for blood infusion because the ionized calcium in lactated Ringer's solution can interact with the citrate anticoagulant (CPDA-1) in bank blood, potentially leading to clot formation (Sheldon &

Table 9-9 Characteristics and electrolyte content (mEq/L) of various crystalloid solutions

Product and distributor	Osmolality (mOsm/L)	pH	Na$^+$	Cl$^-$	Mg^{++}/Ca^{++}	K$^+$	Buffers		
							Lactate	Gluconate	Acetate
0.9% NaCl—normal saline (Abbott, Baxter, Kendall McGaw)	308	5.7	154	154	0/0	0	0	0	0
Lactated Ringer's solution (Abbott, Baxter, Kendall McGaw)	272	6.7	130	109	0/3	4	28	0	0
Plasma-Lyte A (Baxter)	294	7.4	140	98	3/0	5	0	23	27
Plasma-Lyte 148 (Baxter)	294	4-6.5	140	98	3/0	5	0	23	27
Normosol-R pH 7.4 (Abbott)	295	7.4	140	98	3/0	5	0	23	27
Isolyte S pH 7.4 (Kendall McGaw)	295	7.4	141	98	3/0	5	0	23	27

Note. Modified from *Facts and Comparisons* (p. 50) by Walters Kluwer, Inc., 1991, St. Louis; and from *The ICU Book* (p. 655) by P.L. Marino, 1991, Philadelphia: Lea & Febiger.

Collins, 1987; Walker, 1990). It has been found that 25% of electrolyte solution used to prime blood tubing remains in the tubing after 10 minutes and 10% after 30 minutes (Ryden & Oberman, 1975). Sustained use of normal saline can lead to hyperchloremic metabolic acidosis; therefore serum electrolytes should be carefully evaluated. The lactate in lactated Ringer's solution may be incompletely cleared in the presence of hepatic failure.

Hypertonic solutions Hypertonic solutions are hyperosmolar, highly concentrated saline solutions that are designed to allow the use of smaller resuscitation volumes with similar or greater effects than isoosmotic solutions. The high osmolarity of 7% NaCl (2400 mOsm) has a significant effect on drawing fluid from the intracellular space into extracellular spaces. This effect has been considered "unphysiologic" to the cells by some, but in reality, it simulates the body's "homeostasis" in times of exertion and hemorrhage (Shackford, 1989). The hemodynamic effects of hypertonic solutions include increased microcirculation, cardiac output, mesenteric and coronary blood flow, and vasodilation (hyperemia) and improved myocardial contractility and oxygen transport (Mattox et al., 1991; Velasco, Pontieri, Rocha, Silva, & Lopes, 1980). The risks include excessive serum osmolality, hypernatremia, hypokalemia, and altered thermal regula-

tory set points. Angiotensin II was suppressed in postoperative cardiac surgery patients receiving 1.8% hypertonic saline, which may be beneficial in perfusing the kidney, heart, and intestines (Cross et al., 1989). Mattox et al. (1991) found in a three-center, prospective, randomized study of hypotensive trauma patients that the infusion of 250 ml of hypertonic (7.5%) saline in 6% dextran 70 (HSD) was safe in that no episodes of seizures, blood crossmatching difficulties, or anaphylactoid reactions occurred. The incidence of adult respiratory distress syndrome, renal failure, and coagulopathies was higher in the standard crystalloid group. Patients receiving HSD showed a more rapid initial rise in BP in comparison with the crystalloid group. Survival was not significantly different for blunt versus penetrating injuries, but for patients requiring surgery, a significant treatment effect in favor of HSD was shown. However, in experimental studies of normal saline versus hypertonic saline (HTS) in controlled and uncontrolled hemorrhagic shock, treatment with HTS resulted in a dramatic drop in MAP and early mortality in the uncontrolled hemorrhage group compared with the controlled hemorrhage group with HTS that showed a steep rise in MAP over the 3-hour observation (Gross, Landau, Assalia, & Krausz, 1988).

Colloids Colloid solutions are large, molecular-weight substances that do not readily cross through capillary walls and therefore do not normally pass between the tissue compartments as crystalloids can. Colloids within the intravascular space exert an osmostic force to retain fluid (colloid osmotic pressure [COP]). The normal plasma COP is 20 mm Hg. These solutions include human serum albumin (COP = 20), polysaccharides (dextran [COP = 40/72 for dextran 40/70]), and 6% hydroxyethyl starch (hetastarch [COP = 35]) (Halvorsen, Blaisdell, & Holcroft, 1990; Marino, 1991). Colloids such as dextran 70 when added to hypertonic saline prolong the duration of action and expand plasma volume to a greater degree. Their disadvantages include a potential for coagulopathy and a rare incidence of allergic reactions. Hetastarch will artificially raise the serum amylase level. Dextrans can interfere with the crossmatching of blood. Although some centers use colloids as the preferred resuscitative fluid, most use crystalloid, which is less expensive, and add colloid and blood products as physiologic changes dictate.

Velanovich (1989) statistically analyzed published articles that reported the effects of colloid versus crystalloid fluids. Velanovich analyzed mortality in relation to crystalloid versus colloid and found an overall pooled treatment effect in favor of crystalloid, but also reported that trauma and nontrauma populations may not be comparable because of the common permeability state in trauma that allows the extravasation of colloids. For trauma patients only, the treatment effect still favored crystalloid, whereas nontrauma patient groupings favored colloid.

Transfusion Traumatic injury is heavily focused on hemorrhagic volume loss that requires replacement. Many options exist today to maximize oxygen delivery while limiting the amount of blood products required.

Anemia Cardiac output increases in anemia because of decreased resistance to flow of anemic blood (dilutional effect), which allows a basically work-free increase in flow to counter the decrease in oxygen content. This benefit is limited, however, since the accelerated circulation can cancel the effect of increased oxygen delivery by not allowing adequate time for diffusion (Bryan-Brown, 1988). Red cells have an autoregulatory function, increasing 2,3-diphosphoglyceric acid (2,3-DPG), which reduces the affinity of hemoglobin for oxygen, which then facilitates release of oxygen in the capillary bed. An adequate Hgb level does not

ensure adequate tissue oxygenation. The presence of shock, preexisting cardiopulmonary disease, and sepsis will likely alter the tolerance to anemia, and individualization is the key to transfusion practice. The actual Hct threshold for optimal initiation of transfusion therapy in individuals who are stable and under limited stress is 20%.

ERYTHROPOIETIN The marrow is stimulated after acute hemorrhage to produce erythrocytes. The hormone erythropoietin regulates the production of RBCs. Red blood cell replacement generally takes up to 60 days, since only 15 to 50 ml of cell volume is produced daily (Marino, 1991). Because the process is time-consuming and erythropoietin activity can be depressed by inhibitory factors in thermal burns, patients with acute hemorrhage usually require transfusion to survive this period of RBC reproduction. However, inherent risks exist in transfusion, such as disease transmission, and some patients regard transfusion of blood as against their beliefs. For these individuals, stimulation of RBC production is desired. Human recombinant erythropoietin (EPO) is currently approved for use in patients with chronic renal failure and patients with human immunodeficiency virus (HIV) who are treated with zidovudine (AZT). Caution must be taken to modify the dose to avoid increased viscosity, which can lead to vascular complications. Clinical trials are in progress to evaluate the use of EPO for anemia of prematurity, cancer, and rheumatoid arthritis, as well as to increase red cell procurement in presurgical autologous donation and as a perisurgical adjuvant to reduce transfusion requirements (Abels & Rudnick, 1991). Case studies report use of EPO for a patient whose faith is Jehovah's Witness, who refused homologous transfusion after a burn injury; and for a patient involved in a motor vehicle crash and sustained multiple fractures, whose Hct was 13% by the third day (Boshkov, Tredget, & Janowska-Wieczorek, 1991; Koestner, Nelson, Morris, & Safcsak, 1990). Erythropoietin substantially increased packed cell volume, Hgb levels, and reticulocyte counts, thereby providing an alternative therapy for life-threatening anemia. Treatment in humans after acute blood loss is expected to reduce the need for homologous transfusion.

Blood products Blood products are an important commodity when treating traumatic shock. The processing of blood for transfusion has changed over time, with the current focus on component therapy so that only that which is needed is given. Newer additive solutions have been developed that lengthen the red cell life span, dilute the red cell volume to a more reasonable hematocrit, and improve the energy component of the blood, 2,3-DPG. These are all beneficial changes for the recipient and allow for greater utilization of a scarce resource. Certain risks remain with the transfer of blood from one person to another, although it presents far less danger than that of the late 1800s when transfusion of milk was attempted (Miale, 1972). In 1901 the three types of blood (A, AB, and O) were identified. This is the most important aspect of transfusion today, ensuring the compatibility of units with the recipient's blood, as well as assuring the necessity of the transfusion. One unit of red blood cells increases the hemoglobin concentration by approximately 1 g/dl (Menitove, 1991) and hematocrit by 3%.

BLOOD TYPES AND REACTIONS   Blood is classified by the type of antigen it carries; e.g., type A blood has A antigen but not B, and vice versa. The antigen will react with its antibodies if contact is made. It is most serious to have an A, B, or O incompatibility because the antibodies are primed to defend. When noncompatible red cells are given, the donor antigen can be bombarded by the recipient's vast supply of antibody within his or her plasma. On the other hand, if plasma is given to the wrong recipient, the incorrect transfused antibody will be promptly diluted by the recipient's blood volume. Minor reactions such as these can cause a transfusion reaction, but it would generally be delayed and would normally not be hemolytic in nature. This is the rationale behind the "universal donor" of group O blood. Type O blood has no antigen for the recipient to react against, and the dilutional effect renders the antibody harmless. However, it is much safer to consider type O packed cells as a universal donor than type O whole blood, which contains much more plasma. In an effort to create greater availability of O cells, researchers have biomechanically manipulated the RBCs by enzymatic conversion (from B to O) and transfused these converted cells to volunteers with positive results (Lenny, Hurst, Goldstein, Benjamin, & Jones, 1991).

Delayed reactions can occur in relation to the D Ag (Rh factor). Although Rh-positive blood has been infused to Rh-negative patients in emergencies and in situations of shortage, it primes the person to develop a delayed reaction when resensitized to the Rh antigen. Rh-positive blood should be avoided in women of child-bearing age; RhoGAM is ineffective for handling significant infusion, since one vial only affords passive immune suppression for 15 ml of blood. After infusion of 200 ml or more of Rh-positive red cells, 80% of recipients had detectable anti-Rh in their plasma after a few months (Mollison, 1983). Signs and symptoms of delayed transfusion reactions are jaundice, increased bilirubin, fever, decreased Hgb level, hemoglobinuria, and a positive Coombs' test. Renal failure rarely accompanies delayed reactions. A hemolytic transfusion reaction is rare but has a mortality of about 10% as a result of initiation of renal failure and disseminated intravascular coagulation (DIC) from a major incompatibility. Signs and symptoms include chest pain, anxiety, hypotension, flushed appearance, nausea, and abdominal and flank pain. When the patient is under anesthesia, a hemolytic transfusion reaction may be detected by abnormal oozing of blood or by hemoglobinuria (Huestis, Bove, & Busch, 1981). Prompt discontinuation of the unit and consultation with the transfusion service are essential. Usually, acute hemolytic reactions are the result of inaccurate handling of a blood specimen, either the improper identification of the recipient or the misidentification of the donor. It is imperative that personnel adhere to the principle that the patient *must* be wearing an identifying tag before any specimen for laboratory work pertinent to transfusion is drawn, and before administration of blood products.

COMPATIBILITY TESTING   The typical laboratory testing for transfusion compatibility involves typing the patient's blood for ABO and Rh, screening it for antibodies, and performing a major crossmatch of the patient's serum and the donor red cells. However, in the trauma patient, time is of the essence. The standard is to do an immediate spin saline crossmatch (ISXM), which only verifies no gross ABO incompatibility. If blood is needed immediately, O-negative packed cells are given. Blood specimens take 5 to 10 minutes to clot before ABO and Rh typing can proceed, but methods to allow removal of cells before clotting are available, which allow ABO and Rh typing within about 5 minutes. Eventually the serum is needed to do an antibody screen, which takes at least 25 minutes. Type-specific, uncrossmatched blood can usually be delivered to a department within 15 minutes. Studies have shown that ISXM does not always detect ABO incompatibility, but the incidence is very low and does not usually result in life-threatening hemolytic reactions when limited volume is given. It is even suggested that computerized testing from blood bank records to demonstrate donor-recipient ABO incompatibility would be as effective as ISXM (Judd, 1991). Although significant effort goes into the testing phases, it must be remembered that fatal reactions are not usually the result of imperfect serologic testing but, rather, imperfect patient identification. Blood substitutes that would avoid the need for compatibility testing and significantly reduce risks of transfusion are undergoing continued testing, but none are in widespread use.

Massive transfusion   The most common definition of massive transfusion is the replacement of one half of the patient's blood volume at one time or the complete replacement of the patient's blood volume over 24 hours (Harris, 1985; Huestis et al., 1981). Others have defined it as greater than 12 units in 12 hours (Reed et al., 1986). In the ED or receiving resuscitation area, protocols for handling patients with massive transfusion needs are recommended. Aspects included are access to O-negative and uncrossmatched blood, specimen procurement, storage of blood, documentation issues, and associated complications. Most trauma centers do not permanently store blood products outside of their transfusion department because of rigorous standards for monitoring. It is also unnecessary, since rapid access can be obtained in other ways, such as a transfusion technician maintained on the major trauma team paging system. This allows early awareness of blood needs, and the technician can arrive in the resuscitation area before the patient, with a "bucket" or cooler of O-negative blood. This cooler should then be labeled with the trauma alias name and number. Devices within the cooler indicate whether the units of blood are remaining cool enough for safe return to the blood bank. Generally, once a cooler of O-negative uncrossmatched blood is left in the patient area, type-specific products, although available, are often not used to avoid accidental delivery of type-specific products to another trauma patient in the same area. Specific protocols will vary, but the

team must understand their rationale and how to work within the system. A system of transferring the blood bucket to diagnostic areas and the operating room for critical patients should be in place. Another area of caution relates to prehospital use of blood. Some critical care ground and flight programs carry and administer blood from the referring hospital or carry O-negative cells. It is crucial that the blood units be accounted for and that a plan exists for conversion to in-house units.

The first nursing responsibility is to ensure that the patient is properly and permanently identified. An alias armband with a trauma medical record number works effectively and can be part of a prestamped trauma packet. This number should remain with the patient throughout the current hospital stay to assist the transfusion service in tracking and verifying urgent requests for more blood products. Documentation of each blood unit number on the trauma data base is important in case the blood bank needs to track the unit; e.g., the donor later develops a positive HIV test, or hemolysis is detected. The volume of blood infused should be recorded separate from the crystalloid, and the blood unit number can easily be entered. Each unit of PRBCs, despite variation in actual volume, is typically recorded as 250 ml. This may be an issue in facilities that routinely use PRBCs with additives that increase the volume to 350 ml. For pediatric patients, it is very important to take into account the Hct of the unit if possible, since a 15 ml/kg bolus of a unit with Hct of 65% versus 80% would result in varying amounts of actual RBC delivery. The younger the child, the more important this becomes.

Complications of massive transfusion relate to the speed of administration, the effectiveness of warming fluids, and the characteristics of the products delivered. Bank blood, which is stored at 4° C, is not only cold, but depending on its shelf time (generally up to 42 days), contains particulate matter; a lower level of erythrocyte 2,3-DPG, which decreases the efficiency of oxygen release to the tissues; elevated potassium levels; and excess citrate. These changes can cause complications in patients receiving large amounts of blood over a short time. Significant citrate levels can lead to depressed myocardial contractility caused by hypocalcemia from the binding of calcium with the citrate. Normally this is a problem only in cold patients with poorly functioning livers.

Most people can tolerate the citrate load when receiving even one unit every 5 minutes without
needing supplemental calcium (Collins, 1976;
Huestis et al., 1981). The coagulation factors
have been removed in most blood units, and any
remaining factors, as well as platelets, do not
maintain their function in storage. Hypothermia
is another high risk in high-volume infusion,
since it alters coagulation and shifts the oxyhemoglobin curve.

BLOOD DELIVERY SYSTEMS   Reports of fluid warmer
efficiency are somewhat difficult to compare because fluid warmer performance is linked to the
type of infusate tested, e.g., cold PRBC, diluted
PRBC, crystalloid (Presson, Hillier, & Haselby,
1991). Systems like the Level I 250 or 500 series
fluid warmers are sufficient to warm fluid for
some patients (Figure 9-19). It is simple to set up,
can be set up quickly (30 sec), and can infuse by
gravity during transport. Fluid is warmed through
a heat exchanger with a water bath temperature of
40° C. When fluid was infused at a flow rate of
225 ml/min through the Level I, the output temperature was 33.6° C; however, by 400 ml/min,
the outflow temperature was 24.2° C, too cool to
be as effective (Presson, 1990). Therefore fluid
warmers must be selected for the rate of flow expected. Actually, the Level I when combined
with an automated pressure inflation/deflation device can infuse the fluid faster than one person
can spike and change the units. One additional
disadvantage to this device is that basically one
type of blood product, i.e., PRBC, is infusing at a
time, which is not as physiologic as blood product
mixtures or "cocktails" allowed by other systems.

The Haemonetic rapid infusion system (RIS) is
used in some trauma resuscitation areas and
mainly by anesthesia personnel in the operating
suite (Figure 9-20). This device has a quick set-up
process (5 minutes), a clear control panel allowing fingertip changes in flow rate and pressure,
significant air filter/elimination checks, and the
ability to infuse multiple products into a reservoir
for combined administration. Even the Haemonetic cell saver system from the operative field can
be attached to the RIS, allowing combined autotransfusion of processed RBCs. Bank blood can
be processed through the cell saver to eliminate
particulate matter and then warmed and delivered
via the RIS. Flow rates of up to 1500 ml/min
(one fourth of the body's blood volume) can be

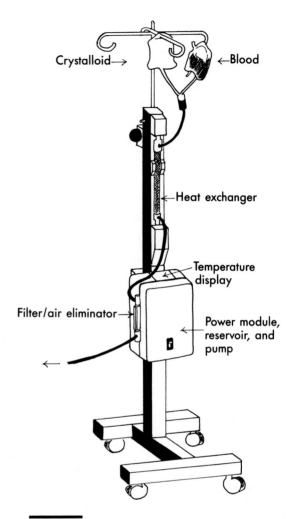

Figure 9-19   Level I System 250 fluid warmer unit.

obtained while maintaining a normothermic intraoperative temperature. The unit will alarm and
not allow infusion if fluids are less than 34° C.
Fluid boluses are also easy to deliver. With devices such as these, there is truly no excuse for intraoperative hypothermia. A comparison of conventional fluid administration and use of the RIS
in major trauma patients showed a significant reduction in pneumonia and hospital costs and a
trend of decreased ICU and ventilator days (Dunham et al., 1989). Major liver transplant cases
have also had excellent results with the use of the
RIS.

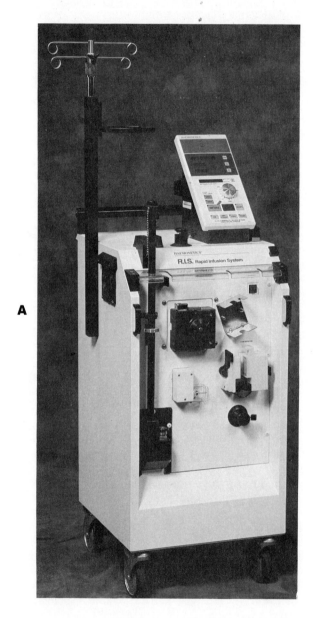

Figure 9-20 Rapid Infusion System for rapid fluid delivery and fluid warming. **A,** View of machine, with rate and pressure control. (*Note.* Courtesy Haemonetics Life Support Division, Braintree, MA.)

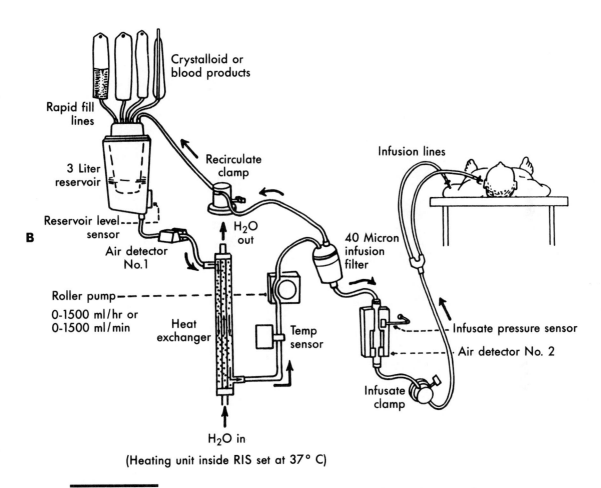

B

Crystalloid or
blood products

Rapid fill
lines

Recirculate
clamp

3 Liter
reservoir

Infusion lines

Reservoir level
sensor

H_2O
out

Air detector
No.1

40 Micron
infusion
filter

Roller pump

0-1500 ml/hr or
0-1500 ml/min

Heat
exchanger

Temp
sensor

Infusate pressure sensor

Air detector No. 2

Infusate
clamp

H_2O in

(Heating unit inside RIS set at 37° C)

Figure 9-20, cont'd   B, Schematic of tubing path from reservoir through heater, air detectors, air eliminator, and filter.

AUTOTRANSFUSION Autotransfusion is implemented to reinfuse shed blood into the patient. This allows rapid cellular and volume replacement and decreased risk of disease transmission from homologous blood. The concept is implemented intraoperatively to return surgical field blood, postoperatively in orthopedic cases, and in emergent trauma in the presence of hemothorax. The nurse is involved in autotransfusion through the anticipation of need, and proper and efficient set-up and reinfusion. The use of autotransfusion has been questioned when bank blood is immediately available. No studies have evaluated the relative safety of bank blood (in terms of the risk of disease transmission, alloimmunization, incompatibility, and storage-related deficits) versus autotransfusion (risk of contamination, inappropriate anticoagulant ratio) in apparent thoracic trauma. Combined thoracic and abdominal trauma may result in infusion of contaminated blood, but it has been reported to be administered without adverse effects. Autotransfusion is indicated for patients with suspected hemothorax, which is amenable to placement of tube thoracostomy and drainage and reinfusion of shed blood. For autotransfusion to be effective, the special container must be prepared before final chest tube placement; otherwise significant quantities of blood are lost to the basic chest drainage unit chamber. In major thoracic hemorrhage, it has been questioned whether thoracostomy and drainage might hasten exsanguination. However, when the patient is not immediately ready for surgery or the extent of the injury is not apparent from chest x-ray and clinical examination, autotransfusion can be a helpful adjunct.

Nursing issues include the appropriate use of anticoagulant to avoid clot formation and the appropriate use of filters. Some centers administer autotransfused blood without anticoagulant. The use of macrofilters as provided with regular blood tubing will screen for gross particulate matter; however, some transfusion services recommend a micropore filter for reinfusion of autotransfused blood. Each autotransfusion set should be used for only 4 hours to avoid bacterial contamination. Volume infused should be recorded separately from the usual documentation of blood product transfusion.

COAGULOPATHY Microvascular bleeding can occur as a result of dilutional thrombocytopenia during and after massive transfusion, as well as from consumption of platelets. Abnormal coagulopathy with or without DIC is also associated with severe head injury in 50% of cases (Goodnight, Kenoyer, & Rappaport, 1974; Popp & Bourke, 1985). The brain has a very high tissue thromboplastin concentration, which can be released into the bloodstream after cerebral injury, initiating hypercoagulation. The prophylactic administration of platelets and fresh frozen plasma has not been shown to be effective for prevention of microvascular bleeding; therefore routine administration is contraindicated (Reed et al., 1986; Winter, Plummer, Bottini, Rockswold, & Ray, 1989). Close monitoring of prothrombin, partial thromboplastin time, platelet levels, and fibrinogen or fibrin degradation products should guide administration of platelets and fresh frozen plasma. Further discussion is found in Chapter 19.

ASSESSMENT AND INTERVENTIONS RELATED TO SPECIFIC INJURIES
General Therapeutic Decisions
Frank-Starling curve*

The Frank-Starling curve demonstrates the relationship between preload and ventricular output (cardiac output). Essentially, the curve shows that as preload increases, so too does the cardiac output. This is possible because when faced with an increased volume load, the heart responds by increasing its peak systolic ventricular pressure and thus its cardiac output.

In addition to preload, contractility plays an important role in establishing cardiac output. Figure 9-21 shows three curves that represent three different cardiac contractilities. As can be seen, for a given preload, the cardiac output decreases when contractility decreases. Similarly, to maintain a given cardiac output, preload must be increased as contractility decreases.

In all three curves (representing three different cardiac contractilities), point A represents hypovolemia. An increase in volume (preload) will place the patient's hemodynamic status at a point further along the curve and with increased cardiac output—a successful intervention. It can be noted that for each curve, cardiac output was increased simply by increasing preload and without any change in contractility.

When the hemodynamic status reveals normo-

---

*This section contributed by Margaret J. Neff, B.S.

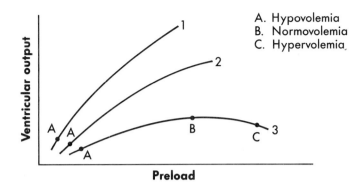

A. Hypovolemia
B. Normovolemia
C. Hypervolemia

Figure 9-21   Frank-Starling curves in relation to hemodynamic changes. Demonstrates effect of low and excessive preload and poor contractility on ventricular output. Curve *1* represents hypercontractility; curve *2*, normal contractility; curve *3*, hypocontractility. (*Note.* Modified from *Intensive Care Manual for Physicians* by T. Feeley, F. Mihm, R. Pearl, T. Raffin, and M. Rosenthal, 1990, Stanford, CA: Stanford University Medical Center, Department of Anesthesiology.)

volemic hypocontractility (point B), measures to increase cardiac output must be aimed at increasing contractility, since fluid resuscitation (increasing preload) will have no beneficial effect. In this case, arterial dilators and inotropes can be used to increase contractility. For the same preload, cardiac output is greater as a result of the increased contractility.

The final condition demonstrated on Figure 9-21 is that of hypervolemia (point C). In this case, the therapeutic measures needed to increase cardiac output must be aimed at decreasing the preload (volume) and thus bringing the patient's hemodynamic status back "up" the curve to point B. This decrease in volume can be effected with venodilators or diuretics.

Viability of emergent thoracotomy

The issue of emergent thoracotomy has been hotly debated for some time. Most discussions center around ultimate patient outcome in light of the presence of penetrating or blunt trauma. Medical examiners raise the issue that the patients are transported dead to the hospital; they would prefer that patients be left at the scene to facilitate medical and legal investigation. So who is the right candidate for emergent thoracotomy? There are no clear-cut answers, but some criteria are helpful. Emergency medical services are also reviewing the value of paramedic resources in providing advanced life support and code 3 (lights and sirens) transport of nonviable patients. This

has resulted in development of new guidelines for determination of death in the field. Prehospital training in very careful detection of vital signs and signs of life is essential to avoid missed diagnosis. Signs of life refer to an auscultated heartbeat, pupillary activity, respiratory effort (gasp), motor function (any movement), or other signs of viability in contrast to the usual vital sign parameters. Cases have occurred where law enforcement personnel determined death and prevented paramedic intervention, only to learn that the patient was alive. Field situations are difficult because of noise, weather, multiple priorities, and safety issues, but safe determination of death should be possible with base physician direction as required.

Protocols are appearing that limit field intervention based on length of down time and/or expected transfer time to a trauma center, varying from 5 to 20 minutes. It seems that patients deserve the benefit of the doubt, since data are still somewhat limited. Incidents involving violence and angry crowds sometimes set the tone for resuscitation efforts and transfer as well.

Criteria for ED thoracotomy often include (1) loss of vital signs in the ED, and patient remains unresponsive to volume plus blood resuscitation; (2) loss of vital signs en route to the trauma center, and patient has ongoing CPR for less than 15 minutes; and (3) patient without vital signs in the field, but with signs of life and have ongoing CPR for less than 15 minutes. The consensus is that patients with penetrating injury in full arrest or in extremis have a better potential outcome from thoracotomy than patients with blunt injury. Stab wounds in comparison with gunshot wounds have a greater survival rate, since the extent of destruction is often less. Status on ED arrival is one factor to guide surgical decision-making in that patients arriving with relatively stable vital signs have a higher percent of "saves" than those in extremis, but patients in extremis are saved. In fact, Baker, Thomas, and Trunkey (1980) reported a 50% survival rate of patients arriving with no signs of life after cardiac injuries. Crawford (1991) reports that patients with the greatest salvage rate are not those who arrive in extremis or deteriorate shortly after arrival, but those who cannot be stabilized with normal resuscitation. A classification system can be useful in evaluating efficacy of ED thoracotomy and approximately corresponds with the amount of blood loss (Roberge, Ivatury, Stahl, & Rohman, 1986). These include (1) profound shock, (2) agonal, (3) "dead" on arrival, and (4) "dead" on the scene. The authors further define these and encourage inclusion of field transportation data and neurologic status of survi-

vors in studies of ED thoracotomy. Patients with hemorrhagic abdominal or pelvic injuries may also benefit from thoracic access allowed by emergent thoracotomy to occlude the descending aorta, diverting blood from the bleeding source and to essential organs, such as the heart and brain (Holcroft & Blaisdell, 1991) (Figure 9-22). Back pressure can develop, which may eventually increase the abdominal or pelvic bleeding. The incision is usually a left thoracotomy at the fourth or fifth intercostal space or a median sternotomy. Extension to the right mediastinum may be made, requiring a sternal saw or Lebsche sternal chisel and mallet. Specialized equipment, such as vascular clamps and rib retractors, is routinely used, and the nurse must be familiar with its function to assist the surgeon during this sudden ED operative procedure.

Interventions Related to Specific Injuries

Hemothorax
Fluid volume deficit
Impaired gas exchange
Altered tissue perfusion
High risk for hypothermia

Penetrating or blunt injury can result in a he-

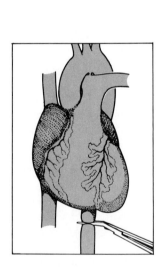
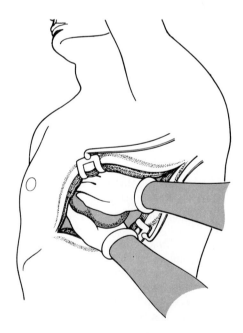

Figure 9-22 Emergency left thoracotomy site with internal cardiac massage. Descending aorta is shown cross-clamped with vascular clamp.

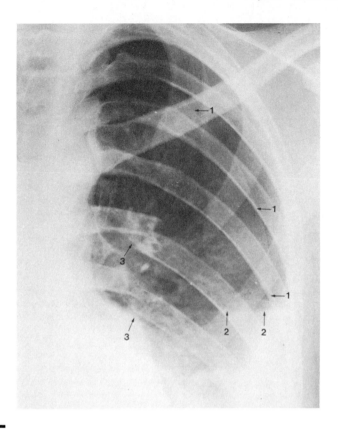

Figure 9-23   Chest x-ray of 42-year-old woman in MVC. *1,* Edge of partially collapsed left lung (pneumothorax). *2,* Fluid level in pleura, which in this case is due to blood (hemothorax). *3,* Fractures of left seventh and eighth ribs. (*Note.* From *Self-assessment in Radiology and Imaging: Cardio-Thoracic Imaging* (p. 16) by M.B. Rubens, 1989, St. Louis: Mosby–Year Book, Inc.)

mothorax, which is a collection of blood in the pleural space. As this enlarges, the lung begins to collapse, leading to altered gas exchange. In addition, the hemorrhage involved can amount to significant volumes, leading to hemodynamic instability. Hemothorax is often found in conjunction with pneumothorax. Rib fractures may result in damage to the intercostal arteries or veins (Figure 9-23). Therapy requires placement of a chest tube (36 or 40 French for an adult) and placement to suction. Autotransfusion may be desired. Chest drainage units with dry water seal and/or dry suction control allow for more rapid assembly. The tubing should be coiled at bed height and not allowed in a dependent position to facilitate maximal drainage and to prevent accidental dislodgement. Large mediastinal or pleural hemorrhage

(1500 to 2000 ml) and sustained rates of 150 to 200 ml/hr indicate a need for operative intervention.

Vessel injury   Fluid volume deficit
High risk for altered tissue
  perfusion
High risk for sensory/perceptual
  alterations
Decreased cardiac output
Pain

The great vessels include the inferior and superior venae cavae, brachiocephalic and subclavian vessels, carotid arteries, and pulmonary arteries. The aorta is a high-flow vessel with anatomic properties that explain injury at specific sites. See Figure 9-24 for illustration of types of vascular

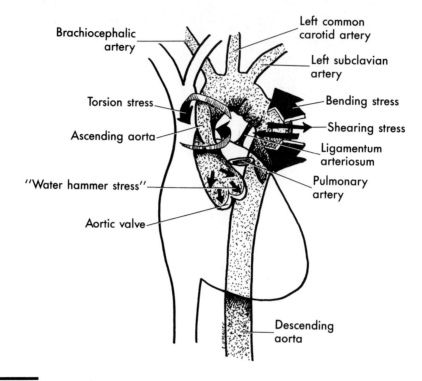

Figure 9-24 Diagram of cardiac and great vessel anatomy and sites of torsion, bending, shearing, and "water hammer" stress.

stress that were discussed in the blunt mechanism section of this chapter. The most common site for blunt aortic injury is at the level of the ligamentum arteriosum, just distal to the left subclavian artery branch (Figure 9-25). This area is also called the *aortic isthmus*, the point where the arch and descending aorta attach, and is at great risk from deceleration stress. The heart and ascending aorta are relatively mobile structures, whereas the isthmus area becomes fixed by the ligament and pleural reflections and the intercostal and left subclavian arteries. The descending portion is also relatively mobile. The fixed points are at risk of tears to the intima, media, and/or adventitial layer. When the adventitia remains intact, its tensile strength can allow survival from a contained hematoma and pseudoaneurysm. Tears in the ascending aorta result in massive intrapericardial tamponade, and most of these injuries result in immediate death. Ascending tears are more likely to occur with direct blunt trauma and are associated with skeletal injury of the clavicle or first rib (Sabiston, 1991).

Signs and symptoms of aortic injury include evidence of mediastinal hemorrhage. The resultant mediastinal widening on chest x-ray film is not definitive for aortic injury, since other mediastinal vessel hemorrhage, such as sternal and rib fractures, fractures of the lower cervical and thoracic spine, and small thoracic arteries and veins, may result in a similar sign. Other signs and symptoms include tracheal deviation and nasogastric tube displacement to the right from an expanding hematoma on the left, contributing to dyspnea and dysphagia respectively. Hoarseness may develop because the left recurrent laryngeal nerve is in proximity of the ligamentum arteriosum. Chest pain is often present, radiating posteriorly to the scapula area.

Ascending aorta injury can result in damage to the aortic valve with auscultatory changes and may affect right cerebral and right upper extremity flow. Further distal aortic injury affects the left common carotid and subclavian artery, which can account for differences in pulse strength and blood pressure in the left versus right arm. If aor-

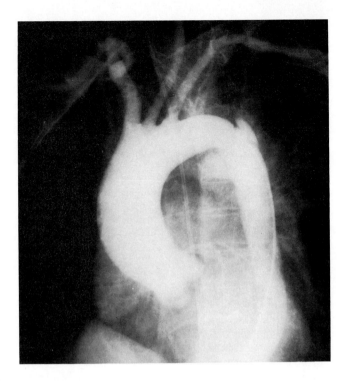

Figure 9-25   Arch aortogram with extravasation at level of ligamentum arteriosum. (*Note*. From *Thoracic Surgery: Surgical Management of Chest Injuries* [Vol. 7] [p. 207] by W.R. Webb and A. Besson, 1991, St. Louis: Mosby–Year Book, Inc.)

tic coarctation occurs as a result of narrowing of the lumen from a clot or vascular flap, proximal hypertension may develop with resulting upper extremity BP significantly exceeding lower extremity BP. Creation of a false lumen from dissection results in severe, tearing chest pain. Hematoma formation and dissection cause narrowing of the arterial lumen, which increases intravascular pressure, further stressing the vessel and thereby leading to a vicious cycle. Definitive diagnosis is by thoracic aortography followed by surgical intervention.

Cardiac perforation/rupture   Fluid volume deficit
Decreased cardiac output

Penetrating injury to the chest, back, neck, or upper abdomen should be considered to produce a possible cardiac perforation until proven otherwise. The right ventricle is most commonly affected by stab wounds because of its anterior posi-

tion in the thorax. Blunt cardiac rupture can also occur from direct compressive injury, or blast effect, but the incidence is rare. Pericardial tears are not common in blunt trauma in comparison with penetrating trauma (Turney & Rodriguez, 1990). Hemorrhage from injuries to the atrium can be controlled by finger pressure or traction on a Foley catheter balloon inserted through the defect and inflated. Direct suturing can be accomplished with use of a vascular clamp and pledgeted Teflon closure. The atrium is a low-pressure system allowing easier control. Ventricular injuries most often occur in the right ventricle; however, gunshot wounds are less preferential. Careful assessment for murmurs and conduction defects should be ongoing to detect rare valvular or septal defect. Surgical intervention is required.

Cardiogenic shock   Decreased cardiac output

Cardiogenic shock in trauma usually results from ischemic injury related to coronary artery contusion with thrombus, ischemia related to hypotension and atherosclerotic disease, or changes in contractility associated with cardiac contusion.

Cardiac contusion   Decreased cardiac output
Altered tissue perfusion
(general)
Activity intolerance

It is commonly difficult to diagnose myocardial contusion because no benchmark exists; multiple definitions and diagnostic tests are listed in the literature. Various studies have questioned the necessity of diagnosing this condition, since the implications are unclear (Healey, Brown, & Fleiszer, 1990; Miller & Shumate, 1989). Wisner, Reed, and Riddick (1990) conducted a significant review of 3010 patients with blunt trauma for evidence of sequelae attributable to myocardial contusion. Their focus was to determine clinically significant sequelae of blunt chest injury rather than attempt to define the phenomenon. All patients with suspected contusion received cardiac monitoring for 48 hours or until echocardiography was done with results indicating no suspected contusion. No patients were readmitted to the ICU because of cardiac events. It was rare for patients with rule-out myocardial contusion as a diagnosis to develop heart failure. Arrhythmias occurred in this group within 48 hours of admission in 20% of patients. Figure 9-26 is the algorithm developed for management of patients with blunt chest trauma. Conduction abnormalities on admission electrocardiogram did predict serious arrhythmias, whereas echocardiography and creatine phosphokinase isoenzyme levels did not predict morbidity. Supportive therapy for cardiac failure includes positive inotropes, vasodilators, and careful fluid management. Arrhythmias are treated following the advanced cardiac life support standards.

Distributive shock   Fluid volume deficit
(relative)
Spinal—ineffective
thermoregulation;
sensory/perceptual
alterations
Septic—cardiac output
(varied)
Hyperthermia
Anaphylactic—ineffective
airway clearance

Distributive shock results from a relative decrease in intravascular volume. In trauma this may occur in spinal shock, septic shock, or anaphylactic shock. Neurogenic shock is treated with

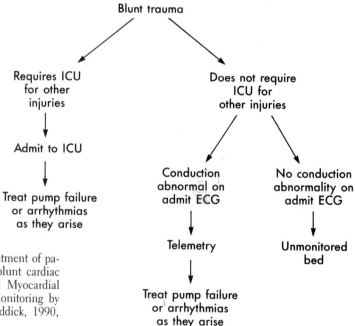

Figure 9-26 Algorithm for triage and treatment of patients with blunt trauma and suspected blunt cardiac injury. (*Note.* Redrawn from "Suspected Myocardial Contusion: Triage and Indications for Monitoring by D.H. Wisner, W.H. Reed, and R.S. Riddick, 1990, *Annals of Surgery, 212* (1), pp. 82-86).

volume, as well as vasoconstrictors. In this case, a pulmonary artery catheter is not necessary (Sabiston, 1991). Spinal shock is discussed in Chapter 11. In septic shock, hypovolemia and hypermetabolism occur and as the process progresses, inflammatory mediators disrupt microvascular endothelium, leading to permeability and decreased cardiac output. Patients in septic shock are optimally treated with the advantage of a pulmonary artery catheter and SvO_2 monitoring. Inadequate splanchnic perfusion and pulmonary compromise lead to multiple organ failure, which is discussed in Chapter 19. It should be remembered that another form of distributive shock, anaphylactic shock, can occur in trauma patients from the administration of dyes and agents used for contrast radiographic study.

Obstructive shock	Decreased cardiac output
	Altered tissue perfusion
	Tamponade—decreased cardiac output
	Tension pneumothorax— impaired gas exchange
	Embolus—impaired gas exchange; sensory/perceptual alterations

Obstructive shock occurs when the stroke volume is impacted by restrictive forces: pressure within the pericardial sac from tamponade, mediastinal pressure from a tension pneumothorax, or air embolism with trapping of air in the ventricle.

Cardiac tamponade

Cardiac tamponade may be associated with aortic injury or blunt and penetrating injury to the heart itself. Injury to the ascending aorta results in a hematoma that may extend into the pericardium and is a major cause of death in aortic dissection. An understanding of the signs of tamponade according to Beck's triad should improve recognition of cardiac compression (Sternbach, 1988). The rise in intrapericardial pressure produces distinct clinical signs. Acute collection of blood in the pericardial sac will show only a slight increase in cardiac silhouette. A fall in arterial pressure, a rise in venous pressure, and muffled heart tones may be appreciated. However, the symptoms of tamponade can be duplicated by extracardial hematoma (Martin, Mavroudis, Dyess, Gray, & Richardson, 1986). Elevated venous pressure may also be caused by tension pneumothorax, shivering, or an obstructed or kinked CVP line. Treatment and diagnosis are initially provided by pericardiocentesis (needle and syringe tap of pericardial sac to remove any unclotted blood). If fluid is drained, a substantial improvement in the patient's condition is expected. A pericardial window may also be done in the ED or the operating room and involves a subxyphoid surgical approach for better visualization. If tamponade is diagnosed, a cardiac injury is suspected and cardiac surgery warranted (Figure 9-27). The patient is maintained with fluid replacement until emergent operative intervention.

Special Considerations

Bullet embolism must be considered when gunshot wounds have been sustained. The bullet or its fragments can travel through the vascular system, lodging in areas of decreased vessel lumen size or flow. Distant perfusion is important to evaluate, and x-ray films to determine bullet location are useful, especially when an odd number of entrance/exit wounds exists. Impalement is a special category of penetrating injury and deserves mention in terms of immediate action. The general practice is to avoid removal of a penetrating object until definitive location is clearly demonstrated on CT scanning or by visual examination intraoperatively where a team is readily available for prompt intervention. Significant hemorrhage may occur on removal of the object once the object no longer is tamponading the laceration.

Complications
End organ failure

This chapter has reviewed the effects of inadequate perfusion on end organs, such as the kidneys, liver, and lungs. Critically ill patients who progress to multiple organ failure (MOF) and survive may have permanent damage requiring long-term treatment, such as supplemental oxygen, or hemodialysis. MOF is discussed further in Chapters 18 and 19.

Deep vein thrombosis and pulmonary embolism*

One complication specific to perfusion that trauma patients may suffer is the development of

---

*This section contributed by Margaret J. Neff, B.S.

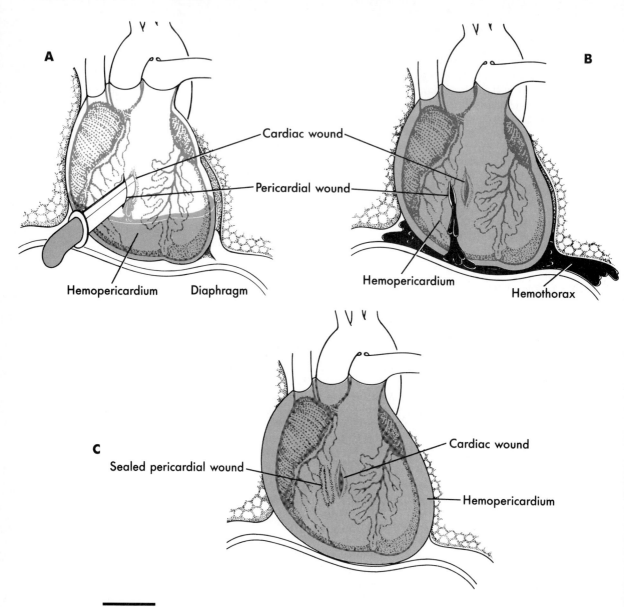

Figure 9-27 **A,** Cardiac injury with pericardial disruption. **B,** Bleeding from heart through pericardial tear into pleural space. **C,** Self sealing of pericardial wound resulting in pericardial tamponade.

venous thrombosis with the potential complication of pulmonary embolus. Other types of emboli, including fat and air, also present risk to the trauma patient, but the focus here will be on venous thrombus and embolus.

Studies vary regarding the estimated risk (20% to 90%) of venous thrombosis in the trauma patient (Shackford et al., 1990). General risk factors include obesity, immobility, venous trauma, estrogens, hypercoagulability, and a history of venous thrombosis. A study by Shackford et al. evaluated the risk of venous thrombus by categorizing trauma patients into low- and high-risk categories. Their high-risk factors included stasis, local venous injury, hypercoagulability, and age greater than 45 years. They showed no cases of venous thrombosis in the low-risk group and a 7% rate in the high-risk group.

Diagnosis of venous thrombosis has in the past relied on clinical signs and symptoms (calf swelling, tenderness, pedal edema, and warmth) with confirmation by venography. Venography, however, is invasive and has its own associated risks. Recently the emphasis has been more on Doppler studies and magnetic resonance imaging (MRI). Doppler scans and MRI are both very good at identifying pelvic and thigh deep vein thrombosis (DVT). However, Doppler scan is less proficient at detecting calf DVT, and there have not been enough studies to know the effectiveness of MRI in identifying calf DVT (Vukov, Berquist, & King, 1991).

Prophylaxis is clearly the goal, particularly in the high-risk patients. Mechanical methods include compression stockings and sequential gradient compression (SCD). Even if the injured leg is not amenable to mechanical prophylaxis, application of these methods to the uninjured leg may be beneficial through the increase in systemic fibrinolytic activation (Shackford et al., 1990). Pharmacologic intervention includes anti-platelet therapy (e.g., aspirin), anticoagulation (e.g., heparin and warfarin), and volume expansion with dextran (Caprini & Natonson, 1989).

The goal of prophylaxis is the prevention of not only DVTs but also their potential progression to pulmonary embolus. The diagnosis of pulmonary embolus is made primarily clinically. A patient presenting with risk factors for a DVT, having signs and symptoms of a DVT, and complaining of shortness of breath, pleuritic chest pain, and hemoptysis is highly suggestive of having a pulmonary embolus. Unfortunately, laboratory data and chest radiograph are not specific for pulmonary embolus. In fact, in most cases the chest x-ray film will look completely normal. Diagnostic strategies generally include an attempt to identify the presence of a DVT (to establish cause), as well as a ventilation/perfusion scan ($\dot{V}/\dot{Q}$ scan) to document an area of good ventilation and poor perfusion (consistent with pulmonary embolus). However, the $\dot{V}/\dot{Q}$ scan may often be read as "indeterminate." At this point the decision must be made to either treat empirically or proceed to the only truly diagnostic study for pulmonary embolus: a pulmonary angiogram.

Treatment includes the same entities seen in DVT prophylaxis—namely mechanical compression (except in a leg with evidence of DVT and venous congestion) and anticoagulation. The anticoagulation is started with heparin and then continued with warfarin for up to 6 months. Additional treatment modalities may be employed depending on the severity of the thrombosis and embolus and on the patient's ability to undergo prolonged anticoagulation. For instance, a massive pulmonary embolus, such as a saddle embolus, would likely lead to surgical intervention to remove the clot. Use of anticoagulants in trauma can be problematic when hemorrhagic sites are present. Trauma-induced bleeding must be controlled before the use of agents that will accentuate the potential for bleeding caused by changes in coagulation processes (Office of Medical Applications of Research, 1986). Anticoagulants have not generally been used in patients with acute head injury.

Another therapy is placement of a filter in the inferior vena cava (IVC). This essentially replaces the older method of IVC ligation, which is now only rarely used. Indications for placement of an IVC filter include the following: contraindications to anticoagulation therapy; failure of anticoagulation (recurrent pulmonary embolus or hemorrhage); a massive pulmonary embolus; a large, free-floating thrombus; and tumor patients with DVT. With the placement of an IVC filter, there is an approximate 5% risk of recurrent pulmonary embolus and also of IVC occlusion (Wittich, 1992).

In addition to the myriad of problems encountered by the trauma patient, the risk of DVT formation and subsequent pulmonary embolus must be kept in mind. Identifying patients at high risk and using appropriate prophylactic measures will help decrease the incidence of DVT. However, prophylaxis will not prevent all occurrences of DVT and is not possible in an estimated 14% of trauma patients (Shackford et al., 1990). Clinical signs and symptoms, as well as diagnostic tests, must be used to diagnose a suspected DVT or pulmonary embolus, and then the best possible therapy employed.

Table 9-10 reviews therapeutic and diagnostic modalities common to perfusion deficit and is useful in orientation of inexperienced trauma nurses. The table on pp. 250-253 lists the nursing diagnoses, interventions, and evaluative criteria pertinent to the trauma patient with altered perfusion.

Table 9-10 Therapeutic and diagnostic modalities related to perfusion

Interventions	Indications	Equipment
Nursing diagnoses: Impaired gas exchange; Ineffective breathing pattern		
Pleural decompression	Pneumothorax by chest x-ray examination or clinical findings	*Tube thoracostomy* Chest drainage unit, distilled water or NS (500 ml), wall suction, chest tube tray, chest tube (adult: 28 to 36 Fr), antiseptic solution, 2-inch pink tape, gauze
	Evidence of tension pneumothorax	*Needle thoracostomy* 14- to 16-gauge IV Angiocath, syringe prn
	Hemothorax	Above equipment for tube thoracostomy (adult: 36 to 40 Fr) plus autotransfusion device, CPD or ACD anticoagulant (30 ml to start; 8:1 ratio), micropore filter, blood tubing, pressure bag, back-up blood available
Nursing diagnoses: High risk for fluid volume deficit; Altered tissue perfusion; Decreased cardiac output		
Venous access	Prophylactic	*Peripheral* Site prep pads, tourniquet, catheters: (adult: 14- to 16-gauge [1 or 2]), transparent dressings, and blood tubes for concurrent laboratory specimens
	Monitoring/difficult access	*Central* Percutaneous sheath introducer set, percutaneous catheter introducer 8 Fr, manometer or transducer, transparent dressing, central venous or pulmonary artery catheter
	Difficult access	*Cutdown* Cutdown tray, Betadine prep, feeding tube or Angiocath *Intraosseous* Intraosseous needle, Betadine prep, stabilizing dressings
Rapid fluid infusion	Hypovolemia	Pressure bags, blood tubing, or Level I fluid infusor set-up or Rapid Infusion System (see hypothermia), uncrossmatched blood bucket

Table 9-10 Therapeutic and diagnostic modalities related to perfusion—cont'd

Interventions	Indications	Equipment
Nursing diagnoses: High risk for fluid volume deficit; Altered tissue perfusion; Decreased cardiac output—cont'd		
Arterial line	Unstable VS, ABG monitoring	Arterial line set-up, portable invasive BP monitor, or Tycos manometer (for MAP) and additional stopcock
Thoracotomy (open chest)	Traumatic arrest, suspected major thoracic vessel disruption, rapid deterioration after significant mechanism	Open cavity tray, suction, warm NS irrigation, Betadine, and special equipment as indicated: Internal defibrillation paddles (specific to monitor in use); Lebsche sternal chisel and mallet, double-armed suture with Teflon pledgets, extra vascular clamps, toothed tissue forceps, rib shears, Foley catheter (for balloon hemostasis technique)
Pericardiocentesis	Tamponade	Pericardiocentesis tray and ECG machine, or 18-gauge spinal needle and 30-ml syringe
Diagnostic peritoneal lavage (DPL)	Suspected intraabdominal hemorrhage	DPL tray, 1000 ml warm NS, adjuncts: Lidocaine with epinephrine, IV macrotubing without filter, or bladder irrigation tubing, suture, peritoneal dialysis catheter
Nursing diagnoses: Hypothermia; High risk for altered body temperature; Ineffective thermoregulation		
Heat delivery	All patients, especially those experiencing exposure, burns; pediatric and elderly patients	Warm fluids: *Already warmed* IV, DPL, open chest, wound care *Level I fluid infusor/warmer* Machine plus tubing with large-bore extension and spare filter *Rapid Infusion System* Machine, tubing, attendant; Heat lamps, warm blankets and heat retention drape, heated ventilator
Monitoring		Core temperature measurement device: tympanic and bladder or pulmonary artery for continued assessment

Nursing diagnosis	Nursing intervention	Evaluative criteria
Fluid volume deficit Related to hemorrhage, fluid shifts, capillary permeability, decreased vascular tone As evidenced by altered mental status, changes in skin signs, abnormal vital signs, external hemorrhage, internal hemorrhage as demonstrated by DPL, CT scan, or skeletal fractures, low SVR	**Assess oxygenation** Obtain arterial blood gas. Apply pulse oximeter or tissue oxygen indicator devices (e.g., Ptco$_2$, Pcjo$_2$). Apply high-flow oxygen. Assist ventilation as needed. **Control hemorrhage** Apply pressure: manual, dressings, tourniquet, MAST (for pelvic bleeding). Stabilize fractures. Assist with prompt transfer to angiography for embolization. Facilitate rapid transfer to OR for definitive repair—use portable monitor; keep O-negative blood bucket with patient. Prepare for emergent thoracotomy with aortic cross clamping. **Obtain IV access** Place large-bore, short peripheral catheters with trauma blood tubing; assist MD with cutdown and central line procedures. **Increase preload** Measure CVP; anticipate pulmonary artery catheter in ICU. Administer fluid: • Crystalloid, 1 to 2 liters. Evaluate effect: • transfuse with PRBCs for sustained hemodynamic instability unaltered by crystalloid and for Hct <20%; • use a rapid infusor; • consider vasoconstrictors for spinal shock only. Set up autotransfusor for patients with severe intrathoracic injury or evidence of hemothorax.	Mental status (GCS) will improve. Skin will be warm and dry. Pulses will be palpable. Pulse pressure will be ≥30. MAP will be 70 to 100 mm Hg. CVP will be 3 to 11 mm Hg. CO will be 4 to 8 L/min. CI will be 2.7 to 4.5 L/min/m^2. SVR will be 850 to 1400 dynes/sec/cm^5. Hct will increase and stabilize. Chest tube output will decrease. IVs will remain patent and allow rapid infusion. Team will be aware of total crystalloid and blood volumes infused. Volume will be documented with PRBC numbers. Neurovascular status distal to pressure will not deteriorate.
Decreased cardiac output Related to intravascular volume loss, reduced contractility, myocardial depressant factor, change in vascular tone, decreased preload As evidenced by abnormal vital signs, low cardiac index, and abnormal hemodynamic parameters	**Optimize fluid volume** Evaluate fluid volume status and contractility with Frank-Starling curve in relation to therapy. Detect signs of anaphylaxis, and treat with diphenhydramine, epinephrine, fluid as ordered. **Optimize cardiac output** Administer inotropic and vasoactive agents as ordered, monitoring their influence on CI, VO$_2$, and renal function. Improve stroke volume and reduce afterload: • assist with pericardiocentesis for suspected tamponade;	Changes in preload will optimize cardiac index. Urine output will be 0.5-1.0 ml/kg/hr. Pericardial tamponade and tension pneumothorax will be quickly diagnosed and treated. PAOP will be 6 to 12 mm Hg. SVR will be 850 to 1400 dynes/sec/cm^5. PAP will be 15-30/8-16 mm Hg. CI will be 2.7 to 4.5 ml/min/m^2. VO$_2$ will be 180 to 280 ml/min. Svo$_2$ will be 65% to 78%. Spo$_2$ will be >90%.

Nursing diagnosis	Nursing intervention	Evaluative criteria
	• detect hyperresonance, decrease in breath sounds, and tracheal shift consistent with tension pneumothorax, and assist with needle decompression and eventual tube thoracostomy; • avoid venous air embolism by use of Luer-Lok IV attachments; and tape lines securely; place patient on left side if venous air embolism suspected, and assist with withdrawal of blood from the right heart; • detect arm BP differences or upper extremity hypertension as indicator of aortic injury, which could obstruct aortic outflow.	
High risk for hypothermia and ineffective thermoregulation Related to radiant, convective, and evaporative heat loss from exposure, low ambient temperature, cold fluid administration, cool ventilated air, and anesthetic agent effects	**Monitor core temperature** Use tympanic, bladder, or pulmonary artery thermister. **Reduce heat loss** Keep patient covered to avoid convective loss as possible. Keep skin surfaces dry. Administer fluids at or near body temperature by rapid infusion warmer systems: Use warm fluids for wound cleaning and peritoneal lavage. **Supply heat sources** Use heated ventilator air. Use warm blankets and thermal covers. Increase room air temperature. Use overhead radiant heat lamps.	Core temperature optimally will be 37° C or at least >35° C. Patient will not shiver or complain of feeling cold.
High risk for injury: pulmonary embolism Related to immobility, positioning, venous stasis, long-term indwelling femoral IV lines contributing to development of deep vein thrombosis	**Reduce venous stasis** Teach and encourage flexion/extension exercises of lower legs. Avoid sustained positions with hip flexion. Use pneumatic compression devices. Encourage and assist with activity out of bed. Monitor IV sites for signs of phlebitis; discontinue at first evidence. Encourage shifting of central lines to peripheral sites as soon as patient condition indicates. Closely assess lower extremities for heat, redness, tenderness, or swelling. Monitor circumference of extremities after venous repair. Position extremities carefully intraoperatively.	Patient will actively exercise as allowed. Compression devices will be consistently used. Extremities will show no evidence of redness, swelling, or tenderness, other than that associated with injuries. No DVT or pulmonary embolism will develop.

CASE STUDY A 21-year-old helmeted male motorcycle rider struck a stationary vehicle and was found face down on an embankment. He was combative at the scene with a loss of consciousness; the paramedics obtained a HR in the 90s and palpated an SBP at 110. The patient was placed in C-spine precautions, oxygen was started, and a 14-gauge IV line was placed. The patient had received 400 ml of IV fluids on helicopter arrival.

On arrival of the flight team, the patient had labored respirations of 30/min, intermittent consciousness with a GCS of 4, BP was 101/68, and HR was 96. He was intubated before take-off after rapid sequence induction with in-line neck stabilization. Blood was suctioned from his endotracheal tube. His Spo_2 monitor could not capture a strong pulse signal, and fluids were infusing wide open. His exit from the helicopter was a "hot" off-load because of his condition.

What information from the flight team is helpful?
First, a summary of prehospital fluid delivery is needed. In this case, the total crystalloid from paramedics and flight crew equaled 1200 ml. Learning the location of family is helpful, and the flight crew informs you that the highway patrol and fire personnel at the scene are attempting to reach relatives by using information in the patient's wallet.

On arrival in the ED, his BP is 76/palpable; HR is 68; and respirations are assisted, with bilateral breath sounds. He is given 2500 to 3000 ml crystalloid and 4 units of O-negative PRBCs with an initial Hct of 14.9%, Hgb of 5.2 g/dl, and a clinical finding of a tense abdomen and altered conscious-

ness. A nasogastric tube and temperature Foley (hematuria noted) are placed, and chest, C-spine, pelvis, and left knee x-ray films are obtained. He is given IV antibiotics and a tetanus vaccination and taken to OR within 14 minutes.

Why is CT scan or DPL not done?
The patient's status is too critical for CT scan, and clinical examination reflects an abdominal source of the hypotension, so emergent laparotomy is planned. His chest x-ray film does not show any evidence of mediastinal hemorrhage.

What expected diagnostic examination is not done?
In the presence of altered level of consciousness, normally a head CT scan would be done. However, there is not time to do one, so the neurosurgeon plans to reassess after the emergent surgery.

Intraoperatively, the laparotomy reveals a large laceration to the spleen just inferior to the hilum, a 10-cm laceration of the left lobe of the liver, and a 4-cm laceration to the right lobe. The cell saver and a rapid infusion system are used to infuse 16 units PRBC, 10 units platelets, and 6 units FFP. A splenectomy is done to allow attention to focus on the liver injuries. The liver is tamponaded, argon coagulation used, and packed with 9 lap packs. The patient's estimated blood loss is 4800 ml. Concurrently, an orthopedic surgeon examines the left knee, which has no fracture but a laceration that comunicates with the joint. Irrigation and debridement are done, and a cast is applied after repair of a quadricep tendon laceration.

Immediately after surgery the patient has a

head CT scan, which reveals a 2-cm right parietal intraparenchymal hematoma and right parietal and left temporal and frontal contusions with no midline shift. His abdomen is also scanned to discern the degree of injury to his left kidney. A focal perirenal hematoma is found. On admission to the ICU, his temperature is 35.6° C, not hypothermic.

What laboratory results are particularly interesting in a hypovolemic patient with significant head injury?

The coagulation studies are especially important, since head injury can contribute to altered coagulation, and prolonged bleeding times could place the patient at risk of greater intracranial bleeding. On ED arrival, his PT is 16.9 sec and APTT is 66.2 sec (prolonged). The neurosurgeon requests aggressive treatment with fresh frozen plasma for any PT >13 sec.

Monitoring in the intensive care revolves around the patient's tenuous liver laceration with a high risk for continued bleeding and a desire to keep the patient "dry" because of his head injury. The neurosurgeon desires hyperventilation, a serum sodium of 145 to 150 mEq/L, and a BUN/creatinine ratio >20:1. Research has shown that an alternate approach is to maintain cerebral perfusion pressure with volume expansion and even catecholamine infusions to increase SBP, and use of mannitol and CSF drainage to maintain a reasonable ICP. The overall goal in multiple trauma is to reduce secondary injury to the brain while maintaining the perfusion to other organs.

What follow-up studies are expected?

A repeat head CT scan is indicated and is done the following morning, revealing a significant enlargement of the right intraparenchymal clot, so the patient is taken to OR for evacuation of the clot. At this time, a Camino intracranial pressure device is placed in the subdural space and a repeat exploratory laparotomy undertaken to evaluate the liver packing. A moderate amount of blood is present in the abdomen, but otherwise, hemostasis is reasonable.

The patient is receiving low-dose dopamine (2.8-4.9 mcg/kg/min) to optimize renal perfusion. He requires sedation and chemical paralysis for a P/F ratio of 115 related to pulmonary contusions. He is transfused to maintain a Hct of approximately 30% due to his head and pulmonary injuries. Despite FFP, his PT is 13.5 to 14.4/sec, but there is no increase in the intracerebral drain output. A pulmonary artery catheter is placed with a

mixed venous oxygen saturation device. By the third postoperative day his DO_2 is 1054; VO_2, 206; CO, 7.5 ml/min; SVR, 996 dynes/sec/cm^5; and CVP is 17 to 10 mm Hg after receiving furosemide. No PAOP is obtained because the catheter will not wedge, but it had correlated with his CVP earlier. His serum osmolality ranges from 277 to 313 mOsm; Spo_2, 98%; Svo_2, 78%; and CPP, 70 to 90. Overall, he is stable, but requires frequent reevaluation of fluid and ventilatory parameters.

By the seventh to eighth postoperative day, his pulmonary artery catheter and ICP monitor are discontinued and he is extubated by the ninth day. He is transferred to the floor on the twelfth day and to the rehabilitation unit on the fifteenth day, with left hemiplegia from the brain injury and cognitive deficits of immediate memory, abstractions, judgment, and calculations. He requires physical therapy for his left thigh and knee injury and to ensure safe mobilization in his less inhibited state.

What protection should the nurse ensure related to his abdominal injuries?

His activity is limited because of the severe liver laceration; he should receive the pneumococcal vaccination because of the splenectomy. His platelets by the rehabilitation admit date are 1.3 million, related to increased marrow output secondary to his asplenia. Careful attention to avoid development of DVT is essential because of the increased blood viscosity.

RESEARCH QUESTIONS

- What clinical findings are associated with inaccurate noninvasive blood pressure readings?
- What are the differences in patient outcomes in using immediately available uncrossmatched bank blood versus autotransfusion?
- Does administration of erythropoeitin postoperatively in the elderly trauma patient with Hct <25% improve mobility, endurance, and feeling of wellness?
- Do comparisons of hematocrit and osmolality assist in evaluating the effect of dilution versus blood loss in the presence of decreased hematocrit?
- What parameters are the earliest and most reliable indicators of acute blood loss?
- What are the temporal relationships between compensatory responses and shock?

▪ Does a decrease in the waveform output on pulse oximeters signal decreasing perfusion? How does it correlate with more invasive measures?

RESOURCES

American Association of Blood Banks (AABB)
8101 Glenbrook Rd.
Bethesda, MD 20814
(703) 528-8200

American National Red Cross (ANRC)
National Headquarters
Washington, DC 20006
(202) 639-3004

Council of Community Blood Centers (CCBC)
725 15th St. NW, Suite 700
Washington, DC 20005
(202) 393-5725

National Heart, Lung, and Blood Institute (NHLBI)
Division of Blood Diseases and Resources
Building 31, 9000 Rockville Pike
Bethesda, MD 20892
(301) 496-4868

International

International Federation of Blood Donor Organizations
30, rue du Boichot
F-39100 Dole, France
PH 84 723494

International Society of Blood Transfusion
Boite Postate 100
F-91943 Les Ulis Cedex, France
PH 69 072040

League of Red Cross and Crescent Societies
17, Chemin des Crets
Boite Postale 372
Petit-Saconnex
CH-1211 Geneva 19, Switzerland
PH 22 7345580

ANNOTATED BIBLIOGRAPHY

Bryan-Brown, C.W. (1988). Blood flow to organs: Parameters for function and survival in critical illness. *Critical Care Medicine, 16* (2), 170-178.
Article that reviews the concepts pertinent to organ flow in supply-dependent and supply-independent organs. It covers blood volume, blood pressure, and oxygen content and applies it to critical care. The content is well referenced and is well worth reading.

Capan, L.M., Miller, S.M., & Turndorf, H. (1991). *Trauma anesthesia and intensive care.* Philadelphia: J.B. Lippincott.
A comprehensive, clearly written, in-depth book that is heavily focused toward the rationale for assessment findings and recommended interventions. The sections on anesthetic implications are of interest from a nursing perspective as well. Multiple calculations and formulas are explained and demonstrated by application to clinical scenarios.

Maull, K.I., Cleveland, H.C., Strauch, G.O., & Wolferth,

C.C. (Eds.) (1990). *Advances in trauma* (Vol. 5). St. Louis: Mosby–Year Book, Inc.
A volume in a series on trauma care that reflects current issues in a concise format. Supportive graphics are of educational value, and content is easy to find.

Gosling, J.A., Harris, P.F., Humpherson, J.R., Whitmore, I., & Willan, P.L.T. (1985). *Atlas of human anatomy with integrated text.* Philadelphia: Gower Medical Publishing, J.B. Lippincott.
A text that is an exquisite source of anatomic description. The use of photographs of cadaver specimens that have been carefully dissected to focus on selected aspects of anatomy in conjunction with matched, labeled drawings is effective in conveying the complexities of anatomy. The interrelationships between structures are clear and can be applied to clinical and operative scenarios. This book is useful for the clinician who wants to understand procedures, operative techniques, or mechanism of injury and is also valuable in teaching health professionals the anatomic factors related to their practice, i.e., vascular access in relation to arteries, veins, and nerves or the inherent risks in placing a nasogastric tube in a patient with head and facial trauma.

REFERENCES

Abels, R.I., & Rudnick, S.A. (1991). Erythropoietin: Evolving clinical applications. *Experimental Hematology, 19,* 842-850.

American Association of Blood Banks. (1985). *Technical manual* (9th ed.). Arlington, VA: Author.

American Heart Association. (1987). *Recommendations for human blood pressure determination by sphygmomanometers.* Dallas: Author.

Andrews, J. (1989). Difficult diagnoses in blunt thoracoabdominal trauma. *Journal of Emergency Nursing, 15* (5), 399-404.

Armstrong, P. (1989). Chest. In T.E. Keats, (Ed.), *Emergency Radiology* (2nd ed.) (pp. 149-240). Chicago: Mosby–Year Book, Inc.

Baker, C.C., Thomas, A.N., & Trunkey, D.D. (1980). The role of emergency room thoracotomy in trauma. *Journal of Trauma, 20,* 848.

Baldwin, J.F., & Smit, S. (1988). Fluid replacement for shock. In J.E. Campbell (Ed.), *Basic trauma life support: Advanced prehospital care* (2nd ed.) (pp. 238-245). Englewood Cliffs, NJ: Prentice Hall-Brady.

Barker, S.J., & Tremper, K.K. (1987). The effect of carbon monoxide inhalation on pulse oximetry and transcutaneous PO_2. *Anesthesiology, 66,* 677-679.

Bates, B. (1987). *A guide to physical examination and history taking* (4th ed.). Philadelphia: J.B. Lippincott.

Berne, R.M., & Levy, M.N. (1986). *Cardiovascular physiology* (5th ed.). St. Louis: Mosby–Year Book, Inc.

Bickell, W.H., Shaftan, G.W., & Mattox K.L. (1989). Intravenous fluid administration and uncontrolled hemorrhage (letter). *Journal of Trauma, 29* (3), 409.

Bivins, H.G., Knopp, R., & Tiernan, C. (1982). Blood volume displacement with inflation of antishock trousers. *Annals of Emergency Medicine, 11,* 409-412.

Blumenthal, S. et al. (1977). Report of the task force on blood pressure control in children. *Pediatrics 59* (5)(Suppl.), 797-820.

Bonica, J.J. (1981). Maternal physiologic and psychologic alterations during pregnancy and labor. In E.V. Cosmi, (Ed.), *Obstetric anesthesia and perinatology*, New York: Appleton-Century-Crofts.

Borst, C., & Karemaker, J. (1983). Time delays in the human baroreceptor reflex. *Journal of the Autonomic Nervous System*, 9, 399-409.

Borst, C. van Brederode, F.M., Wieling, W., Von Montfrans, G.A., & Dunning, A.J. (1984). Mechanisms of initial blood pressure response to postural change. *Clinical Science*, 67, 321-327.

Borst, C., Wieling, W., van Brederode, J.F., Hond, A., deRyk, L.G., & Dunning, J. (1982). Mechanisms of initial heart rate response to postural change. *American Journal of Physiology*, 243 (12), H676-681.

Boshkov, L.K., Tredget, E.E., & Janowska-Wieczorek, A. (1991). Recombinant human erythropoietin for a Jehovah's Witness with anemia of thermal injury. *American Journal of Hematology*, 37, 53-54.

Bridges, N., Parvin, N.M., & vanAssendelft, O.W. (1987). Evaluation of a new system for hemoglobin measurement. *American Clinical Products Review*, 6 (2), 22-25.

Brown, B.R., Jr. (1988). *Anesthesia in hepatic and biliary tract disease*. Philadelphia: F.A. Davis.

Brunette, D.D., Fifield, G., & Ruiz, E. (1987). Use of pneumatic antishock trousers in the management of pediatric pelvic hemorrhage. *Pediatric Emergency Care*, 3 (2), 86-90.

Bryan-Brown, C.W. (1988). Blood flow to organs: Parameters for function and survival in critical illness. *Critical Care Medicine*, 16 (2), 170-178.

Butman, A.M., & Paturas, J.L. (Eds.). (1986). *Prehospital trauma life support*. Akron, OH: Educational Direction, Inc.

Cammack, K., Rapport, R.L., Paul, J., & Baird, C. (1959). Deceleration injuries of the thoracic aorta. *Archives of Surgery*, 79, (2), 244-251.

Cannon, W.B., Fraser, J., & Cowell, E.M. (1918). The preventive treatment of wound shock. *Journal of the American Medical Association*, 70 (9), 618-621.

Caprini, J.A., & Natonson, R.A. (1989). Postoperative deep vein thrombosis: Current clinical considerations. *Seminars in Thrombosis and Hemostasis*, 15 (3), 244-249.

Chyun, D. (1985). A comparison of intra-arterial and auscultatory blood pressure readings. *Heart & Lung*, 14, (3), 223-228.

Cogbill, T.H., Moore, E.E., Jurkovich, G.J., Morris, J.A., Mucha, P., Jr., Shackford, S.R., Stolee, R.T., Moore, F.A., Pilcher, S., LoCicero, R., Farnell, M.B., & Molin, M. (1989). Nonoperative management of blunt splenic trauma: A multicenter experience. *Journal of Trauma* 29, (10), 1312-1317.

Collins, J.A. (1976). Massive blood transfusion. *Clinics in Haematology*, 5, 201-222.

Comroe, J.H., Jr. (1965). *Physiology of respiration*. Chicago: Mosby–Year Book, Inc.

Cotter, C.P., Hawkins, M.L., Kent, R.B. III, & Carraway, R.P. (1989). Ultrarapid diagnostic peritoneal lavage. *Journal of Trauma*, 29 (6), 615-616.

Crawford, F.A., Jr. (1991). Penetrating cardiac injuries. In D.C. Sabiston, Jr. (Ed.), *Textbook of surgery: The biological basis of modern surgical practice* (14th ed.) (1851-1855). Philadelphia: W.B. Saunders.

Cross, J.S., Gruber, D.P., Burchard, K.W. Sig-ngh, A.K., Moran J.M., & Gann, D.S. (1989). Hypertonic saline fluid therapy following surgery: A prospective study. *Journal of Trauma*, 29 (6), 817-826.

Cutler, B.S., & Daggett, W. (1971). Application of the G-suit to the control of hemorrhage in massive trauma. *Annals of Surgery*, 173, 511-514.

Demling, R.H. (1989). Trauma and burns. *Bulletin of the American College of Surgeons*, 74 (1), 48-54.

DeMuth, W.E., Jr. (1966). Bullet velocity and design as determinants of wounding capability: An experimental study. *Journal of Trauma*, 2, 222-232.

DeMuth, W.E., Jr. (1968). High velocity bullet wounds of the thorax. *American Journal of Surgery*, 115, 616-625.

Dick, T. (1988). Turbobulb: Oversized inflator streamlines blood pressures. *Journal of Emergency Medical Services*, 13 (8), 37.

Donovan, P.J., Cline, D.M., Whitley, T.W., Foster, C., & Outlaw, M. (1989). Prehospital care by EMTs and EMT-Ps in a rural setting: Prolongation of scene times by ALS procedures. *Annals of Emergency Medicine*, 18 (5), 495-500.

Dorlas, J.C., Nijboer, J.A., Butijn, W.T., van der Hoeven, G.M.A., Settels, J.J., & Wesseling, K.H. (1985). Effects of peripheral vasoconstriction on the blood pressure in the finger, measured continuously by a new noninvasive method (the Finapres). *Anesthesiology*, 62, 342-345.

Dries, D., & Waxman, K. (1991). Adequate resuscitation of burn patients may not be measured by urine output and vital signs. *Critical Care Medicine*, 19 (3), 327-329.

Drucker, R.B. (1987). Fluid therapy. In J.H. Davis, W.R. Drucker, R.S. Foster, Jr., R.L. Gamelli, D.S. Gann, B.A. Pruitt, Jr., & G.F. Sheldon, *Clinical surgery* (Vol. 1) (pp. 847-859). St. Louis: Mosby–Year Book, Inc.

Duncan, A.O., Phillips, T.F., Scalea, T.M., Maltz, S.B., Atweh, N.A., & Sclafani, S.J.A. (1989). Management of transpelvic gunshot wounds. *Journal of Trauma*, 29 (10), 1335-1340.

Dunham, C.M., Belzberg, H., Lyles, R., Weireter, L., Skurdal, D., Sullivan, G., Esposito, T., & Namini, M. (1989). The rapid infusion system: A superior method for the resuscitation of hypovolemic trauma patients. (Handout). Baltimore: Maryland Institute for Emergency Medical Services Systems.

Dutky, P.A. Stevens, S.L., & Maull, K.I. (1989). Factors affecting rapid fluid resuscitation with large-bore introducer catheters. *Journal of Trauma*, 29 (6), 856-860.

Eichelberger, M.R., & Anderson, K.D. (1988). Sequelae of thoracic injury in children. In M.R. Eichelberger & G.L. Pratsch (Eds.), *Pediatric trauma care* (pp. 59-68). Rockville, MD: Aspen Publishers.

Elboim, C.M. (1985). Hemorrhagic shock and trauma. *Comprehensive Therapy*, 11 (2), 6-12.

Fagan, M.J., (1988). Relationship between nurses' assessments of perfusion and toe temperature in pediatric patients with cardiovascular disease. *Heart & Lung*, 17 (2), 157-165.

Feldman, R. (1986). IV line placement: A time study for prehospital providers. *Journal of Emergency Medical Services (JEMS)*, August, 43-45.

Fink, M.P. (1989). Clinical care in the ICU. In A. Marston, G.B. Bulkley, R.G. Fiddian-Green, & U.H. Haglund

(Eds.), *Splanchnic ischemia and multiple organ failure*. St. Louis: Mosby–Year Book, Inc. An Edward Arnold publication.

Finley, P.R. (Ed.). (1992). *Clinical laboratory handbook* (8th ed.). Tucson, AZ: Dept. of Pathology, Univ. of Arizona Health Science Center.

Fischbach, F.T. (1988). A *manual of laboratory diagnostic tests* (3rd ed.). Philadelphia: J.B. Lippincott.

Flaherty, L., & Jurkovich, G.J. (1991). Minor splenic injuries: Associated injuries and transfusion requirements. *Journal of Trauma, 31* (12), 1618-1621.

Flancbaum, L., Trooskin, S.Z., & Pedersen, H. (1989). Evaluation of blood-warming devices with the apparent thermal clearance. *Annals of Emergency Medicine, 18* (4), 355-359.

Frykberg, E.R., Crump, J.M., McLellan, G.L., Vines, F.S., Brunner, R.G., Dennis, I.W., & Alexander, R.H. (1989). A reassessment of the role of arteriography in penetrating proximity extremity trauma: A prospective study. *Journal of Trauma, 29* (8), 1041-1052.

Gaffney, F.N., Thal, E.R., Taylor, W.F., Bastian, B.C., Weigelt, J.A., Atkins, J.M., & Blomquist, C.G. (1981). Hemodynamic effects of medical anti-shock trousers. *Journal of Trauma, 21,* 931-937.

Ganong, W.F. (1983). *Review of medical physiology* (11th ed.). Los Altos, CA: Lange Medical Books.

Giard, D.A., & Ross, C.S. (1989). The use of pulse oximetry in prehospital treatment and transport. *Ohmeda educational pamphlet*. Louisville, CO: The BOC Group.

Goerke, J., & Mines, A.H. (1988). *Cardiovascular physiology*. New York: Raven Press.

Goldsmith, S. (1983). Comparative hemodynamic effects of anti-shock suit and volume expansion in normal human beings. *Annals of Emergency Medicine, 12* (6), 348-350.

Goodnight, S.H., Kenoyer, G., Rappaport, S.I., Patch, M.J., Lee, J.A., & Kurze, T. (1974). Defibrination after brain tissue destruction: a serious complication of head injury. *New England Journal of Medicine, 290,* (19), 1043-1047.

Gorback, M.S., Quill, T.J., & Lavine, M.L. (1991). The relative accuracies of two automated noninvasive arterial pressure measurement devices. *Journal of Clinical Monitoring, 7,* 13-22.

Gosling, J.A., Harris, P.F., Humpherson, J.R., Whitmore, I., & Willan, P.L.T. (1985). *Atlas of human anatomy with illustrated text*. London: Gower Medical Publishing.

Gregory, J., Flancbaum, L., Townsend, M., Cloutier, C., & Jonasson, O. (1991). Incidence and timing of hypothermia in trauma patients undergoing operations. *Journal of Trauma, 31* (6), 795-800.

Grisham, M.B., & Granger, D.N. (1989). Free radicals: Reactive metabolites of oxygen as mediators of postischemic reperfusion injury. In A. Marston, G.B. Bulkley, R.G. Fiddian-Green, & U.H. Haglund (Eds.), *Splanchnic ischemia and multiple organ failure* (135-144). St. Louis: Mosby–Year Book, Inc. An Edward Arnold publication.

Gross, D., Landau, E.H., Assalia, A., & Krausz, M.M. (1988). Is hypertonic saline resuscitation safe in "uncontrolled" hemorrhagic shock? *Journal of Trauma, 28* (6), 751-756.

Guyton, A.C. (1987). *Human physiology and mechanisms of disease* (4th ed.). Philadelphia: W.B. Saunders.

Haglund, U.H. (1989). Myocardial depressant factors. In A. Marston, G.B. Bulkley, R.G. Fiddian-Green, & U.H.

Haglund (Eds.), *Splanchnic ischemia and multiple organ failure* (229-236). St. Louis: Mosby–Year Book, Inc. An Edward Arnold Publication.

Halpern, J.S. (1987). Clinical notebook: Assessment of orthostatic hypotension. *Journal of Emergency Nursing, 13* (3), 170-171.

Halpern, J.S. (1989). Mechanisms and patterns of trauma. *Journal of Emergency Nursing, 15* (5), 380-388.

Halvorsen, L., Blaisdell, F.W., & Holcroft, J.W. (1990). Recent advances in prehospital fluid resuscitation: Hypertonic saline. In K.I. Maull, K.C. Cleveland, G.O. Strauch, & C.C. Wolferth (Eds.), *Advances in Trauma* (Vol. 5) (pp. 1-16). St. Louis: Mosby–Year Book, Inc.

Hardy, G.R. (1988). Svo$_2$ continuous monitoring techniques. *Dimensions in Critical Care Nursing, 7* (1), 8-17.

Harman, P.K., & Floten, H.S. (1991). Penetrating wounds. In W.R. Webb & A. Besson (Eds.), *Thoracic surgery: Surgical management of chest injuries* (Vol. 7) (pp. 269-278). St. Louis: Mosby–Year Book, Inc.

Harris, E. (1985). Massive transfusion. In R.C. Rutman & W.V. Miller, *Transfusion therapy: Principles and practice* (2nd ed.) (pp. 289-299). Rockville, MD: Aspen Publishers.

Hartling, R.P., McGahan, J.P., Blaisdell, F.W., & Lindfors, K.K. (1987). Stab wounds to the extremities: Indications for angiography. *Radiology, 162* (2), 465-467.

Healey, M.A., Brown, R., & Fleiszer, D. (1990). Blunt cardiac injury: Is this diagnosis necessary? *Journal of Trauma, 30* (2), 137-146.

Henneman, E.A., & Henneman, P.L. (1989). Intricacies of blood pressure measurement: Reexamining the rituals. *Heart & Lung, 18* (3), 263-273.

Henneman, P.L., Greenfield, R.H., & Bessen, H.A. (1989). The effect of acute blood loss and intravenous crystalloid administration on hematocrit. *Annals of Emergency Medicine, 18* (9), 918. (Abstract)

Holcroft, J.W., & Blaisdell, F.W. (1991). Shock: Causes and management of circulatory collapse. In D.C. Sabiston, Jr. (Ed.), *Textbook of surgery* (14th ed.). Philadelphia: W.B. Saunders.

Holland, P.V. (Ed.). (1989). *Standards for blood banks and transfusion services* (13th ed.). Arlington: American Association of Blood Banks.

Huestis, D.W., Bove, J.R., & Busch, S. (1981). *Practical blood transfusion* (3rd ed.). Boston: Little, Brown.

Jameson, L. (1990). Hypercalcemic death during use of high capacity fluid warmer for massive transfusion. *Anesthesiology, 73,* 1050-1052.

Jeffrey, R.B., Jr., & Federle, M.P. (1988). The collapsed inferior vena cava: CT evidence of hypovolemia. *American Journal of Roentgenology, 150,* 431-432.

Johnson, R.P., & Mellors, J.W. (1988). Arteriolization of venous blood gases: A clue to the diagnosis of cyanide poisoning. *The Journal of Emergency Medicine, 6,* 401-404.

Johnson, S.L. (1970). *The history of cardiac surgery: 1896-1955*. Baltimore: The Johns Hopkins University Press.

Jones, S.E., Nesper, T.P., & Alcouloumre, E. (1989). Prehospital intravenous line placement: A prospective study. *Annals of Emergency Medicine, 16,* 244-246.

Judd, W.J. (1991). Are there better ways than the crossmatch to demonstrate ABO incompatibility? *Transfusion, 31* (3), 192-194.

Judkins, D., & Iserson, K.V. (1991). Rapid admixture blood warming. *Journal of Emergency Nursing, 17* (3), 146-152.

Kandel, G., & Aberman, A. (1983). Mixed venous oxygen saturation. *Archives of Internal Medicine, 143,* 1400-1402.

Kelley, S.I. (1988). *Pediatric emergency nursing.* Norwalk, CT: Appleton & Lange.

Kirkendall, W.M., Feinleib, M., Freis, E.D., & Mark, A.L. (1980). Recommendations for human blood pressure determination by sphygmomanometers: Subcommittee of the AHA Postgraduate Education Committee. *Circulation, 62,* 1145A-1155A.

Kirklin, J.K., Blackstone, E., Kirklin, J.W., McKay, R., Pacifico, A., & Bargeron, L. (1981). Intracardiac surgery in infants under age 3 months: Predictors of postoperative in-hospital death. *American Journal of Cardiology, 48,* 507-512.

Knopp, R., Claypool, R., & Leonardi, D. (1980). Use of the tilt test in measuring acute blood loss. *Annals of Emergency Medicine, 9,* 72-75.

Koestner, J.A., Nelson, L.D., Morris, J.A., Jr., & Safcsak, K. (1990). Use of recombinant human erythropoietin (r-HuEPO) in a Jehovah's Witness refusing transfusion of blood products: Case report. *Journal of Trauma, 30* (11), 1406-1408.

Koziol-McLain, J., Lowenstein, S., & Fuller, B. (1991). Orthostatic vital signs in emergency department patients. *Annals of Emergency Medicine, 20* (6), 606-610.

Kram, H.B., & Shoemaker, W.C. (1985). Conjunctival oxygen tension in experimental and clinical conditions: Tissue oxygen metabolism in hyperoxia, hypoxia and hemorrhagic shock, *Acute Care, 11,* 89-99.

Kramer, G.C., Perron, P.R., Lindsey, D.C., Ho, H.S., Gunther, R.A., Boyle, W.A., & Holcroft, J.W. (1986). *Surgery, 100* (2), 239-246.

Lange, S. (1990). *Radiology of chest disease.* New York: Thieme Medical Publishers.

Lemos, M.J., & Clark, D.E. (1988). Scalp lacerations resulting in hemorrhagic shock: Case reports and recommended management. *Journal of Emergency Medicine, 6* (5), 377-379.

Lenny, L.L., Hurst, R., Goldstein, J., Benjamin, L.J., & Jones, R.L. (1991). Single-unit transfusions of RBC enzymatically converted from group B to group O to A and O normal volunteers. *Blood, 77* (6), 1383-1388.

Levine, E.A., Rosen, A.L., Sehgal, L.R., Gould, S.A., Egrie, J.C., Sehgal, H.L., & Moss, G.S. (1989). Treatment of acute postoperative anemia with recombinant human erythropoietin. *Journal of Trauma, 29* (8), 1134-1139.

Levitt, M.A., Lieberman, M., & Lopez, B. (1989). Evaluation of the tilt test in an emergency department population. *Annals of Emergency Medicine, 18* (4), 439 (abstract).

Little, R.A. (1989). 1988 Fitts lecture: Heart rate changes after haemorrhage and injury: A reappraisal. *Journal of Trauma, 29* (7), 903-906.

Malangoni, M.A. (1990). Splenic salvage: Current expectations and results. In K.I. Maull, H.C. Cleveland, G.O. Strauch, & C.C. Wolferth (Eds.), *Advances in trauma* (Vol. 5) (pp. 123-143). St. Louis: Mosby–Year Book, Inc.

Mangubat, E.A., & Eichelberger, M.R. (1988). Hypovolemic shock in the pediatric patient. In M.R. Eichelberger & G.L. Pratsch, *Pediatric trauma care* (pp. 69-77). Rockville, MD: Aspen Publishers.

Marino, P.L. (1991). *The ICU book.* Philadelphia: Lea & Febiger.

Martin, L.F., Mavroudis, C., Dyess, D.L., Gray, L.A., Jr., & Richardson, J.D. (1986). The first 70 years experience managing cardiac disruption due to penetrating and blunt injuries at the University of Louisville. *American Surgeon, 52,* 14-19.

Martinez, R. (1989). *Injuries: Patterns and Prevention.* Dallas: American College of Emergency Physicians.

Matthay, R.A., & Sostman, H.D. (1990). Chest imaging. In R.B. George, R.W. Light, M.A. Matthay, & R.A. Matthay (Eds.), *Chest medicine: Essentials of pulmonary and critical care medicine* (pp. 81-100). Baltimore: Williams & Wilkins.

Mattox, K.L., Bickell, W., Pepe, P.E., Burch, J., & Feliciano, D. (1989). Prospective MAST study in 911 patients. *Journal of Trauma, 29* (8), 1104-1112.

Mattox, K.L., Maningas, P.A., Moore, E.E., Mateer, J.R., Marx, J.A., Aprahamian, C., Burch, J.M., & Pepe, P.E. (1991). Prehospital hypertonic saline/dextran infusion for post-traumatic hypotension: The U.S.A. Multicenter Trial. *Annals of Surgery, 213* (5), 482-491.

Mauro, A.M.P. (1988). Effects of bell versus diaphragm on indirect blood pressure measurement. *Heart & Lung, 17* (5), 489-494.

McFarland, M.B., Grant, M.M., & Schumacher, J.L. (1988). *Nursing implications of laboratory tests* (2nd ed.). New York: John Wiley & Sons.

McSwain, N. (1984). To manage multiple injury. *Emergency Medicine, 16* (4), 57-92.

Meeker, M.H., & Rothrock, J.C. (1991). *Alexander's care of the patient in surgery* (9th ed.). St. Louis: Mosby–Year Book, Inc.

Melton, J.D., Heller, M.B., Kaplan, R., & Mohan-Klein, K. (1989). Occult hypoxemia during aeromedical transport: Detection by pulse oximetry. *Prehospital and Disaster Medicine, 4* (2), 115-121.

Memmer, M.K. (1988). Acute orthostatic hypotension. *Heart & Lung, 17* (2), 134-141.

Menitove, J.E. (1991). Transfusion practices in the 1990s. *Annual Review of Medicine, 42,* 297-309.

Miale, J.B. (1972). *Laboratory medicine: Hematology* (4th ed.). St. Louis: Mosby–Year Book, Inc.

Miller, F.B., & Shumate, C.R. (1989). Myocardial contusion: When can the diagnosis be eliminated? *Archives of Surgery, 124,* 805-808.

Mines, A.H. (1986). *Respiratory physiology* (2nd ed.). New York: Raven Press.

Mize, J., Koziol-McLain, J., & Lowenstein, S. (1991). Temperature: The forgotten measurement in trauma patients. *Journal of Emergency Nursing, 17* (6), 430.

Mollison, P.L. (1983). *Blood transfusion in clinical medicine* (7th ed.). Oxford: Blackwell Scientific Publications.

Moodie, D.S. (1980). Measurements of cardiac output by thermodilution in pediatric patients. *Pediatric Clinics of North America, 27,* 513-523.

Moore, E.E., Shackford, S.R., Pachter, H.L., McAninch, J.W., Browner, B.D., Champion, H.R., Flint, L.M., Gennarelli, T.A., Malangoni, M.A., Ramenofsky, M.L., & Trafton, P.G. (1989). Organ injury scaling: Spleen, liver, and kidney. *Journal of Trauma, 29* (12), 1665-1666.

Moore, K.I., & Newton, K. (1986). Orthostatic heart rates and blood pressures in healthy young women and men. *Heart & Lung, 15* (6), 611-617.

Moylan, J.A. (Ed.). (1988). *Trauma surgery*. Philadelphia: J.B. Lippincott.

Muhr, W.F., Jr., Teplick, S.K., & Wolferth, C.C., Jr. (1990). The role of interventional radiology in the complications of blunt abdominal trauma. In K.I. Maull, H.C. Cleveland, G.O. Strauch, & C.C. Wolferth (Eds.), *Advances in trauma* (Vol. 5) (pp. 197-213). St. Louis: Mosby–Year Book, Inc.

Neff, J., & Shaver, J. (1987). Hypothermia in emergency trauma center patients. *Journal of Emergency Nursing, 13*, (6), 382.

Norris, A.H., Shock, N., & Yiengst, M. (1953). Age changes in heart rate and blood pressure responses to tilting and standardized exercise. *Circulation, 8* (10), 521-526.

Office of Medical Applications of Research, National Institutes of Health. (1986). Consensus conference: Prevention of venous thrombosis and pulmonary embolism. *Journal of the American Medical Association, 256* (6), 744-749.

Palve, H., & Vuori, A. (1991). Minimum pulse pressure and peripheral temperature needed for pulse oximetry during cardiac surgery with cardiopulmonary bypass. *Journal of Cardiothoracic and Vascular Anesthesia, 5* (4), 327-330.

Parati, G., Mutti, E., Ravogli, A., Trazzi, S., Villani, A., & Mancia, G. (1990). Advantages and disadvantages of non-invasive ambulatory blood pressure monitoring. *Journal of Hypertension, 8* (Suppl. 6), S33-S38.

Parati, G., Pomidossi, G., Casadei, R., & Mancia G. (1985). Lack of alerting reaction to intermittent cuff inflations during non-invasive blood pressure monitoring. *Hypertension, 7*, 597-601.

Parrillo, J.E. (1991). Shock. In J.D. Wilson, E. Braunwald, K.J. Isselbacher, R.G. Petersdorf, J.B. Martin, A.S. Fauci, & R.K. Root, *Harrison's principles of internal medicine* (12th ed.) (pp. 232-242). New York: McGraw-Hill.

Perlroth, M.G. (Fall, 1989). *Cardiovascular physiology.* [Physiology 200 syllabus, 483-495]. Stanford, CA: Stanford University School of Medicine.

Pickhardt, B., Moore, E.E., Moore, F.A., McCroskey, B.L., & Moore, G.E. (1989). Operative splenic salvage in adults: A decade perspective. *Journal of Trauma, 29* (10), 1386-1391.

Popp, A.J., & Bourke, R.S. (1985). Pathophysiology of head injury. In R.H. Wilkins & S.S. Rengachary (Eds.), *Neurosurgery* (pp. 1536-1543). New York: McGraw-Hill.

Popp, J., Vouekw, E.A. (1984). Pathophysiology of head injury. (1536-1543), In R.H. Wilkins & S.S. Rengachary (Eds.), *Neurosurgery* (pp. 1536-1543). New York: McGraw-Hill.

Poppers, P.J., Epstein, R.M., & Donham, R.J. (1971). Automatic ultrasound monitoring of blood pressure during induced hypotension. *Anesthesiology, 35*, 431-435.

Pratt, R.S. (1980). Hypothermia: The chill that need not kill. *Bulletin of the American College of Surgeons, 65*(10), 28-35.

Presson, R.G., Jr., Haselby, K.A., Bezruczko, A.P., and Barnett, E. (1990). Evaluation of a new high efficiency blood warmer for children. *Anesthesiology, 73*, 173-176.

Presson, R.G., Jr., Hillier, S.C., & Haselby, K.A. (1991). Blood or fluid warmers? [Correspondence], *Anaesthesia, 46* (4), 319.

Quaal, S.J. (1988). Hemodynamic monitoring: A review of the literature. *Applied Nursing Research, 1* (2), 58-67.

Ramanathan, S., & Porges, R.M. (1991). Anesthetic care of the injured pregnant patient. In L.M. Capan, S.M. Miller, & H. Turndorf (Eds.), *Trauma anesthesia and intensive care* (pp. 599-627). Philadelphia: J.B. Lippincott.

Reed, R.L., Ciavarella, D., Heimbach, D.M., Baron, L., Pavlin, E., Counts, R.B., & Carrico, C.J. (1986). Prophylactic platelet administration during massive transfusion. *Annals of Surgery, 203* (1), 40-48.

Reines, H.D., Barlett, R.L., Chudy, N.E., Kiragu, K.R., & McKnew, M.A. (1988). Is advanced life support appropriate for victims of motor vehicle accidents: The South Carolina highway trauma project. *Journal of Trauma, 28* (5), 563-570.

Rhea, J.T., Novelline, R.A., Lawrason, I., Sacknoff, R., & Oser, A. (1989). The frequency and significance of thoracic injuries detected on abdominal CT scans of multiple trauma patients. *Journal of Trauma, 29* (4), 502-505.

Rhodes, M., Brader, A., Lucke, J., & Gillott, A. (1989). Direct transport to the operating room for resuscitation of trauma patients. *Journal of Trauma, 29*, (7), 907-915.

Richardson, J.D., Polk, H.C., Jr., and Flint, L.M. (Eds.) (1987). *Trauma: Clinical care and pathophysiology*, Chicago: Mosby–Year Book, Inc.

Rivkind, A.I., Siegel, J.H., & Dunhan, M. (1989). Patterns of organ injury in blunt hepatic trauma and their significance for management and outcome. *Journal of Trauma, 29* (10), 1398-1415.

Roberge, R.J., Ivatury, R.R., Stahl, W., & Rohman, M. (1986). Emergency department thoracotomy for penetrating injuries: Predictive value of patient classification. *American Journal of Emergency Medicine, 4*, 129-135.

Robertson, L.S. (1985). Motor vehicles. In J.J. Alpert & B. Guyer (Eds.). *The Pediatric Clinics of North America: Injuries and injury prevention, 32* (1), 87-94.

Ros, S.P., McMannis, S.I., Kowal-Vern, A., Zeller, W.P., & Hurley, R.M. (1991). Effect of intraosseous saline infusion on hematologic parameters. *Annals of Emergency Medicine, 20* (3), 243-245.

Ryden, R.E., & Oberman, H.A. (1975). Compatibility of common intravenous solutions with CPD blood. *Transfusion, 15*, 250-255.

Sabiston, D.C., Jr. (Ed.) (1991). *Textbook of surgery: The biological basis of modern surgical practice* (14th ed.). Philadelphia: W.B. Saunders.

Savage, R.A. (1987). Hematology quality control practices may be weak. *CAP Today, 1*, 21.

Scalea, T.M., & Sclafani, S.J.A. (1991). Angiographically placed balloons for arterial control: A description of a technique. *Journal of Trauma, 31* (12), 1671-1677.

Schneider, P.A., Mitchell, J.M., & Allison, E.J., Jr., (1989). The use of military antishock trousers in trauma: A reevaluation. *Journal of Emergency Medicine, 7*, 497-500.

Schriger, D.S., & Baraff, L.J. (1988). Defining normal capillary refill: Variation with age, sex, and temperature. *Annals of Emergency Medicine, 17*, 932-935.

Schriger, D.S., & Baraff, L.J. (1990). The distribution of orthostatic vital sign changes in a normal adult population and the variation of these changes with age. *Annals of Emergency Medicine, 19*, 471.

Schriger, D.S., & Baraff, L.J. (1991). Capillary refill: Is it a useful predictor of hypovolemic states? *Annals of Emergency Medicine, 20*, 601-605.

Schulte, D.M. (1986). A comparison of time intervals after posture change when measuring pulse and blood pressure in healthy elderly and nonelderly subjects. Unpublished Master's thesis. University of Colorado, Denver, CO.

Scientific Committee. (1990). Consensus document on non-invasive ambulatory blood pressure monitoring. *Journal of Hypertension*, 8 (Suppl. 6), S135-S140.

Sedlak, S.K., & Mace, D. (1989). Hidden problems with bleeding in trauma patients. *Journal of Emergency Nursing*, 15 (5), 422-428.

Shackford, S.R. (1989). Hypertonic saline for postoperative fluid therapy: Salient features [Editorial]. *Journal of Trauma*, 29 (6), 894-895.

Shackford, S.R., Davis, J.W., Hollingsworth-Fridlund J., Brewer, N.S., Hoyt, D.B., & Mackersie, R.C. (1990). Venous thromboembolism in patients with major trauma. *American Journal of Surgery*, 159 (4), 365-369.

Shapiro, B.A., Harrison, R.A., Cane, R.D., & Templin, R. (1989). *Clinical application of blood gases* (4th ed.). Chicago: Mosby–Year Book, Inc.

Sheldon, G.F., & Collins, M.L. (1987). Transfusion therapy. In J.H. Davis, W.R. Drucker, R.S. Foster, Jr., R.L. Gamelli, D.S. Gann, B.A. Pruitt, Jr., & G.F. Sheldon, *Clinical surgery* (Vol. 1). St. Louis: Mosby–Year Book, Inc.

Sherman, J.C., Delaurier, G.A., Hawkins, M.L., Brown, L.G., Treat, R.C., & Mansberger, A.R., Jr. (1989). Percutaneous peritoneal lavage in blunt trauma patients: A safe and accurate diagnostic method. *Journal of Trauma*, 29 (6), 801-805.

Shippy, C.R., & Appel, P.R. (1984). The influence of colloid and crystalloid infusion on blood volume in critically ill adults. *Critical Care Medicine*, 12, 107-112.

Shoemaker, W.C. (1982). Pathophysiology and therapy of hemorrhage and trauma states. In R.A. Cowley & B.F. Trump (Eds.), *Pathophysiology of shock, anoxia, and ischemia* (pp. 439-446). Baltimore: Williams & Wilkins.

Shoemaker, W.C., Appel, P.L., Kram, H.B., Waxman, K., & Lee, T. (1988). Prospective trial of supranormal values of survivors as therapeutic goals in high-risk surgical patients. *Chest*, 94, 1176-1186.

Siegal, J.H., Linberg, S.E., & Wiles, C.E. (1987). Therapy of low-flow states. In J.H. Siegal (Ed.), *Trauma: Emergency surgery and critical care* (pp. 201-283). New York: Churchill Livingstone.

Simpson, E. (1989). Hct/Hb ratio [Letter to the editor]. *CAP Today*, 4, 26.

Smith, J.J., & Kampine, J.P. (1980). *Circulatory physiology: The essentials.* Baltimore: Williams & Williams.

Smith, J.P., Bodai, B.I., Hill, A.S., & Frey, C.F. (1985). Prehospital stabilization of critically injured patients: A failed concept. *Journal of Trauma*, 25 (1), 65-70.

Snyder, H.S., & Dresnick, S.J. (1989). Lack of a tachycardic response to hypotension in penetrating abdominal injuries. *Journal of Emergency Medicine*, 7 (4), 335-339.

Stamler, K.D. (1989). Effect of crystalloid infusion on hematocrit in nonbleeding patients, with applications to clinical traumatology. *Annals of Emergency Medicine*, 18 (7), 747-749.

Stein, P.D., Sabbah, H.N., Hawkins, E.T., White, H.J., Viano, D.C., & Vostal, J.J. (1983). Hepatic and splenic injury in dogs caused by direct impact to the heart. *Journal of Trauma*, 23 (5), 395-403.

Sternbach, G. (1988). Claude Beck: Cardiac compression triads. *Journal of Emergency Medicine*, 6, 417-419.

Stivelman, R.C., Glaabitiz, J.P., & Crampton, R.S. (1963). Laceration of the spleen due to nonpenetrating trauma: One hundred cases. *American Journal of Surgery*, 106, 888-891.

Sutcliffe, A. (1987). Emergency anaesthesia. In T.H. Taylor & E. Major (Eds.), *Hazards and complications of anaesthesia.* (pp. 437-445). Edinburgh: Churchill Livingstone.

Szaflarski, N.L., & Cohen, N.H. (1989). Use of pulse oximetry in critically ill adults. *Heart & Lung*, 18 (5), 444-453.

Tait, A.R., & Larson, L.O. (1991). Resuscitation fluids for the treatment of hemorrhagic shock in dogs: Effects on myocardial blood flow and oxygen transport. *Critical Care Medicine*, 19 (12), 1561-1565.

Tremper, K.K., Barker, S.J., Hufstedler, S.M., & Weiss, M. (1989). Transcutaneous and liver surface PO_2 during hemorrhagic hypotension and treatment with phenylephrine. *Critical Care Medicine*, 17 (6), 537-540.

Turney, S.Z., & Rodriguez, A. (1990). Injuries to the great thoracic vessels. In S.Z. Turney, A. Rodriguez, & R.A. Cowley, *Management of cardiothoracic trauma* (pp. 229-260). Baltimore: Williams & Wilkins.

Underhill, S.L. (1986). Assessment of cardiac function. In Patrick, M.L., Woods, S.L., Craven, R.F., Rokosky, J.S., & Bruno, P.M., *Medical surgical nursing* (pp. 470-487). Philadelphia: J.B. Lippincott.

Vary, T.C., & Linberg, S.E. (1988). Pathophysiology of traumatic shock. In V.D. Cardona, P.D. Hurn, P.J.B. Mason, A.M. Scanlon-Schilpp, & S.W. Veise-Berry, *Trauma nursing: From resuscitation through rehabilitation* (pp. 127-159). Philadelphia: W.B. Saunders.

Velanovich, V. (1989). Crystalloid versus colloid fluid resuscitation: A metaanalysis of mortality. *Surgery*, 105 (1), 65-71.

Velasco, I.T., Pontieri, V., Rocha, M., Silva, E., Jr., & Lopes, O.U. (1980). Hyperosmotic NaCl and severe hemorrhagic shock. *American Journal of Physiology*, 239 (5), H664-H673.

Venus, B., Mathru, M., Smith, R.A., & Pham, C.G. (1985). Direct versus indirect blood pressure measurements in critically ill patients. *Heart & Lung*, 14 (3), 228-231.

Vukov, L.F., Berquist, T.H., & King, B.F. (1991). Magnetic resonance imaging for calf deep venous thrombophlebitis. *Annals of Emergency Medicine*, 20 (5), 497-499.

Walker, R.H. (Ed.). (1990). *Technical manual* (10th ed.). Arlington: American Association of Blood Banks.

Weil, M.H., Grundler, W., Yamaguchi, M., Michaels, S., & Rackow, E.C. (1985). Arterial blood gases fail to reflect acid-base status during cardiopulmonary resuscitation: A preliminary report. *Critical Care Medicine*, 13 (11), 884-885.

West, J.B. (1979). *Respiratory physiology: The essentials* (2nd ed.). Baltimore: Williams & Williams.

White, S., Hamilton, W., & Veronesi, J. (1991). A comparison of field techniques used to pressure-infuse intravenous fluids. *Prehospital and Disaster Medicine*, 6 (2), 129-134.

Wieling, W., & Dambrent, J. (1984). Cardiovascular effects of rising suddenly [Letter to the editor]. *New England Journal of Medicine*, 310 (18), 1189.

Winter, J.P., Plummer, D., Bottini, A., Rockswold, G.R., & Ray, D. (1989). Early fresh frozen plasma prophylaxis of abnormal coagulation parameters in the severely head-injured patient is not effective. *Annals of Emergency medicine, 18* (5), 553-555.

Wisner, D.H., Reed, W.H., & Riddick, R.S. (1990). Suspected myocardial contusion: Triage and indications for monitoring. *Annals of Surgery, 212* (1), 82-86.

Wittich, (1992). *Interventional radiology* Lecture in a series on diagnostic radiology. Stanford, CA: Stanford University School of Medicine.

Zorko, M.F., & Polsky, S.S. (1986). Rapid warming and infusion of packed red blood cells. *Annals of Emergency Medicine, 15,* 907-910.

Sensory/Perceptual

Responsiveness and vision

■■

Michelle Lucatorto

Joe E. Taylor

OBJECTIVES

❑ Describe the pathophysiologic mechanisms of primary and secondary head injury.

❑ Relate the pathophysiologic processes of head injury with assessment data.

❑ Analyze assessment data in the patient with altered responsiveness for the formulation of nursing diagnoses appropriate to the individual patient.

❑ Outline interventions appropriate to nursing care of the patient with altered responsiveness.

❑ Integrate assessment data for the patient with an eye injury into an appropriate plan of care.

INTRODUCTION This chapter discusses those traumatic injuries that affect responsiveness and vision. The chapter is presented in two sections: one deals specifically with head injury, and the other deals specifically with injury to the eye. Realistically, many patients who have sustained a head injury may have sustained an eye injury also. Injury to the eye may result in alteration or loss of vision. Injury to the brain may impair responsiveness as the result of disruption in sensory and cognitive processing. Therefore it is logical to include both in a chapter discussing alterations in sensory perception.

Vision is usually not fully appreciated until it is threatened by disease or trauma. The clinical topic of eye injury is included with head injury because 67% of patients sustaining blunt maxillofacial trauma will also sustain ocular or orbital injury (Holt & Holt, 1988). In addition, head injury may result in impaired vision as a result of optic, oculomotor, trigeminal, or abducens nerve injury. Individuals with impaired vision are also

at risk to sustain head injury caused by falls, motor vehicle accidents, and occupational and recreational accidents.

This chapter reviews mechanisms of injury, pathophysiology, nursing diagnoses, interventions, and evaluation of treatment.

CASE STUDY Jim is a 23-year-old who was helping his father load and transport sacks of lime in the back of a pickup truck. The truck hit a tree stump in the field while traveling at 30 mph. Jim was thrown 20 feet away from the truck.

The medics inform the ED staff that Jim was found under broken sacks of lime. Initially he would open his eyes to voice, localize to painful stimuli bilaterally, and answer questions inappropriately. His pupils were 3 mm, round, and reactive to light. BP was 120/90; pulse, 90; respirations, 16. After a few moments he regained complete consciousness and orientation. Jim was taken to the ED, where initial assessment findings include a Glasgow coma scale (GCS) score of 15; pupils 3 mm, round, equal, and reactive to light; BP, 116/70; pulse, 98; and respirations, 18. He is complaining of burning eyes and a headache.

Eye irrigations with normal saline and neurologic checks every 15 minutes are prescribed by the physician. A computerized tomography (CT) scan is scheduled after eye irrigations are completed.

During the eye irrigations, the nurse observes that the patient is less responsive. The nurse assesses Jim's neurologic status and finds he is confused about the day and place and his right pupil is 1 mm larger than his left, with both having a brisk response to light. The nurse reports these findings to the neurosurgeon, and a CT scan is performed, which shows a right temporal epidural hematoma causing compression and a midline shift. Jim is taken to the operating room for evacuation of an epidural hematoma.

What was Jim's initial GCS score, based on the medic's description of the neurologic assessment?

Jim's initial GCS score was 11. He scored 3 points on the eye-opening scale for opening his eyes to speech; 3 points on the verbal response scale for answering questions inappropriately; and 5 points on the motor response for localizing pain.

In addition to deterioration in Jim's GCS score, what other assessment parameters would indicate increasing intracranial pressure (ICP) in a neurologically injured patient?

Pupillary size, shape, and reactivity changes provide important assessment parameters for increasing ICP. Muscle strength should be assessed because the presence of an arm drift or weakness of an extremity or hemiparesis is an important sign. Rate and character of respirations also provide clinical evidence for increasing intracranial pressure. Vital signs reflect later stages of increased ICP: increased BP with a widened pulse pressure and bradycardia.

What intervention should the nurse be prepared for, in the event of increasing ICP?

Clinical evidence of deterioration in neurologic status was demonstrated by a right pupillary change, which indicates oculomotor (third cranial nerve) compression with impending herniation. This warrants immediate diagnostic testing to determine the cause. This is shown in the case study because time is taken for a CT scan. Concurrent treatment (administered as the nurse prepares for test transport or at the testing site) may include administration of osmotic diuretics, furosemide, steroids, and anticonvulsants. Maintenance of adequate airway and blood pressure is critical and may require invasive monitoring. The nurse should therefore prepare for line insertion, pulmonary artery and ICP monitoring, continuous pulse oximetry, and medication administration. Emergency airway equipment, a portable monitor, anticonvulsants, and mannitol should be taken to diagnostic testing areas.

What are the pathophysiologic differences between acid and alkali burns to the eye?

Acidic substances are neutralized by by-products of damaged cells, and the injury is usually superficial. Alkaline substances penetrate deeply into the eye and usually cause necrosis and scarring regardless of treatment. Lime is an alkaline agent.

RESPONSIVENESS

Responsiveness refers to one's ability to interact with one's environment and reflects functions controlled by the brain. To understand the impact of head injury on responsiveness and behavior, a review of brain functions is essential. Although a complete discussion of brain anatomy and physiology is beyond the scope of this chapter, a basic review of concepts is presented. Pathophysiologic aspects of intracranial pressure and cerebral blood flow dynamics are also presented as an introduction to head injury.

Anatomic and Physiologic Considerations

The brain contains centers for cognitive processing located in the cerebral hemispheres. Centers for processing specific information are divided by function into the lobes of the brain (Figure 10-1). It must be remembered that the brain is a complex organ with multiple interconnections; therefore no area of the brain functions alone. The frontal lobe contains centers for voluntary movement, higher thought process, and speech production and influences cranial nerve function. The parietal lobe interprets and analyzes sensory information, provides for spacial orientation, and contributes to awareness of body parts. The temporal lobe interprets and analyzes the auditory information, including speech. The occipital lobe interprets and analyzes visual information. Memory pathways are located in the frontal and temporal areas. Deep within the cerebral hemispheres, the basal ganglia exert an involuntary influence over the production, rate, and muscle

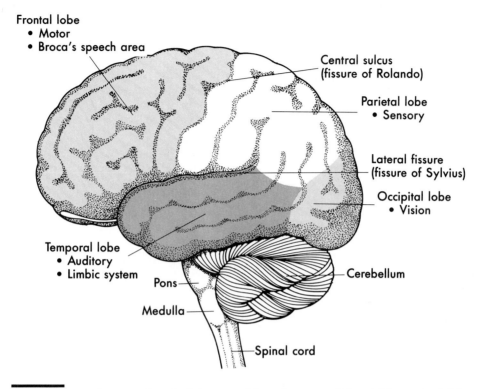

Figure 10-1   Localization of cerebral function. Major functions of frontal lobe, parietal lobe, temporal lobe, and occipital lobe are indicated.

tone aspects of movement. The diencephalon contains the hypothalamus, which monitors the physiologic environment to influence water balance, hormone regulation, and physiologic responses to emotional states. The thalamus is also located in the diencephalon. The thalamus is a relay center for sensory impulses and a component of the reticular activating system. The brainstem (midbrain, pons, and medulla) contains nuclei for the cranial nerves with the exception of the olfactory and optic nerves (Table 10-1). The midbrain serves as a center for auditory and visual reflexes and contains the nuclei of cranial nerves III and IV. The pons (bridge) functions to connect the brainstem to the cerebellum and impacts respiratory rate when nuclei within it are stimulated. The pons also contains nuclei of cranial nerves V through VIII. The medulla contains neurons essential to vital functions, such as respiratory and heart rates, vomiting, coughing, swallowing, and vasoconstriction and contains nuclei of cranial nerves IX through XII.

Transmission pathways for sensory and motor impulses also travel through the brainstem. Part of the reticular activating system is located in the brainstem and with the thalamus is responsible for maintaining attention and wakefulness (Edelsohn, 1986) (Figure 10-2).

The cerebellum controls coordination of skeletal muscle movement, controls fine movement, and contributes to balance, mediating responses that are outside the conscious level. The cerebellum is connected to the brainstem by three groups of white matter, called the *cerebellar peduncles*, and is separated from the cerebral hemispheres by a strong membrane called the *tentorium cerebelli*.

Injury to the brain may produce focal neurologic damage resulting in a deficit, which may be explained by the corresponding anatomic structure. For example, damage to the frontal cortex or motor pathways produces hemiparesis or hemiplegia. Injury to the brain may also produce global or nonfocal damage as the result of wide-

Table 10-1 Motor and sensory function of the cranial nerves

Nerve	Function
I Olfactory	Sense of smell
II Optic	Central and peripheral vision
III Oculomotor	Motor to medial, superior, and inferior rectus muscles and the inferior oblique muscle (up, down, and inward eye movements), and levator palpebrae súperioris muscles (elevates eyelid) Pupil constriction in response to light and accommodation
IV Trochlear	Motor to superior oblique muscles of eye (downward and inward eye movements)
V Trigeminal	Sensation to face Motor to muscles of mastication Afferent arc of corneal reflex
VI Abducens	Motor to lateral rectus muscles of eye (lateral eye movements)
VII Facial	Motor to muscles of face and eyelid closure Taste to anterior two thirds of tongue Autonomic to lacrimal and salivary glands
VIII Acoustic	Sense of hearing Sense of equilibrium
IX Glossopharyngeal	Sensory and motor to pharyngeal muscles (elevates pharynx during swallowing and speech) Autonomic to parotid and salivary glands Taste to posterior one third of tongue
X Vagus	Sensory and motor to pharynx and larynx Autonomic innervation to heart, lungs, great vessels, and GI tract
XI Spinal Accessory	Motor to sternocleidomastoid and trapezius muscles
XII Hypoglossal	Motor to tongue

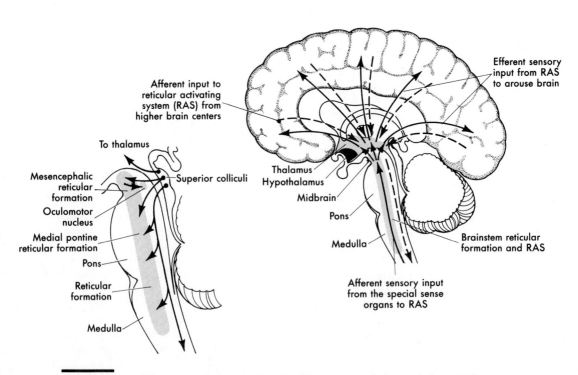

Figure 10-2 Reticular activating system (RAS) of brainstem and diencephalon. RAS activates higher brain centers and plays key role in maintaining attention.

spread insult. For example, hypoxia or hypotension may result in global injury.

Intracranial pressure and cerebral blood flow dynamics

Intracranial pressure represents the sum of the pressures exerted by the three intracranial components: brain volume, blood volume, and cerebral spinal fluid (CSF) volume. According to the Monro-Kellie theory, the intracranial contents fill the rigid cranial vault and are therefore incompressible. An increase in the volume, or added volume (i.e., epidural or subdural hematoma), to one of these components results in an increase in ICP unless a reduction occurs in the volume of one or more of the other components. The reduction in the volume of one or more of the intracranial components in response to an increase in another compartment is referred to as *compensation*. Compensatory mechanisms include the shunting of intracranial CSF to the spinal subarachnoid space, an increased outflow of venous sinus blood from the brain, and an increased CSF reabsorption rate in response to pressure elevation (Muwaswes, 1985). As compensatory mechanisms reach their maximal limits, pressure

rises rapidly with additional volume increases. The process of compensation in response to increasing intracranial content is presented by the volume pressure curve (Figure 10-3). The pressure plateau phase in response to increasing volume represents compensation. The sharp rise in intracranial pressure with further additions of volume occurs as compensatory mechanisms are exhausted (Maset et al., 1987).

The brain receives 15% to 20% of the cardiac output to perform its complex activities. The brain requires more energy per kilogram of weight of cells than any other organ in the body (Plum & Posner, 1985). Cerebral blood flow (CBF) depends on cerebral perfusion pressure (CPP) and cerebral vessel diameter, which depends on autoregulation. Autoregulation refers to the ability of the brain to regulate cerebral vessel diameter and therefore cerebral blood flow in response to tissue demands over a range of mean arterial pressures from 60 to 150 mm Hg (Aaslid, Lindegaard, Sorteberg, & Nornes, 1989). The CPP value is calculated as mean systemic arterial pressure (MAP) in millimeters of mercury (mm Hg) minus ICP in mm Hg. The CPP in a patient with a mean arterial pressure of 90 mm Hg and an ICP

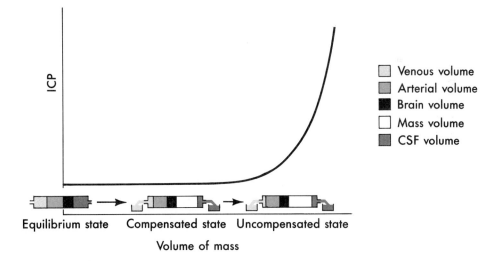

Figure 10-3 Intracranial pressure response to increasing intracranial volume. Initially, small additions of volume can be compensated and relatively normal pressures maintained. As compensation mechanisms become exhausted, additional volume will result in large pressure increases. (*Note*. Redrawn from Intracranial Pressure Monitoring [955-959] by J.D. Ward and D.P. Beeker. In W.C. Shoemaker, W.L. Thompson, and P.R. Holbrook [Eds.],1984, *Textbook of Critical Care*, Philadelphia: W.B. Saunders.)

of 10 mm Hg is 80 mm Hg. The formula for calculation of CPP reflects the contribution of both arterial pressures and intracranial pressures in cerebral perfusion.

Increased ICP produces secondary damage through reduction of CPP and therefore CBF. Normal CPP is between 80 and 100 mm Hg (Andrus, 1991). In head injury with altered autoregulation, CBF declines with CPP and results in ischemia (Bruce et al., 1973). Cerebral perfusion pressures less than 40 mm Hg are associated with electroencephalogram changes and a CBF of 65% of normal (Mitchell, 1986). Serial readings of ICP and CPP are more informative than a single reading. Changaris et al. (1987) reported a high likelihood of death in those patients with drops in CPP below 50 mm Hg in more than 33% of the measurements. Rosner and Becker (1984) reported generation of pathologic intracranial pressure waves associated with the reduction in CPP as a result of decline in aterial pressure. A critical reduction in CBF occurs when ICP is within 40 mm Hg of the MAP, which results in a CPP of 40 mm Hg, although the exact degree of increased ICP producing irreversible changes is controversial (Plum & Posner, 1985). Pathologic intracranial pressure waves have been recorded with CPP in the range of 60 to 70 mm Hg (Rosner, 1987).

Increased ICP is thought to have a deleterious effect on cerebral blood vessel autoregulation by causing an uncoupling of the brain's metabolic needs and CBF. This disruption of autoregulation may further contribute to increased ICP through an increase in cerebral blood volume. The role of autoregulation in the maintenance of cerebral homeostasis is discussed next.

The ratio between cerebral metabolic rate of oxygen ($CMRO_2$) and CBF can be measured as the difference between the oxygen content of arterial and jugular venous blood, expressed as $AVDO_2$.

$$AVDO_2 = \frac{CMRO_2}{CBF}$$

Recent investigations using CBF and $AVDO_2$ monitoring provide evidence for a hyperemic state in response to head injury. Normal or elevated CBF with a reduced $CMRO_2$ (low $AVDO_2$) has been correlated with increased ICP. This uncoupling of metabolic supply and demand may repre-

sent failure of cerebral autoregulation (Obrist, Langfitt, Jaggi, Cruz, & Gennarelli, 1984). Animal experiments demonstrate sustained vessel dilation with percussion impact to the head (Proctor, Palladino, & Fillipo, 1988). This hyperemic state is also referred to as *luxury perfusion*, because cerebral blood flow is greater than tissue needs. Luxury perfusion causes a relative increase in cerebral blood volume and may be a mechanism that contributes to an increased ICP (Marmarou et al., 1987). Although luxury perfusion is associated with increased ICP, the relative degree of hyperemia as yet has not been proven to be predictive of ICP (Muizelaar et al., 1989; Obrist et al., 1984). The relationship between cerebral perfusion pressure and $AVDO_2$ measurements may have future implications for monitoring and interventions. The variables of time after injury and specific pathophysiologic processes may impact the development of an ischemic versus hyperemic state (Marion, Darby, & Yonas, 1991). Implications are discussed as related to clinical management in the general interventions section.

In addition to cerebral blood vessel autoregulation in response to metabolic tissue demands, cerebral vessel diameter responds to systemic P_{CO_2} levels. High levels of P_{CO_2} result in cerebral vessel dilation, and low levels result in cerebral vessel constriction. It has been shown that the autoregulatory response to Pa_{CO_2} is well preserved until the very late stages of increased ICP (Enevoldsen & Finn, 1978). Autoregulatory response to Pa_{CO_2} will be considered later as a treatment modality.

Cerebral edema contributes to increased ICP by increasing the brain volume of the intracranial contents. Mechanisms resulting in cerebral edema may be vasogenic or cytotoxic. In vasogenic edema a disruption occurs in capillary permeability, which allows for the leakage of plasma proteins into the extravascular space. Vasogenic edema accumulates primarily in the white matter of the brain. The rise in extravascular oncotic pressure results in a fluid shift. Vasogenic edema is attributed to disruption in the blood-brain barrier after trauma. In cytotoxic edema, cellular injury results in the failure of the sodium-potassium pump. Sodium leaks into the cells, resulting in cellular edema. The mass effect of hematomas leads to tissue compression and cerebral edema, which increases the mass effect and further increases edema. Cytotoxic edema occurs more frequently in gray matter and is attributed to cellular hypoxia and immediate neuronal trauma (Overgaard & Tweed, 1976). Increased ICP can be caused also by an increase in volume of CSF (hydrocephalus). Mass lesions obstructing CSF outflow or reabsorption can result in an increased CSF volume. Blood (as a result of subarachnoid hemorrhage) or white blood cells (caused by infection) can also disrupt the mechanisms for reabsorption of CSF and therefore increase CSF volume.

General Assessment

Assessment of the patient with altered responsiveness begins with a history of events leading up to transport to the ED. The nature of the injury and progression of neurologic events are important to determine. The patient's past medical history and current medications should also be obtained if possible. The value of the history should be recognized, because significant data, such as a patient who is in a Coumadin regimen and has an increased potential for bleeding, could be overlooked. Initial physical assessment of the head-injured patient focuses on the ABCs (airway, breathing, circulation), as well as the neurologic assessment. Hypoxemia often occurs in the patient with a head injury, because the traumatic event may result in blunt or penetrating injury to the chest wall or airway compromise. A reduction in responsiveness may result in hypoventilation and risk for aspiration. Neurogenic pulmonary edema may occur with massive alpha adrenergic discharge, which alters both the pulmonary and systemic circulation (Baigelman & O'Brien, 1981; Crittenden & Beckman, 1982). Blood loss, shock, and myocardial trauma may result in hypotension, which should be treated aggressively to reduce secondary brain injury. Head injury itself may result in a hyperadrenergic state, manifesting as either sustained or labile hypertension (Clifton et al., 1983). Both hypotension and hypertension are dangerous in the face of head injury and impaired cerebral autoregulation; therefore monitoring of blood pressure is imperative. An arterial line is usually inserted in the ED or neuroscience intensive care unit to facilitate diagnosis of blood pressure alterations and monitor hemodynamic interventions. A central venous or pulmonary artery catheter also may be inserted to monitor hemodynamic status. Laboratory studies to detect such toxic substances as ethanol, narcotics, and barbiturates and such metabolic states as hypo-

glycemia, uremia, and hyponatremia provide insight to neurologic status and also guide treatment (e.g., a patient found unresponsive after a fall who has a blood glucose level of 43 mg/dl).

Neurologic assessment

Bedside neurologic assessment of the head-injured patient is a critical interdisciplinary process. Baseline assessment is made as soon as possible, and subsequent assessments are compared with the baseline assessment to detect early indications of progress in response to therapy or deterioration in spite of therapy. Aspects of neurologic assessment and monitoring that are discussed include level of consciousness using the Glasgow coma scale, pupillary assessment, oculocephalic/oculovestibular reflex testing, respiratory pattern assessment, and intracranial pressure monitoring. Integration of the physical assessment findings into herniation syndromes will be presented also.

Level of consciousness assessment using the Glasgow coma scale The most common tool used in the neurologic assessment of the head-injured patient is the Glasgow coma scale. The GCS is divided into three subscales: the eye opening scale, the verbal scale, and the motor scale (Table 10-2). The sum of the three subscales is the GCS score. On all three subscales, the score is determined by the best response. Although the total GCS score is the value referred to in research

---

Table 10-2 The Glasgow coma scale (GCS)

Subscale	Description	Score
Eye opening	Spontaneously	4
	To speech	3
	To pain	2
	Do not open	1
Best verbal response	Oriented	5
	Confused	4
	Inappropriate speech	3
	Unintelligible speech	2
	No verbalization	1
Best motor response	Obeys command	6
	Localizes pain	5
	Withdraws from pain	4
	Abnormal flexion	3
	Abnormal extension	2
	No motor response	1

Note. Best total score = 15; E4, V5, M6. Worst score = 3.

protocols, triage criteria, and other decision schemes, a separate value for each component—eye, verbal, and motor—must be documented.

When a patient is scored on the eye opening scale, a 4 is given if the patient opens the eyes without stimulation; a 3 is given if the patient opens the eyes in response to speech (e.g., calling the patient's name); a 2 is given if the patient opens the eyes to painful stimuli; and a 1 is given if the eyes do not open to pain. Difficulty assessing the eye opening scores can occur in the trauma patient who has sustained eye injuries with periorbital edema or eye dressings. If eye opening can not be assessed, it should be considered untestable and coded ES (eyes swollen). This will eliminate conflicting scores that may occur if one nurse scores this as a 1, while another nurse scores the patient as a 3 for eyebrow elevation in response to voice (Ingersoll & Leyden, 1988).

When a patient is scored on the verbal scale, a 5 is given for orientation to person, place, and time; a 4 is given for answering questions but with disorientation (e.g., patient describes left leg discomfort but doesn't know the year); a 3 is given if the patient speaks in words and phrases that do not make sense; a 2 is given for incomprehensible sounds that are usually moans or groans; and a 1 is given if the patient makes no verbalizations. Intubation or the presence of a tracheostomy, which prevents speech, poses a problem with scoring the verbal scale and, as in the eye opening scale, should be considered untestable. An endotracheal tube may be coded ET, and a tracheostomy tube coded TR. In this case, the total GCS score may be documented as 10ET. The verbal scale is also untestable in an aphasic patient and is generally considered unreliable for patients with receptive or expressive aphasia.

When a patient is scored on the motor scale, a 6 is given if the patient obeys verbal motor commands (e.g., squeezes and releases the examiner's hands or shows two fingers); a 5 is given if the patient localizes pain (e.g., tries to push examiner's hand away); a 4 is given if the patient withdraws to pain (pulls arm away from pain); a 3 is given if the patient demonstrates abnormal flexion posturing (i.e., flexes arm at wrist and elbow and extends and internally rotates legs); a 2 is given if the patient demonstrates extension posturing (i.e., internally rotates the arm, extends arm and wrist, and extends and internally rotates legs); and a 1 is

given if no motor response to pain occurs. One problem with scoring is that the pattern of the motor response may vary with the site of pain application. A sternal rub may produce extension posturing, whereas nail bed pressure may result in a flexion response (Fisher, 1969). Therefore a consistent method of applying pain to determine a motor response should be employed. Another problem is that a patient may develop left hemiparalysis (paralysis of half of the body) and move the right leg to command and still score a 6 on the motor scale. The motor subscale is not designed to detect changes in motor strength. Testing the upper extremities for hand pronation or arm drift with the patient's arm extended at shoulder height, palms up, and eyes closed may reveal mild hemiparesis (weakness of half of the body). Testing the upper extremity for resistance to opposing force and grading the extremity should also be done in the motor evaluation. Testing the lower extremity for strength and grading the extremity is done by having the patient lift one leg off the bed at a time against the examiner's resistance. (Table 10-3). The presence of casts, traction, or other limb-restraining equipment also presents difficulty with assessment. The GCS may be used also in the initial grading of the severity of a traumatic brain injury (Table 10-4).

Although the GCS is the most commonly used assessment tool for the head-injured patient, other tools are available. The Maryland coma scale (MCS) (Salcman, Schepp, & Ducker, 1981), the reaction level scale (RLS85) (Starmark, Stalhammer, Holmgren, & Rosander, 1988), and the clinical neurologic assessment tool (CNA) (Crosby & Parsons, 1989) are three examples. The content of these tools includes areas assessed by the GCS. The MCS also includes medication information, vital signs, the oculovestibular reflex, facial grimacing, the corneal reflex, and seizure activity. The MCS was designed to include parameters that are often considered in diagnostic and treatment decisions when using the GCS. The CNA assesses verbal, motor, and cognitive functions in greater detail than the GCS. The CNA also evaluates muscle tone and observations of chewing and yawning behavior. The CNA was designed to capture more subtle changes in level of consciousness than can be done with the GCS.

The GCS has been shown to predict death in 77% of patients with acute head injury with scores below 7 (Rocca et al., 1989). Research is

Table 10-3 Voluntary motor grading scale

Motor score	Examiner's test	Patient's response
5	Ask the patient to extend arms in a 90-degree angle to the trunk, turn palms toward the ceiling, and close eyes for 10-20 seconds. Watch for drifting of the arm or pronation of the hand. Ask the patient to keep the arms extended (eyes open) and resist your opposing force as you try to push the patient's arms down. Ask the patient to lift the legs off the bed, one at a time, and hold the position for 10-20 seconds. Watch for drifting downward toward the bed. Have the patient keep the leg off the bed as you apply opposing force.	Patient holds the extremity in the starting position against gravity and *full* opposing force.
4	Same as above	Patient holds the extremity in the starting position against gravity and *some* force. Resistance to force, however, is overcome by the examiner.
3	Same as above	Patient holds the extremity in the starting position against gravity, but offers no resistance to mild opposing force by the examiner.
2	Same as above	The patient cannot lift arms and/or legs up against gravity, but can flex and extend them through full range of motion.
1	Same as above	Muscle contraction is present in the arms and/or legs, but no significant movement of the extremity occurs.
0	Same as above	No muscle contraction or movement of the extremity occurs.

in progress in the development of head-injury scales that measure ongoing clinical neurologic status, as well as predict outcome. The major advantage for using the GCS is that previous research reports with mortality and treatment results provide clinical data in terms of GCS score. The GCS is the most widely used assessment tool and is used by the traumatic coma data bank (TCDB) (Marshall et al., 1988a). The TCDB is a collaborative project developed to study the nature of head injury. The major goals of the TCDB are to (1) characterize preinjury and postinjury periods of head injury, (2) assess the influence of a variety of factors on outcome, and (3) examine whether therapy for increased ICP affects outcome (Marshall et al., 1988a). The results of the development of the TCDB include the generation of questions and hypotheses related to head injury. Future nursing research endeavors will be guided by the efforts of the TCDB. Use of consistent terminology allows for a broader base of information sharing.

Pupillary assessment Pupillary response is not included in the GCS; however, it is a key parameter to follow in neurologic patients, because the size, shape, and reactivity of the pupils have clinical significance in localizing injury (Table 10-5). For examination of the pupillary response to light, the room should be darkened and a bright light should be used. The normal range of pupil size is 1.5 to 6.0 mm, with an average of 3.5 mm. Both pupils should be round and briskly constrict in response to the light stimulus in one eye. Bilateral response is referred to as *direct* and *consensual light response*. Consensual response refers to the constriction of the pupil opposite to the one exposed to the light stimulus. The size of each pupil should be documented in millimeters. Wilson, Amling, Floyd, and McNair (1988) demonstrated that nurses working in a neurologic set-

Table 10-4 Head injury grading scale

	Grade 0	Grade 1	Grade 2	Grade 3	Grade 4
Glascow coma score	15	15	12-14	9-11	8 or less
Clinical features	Patient has no history of loss of consciousness. Patient is alert and oriented. Patient does not experience posttraumatic amnesia.	Patient may have mild alteration in responsiveness or history of loss of consciousness or mild posttraumatic amnesia, but eyes open spontaneously, the patient is oriented, and no focal deficits are present. Patient may complain of headache/nausea/vomiting.	Patient has some alteration in responsiveness, but can follow at least simple commands and no focal neurologic deficits are present; or the patient has no alteration in responsiveness, but a focal deficit is present.	Patient has significant alteration in responsiveness and does not follow commands, but responds appropriately to painful stimuli. Focal deficit is usually present.	Patient has severe alteration in responsiveness and does not respond appropriately to pain. Patient may have no evidence of brain function.

Note. Adapted from Emergency Room Management of the Head-Injured Patient. (pp. 23-66) by R.K. Narayan. In D.P. Becker & S.K. Gudeman (Eds.), *Textbook of Head Injury*, 1989, Philadelphia: W.B. Saunders.

Table 10-5 Clinical significance of pupillary changes

Description	**Clinical significance**
Ipsilateral miosis (Horner's syndrome): one pupil is smaller. Ptosis of the eyelid occurs, as well as anhidrosis of the face ipsilateral to the small pupil.	Occurs with downward displacement of the hypothalamus with herniation. May also occur with internal carotid artery occlusion.

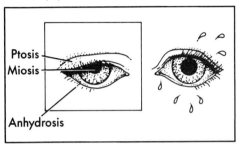

Bilateral miosis: light reaction may be seen with magnifying glass. Pupils are both small or "pinpoint" (2 mm).	Continued herniation or hemorrhage into the pons. Other causes include ophthalmic miotic drugs (acetylcholine, pilocarpine, physostigmine, and edrophonium), opiates, and metabolic encephalopathies.

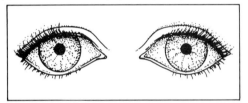

Ipsilateral mydriasis (hutchinsonian pupil): one pupil is larger than the other. The larger pupil is unreactive to light (often referred to as a *blown pupil*).	Occurs in rapidly progressing intracranial hypertension as the result of compression of the third cranial nerve.

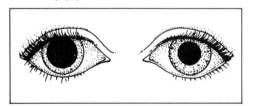

Bilateral midposition: both pupils (4-5 mm) are unreactive to light (referred to as *fixed and dilated*).	Occurs with midbrain compression from transtentorial/central herniation. Other causes include high doses of dopamine (30 mcg/kg/min) in the presence of shock; drugs (amphetamines, cocaine, atropine, and scopolamine); severe anoxia; and brain death.

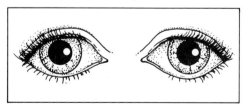

Bilateral mydriasis: both pupils are >6 mm and unreactive to light.	Terminal stages of herniation. Other causes include atropine, hypothermia, and severe barbiturate intoxication.

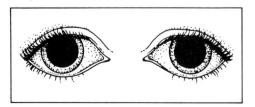

Note. Adapted from "Pathologic Papillary Signs: Self-Learning Module (Part 2) by B.S. Bishop, 1991, *Critical Care Nurse, 11* (7), pp. 58-67. *Miosis,* Constricted; *mydriasis,* dilated; *ptosis,* drooping upper eyelid; *anhidrosis,* lack of sweat.

ting could accurately describe pupillary size without the aid of a measurement tool. Nurses new to the neurologic specialty may benefit from using a measurement tool, which can be constructed by cutting a standard pupil gauge off a neurologic flow sheet and taping it to a tongue depressor or flashlight. Pupillary reaction should be documented as brisk, sluggish, or nonreactive. A sluggishly reactive pupil may indicate early third cranial nerve compression. Wilson et al. (1988) found that even experienced nurses have difficulty with evaluation of pupillary reaction; it is more subjective than size. Recent research indicates that the shape of the pupil is an important clinical assessment parameter because oval-shaped pupils have been associated with ICP levels of 15 to 20 mm Hg in patients with posterior frontal or anterior temporal lesions and contusions (Marshall et al., 1988b).

Oculocephalic and oculovestibular reflex testing Brainstem reflexes may also be followed in the severely head-injured comatose patient. Normal oculocephalic and oculovestibular reflexes indicate the presence of brainstem function. The oculocephalic reflex (doll's eyes) is tested by rotating the patient's head side to side or up and down. The normal response is for the eyes to move in the direction opposite to the direction the head is turned. Loss of the oculocephalic reflex is seen as eyes moving in the direction of the head turning (Figure 10-4). The oculocephalic reflex should not be tested until a cervical spine fracture is ruled out. The oculovestibular reflex (iced caloric) is performed by a physician. The head of the patient's bed is elevated 30 degrees, and the external auditory canal is irrigated with 120 ml 30° C (86° F) water. In the comatose patient, a normal response is conjugate deviation of the eyes toward the stimulus (Figure 10-4). The oculovestibular reflex should not be performed until examination assures that the tympanic membrane is intact. The oculovestibular reflex may be blocked by barbiturates, phenytoin, and succinylcholine. These reflexes should be tested only by experienced practitioners; however, health team members should be aware that loss of these reflexes may indicate a pathologic condition of the brainstem.

Respiratory patterns The respiratory pattern, like the pupillary response, is another clinical indicator of a pathologic condition of the brain that should be assessed in the head-injured patient (Table 10-6). Respiratory patterns are not as reliable as indicators of damage as the pupillary responses because they are often influenced by pulmonary disease and metabolic disturbances. Respiratory patterns are more difficult to assess in the patient with mechanical ventilation.

Intracranial pressure monitoring

Intracranial pressure monitoring is used to evaluate neurologic responses to injury and to guide therapy. Important information regarding the patient's individual ICP and CPP responses to injury and therapy can be obtained. In addition, specific levels of ICP and CPP can be treated and evaluated with a standardized protocol based on previous research findings. Saul and Ducker (1982) reported a significant reduction in mortality with the institution of a protocol based on ICP level.

Methods available for ICP monitoring include pressure recordings from the intraventricular, subarachnoid, epidural, and intraparenchymal areas. Table 10-7 describes anatomic placement and lists advantages and disadvantages associated with each of these devices. All of these devices permit measurement of ICP and calculation of CPP. The ICP monitoring system is similar to other invasive hemodynamic monitoring systems (e.g., arterial pressure) with a few important exceptions. Only sterile, preservative-free normal saline can be used to prime the tubing. The transducer system must be flushless, or the flush device removed and the tubing for attaching flush solutions capped. Only povidone-iodine (Betadine) can be used to clean ports for injection of medications or withdrawal of CSF samples. The zero point for leveling the transducer is located at the external auditory canal.

The intraventricular catheter allows for additional diagnostic testing via the volume-pressure response. The volume-pressure response test is conducted by a physician only and consists of adding 1 ml of sterile, preservative-free normal saline or withdrawing 1 ml of CSF while monitoring for a change in ICP. The normal response is a 2 mm Hg or less change in ICP (Maset et al., 1987). Values above this indicate that the extent of injury has exhausted compensation mechanisms and is at a dangerous point on the volume-pressure curve. Volume-pressure testing may

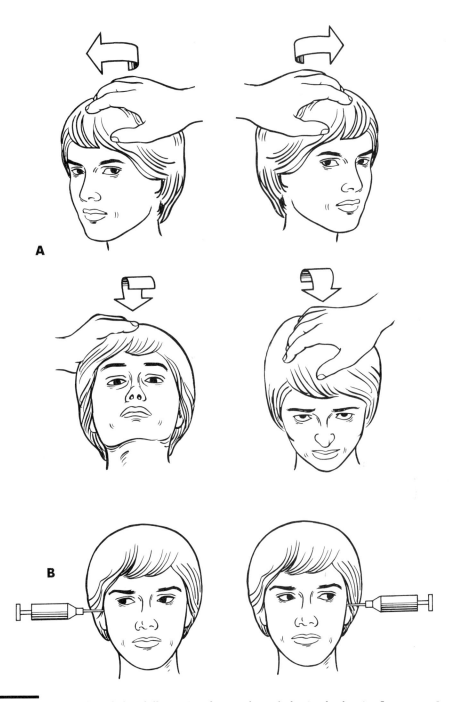

Figure 10-4   **A,** Oculocephalic (doll's eyes) and **B,** oculovestibular (iced caloric) reflex testing. In oculocephalic test, head is rotated side to side or up and down. Eyes moving in direction opposite to direction head is turned indicates reflex is intact. In oculovestibular test, external auditory canal is irrigated with iced saline. Eyes moving toward direction of irrigation indicates reflex is intact.

Table 10-6 Abnormal respiratory patterns associated with coma

Type	Neuroanatomic lesion	Description	Respiratory pattern
Cheyne-Stokes respiration	Usually bilateral in cerebral hemispheres Cerebellar sometimes Midbrain Upper pons	A rhythmic waxing and waning in the depth of respiration, followed by apnea. Secondary to (1) an increased sensitivity to $Paco_2$, increasing the depth and rate of respirations, and (2) decreased stimulation from the cerebral hemispheres, resulting in the apneic phase.	
Central neurogenic hyperventilation	Low midbrain Upper pons	Sustained and rapid respirations with normal Pao_2, low $Paco_2$, and elevated pH with no evidence of pulmonary dysfunction.	
Apneustic breathing	Midpons Low pons	Prolonged or brief pauses at full inspiration. May alternate with expiratory pauses.	
Cluster breathing	Low pons High medulla	Clusters of irregular breathing with periods of apnea at irregular intervals.	
Ataxic breathing	Medulla	Unpredictable breathing patterns with pausing and alternating periods of deep and shallow respirations.	

One minute

Note. From "Abnormal Respiratory Patterns in the Comatose Patient Caused by Intracranial Dysfunction" by R.R.M. Gifford and M.R. Plant, 1975, Journal of Neurosurgical Nursing, 7 (1), 58; and The Clinical practice of Neurological and Neurosurgical Nursing (p. 138) by J.V. Hickey, 1986, Philadelphia: J.B. Lippincott.

Table 10-7 Comparison of methods for monitoring intracranial pressure

Description	Advantages	Disadvantages
Intraventricular catheter		
Catheter placed in anterior horn of lateral ventricle	Can drain CSF Provides access to administer medication Provides access to test volume-pressure response Provides access to obtain CSF for laboratory/culture specimens	Placement difficult with shifted or small ventricles Tissue damage/hemorrhage with insertion Infection rate 8% at 5 days; 40% at 12 days (Ward et al., 1987)
Subarachnoid screw		
Catheter placed in subarachnoid space	Easier to place than intraventricular catheter Does not penetrate brain parenchyma Small quantity of CSF may be obtained for laboratory/culture specimens (Lehman, 1990)	Volume pressure response cannot be tested CSF drainage cannot be done Infection rate 6.9% (Franges & Beideman, 1988)
Epidural sensor		
Sensor placed above dura	Ease of placement Noninvasive Infection rate less than other two methods	Cannot sample or drain CSF Cannot test volume pressure response May not be as reliable or accurate as other methods, especially when ICP in range above normal
Fiberoptic transducer		
Fiberoptic transducer–tipped catheter, which can be placed in subarachnoid space, lateral ventricles, and brain parenchyma (Hollingsworth-Fridlund, Vos, & Daily, 1988)	Smaller catheter; therefore smaller burr holes required for placement Kinking, dampening, and movement artifact associated with fluid column pressure transmission are eliminated Calibrated one time only—done before insertion ICP waveform remains accurate during CSF drainage with ventricular placement Theorized to have reduced infection risk as compared with fluid-filled systems	Bending and manipulation of catheter may damage sensing fibers; once damaged, catheter must be replaced Zero reference cannot be checked after insertion ICP peak pressures may be read as higher when compared with fluid-filled subarachnoid and ventricular system

cause a significant elevation in ICP and increases the risk of infection (Price, 1981).

Nursing assessment of cerebral perfusion pressure and the ICP waveform Assessment of ICP, CPP, and the ICP waveform characteristics is an important nursing responsibility. The nurse should focus on both the absolute values of ICP and CPP and trends in the pressures. Normal intracranial pressure is less than 15 mm Hg. Intracranial pressure can be determined by a manometer or a transducer attached to an oscilloscope. The waveform displayed on the oscilloscope provides valu-

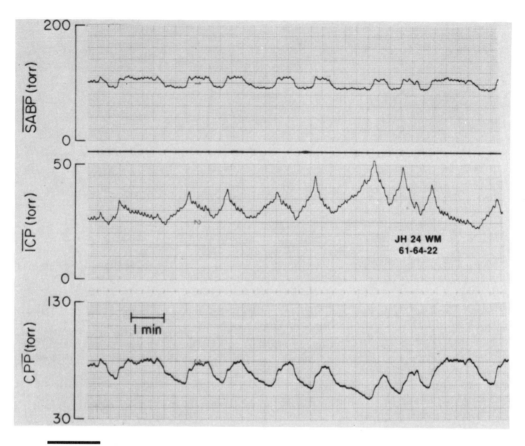

Figure 10-5   Intracranial pressure B wave generation associated with alterations in systemic arterial blood pressure (SABP) and cerebral perfusion pressure (CPP). This patient has elevated baseline ICP and is developing increasingly elevated pressure peaks in response to reductions in SABP. These sharp increases occurring every 1 to 2 minutes indicate reduction in intracranial compliance. (*Note.* From Cerebral Perfusion Pressure: Link between Intracranial Pressure and Systemic Circulation [p. 440] by M.J. Rosner. In J.H. Wood [Ed.], *Cerebral Blood Flow: Physiologic and Clinical Aspects*, 1987, New York: McGraw-Hill. *Note.* Torr = mm Hg.

able information. Characteristic waveforms can be seen with trend recording. These waveforms were initially described by Lundberg (1960) and are called A, B, and C waves. A waves are also referred to as *plateau* waves. A waves are a significant indicator of ICP decompensation and occur in patients with an elevated baseline ICP. The ICP may increase to 50 to 100 mm Hg and remain sustained for 5 to 20 minutes. A waves may be correlated with arterial blood pressure changes if a simultaneous strip of both can be obtained. It is theorized that a reduction in CPP initiates an intracranial vasodilation cascade, which increases cerebral blood volume (CBV) and therefore ICP

(Rosner & Becker, 1984). B waves are sharper and more rhythmic oscillations in ICP, which may range from 0 to 50 mm Hg and occur every 30 seconds to 2 minutes. B waves do not necessarily occur on an elevated baseline ICP, but their appearance, especially if increasing in frequency, may indicate early decompensation. B waves also correlate with changes in blood pressure. The major difference between A and B waves is that the degree and duration of ICP response is less severe with B waves. Pathologic ICP waveforms correlated with arterial blood pressure and CPP reduction are shown in Figure 10-5. C waves may occur 4 to 8 times per minute and are mild

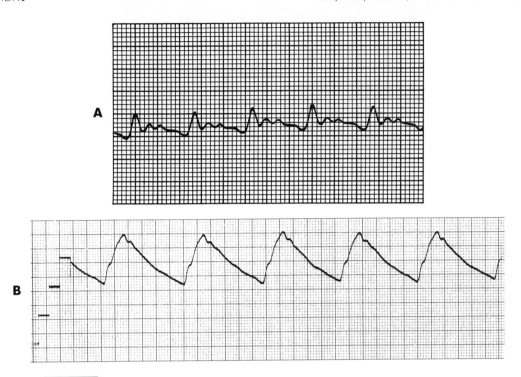

Figure 10-6   Analysis of ICP pulse wave characteristics. **A,** At normal intracranial pressures, appearance of ICP pulse wave is saw-toothed. **B,** As ICP rises and intracranial compliance is reduced, ICP pulse wave becomes more rounded.

fluctuations in ICP with an amplitude up to 20 mm Hg. C waves may correspond to respiratory or blood pressure fluctuations but are considered physiologic in nature and not dangerous.

Nursing assessment of the ICP pulse wave   The characteristic of the individual pulse wave, as well as the trending information described, is an important area for nursing assessment. The normal ICP pulse wave consists of three arterial components and occasionally several retrograde venous pulsations. The ICP waveform is a saw-toothed pattern at normal values, but begins to become more rounded as ICP increases (Figure 10-6). It is theorized that the ICP pulse wave configuration change indicates a reduction in intracranial compliance. Patients with head injury experience variation in adaption ability at the same ICP value; therefore waveform interpretation is another tool for nursing assessment (Germon, 1988).

Herniation syndrome   The term *herniation* refers to brain tissue shifting laterally or downward as the result of increasing intracranial pressure.

The described patterns of herniation are theorized to occur as intracranial mass is dispersed from an area of higher pressure to an area of lower pressure. Herniation patterns have been categorized into syndromes based on the direction of tissue movement and clinical findings associated with compression of different brain areas. Lateral herniation of the cingulate gyrus of one cerebral hemisphere under the falx cerebri (fold of dura matter that lies between the cerebral hemispheres) is referred to as *cingulate* herniation. This lateral displacement of tissue is the result of increasing pressure in one cerebral hemisphere. Herniation of tissue as evidenced by horizontal displacement of the pineal gland on CT scan has been associated with a depressed level of consciousness (Ropper, 1986).

Downward displacement of tissue compressing first the diencephalon and then brainstem structures occurs as the result of cerebral hemisphere increases in ICP. This downward displacement is referred to as *central* or *transtentorial* herniation. In the presence of an expanding unilateral mass, central herniation may be preceded by cingulate herniation. Initial pressure on the diencephalon may produce the clinical picture of impaired consciousness, Cheyne-Stokes respirations, and small, reactive pupils. Oculocephalic and oculovestibular reflexes remain intact, and abnormal flexion posturing occurs. Further compression onto the upper brainstem results in midposition and light-fixed pupils, impaired oculocephalic and oculovestibular reflexes, and extension posturing. As the lower brainstem is compressed, the pupils dilate and remain light-fixed. Lower brainstem compression also causes loss of oculocephalic and oculovestibular reflexes. The patient may become motionless, although a flexor withdrawal response may occur in the legs with plantar stimulation (Plum & Posner, 1985).

Unilateral displacement of the medial temporal lobe laterally and downward over the edge of the tentorium (fold of dura mater between the cerebral hemispheres and the cerebellum) and onto the brainstem is referred to as *uncal* herniation. Tissue impaction between the tentorium and the brainstem causes bilateral midbrain compression. Pressure on the third cranial nerve results in a dilated, unreactive pupil usually associated with a depressed level of consciousness. Oculocephalic and oculovestibular reflexes may show disruption if tested in the comatose patient. Further tissue displacement results in bilateral brainstem compression with clinical findings as described above in the brainstem involvement with central herniation (Plum & Posner, 1985). Figure 10-7 shows the uncal herniation with accompanying signs.

Assessment and Interventions Related to Specific Injuries

Neurologic damage as the result of head injury can be attributed to both primary and secondary mechanisms of injury. Primary injury occurs with the movement of the semifluid brain within the

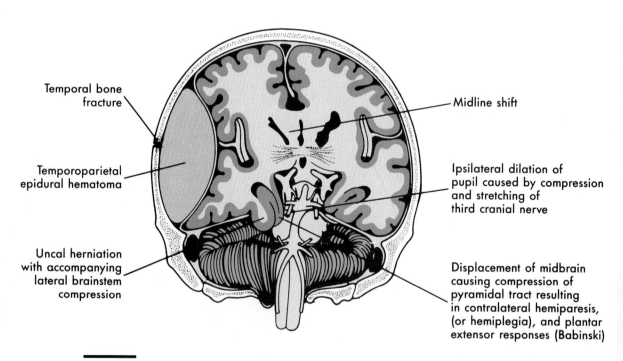

Temporal bone fracture

Temporoparietal epidural hematoma

Uncal herniation with accompanying lateral brainstem compression

Midline shift

Ipsilateral dilation of pupil caused by compression and stretching of third cranial nerve

Displacement of midbrain causing compression of pyramidal tract resulting in contralateral hemiparesis, (or hemiplegia), and plantar extensor responses (Babinski)

Figure 10-7 Cross section showing herniation of lower portion of temporal lobe (uncas) through tentorium caused by temporoparietal epidural hematoma. Herniation may occur also in cerebellum. Note mass effect and midline shift. (*Note.* Redrawn from *Advanced Concepts in Clinical Nursing* [2nd ed.] by K.C. Kintzel [Ed.], 1977, Philadelphia: J.B. Lippincott.)

rigid skull, producing disruption in neuronal function, formation of hematomas, shearing of tissue and blood vessels, and disruption in skull integrity. Secondary injuries may occur as a physiologic response of the brain to primary injuries. Secondary injuries include increased intracranial pressure (ICP), cerebral edema with alterations in normal cerebral blood flow, and systemic responses to cerebral injury (Manifold, 1986). Hypoxia and hypotension contribute to the development of secondary injuries by causing cerebral anoxia. Aggressive evaluation and treatment are aimed toward minimizing the effects of primary injury and preventing or reducing the effects of secondary injury. The pathophysiology of secondary injuries relates to the previous discussion of ICP and cerebral blood flow. A discussion of the pathophysiologic mechanisms of primary injury with associated nursing diagnoses follows.

Concussion   Pain (headache)

Temporary cessation of neuronal function on impact results in concussion injury. Concussion manifests as a brief loss of consciousness associated with either antegrade amnesia (posttraumatic), retrograde amnesia (events before the injury), or both. Neurologic assessment, skull films, and CT scan may be performed upon arrival at the hospital. Skull films have been cited as being neither cost effective nor clinically useful in the diagnosis of potential deterioration in mild head injury (Cooper & Ho, 1983; Miller, Murray, & Teasdale, 1990). Patients with normal CT scan and neurologic examination can usually be safely triaged home from the ED (Livingston, Loder, Koziol, & Hunt, 1991). A GCS score of less than 15 or abnormal films may warrant a 24- to 48-hour observation in the hospital. Neurologic deterioration requiring neurosurgical intervention occurs in 2% to 3% of these cases, as compared with a 1:6000 risk with normal films and examination (Dacey, Alves, Rimel, Winn, & Jane, 1986). Minor head injury is defined as a loss of consciousness for 20 minutes or less, GCS score of 13 to 15, no mass lesions, and hospitalization for less than 48 hours. Minor head injury represents 72% to 73% of all head injuries (Kay, 1988). Of all patients with the clinical criteria of mild head injury, 80% are diagnosed with concussion (Kraus & Nourjah, 1988). Before discharge, patients diagnosed with minor head injury should be in-

formed that they may experience a postconcussion syndrome, which can include neurologic symptoms of headache, restlessness, irritability, and distractibility, and disruption in sleep (see box, p. 282). Neuropsychologic testing demonstrates that reaction time with information-processing tasks may be impaired for as long as 3 months after injury (Hugenholtz, Stuss, Stethem, & Richard, 1988). At home this may be experienced as difficulty thinking with multiple stimuli (e.g., environmental noise during tasks) and feelings of stress and fatigue. The symptoms of the postconcussion syndrome may lead to disruptions in interpersonal relationships, self-perception, and work abilities. Cognitive and behavioral therapy may be indicated for these symptoms, especially if the patient experiences prolonged posttraumatic amnesia (Levin & Eisenberg, 1988). The patient must realize not only the presence of neurologic symptoms, but also that there is treatment available. See Chapter 24, for further discussion.

Contusion   High risk for altered cerebral tissue perfusion

To understand contusion injury, it is helpful to think of the brain as a semiliquid substance, such as gelatin, in a hard container (the skull) exposed to impact or force. The impact of brain against the skull causes tissue damage, characterized by extravasation of blood and tissue death. Contusions are caused by impact of the brain against the bony surface of the skull (Figure 10-8). This occurs particularly over the frontal and temporal lobes because the inner surfaces of the frontal and temporal bones are irregular (Jorden, 1983). Injuries located directly under the area of impact are referred to as *coup* injuries. *Contrecoup* injuries are the result of brain movement, often against the opposite surface. Contrecoup injuries may occur also as brain tissue is pulled away from the skull with the initial movement. After a contusion injury, patients may initially experience a depressed level of consciousness. The duration of the alteration in consciousness and neurologic outcome depend on the extent and depth of the injury, with brainstem contusions having the worst prognosis (Levin et al., 1988). Patients with contusions may have normal initial CT scans and then develop hemorrhage or edema within the first 72 hours. Recent experience with magnetic resonance imaging (MRI) demonstrates

Discharge instructions for patient with minor head injuries

You are being discharged to home after your head injury. We do not anticipate that you will develop significant problems at home. If problems do occur, it is most likely to be in your first 24 to 48 hours at home.

You or your family member or friend should call your doctor, or you should return to the emergency department if any of the following occur:

1. Excessive sleepiness or difficulty waking the injured person
2. Increasing or severe headache
3. Difficulty walking, including weakness, stumbling, or unsteadiness
4. Uncoordination, weakness, or inability to move the arms or legs
5. Clear or bloody fluid coming out of the nose or the ears
6. Blurred vision or unequal pupils (the black part of the eye)
7. Uncontrollable shaking movement of the arms or legs with or without changes in wakefulness
8. Confusion or change in the injured person's behavior
9. Nausea and/or vomiting
10. Change in breathing pattern
11. Any new or worrisome symptom
    - *Minor* headache and memory problems are common after a mild head injury. If these occur, call and discuss these with your doctor during normal office hours.
    - Keep any follow-up doctor or rehabilitation appointments that have been scheduled for you.
    - Do not drink any alcoholic beverages for 2 or 3 days. Do not take any pain medication stronger than Tylenol or aspirin unless it is prescribed by your doctor.

Note. Adapted from "Restoring Social Competence in Minor Head Injury Patients" by J.L. Hinkle, S.M. Alves, R.W. Rimel, and J.A. Jane, 1986, *Journal of Neuroscience Nursing, 18* (5), pp. 268-271; and Emergency Room Management of the Head Injured Patient (pp. 23-66) by R.K. Narayan. In D.P. Becker and S.K. Gudeman (Eds.), 1989, *Textbook of Head Injury*, Philadelphia: W.B. Saunders.

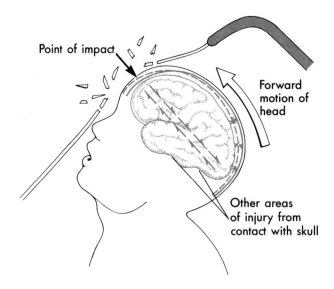

Figure 10-8   Closed blunt injury. Skull molding occurs at impact. Stippled line, preinjury contour; Solid line, contour moments after impact. Subdural veins torn as brain rotates forward. Shearing strains throughout brain. Trauma to inferior temporal and frontal lobes over floors of middle and anterior fossae occur, causing coup and contrecoup injury. (*Note.* Redrawn from *Neurological Pathophysiology* [p. 293] by S.G. Eliasson, A.L. Prensky, and W.B. Hardin Jr. (eds.), 1974, New York: Oxford University Press.)

that perifocal edema in the frontal and temporal lobes is associated with the development of delayed traumatic intracerebral hematoma (Tanaka et al., 1988). MRI is superior to CT scanning in the detection of cerebral contusion injury and associated edema (Snow, Zimmerman, Gandy, & Deck, 1986). Steroids may be used if edema is present with diagnostic imaging. Prophylactic anticonvulsants may be started, because contusions are associated with posttraumatic seizures. The presence of extravascular blood is a contributing factor to epileptogenesis (Dodson & Ferrendelli, 1987).

Epidural hematoma   High risk for altered
cerebral tissue perfusion

An epidural hematoma is an accumulation of blood between the cranium and the dura mater. Epidural hematomas account for approximately 2% of all head injury (Hickey, 1986). Loss of consciousness usually occurs at the time of injury, and 15% to 20% of these patients will regain consciousness again for a brief period before deterioration (Plum & Posner, 1985). The source of bleeding is often a laceration of the middle meningeal artery, which lies in the groove of the tem-poral bone, sustained from a fracture. Arterial bleeding results in a rapid accumulation of blood with compression and shifting of intracerebral contents. Rapid accumulation of blood over the cerebral hemisphere or into the temporal fossa can result in an uncal herniation syndrome as the lower portion of the temporal lobe (uncus) compresses the brainstem and the third cranial nerve, resulting in ipsilateral pupil dilation (see Figure 10-7). Epidural hematomas located above the cerebellum and brainstem (supratentorial) are associated with a 9% to 36% mortality. Less commonly, fracture of the occipital bone may lacerate venous vessels in the transverse sinus. Epidural hematomas extending into the cerebellar and brainstem areas (infratentorial) comprise 0.3% of all head injuries and are associated with a 30% to 50% mortality. This high mortality is attributed to compression of the brainstem vasomotor, respiratory, and consciousness centers (Brambella, Rainoldi, Gipponi, & Paoletti, 1986).

Epidural hematomas are diagnosed by CT scan (Figure 10-9) and are treated by surgical evacuation. If CT scanning is not available or the patient is not stable enough to be moved, burr holes may be placed into the skull for emergency decompression of the hematoma (Figure 10-10)

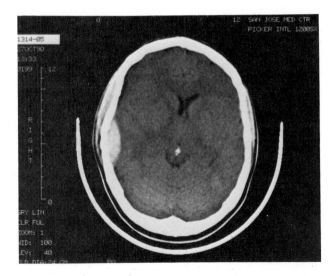

Figure 10-9   CT scan of head showing lenticular (lens)-shaped parietal epidural hematoma with effacement of ventricular system and slight mass effect, requiring craniotomy and evacuation of hematoma. (Courtesy Mark Eastham, MD, Department of Neurosurgery, San Jose Medical Center, San Jose, CA.)

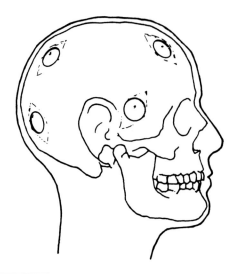

Figure 10-10 Locations of burr holes necessary to provide complete exploration for epidural hematoma. (*Note.* From "Emergency Burr Holes: Current Role in Neurosurgical Acute care" by J.E. Wilberger, 1990, *Topics in Emergency Medicine,* 11 [4], p. 70.)

(Wilberger, 1990). The major indication for burr hole decompression of an epidural hematoma in the ED is an acute deterioration in the patient's level of consciousness. Definitive treatment of the epidural hematoma that is causing compression and pathologic neurologic signs is craniotomy for evacuation. Postsurgical treatment focuses on management of increased ICP and maintenance of adequate CBF.

Subdural hematomas   High risk for injury
                                      Altered cerebral tissue
                                        perfusion

Subdural hematomas (SDH) are collections of blood between the meningeal layers of the dura mater and arachnoid in the brain (Figure 10-11, A). They comprise 17% to 29% of all head injuries (Gennarelli, 1982). The bleeding source is usually venous, caused by injury to the subcortical bridging veins. Elderly and alcoholic patients with cortical atrophy are predisposed to SDHs because of the tension placed on the cortical bridging veins as the cerebral tissue is pulled away from the dura mater. SDHs may occur after a mild injury in these patients. Patients may be unable to account for the injury that produced the SDH. They may demonstrate progressive changes in cognition and motor strength over weeks or months.

SDHs are usually found over the frontal and temporal lobes. SDHs are classified according to the onset of symptoms: acute SDHs present in 24 to 72 hours; subacute SDHs present in 72 hours to 10 days; chronic SDHs may not present for as long as several months (Gennarelli, 1982). Presentation includes a decreased level of consciousness, and patients may have focal signs of brain dysfunction resulting from compression. In acute SDHs, like epidural hematomas, rapid accumulation of blood may cause compression and shifting of intracranial contents. SDHs are diagnosed by CT scan (Figure 10-11, *B*). CT scanning may be helpful in determining the relative age of the SDH. Acute SDHs are likely to appear as high attenuations; subacute SDHs appear isodense; and chronic SDHs appear hypodense (Markwalden, 1981). Prophylactic anticonvulsants and antibiotics are started, and the hematoma is surgically evacuated. Chronic SDHs may be treated surgically with a craniotomy, followed by catheter insertion for drainage.

Intracerebral hematomas   High risk for altered
                                         cerebral tissue
                                         perfusion

Intracerebral hematomas represent 4% of all head injuries. Bleeding into the brain parenchyma may be acute or delayed. Acute hematoma is caused by vessel rupture with tissue shearing in blunt trauma and vessel laceration in penetrating injuries. Laceration of cerebral vessels from a depressed skull fracture can also result in an acute intracerebral hematoma formation. Traumatic intracerebral hematoma is associated with contusion injury and is therefore often located in the frontal and temporal lobes. Large intracerebral hematomas with a 15 mm or greater shift in brain structures or absence of basal cisterns on CT scanning are associated with poor outcome even with surgical intervention (Toutant et al., 1984). The presence of intraventricular hemorrhage is also associated with poor outcome. Traumatic aneurysm may result from weakening of a vessel wall with shearing forces and may result in an intracerebral hematoma or subarachnoid hemorrhage as long as 3 weeks after injury (Aarabi, 1988). Prophylactic anticonvulsants are

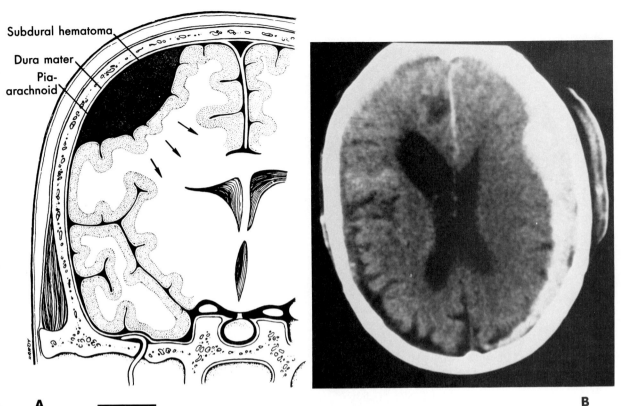

A   **B**

Figure 10-11 **A,** Subdural hematoma causing increased intracranial pressure with shifting of tissue and **B,** Acute subdural hematoma as seen on computed axial tomography. (**A,** From *The Practice of Emergency Care* (2nd ed.) (p. 331) by J.H. Cosgriff, Jr., and D.L. Anderson, 1984, Philadelphia: **B,** From Department of Radiology, Shadyside Hospital, Pittsburgh, PA.).

started for prevention of seizures. Surgery may be indicated if the hematoma is larger than 3 cm, the patient's neurologic condition deteriorates, and the hematoma is surgically accessible.

Skull fractures   High risk for infection

Cranial bones have three layers: the outer table, which lies next to the scalp; the middle, or diploetic, layer; and the inner table, which lies next to the brain. Disruption in the integrity of the cranial bones is common in head injury (Gardner, 1986). The fractures may be caused by force with impact or penetration. Skull fractures are classified as linear, depressed, or basilar (Nikas, 1987). Linear fractures may involve either the inner or outer tables of the cranial bones without bone displacement. The danger with lin-

ear fractures is that laceration of vessels lying in the grooves of the inner table of the cranium may occur. The most common site for a linear fracture is the temporal and parietal bones transversing the middle meningeal artery, leading to an epidural hematoma formation. Occipital fractures may extend into the skull base, producing hematoma with brainstem compression, cranial nerve injury, and cerebrospinal fluid (CSF) leaks (Young & Schmidek, 1982). In depressed fractures, the outer table of the cranium is displaced below the inner table. If a scalp laceration exists that allows communication with the environment, the fracture is classified as *open*; surgical removal of some of the contaminated bone fragments may be indicated (Figure 10-12). Often, bone fragments can be replaced (Figure 10-13).

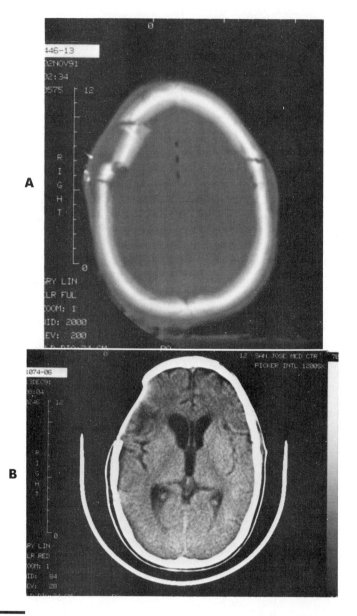

Figure 10-12 CT scan of severe blunt trauma to head. **A,** Bilateral skull fractures and open depressed fracture manifested by intracranial air (dark spots). Underlying brain is severely lacerated. **B,** Craniectomy defect at site of prior open depressed fracture after 6 weeks with underlying encephalomalacia and slight ventricular enlargement. (Courtesy Mark Eastham, MD, Department of Neurosurgery, San Jose Medical Center, San Jose, CA.)

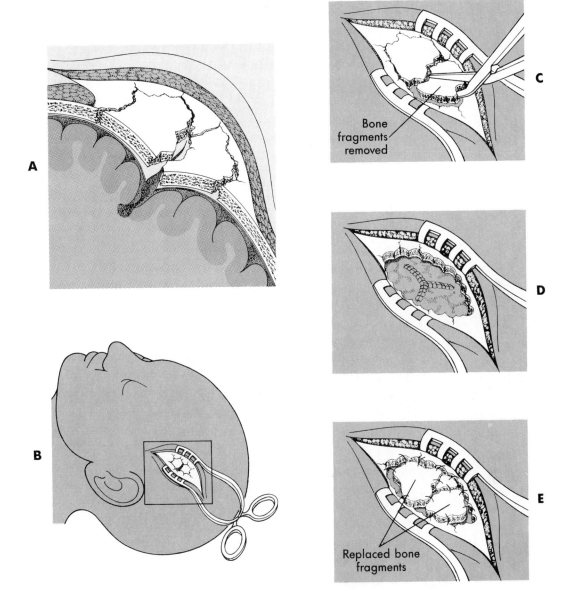

Figure 10-13 Treatment of compound depressed fracture of skull. **A,** Depressed skull fracture and scalp injury. **B,** Incision to expose fracture and remove devitalized scalp. **C,** Removal of impacted bone by burr hole to locate and identify normal dura, followed by resection of bone fragments. **D,** Watertight closure of dura after brain debridement. **E,** Replacement and fixation of bone fragments. (*Note.* Redrawn from Diagnosis and Treatment of Head Injury (pp. 2017-2148) by D.P. Becker, G.F. Gade, H.F. Young, and T.F. Fewerman. In *Neurological Surgery* [3rd ed.] by J.R. Youman [Ed.], 1990, Philadelphia: W.B. Saunders.)

If the bone has been shattered into pieces (comminuted), a synthetic flap may be used to protect the brain after the period of acute injury has passed. A depressed fracture may lacerate the brain parenchyma or a venous sinus and produce hemorrhage.

Basilar skull fractures   Basilar skull fractures are linear fractures occurring at the base of the brain. These fractures are the result of tension exerted on the fragile bones at the base of the skull at the time of impact (Figure 10-14). The major complications of a basilar skull fracture are cranial

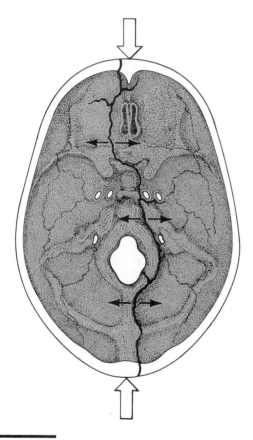

Figure 10-14   Fracture mechanism at base of skull. Bone is more resistant to compression than to tension. Impact forces compress outer skull and generate tension along fragile bones at base of skull. These tension forces result in linear fractures that may extend across entire skull base. (Note. *Open arrows*, Compressive forces; *solid arrows*, tension.) Redrawn from "Head Injuries: Biomechanical Principles" by S. Lingren, 1986, *Acta Neurochirurgica, Supplementum 36*, p. 29.)

nerve injury and dural tears, leading to CSF leaks and meningitis. Refer to Table 10-1 for review of cranial nerves.

Basilar skull fractures may begin in the squamous portions of the temporal bone and may extend anteriorly, medially, or posteriorly. Fractures may extend anteriorly, causing damage to the first cranial nerve (olfactory), and pierce the arachnoid to produce a CSF leak from the nose (CSF rhinorrhea). Anterior fractures may also damage venous sinuses and cause blood to leak into periorbital tissues, producing ecchymoses or raccoon's eyes. Fractures extending medially may damage the seventh (facial) and eighth (acoustic) cranial nerves and result in bleeding behind the tympanic membrane (hemotympanum). Cerebrospinal fluid may also collect behind the tympanic membrane. If the tympanic membrane is disrupted, CSF may leak out of the ear (CSF otorrhea). Posterior extension of the fracture may damage the sigmoid sinus and cause bleeding into the mastoid air cells, resulting in postauricular swelling and ecchymoses, described as Battle's sign. Battle's sign will appear in 24 to 48 hours after injury, although it may be seen earlier (Figure 10-15). Laceration of the portion of the internal carotid artery that lies in the cavernous sinus behind the orbit can result in a carotid-cavernous fistula. Engorgement of the venous cavernous sinus with arterial blood results in exophthalmos (protrusion of the eye), chemosis (conjunctival edema), and an orbital bruit that diminishes with carotid compression. Laceration or contusion of the brainstem with basilar skull fractures can result in immediate death (Friedman, 1983).

Nursing care of the patient with a basilar skull fracture includes monitoring for CSF leaks and central nervous system (CNS) infection. If CSF is mixed with blood, the halo sign test can be used, which is performed by placing the fluid on a piece of filter paper or linen. The test results are positive when the blood forms a circle in the center with a yellow or clear ring of CSF around the circle. If clear fluid drains out of the ear or nose, a dextrose stick can be used for testing. Cerebrospinal fluid normally contains glucose and will therefore test positive. If nasal bleeding is present, this testing method will not be valid because blood also contains glucose. When nasal drainage is tested for CSF, false-positive rates can be as high as 75%. A clinical indicator is that nasal

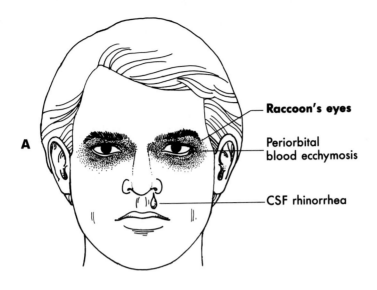

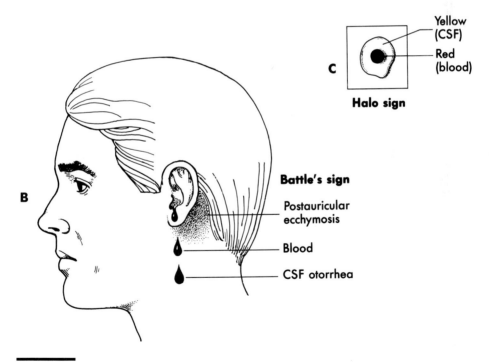

Figure 10-15 Clinical findings associated with basilar skull fracture. Anterior extension of fracture may pierce arachnoid and cause nasal leakage of CSF (CSF rhinorrhea), or damage venous sinuses causing blood to accumulate in periorbital tissues (raccoon's eyes) (**A**). Medial extension of fracture may result in blood leakage or CSF leakage from ear (CSF otorrhea). Posterior extension of fracture may cause venous bleeding into mastoid air cells, producing postauricular swelling and ecchymoses (Battle's sign) (**B**). Halo sign or bull's eye test to detect presence of CSF (**C**).

drainage has a stringy, mucous characteristic not found with CSF (Katz & Kaplan, 1985). If the patient is alert, he or she may report the salty taste of CSF. The patient with a CSF leak is usually kept lying with the head slightly elevated to promote dural healing, which usually occurs spontaneously within 7 to 10 days. A gauze 4×4 may be loosely taped like a sling under the nose or across the ear, but the nose and ear should not be packed, because glucose-rich CSF may increase risk of infection. The patient should not blow the nose and should avoid coughing and sneezing. Signs and symptoms of meningeal irritation may indicate CNS infection or subarachnoid hemorrhage. Signs and symptoms of meningeal irritation include a stiff neck (nuchal rigidity), headache, photophobia, fever, nausea, and vomiting.

Diffuse axonal injury   High risk for impaired
social interaction

Diffuse axonal injury (DAI) is a common finding in severe head injury. As the terminology suggests, diffuse axonal injury is a widespread pathophysiologic process involving the axonal component of neuronal continuity. Rotational and acceleration/deceleration forces causing tissue movement and shearing injury have been proposed as primary pathophysiologic mechanisms. Evidence that the injury is common at gray-white tissue interfaces supports that theory (Blumberg, Jones, & North, 1989). Another theory of pathogenesis is that DAI occurs as a secondary injury in response to hypoxia, edema, and herniation, because generalized brain swelling is a commonly associated finding. Clinical-pathologic study of DAI reveals macroscopic evidence of hemorrhagic foci in the corpus callosum and dorsolateral brainstem, and microscopic evidence of axonal retraction balls in white matter areas (Sahuquillo et al., 1989). Diffuse axonal injury is categorized into grades by severity and characteristics of injury. In grade I (mild), white matter injury is evident in the cerebral hemispheres, brainstem, and/or cerebellum. Often subarachnoid hemorrhage is evident. In grade II, characteristics of grade I may be found in association with a focal lesion (e.g., hemorrhage) in the white matter of the cerebral hemispheres and/or intraventricular hemorrhage. In grade III, characteristics of grades I and II may be present in association with a focal lesion of the brainstem (Adams et al., 1989).

Initial diagnosis is made by clinical examination and possible CT scan findings of associated features, such as subarachnoid, intraventricular, and cerebral white matter hemorrhage, and acute brain swelling (Takenaka et al., 1990) (Figure 10-16). By 1 month after injury, evidence of ventricular enlargement on CT scan and corpus callosal atrophy on MRI are suggestive of DAI (Levin et al., 1990). MRI scanning demonstrates the diffuse white matter involvement better than CT scanning (Figure 10-17).

The clinical course for a patient with a severe DAI is often that of immediate and prolonged coma leading to a persistent vegetative state. (Parker, Parker, & Overman, 1990). The prognosis for functional recovery after DAI is inversely proportional to the degree of injury and amount of secondary insult. Management of DAI is directed at control of cerebral edema, increased ICP, and systemic complications.

Penetrating injuries   High risk for infection

Penetrating injury is usually produced as a missile enters the intracranial cavity. The missile often travels through the brain in a straight pathway and exits the cranium. The missile may ricochet off bone, however, and at times produces secondary smaller missiles after contact with bone (Ordog, Wasserberger, & Balasubramanian, 1988). The missile produces brain damage through three major mechanisms: direct damage, shock wave generation, and cavitation. Direct damage results in tissue disruption and artery laceration as the missile moves through the brain. Pressure waves are generated from the missile during movement through tissue. These pressure waves travel far from the missile pathway (Carey, Tutton, Strub, Black, and Tobey, 1984). A cavity often much larger than the diameter of the missile occurs in the path of the missile as the result of transfer of kinetic energy. This cavity may move inward and back outward several times, creating a large rise in the intracranial pressure (Carey, Sarna, Farrell, & Happel, 1989). As the missile enters the brain, debris such as bone fragments and hair often is driven into brain tissue. Occasionally a missile may not penetrate the cranial cavity, but fracture the skull, driving bone fragments into the brain.

The diagnosis of a missile injury is initially made by examination of the head for an entry and exit wound. Skull films are obtained to determine the extent of bony injury. A CT scan is

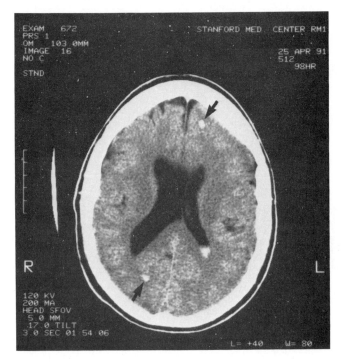

Figure 10-16 CT scan of head after blunt head trauma in skier who hit tree at high speed. Intraventricular hemorrhage is evident in tip of left ventricle and focal intracerebral hemorrhage in two locations *(see arrows)*. Focal hemorrhage is indicative of diffuse axonal injury, or shear effect. (Courtesy Lawrence M. Shuer, MD, Department of Neurosurgery, Stanford University Medical Center, Stanford, CA.)

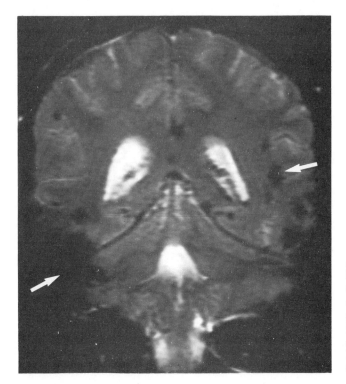

Figure 10-17 Magnetic resonance imaging of brain with diffuse axonal injury. 26-year-old man with traumatic brain injury. MRI shows axonal shear injury of the temporal lobes bilaterally, as noted by dark areas *(see arrows)*. (Courtesy Dieter E. Enzmann, MD, Department of Radiology, Stanford University Medical Center, Stanford, CA.)

Figure 10-18 Gunshot wound to head. **A,** Brain window of CT scan shows spray of bullet fragments, reflecting the direction of bullet. Arrow shows site and angle of entrance of bullet. **B,** Bone window of CT scan shows exit site with lifting of skull and fracture from significant energy released. (Courtesy Lawrence M. Shuer, MD, Department of Neurosurgery, Stanford University Medical Center, Stanford, CA.)

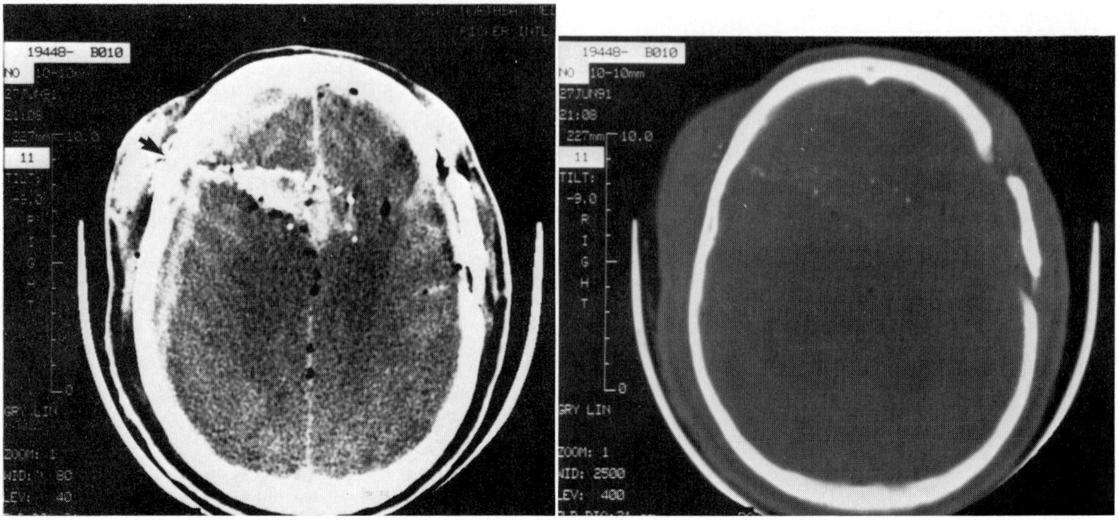

done to determine the trajectory of the missile pathway(s). The CT scan will also detect associated injuries, such as hematoma formation and cerebral edema (Rosenwasser, Andrews, & Jimenez, 1991) (Fig 10-18).

Treatment of missile injuries includes control of ICP, management of associated injuries, and debridement. The extent of surgical debridement may be limited by high ICP and risk of secondary injury as a result of the debridement. Systemic antibiotics are administered to reduce the risk of infection and abscess formation, which may not develop for 6 to 8 weeks after injury (Aarabi, 1987; Brandvold, Levi, Feinsod, & George, 1990). Anticonvulsants are started because of the high risk for the development of epilepsy after missile injury (Rosenwasser et al., 1991).

General Interventions

In the acute phase of head injury, nursing care is focused on safe and rapid execution of medical prescriptions for therapy, preparation and transport of the patient for diagnostic testing or surgery, and neurologic assessment. Throughout this period, nursing interventions directed at minimizing the secondary injuries caused by increased ICP are critical. A summary of nursing diagnoses, interventions, and evaluation criteria are found in the table on pp. 293-294.

Nursing diagnosis	Nursing intervention	Evaluative criteria
Altered cerebral tissue perfusion Related to cerebral edema, decreased cerebral perfusion As evidenced by change in level of responsiveness, motor changes, pupillary abnormalities	**Maintain oxygenation** Provide suctioning to maintain adequate airway. Limit each suctioning attempt to 15 seconds. Provide preoxygenation by bagging with 100% oxygen for 1 minute before initial suctioning attempt and 1 to 5 minutes between attempts. Consult with the physician regarding lidocaine administration to reduce the cough reflex.	Patient's Pao_2 will remain above 80 mm Hg.
	Maintain ventilation Provide hyperventilation as prescribed. Maintain hypocapnia during transfer with manual bagging.	Patient's $Paco_2$ will remain between 25 and 30 mm Hg.
	Reduce cerebral edema with pharmacologic intervention Give mannitol intravenously at doses of 0.5 to 2 g/kg over 10-20 minutes; monitor serum osmolality and report values above 320 mOsm/L. Give Lasix intravenously at doses of 20-60 mg. Maintain fluid restriction as prescribed by the physician.	ICP will remain below 15 mm Hg, and the CPP will remain above 60 mm Hg.
	Avoid increases in ICP by nonpharmacologic means Maintain normothermia or hypothermia if prescribed by the physician by: • monitoring patient's temperature and reporting elevations; • if hypothermia is prescribed, obtaining a cooling mattress; • monitoring for shivering; if shivering occurs, consulting the physician regarding use of chlorpromazine; • monitoring EKG for cardiac arrhythmias; • monitoring skin condition to prevent cold burns and skin breakdown. Turn and position appropriately, remembering to: • avoid neck flexion, extension, and rotation; • avoid extreme hip flexion;	Patient will remain afebrile (or temperature $< 38°$ C). Patient will not shiver. Patient will remain without arrhythmias. Patient will remain without skin breakdown. Patient will not experience ICP >15 mm Hg or CPP <60 mm Hg related to position.

Continued.

Nursing diagnosis	Nursing intervention	Evaluative criteria
Altered cerebral tissue perfusion—cont'd	• raise the head of the bed 30-45 degrees unless patient is hypotensive or clinical condition deteriorates with the head of the bed elevated; • use the drawsheet to pull the patient up in bed and have patient exhale, avoiding Valsalva's maneuver; • avoid having the patient hold on to the side rails during turning. Ensure appropriate stimulation by: • avoiding clinical conversation at the bedside related to injury or prognosis; • providing brief, simple explanations to the patient accompanied by gentle touch; • avoiding activities that are associated with abnormal flexion or extension responses.	Patient will not experience ICP >15 mm Hg related to stimulation.
	Prevent increased intrathoracic and intraabdominal pressure by: • consulting physician regarding bowel program using softeners, fiber, or stimulants, based on the consistency of stool, effort required to evacuate stool, and frequency of bowel movements; monitoring for daily or every-other-day bowel movements.	Patient will not experience ICP >15 mm Hg while evacuating stool. Bowel content consistency will not require straining.
	Prevent seizure activity Administer anticonvulsant therapy as prescribed. Administer anticonvulsant therapy in status epilepticus cases as indicated; specific agents include: • *phenytoin, 15-20 mg/kg* • *phenobarbital, 15-20 mg/kg* • *diazepam, 10-40 mg*	Patient will be seizure free, or seizures will be controlled rapidly once evident.
	If seizure activities occur, protect airway, support breathing, supply oxygen, and place in side-lying position when feasible. Plan for possible intubation, especially if large doses of anticonvulsant are needed.	Patient will be without injury related to seizures. SpO_2 will not decrease for an extended period.
	Assess and report the character of the seizure activity including: • presence and nature of aura; • presence of tonic/clonic activity; • body parts where movement began; • presence of diaphoresis, abnormal respiratory patterns, and incontinence; • presence of eye deviation.	Character of seizure will be fully recorded.

Nonpharmacologic therapy

Hyperventilation/ventilation Experimental research has shown that (1) the immediate response to head injury is cerebral vessel dilation and (2) a state of relative hyperemia with uncoupling of the tissue metabolic needs and CBF results. It has also been shown that CO_2 responsiveness of the brain remains intact in all but the most severe head injuries. The advent of $AVDO_2$ monitoring may help diagnose ischemic and hyperemic states and guide the titration of hyperventilation in relation to CBF and tissue metabolic needs. (Walleck, 1989).

Hyperventilation makes use of CO_2 reactivity to decrease cerebral blood volume, thereby decreasing ICP in hyperemic states (Spielman, 1981). Controlled ventilation with intubation is instituted to maintain a $Paco_2$ of 25 to 30 mm Hg acutely (Geisler & Salcmam, 1987). Reduction of $Paco_2$ to 25 to 30 mm Hg produces cerebral vasoconstriction to reduce CBV and therefore reduce ICP. Reduction in $Paco_2$ below 20 mm Hg may result in severe vasoconstriction and ischemia (Jagger & Bobovsky, 1983). The effects of hyperventilation on cerebral vessel diameter may last only 3 to 4 hours before adaption occurs. Hyperventilation should never be discontinued abruptly, because rebound cerebral vessel dilation may occur (Geisler & Salcman, 1987). In addition to hyperventilation for Pco_2, adequate oxygenation should also be assured to maintain PO_2 greater than 80 mm Hg, because hypoxemia can result in cerebral vessel dilation.

Maintenance of an adequate airway in the intubated patient requires suctioning for removal of secretions. In the ED, hyperventilation may be initiated by manual bagging until intubation is performed. Hyperextension of the neck to open the airway is contraindicated until a cervical spine fracture is ruled out. Although suctioning to maintain an airway is necessary, suctioning has been correlated with increases in ICP. Theories regarding the cause of ICP elevation during suctioning include cerebrovascular dilation in response to hypoxemia or hypercarbia and prevention of cerebral venous outflow as a result of increasing intrathoracic pressure with coughing (Rudy, Baun, Stone, & Turner, 1986). Exaggerated ICP responses to suctioning have been reported for a group of patients with various ICP values (Tsementzis, Harris, & Loizou, 1982). A review of the literature reveals disparity in the degree of ICP rise with suctioning, the mechanism for rise in ICP, and preventive treatment (Kocan, 1988). Until research provides a clearer basis, some potential interventions include careful monitoring of the patient's own baseline, performing suctioning for secretion control only, limiting suction time to 15 seconds, and hyperoxygenating and reducing $Paco_2$ by bagging the patient with 100% oxygen before each suction catheter pass (Parsons & Shogan, 1984). Research indicates that reduction of the cough reflex may prevent increases in ICP that occur with suctioning (Rudy et al., 1986). Lidocaine (1.5 mg/kg) may be given prophylactically to prevent ICP elevations in response to suctioning (Yano et al., 1986). In the unconscious patient, extra care must be taken to provide an adequate airway. A side-lying position may prevent aspiration of pooled secretions.

Hypothermia Hypothermia reduces the cerebral metabolic rate by 7% per degree centigrade (Ward, Moulton, Muizelaar, & Marmarou, 1987). Hypothermia is used as an adjunctive method to decrease ICP. The rectal or core temperature may be reduced to approximately 31° C (88° F) with a cooling blanket. Shivering may occur with hypothermia and may be treated with chlorpromazine 5 to 25 mg IV every 8 hours or 50 mg IM every 6 to 8 hours (Jagger & Bobovsky, 1983). Use of hypothermia as a treatment requires continuous EKG monitoring because cardiac dysrhythmias may occur. Nursing management also includes skin assessment to prevent cold burns and altered tissue integrity.

Cerebrospinal fluid drainage If an intraventricular catheter is used to monitor ICP, CSF drainage can be used as treatment for increased ICP. Drainage of CSF decreases total volume in the brain, which reduces ICP. It is theorized that removal of CSF also promotes the movement of white matter edema into the ventricles, providing a continuous and prolonged effect on ICP (Jagger & Bobovsky, 1983). The nurse must secure the CSF collection chamber to an IV pole to prevent rapid lowering (i.e., dropping to the floor), which results in rapid fluid drainage and ICP changes, which can cause tissue shifting and hemorrhage.

Drainage of CSF is usually done according to a specific prescription written by the neurosurgeon. Drainage is usually conducted against a pressure gradient of 15 to 20 cm CSF, which corresponds to an ICP pressure gradient of 11 to 15 mm Hg (1 cm = 1.36 mm Hg). This pressure gradient is established by raising the CSF collection chamber 15 to 20 cm above the patient's external auditory canal. Monitoring the ICP waveform is usually done continuously, and drainage is conducted intermittently for specific ICP values. An example of this is draining (often referred to as venting) CSF if ICP >15 mm Hg for 3 minutes. Intermittent drainage is done briefly to prevent rapid CSF removal and ventricular collapse. After venting CSF, the nurse should reevaluate the ICP waveform and the amount of CSF drainage.

Turning and positioning Nurses caring for patients who have ICP monitoring devices placed have often noted various individualized ICP responses to such interventions as changing the elevation of the head of the bed, turning the patient, performing range of motion, changing dressings, performing physical assessments, and conversing with the patient. Several investigations have been conducted for the purpose of creating definitive statements about the effects of these interventions. These studies have used small samples, patients with different pathologic processes, and varied research methodologies, making global statements difficult to develop.

The findings of early investigations examining the relationship between head elevation and ICP have indicated that ICP may be lowered with head elevation (Kenning, Toutant, & Saunders, 1981; Parsons & Wilson, 1984; Synder, 1984). Promotion of cerebral venous drainage was theorized to account for the reduction in ICP (Mitchell, 1986). This theory has been challenged by Rosner and Coley's (1986) finding that although ICP decreases with head elevation, CPP also significantly decreases as the result of arterial blood pressure decline, and that these CPP reductions are associated with the generation of pathologic ICP waves. Rosner and Coley hypothesize that patients with elevated ICP have already used cerebral venous blood displacement to the maximal capacity in an effort to compensate for the increase in the intracranial contents and are therefore the least likely to benefit from head elevation. March, Mitchell, Grady, and Winn (1990) found that the CPP and ICP response to head elevation varies for each patient. A practical approach to decision making for the patient without an ICP monitoring device includes analyzing

blood pressure and clinical neurologic response to head elevation. Patients who are dehydrated, in myocardial or septic shock, on mechanical ventilation, or who have received medications that cause hypotension may be at greatest risk to experience a reduced CPP from head elevation.

Mitchell and Mauss (1978) and Mitchell, Ozuna, and Lippe (1981) found that head-injured patients tend to experience an increase in ICP associated with being turned in bed but that the degree is individualized. Boortz-Marx (1985) also reported ICP elevations with turning, but these increases were not significant. Parsons and Wilson (1984) studied a group of patients with ICP ≤15 mm Hg and CPP ≥50 mm Hg and concluded that these patients may be safely turned. Head rotation and neck flexion/extension have consistently been demonstrated to increase ICP (Hulme & Cooper, 1976; Shalit & Umansky, 1977; Mitchell & Mauss, 1978; Parsons & Wilson, 1984; Boortz-Marx, 1985). Patients should be turned to minimize pulmonary and skin complications unless turning results in clinical deterioration, significant increases in ICP, or increases in ICP that do not return to baseline within a few minutes. Some practical suggestions are to make the turn as comfortable as possible by having enough assistance, turning the patient gently and slowly, and avoiding manipulation of limbs with fractures, pressure on wounds or injuries, tension on tubing or equipment (e.g., ventilator, indwelling catheter), and neck flexion/extension or head rotation during the turn. The same principles apply for other nursing care activities. In addition, routine nursing care should be planned to allow for rest periods. Mitchell et al. (1981) found that a cumulative increase in baseline ICP occurred when activities were spaced at 15-minute intervals. No baseline ICP increase occurred when activities were spaced at 1-hour intervals.

Pharmacologic therapy

Diuretics Osmotic diuretics reduce total body water content by establishing an osmotic gradient. It is theorized that extraction of tissue water across the blood-brain barrier reduces total intracranial volume to reduce pressure and increase compliance (Cascino et al., 1983). Mannitol may be given as a rapid infusion in emergency situations or infused over 10 to 20 minutes as a maintenance drug. The onset of action occurs in 10 to 15 minutes with a duration of 2 to 3 hours. Mannitol may also decrease blood viscosity and therefore improve perfusion as fluid shifts from the tissue to the vascular compartment (Muizelaar, Lutz, & Becker, 1984). Mannitol is the osmotic diuretic most commonly used for the treatment of increased ICP. The usual dose for mannitol is 0.5 to 2 mg/kg every 4 to 6 hours; however, it is titrated to individual needs. Mannitol is excreted by the kidneys, and because it reduces total body water content, it changes serum electrolytes and osmolality. Laboratory values are obtained frequently to monitor for hypernatremia, hyperosmolality, and elevation in blood urea nitrogen and creatinine (Heinemeyer, 1987). Therapy may be discontinued for a serum osmolality greater than 320 mOsm/L to prevent renal failure. Lasix (furosemide) may be given to lengthen the time between mannitol doses to prevent hyperosmolarity (Ward, Moulton, Muizelaar, & Marmarou, 1987). Renal failure has been reported in patients with increased serum osmolality (Goldwasser & Fotino, 1984). Mannitol is usually decreased gradually, while monitoring the patient's neurologic status for rebound edema.

Furosemide is used as an adjunct to osmotic diuresis. Furosemide reduces total body water by inhibiting renal tubular reabsorption of sodium and chloride. Furosemide may also decrease secretion of CSF (Buhrley & Reed, 1972). Unlike mannitol diuresis, furosemide produces an isotonic water loss, which may be less effective in reducing ICP (Cascino et al., 1983). Furosemide and mannitol are often used in combination. Animal experiments suggest that combination therapy may be more effective in reducing ICP (Millson, James, Shapiro, & Laurin, 1981).

Barbiturates It is theorized that barbiturates reduce ICP and protect the brain from ischemic injury by reducing metabolic tissue demands and oxygen consumption. It is theorized also that barbiturate therapy provides diversion of blood flow to ischemic areas and stabilizes neuronal membranes (Piatt & Schiff, 1984). Pentobarbital may be given as an initial bolus dose of 5 to 10 mg/kg and then titrated to a blood level of 35 to 45 mg/dl. Barbiturate therapy is used in conjunction with other therapies geared toward decreasing ICP. In some centers it is used only for high ICP levels that have not responded to other interventions (Bowers & Marshall, 1982). Barbiturate therapy in intracranial hypertension not responsive to other therapies has been shown to decrease

ICP (Eisenberg, Frankowski, Contant, Marshall, & Walker, 1988). In a randomized study comparing barbiturate therapy with mannitol therapy, no significant effect on outcome occurred for either therapy (Schwartz et al., 1984). It has been suggested that barbiturate therapy is best instituted as part of a combination therapy approach (James, 1980). It must be remembered that administration of barbiturates will result in an unreliable bedside neurologic assessment, as well as cause difficulty in determining brain death. In addition, barbiturates may cause hypotension that requires fluid or vasopressor therapy.

Recently, interest has been shown in the role of narcotic sedation to decrease metabolic tissue demands. The effect of narcotic sedation on cerebral blood vessel diameter is not known (Walleck, 1989). Further research is needed to clarify the role of barbiturate therapy and narcotic sedation in head injury.

Steroids Dexamethasone has been used routinely in the treatment of cerebral edema. Evidence of effectiveness is established in reducing focal cerebral edema caused by primary and metastatic brain tumors. Doses of 1 to 2 mg/kg/day are recommended to reduce ICP (Heinemeyer, 1987). Recently, questions have been raised as to the efficacy of steroids in reducing generalized ICP that occurs with head injury (Clifton, 1986). Studies of both low- and high-dose steroids in preventing cerebral edema associated with head injury have failed to demonstrate benefit. Administration of steroids may result in infection, syndrome of inappropriate antidiuretic hormone release (SIADH), and hyperglycemia (Harper, 1988). Research regarding the appropriate dosage and timing of initial dose on the reduction of edema in head injury is needed (Braughler & Hall, 1985).

Anticonvulsants The role of anticonvulsants in the prevention of posttraumatic seizures is a controversial issue. Conditions that place a patient in a high-risk-for-seizure category are (1) early (first week) seizures, (2) intracranial hematomas, and (3) depressed skull fracture (Narayan, 1989). Penetrating injuries, injuries involving the motor cortex, and genetic predisposition to seizure disorders also place the patient in a high risk category (Caveness et al., 1979).

If anticonvulsants are prescribed, the nurse must be knowledgable in administration. Phenytoin may be administered as a loading dose of

1000 mg and maintenance dosage of 300 to 400 mg/day to achieve a blood level of 10 to 20 mg/dl. Phenytoin may not be administered intravenously at a rate exceeding 50 mg/minute. Intravenous phenytoin is compatible in normal saline only. Phenobarbital may not be administered intravenously at a rate exceeding 60 mg/minute.

Complications of Head Injury

Survivors of head injury are often faced with a long and difficult recovery in rehabilitation. Sustained neurologic deficits alter the life of the patient and significant others. The most extreme cases of poor neurologic outcome after head injury are found in those patients in the persistent vegetative state and those who are brain dead.

Persistent vegetative state

The syndrome of the persistent vegetative state (PVS) is the result of severe brain damage. The PVS may occur weeks after both traumatic and nontraumatic brain injury. The patient in a PVS appears to be awake, because the eyes open spontaneously and demonstrate random movement, although they do not demonstrate purposeful visual pursuit. Motor responses consist of primitive and reflex movements seen as withdrawal or posturing responses (Zegeer, 1981). These motor patterns may occur spontaneously or in response to pain and loud environmental noise. The patient does not make meaningful verbalizations, but may groan. Respiratory patterns may vary and become increasingly labored and noisy with stimulation. The patient may have periods of sleep and relative awakeness. Thus, although the patient may appear to be awake, no neurologic signs suggest cognitive function or meaningful awareness (Berrol, 1986).

The continuation of aggressive medical and nursing interventions for the patient in the PVS poses a difficult ethical dilemma for caregivers and significant others (Flaherty, 1982). Thomasma and Brumlik (1984) propose that case-by-case decisions rather than universal policy be used for decision making. Health care professionals and families may benefit from advice and support that can be obtained through discussion with members of a bioethical committee.

Brain death

Despite health team interventions, some patients will not survive a head injury and brain death will occur. Most states have statutes or judicial decisions that allow physicians to determine death based on clinical evidence of irreversible cessation of brain function. Statutes do not usually list the criteria for determination of brain death, but rather require that the practitioners use accepted medical standards in decision making (Guidelines for the Determination of Death, 1981). The practice of neurologists and neurosurgeons varies greatly regarding the declaration of brain death, particularly in the assessment of brainstem function (Black and Zervas, 1984). The determination of brain death, however, requires three major criteria: a known cause for coma is established; the metabolic and toxic causes for coma are explored and ruled out; and no evidence of brainstem functioning exists (Pitts, 1984). Two separate clinical assessments, separated by a designated period of time, are required for the determination of brain death. Brainstem reflex responses used to determine brain death are listed in Table 10-8. Diagnostic tests that may be

---

Table 10-8 Brainstem reflex responses used to determine brain death

Reflex	Finding supportive of brain death
Pupillary light	No pupil constriction to light stimulus
Oculocephalic	No eye movement when head is briskly rotated to either side or when the neck is flexed or extended
Oculovestibular	No eye movement to ice water irrigation of either ear
Cough	No cough in response to endotracheal suctioning
Gag	No soft palate elevation and pharyngeal contraction in response to pharyngeal stimulation
Corneal	No eyelid closure in response to irritation of the cornea with a moist cotton swab
Respiratory	Refer to apnea testing in the box on p. 300.

Table 10-9 Diagnostic tests used to support or confirm brain death

Test	Finding
Electroencephalography (EEG)	Absence of electrical activity; however, artifact-free EEGs difficult to obtain in ICU
Cerebral angiography	Absence of cerebral blood flow
Intracranial pressure monitoring	Cerebral perfusion pressure equal to zero
Radioisotope brain scan	Absence of cerebral blood flow
Transcranial Doppler studies	Absence of cerebral blood flow
Brainstem auditory evoked potentials	Loss of all but wave I; test not reliable when damage to hearing occurs with injury or was present before injury

used to support or confirm the determination of brain death are listed in Table 10-9. A complete example of a brain death protocol is found in the box on p. 300 (Barelli et al., 1990; Belsh, Blatt, & Schiffman, 1986; Earnest, Beresford, & McIntyre, 1986; Kaufman & Lynn, 1986; Outwater & Rockoff, 1984).

According to the Mandatory Donation Request Act, in most states the next of kin must be approached for organ donation. This may be done by the primary physician, although in some states the request may not be elicited by the physician pronouncing brain death. Acceptance by the general public, as well as health care providers, of the organ donation process lags behind the requirements of the Mandatory Donation Request Act (Ross, Nathan, & O'Malley, 1990). Organ donations can be lost in any one of several stages of the organ donation process. The greatest number are lost because the family denies consent; next, consent to donate is not requested of the family; and finally, the state of brain death goes unrecognized or undeclared by health professionals (The Partnership for Organ Donation, 1991). Research by the Kentucky Organ Donor Affiliates indicates that the timing and sequence of information given to families impact their decision.

The process of "decoupling," or separating the request for donation from the notification of death, has improved the consent rates (see Appendix D). The coordinated efforts of physicians, nurses, social workers, chaplains, and organ donor organization representatives are of utmost importance to family integrity and successful organ donation. The members of the organ procurement team have much experience in tactful, objective discussion with family and are a useful resource for health team members, as well as family.

VISION

This section of the chapter deals with specific injuries to the eye that cause cellular damage, pain, and loss of vision, either permanently or temporarily. Disorders that are discussed are blow-out and blow-in fractures; penetrating injuries/globe rupture and enucleation; hyphema; and burns to the eye.

Mechanism of Injury

The eye and its many components can be injured by several mechanisms of injury. In general, these injury mechanisms are categorized into groups related to cause of the injury. The groups are mechanical, light/heat, and chemical, as they relate to causal energy sources. Mechanical energy sources account for the majority of eye injuries. This category can be further divided into three subcategories: blunt trauma, penetrating trauma, and foreign bodies. Blunt trauma mechanisms of injury are characterized by either flat or rounded objects hitting the orbit with damaging speed, or the head itself coming in contact with a stationary object at a damaging speed. Blunt injuries may include direct injury to the globe or to the surrounding bony and muscular structures of the orbit. A stray baseball striking a person in the eye could be termed a blunt trauma. Penetrating injuries include those injuries in which the orbit is actually entered by a sharp object or projectile. An example of a penetrating injury is an ice pick deliberately stabbed into the globe of a person during an altercation. Foreign bodies, especially glass fragments from a motor vehicle crash, can cause damage to the eye by scraping or abrading the corneal surfaces or even damaging the internal structures of the eye.

The eye is very sensitive to intense light sources, such as the sun and welding machines. It

Protocol for the diagnosis of brain death

The brain death examination should be performed only after the patient has been observed in the hospital for a minimum of 6 hours and meets all criteria listed in Treatable Causes of Coma Assessment (section A below). Two clinical examinations of responsiveness and brainstem reflexes (sections B & C below) are required and must be performed by separate examiners. The examinations must be a minimum of 2 hours apart. Apnea testing (section D below) must be performed once.

Mandatory testing	Clinical evaluations	
	#1	#2
A. Treatable causes of coma assessment		
1. Etiology of coma known	_____	_____
2. Serum electrolytes, glucose, and pH within normal limits	_____	_____
3. Body temperature above 32.2° C (90° F)	_____	_____
4. Systolic blood pressure above 90	_____	_____
5. Absence of drugs or alcohol, which would impair responsiveness	_____	_____
B. Responsiveness		
1. No spontaneous movements and no evidence of posturing or shivering	_____	_____
2. No response to painful stimulation (supraorbital pressure)	_____	_____
C. Brainstem reflexes and responses		
1. Light-fixed pupils	_____	_____
2. Absent corneal reflexes	_____	_____
3. Absent gag with pharyngeal stimulation	_____	_____
4. Absent cough with tracheal stimulation	_____	_____
5. Absent ocular response to head turning (no eye movement)	_____	_____
6. Absent ocular response to irrigation of ears with 50 ml iced water (no eye movement)	_____	_____
D. Apnea testing		
1. Absent spontaneous respiratory effort when $Paco_2$ greater than 60 torr* $Paco_2$ at end of apnea test		_____

*Before testing, an effort should be made to normalize blood gases based on the patient's history. Monitor oxygen saturation with continuous pulse oximetry. Disconnect patient from ventilator; administer oxygen at 12 L/min via endotracheal catheter. Observe for respiratory efforts for a maximum of 10 minutes. Place patient back on ventilator if cardiac rhythm changes, if any spontaneous respiratory efforts occur, or if 10 minutes has elapsed. Draw arterial blood gases before replacing patient on ventilator.

Nonmandatory testing

	#1	#2
A. Additional supporting laboratory investigations (not required)		
1. EEG shows electrocerebral silence.	_____	_____
2. Dynamic nuclear brain scan shows absence of cerebral blood flow.	_____	_____
3. Angiogram shows absence of cerebral blood flow.	_____	_____
4. Evoked potentials are absent.	_____	_____
B. Comments:		

is also vulnerable to injury from intense heat sources, such as flash burns and explosions. Although heat and light are grouped together for discussion, intense light may cause damage to the cornea and retina, whereas heat sources usually account for external tissue damage and corneal trauma.

Chemicals that are corrosive in nature can have an effect on the outer corneal layer of the eye. Strong acids or bases may emulsify or damage these sensitive tissues, as well as the soft tissues surrounding the globe itself. These injuries usually happen as a result of chemical spills or splashes. Many of these injuries take place in industrial or home settings.

Anatomic and Physiologic Considerations
External eye

Many of the structures of the eye that are readily visible on assessment are protective mechanisms for the eye itself. The entire orbit is surrounded by the lids and soft tissue, which protect the globe from small foreign bodies and mild blunt trauma. The eyelashes also serve to keep out unwanted small particles, such as dirt and small glass fragments. The lacrimal glands lubricate the eyes with tears, which also can flush out foreign bodies that have gotten past the lids and

lashes. The bony orbital rims provide protection for the globes by forming a "shield" around the eye. The bony rims protect the eyes from more formidable blunt trauma than the soft tissue. It must be noted that these bony rims are often fractured in blunt trauma. Because the muscles involved in movement for the eye are attached here, eye motion and position may be impaired when injuries occur (Figure 10-19).

The cornea is the outer lining of the globe itself. It is very sensitive to tactile stimulation. Nerve endings in the cornea and the lids initiate the blink reflex when stimulated—another protective mechanism. The cornea is often the point of injury in many mechanisms of injury. The conjunctiva rests on top of the cornea to provide an extra measure of protection.

Internal eye

The internal structures of the eye are primarily responsible for vision. Light passes through the cornea, anterior chamber, iris and pupil, lens, and the posterior chamber to be projected onto the retina, which senses the image. The image is then transmitted to the brain via the optic nerve. The iris is the colored part of the eye, which acts as a shutter to control the amount of light entering the eye. The lens expands and contracts un-

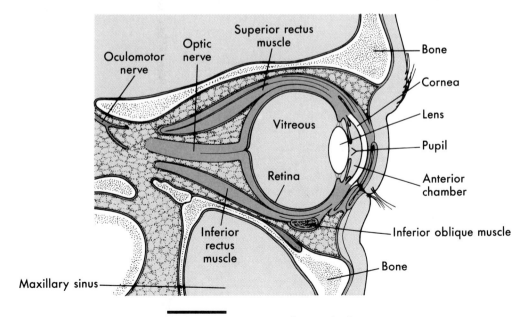

Figure 10-19 Anatomy of eye and orbit.

Table 10-10 Functions of the ocular muscles

Muscle	Primary action	Secondary action
Lateral rectus	Abduction	None
Medial rectus	Adduction	None
Superior rectus	Elevation	Adduction, intorsion
Inferior rectus	Depression	Adduction, extorsion
Superior oblique	Depression	Intorsion, abduction
Inferior oblique	Elevation	Extorsion, abduction

Note: From *General Ophthalmology* (8th ed.) (p. 195) by D. Vaughn and T. Asbury, 1977, Los Altos, CA: Lange Medical Books.
Intorsion, Inward rotation; *extorsion,* outward rotation.

Table 10-11 Paired primary muscle movements responsible for the six cardinal directions of gaze.

Cardinal direction of gaze	Paired response "yoke" muscles
Eyes up, right	Right superior rectus and left inferior oblique
Eyes right	Right lateral rectus and left medial rectus
Eyes down, right	Right inferior rectus and left superior oblique
Eyes down, left	Right superior oblique and left inferior rectus
Eyes left	Right medial rectus and left lateral rectus
Eyes up, left	Right inferior oblique and left superior rectus

Note. From *General ophthalmology* (8th ed.) (p. 195) by D. Vaughn and T. Asbury, 1977, Los Altos, CA: Lange Medical Books.
Straight up or down gaze is not considered a cardinal direction, since no single pair of yoke muscles are involved.

der muscular control to focus the image on the retina. The canal of Schlemm is responsible for maintaining adequate pressures within the anterior chamber (aqueous humor). Many penetrating injuries are responsible for providing a passage for leakage of aqueous humor or vitreous humor. This pressure-regulating system may also be damaged in blunt trauma. Vision loss may be attributed to injuries to these functional areas of the eye, as well as nerve injuries, such as a hematoma within the optic nerve sheath or other injuries.

The orbit is pyramidal in shape and contiguous with many sinuses. It is completely formed between 7 years of age and puberty. The eye itself constitutes approximately one third of the orbital volume (Rootman, 1988). The major arterial supply to the orbit is the ophthalmic artery, which arises from the internal carotid artery near the optic nerve. Injury to the cavernous sinus can lead to a carotid-cavernous arteriovenous fistula from a penetrating injury that nicks the carotid artery, or from blunt trauma with basillar skull fracture (Rootman & Graeb, 1988). Posterior orbital injury can result in CSF leaks, since its periosteum is continuous with the dura. Within the orbit six striated extraocular muscles exist, which work together to allow the six cardinal directions of gaze. Each movement of the eye depends on the cooperative function of all the muscles; however, it is helpful to know the primary and secondary actions of the muscles and understand the coordinated paired primary movements that contribute to a full range of eye motion (Tables 10-10 and 10-11).

General Assessment

Nursing assessment measures for the patient with an eye injury include a description of the injury by the patient and a description of the eye, including redness, swelling, position of the globe, movements of the eye, shape of the pupil, presence of opacities or penetrating objects, and condition of the lid. Any bleeding or discharge from the eye should be described. Sensation to the face should also be assessed to detect fifth nerve damage. The patient should be asked to describe any eye pain or irritation and provide a description of visual impairments. Visual acuity is a key assessment parameter.

The nurse should also assess for the presence of hard or soft contact lenses or foreign bodies by looking at the eye tangentially with a light. Hard contacts may be removed by suction or by widely opening the patient's eyes and then closing them with mild pressure around the contact. Suction is the preferred method if foreign bodies or penetrating injury is suspected. Soft contacts may be lifted off the eye by grasping the lens with the index finger and thumb. The nurse should follow the assessment parameters as therapy is instituted.

Diagnostic and Monitoring Procedures

Three diagnostic procedures that the emergency nurse should be able to perform with competence are visual acuity readings, fluorescein staining, and intraocular pressure readings with a tonometer.

Visual acuity

Visual acuity readings are necessary to provide a baseline for the patient assessment in the emergency setting and should be performed as soon as possible within the nursing assessment. In certain cases the visual acuity reading may not be practical—as in a severe penetrating injury. However, the baseline should be established when feasible.

The acuity can be measured by distant, near, or gross vision testing. For distant vision the Snellen eye chart is used to determine visual functioning compared with normal vision at 20 feet. The chart is read by the standing or seated patient at a 20-foot distance. If the patient can read at 20 feet what the normal eye can read at 40 feet, the visual acuity is 20/40. Acuity is measured in each eye separately and then together. Near vision is measured with a pocket chart, such as the Rosenbaum vision screener, which functions in the same manner as the Snellen chart, but is adapted for use at 14 inches from the nose. This is useful when standing is contraindicated or if the patient cannot safely or reasonably be transported to a distant vision chart (Seidel, Ball, Dains, & Benedict, 1990). Gross visual testing is used when the patient is not successful with near or distance testing or when equipment or time does not allow use of such charts. It is also useful in penetrating injury or suspected globe rupture because it allows limited vision testing without further accommodation and eye movement, which might be detrimental to the eye (Neff, 1991). The box (upper right) demonstrates the methods for documenting visual acuity.

Fluorescein staining

In contrast to visual acuity readings, fluorescein staining is used to diagnose abrasions, small cuts, burns, or small ulcers on the cornea. The deformities on the cornea will absorb the stain and be visible as bright yellowish green areas when a cobalt blue light is directed toward the stained eye. To optimally perform the procedure, the nurse should request an order to topically

---

Methods of documenting visual acuity (Va) testing

$$Va \; \overline{sc} \; 20 \Big/ \frac{30 - 1}{50 + 2}$$

- Va without correction at 20 feet
- Right eye (OD) 30-foot equivalent, missed 1
- Left eye (OS) 50-foot equivalent, plus 2 correct from next smallest line 20/40

$\overline{cc}$ = with correction (glasses/contacts)
$\overline{c}$ PH = with pinhole correction
CF @ 5 feet = Right eye can count fingers at 5-foot distance
HM @ 2 feet = Hand motion detected at 2-foot distance
LP = Light perception present

Note. From "Patient Care Guidelines: Visual Acuity Testing by J. Neff, 1991, *Journal of Emergency Nursing*, 17 (6), 431-436.

OD, Right eye; *OS,* left eye; *OU,* both eyes; *CF,* count fingers; *HM,* hand motion; *LP,* light perception.

---

anesthetize the injured eye. A fluorescein strip is removed from its sterile, single-use package, and the end of the strip is moistened with sterile saline. The lower lid is pulled down slightly, and the strip is touched to the inner sac of the lower eyelid. The patient is asked to blink to distribute the stain. The examination is performed in a darkened room with the cobalt blue light.

Intraocular pressure

Intraocular pressure is measured using a tonometer. Tonometers come in two versions—the manual type, in which a manual plunger is touched to an anesthetized cornea; and an electronic type, in which the end of an electronic sensor is touched to the anesthetized cornea. Great care must be taken by the person performing the examination because of the possibility of injuring the eye. After the eye is anesthetized, the examiner should explain the procedure to the patient and place the patient in a reclining position. The sterile tonometer should be touched gently to the eye until a reading can be ascertained. The mechanical type of tonometer, such as the

Schiøtz measurement of indentation, is read by looking at the pointer/scale apparatus and converting the reading to millimeters of mercury (mm Hg). The electronic tonometer gives a digital reading. A normal reading is between 11 and 22 mm Hg (Kanski, 1989).

The nurse must be familiar with each of these diagnostic procedures to provide information for the nursing assessment, as well as the medical examination.

General diagnostic studies for orbital/ophthalmologic injury include basic plain film radiographs, including Caldwell and Waters views of the orbits and a lateral view for foreign body detection and assessment of bony defects. These are important, since clinical signs and symptoms may suggest fracture but may reflect only edema and hemorrhage (Rootman & Neigel, 1988). The continued improvement in computed tomography imaging and the lesser radiation dose and greater soft tissue definition in comparison with regular tomograms have made CT the imaging choice for orbital bone and soft tissue anatomy. Orbital vascular structures can be seen without intravenous contrast, but contrast may be requested. Angiography is essential for evaluation of arteriovenous fistulas. Magnetic resonance imaging is costly but is noninvasive, allows a variety of views without patient repositioning, and is less affected by artifact from such items as dental fillings (Nugent, Rootman, & Robertson, 1988).

Assessment and Interventions Related to Specific Injuries
Blunt injuries

Blunt injury to the eye may create superficial or deep hematomas, abrasions, and structural damage to the surrounding bone, muscle, and the eye itself. The most severe blunt damage may occur from injuries that result in accompanying fractures or significant hemorrhage.

Blow-out/Blow-in fractures	Sensory/perceptual alteration, visual
	Pain
	Anxiety
	High risk for infection

Blow-out fractures result from forceful, indirect, blunt trauma to the orbital soft tissue. The sudden rise in orbital hydraulic pressure generated by the trauma results in herniation of periorbital tissue through the weakest part of the orbital rim, the orbital floor, and into the maxillary sinus (Holt & Holt, 1988). The mechanism of injury is depicted in Figure 10-20. Muscle, nerve, and blood vessel damage may be produced by tissue shifts and bone fragments. Also, hematoma formation and edema around the optic nerve may impair vision. However, surgical decompression of the optic nerve sheath has been demonstrated to restore vision in some cases (Guy, Sherwood, & Day, 1989)

The typical clinical picture of a severe blow-out fracture includes enophthalmos (recession of the eye into the orbit), paralysis of upward gaze, numbness over the cheek, and ipsilateral nose bleeding (Elkington & Khaw, 1988) (Figure 10-21). Patients with minor blow-out fractures may not have these signs and symptoms and hemorrhage may temporarily mask enophthalmos. The only symptom a patient with a minor blow-out fracture may have is abrupt inflation of periorbital tissue with air upon nose blowing (Forrest, Schuller, & Strauss, 1989). Enophthalmos occurs as a result of herniation or fibrosis of the supportive periorbital fat tissue or increase in orbit capacity caused by outward movement of the walls (Rowe, 1984). Paralysis of upward gaze occurs with entrapment or laceration of the inferior rectus muscle. Restriction of eye movements causes diplopia (double vision), because the eyes "see" two different objects at one time. Damage to the infraorbital nerve, which passes through the floor of the orbit, results in sensory changes over the cheek. The diagnosis of a blow-out fracture can be made by x-ray studies in 90% of the cases (Melamed, 1988). Nursing assessment includes evaluation of visual acuity, as well as observation for the clinical indicators just described. The patient with a suspected blow-out fracture should be cautioned against nose-blowing, which raises intraocular pressure and can cause further damage.

Surgical repair for blow-out fractures is indicated when eye movement is restricted and when extensive bony fragments cause significant movement of the globe or diplopia. The need for surgical repair is decided 5 to 15 days after the injury, when tissue edema has subsided. A forced reduction maneuver, in which the eye is anesthetized and the globe manually elevated, is per-

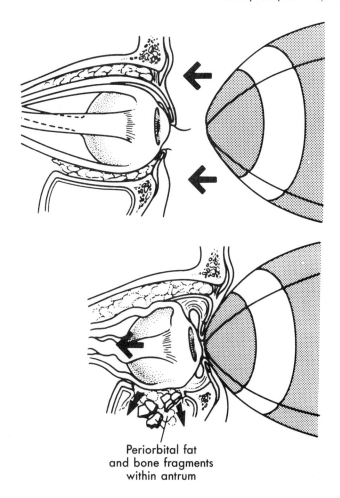

Periorbital fat
and bone fragments
within antrum

Figure 10-20 Blunt trauma produces sudden increase in pressure that forces soft tissue through weak bony floor of orbit into maxillary sinus. (*Note.* From *Otolaryngology: Head and Neck Surgery* [7th ed.] [p. 218] by D.D. DeWeese, W.H. Saunders, D.E. Schuller, and A.J. Schleuning II, 1988, St. Louis: Mosby–Year Book, Inc.)

formed. Restriction of eye movement indicates that bony fragments or tissue continues to cause compression, whereas a freely elevated eye indicates that a nerve palsy occurred. Enophthalmos (inward protrusion) greater than 2 mm requires surgical manipulation of the posterior orbit to prevent/reduce damage to the optic nerve (Deutsch & Feller, 1985).

A much rarer type of blunt injury to the eye is "blow-in" fracture, which, in contrast to the blow-out fracture, is commonly the result of high-velocity blunt trauma to the bony orbital rim

(Antonyshyn, Gruss, & Kassel, 1989; Chirico, Mirvis, Kelman, & Karesh, 1989). The result of high-velocity trauma to the orbit is inwardly displaced bone fragments, which cause increased pressure in the orbital cavity, leading to exophthalmos. Although most blow-in fractures occur from traumatic fractures of the orbital roof, several cases of blow-in fractures have been documented from medial orbital rim and orbital floor fractures. The primary differences between blow-in and blow-out fractures involve the high-velocity impact and the inwardly displaced bone fragments, which can

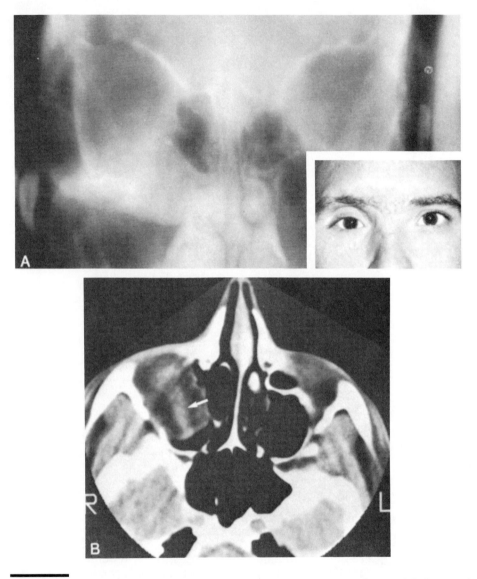

Figure 10-21 Signs of blow-out fracture. Clinical photograph shows right enophthalmos and globe ptosis. Upper polytomography film shows blow-out fracture. Lower axial CT scan shows inferior rectus muscle and surrounding fat herniating through defect *(arrow).* (*Note.* From The Clinical Evaluation and Pathology of Tumors of the Eye, Orbit and Lacrimal Apparatus by J. Rootman. In S.E. Thawley [Ed.], *Comprehensive Management of Head and Neck Tumors* [Vol. 2], 1987, Philadelphia: W.B. Saunders.)

result in a higher incidence of globe injuries, including globe rupture and optic nerve damage. Antonyshyn et al. (1989) found that approximately 12% of patients with blow-in fractures incurred globe rupture. Of these, 12% subsequently required enucleation as a result of complications.

Orbital roof fractures are dangerous because they are more associated with intracranial hemorrhage, CSF leakage, and optic nerve damage. The associated force often results in brain concussion or laceration, necessitating a combined team approach (ophthalmology and neurosurgery). Optic nerve trauma may be the result of contusion, deceleration, fracture, compression, or even intracranial damage. Visual loss and pupillary reaction are important to monitor, since immediate loss is usually irreparable, whereas delayed or progressive loss may respond to steroids and/or decompression (Rootman & Neigel, 1988).

Hyphema   Sensory/perceptual alteration, visual
　　　　　　　Pain
　　　　　　　Anxiety
　　　　　　　High risk for infection

Hyphema refers to blood accumulation in the anterior chamber of the eye in front of the iris (Figure 10-22). Hyphema is produced by vessel rupture with both blunt and penetrating eye injuries. It may appear as a crescent-shaped hemorrhage in the bottom of the eye if the patient is in a sitting position or may spread over the eye if the patient is supine. Small hemorrhages may resolve in days without treatment. Larger hemorrhages cause compression damage and require bedrest and immobilization of the eyes by patching. Surgical evaluation may be required. Blood breakdown products may raise intraocular pressure by disrupting the filtering system of the eye and therefore result in vision loss (Holt & Holt, 1988). If hyphema accompanies a penetrating injury, bleeding may increase because of pupillary dilation during inspection for foreign bodies.

Bleeding between the conjunctiva (mucous membrane lining of the eye and reflected onto the eye) and the eye itself is termed *subconjunctival hemorrhage*. Subconjunctival hemorrhage, unlike hyphema, does not change patterns with position changes and does not obscure the iris. Subconjunctival hemorrhage occurs commonly with eye injury, but rarely leads to further damage unless it is associated with a large hematoma ele-

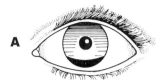

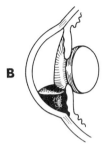

Figure 10-22   Typical hyphema. **A,** Anterior view showing meniscus-like appearance. **B,** Sagittal view of typical hyphema. (*Note.* From *Essentials of Emergency Medicine,* [p.559] by P. Rosen, R. Barkin, and G. Sternbach, 1990, St. Louis: Mosby–Year Book, Inc.)

vating the lid from the eye. Eye lubrication is then implemented to prevent corneal dryness and irritation.

Penetrating injuries

Penetrating eye injuries carry a great risk for some degree of permanent vision loss as a result of mechanical injury, inflammation, or infection. LaRoche, McIntyre, and Schertzer (1988) found that in the pediatric population, penetrating injuries resulted in some degree of blindness in 40% of the cases. In the pediatric population, eye injury is often caused by unsafe toys or unsafe play. In the adult population, penetrating injuries can be related to occupational injuries (welding, hammering metal) or violence (poker, the nail of a thumb in the eye, the ring on the first finger). Penetrating injuries may occur also with motor vehicle accidents and gunshot wounds (Figure 10-23).

Creative eye patching may be necessary when objects are impaled in or near the eye. An elevated container, such as a paper cup, may need to be secured over the object, and both eyes may need to be patched. A semipressure patch should not be used if a foreign body is present or suspected (Karesh, 1989; Newell, 1985).

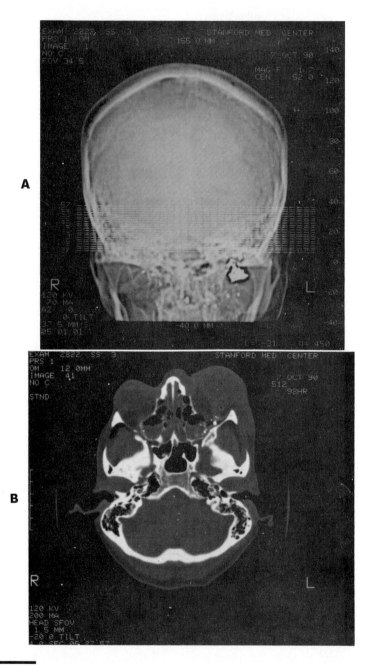

Figure 10-23 Penetrating injury from gunshot wound of right cheek and palate with bullet lodging behind left eye. **A,** Frontal view of head and face showing bullet fragments in left orbit area. **B,** CT scan showing extreme exophthalmus (protrusion) of left eye caused by edema and hemorrhage with intact globe. (Courtesy Stanford Trauma Service, Stanford University Hospital, Stanford, CA.)

If the entry wound is small, it may be concealed by subconjunctival hemorrhage; therefore careful history taking is essential. If the patient is unconscious, a wound through the eyelid should raise clinical suspicion of a penetrating injury. In some instances the object may protrude from the eye or the iris may protrude from the wound. In cases of shotgun wounds to the eye, Ford and Barr (1990) cite pellet fragmentation as a significant consequence. The authors note that in these cases, one entrance wound and more than one exit wound are noted on detailed surgical inspection of the globe. Although this type of injury is rare, detailed surgical inspection is imperative.

Globe rupture   Sensory/perceptual alteration,
                                     visual
                                 Pain
                                 High risk for injury
                                 High risk for infection
                                 High risk for body image
                                     disturbance

In penetrating injuries, the danger always exists that a foreign body is lodged deeply within the eye or that the globe has been ruptured. Proper immobilization of both eyes by patching is a priority in early management. On careful examination, seepage of aqueous fluid from the anterior chamber may be noted (Figure 10-24). If the patient is alert, he or she will complain of vision loss in the affected eye and severe pain, and the pupil may be distorted because of loss of eye substance. After dilating the pupil to examine for foreign objects, the ophthalmologist may palpate the globe to assess for softness of the eye, which suggests globe rupture. Surgical removal of penetrating fragments may be required. In some cases, small metallic fragments may be removed with a 20-gauge intraocular, electromagnetic-tipped instrument through a pars planar scleral incision (May, Noll, & Muno, 1989). Infectious endophthalmitis (intraocular infection) after penetrating injury is a great threat to any remaining vision because of inflammation and retinal necrosis. Penetrating injuries are usually treated with prophylactic antibiotics (Schemmer & Driebe, 1987).

Globe rupture may result in vitreous humor herniation and prolapse of the eye. The vitreous humor that is no longer contained may cause irritation of nerves not only of the injured or "exciting" eye, but also the unaffected or "sympathizing" eye. Sympathetic ophthalmia refers to the inflammation of the nerves of the unaffected eye and is a form of uveitis. Sympathetic ophthalmia usually occurs from 5 days to 2 months after globe rupture, but may take years to manifest. Early evidence (within 10 days) of sympathetic ophthalmia in a patient with a severely injured sightless eye requires enucleation of the injured eye to spare vision of the uninjured eye. Once inflammation in the sympathizing eye is advanced, enucleation is not recommended, because the injured eye may retain greater visual acuity than the sympathizing eye (Asbury, 1989); Yanoff and Fine, 1989).

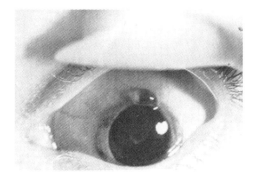

Figure 10-24 Aqueous fluid seeping from anterior chamber after penetration by foreign body. (*Note.* From *Emergency Nursing: A Comprehensive Review* [p. 349] by M.K. Fincke and N.E. Lanros (Eds.), 1986, Rockville, MD: Aspen Publishers.)

Foreign bodies   Pain
                                   High risk for infection

Cinders, dirt, glass, or dust may lodge in the conjunctiva or cornea. The patient will complain of discomfort that is aggravated by movement of the eyelid. The patient also may experience lacrimation or blepharospasm. Superficial debris may be detected by (1) darkening the room, (2) having the patient close the eyes, and (3) gently placing a penlight on the eyelid to look for foreign bodies. The foreign material will show up as black shadows. Superficial debris may be detected also by everting the upper or lower eye lid (Figure 10-25). The nurse should also inspect the eyebrows and hair line for foreign bodies that may fall into the eyes. Superficial debris can be removed by irrigation with normal saline, gentle re-

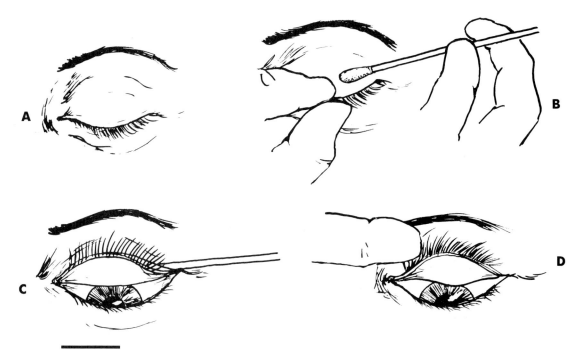

Figure 10-25 Method for lid eversion to inspect eye and remove foreign bodies. **A,** Eyelid closed. **B,** Placement of cotton swab (eyelashes pulled down and back over swab). **C,** Eyelid everted over swab. **D,** Examination of inside of eyelid and eye.(*Note.* From *Emergency Nursing: Principles and Practice* [ed 3] by S.B. Sheehy, 1992, St. Louis: Mosby–Year Book, Inc.)

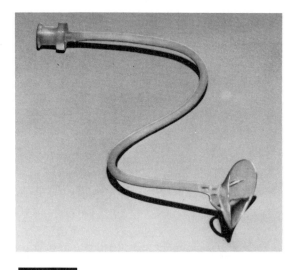

Figure 10-26 Morgan therapeutic lens with molded scleral cup and tubing that can be attached to continuous irrigation system. (Courtesy MorTan, Inc., Missoula, MT.)

moval with a moistened cotton swab, or powerful small vacuum. A commercial irrigation system, the Morgan lens, is available for sustained eye irrigations, once obvious debris is removed (Figure 10-26). This device is a molded scleral lens (like a contact lens) with attached silicone tubing through which irrigation fluid can be delivered. This system allows for continuous irrigation at a constant flow rate. Rubbing of the eye by either the patient or the nurse should be avoided to prevent corneal abrasion. If foreign bodies are not easily removed by irrigation, an ophthalmologist should be consulted, because the material may be embedded in the cornea.

Corneal abrasion is the major complication of foreign body removal. Eye patching may be necessary once it is assured that no foreign particles or substances remain. Semipressure patches are used to reduce irritation. Both eyes should be patched, because movement in one eye causes involuntary reciprocal movement in the other. Tape or an elastic headband is used to secure the patches.

Burns Pain
Sensory/perceptual alteration, visual
High risk for injury
Anxiety
High risk for body image disturbance

Burns to the eye may occur from ultraviolet radiation exposure or from contact with physical and chemical agents. Common sources of ultraviolet radiation exposure are welding, home sunlamps, tanning salons, or the sun itself. Long-term ultraviolet light exposure can lead to permanent thinning of the corneal epithelium (Walters & Kelley, 1987). Physical agents such as a flame or a curling iron may cause thermal injuries, which are often limited to the corneal epithelium (Bloom, Gittinger, & Kazarian, 1986). Chemical injuries to the eye may be produced by occupational exposure, housecleaning (e.g., splashing cleaning agents), or abusive incidents. Acidic substances are neutralized by the by-products of the damaged cell; therefore the injury is superficial but may result in altered vision. Alkaline substances cause much more damage to the eye than acidic substances, because they are not readily neutralized. Alkaline substances penetrate deeply in the eye causing necrosis. Scarring usually results regardless of treatment. In addition, the damage can worsen days after the injury (Melamed, 1988). Alkali burns result in corneal ulceration seen as an opacified lesion.

Treatment of corneal injury caused by ultraviolet exposure is symptomatic. Pressure patching is done to prevent further irritation of the cornea with eyelid movement. Prophylactic antibiotic and anesthetic eyedrops may be prescribed for a few days. Cycloplegic eyedrops, which can paralyze the ciliary muscle, may be given to prevent iris adhesions that may adhere to the lens (Bloom et al., 1986). The treatment of physical injuries secondary to thermal contact is similar to that for ultraviolet exposure. Eye exposure to chemical agents should be treated with copious irrigation. Normal saline is the preferred treatment and is used in the hospital setting, but any source of available water (e.g., water fountain, sink) should be used in the field. The eyelids should be held apart during irrigation. Sources differ on the length of time needed for irrigation, but indicate that 2 hours may be required (Pfister & Koski, 1982). Newer irrigation systems, such as the molded scleral lens, allow for irrigations to be continued for up to 24 hours or longer. In addition, the molded scleral lens allows for more complete irrigation of the eye than manual methods (Figure 10-27). Topical anesthetics are given to reduce discomfort and facilitate compliance (Deutsch & Feller, 1985).

General Interventions
Protection and prevention

Primary prevention of eye injuries is an important nursing goal, because many eye injuries may be caused by lack of knowledge by the public. Protective sunglasses that prevent ultraviolet radi-

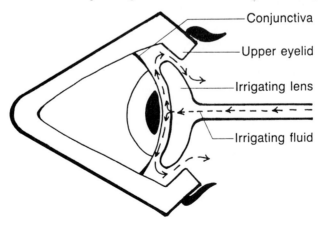

Figure 10-27   Eye irrigation with molded scleral lens. (*Note.* From Eye Irrigation [p. 412] by J. Neff. In M.E. Mancini and J. Klein (Eds), *Decision Making in Trauma Management*, 1991, Philadelphia: B.C. Decker.)

ation should be worn during exposure with tanning and outdoors activities. Although many people may be aware of the discomfort caused by ultraviolet radiation, they may not realize the damaging effects of long-term exposure. Parents should be cautioned to prevent their children's exposure to toys with sharp edges, as well as aggressive play activities near the face. It has been suggested that dangerous play objects carry a developmentally appropriate warning label (like the *Mr. Yuck* sticker, which is placed on harmful chemicals) to aid consumers in choosing toys (LaRoche et al., 1988). Occupational health nurses should inform employees of risks to chemical, thermal, or particulate exposure and develop policies and procedures that include appropriate protective eye wear. In the ED, however, nursing measures are directed at educating those patients to be discharged and promoting comfort and safety.

Patient education	Knowledge deficit related to discharge instructions
	Pain, related to eye injury
	Sensory/perceptual alteration, visual

Patients who will be wearing pressure patches require demonstration and return demonstration of the patch application because too much pressure can lead to further irritation and too little pressure can result in eye opening and rubbing against the patch (Figure 10-28). Patients should be taught that patching of one eye results in loss of depth perception, which may affect safe driving and ambulation. Analgesic eyedrops are avoided before examination because they may mask symptoms or cause damage with open fractures. The correct technique for instilling eyedrops should also be taught by demonstration and return demonstration. Eye pain may be reduced by administering systemic analgesics and by the use of cycloplegic agents, which reduce the pain of ciliary body inflammation. Administration of topical anesthetics promotes comfort, but patients should be instructed to avoid continued use of these after discharge, since healing is delayed, protective reflexes are hindered, and symptoms of further damage may be masked. Controlling the environment by reducing the light in the room will also promote comfort. Nursing interventions are presented in detail in the table on pp. 313-314.

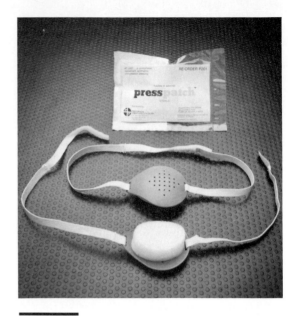

Figure 10-28   Commercial eye patch system that consists of soft inner pad and hard cover. System is held in place by elastic headband. It is useful in unconscious trauma patients or those with corneal abrasions, but pressure patch should not be used in presence of hyphema, penetrating injury, or undiagnosed eye injury. (Courtesy Precision Therapeutics, Inc., Las Vegas.)

If permanent vision loss occurs as the result of the eye injury, the patient may need referral to the American Association for the Blind for rehabilitation and support services. The loss of vision is an anxiety-producing event, and nursing support may help ease the stress. Patient care during hospitalization will likely require significant referral to and consultation from community resources because acute blindness is not a common condition.

Complications
Impaired vision

Eye injuries may lead to complications that are severe and permanent in nature, although many injuries have less devastating effects. Of course the major complication that results from eye injury is loss of vision. Loss of vision can be defined on a continuum anywhere from a slight acuity or visual field deficit to total blindness. Loss of vision can be caused by damage to the cornea, which is irreparable, and by injury to the lens sys-

The trauma patient with sensory/perceptual alteration (visual)

Nursing diagnosis	Nursing intervention	Evaluative criteria
Sensory/perceptual alteration, visual Related to disruption of optic nerve, disruption of cornea or retina, release of vitreous humor, entrapment of ocular muscle As evidenced by decreased visual acuity, nonintact extraocular movement, visible foreign body or substance, puncture wounds, tissue destruction	**Maintain visual acuity** Instruct patient to lie still, thus preventing further injury. Stabilize injured eye by using protective patch or other method. Use hearing and touch as methods of communicating information to the patient.	Visual acuity will be maintained at baseline or above. Patient will gain information through use of other senses.
	Remove superficial foreign bodies Irrigate eye with saline for 5 to 15 minutes, and longer if chemical exposure. Lift the foreign body off the eye with a moistened swab or by the use of suction. Evert the lid by grasping the lashes of the upper lid, exerting a downward pull while gently applying pressure on upper lid with a cotton swab and pulling the eye lid over the cotton swab. If the foreign body is not easily removed, place an elevated cover (i.e., cup) over the eye to prevent any pressure until an ophthalmologist examines the patient. If an object is impaled into the eye, immobilize both eyes immediately and place an elevated cover over the eyes. Have fluorescein strips available for staining and ultraviolet light for visualization.	Sources of injury will be eliminated. Eye will be thoroughly and completely assessed.
High risk for injury Related to inappropriate eye movement, swelling, intraocular pressure changes, foreign substances, altered depth perception, loss of visual field	**Promote stabilization of injured eye** Properly patch or stabilize injured eye as ordered/appropriate. Keep patient still during procedures. Keep side rails up and call light within reach in a standard place. Have significant other stay in room with patient. Apply ice compresses first 24 hours. Teach patient about loss of depth perception with monocular vision. Caution against use of continued anesthetic drops at home. Instruct regarding eye patch application.	Visual acuity will not decrease below baseline. Eye will have no obvious further injuries. Patient will not experience physical injury as the result of altered vision.

Continued.

Nursing diagnosis	Nursing intervention	Evaluative criteria
High risk for infection Related to manipulation of eye, exposure to solutions, contamination from the scene and/or instrument of injury	**Maintain aseptic precautions** Use sterile irrigation solutions and setups. Use sterile instruments. Use sterile bandaging/patching techniques when possible. Use good hand-washing techniques. Instruct patient to keep hands away from injured eye. Administer antibiotics as ordered. Administer tetanus prophylaxis as ordered. Provide instructional resources to teach patient or significant other techniques for eyedrop or ointment administration.	Injured eye will not become contaminated. No infection will develop. Injured eye will have no drainage, edema, redness. Patient will give return demonstration of correct technique for administration of eye medications.
High risk for pain Related to ocular pressure, irritation, nerve entrapment, tissue swelling	**Promote comfort** Stabilize injured eye. Apply ice, if ordered. Keep patient's head elevated slightly. Reduce environmental light when possible. Ask patient to lie still. Anesthetize eye with ophthalmic solution, if ordered; warn the patient that some pain will return once the effects of the topical agents wear off. Administer ordered antiinflammatory agents, analgesics, and cycloplegic agents.	Patient will report a decrease in pain. Patient will demonstrate increased relaxation, as evidenced by facial expression, normal heart rates and respiratory rates. Patient will report decreased photophobia. Patient will develop greater tolerance of irrigation with less squinting and blinking.
High risk for anxiety, powerlessness Related to cause of injury, long-term visual prospects, current altered visual acuity	**Promote relaxation and support understanding of status and procedures by patient** Speak to patient in mild voice tone. Keep room lighting dim. Involve appropriate significant others in care. Explain procedures thoroughly. Decrease pain by administering topical anesthetics and analgesics if ordered. Ensure clear understanding of short-term and long-term visual acuity status.	Patient will report a decrease in anxiety. Patient will demonstrate a calm and composed state. Patient will demonstrate involvement in care and instigate discussions.

tem or collection of blood within the anterior or posterior chamber. Loss of vision can be caused by injury to the retina or by injury to the optic nerve. Complete visual impairment can also be caused by acute head injury or a pathologic condition in which the optic centers are affected. Visual anomalies such as diplopia can be caused by damage to the bony or muscular structures of the orbit. Globe rupture, sympathetic ophthalmia, and traumatic enucleation can completely destroy vision in the injured eye.

Blunt and penetrating trauma to the eye can also involve injury to Schlemm's canals, which regulate intraocular pressures. Any blockage or impairment of these canals may cause increased intraocular pressure. When intraocular pressure is sufficiently elevated to cause visual damage, glaucoma exists. Patients who have glaucoma as a complication of injury may require surgery and/or long-term medication therapy (Vaughan, 1989).

Cataracts may be caused by lens damage from an intraocular foreign body or, less commonly, from contusion, heat, or radiation exposure. They may also occur when blood staining persists from vitreous hemorrhage. An acute vitreous bleed can be detected by slit lamp examination and should be monitored. The vitreous is inelastic, and even a contusion can result in acute or long-term retinal tears or detachment.

Infection

The risk of infection is always a concern when related to eye injury. The more severe the injury, the greater the chance of infection. Also, the immune system is compromised increasingly as more body systems are added to the injury list. In short, the patient is at a double risk of infection, because the primary defense to pathogens, the epithelium, has been broken and the immune system may be compromised to a greater or lesser extent. Many potential infection sources are encountered by the patient even before arrival in the treatment area. However, the nurse can lessen the chances of infection by observing good aseptic technique and hand-washing procedures. Instruments must be sterile in all situations. Prophylactic antibiotics may be ordered topically, orally, or intravascularly—depending on the physician's preference and the extent of the injury. The major pathogens involved in eye infections are bacteria such as *Staphylococcus* and *Psuedomonas*. However, herpesvirus infections have also been transmitted to patients with eye injuries.

SUMMARY Numerous complications may result from injuries that impact responsiveness—from infection and seizures to brain death. The risk of persistent vegetative states and the significant rehabilitative issues surrounding injury to the brain evoke the critical need for professional, informed nursing care.

Significant life-style changes can result from impairment of responsiveness and vision. Both the brain and the eye are at risk of damage from blunt and penetrating trauma to the head or face. Utmost attention must be given to their protection and support during trauma assessment and intervention.

COMPETENCIES

The following clinical competencies pertain to **caring for the patient with traumatic injury affecting responsiveness and/or vision.**

☑ Identify signs of a malfunctioning intracranial pressure monitoring system and the actions to be taken to correct the malfunction, using the policies and procedures of the individual organization.

☑ Describe or demonstrate interventions that will protect the patient in status epilepticus, using the organization's nursing care standards.

☑ Demonstrate psychosocial skills in crisis intervention when interacting with the family/significant other(s) of the patient with a head injury.

☑ Provide accurate and complete information regarding the signs and symptoms requiring immediate action on the part of the patient/family/significant other when discharging a patient from the ED, using the guidelines developed by the individual organization.

☑ Identify priority interventions in the patient with acute intracranial hypertension, based on clinical knowledge of interventions and rationale, standing orders or written protocol, and the nurse practice act.

☑ Recognize the signs and symptoms of neurologic deterioration, including pupillary size, shape, and reactivity; level of consciousness; motor and cranial nerve assessment; respiratory patterns; ICP and CPP trends and abnormal values; and vital sign trends and abnormal values for the patient.

☑ Perform a visual acuity examination, using both the Snellen eye chart and the pocket chart.

☑ Properly patch an injured eye.

☑ Instill ophthalmic solutions and ointments according to physician orders.

☑ Irrigate/flush an eye using normal saline or other solution.

☑ Adapt patient education/discharge instructions to facilitate compliance by the visually impaired patient.

CASE STUDY A A 21-year-old man was working at a construction site and fell through the flooring, impaling himself on a 1-inch, uncapped, reinforced steel bar (rebar) below the flooring and was left hanging from the second floor level. The rebar penetrated his jaw and face and exited through his right orbit. After a lengthy extrication that required sawing the rebar to free him, the patient was flown to a trauma center. His pulse is 54; BP, 148/80; and RR, 20 with fair depth. He is awake, but quiet with a GCS score of 15 (Figure 10-29, A).

What are the most important areas for concern?

Airway patency is most important because of the proximity of the rebar to the patient's neck and the potential for hematoma expansion, plus the oral bleeding from the impaled rebar and the risk of loose teeth. He is awake and breathing spontaneously, but is electively intubated by fiberoptic laryngoscope prophylactically. The movement of the rebar with deep breathing causes pain from the rebar, since each respiration raises his chest and torques the rebar within his face. A respiratory therapist adjusts the ventilator settings for the appropriate rate and tidal volume, and the patient is mildly sedated before and after the intubation. He receives an analgesic once the primary survey and CT scan is complete.

His cervical spine is not in alignment, but is maintained stable by the rebar, which extends from above his orbit to midchest level. Lateral cervical spine films are obstructed by the rebar.

The potential for intracranial injury must be ruled out. A quick view of the head by CT scan is done, and no intracranial involvement is demonstrated. The scan is suboptimal because of artifact from the rebar.

The cause of the patient's bradycardia is evaluated; the possibility of a vasovagal attack is considered initially, but his blood pressure is normal. It is considered most likely that the bradycardia is the result of pressure on the carotid artery.

Is immediate ophthalmology consult indicated?

Yes, the patient is stable and will be going to the operating room for removal of the rebar, so early examination of the orbit is indicated while the patient is awake and oriented and before the onset of orbital swelling. An ophthalmologist is part of the team of surgeons, which also includes surgeons who specialize in trauma surgery; ENT, head, and neck surgery; plastic surgery; and neurologic surgery.

Are other diagnostic studies needed?

Yes, angiography is indicated to determine whether vasculature in the neck is involved and to assist in planning removal of the rebar. Later in the hospital course, CT views of the orbits and face will be required.

What special precautions are needed intraoperatively?

Medications that could raise intraocular pressure should be avoided.

C-spine precautions must be maintained. This is provided by applying Gardner-Wells tongs and is especially beneficial in the process of removal of the rebar, which requires significant force. C-spine films are completed postoperatively, as well as further neurologic examination, and injury to the patient's C-spine is ruled out.

Blood products must be available in the event that vessels are injured during the removal of the bar. Discussion ensues about the technique to remove the bar, i.e., whether to pull it straight out or to try to twist it out, since the rebar has some cylindrical markings. A decision is made to use a steady, pulling force; this method proves successful, with no significant blood loss.

Infection is a significant concern because of gross contamination on the rebar, which penetrated through soft tissue and bone. Liberal intraoperative antibiotic flush is used, and systemic antibiotics were initiated in the ED.

How likely is it that the patient's eye will be uninjured, and what complications are possible?

Visual acuity of the right eye with the rebar cannot be ascertained. It is unknown how devastating the injury is. Personnel at the scene thought they saw cornea on the rebar. This leads to considerable discussion about the likelihood that the patient has lost his eye. Once the rebar is removed by the trauma surgeon, the ophthalmologist immediately assesses the orbit and finds that the eye is present and the globe is not ruptured (Figure

10-29, B). This is not uncommon, since the globe will move out of the way of penetrating items, although gunshot wounds and multiple glass shards create a different picture (Sugar, 1984). The surgery team continues to cleanse, drain, and dress the neck wound, and then the team focuses on the patient's eye. A complete examination is done and the lid lacerations sutured. By discharge, his vision is normal except for diplopia.

Had his eye been perforated or a foreign body retained, the potential for bilateral uveitis (sympathetic ophthalmia) and resulting blindness would exist.

Incidents such as these create a great deal of community interest. The local television station was in contact with the hospital news bureau and gained access to the patient and his family the following day to highlight his narrow escape from death and his amazing retention of vision. The patient has since had multiple reconstructive surgeries for the jaw and face and may have further plastic surgery on the eye, since it is slightly lower than the left (Figure 10-29, C). He has started training for a new career outside of construction site work and considers each birthday a "rebirthday."

CASE STUDY B Mary was an 83-year-old unrestrained passenger of a vehicle when it was involved in an accident. The vehicle was traveling at a speed of 25 mph when it hit a large oak tree on the side of the road. Medics report Mary was found fully alert and conscious and was complaining of severe right eye pain. On arrival to the ED she has blurred vision of her right eye and is now complaining of double vision. On inspection of the eye, the nurse finds that the right pupil and iris are difficult to differentiate because of hazy, red fluid in the anterior chamber of the eye. Mary's neurologic status deteriorates while on an in-patient unit 12 hours after injury.

What type of head injury does the mechanism of injury suggest in this case?

The age of the patient and delayed deterioration of neurologic status suggests acute subdural hematoma; however, epidural hematomas and contusions may present with delayed neurologic deterioration. Absence of open skull fracture or penetrating object suggests closed head injury.

What preventive measures should the nurse take when the patient arrives in the ED?

The nurse should prevent further injury by immobilizing the cervical spine until a fracture is ruled

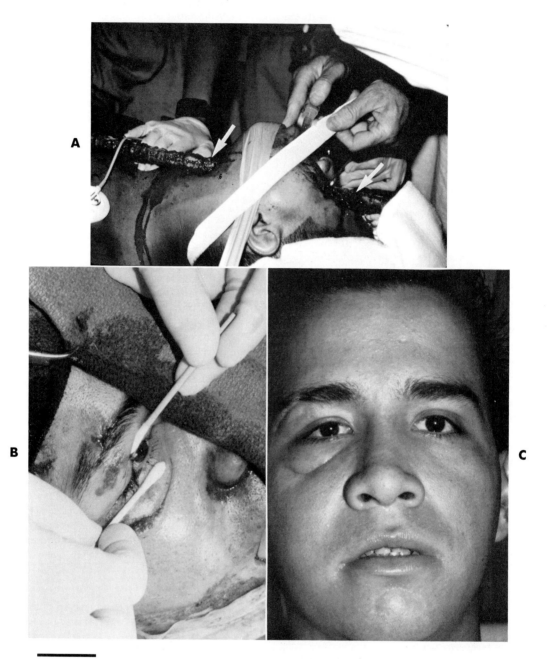

Figure 10-29 **A,** Impalement of right orbit by reinforced steel bar (rebar) after construction accident. Arrows point to rebar. (Gloves should be worn.) **B,** Intraoperative discovery of intact globe. **C,** Patient following rebar injury after hospital discharge. (Courtesy Stanford University Trauma Service, Stanford, CA.)

out by x-ray study. The patient's head should be elevated after spinal clearance to lower intraoccular pressure and possible increased ICP. Both eyes should be patched.

When should visual acuity evaluation be performed?

A visual acuity evaluation should be performed as soon as possible, but it should not interfere with prompt intervention. If the patient has an immobilized cervical spine, a pocket eye chart may be used, or gross visual acuity at a minimum.

RESEARCH QUESTIONS
Responsiveness

- Does a video displaying actual pathologic assessment findings (posturing, sluggish pupils) result in greater interrater reliability in nursing assessment than lecture with slides of abnormal assessment findings?
- Do audio taped recordings of familiar voices result in similar ICP changes as actual presence of familiar persons talking to the patient?
- Does the speed with which the patient is turned affect changes in ICP?
- Does implementation of a mild head injury support group/outpatient assessment clinic referral on discharge from the ED improve psychosocial adjustment?
- What is the most effective method(s) of community-based head injury prevention to reduce the incidence of head injury?

Vision

- Is instillation of antibiotic/analgesic eyedrops similar for patients with the head of the bed flat, elevated 15 degrees, and elevated 45 degrees?
- How frequently should an eye patch be removed for further assessment in the first 24 hours after injury?
- How does the patient with a visual loss perceive touch, smells, and hearing in the ED?
- How much pressure is generated to the eye with application of an eye dressing?
- Compare new premade eye patches with patches with tape.
- Does warmed eye irrigation solution, in contrast to room temperature solution, reduce the need for topical anesthetic?

RESOURCES
Responsiveness

American Association of Neuroscience Nurses
224 North Des Plaines, Suite 601
Chicago, IL 60661
(312) 993-0043

American Paralysis Association
7655 Old Springhouse Rd.
McLean, VA 22101
(703) 556-7782

American Speech-Language-Hearing Association
10801 Rockville Pike
Rockville, MD 20852

Epilepsy Foundation of America
4351 Garden City Dr.
Landover, MD 20785
(310) 459-3700

Family Survival Project for Brain-Damaged Adults
1736 Divisadero St.
San Francisco, CA 94115
(415) 921-5400

National Head Injury Foundation
18A Vernon St.
Framingham, MA 01701
(617) 879-7473

National Institute of Handicapped Research
U.S. Department of Education
Mail Stop 2305
Washington, DC 20202

Office of Scientific and Health Reports
National Institute of Neurological and Communicative
    Disorders and Stroke
Building 31, Room 8A06
National Institutes of Health
Bethesda, MD 20205
(310) 496-5751

Vision

American Foundation for the Blind
1100 17th St. NW
Washington, DC 20036

American Society of Ophthalmic Registered Nurses
PO Box 193030
San Francisco, CA 94119
(415) 561-8513

National Institute for Occupational Safety and Health
Robert A. Taft Laboratories
4676 Columbia Pkwy.
Cincinnati, OH 45226

ANNOTATED BIBLIOGRAPHY
Responsiveness

Cooper, P. (1987). *Head injury* (2nd ed.). Baltimore: Williams & Wilkins.
    Comprehensive reference on the subject of head injury. As Dr. Cooper states in the preface, the book is primarily directed to the practicing neurosurgeon; however, it is also a valuable reference for the practicing neuroscience nurse. Of special interest to the emergency nurse is the chapter on emergency care, which provides an excellent overview of the

initial assessment of the head-injured patient and a review of the role of hypoxia and shock in the contribution to secondary injury. This book is an extremely valuable reference for intracranial pressure monitoring because it contains three chapters devoted to the subject. The pathophysiology, diagnosis, and medical and surgical interventions, along with their rationale for the scope of practice related to acute care management of head injury, are well covered in this book. The authors seem to represent both academic and direct patient care points of view. Nursing care is not clearly delineated, but advanced concepts related to the interdependent aspects of clinical practice are easily inferred from the content of most chapters. This book is a "must" reference for nurses practicing in the trauma setting.

Hickey, J.V. (1986). *The clinical practice of neurological and neurosurgical nursing (2nd ed).* Philadelphia: J.B. Lippincott.

Book that contains information appropriate for basic reading. Includes a chapter on craniocerebral trauma and the multitrauma patient. Nursing care is detailed throughout the chapters and outlined in table format. The book also contains a chapter on anatomy and physiology and a chapter on assessment. The reference lists for these chapters reflect both nursing and medical literature.

Wirth, F.P., & Ratcheson, R.A. (Eds.) (1987). *Neurosurgical Critical Care: Vol. 1. Concepts in neurosurgery.* Baltimore: Williams & Wilkins.

Excellent reference for the neurotrauma nurse. The book is organized in a systems approach rather than neurosurgical diagnoses. The chapters are written by experts in the field of neurotrauma and provide both theoretical and clinical information. The reference lists for each chapter are extensive and provide opportunities for continued exploration of the topics. This text assumes understanding of neuroscience anatomy and physiology, as well as clinical experience in the field of neurosurgery, and therefore is challenging reading.

Vision

Deutsch, T.A. & Feller, D.B. (1985). Injuries of the eyes, lids and orbit. In Zuidema, G.D., Ruthford, R.B., & Ballinger, W.F. (Eds.), *Management of trauma (4th ed.).* Philadelphia: W.B. Saunders.

Extensive overview of eye injuries. This chapter contains the "A to Z" of eye injuries with detailed anatomic diagrams, radiographic pictures, and actual patient photographs. Medical and surgical management is discussed clearly and extensively. The chapter is an excellent reference for the trauma nurse. Nursing care, however, is not discussed as an entity of itself, and specific nursing interventions must be extrapolated from the content of the chapter. The reference list is limited for the content provided, but much of the chapter content seems to be based on both theoretical and clinical experience. This chapter provides a detailed overview worth reading.

REFERENCES

Aarabi, B. (1987). Comparative study of bacteriological contamination between primary and secondary exploration of missile head wounds. *Neurosurgery, 20,* 610-616.

Aarabi, B. (1988). Traumatic aneurysms of the brain due to high velocity missile head wounds. *Neurosurgery, 22* (6), 1056-1062.

Aaslid, R., Lindegaard, K.F., Sorteberg, W., & Nornes, H. (1989). Cerebral autoregulation dynamics in humans. *Stroke, 20* (1), 45-52.

Adams, J.H., Doyle, D., Ford, I., Gennarelli, T.A., Graham, D.I., & McLellan, D.R. (1989). Diffuse axonal injury in head injury: Definition, diagnosis, and grading. *Histopathology, 15,* 49-59.

Andrus, C. (1991). Intracranial pressure: Dynamics and nursing management. *Journal of Neuroscience Nursing, 23* (2), 85-92.

Antonyshyn, O., Gruss, J.S., & Kassel, E.E. (1989). Blow-in fractures of the orbit. *Plastic and Reconstructive Surgery 84,* 10-20.

Asbury, T. (1989). Uveal tract. In D. Vaughan, T. Asbury, & K. Tabbara (Eds.), *General ophthalmology* (12th ed.) (pp. 130-143). Norwalk, CT: Appleton & Lange.

Baigelman, W., & O'Brien, J.C. (1981). Pulmonary effects of head trauma. *Neurosurgery, 9,* 729-735.

Barelli, A., DellaCorte, F., Calimici, R., Sandroni, C., Proietti, R., & Magalini, S.I. (1990). Do brainstem auditory evoked potentials detect the actual cessation of cerebral functions in brain dead patients? *Critical Care Medicine, 18*(3), 322-323.

Belsh, J.M., Blatt, R., & Schiffman, P.L. (1986). Apnea testing in brain death. *Archives of Internal Medicine, 146,* 2385-2388.

Berrol, S. (1986). Considerations for management of the persistent vegetative state. *Archives of Physical Medicine and Rehabilitation, 67,* 283-285.

Bishop, B.S. (1991). Pathologic pupillary signs: Self-learning module (Part 2). *Critical Care Nurse, 11* (7), 58-67.

Black, P.M., & Zervas, N.T. (1984). Declaration of brain death in neurosurgical and neurological practice. *Neurosurgery, 15*(2), 170-174.

Bloom, S.M., Gittinger, J.W., & Kazarian, E.L. (1986). Management of corneal contact thermal burns. *American Journal of Ophthalmology, 102* (4), 536.

Blumberg, P.C., Jones, N.R., & North, J.B. (1989). Diffuse axonal injury in head trauma. *Journal of Neurology, Neurosurgery, and Psychiatry, 52* 838-841.

Boortz-Marx, R. (1985). Factors affecting intracranial pressure: A descriptive study. *Journal of Neuroscience Nursing, 17,* 89-94.

Bowers, S.A., & Marshall, L.F. (1982). Severe head injury: Current treatment and research. *Journal of Neurosurgical Nursing, 14,* (5), 210-218.

Brambella, G., Rainoldi, E., Gipponi, D., & Paoletti, P. (1986). Extradural hematoma of the posterior fossa: A report of eight cases and review of the literature. *Acta Neurochirurgica, 80,* 24-29.

Brandvold, B., Levi, L., Feinsod, M., & George, E.D. (1990). Penetrating craniocerebral injuries in the Israeli involvement in the Lebanese conflict, 1982-1985, *Journal of Neurosurgery 72,* 15-21.

Braughler, J.M., & Hall, E.D. (1985). Current application of "high dose" steroid therapy for CNS injury. *Journal of Neurosurgery, 62,* 806-810.

Bruce, D.A., Langfitt, T.W., Miller, D., Schutz, H., Vapalahti, M.P., Stanek, A., & Goldberg, H.I. (1973). Regional cerebral blood flow, intracranial pressure, and brain metabolism in comatose patients. *Journal of Neurosurgery, 38,* 131-144.

Buhrley, L.E., & Reed, D.J. (1972). The effect of furosemide on sodium-22 uptake into cerebrospinal fluid and brain. *Experimental Brain Research, 14,* 503-510.

Carey, M.E., Sarna, G.S., Farrell, J.B., & Happel, L.T. (1989). Experimental missile wound to the brain, *Journal of Neurosurgery, 71,* 754-764.

Carey, M.E., Tutton, R.H., Strub, R.L., Black, F.W., & Tobey, E.A. (1984). The correlation between surgical and CT estimates of brain damage following missile wounds. *Journal of Neurosurgery, 60,* 947-954.

Cascino, T., Baglivo, J., Conti, J., Szewczykowski, J., Posner, J.B., & Rottenberg, D.A. (1983). Quantitative CT assessment of furosemide- and mannitol-induced changes in brain water content. *Neurology, 33,* 898-903.

Caveness, W.F., Meirowsky, A.M., Berkeley, L.R., Mohr, J.P., Kistler, J.P., Dillon, J.D., & Weiss, G.H. (1979). The nature of posttraumatic epilepsy. *Journal of Neurosurgery, 50,* 545-553.

Changaris, D.G., McGraw, P.C., Richardson, J.D., Garretson, H.D., Arpin, E.J., & Shields, C.B. (1987). Correction of cerebral perfusion pressure and Glasgow coma scale to outcome. *Journal of Trauma, 27* (9), 1009-1011.

Chirico, P.A., Mirvis, S.E., Kelman, S.E., & Karesh, J.W. (1989). Orbital "blow-in" fractures: Clinical and CT features, *Journal of Computer Assisted Tomography, 13,* 1017-1022.

Clifton, G.L. (1986). Controversies in the medical management of head injury. In J. Little (Ed.), *Clinical neurosurgery: Proceedings of the Congress of Neurological Surgeons* (pp. 587-603). Baltimore: Williams & Wilkins.

Clifton, G.L., Robertson, C.S., Kyper, K., Taylor, A.A., Dhekne, R.D., & Grossman, R.G. (1983). Cardiovascular response to severe head injury. *Journal of Neurosurgery, 59* 447-454.

Cooper, P.R., & Ho, V., (1983). Role of emergency skull x-ray films in the evaluation of the head-injured patient: A retrospective study. *Neurosurgery, 13,* 136-139.

Crittenden, B.J., & Beckman, D.L. (1982). Traumatic head injury and pulmonary damage. *Journal of Trauma, 22,* 766-769.

Crosby, L., & Parsons, L.C. (1989). Clinical neurologic assessment tool: Development and testing of an instrument to index neurologic status. *Heart & Lung, 18,* 121-129.

Dacey, R.G., Alves, W.M., Rimel, R.W., Winn, R., & Jane, J.A. (1986). Neurosurgical complications after apparently minor head injury: Assessment of risk in a series of 610 patients. *Journal of Neurosurgery, 65,* 203-210.

Deutsch, T.A., & Feller, D.B. (1985). Injuries of the eyes, lids, and orbit. In G.D. Zuidema & R.B. Rutherford (Eds.), *The management of trauma* (4th ed.) (pp. 243-284). Philadelphia: W.B. Saunders.

Dodson, W.E., & Ferrendelli, J.A. (1987). Convulsive disorders and their management. In F.P. Wirth and R.A. Ratcheson (Eds.), *Neurosurgical critical care: Concepts in neurosurgery* (Vol. 1) (pp. 169-185). Baltimore: Williams & Wilkins.

Earnest, M.D., Beresford, H.R., & McIntyre, H.B. (1986). Testing for apnea in suspected brain death: Methods used by 129 clinicians. *Neurology, 36,* 542-544.

Edelsohn, L. (1986). Coma. *Primary Care, 13,* 63-69.

Eisenberg, H.M., Frankowski, R.F., Contant, C.F., Marshall, L.F., & Walker, M.D. (1988). High-dose barbiturate control of elevated intracranial pressure in patients with severe head injury. *Journal of Neurosurgery, 69,* 15-23.

Elkington, A.R., & Khaw, P.T. (1988). ABCs of eyes: Injury to the eye. *British Medical Journal, 297,* 122-125.

Enevoldsen, E.M., & Finn, T.J. (1978). Autoregulation and CO_2 responses of cerebral blood flow in patients with acute severe head injury. *Journal of Neurosurgery, 48,* 689-703.

Fisher, C.M., (1969). The neurologic examination of the comatose patient. *Acta Neurologic Scandinavica Supplementum 36,* 4-56.

Flaherty, M.J. (1982). Care of the comatose: Complex problems faced alone. *Nursing Management, 13,* 44-46.

Ford, J.G., & Barr, C.C. (1990). Penetrating pellet fragmentation: A complication of ocular shotgun injury. *Archives of Ophthalmology, 108,* 48-50.

Forrest, L.A., Schuller, D.E., & Strauss, R.H. (1989). Management of orbital blow-out fractures: Case reports and discussion. *American Journal of Sports Medicine, 17* (2), 217-220.

Franges, E.Z., & Beideman, M.E. (1988). Infections related to intracranial pressure monitoring. *Journal of Neuroscience Nursing, 20* (2), 94-103.

Friedman, W.A. (1983). Head injuries. *Clinical Symposia, 35* (4), 1-32.

Gade, G.F., Becker, D.P., Miller, J.D., & Dwan, P.S. (1990). Pathology and pathophysiology of head injury. In J.R. Youmans (Ed.), *Neurologic Surgery.* Philadelphia: W.B. Saunders.

Gardner, D. (1986). Acute management of the head injured adult. *Nursing Clinics of North America, 21* (4), 555-562.

Geisler, F.H., & Salcman, M. (1987). Respiratory system: Physiology, pathophysiology, and management. In F.P. Wirth & R.A. Ratcheson (Eds.), *Neurosurgical critical care: Concepts in neurosurgery* (Vol. 1) (pp. 1-50). Baltimore: Williams & Wilkins.

Gennarelli, T.A. (1982). Influence of the type of intracranial lesion on outcome from severe head injury. *Journal of Neurosurgery, 56,* 26-32.

Germon, K. (1988). Interpretation of ICP pulse waves to determine intracerebral compliance. *Journal of Neuroscience Nursing, 20,* 344-349.

Goldwasser, P., & Fotino, S. (1984). Acute renal failure following mannitol infusion: Appropriate response of tubuloglomerular feedback? *Archives of Internal Medicine, 144,* 2214-2216.

Guidelines for the determination of death. Report of the medical consultants on the diagnosis of death to the President's commission for the study of ethical problems in medicine and biomedical and behavioral research (1981). *Journal of the American Medical Association, 246,* 2184-2186.

Guy, G., Sherwood, M., & Day, A. (1989). Surgical treatment of progressive visual loss in traumatic optic neuropathy. *Journal of Neurosurgery, 70,* 799-801.

Harper, J. (1988). Use of steroids in cerebral edema: Therapeutic implications. *Heart and Lung, 17* (1), 70-75.

Heinemeyer, G. (1987). Clinical pharmacokinetic considerations in the treatment of increased intracranial pressure. *Clinical Pharmacokinetics, 13,* 1-25.

Hickey, J.V. (1986). *The clinical practice of neurologic and neurosurgical nursing* (2nd ed.). Philadelphia: J.B. Lippincott.

Hollingworth-Fridlund, P., Vos, H., & Daily, E.K. (1988).

Use of fiberoptic pressure transducer for intracranial pressure measurements: A preliminary report. *Heart and Lung, 17,* 111-119.

Holt, G.R., & Holt, J.E. (1988). Management of orbital trauma and foreign bodies. *Otolaryngologic Clinics of North America, 21* (1), 35-52.

Hugenholtz, H., Stuss, D.T., Stethem, L.L., & Richard, M.T. (1988). How long does it take to recover from a mild concussion? *Neurosurgery, 22* (5), 853-857.

Hulme, A., & Cooper, R. (1976). The effects of head position and jugular vein compression on intracranial pressure: A clinical study. In J.W.F. Beks, D.A. Bosch, & M. Brock (Eds.), *Intracranial pressure II* (p. 259-263). New York: Springer-Verlag.

Ingersoll, G.L., & Leyden, D.B. (1988). The Glasgow coma scale for patients with head injuries. *Critical Care Nurse, 7* (5), 26-32.

Jagger, J.A., & Bobovsky, J. (1983). Nonpharmacologic therapeutic modalities. *Critical Care Quarterly, 5,* 1-11.

James, H.E. (1980). Combination therapy in brain edema. In J. Cervós-Navarro & R. Ferszt (Eds.), *Advances in neurology: Brain edema* (Vol. 28) (pp. 491-501). New York: Raven Press.

Jorden, R.C. (1983). Pathophysiology of brain injury. *Critical Care Quarterly, 5,* 1-12.

Kanski, J.J. (1989). *Clinical ophthalmology: A systematic approach* (2nd ed.). London: Butterworth.

Karesh, J.W. (1989). Ocular and periocular trauma. *Emergency Medical Service, 18*(6), 46-55.

Katz, R.T., & Kaplan, P.E. (1985). Glucose oxidase sticks and cerebral fluid rhinorrhea. *Archives of Physical Medicine and Rehabilitation, 66,* 391-393.

Kaufman, H.H., & Lynn, J. (1986). Perspectives on neurosurgical practice: Brain death. *Neurosurgery, 19*(5), 850-856.

Kay, T. (1988). Mild head injury: An overview of clinical manifestations and research agenda. *Trends in Rehabilitation, 3,* (3), 10-17.

Kenning, J.A., Toutant, S.M., & Saunders, R.L. (1981). Upright patient positioning in the management of intracranial hypertension. *Surgical Neurology, 15,* 148-152.

Kocan, M.J. (1988). *Effects of endotracheal suctioning in patients with intracranial hypertension.* Unpublished manuscript, University of Pennsylvania, School of Nursing, Philadelphia.

Kraus, J.F., & Nourjah, P. (1988). The epidemiology of mild, uncomplicated brain injury. *Journal of Trauma, 28* (2), 1637-1643.

LaRoche, G.R., McIntyre, L., & Schertzer, L. (1988). Epidemiology of severe eye injuries in childhood. *Ophthalmology, 95* (12), 1603-1607.

Lehman, L.B. (1990). Intracranial pressure monitoring and treatment: A contemporary view. *Annals of Emergency Medicine, 19,* 295-303.

Levin, H.S., & Eisenberg, H.M. (1988). Postconcussional syndrome. *Neurotrauma Medical Report, 2* (4), 1-3.

Levin, H.S., Williams, D.H., Crofford, M.J., High, W.M., Eisenberg, H.M., Amparo, E.G., Guinto, F.C., Kalisky, Z., Handel, S.F., & Goldman, A.M. (1988). Relationship of depth of brain lesions to consciousness and outcome after closed head injury. *Journal of Neurosurgery, 69,* 861-866.

Levin, H.S., Williams, D.H., Valastro, B.S., Eisenberg, H.M., Crofford, M.J., & Handel, S.F. (1990). Corpus callosal atrophy following closed head injury: Detection with magnetic resonance imaging. *Journal of Neurosurgery, 73,* 77-81.

Livingston, F.H., Loder, P.A., Koziol, J., & Hunt, C.D. (1991). The use of CT scanning to triage patients requiring admission following minimal head injury. *Journal of Trauma, 31,* 483-487.

Lundberg, N. (1960). Continuous recording and control of ventricular fluid pressure in neurosurgical practice. *Acta Psychiatrica Scandinavica, 36* (Supp. 149), 1-193.

Manifold, S.L. (1986). Craniocerebral trauma: A review of primary and secondary injury and therapeutic modalities. *Focus on Critical Care, 13* (2), 22-35.

March, K., Mitchell, P., Grady, S., and Winn, R. (1990). Effect of back rest position on intracranial and cerebral perfusion pressures. *Journal of Neuroscience Nursing. 22,* 375-381.

Marion, D.W., Darby, J. & Yonas, H. (1991). Acute regional cerebral blood flow changes caused by severe head injuries. *Journal of Neurosurgery, 74,* 407-414.

Marmarou, A., Maset, A.L., Ward, J.D., Choi, S., Brooks, D., Lutz, H.A., Moulton, R.J., Muizelaar, P., DeSalles, A., & Young, H.F. (1987). Contribution of CSF and vascular factors to elevation of ICP in severely head-injured patients. *Journal of Neurosurgery, 66,* 883-890.

Marshall, S.B., Cayard, C., Foulkes, M.A., Hults, K., Gautille, T., Charlebois, D.B., Tisdale, N.A., & Turner, H. (1988a). The traumatic coma data bank: A nursing perspective (Part 1). *Journal of Neuroscience Nursing, 20* (4), 253-257.

Marshall, S.B., Cayard, C., Foulkes, M.A., Hults, K., Gautille, T., Charlebois, D.B., Tisdale, N.A., & Turner, H. (1988b). The traumatic coma data bank: A nursing perspective (Part 2). *Journal of Neuroscience Nursing, 20* (5), 290-295.

Maset, A.L., Marmarou, A., Ward, J.D., Choi, S. Lutz, H.A., Brooks, D., Moulton, R.J., DeSalles, A., Muizelaar, J.D., Turner, H., & Young, H.F. (1987). Pressure volume-index in head injury. *Journal of Neurosurgery, 67,* 832-840.

May, D.R., Noll, F.G., & Muno, Z.R. (1989). A 20-Gauge intraocular electromagnetic tip or simplified intraocular foreign-body extraction. *Archives of Ophthalmology, 107,* 281-282.

Melamed, M. (1988). The injured eye at first sight. *Emergency Medicine, 20* (17), 18-22.

Miller, J.D., Murray, L.S., & Teasdale, G.M. (1990). Development of a traumatic intracranial hematoma after a "minor" head injury. *Neurosurgery, 27,* 669-673.

Millson, C., James, H.E., Shapiro, H.M., & Laurin, R. (1981). Intracranial hypertension and brain edema in albino rabbits. Part 2: Effects of acute therapy with diuretics. *Acta Neurochirurgica, 56,* 167-181.

Mitchell, P.H. (1986). Intracranial hypertension: Influence of nursing care activities. *Nursing Clinics of North America, 21* (4), 563-576.

Mitchell, P.H., & Mauss, N.K. (1978) The relationship of patient and nurse activity to intracranial pressure variations. *Nursing Research, 27,* 4-10.

Mitchell, P.H., Ozuna, J. & Lippe, H.P. (1981). Moving the patient in bed: effects on intracranial pressure. *Nursing Research, 30,* 212-218.

Muizelaar, J.P., Lutz, H.A., & Becker, D.P. (1984). Effect of mannitol on ICP and CBF and correlation with pressure autoregulation in severely head-injured patients. *Journal of Neurosurgery, 61,* 700-706.

Muizelaar, J.P., Marmarou, A., DeSalles, A.F., Ward, J.D., Zimmerman, R.S., Zhongchao, L., Choi, S.C., & Young, H.F. (1989). Cerebral blood flow and metabolism in severely head-injured children. *Journal of Neurosurgery, 71,* 63-71.

Muwaswes, M. (1985) Increased intracranial pressure and its systemic effects. *Journal of Neuroscience Nursing, 17* (4), 238-243.

Narayan, R.K. (1989) Emergency room management of the head-injured patient. In D.P. Becker & S.K. Gudeman (Eds.), *Textbook of head injury* (pp. 23-66). Philadelphia: W.B. Saunders.

Neff, J. (1991). Eye irrigation. In M.E. Mancini & J. Klein (Eds.), *Decision making in trauma management* (p. 412). Philadelphia: B.C. Decker.

Neff, J. (1991). Patient care guidelines: Visual acuity testing. *Journal of Emergency Nursing, 17* (6), 431-436.

Newell, S.W. (1985). Management of corneal foreign bodies. *American Family Physician, 31*(2), 146-156.

Nikas, D.L. (1987). Critical aspects of head injury. *Critical Care Nursing Quarterly, 10* (1), 19-44.

Nugent, R., Rootman, J., & Robertson, W. (1988). Applied investigative anatomy. In J. Rootman, *Diseases of the orbit,* (pp. 35-48). Philadelphia: J.B. Lippincott.

Obrist, W.D., Langfitt, T.W., Jaggi, J.L., Cruz, J., & Gennarelli, T.A. (1984). Cerebral blood flow and metabolism in comatose patients with acute head injury. *Journal of Neurosurgery, 61,* 241-253.

Ordog, G.J., Wasserberger, J., & Balasubramanian S. (1988). Shotgun wound ballistics. *Journal of Trauma, 28,* 624-631.

Outwater, K.M., & Rockoff, M.A. (1984). Apnea testing to confirm brain death in children. *Critical Care Medicine, 12*(4), 357-358.

Overgaard, J., & Tweed, W.A. (1976). Cerebral circulation after head injury. Part 2: The effects of traumatic brain edema. *Journal of Neurosurgery, 45,* 292-300.

Parker, J.R., Parker, J.C., & Overman, J.C. (1990). Intracranial diffuse axonal injury at autopsy. *Annals of Clinical and Laboratory Science, 20,* 220-224.

Parsons, L.C., & Shogan, J.S.O. (1984). The effects of the endotracheal tube suctioning/manual hyperventilation procedure on patients with severe closed head injury. *Heart and Lung, 13* (4), 372-308.

Parsons, L.C., & Wilson, M.M. (1984). Cerebrovascular status of severe closed head injured patients following passive position changes. *Nursing Research, 33,* 68-75.

Pfister, R.R., & Koski, J. (1982). Alkali burns of the eye: Pathophysiology and treatment. *Southern Medical Journal, 75*(4), 417-22.

Piatt, J.H., & Schiff, S.J. (1984). High-dose barbituate therapy in neurosurgery and intensive care. *Neurosurgery, 15* (3), 427-444.

Pitts, L.H. (1984). Determination of brain death. *Western Journal of Medicine, 140,* 628-631.

Plum, F., & Posner, J.B. (1985). The diagnosis of stupor and coma (4th ed.). Philadelphia: F.A. Davis.

Price, M.P. (1981). Significance of intracranial pressure waveform. *Journal of Neurosurgical Nursing, 13,* 202-206.

Proctor, H.J., Palladino, G.W., & Fillipo, D. (1988). Failure of autoregulation after closed head injury: An experimental model. *Journal of Trauma, 28* (3), 347-352.

Rocca, B., Martin, C., Viviand, X., Pierre-Francois, B., Saint-Gilles, H.L., & Chevalier, A. (1989). Comparison of four severity scores in patients with head trauma. *Journal of Trauma, 29*(3), 299-305.

Rootman, J. (1988). *Diseases of the orbit: A multidisciplinary approach.* Philadelphia: J.B. Lippincott.

Rootman, J., & Graeb, D.A. (1988). Vascular lesions. In J. Rootman (Ed.), *Diseases of the orbit: A multidisciplinary approach* (pp. 525-568). Philadelphia: J.B. Lippincott.

Rootman, J. & Neigel, J. (1988). Structural lesions: Trauma. In. J. Rootman (Ed.), *Diseases of the orbit: A multidisciplinary approach* (pp. 504-523). Philadelphia: J.B. Lippincott.

Ropper, A.H. (1986). Lateral displacement of the brain and level of consciousness in patients with an acute hemispheral mass. *New England Journal of Medicine, 314,* 953-958.

Rosenwasser, R.H., Andrews, D.W., & Jimenez, D.F. (1991). Penetrating craniocerebral trauma. *Surgical Clinics of North America, 71,* 305-316.

Rosner, M.J. (1987). Cerebral perfusion pressure: Link between intracranial pressure and systemic circulation. In J.H. Wood (Ed.), *Cerebral blood flow: Physiologic and clinical aspects* (pp. 425-448). New York: McGraw-Hill.

Rosner, M.J., & Coley, I.B. (1986). Cerebral perfusion pressure, intracranial pressure, and head elevation. *Journal of Neurosurgery, 65,* 636-641.

Rosner, M.J., & Becker, D.P. (1984). Origin and evolution of plateau waves. *Journal of Neurosurgery, 60,* 312-324.

Ross, S.E., Nathan, H., & O'Malley, K.F. (1990). The impact of a required request law on vital organ procurement. *Journal of Trauma, 30* (7), 820-823.

Rowe, N.L. (1984). Fractures of the zygomatic complex and orbit. In N.L. Rowe & J.L. Williams (Eds.), *Maxillofacial injuries* (Vol. 1) (pp. 435-537). New York: Churchill Livingston.

Rudy, E.B., Baun, M., Stone, K., & Turner, B. (1986). The relationship between endotracheal suctioning and changes in intracranial pressure: A review of the literature. *Heart and Lung, 15* (5), 488-494.

Sahuquillo, J., Vilalta, J., Lamarca, J., Rubio E., Rodriquez-Pazon, M., & Salva, J.A. (1989). Diffuse axonal injury after severe head trauma: A clinico-pathological study. *Acta Neurochirurgica, 101,* 149-158.

Salcman, M., Schepp, R.S., & Ducker, T.B. (1981). Calculated recovery rates in severe head trauma. *Neurosurgery, 8* (3), 301-308.

Saul, T.G., & Ducker, T.B. (1982). Effect of intracranial pressure monitoring and aggressive treatment on mortality in severe head injury. *Journal of Neurosurgery, 56,* 498-503.

Schemmer, G.B., & Driebe, W.T. (1987). Post-traumatic bacillus cereus endopthalmitis. *Archives of Ophthalmology, 105,* 342-344.

Schwartz, M.L., Tator, C.H., Rowed, D.W., Reid, S.R., Meguro, K., & Andrews, D.F. (1984). The University of Toronto head injury treatment study: A prospective randomized comparison of phenobarbital and mannitol. *Canadian Journal of Neurological Sciences, 11* (4), 434-440.

Seidel, H.M., Ball, J.W., Dains, J.E., & Benedict, W.

(1991). *Mosby's guide to physical examination* (2nd ed.). St. Louis: Mosby–Year Book, Inc.

Shalit, M.N., & Umansky, F. (1977). Effects of routine bedside procedures on intracranial pressure. *Israel Journal of Medical Science, 13,* 881-886.

Snow, R.B., Zimmerman, R.D., Gandy, S.E., & Deck, M.D.F. (1986). Comparison of magnetic resonance imaging and computed tomography in the evaluation of head injury. *Neurosurgery, 18,* 45-52.

Spielman, G. (1981). Coma: A clinical review. *Heart and Lung, 10,* 700-707.

Starmark, J.E., Stalhammer, D., Holmgren, E., & Rosander, B. (1988). Comparison of the Glasgow coma scale and the reaction level scale (RLS85). *Journal of Neurosurgery, 69,* 699-706.

Sugar, J. (1984). Chemical, thermal, and penetrating injuries of the anterior segment of the eye. In J.T. Wilensky & J.E. Read (Eds.), *Primary ophthalmology* (pp. 53-60). Orlando: Grune & Stratton.

Synder, M. (1984). Relation of nursing activities to increases in intracranial pressure. *Journal of Advanced Nursing, 8,* 273-279.

Takenaka, N., Mine, T., Suga, S., Tamura, K., Sagou, M., Hirose, Y., Ogino, M., Okuno, T., & Enomotu, K. (1990). Interpeduncular high-density spot in severe shearing injury. *Surgical Neurology, 34,* 30-38.

Tanaka, T., Sakai, T., Uemura, K., Teramura, A., Fujishima, I., & Yamamoto, T. (1988). MR imaging as a predictor of delayed post-traumatic cerebral hemorrhage. *Journal of Neurosurgery, 69,* 203-209.

Thomasma, D.C., & Brumlik, J. (1984). Ethical issues in the treatment of patients with a remitting vegetative state. *American Journal of Medicine, 77,* 373-377.

Toutant, S.M., Klauber, M.R., Marshall, L.F., Toole, B.M., Bowers, S.A., Seelig, J.M., & Varnee, J.B. (1984). Absent or compressed basal cisterns of first CT scan: Ominous predictors of outcome in severe head injury. *Journal of Neurosurgery, 61,* 691-694.

Tsementzis, S.A., Harris, P., & Loizou, L.A. (1982). The effect of routine nursing care procedures on the ICP in severe head injuries. *Acta Neurochirurgica, 65,* 153-166.

Vaughan, D. (1989). Glaucoma. In D.Vaughan, T. Asbury, and K.F. Tabbara (Eds.), *General ophthalmology* (12th ed.) (pp. 190-205). Norwalk, CT: Appleton & Lange.

Walleck, C.A. (1989). Controversies in the management of the head-injured patient. *Critical Care Clinics of North America, 1,* 67-74.

Walters, B.L., & Kelley, T.M. (1987). Commercial tanning facilities: A new source of eye injury. *American Journal of Emergency Medicine, 5,* 386-389.

Ward, J.D., Moulton, R.J., Muizelaar, J.P., & Marmarou, A. (1987). Cerebral homeostasis and protection. In F.P. Wirth & R.A. Ratcheson (Eds.), *Neurosurgical critical care: Concepts in neurosurgery* (Vol. 1) (pp. 187-213). Baltimore: Williams & Wilkins.

Wilberger, J.E. (1990). Emergency burr holes: Current role in neurosurgical acute care. *Topics in Emergency Medicine, 11* (4), 69-74.

Wilson, S.F., Amling, J.K., Floyd, S.D., & McNair, N.D. (1988). Determining interrater reliability of nurses' assessments of pupillary size and reaction. *Journal of Neuroscience Nursing, 20* (3), 189-192.

Yano, M., Nishiyama, H., Yokota, H., Kato, K., Yamamoto, Y., & Otsuka, T. (1986). Effect of lidocaine on ICP response to endotracheal suctioning. *Anesthesiology, 64,* 651-653.

Yanoff, M. & Fine, B. (1989). *Ocular pathology: A text and atlas* (3rd ed.). Philadelphia: J.B. Lippincott.

Young, H.A., & Schmidek, H.H. (1982). Complications accompanying occipital skull fracture. *Journal of Trauma, 22* (11), 914-920.

Zegeer, L.J. (1981). The patient in the persistent vegetative state. *Journal of Neurosurgical Nursing, 13,* 243-247.

11 Mobility

Spinal and musculoskeletal injuries

Jean A. Proehl

OBJECTIVES

❏ Differentiate between complete and incomplete, permanent and temporary spinal cord injuries.

❏ Describe the emergency nursing management of the patient with an actual or potential spinal cord injury.

❏ Assess a patient with musculoskeletal injuries, and determine nursing care priorities based on this assessment.

❏ Identify patients at risk for compartmental syndrome or fat embolus, and describe assessment findings associated with these complications.

❏ Discuss recent research and current controversies pertinent to the care of the patient with spinal or musculoskeletal injuries.

INTRODUCTION With the exception of high spinal cord trauma and massive pelvic damage, injuries to the spinal cord and musculoskeletal system are usually not life threatening. However, because these injuries may temporarily or permanently alter a patient's mobility, they are a major source of disability. Thus they require early and appropriate care to prevent permanent complications and to achieve optimal outcomes.

CASE STUDY A 16-year-old male is brought to the hospital by friends after a dirt bike accident. On arrival he is alert and oriented and complaining of severe left thigh pain. BP is 140/90; HR, 112; and respirations, 28. His skin is warm, pink, and dry. The nurse notes abrasions to both hands and forearms and a deformed left thigh with bone ends protruding. No other injuries are present.

Should this patient's cervical spine be immobilized?
    Yes, the mechanism of injury indicates that he is at risk for neck trauma even though he is not complaining of neck pain.

How should his left leg be immobilized?
    A traction splint should be used for femur fractures even in the presence of an open wound. If possible, the wound should be irrigated briefly to remove gross contamination; then a sterile dressing should be placed over the wound. The nurse should check distal neurovascular status before and after splint application.

What laboratory studies are indicated for this patient?
    Hemoglobin and hematocrit values should be monitored to assess blood loss. The patient should be typed and crossmatched for at least 4 units of blood, since he will require surgical intervention and probably need blood product replacement. The open wound should be swabbed for a culture and sensitivity before it is covered with a sterile dressing.

What medications will the physician order?
    Tetanus prophylaxis will be administered if the patient's immunizations are not current. Antibiotics, usually an intravenous cephalosporin, are indicated for all open fractures. Analgesics may be or-

325

dered if not contraindicated by other injuries or conditions.

SPINAL INJURIES

Approximately 10,000 spinal injuries are sustained each year in the United States, with young men the group most frequently injured and elderly women the next most frequently injured (Metcalf, 1986; Richmond, 1985; Riggins & Kraus, 1977). Most complications occur before the patient reaches the hospital, so early recognition of potential spinal injuries is crucial for proper management (Cloward, 1980). A decrease in the number of patients admitted with complete lesions was noted between 1972 and 1981 in one study (Nikas, 1986) and is probably attributable to improved prehospital care and immobilization.

Mechanism of Injury

Motor vehicle accidents are the leading cause of spinal injury in all populations, followed by falls, gunshot wounds, and diving accidents (Metcalf, 1986; Richmond, 1985; Riggins & Kraus, 1977). Although motor vehicle accidents are responsible for the greatest number of cervical spine injuries, falls are associated with a higher relative risk of cervical spine injury (Roberge et al., 1988; Jacobs & Schwartz, 1986). The potential for permanent injury is great if spinal injuries are not properly immobilized early; therefore any patient with a suspicious mechanism of injury must be immobilized until spinal injury is ruled out. There is debate regarding whether spinal injury can be ruled out clinically without radiographic examination. However, the most foolproof way of ruling out spinal injury is by x-ray examination. Cervical spine (c-spine) injury should always be suspected in the patient with a head injury, because the two frequently occur together (Nikas, 1986). Forces that may cause spinal injury include flexion, extension, axial loading, rotational forces, and penetrating trauma.

Flexion occurs when the head is forced forward until the chin strikes the chest or another object. This occurs with dives into shallow water or sudden deceleration in motor vehicle accidents. Flexion may result in anterior subluxation, bilateral interfacetal dislocation, simple wedge fracture, or a flexion teardrop fracture (Adelstein & Watson, 1983; Knezevich, 1986).

Extension results when the head is forced backward; it occurs with falls or as a result of sudden deceleration, where the head first flexes forward and then is hyperextended backward (whiplash). Properly adjusted headrests in motor vehicles can help prevent hyperextension of the head. Hyperextension may result in an extension teardrop fracture, hangman's fracture (bilateral fractures of posterior arches of C2), or posterior arch fractures (Adelstein & Watson, 1983; Knezevich, 1986).

Axial loading, also known as *vertical compression*, is a force transmitted straight down the spine as with diving injuries, an object landing on top of the head, or the head striking the roof of a car. This may result in bilateral fractures to the anterior and posterior arches of C1 (Jefferson fracture) or burst fractures of the lower cervical vertebrae (Adelstein & Watson, 1983; Knezevich, 1986).

Rotational or twisting forces may complicate any of the above mechanisms and are commonly involved in extension injuries (Adelstein & Watson, 1983). Ligamentous injury should be suspected when rotational forces have been involved.

Penetrating trauma to the spine occurs most commonly with gunshot wounds and stabbing injuries but may result also from impalement. In addition to the direct trauma to the cord, damage to surrounding structures may occur also, most notably the esophagus and great vessels. This patient is also at risk for a central nervous system infection, such as meningitis or encephalitis caused by direct contamination of the cerebral spinal fluid.

Spinal injuries are rare in children (Jaffe, Binns, Radkowski, Barthel, & Engelhard, 1987) even though the head is relatively larger and heavier in young children and the neck muscles and ligaments are weaker than those of an adult. Cervical and head injuries may occur as a result of being "shaken" by a parent or caregiver (Stauffer & Mazur, 1982). One study found the following variables to be significantly associated with cervical spine injury in children: neck pain; neck tenderness; limitation of neck mobility; history of trauma to the neck; abnormal reflexes, strength, and sensation; and altered mental status (Jaffe et al., 1987).

The elderly or patients with chronic diseases may have osteoporotic or rheumatoid degeneration that weakens the vertebral bodies. In this case seemingly insignificant trauma, a simple fall from fainting, for example, may cause serious fractures and spinal cord damage.

With these factors in mind, the nurse should attempt to determine the circumstances surrounding the injury. If a motor vehicle accident caused the injury, where was the patient inside the vehicle? Were seat/lap belts, headrests, or a car seat used and used correctly? Was the patient ejected from the vehicle? If the patient fell, how far was the fall? What kind of surface did the patient land on? What part of the patient's body hit first?

Anatomic and Physiologic Considerations

The spine is composed of 33 vertebrae: 7 cervical, 12 thoracic, 5 lumbar, 5 sacral (fused in the adult), and 3 to 5 coccygeal vertebrae fused together to form the coccyx (Figure 11-1). The bony vertebrae are connected by ligaments, which hold them in close approximation to one another. Between the vertebrae are fibrocartilaginous disks, which cushion the movements of the vertebrae. Damage to these structures may coexist with vertebral fractures or may occur without simultaneous bony injury.

The cervical vertebrae are the smallest and most mobile and therefore at greatest risk of injury. The skull rests directly on C1, the atlas, a modified vertebra with no spinous processes. The atlas pivots on a tooth-like projection of C2, the odontoid.

The thoracic vertebrae that are lower in the spinal column are larger than those above. The thoracic spine is relatively immobile because of the attached rib cage, and fractures here should always make one suspicious of concurrent thoracic trauma.

The lumbar vertebrae are the largest and strongest in the spine, yet they are fairly mobile because the supporting muscles are relatively short and weak. As a result, the lumbar area is frequently injured.

The fused sacrum and coccyx are relatively immobile. The sacrum is rarely injured in isolation—significant pelvic fractures usually are present also. The coccyx is only slightly mobile and is usually injured as a result of vertical loading forces where the patient lands on the buttocks.

The spinal cord lies within the spinal canal from the base of the skull to the level of L2. The canal is widest in the high cervical and lumbar

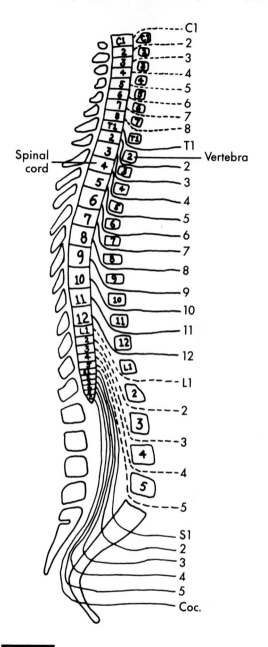

Figure 11-1 Alignment of spinal nerves with vertebrae. (*Note.* From *Neuroanatomy Made Ridiculously Simple* [p. 5] by S. Goldberg, 1979, Miami: MedMaster.)

regions to allow the spinal nerve roots to enter. Relatively more displacement of a fracture or dislocation at these levels is required to injure the cord within the canal. The cord is enclosed in the

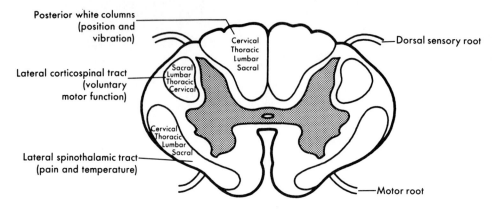

CROSS SECTION OF CERVICAL SPINAL CORD

Figure 11-2   Cross section of cervical spinal cord. (*Note.* From *Emergency Medicine: Concepts and Clinical Practice* [2nd ed.] [p. 464] by P. Rosen, F.J. Baker II, R.M. Barkin, G.R. Braen, R.H. Dailey, & R.C. Levy [1987], St. Louis: Mosby–Year Book, Inc.)

meninges and a layer of epidural fat, both of which serve to cushion the cord and protect it from injury.

The spinal cord is composed of a central H-shaped area of gray matter surrounded by white matter (myelin), as illustrated in Figure 11-2. The anterior horns of the gray matter contain the motor (efferent) neurons. The posterior horns of the gray matter contain the sensory (afferent) neurons.

General Assessment

Pain or tenderness of the neck is a frequent complaint of patients with spinal cord injuries (Ringenberg, Fisher, Urdaneta, & Midthun, 1988). Muscle spasm may also be present, which provides some splinting of the injured spine (Aprahamian, Thompson, Finger, & Darin, 1984). For this reason, care should be taken with any patient receiving paralytic agents (e.g., curare derivatives, succinylcholine) to facilitate intubation, because this protective spasm is then lost and fractures or dislocations may be more easily displaced; one source recommends against succinylcholine use in patients with potentially unstable c-spine injuries (Hochbaum, 1986).

The patient may also complain of weakness, paralysis, or paresthesia of the arms and legs. This should alert the nurse to the probability that an injury has occurred to the spinal cord itself.

Did the patient lose consciousness? Loss of consciousness is usually associated with head trauma, and head trauma frequently coexists with cervical spine trauma.

Is the patient under the influence of drugs or alcohol? Frequently, patients struck by motor vehicles are intoxicated and are more likely to sustain chest and spinal injuries than sober pedestrians (Jehle & Cottington, 1988). These substances may alter the data obtained during physical examination because intoxicated patients may not obey commands and may not indicate to the examiner the location of pain. However, focal or localized findings such as weakness or numbness of only one or two extremities do not result from drug or alcohol intoxication.

Does the patient have multiple, severe injuries? Any multiple trauma patient is at high risk for spinal injury (Ringenberg et al., 1988). Patients with multiple trauma may be unconscious or focus on the pain associated with other injuries and not notice neck pain initially (Ringenberg et al., 1988; Sumchai, Sternbach, & Laufer, 1988).

Inspection and palpation

Inspection of the neck and back is difficult to perform on the properly immobilized patient. Palpation frequently precedes inspection in this case until injury of the c-spine is ruled out radiographically. Although inspection may be deferred until x-ray films are obtained and injury ruled out, at some point in the physical examination the examiner should visually inspect the patient's back for open wounds, deformity, or impaled objects. If major wounds are suspected because of blood loss or mechanism of injury, the patient may be carefully logrolled before x-ray films are obtained.

The examiner should palpate the entire spinal column for tenderness and deformities. If palpation is performed on areas that cannot be seen, the examiner should wear gloves to protect against contact with hidden blood or body fluids. The examiner should palpate carefully in this situation, because broken glass and other sharp objects frequently accompany the patient from the accident scene. A sudden "stepping off" felt while palpating a bony prominence is known as a *step defect* and alerts the examiner to the probability of an underlying fracture or dislocation. Muscle spasm may also be noted as a loss of the normal curvature of the spine, particularly in the normally lordotic cervical and lumbar areas.

Sensory function

Assessment of sensory function helps to determine the presence and location of spinal cord injury. If any sensory sparing exists below the level of the lesion, there is a 50% chance the patient will walk within 1 year (Cerullo & Quigley, 1985). Sensation is evaluated by the patient's ability to discriminate sharp from dull on pinprick. Referral to a dermatome chart will help establish the level of the spinal cord lesion. In general, C4 is at the top of the shoulders, T4 at the nipple line, and T10 at the umbilicus. The lowest segment, S4, innervates the perineal area and **not** the sole of the foot (the lowest part of the body). Proprioception (position sense), vibratory sensation, and deep tendon reflexes also may be evaluated.

A rectal examination should always be performed to check for sacral sparing, indicated by the presence of sphincter tone and the anal wink reflex after pricking of the perineal skin. Sacral sparing indicates that the lesion of the cord is incomplete, and maximal attention must be paid to proper immobilization so that the injury is not converted to a complete one. Patients with complete lesions rarely have any recovery of function (Cerullo & Quigley, 1985).

The bulbocavernosus reflex, exhibited by rectal sphincter contraction with gentle tugging at the penis or clitoris, is a very primitive spinal arc reflex and will be one of the first to return after spinal shock resolves, usually within 24 hours after injury (Meyers, 1984). The presence of the bulbocavernosus reflex does not indicate sacral sparing (Cerullo & Quigley, 1985). Instead, it indicates that voluntary sensation and muscle control are absent and confirms that the lesion is complete (Meyers, 1984).

Motor function

Assessment of motor strength and movement provides valuable information. The examiner compares the patient's strength with what is normal for a patient of similar size and age. The spinal cord assessment record in Figure 11-3 describes the movements used to assess the level of cord functioning. Myotome charts map out motor innervation (like dermatome charts map out sensory innervation) and may be used also. Injuries are labeled by the last functioning level, and it is not unusual to find a "sensory" level one or two segments below the "motor" level (Cerullo & Quigley, 1985). Also, the level of the bony fracture may not correspond exactly with the level of the cord injury. The spinal cord and the vertebral column grow at different rates, so in adults the cord segments are displaced upward from their corresponding vertebrae. This becomes more pronounced caudally down the cord.

Diagnostic and Monitoring Procedures
Radiographic studies

Many sources believe that x-ray examinations are essential to the thorough evaluation of spinal injuries because history and physical examination findings may be lacking even in the presence of significant fractures (Jacobs & Schartz, 1986; Mace, 1985). One study found that fractures could not be predicted on the basis of the history and physical examination 50% of the time (Jacobs & Shartz, 1986). Another study found no cervical fractures in alert adult patients with no neck pain or tenderness (Roberge et al., 1988). However, the absence of a fracture on x-ray film does not rule out spinal cord injury. Of traumatic c-spine injuries, 10% to 17% have no overt radiologic evidence of fracture. Frequently these injuries present as the incomplete central cord syndrome (Cerullo & Quigley, 1985; Riggins & Kraus, 1977). Congenital abnormalities or developmen-

MOTOR ASSESSMENT		DATE																											
		TIME																												
MOTOR STRENGTH			R	L	R	L	R	L	R	L	R	L	R	L	R	L	R	L	R	L	R	L	R	L	R	L	R	L	R	L
SHOULDER	FLEX	C4,5																												
ELBOW	EXT	C7																												
	FLEX	C5,6																												
WRIST	EXT	C7																												
	FLEX	C7,8																												
FINGER	ABD	C8,T1																												
HIP	ABD	L4,5																												
	FLEX	L2,3																												
KNEE		L3,4																												
ANKLE		L5,S1																												
PLANTAR		S1,2																												
VITAL CAPACITY																													
EXAMINER INITIALS																													

SENSORY ASSESSMENT		DATE							
		TIME							
SENSORY TO PINPRICK			R	L	R	L	R	L	R	L
UPPER LATERAL ARM	C5								
POSTERIOR ASPECT—THUMB	C6								
POSTERIOR ASPECT—3RD FINGER	C7								
POSTERIOR ASPECT—PINKY	C8								
NIPPLE LINE	T4								
UMBILICUS	T10								
GROIN	L1								
ANTERIOR THIGH	L2								
SOLE OF FOOT	S1								
PERIANAL	S3,4,5								
POSITION SENSE	BIG TOE								
	INDEX FINGER								
DEEP PAIN	BIG TOE								
EXAMINER INITIALS									

INITIALS	SIGNATURE	INITIALS	SIGNATURE

MOTOR ASSESSMENT SCALES

MOTOR STRENGTH
0 = NO MOVEMENT
1 = FLICKER OR TRACE OF MOVEMENT
2 = INCOMPLETE ROM
3 = FULL ROM = RESISTANCE
4 = FULL ROM AGAINST SLIGHT RESISTANCE
5 = FULL ROM AGAINST MAXIMUM RESISTANCE

SENSORY ASSESSMENT SCALES

SENSORY TO PINPRICK
N = NORMAL SENSATION
↓ = HYPOAESTHESIA
↑ = HYPERAESTHESIA
O = ABSENT SENSATION
P = PARAESTHESIA

POSITION SENSE
+ = TOTAL ACCURACY IN DETERMINING POSITION OF TOE/FINGER
− = UNABLE TO TELL POSITION OF TOE/FINGER
± = CAN DETERMINE POSITION OF TOE/FINGER AT TIMES

DEEP PAIN
+ = ELICITS SEVERE PAIN
− = FEELS NOTHING

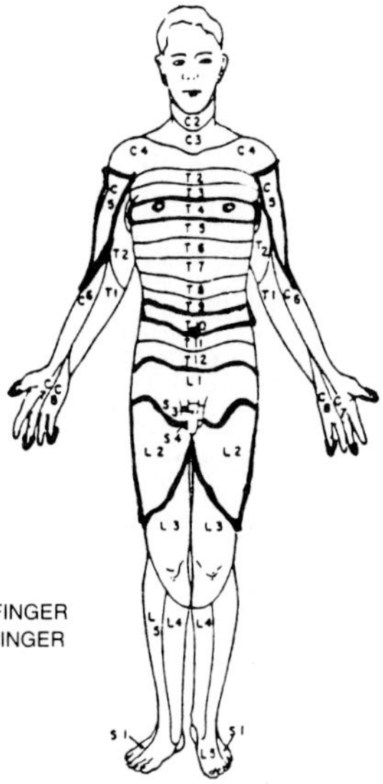

PT. NO.

NAME

D.O.B.

UNIVERSITY OF WASHINGTON MEDICAL CENTERS
HARBORVIEW MEDICAL CENTER
UNIVERSITY OF WASHINGTON MEDICAL CENTER
SEATTLE, WASHINGTON

SPINAL CORD ASSESSMENT RECORD

HMC 0222   JUN 89

Figure 11-3 Spinal cord assessment record. (Courtesy Harborview Medical Center, Seattle.)

Motor Assessment

1) The motor functions tested are representative of various levels of the spinal cord.

2) All motor functions should be tested bilaterally.

3) Rate motor movements with the 0–5 scale on the front of the sheet.

4) For correct assessment technique use both hands — one to support and/or apply resistance to the extremity and one to feel for the muscle contraction. Specific muscle group assessment is described in the following. (For additional reference, see the pictorial guide in your unit or in Nursing Educational Office or contact a Neuroscience CNS.)

Shoulder Flexion

(Cord level C4, 5)

—Examiner places hand on anterior aspect of upper arm and asks patient to raise entire arm straight up in front of them.

Elbow Flexion

(Cord level C5, 6)

—Examiner places one hand on the upper arm of patient and the other hand on the patient's forearm. Ask patient to flex (bend) the elbow up from a supine position.

Elbow Extension

(Cord level C7)

—Examiner places the arm up and across the patient's chest. Examiner places one hand on the back of the upper arm and the other hand on the back of the forearm. The patient is asked to extend the elbow.

Wrist Flexion

(Cord level C7, 8)

—Examiner places one hand on the anterior wrist and the other hand just lightly supports the patient's hand. Ask the patient to flex wrist.

Wrist Extension

(Cord level C7)

—Examiner places one hand on anterior wrist and the other hand tightly supports the patient's hand. Ask the patient to extend wrist.

Hip Flexion

(Cord level L2, 3)

—Examiner places one hand on the anterior thigh and the other hand is placed at the foot. Ask the patient to flex the hip and lift the whole leg.

Hip Abduction

(Cord level L4, 5)

—Examiner places hand on the lateral aspect of the thigh. Ask patient to abduct entire leg.

Finger Abduction

(Cord level C8, T1)

—Examiner places the palm of their hand against the bottom side of the patient's fingers. Examiner then gently closes fingers around the patient's and asks the patient to spread their fingers apart.

Knee Extension

(Cord level L3, 4)

—Examiner places one hand under the leg and rests hand over the opposite knee. Examiner then places a hand over patient's lower leg. Ask the patient to extend the knee.

Ankle Flexion

(Cord level L5, S1)

—Examiner places hand across anterior aspect of the foot close to ankle. Ask patient to flex foot toward chest.

Plantar

(Cord level S1, 2)

—Examiner places hand underneath ball of patient's foot. Ask patient to press down with foot as if pressing on a gas pedal.

Figure 11-3, cont'd   For legend see opposite page.

tal differences in children may mimic cervical fractures or subluxations on x-ray films. When the examiner is in doubt, the child must be kept immobilized until this is ruled out (Stauffer & Mazur, 1982).

Cross-table lateral films of the cervical spine should be obtained and cleared by a physician before the patient is moved to obtain subsequent x-ray films. However, 17% to 25% of cervical spine fractures may be missed with cross-table lateral films alone (Mace, 1985). Therefore a complete series of films is necessary. The cervicothoracic junction (C7-T1) must be visualized on the cross-table lateral films since 18% of c-spine injuries occur here (Cerullo & Quigley, 1985). Although controversial, Swimmer's views (extending the arm that is closest to the x-ray tube above the patient's head), downward traction on the shoulders, and/or tomograms may be necessary for complete visualization in people with large or muscular shoulders. Asking cooperative patients to "blow out" while they reach for their toes may be helpful. Frequently the emergency physician will review and clear films initially, but early consultation with a radiologist is helpful and was found to expedite patient care and improve detection of abnormal findings on x-ray films in one study of trauma patients (Daffner & Diamond, 1988). Clothing should be cut off or repositioned without moving the patient if it will obscure the x-ray films. Gentle manual traction may be required to maintain immobilization while obtaining x-ray films if the patient is not fully cooperative and the immobilization devices are not radiopaque (such as sandbags). Anteroposterior, lateral, and oblique views of the remaining vertebrae and an open mouth view to visualize the odontoid are then obtained.

Fractures are most often seen where a relatively immobile segment meets a relatively mobile segment of the spinal column. For this reason C4 to C6 and T11 to L1 are the most commonly injured areas (Meyer & Sullivan, 1984). Certain areas of the spinal column are difficult to evaluate because of overlying bony structures, such as the skull, clavicles, and upper ribs. These areas—C1, C2, C7, and T1—should be carefully scrutinized to avoid overlooking an injury (Meyer & Sullivan, 1984). Because noncontiguous vertebral injuries are present in about 5% of patients (Calenoff, Chessare, Rogers, Toerge & Rosen, 1978), x-ray studies should be done on the entire spine if

any injury is found (Cerullo & Quigley, 1985; Meyer & Sullivan, 1984; Ringenberg et al., 1988). Many patients have thoracic or lumbar fractures without concurrent cervical fractures. For this reason doing an x-ray examination of the entire spine of multiple trauma patients should be considered (Pal, Mulder, Brown, & Fleiszer, 1988).

If adequate films cannot be obtained, the patient must remain immobilized until the spine can be radiographically cleared. This may mean sending the patient to surgery or the intensive care unit on a backboard with cervical collar in place. It also presents a difficult problem should the patient vomit. Suction should be ready and the patient secured to the backboard so that turning can be quickly accomplished with a minimal amount of movement. At least three people are needed to logroll the average adult safely (if not secured to a backboard). Proper immobilization technique will be discussed later in the chapter.

Computerized tomography

Computerized tomography (CT) scans are more sensitive and may be necessary for some patients with questionable x-ray findings. These scans are superior to plain radiographs for fracture detection. In one study CT scanning eliminated both false negatives (20%) and false positives (40%) (Mace, 1985). However, patient movement onto the CT table is difficult when c-spine injury is suspected. If the scan cannot be performed with the patient on the backboard, a physician should supervise the move to the table and stabilize the head and neck during the move. A slider board can facilitate smooth movement of the patient. The physician and nurse must assure safe handling during the awkward process of repositioning the patient onto the CT table.

Tomograms are sectional radiographs that can show more detail in a selected plane of an injured area.

Magnetic resonance imaging

Magnetic resonance imaging (MRI) is also useful in the evaluation of a spinal injury. A drawback with the older units is the restriction of metal objects in the room because of the fringe magnetic fields. This restriction prevents the use of much of the life support equipment that the patient may require. The newer units practically eliminate fringe magnetic fields, and more patients can benefit from MRI (Teresi, Lufkin, & Hanafee, 1988). MRI does not require the patient to be moved from the horizontal position and images the spinal cord and any fracture fragments noninvasively (Gebarski et al., 1985).

Assessment and Interventions Related to Specific Injuries

Vertebral injuries — Impaired physical mobility
Pain

The vertebrae may be fractured, dislocated, or subluxed (partially dislocated). The ligaments supporting the vertebrae may be torn or otherwise injured. A variety of combinations of these injuries may occur also. A phenomenon known as *pseudosubluxation* may be observed in pediatric cervical spine x-ray films. In pseudosubluxation, C2 appears to be subluxed onto C3 as a result of normal range of motion because of the laxity of pediatric ligaments (Stauffer & Mazur, 1982). Subluxations may also spontaneously reduce before x-ray studies are done, causing damage to the spinal cord and neurologic deficits with no apparent bony deformity.

Spinal cord injuries — Impaired physical mobility
High risk for ineffective airway clearance
High risk for ineffective breathing pattern

Injury to the spinal cord occurs without concurrent vertebral fracture in 10% to 17% of cases (Cerullo & Quigley, 1985; Riggins & Kraus, 1977), and approximately 14% of spinal fractures and dislocations have an associated spinal cord injury (Aprahamian et al., 1984; Riggins & Kraus, 1977). Fracture-dislocation is the injury most likely to cause spinal cord damage (Aprahamian et al., 1984). In addition to the obvious problems paralysis poses, approximately 10% to 13.8% of patients die within 1 year of acute spinal cord injury, most from respiratory complications (Bracken et al., 1985; Flamm et al., 1985).

The spinal cord may be transected completely or incompletely, contused, and impinged upon by surrounding edema or hematoma. As a result of the complex anatomy of the spinal cord, partial lesions of the cord may result in sparing of some functions and loss of others. These incomplete lesions are summarized in Table 11-1 and illustrated in Figure 11-4. Extreme care must be taken to prevent the conversion of incomplete to complete lesions.

Of those patients with spinal cord injury, about 39% will have complete lesions. This percentage is decreasing as a result of improved prehospital care (Meyer & Sullivan, 1984). Of those with complete lesions, 53% will be quadriplegic and 47% will be paraplegic (Metcalf, 1986). Symptoms of complete lesions include immediate and complete loss of sensation and movement below the injury, poikilothermy (variant body temperature), bladder and bowel dysfunction, and loss of shivering and sweating below the lesion.

Table II-I Incomplete cord syndromes

Lesion	Mechanism of injury	Preserved	Impaired
Anterior cord syndrome (dorsal columns of the spinal cord are spared)	Flexion	Light touch Vibratory sensation Proprioception	Motor function Pain and temperature sensation
Posterior cord syndrome (anterior columns of the cord are spared)	Extension	Motor function Pain and temperature sensation	Light touch Vibratory sensation Proprioception
Central cord syndrome (central gray matter of the cord is injured)	Flexion or extension	Motor function of lower extremities	Motor function of upper extremities
Brown-Séquard syndrome (hemisection of the cord)	Penetrating trauma	Contralateral—pain and temperature sensation Ipsilateral—movement, light touch, proprioception	Contralateral—movement, light touch, proprioception Ipsilateral—pain and temperature

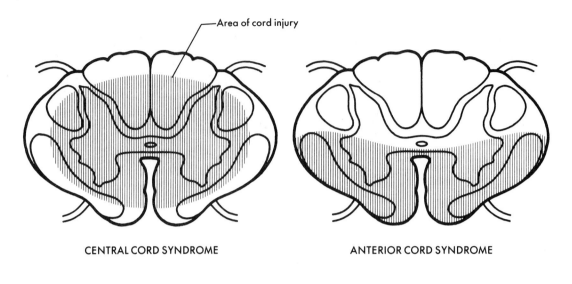

CENTRAL CORD SYNDROME ANTERIOR CORD SYNDROME

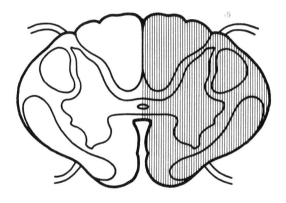

BROWN-SÉQUARD SYNDROME

Figure 11-4 Incomplete spinal cord syndromes. (*Note.* From *Emergency Medicine: Concepts and Clinical Practice* [2nd ed.] [p. 464] by P. Rosen, F.J. Baker II, R.M. Barkin, G.R. Braen, R.H. Dailey, & R.C. Levy [1987], St. Louis: Mosby–Year Book, Inc.)

Functional loss associated with level of spinal cord injury is delineated in the box on p. 335. These patients are also at risk to develop neurogenic shock.

Neurogenic shock Decreased cardiac output

Neurogenic shock usually occurs 30 to 60 minutes after the injury (Richmond, 1985). It results from the isolation of sympathetic nervous system neurons from the supraspinal centers caused by cervical spinal cord injury. As a result, sympathetic impulses cannot reach the thoracic and lumbar areas of the spinal cord from the brain. These sympathetic impulses are responsible for maintaining vascular tone and counteract the slowing effect of the parasympathetic nervous system on the heart. Thus when these impulses are blocked, bradycardia and vasodilation ensue. Hypotension is a result of the vasodilation of peripheral blood vessels. Vasodilation means that the victim's skin will be warm and dry instead of pale and cool as associated with hypovolemic shock.

Level of spinal cord lesion and functional loss

C1 through C4   Quadriplegia with no respiratory function

C4 and C5   Quadriplegia with control of head intact; phrenic nerve is partially spared but may be compromised as a result of edema

C5 and C6   Quadriplegia (incomplete), but gross arm movement intact; phrenic nerve is spared but not intercostals; diaphragmatic breathing is seen

C6 and C7   Quadriplegia (incomplete) with most upper arm and shoulder movement (biceps) intact; phrenic nerve is spared but not intercostals; diaphragmatic breathing is seen

C7 and C8   Quadriplegia (incomplete) with control of upper arms and some of the lower arms (triceps and biceps intact); limited hand movement; intercostals not intact; diaphragmatic breathing is seen

T1 through T6   Paraplegia with loss of all functions below midchest; some impairment of the intercostals is evident

T6 through T12   Paraplegia with loss of motor function below waist; no interference with respiratory function

L1 and L2   Paraplegia with loss of most of the control to legs

Below L2   Paraplegia (incomplete); cauda equina injury with varying degree of motor and sensory loss

Note. From *Quick Reference to Neurological Nursing* (p. 339) by J.V. Hickey, 1984, Philadelphia: J.B. Lippincott.

These patients cannot speed up their heart rate to help maintain cardiac output and so will be bradycardic instead tachycardic, a classic sign of hypovolemic shock. However, because 67% of patients with spinal trauma have concurrent injuries, hypovolemic shock must be ruled out (Nikas, 1986). Neurogenic, or spinal, shock may last for days or months (Metcalf, 1986).

General Interventions

The nursing diagnoses for patients with spinal injuries help to guide and set priorities of care. The interventions for a given nursing diagnosis are specific to the diagnosis, not necessarily the cause of the problem.

Ineffective airway clearance

Airway management is always the first priority in any trauma patient. Because most methods of securing an airway, such as oral intubation, result in movement of the cervical spine, attention to cervical spine immobilization must occur simultaneously. Cervical collars and manual stabilization are sometimes used during airway maneuvers, including oral intubation (Rhee, Green, Holcroft, & Mangili, 1990) but may not provide adequate immobilization (Aprahamian et al., 1984). Manual traction may in and of itself cause significant distraction of the fracture site (Bivins, Ford, Bezmalinovic, Price, & Williams, 1988). If invasive airway management is required before a complete radiologic examination is done, blind nasotracheal intubation or cricothyroidotomy may be performed (Bivins et al., 1988).

In addition to the usual causes of airway obstruction in a multiple trauma patient, retropharyngeal hematomas resulting from cervical fractures may impinge on the airway, necessitating invasive airway management (Tyson, Rimel, Winn, Butler, & Jane, 1979).

With spinal cord injury above the level of C4, the patient will not be able to cough effectively because of diaphragmatic paralysis. Therefore suctioning may be necessary to remove secretions.

Multiple trauma patients and those with spinal cord injuries will ultimately require a nasogastric or orogastric tube to decompress the stomach and help prevent aspiration of gastric contents. Care must be taken not to cause movement of the cervical spine during insertion, and in conscious patients it may be wise to defer tube placement until the cervical spine is cleared or definitively immobilized.

Ineffective breathing pattern

Injuries at the C3-4 level and above result in respiratory arrest as a result of diaphragmatic paralysis. These patients require immediate airway and ventilatory control. Cervical injuries below C5 cause paralysis of the intercostal muscles, and the patient must rely on the diaphragm for respirations. Most patients can manage with diaphragmatic breathing, but an ineffective breathing pattern and hypoventilation may result if other injuries or disease processes are present. Spinal immobilization with belts or wrap-around extrication devices can produce a restrictive effect on the thorax (Bauer & Kowalski, 1988) and may contribute to an ineffective breathing pattern.

Immobilization

Spinal board   Assessment of neurologic function must be ongoing to identify changes. The patient must be reevaluated after any movement, such as placement on a backboard. Edema may manifest as progressive deterioration of neurologic function, whereas the conversion of an incomplete to a complete lesion will result in sudden and dramatic changes.

All patients with potential spinal injury should be immobilized before being moved unless an environmental hazard (e.g., fire, noxious fumes) mandates immediate evacuation of the area (Worsing, 1984). The following steps describe proper immobilization of the spine:

1. With your hands, immediately stabilize the patient's head in the position found, and instruct the patient not to move. Have suction available in case the patient vomits.
2. Perform a brief neurologic examination to include movement and sensation of all extremities.
3. Place the head in a neutral position by applying gentle in-line stabilization. Some authors advocate immobilizing the head and neck in the position found (Buchanan, 1982; Cloward, 1980; Tyson et al., 1979). However, most recent sources (American College of Surgeons, 1989; Meyer & Sullivan, 1984; Rea, 1991) recommend returning the head to a neutral position. One case was reported of complete neurologic recovery after rapid realignment of a complete spinal cord injury (Brunette & Rockswold, 1987).
4. Apply a stiff cervical collar. Soft collars have been shown to be inadequate for immobilization of a potentially injured cervical spine (Aprahamian et al., 1984; Huerta, Griffith, & Joyce, 1987; Podolsky et al., 1983). Several recent studies have focused on the adequacy of various cervical collars in preventing movement. McCabe and Nolan (1986) found Philadel-

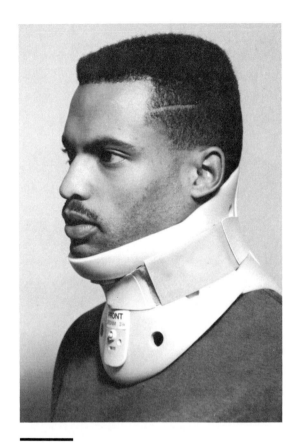

Figure 11-5   Philadelphia collar. (Courtesy DeRoyal Industries, Inc., Powell, TN.)

phia collars (Figure 11-5) equal to stiff collars (Figure 11-6) (Stifneck, California Medical Products; Vertebrace, Jobst) in preventing extension, and stiff collars superior to Philadelphia collars for limitation of flexion and lateral bending. Flexion and lateral bending are the movements most likely to occur with a patient who is immobilized on a backboard. Graziano, Scheidel, Cline, and Baer (1987) found the stiff collars to provide the best overall immobilization. Until recently no stiff collar existed that was suitable for a small child. Now stiff collars are available for infants and small children (Figure 11-7). In addition to function, ease of application and sizing should be assessed when making purchasing decisions, as well as storage capability.

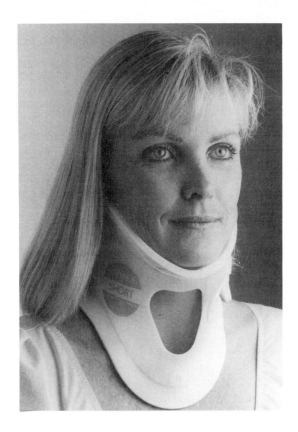

Figure 11-6 Adult Stifneck collar. (Courtesy California Medical Products, Inc., Long Beach, CA.)

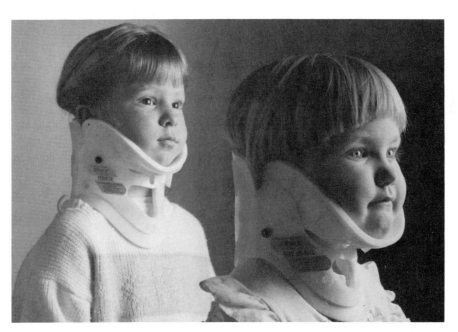

Figure 11-7 Pediatric Stifneck and Baby No-neck collars. (Courtesy California Medical Products, Inc., Long Beach, CA.)

5. Logroll patient to supine position on long backboard with the assistance of at least two other people. One person should move the shoulders and hips, and one should move the legs and assist with the hips. One recent study (N = 10) found that children younger than 7 years actually had cervical spine hyperflexion when placed on standard backboards because of their relatively large occiputs. The authors of this study recommend using a modified backboard with an indentation for the child's head or placing a rolled sheet under the child's shoulders and trunk (Herzenberg, Hensinger, Dedrick, & Phillips, 1989). Adult patients, especially the elderly, may require padding under the head to prevent hyperextension (Butman & Paturas, 1986).

6. Remove jewelry from the neck and ears. Also, at this point helmets should be removed as described in Figure 11-8.

7. Place towel rolls or high-density foam blocks at the sides of the head to help prevent the head from turning side to side. Sandbags are no longer recommended, because they could actually cause movement of the head because of their weight if the patient was turned on the backboard. Also, if the sandbags are narrow, they may slide within the tape, allowing the head to move. This can be avoided by using towels or blankets to form a snug cradle for the head within the tape. Commercially available devices constructed of cardboard are available also (Figure 11-9).

8. Place wide tape across the forehead (Figure 11-9). The tape must be applied directly to the skin for maximum effect. Avoid taping the hair because immobilization (and comfort) will be compromised. Tape in combination with sandbags at the sides of the head will provide almost total immobilization of the head (Podolsky et al., 1983). Tape should not be placed across the chin, since it may cause airway compromise if vomiting occurs (Knezevich, 1986; Rea, 1991; Sumchai, Sternbach, & Laufer, 1988).

9. Secure the rest of the body to the board with straps or sheets. At a minimum, straps should be placed across the shoulders, hips, and legs just proximal to the knees.

10. Repeat a brief neurologic examination. Immobilization must be maintained until the cervical spine is cleared by a physician. Monitor immobilized patients carefully, because they may vomit and be unable to maintain their own airway! Suction equipment should be hooked up and ready to use at all times, especially in the radiology department.

Spinal immobilization may restrict respiratory capacity in children. This restriction may impair ventilation in children with pulmonary or thoracic injuries. One study using healthy volunteers, ages 6 to 15 years, revealed that forced vital capacity was reduced in the supine position. Type of strapping (cross or lateral) used to immobilize the child on the spineboard did not further reduce forced vital capacity (Schafermeyer, et al., 1991).

Children may be immobilized in their carseats in lieu of removing them from the seat and placing them on a backboard (Gross, 1986). In the event the child needs to be removed from the carseat before x-ray studies are cleared, spinal alignment can be maintained by pulling the child longitudinally from the car seat onto a backboard. Positioning the parents so that they are in the child's direct line of vision may help decrease struggling by a frightened child. Parents can also help hold the head still while comforting their child.

Pregnant patients may become hypotensive in the supine position as a result of compression of the vena cava (refer to Chapter 16). To prevent vena caval compression by the gravid uterus, the patient should be tilted to the left. This may be accomplished by placing wedges or pillows under the right side of the backboard.

Patients with degenerative diseases such as ankylosing spondylitis may require modifications of the above techniques if their spine is chronically deformed. Attempting to immobilize these patients flat on a backboard may lead to movement of fractured areas.

Cervical traction Definitive immobilization of patients with spinal injuries occurs after other life-threatening problems are corrected. One definitive method is placement of cranial tongs, which are then attached to weight via a pulley to provide traction. This procedure may be performed in the

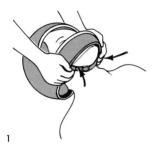

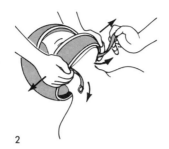

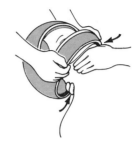

1

One rescuer applies in-line traction by placing his or her hands on each side of the helmet with the fingers on the victim's mandible. This position prevents slippage if the strap is loose.

2

The rescuer cuts or loosens the strap at the D-rings while maintaining in-line traction.

3

A second rescuer places one hand on the mandible at the angle, the thumb on one side, the long and index fingers on the other. With his other hand, he applies pressure from the occipital region. This maneuver transfers the in-line traction responsibility to the second rescuer.

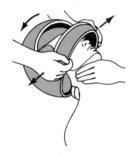

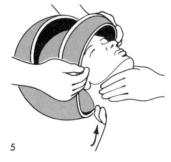

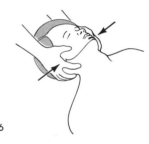

4

The rescuer at the top removes the helmet. Three factors should be kept in mind:
• The helmet is egg-shaped and therefore must be expanded laterally to clear the ears.
• If the helmet provides full facial coverage, glasses must be removed first.
• If the helmet provides full facial coverage, the nose will impede removal. To clear the nose, the helmet must be tilted backward and raised over it.

5

Throughout the removal process, the second rescuer maintains in-line traction from below to prevent head tilt.

6

After the helmet has been removed, the rescuer at the top replaces his hands on either side of the victim's head with his palms over the ears and provides in-line traction until backboard is in place.

Figure 11-8   Helmet removal from injured patients. (*Note.* Redrawn from "Techniques of Helmet Removal from Injured Patients" by American College of Surgeons, Committee on Trauma, 1980. *Bulletin of the American College of Surgeons, 65*, p. 20-21.)

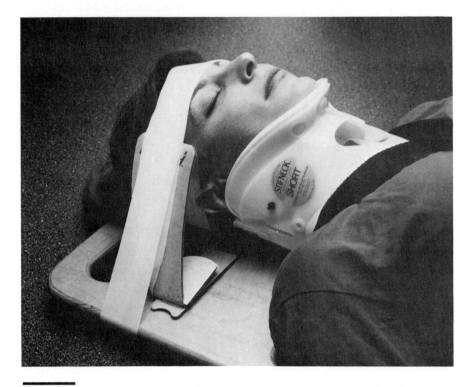

Figure 11-9 Correct patient immobilization. (Courtesy California Medical Products, Inc., Long Beach, CA.)

emergency department by the physician. The older tongs (Crutchfield, Vinke, Blackburn) required burr holes for placement and have for the most part been replaced by spring-loaded tongs such as Gardner-Wells or Heifertz (Cloward, 1980; Sumchai et al., 1988). Placement of cranial tongs (Figure 11-10) requires shaving and prepping the temporal region superior to the ear. The area is then infiltrated with a local anesthetic 1 inch above the ear in line with the pinna. The pinpoints of the tongs are screwed simultaneously through the skin to the skull until 30 pounds of tension is achieved (an indicator will protrude 1 mm from the knob of the screw on Gardner-Wells tongs). Because the skull itself cannot be anesthetized, the patient will experience pain as the pins are tightened (Sumchai et al., 1988). The tongs are attached to weights via a rope and pulley system. Weight is added in 5 pound increments until the desired reduction is obtained as evidenced by x-ray studies. Usually 5 pounds is

needed per disk space, e.g., 15 pounds for a C3 fracture (Cerullo & Quigley, 1985; Cloward, 1980). With some injuries, such as locked facets, considerably more weight may be needed to realign the vertebrae (Cerullo & Quigley, 1985).

Other definitive stabilization techniques are usually performed in the operating room or on the in-patient unit. These techniques include halo jackets; sternal, occiput, and mandible immobilizer (SOMI) braces; and various surgical stabilization procedures. Halo jackets and SOMI braces encircle the thorax and make respiratory assessment difficult and CPR impossible. Nurses caring for these patients should have the tools and knowledge necessary to remove the front portion of the jacket quickly if indicated by cardiac or respiratory compromise. Surgical stabilization is usually deferred for 24 to 48 hours to avoid producing more edema or further compromising the already damaged cord's blood supply (Meyers, 1984).

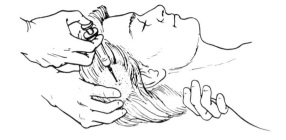

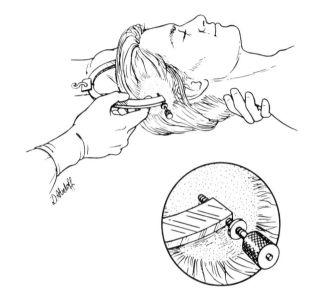

Figure 11-10 Gardner-Wells tong insertion. (*Note.* From *Atlas of Emergency Medicine* [2nd ed.] [p. 153] by P. Rosen and G.L. Sternbach, 1983, Baltimore: Williams & Wilkins.)

Altered tissue perfusion: general

The treatment of neurogenic shock in the acute phase is primarily to keep the patient supine to prevent orthostatic hypotension secondary to vasodilation. On the in-patient unit this is allowed in Stryker frames or Roto-Rest beds, but not in the CircOlectric bed because the patient is upright for a time during the turning phase. Urine output and level of consciousness will determine whether end organ perfusion is adequate. Vasopressors are rarely required (Richmond, 1985). Unless hypovolemia is also present, fluids should be given cautiously to prevent fluid overload in the normovolemic patient.

Altered tissue perfusion: spinal cord

All patients should receive supplemental oxygen because experimentally induced paraplegia has been shown to result in lower tissue oxygen levels in the spinal cord (Tyson et al., 1979).

Pharmacologic therapy

A number of medications have been used to treat spinal cord injuries. Steroids, naloxone, thyrotropin-releasing hormone, and mannitol are among these medications.

Steroids Steroids are used to decrease central hemorrhagic necrosis and surrounding edema (Tyson et al., 1979). Several studies failed to show any improvement in outcome attributable to steroid use (Faden, Jacobs, Patrick, & Smith, 1984; Bracken et al., 1984, 1985). These studies also noted an increase in wound infections and deaths (primarily respiratory-related) when high-dose steroids were used. The recently completed Second National Acute Spinal Cord Injury Study

(NASCIS 2) demonstrated an improvement in neurologic recovery when high-dose methylprednisolone was administered within 8 hours of spinal cord injury. Mortality and major morbidity were similiar in the placebo and steroid groups. The recommended dosing protocol is a 30 mg/kg methylprednisolone bolus followed by a 5.4 mg/kg/hr infusion for 23 hours (Bracken et al., 1990).

Naloxone Naloxone has been used experimentally to improve spinal blood flow (Faden, Jacobs, & Holaday, 1981) and block the effect of endogenous opiates, which are thought to produce some of the histopathologic effects of spinal cord injury (Nikas, 1986). Experimental treatment with high doses of naloxone, 2.7 mg/kg or more, has resulted in improvement of somatosensory evoked potentials in some patients with spinal cord lesions (Flamm et al., 1985). However, NASCIS 2 found no improvement in outcome after a 5.4 mg/kg bolus of naloxone followed by a 4 mg/kg/hr infusion for 23 hours (Bracken et al., 1990). To contrast dosage, the typical initial dose of naloxone for an overdose is 2 mg or about 0.03 mg/kg in a 70 kg patient. One side effect of naloxone use may be an increase in posttraumatic pain because the receptors for both endogenous opiates (endorphins) and exogenous opiates (i.e. morphine) are blocked.

Thyrotropin-releasing hormone Thyrotropin-releasing hormone is a partial opiate antagonist that spares analgesic systems. In experimentally induced spinal cord injuries in cats, thyrotropin-releasing hormone administration resulted in significantly better neurologic recovery than did saline or dexamethasone treatment. This effect is thought to result from an improvement in spinal cord blood flow without the potential for increasing the patient's pain (Faden et al., 1981).

Mannitol Mannitol, an osmotic diuretic, is believed by some to decrease cord edema and improve blood flow to the cord. The recommended dose is 500 ml of a 20% solution infused intravenously over 4 hours (Meyer & Sullivan, 1984).

Fetal astrocytes Research is under way using fetal astrocytes to guide the growth of new cells in the damaged spinal cord (Kluger, 1988). Eventually this may lead to a "cure" for spinal cord injury.

Hyperbaric oxygen therapy Another experimental treatment is the use of hyperbaric oxygen (HBO) to limit the spread of the vascular lesion in the cord (Myers, 1982). Unfortunately, it appears that HBO must be instituted within a few hours of injury to be beneficial (Yeo & Lowry, 1982).

Altered urinary elimination Spinal cord injury results in a loss of the sacral reflexes that normally cause bladder emptying. Therefore a urinary bladder catheter must be inserted to drain the bladder. A Silastic catheter is preferred because it is inert and is associated with fewer infections and less calcium build-up than rubber catheters. Also, Silastic catheters can be left in place for 5 to 6 weeks (Adelstein & Watson, 1983). Catheterization also allows for more precise measurement of urinary output, an important indicator of visceral perfusion. Because of the risk of infection with an indwelling catheter, intermittent catheterization is instituted as soon as is feasible (Richmond, 1985), usually when reflex activity returns (Adelstein & Watson, 1983). Intermittent catheterization not only decreases the chance of infection, it stimulates normal bladder function by permitting intermittent filling and emptying and helps to retrain the bladder to void spontaneously in the presence of an upper motor neuron lesion (Richmond, 1985). Some patients are taught to use the Credé method (a massage technique) to stimulate bladder emptying.

Complications

In addition to the conditions described, other factors may complicate the condition of a patient with a spinal cord injury. Recognition of common complications and therapeutic dilemmas is essential.

Ineffective thermoregulation results in poikilothermy (the body assumes ambient temperature) in patients with spinal cord lesions. Patients with complete lesions cannot sweat or vasodilate below the level of the lesion and so may have elevated temperatures in hot environments. Patients will also lose body temperature in cold environments because they cannot shiver or vasoconstrict (Nikas, 1986; Richmond, 1985).

Fluid volume excess may result from overaggressive fluid resuscitation in patients whose hypotension is caused by vasodilation and not hypovolemia. This excess fluid may result in acute pulmonary edema and respiratory compromise or adult respiratory distress syndrome (ARDS) later in the patient's hospital stay.

Infections frequently occur in paraplegic and quadriplegic patients (Walleck, 1988) and may be life-threatening. The most common pathways for entrance of microorganisms are the various tubes and devices inserted into the patient, such as urinary bladder catheters, endotracheal suction catheters, and intravenous devices. Careful aseptic technique during insertion of invasive equipment will help decrease subsequent infections.

Autonomic dysreflexia is a medical emergency that may occur any time after spinal shock has resolved in a quadriplegic or high paraplegic patient. It is the result of massive sympathetic discharge in response to noxious stimuli below the level of spinal cord injury. A distended bladder is the most common cause, followed by constipation and decubitus ulcers. The onset of autonomic dysreflexia is characterized by a sudden, severe headache and hypertension. The patient may also be flushed and diaphoretic above the level of the spinal cord injury and pale and cool below the lesion. Other signs and symptoms include bradycardia or tachycardia, nasal congestion, and apprehension (Walleck, 1988). The treatment includes elevating the patient's head and removing the offensive stimulus (e.g., drain bladder, evacuate bowel, administer pain medications for wounds). Antihypertensive agents may be used if the previous interventions are not successful.

MUSCULOSKELETAL INJURIES

Musculoskeletal injuries are one of the most frequently occurring types of trauma. Although these injuries often occur in isolation, 85% of multiple trauma patients will have one or more skeletal injuries (Rosenthal, 1984). Musculoskeletal injuries are rarely life threatening but do cause a significant amount of disability that may be lengthy or permanent. This disability may result in high costs to the patient and society as wages are lost and medical expenses incurred. One source found treatment-related costs associated with extremity injuries to be 43% of the total 1-year treatment costs for all trauma patients in the study (MacKenzie, Shapiro, & Siegel, 1988). Because the focus of this book is major trauma, only life- or limb-threatening musculoskeletal injuries and complications will be discussed.

Mechanism of Injury

Obtaining the most complete history possible about the circumstances surrounding the injury helps to predict which injuries the patient is most likely to have sustained. Unrestrained front seat passengers may suffer lower extremity injuries as a result of striking the dashboard with their knees. These injuries may include knee or patellar dislocations, femur fractures, hip fractures or dislocations, and acetabular fractures as a result of the femoral head being pushed through the acetabulum (McSwain, 1980). Adult pedestrians struck by cars also frequently have leg fractures or dislocations. Pelvic fractures are a common outcome of being run over by a vehicle, thrown from or by a vehicle, or falling from a significant height. Gunshot wounds may cause extensive soft tissue trauma, in addition to open fractures.

Children are more frequently involved in pedestrian injuries than adults (Rivara, 1990). They are also more likely to be pulled under the car and run over, thus sustaining multiple injuries. Femur fractures in very young children should always raise the question of abuse in the absence of a consistent mechanism of injury. The normal resiliency of children's bones combined with the relative strength of the normal femur make this an unlikely injury from apparently minor trauma (e.g., falling from a chair). This bony resiliency commonly results in incomplete or greenstick fractures. Greenstick fractures, especially of the femur, may still result in significant blood loss (J. Neff, personal communication, 1989). When the epiphyseal plate is involved, the fracture need not be large to disrupt the normal growth and development of the bone. Elderly patients and those with degenerative bone diseases are at higher risk of fractures because of the loss of bony matrix. Relatively minor falls are frequent precursors of hip fractures or femur fractures in these populations. Fractures may occur spontaneously in osteoporotic bone and *cause* the fall rather than being a *consequence* of the fall.

Anatomic and Physiologic Considerations

The periosteum, which surrounds the bone, contains a dense network of blood vessels that help supply the bone with blood. The medullary cavities inside the long bones of the extremities contain yellow marrow (mostly fat) and some red marrow (responsible for blood cell production). When bones are fractured, blood and fat may be lost from the bone itself. For additional information on the anatomic and physiologic characteristics of muscle, joints & tendons, the reader should refer to an anatomy and physiology textbook or an orthopedic surgery book.

General Assessment

Pain and tenderness on palpation are the most common complaints of a patient with a musculo-skeletal injury. Point tenderness was found to be a good predictor of underlying fracture in one study (Brand et al., 1982). The patient may also complain of limited range of motion or inability to use the injured limb. However, it is a common fallacy among laypeople that a person cannot walk on a broken leg. Frequently adults and older children do use and walk on fractured extremities. With younger children, refusal to ambulate or use the extremity may be the presenting complaint for a musculoskeletal injury. Also, patients may relate having heard a "pop" or actually feeling the bone snap (Rosenthal, 1984).

Inspection and Palpation

Deformity, shortening, or abnormal rotation may be apparent in an injured extremity. In the absence of bilateral injuries, it may be helpful to compare the injured extremity with the normal extremity. Edema and ecchymoses from blood loss into soft tissue are usually also present with fractures. The examiner should carefully note the presence of impaired skin integrity because open fractures are managed differently from closed fractures. Pallor may indicate a disruption of the vascular integrity or poor systemic perfusion. The presence of old scars will alert the examiner to the probability that the area was previously injured.

Palpation of the injured area should be performed gently. The presence of tenderness, point tenderness, and crepitus or bony instability should be noted. Crepitus should never be purposefully elicited because of the potential for damage to surrounding structures by the movement of bone ends. Capillary refill, skin color, and temperature should be checked. The examiner should palpate all pulses distal to the injury and compare with the uninjured extremity if possible. Ongoing pulse checks are easier if an ink mark is made over the pulse when it is found. This is especially helpful for the dorsalis pedis pulse, which may be difficult to find. If the examiner cannot palpate a pulse because of hypotension with altered peripheral tissue perfusion, a Doppler may be helpful. Some patients may congenitally lack a pulse at a certain site. Ten percent of the population lack one or both dorsalis pedis pulses; in these patients the ipsilateral posterior tibial pulse will be stron-ger than usual (Rosenthal, 1984). When a pulse cannot be located, other indicators of tissue perfusion (e.g., capillary refill, skin color, and temperature) or Doppler must be used.

Sensory and motor function

Assessment of peripheral nerve function distal to the injury includes both motor and sensory tests as described in Table 11-2, and Figures 11-11 and 11-12. Sensation is commonly evaluated by the ability to discriminate between sharp and dull stimuli. More sensitive tests include two-point discrimination and vibratory sensation. Motor function evaluation should also include an assessment of strength. Again, comparison with the uninjured extremity can be helpful.

Diagnostic and Monitoring Procedures
Radiographic studies

Plain radiographs are usually sufficient for the emergency department evaluation of skeletal trauma (Cone, 1984). Views should be obtained in two planes, i.e., anteroposterior and lateral, and should include the entire bone and the joint distal and the joint proximal to the bone in question (Rosenthal, 1984). Comparison views of the normal extremity in children are sometimes necessary to differentiate developmental from pathologic findings. In general, comparison views should not be ordered routinely (Cone, 1984).

Using radiotranslucent splints, which will allow x-rays to penetrate, can save the patient a great deal of pain and further tissue damage. Most

---

Table 11-2 Assessment of peripheral nerve function

Nerve	Motor test	Sensory test
Radial	Dorsiflex wrist or extend metacarpal-phalangeal joints	Dorsal web space between the thumb and index finger
Median	Thumb opposition	Pad of index finger
Ulnar	Spread fingers	Pad of little finger
Femoral	Straight leg raise or extend knee	Anterior thigh
Peroneal	Dorsiflex foot	Web space between great toe and second toe
Tibial	Plantar flex foot	Sole of foot

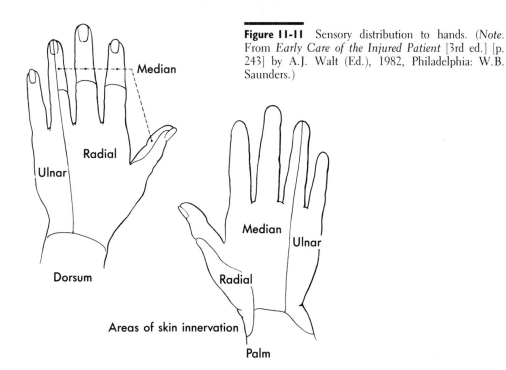

Figure 11-11 Sensory distribution to hands. (*Note.* From *Early Care of the Injured Patient* [3rd ed.] [p. 243] by A.J. Walt (Ed.), 1982, Philadelphia: W.B. Saunders.)

Median

Radial

Ulnar

Dorsum

Median

Ulnar

Radial

Areas of skin innervation

Palm

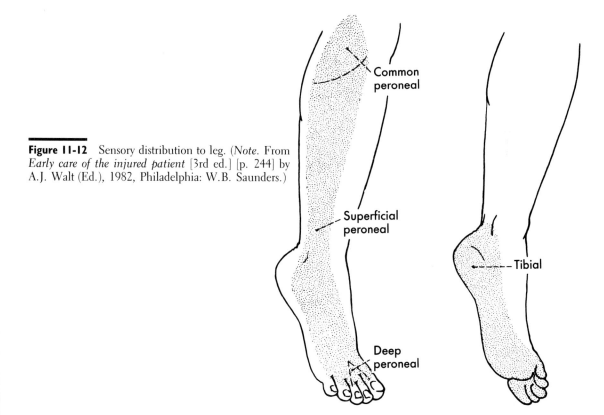

Figure 11-12 Sensory distribution to leg. (*Note.* From *Early care of the injured patient* [3rd ed.] [p. 244] by A.J. Walt (Ed.), 1982, Philadelphia: W.B. Saunders.)

Common peroneal

Superficial peroneal

Deep peroneal

Tibial

commonly used splints are radiotranslucent and do not need to be removed before x-ray examination if correctly applied and no neurovascular compromise is evident. In the event that neurovascular deficits are present, the splint should be removed and the extremity gently repositioned under a physician's direction before x-ray films are obtained. Bulky dressings may make it difficult to obtain clear films and may need to be partially removed. However, open fractures should be kept covered, and a small dressing should not interfere with x-rays. Mobile stretchers with mounted racks for x-ray cassettes are available and allow many films to be taken without lifting, logrolling, or moving the patient from the stretcher. However, many of these stretchers do not yield good quality films, and the radiologist may request that the patient be moved to the regular x-ray table for repeat films. Thus the mechanics and construction of the cassette system is paramount to the success of obtaining x-ray films of patients without changing their position. When purchasing this type of stretcher, the purchaser should consider the composition of the top and the presence of a grid, which are key elements in the quality of subsequent x-rays. The stretcher top should have an aluminum equivalency of 0.8 mm or less. Aluminum equivalency is the thickness of aluminum that would allow the same amount of radiation to pass through as the material being rated. Materials such as polycarbonate and polypropylene allow x-rays to pass but add to scatter, which degrades the quality of the film. An absorber may be incorporated to help absorb some of the scatter. A grid in the stretcher top will also improve the quality of the films and should have an 8:1 ratio with 103 lines per inch for best results (J. Bradcovich, Beta One, personal communication, May 26, 1989). Also the ease of use of the stretcher should be considered: can the cassette holders be adjusted instead of repositioning the patient; can the head be raised far enough to obtain an upright chest film without propping the patient up with a pillow? Trauma rooms with built-in overhead x-ray tubes facilitate doing x-ray examinations in the emergency department and generally result in better quality films than do portable x-ray units.

Arteriograms are helpful if vascular damage is suspected because of diminished or absent pulses, etc. Frequently knee dislocations disrupt the pop-

Table II-3 Potential local blood loss in fractures

Injured area	Liters
Humerus	1.0-2.0
Elbow	0.5-1.5
Forearm	0.5-1.0
PELVIS	**1.5-4.5**
Hip	1.5-2.5
Femur	1.0-2.0
Knee	1.0-1.5
Tibia	0.5-1.5
Ankle	0.5-1.5
Spine/ribs	1.0-3.0

Note. From *Care of the Trauma Patient* (2nd ed.) (p. 372) by G. Shires, 1979, New York: McGraw-Hill; and *Early Care of the Injured Patient* (3rd ed.) (p. 284) by A.J. Walt (Ed.), 1982, Philadelphia: W.B. Saunders.

liteal artery, and arteriograms are done to evaluate vascular patency.

Laboratory studies

The bones have a rich vascular supply (Rosenthal, 1984), and fractures may cause significant blood loss. Measurements of hemoglobin and hematocrit are helpful with multiple fractures or fractures of the pelvis or femur. Potential local blood loss from fractures is outlined in Table 11-3. Type and crossmatch studies are indicated if significant blood loss is present or anticipated.

Urine may be analyzed for myoglobin, a product of muscle breakdown, if severe crushing has occurred or compartmental syndrome is suspected. This is discussed in more detail in the Compartmental Syndrome section.

Assessment and Intervention Related to Specific Injuries
Fractures

A fracture is a disruption in the continuity of a bone. Several classifications of fractures exist; however, the most important determination for initial management is whether the fracture is "open" or "closed."

Closed fractures Closed fractures (formerly called *simple fractures*) have no associated break in skin integrity. Emergent management consists of splinting to prevent soft tissue damage and decrease pain, elevation and ice to decrease edema formation, and referral to an orthopedic surgeon for definitive management.

Open fractures Open fractures (formerly called *compound fractures*) are associated with a break in skin integrity. The examiner should assume that any wound in the vicinity of a fracture communicates with that fracture and should treat it as an open fracture (Rosenthal, 1984). Bacterial contamination may lead to infection of the soft tissue and bone. Ligaments, tendons, and the cartilage within joints are relatively avascular (Iversen & Clawson, 1982), and effective serum antibiotic concentrations in these structures are difficult to achieve. Infection of the bone, osteomyelitis, is also difficult to treat. The formation of pus under pressure within the rigid bony structure compromises the vascular supply and leads to osteocyte destruction (Iversen & Clawson, 1982). Prevention of osteomyelitis is always a primary goal in the treatment of open fractures (Rosenthal, 1984).

Wound cultures should be obtained (Markison, 1984) and a sterile dressing applied (Iversen & Clawson, 1982; Rosenthal, 1984). The accuracy of such cultures in predicting infection is under question. One study found that the best predictive value was from tissue cultures taken in the operating room after debridement was completed (Merritt, 1988). Some sources recommend the dressing be soaked with povidone-iodine solution (Rosenthal, 1984). Tetanus immunization is provided as indicated, and prophylactic antibiotics, usually an intravenous cephalosporin, are administered as soon as possible (Iversen & Clawson, 1982; Trafton, 1984). All open extremity fractures should be examined, irrigated, and debrided in the operating room (Iversen & Clawson, 1982). In the operating room, definitive stabilization is achieved through internal or external fixation devices (Figure 11-13), traction, or plaster or fiberglass casts (Trafton, 1984). Fiberglass casts have the advantage of being lighter and more durable than plaster casts.

Pelvic fractures A large amount of force is required to fracture the pelvis, and severe concomitant injuries are common (Bucholz, 1984). Deformity may not be obvious on inspection, and palpation should include a gentle pelvic rock and pressure on the anterior superior iliac spines and the pubic symphysis to elicit pain or instability. With any pelvic fracture, the rectum and vagina should be examined to check for altered tissue in-

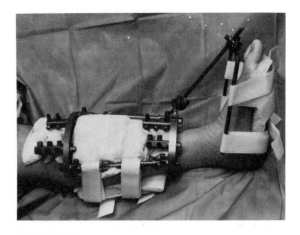

Figure 11-13 External fixation of lower leg. (Courtesy Ace Medical, Los Angeles.)

tegrity (i.e., an open fracture communicating with the vaginal vault or rectum). Open pelvic fractures can result in devastating infections with a high mortality and morbidity (Bucholz, 1984; Trafton, 1984). In male patients a high-riding prostate gland signals an underlying pelvic hematoma, and no catheter should be inserted until a retrograde urethrogram demonstrates urethral patency. Blood at the urinary meatus is also a contraindication to urinary catheter placement (see Chapter 12).

Fluid volume deficit is commonly associated with pelvic fractures because the area is highly vascular and as much as 4.5 liters of blood may be lost into the pelvic space (Walt, 1982). Fracture patterns involving a double break in the pelvic ring are most commonly associated with significant blood loss (Bucholz & Claudi, 1984). This blood accumulates in the retroperitoneal space but may enter the peritoneal space through torn fascial planes and cause a false-positive peritoneal lavage (Bresler, 1988). Large-bore intravenous lines should be established and preparations made to administer blood products if necessary.

Initial splinting of pelvic fractures is usually accomplished with a backboard. However, pneumatic antishock garments may help to stabilize the fracture(s) and tamponade bleeding (American College of Surgeons, 1989; Rosenthal, 1984). Pelvic fractures rarely need operative stabilization

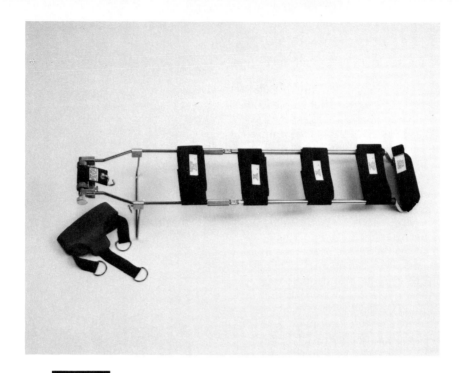

Figure 11-14 Hare traction splint. (Courtesy DYNA MED, Carlsbad, CA.)

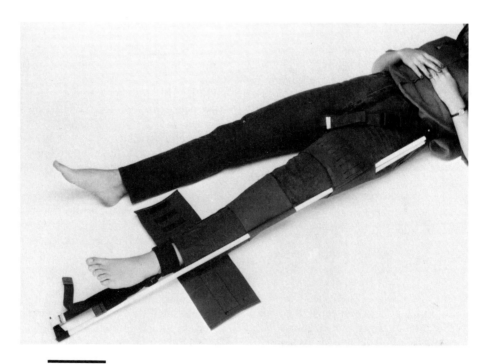

Figure 11-15 Kendrick traction device. (Courtesy Medix Choice, El Cajon, CA.)

and frequently are managed with bedrest, spica casts, or sling traction. In severe cases external fixation devices may be applied.

Femur fractures The femur is the longest and strongest bone in the body and requires a significant amount of force to be fractured. Frequently femur fractures are accompanied by other serious injuries (Trafton, 1984). A fractured femur is usually dramatic in presentation with obvious deformity, shortening, and muscle spasm of the thigh. Conscious patients will complain of severe pain. Swelling of the thigh is a result of underlying blood loss, which may be as much as 2 liters (Walt, 1982).

The need for fluid resuscitation and blood products should be anticipated in all patients with femur fractures. Traction splinting of the femur decreases the pain and soft tissue trauma by preventing muscle spasm. Commercially available traction splints include the Hare (Figure 11-14); Kendrick (Figure 11-15); and Sager (Figure 11-16) brands. A Thomas splint may be employed also (Iversen & Clawson, 1982). The Hare, Kendrick, and Sager splints are easier to apply than a Thomas splint. The Sager and Kendrick models adjust for adults and children; a pediatric-sized version of the Hare splint is available. A Sager model is available that allows both femurs to be splinted with one splint in the event of bilateral fractures. This is difficult (and very uncomfortable for the patient) with the Hare or Thomas splints. Regardless of the type of splint used, the traction should be sufficient to return the leg to its normal length. Measuring the splint on the uninjured leg will facilitate accurate measurement (American College of Surgeons, 1989).

Traction splints should be avoided when the knee, foot, or ankle is injured also. When x-ray films are not yet available to rule out these conditions, the caregiver must make a decision based on clinical assessment of the patient. Traction

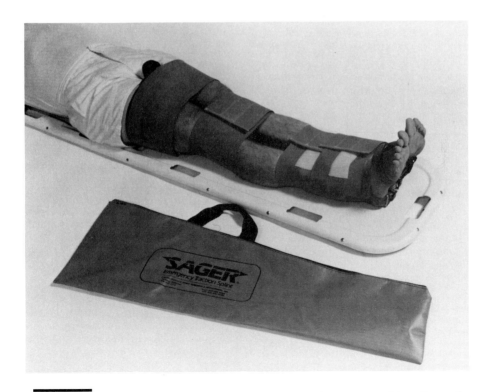

Figure 11-16 Sager Super Bilateral Emergency Traction Splint. (Courtesy Minto Research and Development, Inc., Redding, CA.)

splints may be used in the case of ipsilateral femur and tibia/fibula fractures (known as a *floating knee*).

Most femoral fractures are surgically reduced and stabilized by the placement of an intramedullary nail. This allows the patient to be out of bed on non–weight-bearing status 1 day postoperatively and home in 10 to 14 days—a drastic improvement over the former regimen of 6 weeks of bedrest and traction, with the inherent complications of immobility.

Sternal, rib, and scapular fractures   Fractures of the sternum, ribs, or scapula are rarely significant from a bony perspective but may be associated with life-threatening thoracic injuries. Chapters 8 and 9, on ventilation and perfusion, discuss the management of underlying injuries.

A tremendous amount of force is required to fracture the sternum (Harley & Mena, 1986; Wojcik & Morgan, 1988), and this force is transmitted to the underlying structures. Also, because the usual mechanism of injury is "chest versus steering wheel" (Harley & Mena, 1986; Wojcik & Morgan, 1988), deceleration may play a role in the underlying injuries as well (Harley & Mena, 1986). Sternal fractures with associated rib fractures result in myocardial contusion in 18% of patients, whereas isolated sternal fractures are associated with myocardial contusion in only 6% of the cases (Wojcik & Morgan, 1988).

The upper ribs are well protected by the musculoskeletal framework of the shoulder (American College of Surgeons, 1989; Knezevich, 1986), and fractures are associated with a great deal of force. Usually significant head, neck, or chest trauma accompanies fractures of the first five ribs (American College of Surgeons, 1989).

The scapulas are well protected by surrounding muscle. Although scapular fractures are rare, they may result from significant direct force and are frequently accompanied by life-threatening injuries to other areas (Cooper, 1982).

Dislocations   Pain
High risk for sensory/perceptual
alterations

A dislocation is a disruption of the articulating surfaces of two or more bones. Most dislocations are amenable to reduction and pose no threat to the survival of the limb because neurovascular status is not impaired. One notable exception is a dislocation of the knee (not the patella, but the knee joint itself). Knee dislocations are true orthopedic emergencies because the popliteal artery or nerve is frequently damaged (Campbell, 1982; Worsing, 1984). If no pulse is present, an immediate attempt at closed reduction should be made, without waiting for x-ray studies. Reduction will usually require intravenous sedation to promote muscle relaxation. Postreduction x-ray films are then obtained to rule out concurrent fractures. If a pulse is present, the knee should be carefully splinted in the position found and care should be expedient with close attention to frequent neurovascular assessments.

Amputations   Impaired skin integrity
Impaired tissue integrity
High risk for fluid volume deficit
High risk for body image
disturbance
High risk for impaired physical
mobility

Amputations are devastating injuries in most instances. The loss of a leg or an arm is an obvious cause of disability, but even the loss of a single digit (especially the thumb) may result in the inability to perform previous occupational or recreational activities. For this reason, microsurgical techniques were developed to replant the severed body part so that it will not only survive as viable tissue, but also function. Replantation requires a specialized team and equipment for optimal results, and "replantation centers" have emerged across the country. The role of emergency care providers is to deliver the patient and the severed tissue to such a center as soon as possible after stabilization.

Indications for replantation   In general, the decision to attempt replantation is best left to the microsurgeon. However, several factors should be considered when deciding whether to transfer a patient to a distant replantation center for evaluation.

Specific indications for replantation include "the thumb; all amputations in children; multiple digits, the palm, wrist, and distal forearm levels; an individual digit distal to the superficialis tendon insertion" (Hing, Buncke, Alpert, & Gordon, 1986a, p. 14). The thumb constitutes 40% to 50% of the functional value of the hand because of its role in opposition and grasp. Good functional results are usually achieved with thumb replantation (Hing et al., 1986a; Markison, 1984; O'Hara, 1987). Children have better ability to regenerate transected nerves and will more readily adapt to use of a replanted part than will an adult (Hing et al., 1986a; O'Hara, 1987). Loss of multiple digits will seriously compromise hand function, and an attempt should be made to replant as many digits as possible. Good functional results are usually achieved with distal upper extremity and distal finger replants (Hing et al., 1986a; O'Hara, 1987). Proximal finger replants are occasionally detrimental to the overall function of the hand (Urbaniak, Roth, Nunley, Goldner, & Koman, 1985).

Relative contraindications to replantation include (1) patients with life-threatening injuries or significant systemic disease; (2) excessive "ischemia time;" (3) severely crushed or contaminated injuries; (4) injuries at multiple levels on the same extremity; and (5) psychosocial factors that make patient compliance unlikely (Hing et al., 1986a; O'Hara, 1987). Presence of the "red line sign" is an absolute contraindication to replantation (Markison, 1984). The "red line sign" is the presence of red streaks over neurovascular bundles and reflects "major crush and breakdown of distal vascular integrity, with subsequent extravasation of blood into tissues" (Markison, 1984, p. 106). Reanastomosis of such injuries is unlikely to succeed (Markison, 1984).

Care of amputated tissue "Ischemia time," or the time the severed part is without blood flow, is an important determinant in the likelihood of successful replantation. Fingers contain no muscle and are more resistant to ischemia than muscular tissue. Cooled tissue is also more resistant to ischemia because of decreased metabolism. Uncooled fingers may be successfully replanted 8 to 10 hours after injury; however, cooling the fingers may extend this time up to 28 hours (Hing et al., 1986a, 1986b; O'Hara, 1987). Muscular tissue is best replanted after a maximum of 6 hours of warm ischemia or 10 to 12 hours of cold ischemia (Hing et al., 1986a, 1986b; O'Hara, 1987).

Most references describe the care of the amputated part as gently cleansing or irrigating the part to remove gross contamination, wrapping it in saline or lactated Ringer's solution–moistened sterile gauze, placing it in a sealed plastic bag, and placing the plastic bag on ice, taking care to avoid

direct contact between the ice and the tissue (American College of Surgeons, 1989; Billmire, Neale, & Stern, 1984; Hing et al., 1986a; Knezevich, 1986; Iversen & Clawson, 1982; Markison, 1984; Rea, 1991; Strange, 1987; Wohlstadter, 1979). Many sources caution against immersing the part in saline or lactated Ringer's solution (Billmire et al., 1984; Hing et al., 1986b; Rea, 1991; Wohlstadter, 1979). However, one study (Van Giesen, Seaber, & Urbaniak, 1983) found no difference in viability rates with moistened dressings versus total immersion of experimentally severed rabbit ears. Some sources (O'Hara, 1987; Worsing, 1984) recommend that both the severed part and the stump be wrapped in dry dressings. Moist dressings may increase the potential for both maceration and contamination. Freezing the amputated part should be avoided because the expansion associated with the formation of ice crystals results in cellular damage (Hing et al., 1986b).

Preparation of the patient for replantation The patient must be prepared for a lengthy surgical procedure. Special considerations for replantation include the early administration of an intravenous antibiotic, usually a cephalosporin, and the indicated tetanus prophylaxis (Billmire et al., 1984; O'Hara, 1987). Completely severed vessels do not usually bleed profusely because of smooth muscle constriction. However, partially lacerated vessels, such as in crush injuries, may bleed profusely and require direct pressure and elevation (Hing et al., 1986b; O'Hara, 1987). Tourniquets will only worsen ischemia and should be avoided (Hing et al., 1986b; O'Hara, 1987). Tying or clamping vessels should be avoided, since the tissue that will be reanastomosed may be injured (Hing et al., 1986b; O'Hara, 1987). The replant team will need x-ray studies of the stump and severed part (Hing et al., 1986b; O'Hara, 1987). If a fracture accompanies a partial amputation, the limb should be splinted appropriately. Pain should be managed by intramuscular or intravenous analgesics. Local nerve blocks should not be used because the needle used to inject such blocks may further damage nerves and vessels (Hing et al., 1986b; O'Hara, 1987). Because nicotine causes vasoconstriction, the patient should not be allowed to smoke or chew tobacco or nicotine gum. The patient and significant others should be reassured that all measures are being taken to save the amputated part, but they should not be given false hope. The microvascular surgeon is the most qualified to give the patient a realistic prognosis.

General Interventions

Interventions for musculoskeletal trauma are arranged by nursing diagnoses. The issues of knowledge deficit and fear should be incorporated in nursing care.

Fluid volume deficit

Fluid volume deficits should be anticipated in any patient with multiple fractures or femur or pelvis fractures. Specific interventions include the administration of intravenous fluids and blood products (see Chapter 9 for further information). Splinting may help slow or prevent blood loss; it is discussed in detail in the next section.

High risk for injury

Surrounding soft tissue may be damaged by the movement of bone ends or fragments. Splinting the injured area will help decrease this movement. A variety of devices make effective splints if basic principles are followed:

1. The splint should always immobilize the joint above and below the injury (Rea, 1991; Worsing, 1984).
2. Neurovascular status distal to the injury should be assessed before and after splinting and after every movement of the extremity (American College of Surgeons, 1984; Rea, 1991). Recheck neurovascular status after x-ray films are obtained.
3. Avoid moving the injured area any more than absolutely necessary (Rea, 1991; Worsing, 1984).
4. Remove all clothing and jewelry from the extremity (American College of Surgeons, 1989; Rea, 1991). This facilitates inspection and palpation of the injured extremity, prevents pressure on the extremity from clothing or items in pockets, and improves the quality of subsequent x-ray films.
5. Most deformities may be returned toward anatomic position with gentle traction if necessary to apply the splint (American College of Surgeons, 1989; Iversen & Clawson, 1982, Worsing, 1984). The exceptions are injuries involving joints, espe-

cially the elbow. These injuries should be splinted as found unless the extremity is pulseless (Rea, 1991). In this event, one attempt should be made to reposition the injury to restore circulation before splinting. If the repositioning attempt further compromises neurovascular status or is very painful, splint in the position found.

6. Cover open wounds with a sterile dressing before splinting (American College of Surgeons, 1989; Iversen & Clawson, 1982, Worsing, 1984).
7. Do not force bone ends or soft tissue back into an open wound (Iversen & Clawson, 1982; Rea, 1991). The bone ends may slip back in during repositioning (as with applying a traction splint to a femur fracture) but should not be forced back into the wound (Worsing, 1984).
8. Do not convert a closed fracture to an open fracture. Extremities should be repositioned carefully to prevent violating the skin integrity with the fracture ends. This is most probable with bones that have little overlying soft tissue, such as the tibia.
9. Pad bony prominences inside the splint (Rea, 1991; Worsing, 1984). This will more effectively immobilize the extremity, make the splint more comfortable for the patient, and help prevent pressure sores.

Pain

Musculoskeletal injuries can be very painful. Gentle handling and proper splinting will help decrease the discomfort. Narcotic analgesics are frequently used if not contraindicated by coexisting trauma. Elevation of the splinted extremity and ice packs will help decrease edema formation and the associated discomfort of tissue stretching.

High risk for infection

When skin integrity is impaired, the first line of defense against invading bacteria is gone. Wounds should be covered with sterile dressings. Masks should be worn if the wound is to be exposed for any length of time. Dressings should be removed only *as necessary* for wound observation or treatment. Prophylactic antibiotics are frequently administered preoperatively for open and closed fractures, and all open fractures are cleansed and debrided in the operating room.

Complications

The patient should be monitored for associated fluid volume deficits or impaired gas exchange with serial vital signs, neurologic checks, and laboratory studies as indicated. The injured area should have baseline and ongoing assessments of distal neurovascular status, pain, and edema. Loss of neurovascular function may herald a serious problem requiring prompt intervention to save the limb or its function.

Compartmental syndrome

Compartmental syndrome is ". . . a condition in which increased pressure within a limited space compromises the circulation and function of tissues within that space" (Matsen & Krugmire, 1978, p. 943). Intrinsic compartments are bounded by bone and nonelastic soft tissue, such as fascia, and exist several places in the body (Figure 11-17). Compartmental syndrome commonly results from tibial fractures and other bony or soft tissue injuries (Proehl, 1988). As the pressure within a compartment increases, the metabolic demands can no longer be met because of restricted microvascular flow and cellular injury and dysfunction result. Compartmental syndrome may develop almost immediately or up to 6 days after injury (Matsen, 1980).

Symptoms of compartmental syndrome include (1) severe pain (usually of a severity not explained by the primary injury) that does not respond to medication, (2) pain on passive stretch of the muscles within the involved compartment, (3) hypesthesia of sensory areas innervated by nerves within the involved compartment, and (4) palpable tenseness of the compartmental envelope (Iversen & Clawson, 1982; Matsen & Krugmire, 1978; Proehl, 1988). Pain may be absent or minimal if neural dysfunction coexists (Wright, Bogoch, & Hastings, 1989). Skin color, capillary refill, and distal pulses are unreliable signs. Pulselessness develops late in the syndrome and is an ominous sign (Iversen & Clawson, 1982; Matsen & Krugmire, 1978; Proehl, 1988). A description of assessment findings in compartmental syndrome of the lower leg, forearm, and hand are shown in Table 11-4.

Tissue pressure measurement   Direct measurement of compartmental pressure is often helpful and is necessary in patients who have a confusing clinical presentation or who cannot give reliable

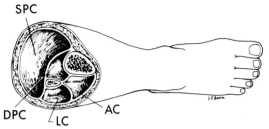

Four compartments of the leg: the anterior compartment (*AC*), the lateral compartment (*LC*), the superficial posterior compartment (*SPC*), and the deep posterior compartment (*DPC*).

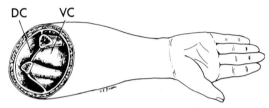

Two compartments of the forearm: the volar compartment (*VC*) and the dorsal compartment (*DC*).

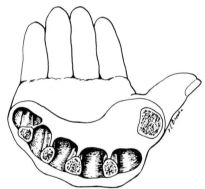

Five interosseous compartments of the hand.

Figure 11-17   Extremity compartments. (*Note*. From *Compartmental syndromes* [p. 82] by F.A. Matsen, 1980, New York: Grune & Stratton.)

responses to sensory tests because of altered mental states or paraplegia. Three methods are available for direct pressure measurements. The Whitesides technique (Figure 11-18) uses commonly available materials: stopcock, saline-filled tubing, syringe, needle, and a mercury manometer (Iversen & Clawson, 1982; Kuska, 1982; White-

Table II-4 Signs and symptoms associated with compartmental syndromes

Compartment	Location of sensory changes	Movement weakened	Painful passive movement	Location of pain/tenseness
Lower leg				
Anterior	First web space	Toe extension	Toe flexion	Along lateral side of anterior tibia
Lateral	Dorsum (top) of foot	Foot eversion	Foot inversion	Lateral lower leg
Superficial posterior	None	Foot plantar flexion	Foot dorsiflexion	Calf
Deep posterior	Sole of foot	Toe flexion	Toe extension	Deep calf—palpable between Achilles tendon and medial malleoli
Forearm				
Volar	Volar (palmar) aspect of fingers	Wrist and finger flexion	Wrist and finger extension	Volar forearm
Dorsal	None	Wrist and finger extension	Wrist and finger flexion	Dorsal forearm
Hand				
Intraosseus	None	Finger adduction and abduction	Finger adduction and abduction	Between metacarpals on dorsum of hand

Note. Adapted from "Compartmental Syndromes: A Unified Concept" by F.A. Matsen, 1975, *Clinical Orthopaedics and Related Research, 113*, p. 10.

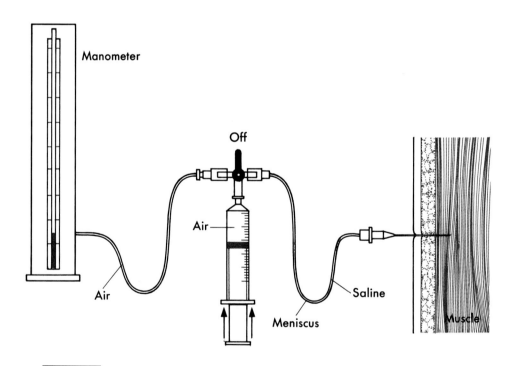

Figure 11-18 Whitesides technique of tissue pressure measurement. Tubing is fitted to mercury manometer tubing and side port. Needle is inserted into muscle through skin, subcutaneous tissue, and fascia. (*Note.* From "Acute Onset of Compartment Syndrome" by B.M. Kuska, 1982, *Journal of Emergency Nursing*, 8[2], p. 78.)

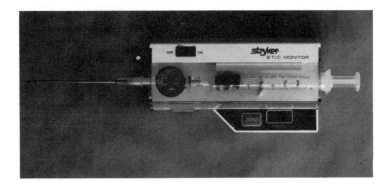

Figure 11-19   Stryker Solid-State Transducer Intra Compartmental (S.T.I.C.) Pressure Monitor System. (Courtesy Stryker, Inc., Kalamazoo, MI.).

sides, Haney, Morimoto, & Harada, 1975). A standard pressure set-up for monitoring arterial pressures, etc. can also be used in conjunction with various needles, catheters, or wicks (Matsen, 1978). A recently introduced instrument, the Stryker Solid-State Transducer Intra Compartmental (S.T.I.C.) pressure monitor system (Figure 11-19), is a simple device for rapid tissue pressure measurements (Proehl, 1988).

Normal tissue pressure is less than 20 mm Hg (Kuska, 1982). Tissue pressures in excess of 30 to 40 mm Hg with suspicious clinical findings are usually an indication for decompression of the compartment by surgical fasciotomy (Iversen & Clawson, 1982; Kuska, 1982; Matsen & Krugmire, 1978; Proehl, 1988; Whitesides et al., 1975). Recent research has indicated that the absolute pressure is not as significant as the relationship of compartmental pressure to mean arterial pressure (Heppenstall et al., 1988). Subtracting compartmental pressure from mean arterial pressure (MAP) (MAP − compartmental pressure = ΔP) will allow a more accurate assessment of metabolic supply and demand. A pressure difference, ΔP, of 30 mm Hg or greater is necessary for metabolic needs to be met in normal tissue and 40 mm Hg or greater in moderately traumatized tissue (Heppenstall et al., 1988).

Fasciotomy   Treatment of a confirmed compartmental syndrome consists of emergency surgical decompression (Matsen & Krugmire, 1978; Whitesides et al., 1975). Research suggests that irreversible damage occurs within 8 to 12 hours after the onset of diminished tissue perfusion (Iversen & Clawson, 1982; Matsen & Krugmire, 1978, Whitesides et al., 1975). Nursing measures include maintaining the limb at heart level, since higher elevation will further compromise the microcirculation and a dependent position will promote edema. Remove all external sources of pressure, such as circumferential dressings or plaster (Matsen & Krugmire, 1978; Proehl, 1988). Also, because of the importance of MAP in maintaining tissue perfusion, systemic blood pressure should be normalized.

Chemical therapy   One new intervention, chemical fasciotomy, is under investigation. Injection of hyaluronidase into the subfascial area leads to the breakdown of hyaluronic acid (one of the components of connective tissue). This allows fluid to escape and the compartmental pressure to decrease. In one dog study, this led to a significant drop in compartmental pressure (Gershuni et al., 1985). However, pressure within the compartment may rise again, necessitating ongoing assessment and perhaps repeated injections.

Myoglobinuria   Myoglobin may be present in the urine as a result of muscle breakdown. To prevent myoglobin from damaging the renal tubules, the kidneys must be flushed well (Iversen & Clawson, 1982). A minimum urine output of 75 to 100 ml/hour should be maintained, and bicarbonate may be given to alkalinize the urine and decrease precipitation of the myoglobin in the tubules (Strange, 1987).

Hyperbaric oxygen therapy   Hyperbaric oxygen

(HBO) has also been suggested as a treatment for compartmental syndrome. Experimental evidence from dog studies demonstrates a reduction in edema and muscle necrosis after treatment with HBO (Skyhar et al., 1986; Strauss, Hargens, Gershuni, Hart, & Akeson, 1986). HBO is not recommended as replacement for surgical fasciotomy in full-blown compartmental syndromes but is recommended as an adjunct and as an intervention in cases where the need for surgical fasciotomy is not clear (Strauss & Hart, 1984).

Fat embolism syndrome

Two major theories exist regarding the pathophysiology of fat embolism syndrome (FES). The first postulates that fat is released directly from the marrow of a fractured bone into the vasculature (Buchan, 1984; Healy, 1986; Knezevich, 1986; Maher, 1986). Others believe that the fat globules actually form within the blood vessels from the free fatty acids that are mobilized during trauma metabolism (Buchan, 1984; Healy, 1986: Knezevich, 1986; Maher, 1986). Regardless of the origin of the fat globules, the outcome is the same: vascular embolization with distal occlusion of blood vessels, especially pulmonary capillaries. The presence of free fatty acids causes diffuse inflammation, and vasoactive amines and histamine are released from these injured vessels and cause vasospasm, edema, and disruption of the capillary alveolar membrane (Buchan, 1984; Luce, Tyler, & Pierson, 1984). These changes result in altered gas exchange as a result of ventilation/perfusion mismatch and respiratory distress. Fat embolism has been implicated as a cause of ARDS (Buchan, 1984).

Signs and symptoms Symptoms of fat embolism are usually seen 12 to 72 hours after trauma (Rea, 1991) but may be seen up to 10 days later (Knezevich, 1986). Some degree of fat embolism is believed to occur in all long bone fractures (Buchan, 1984: Healy, 1986) but is symptomatic in only 5% to 25% of long bone fractures (Healy, 1986). Mortality in diagnosed fat embolism syndrome is 50% (Campbell, 1982; Knezevich, 1986) and is increased with concurrent hypovolemia (Iversen & Clawson, 1982; Knezevich, 1986).

Early symptoms of fat embolism are dyspnea, tachycardia, and fever. As the syndrome progresses, petechiae may be noted across the neck, axilla, chest, and conjunctiva in 25% to 50% of patients. The exact cause of the petechiae is unknown but is thought to be a result of thrombocytopenia or direct involvement of the cutaneous blood vessels. As respiratory compromise occurs, alterations in level of consciousness manifest, progressing from confusion and restlessness to delirium and possibly seizures and coma (Knezevich, 1986).

Laboratory findings consistent with fat embolism include a PaO_2 less than 60 (Iversen & Clawson, 1982; Knezevich, 1986; Maher, 1986) and a platelet count less than 150,000 (Knezevich, 1986). Serum lipase levels may increase, and free fat may be found in the sputum and urine (Knezevich, 1986: Rea, 1991), but these findings are nonspecific (Healy, 1986). Fluffy exudates may be seen on chest x-ray film (Maher, 1986); however, they may not show up for 72 hours after injury (Knezevich, 1986).

The mainstays of therapy are immobilization of the fracture to prevent further release of emboli and respiratory support with high-flow oxygen (Buchan, 1984; Campbell, 1982; Iversen & Clawson, 1982; Knezevich, 1986; Maher, 1986; Rea, 1991). Fluid resuscitation as indicated by the patient's clinical condition will help break up the larger emboli (Maher, 1986). Steroids are frequently employed to decrease the inflammation of the lung tissue surrounding the embolus (Healy, 1986: Iversen & Clawson, 1982; Luce, Tyler, & Pierson, 1984; Knezevich, 1986) and may have prophylactic value as well (Healy, 1986). Other medications endorsed by some sources include heparin, ethyl alcohol, and dextran (Iversen & Clawson, 1982; Knezevich, 1986). One source postulates that heparin is contraindicated in this disorder because heparin activates lipase, which enhances breakdown of neutral fat (Luce et al., 1984). This breakdown of neutral fat liberates fatty acids, which may then cause inflammatory reactions.

SUMMARY Impairment of mobility may have a profound and permanent impact on a person's life. Optimal care in the early hours after trauma may help prevent complications and facilitate healing, thus diminishing the potential disability faced by the patient. The table on pp. 357-358 summarizes nursing diagnoses, their interventions, and evaluation criteria for spinal and musculoskeletal injuries.

Nursing diagnosis	Nursing intervention	Evaluative criteria
Ineffective airway clearance Related to lack of nervous system control As evidenced by decreased respiratory movement, noisy or absent respirations	**Maintain oxygenation** Provide airway adjuncts (oral/nasopharyngeal airway, endotracheal intubation) as indicated, with simultaneous cervical spine immobilization. Carefully insert gastric tube (if no concurrent contraindications) to prevent vomiting/aspiration. Suction carefully to remove secretions—stimulation of the gag reflex may result in retching and head or neck movement and bradycardia. Administer O_2 as ordered.	Patent airway will be achieved without movement of head or neck.
Ineffective breathing pattern Related to lack of intercostal muscle function As evidenced by retractions, shallow respirations, fatigue	**Maintain ventilation** Intubate and ventilate if respirations are absent or fatigue is present or Pao_2 decreases below 60.	Arterial blood gas will be within normal limits.
High risk for injury Related to decreased anatomic stability of vertebrae	**Prevent injury** Instruct patient to lie quietly and not attempt to move head or neck. Maintain clear, supportive communication to reduce fear, anxiety. Immobilize all patients at risk on a backboard with a hard or stiff collar. Use tape and firm supports at each side of the head to prevent flexion, rotation, and lateral movement of the head.	Patient will verbalize understanding of need not to move. No sudden changes will occur in neuromuscular function (swelling may cause gradual changes). Patient will not be able to move head or neck because of proper immobilization.
Altered general tissue perfusion Secondary to neurogenic shock Related to unopposed parasympathetic stimulation As evidenced by signs of distributive shock: flushing of extremities, bradycardia, hypotension	**Maintain circulation** Keep the patient flat. Administer IV fluids as ordered. Administer oxygen as ordered. Measure and record I & O.	Blood pressure will be 90/60 or above. Patient will be alert and oriented if no concurrent injuries resulting in altered levels of consciousness. Urine output will be 1 ml/kg/hr or more. Fluid overload will not occur (lungs clear, no jugular vein distention).
Altered spinal cord tissue perfusion Related to unopposed parasympathetic activity As evidenced by vasodilation, bradycardia	**Support spinal cord perfusion** Provide supplemental oxygen. Administer medications as ordered.	ABG values will be normal. Neurologic status will be stable or improving.
Altered patterns of urinary elimination Related to impaired sensory/motor ability As evidenced by urinary retention (excessive residual when without urinary catheter)	**Promote elimination** Insert an indwelling catheter. Monitor catheter for patency. Measure and record I & O.	No episodes of autonomic dysreflexia will occur (characterized by elevated BP and diaphoresis). BP and heart rate will be within normal limits. No bladder distention will be evident.

Continued.

NURSING DIAGNOSES &
EVALUATIVE CRITERIA   *The patient with altered mobility: spinal and musculoskeletal injuries—cont'd*

Nursing diagnosis	Nursing intervention	Evaluative criteria
Fluid volume deficit Related to vascular blood loss associated with fractures As evidenced by hypotension, abnormal HR, decreased LOC	**Promote musculoskeletal perfusion** Gain intravenous access with large-bore (14- to 16-gauge) IV catheters. Administer crystalloid and blood products as ordered.	Patient will be alert and oriented if no concurrent injuries exist that result in altered levels of consciousness. Urine output will be 1 ml/kg/hr or more.
High risk for injury Related to neurovascular compromise As evidenced by decreased pulse in affected area, coolness of area, decreased motor and sensory function	**Promote stabilization of injured area** Handle injured extremities gently; do not force realignment. Splint injured extremities. Assess neurovascular status of extremities.	Closed fractures will not be converted to open fractures. Neurovascular status will not deteriorate.
Pain, acute Related to tissue destruction and pressure Secondary to fractures or crush As evidenced by request for pain relief, crying, irritation, tachycardia, poor appetite	**Promote comfort** Handle and splint all injured extremities gently. Apply ice pack to injured area. Elevate splinted extremity if no contraindications. Administer pain medication as ordered.	Patient will report a decrease in pain. Increased relaxation will be evident by facial expression, normal respiratory and heart rates (excluding coexisting causes of vital signs alterations). Edema formation will be arrested.
High risk for infection Related to open fracture	**Maintain wound precautions** Cover all open wounds with sterile dressings. Clean and irrigate wound as ordered. Administer antibiotics as ordered. Administer tetanus prophylaxis as indicated.	Clean wounds will not become contaminated. Wound cultures will be negative. No infection will develop as evidenced by lack of purulent drainage, fever, localized erythema or induration.

COMPETENCIES
The following clinical competencies pertain to **caring for the patient with spinal or musculoskeletal injuries.**

☑ *Demonstrate spinal precautions in moving the trauma patient.*

☑ *Perform neurovascular assessment before and after immobilizing extremities.*

☑ *Properly align extremities when applying splinting devices.*

☑ *Monitor the musculoskeletal injury patient for the presence of compartmental syndrome.*

☑ *Intervene appropriately when compartmental syndrome is detected.*

☑ *Assess the spinal injury patient for spinal shock.*

CASE STUDY A 33-year-old male construction worker fell from a 10-foot scaffold onto a concrete sidewalk. He landed on his back with his right leg folded under him. On arrival to the ED he is alert and oriented, immobilized on a backboard with a cervical collar. BP is 110/70, HR is 60, and respirations are 18. Skin is warm, pink, and dry. He has flaccid paralysis of his lower extremities and no sensation or reflexes below the umbilicus. His right lower leg is deformed and swollen but has no open wounds. No other injuries are present.

What examination will be done to determine if the spinal cord lesion is complete?

A rectal examination to check rectal sphincter tone will indicate whether there is sacral sparing, which indicates an incomplete lesion. Absence of rectal sphincter tone indicates a complete spinal cord lesion with very little hope of recovery of function.

How will the examiner determine if a compartmental syndrome is developing in the patient's right lower leg?

Palpation for compartmental tenseness may be performed, but direct tissue pressure measurement is the most accurate parameter, especially in a paralyzed extremity without sensation. Pulses and capillary refill are not reliable indicators.

What x-ray studies will probably be ordered for this patient?

First, a cross-table, lateral cervical spine film will probably be ordered, followed by a complete spinal series, because noncontiguous fractures may exist in the spinal column. Right tibia and fibula films to include the knee and ankle joints may be obtained. Chest x-ray studies are indicated for all multiple trauma patients and also, for this patient, because the mechanism of injury could have caused direct thoracic trauma.

Compartmental pressures are measured in the right lower leg and are normal with the exception of the anterior compartment, where the pressure is 30 mm Hg. The orthopedic surgeon decides to monitor the patient instead of performing a fasciotomy immediately. How should the patient's leg be positioned?

The leg should be positioned at the level of the patient's heart. Elevating it higher may decrease tissue perfusion. Placing the leg in a dependent position will promote edema formation and possibly elevate compartmental pressures.

What is the ΔP for this patient, and is it adequate to meet the metabolic needs of the tissue?

$$\Delta P = MAP - \text{compartmental pressure};$$

$$MAP = \frac{(SBP - DBP)}{3} + DBP$$

$$MAP = \frac{(110 - 70)}{3} + 70 = 13 + 70 = 83$$

$$\Delta P = 83 - 30 = 53$$

A $\Delta P \geq 30$ mm Hg is adequate for normal tissue; a $\Delta P \geq 40$ mm Hg is necessary for moderately traumatized tissue. This patient's ΔP of 53 should be adequate to meet the metabolic needs of the tissue. However, the nurse must monitor him closely to detect deteriorations that may indicate the need for surgical fasciotomy.

RESEARCH QUESTIONS

- Are the initial cultures taken from open fractures cost effective and useful in treating subsequent infections? When is the most effective time to obtain wound cultures? Are tissue cultures or swabs from the wound more accurate?
- What is the best method for preserving amputated tissue for replantation?
- Should mean arterial pressure be measured in the leg when used to calculate ΔP for a potential compartmental syndrome in the leg?
- How effective are motor vehicle headrests in preventing extension injury to the cervical spine?
- Does overzealous fluid resuscitation increase edema in an injured spinal cord?
- What treatment modalities are most effective for fat embolism?

RESOURCES
Spinal Cord Injury

Boston University Hospital
New England Regional Spinal Cord Injury Center
75 E. Newton St.
Boston, MA 02118
(617) 638-7300

Craig Hospital
Rocky Mountain Spinal Cord Injury Center
3425 Clarkson St.
Englewood, CO 80110
(303) 789-8000

Northwestern University Medical Center
Midwest Regional Spinal Cord Injury Care System
230 E. Chicago Ave., Suite 619
Chicago, IL 60611
(312) 908-3425

National Spinal Cord Injury Hotline
2201 Argonne Dr.
Baltimore, MD 21218
(800) 526-3456 or (800) 638-1733 (In MD)

New York University Medical Center
Institute of Rehabilitation Medicine
400 E. 34th St.
New York, NY 10016
(212) 340-6105

Rancho Los Amigos Hospital
7601 E. Imperial Highway
Harriman Building 121
Downey, CA 90242
(213) 940-7048

Thomas Jefferson University
Regional Spinal Cord Injury Center of Delaware Valley
11th & Walnut Streets
Philadelphia, PA 19107
(215) 928-6579

Shepard Center for Spinal Injuries
2020 Peachtree Rd. NW
Atlanta, GA 30309
(404) 332-2020

Wayne State University
Southeast Michigan Spinal Cord Injury System
Rehabilitation Institute of Detroit
261 Mack Blvd.
Detroit, MI 48201
(313) 745-9770

University of Alabama in Birmingham
Spain Rehabilitation Center
Birmingham, AL 35294
(205) 934-3450

University of Rochester Medical Center
Strong Memorial Hospital
601 Elmwood Ave.
Rochester, NY 14642
(716) 275-3271

Texas Regional Spinal Cord Injury System
Institute for Rehabilitation & Research
1333 Moursund Ave.
Houston, TX 77030
(713) 799-5000

University of Michigan
Model Spinal Care Injury Care System
Department of PM&R
RMNI-ZA09-0491
300 North Ingalls Building
Ann Arbor, MI 48109-0491
(313) 763-0971

University of Virginia Medical Center
Box 159
Department of Orthopedics & Rehabilitation
Charlottesville, VA 22908
(804) 928-8578

ANNOTATED BIBLIOGRAPHY

Cerullo, L.J., & Quigley, M.R. (1985). Management of cervical spinal cord injury. *Journal of Emergency Nursing,* *11,* 182-187.
Excellent information on pathophysiology, assessment, and treatment of cervical spinal cord injuries.

Healy, F.T. (1986). Fat embolism syndrome. *Trauma Quarterly, 2*(2), 35-39.
Discussion of fat embolism syndrome pathophysiology, clinical presentation, and treatment, with supporting information from research findings.

Hoyt, K.S. (1990). Pelvic trauma: Assessment and management. *Postgraduate studies in trauma nursing.* Berryville, VA: Forum Medicum.
In-depth discussion of pelvic trauma.

McSwain, N.E., Jr. (1980). Kinematics of orthopedic injury secondary to trauma. *Current Concepts in Trauma Care, 1,* 14-16.
Review of the mechanisms of injury that cause orthopedic trauma in motor vehicle accidents.

O'Hara, M.M. (1987). Emergency care of the patient with a traumatic amputation. *Journal of Emergency Nursing, 13,* 272-277.
Comprehensive article encompassing all nursing aspects of caring for the patient with an amputation in the ED. Based on research and current practice of the Ralph K. Davies Medical Center Microsurgical Replantation Department.

Proehl, J.A. (1988). Compartment syndrome. *Journal of Emergency Nursing, 14,* 283-290.
Overview of compartment syndrome with emphasis on assessment parameters. New developments in treatment and assessment are also discussed.

Richmond, T.S. (1985). A critical care challenge: The patient with a cervical spinal cord injury. *Focus on Critical Care, 12* (2), 23-33.
Brief review of anatomy and physiology of spinal cord injury. Excellent information on nursing care and potential complications in the intensive care or acute care unit.

REFERENCES

Adelstein, W., & Watson, P. (1983). Cervical spine injuries. *Journal of Neurosurgical Nursing, 15,* 65-71.

American College of Surgeons, Committee on Trauma. (1989). *Advanced trauma life support course: Student manual.* Chicago: Author.

Aprahamian, C., Thompson, B.M., Finger, W.A., & Darin, J.C. (1984). Experimental cervical spine injury model: Evaluation airway management techniques. *Annals of Emergency Medicine, 13,* 584-587.

Bauer, D., & Kowalski, R. (1988). Effect of spinal immobilization devices on pulmonary function in the healthy, nonsmoking man. *Annals of Emergency Medicine, 17,* 915-918.

Billmire, D.A., Neale, H.W., & Stern, P.J. (1984). Acute management of severe hand injuries. *Surgical Clinics of North America, 64,* 683-697.

Bivins, H.G., Ford, S., Bezmalinovic, Z., Price, H.M., & Williams, J.L. (1988). The effect of axial traction during orotracheal intubation of the trauma victim with an unstable cervical spine. *Annals of Emergency Medicine, 17,* 25-29.

Bracken, M.B., Collins, W.F., Freeman, D.F., Shepard, M.J., Wagner, F.W., Silten, R.M., Hellenbrand, K.G., Ransohoff, J., Hunt, W.E., Perot, P.L., Grossman, R.G., Green, B.A., Eisenberg, H.M., Rifkinson, N., Goodman, J.H., Meagher, J.N., Fischer, B., Clifton, G.L., Flamm, E.S., & Rawe, S.E. (1984). Efficacy of methylprednisolone in acute spinal cord injury. *Journal of the American Medical Association, 251*, 45-52.

Bracken, M.B., Shepard, M.J., Hellenbrand, K.G., Collins, W.F., Leo, L.S., Freeman, D.F., Wagner, F.C., Flamm, E.S., Eisenberg, H.M., Goodman, J.H., Perot, P.L., Green, B.A., Grossman, R.G., Meagher, J.N., Young, W., Fischer, B., Clifton, G.L., Hunt, W.E., & Rifkinson, N. (1985). Methylprednisolone and neurological function one year after spinal cord injury. *Journal of Neurosurgery, 63*, 704-713.

Bracken, M.B., Shepard, M.J., Collins, W.F., Holford, T.R., Young, W., Baskin, D.S., Eisenberg, H.M., Flamm, E., Leo-Summers, L., Maroon, J., Marshall, L.F., Perot, P.L., Piepmeier, J., Sonntag, V.K.H., Wagner, F.C., Wilberger, J.E., & Winn, H.R. (1990). A randomized, controlled trial of methylprednisolone or naloxone in the treatment of acute spinal cord injury. *New England Journal of Medicine, 322*, 1405-1411.

Brand, D.A., Frazier, W.H., Kohlhepp, W.C., Shea, K.M., Hoefer, A.M., Ecker, M.D., Kornguth, P.J., Pais, M.J., & Light, T.R. (1982). A protocol for selecting patients with injured extremities who need x-rays. *New England Journal of Medicine, 306*, 333-339.

Bresler, M.J. (1988). Computed tomography vs. peritoneal lavage in blunt abdominal trauma. *Topics in Emergency Medicine, 10*, 59-73.

Brunette, D.D., & Rockswold, G.L., (1987). Neurologic recovery following rapid spinal realignment for complete cervical spinal cord injury. *Journal of Trauma, 27*, 445-447.

Buchan, A.S. (1983). Shock. In S. Hughes (Ed.), *The basis and practice of traumatology* (pp. 11-22). Rockville, MD: Aspen.

Buchanan, L.E. (1982). Emergency! First aid for spinal cord injury. *Nursing '82, 12*, 68-75.

Bucholz, R.W. (1984). Injuries of the pelvis and hip. *Emergency Medicine Clinics of North America, 2*, 331-346.

Bucholz, R.W., & Claudi, B. (1984). Complex fractures of the pelvis. In M.H. Meyers, *The multiply injured patient with complex fractures* (pp. 196-209). Philadelphia: Lea & Febiger.

Butman, A.M., & Paturas, J.L. (1986). *Pre-hospital trauma life support*. Akron, OH: Educational Direction.

Calenoff, L., Chessare, J.W., Rogers, L.F., Toerge, J., & Rosen, J.S. (1978). Multiple-level spinal injuries: Importance of early recognition. *American Journal of Roentgenology, 130*, 665-669.

Campbell, E.L. (1982). Lower-extremity injuries. In C. Chipman (Ed.), *Emergency Department Orthopedics* (pp. 97-107). Rockville, MD: Aspen.

Cerullo, L.J., & Quigley, M.R. (1985). Management of cervical spinal cord injury. *Journal of Emergency Nursing, 11*, 182-187.

Cloward, R.B. (1980). Acute cervical spine injuries. *Clinical Symposia, 32*, 1-32.

Cone, R.O. (1984). Clues to initial radiographic examination of skeletal trauma. *Emergency Medicine Clinics of North America, 2*, 245-278.

Cooper, M.A. (1982). Upper-extremity injuries: Shoulder, arm, and wrist. In C. Chipman (Ed.), *Emergency Department Orthopedics* (pp. 13-28). Rockville, MD: Aspen.

Daffner, R.H., & Diamond, D.L. (1988). Trauma radiology: An integrated approach. *Applied Radiology, 17*(1), 51-53.

Faden, A.I., Jacobs, T.P., & Holaday, J.W. (1981). Thyrotropin-releasing hormone improves neurologic recovery after spinal trauma in cats. *New England Journal of Medicine, 305*, 1063-1067.

Faden, A.I., Jacobs, T.P., Patrick, D.H., & Smith, M.T. (1984). Megadose corticosteroid therapy following experimental traumatic spinal injury. *Journal of Neurosurgery, 60*, 712-717.

Flamm, E.S., Young, W., Collins, W.F., Piepmeier, J., Clifton, G.L., & Fischer, B. (1985). A phase I trial of naloxone treatment in acute spinal cord injury. *Journal of Neurosurgery, 63*, 390-397.

Gebarski, S.S., Maynard, F.W., Gabrielson, T.O., Knake, J.E., Latack, J.T., & Hoff, J.T. (1985). Posttraumatic progressive myelopathy: Clinical and radiologic correlation employing MR imaging, delayed CT metrizamide myelography, and intraoperative sonography. *Radiology, 157*, 379-385.

Gershuni, D.H., Hargens, A.R., Lieber, R.L., O'Hara, R.C., Johansson, C.B., & Akeson, W.H. (1985). Decompression of an experimental compartment syndrome in dogs with hyaluronidase. *Clinical Orthopaedics and Related Research, 197*, 295-300.

Graziano, A.F., Scheidel, E.A., Cline, J.R., & Baer, L.J. (1987). A radiographic comparison of prehospital cervical immobilization methods. *Annals of Emergency Medicine, 16*, 1127-1131.

Gross, R.E. (1986). Kid seats and ambulances: Removing and using child restraint seats after collisions. *Journal of Emergency Medical Services, 11*, 34-37.

Harley, D.P., & Mena, I. (1986). Cardiac and vascular sequelae of sternal fractures. *Journal of Trauma, 26*, 553-555.

Healy, F.T. (1986). Fat embolism syndrome. *Trauma Quarterly, 2*(2), 35-39.

Heppenstall, R.B., Sapega, A.A., Scott, R., Sherton, D., Park, Y.S., Maris, J., and Chance, B. (1988). The compartment syndrome: An experimental and clinical study of muscular energy metabolism using phosphorus nuclear magnetic resonance spectroscopy. *Clinical Orthopaedics and Related Research, 226*, 138-155.

Herzenberg, J.E., Hensinger, R.N., Dedrick, D.K., & Phillips, W.A. (1989). Emergency transport and positioning of young children who have an injury of the cervical spine: The standard backboard may be hazardous. *Journal of Bone and Joint Surgery, 71-A*, 15-22.

Hing, D.N., Buncke, H.J., Alpert, B.S., & Gordon, L. (1986a). Indications for replanting amputated parts. *Hospital Physician, 22*(2), 13-17.

Hing, D.N., Buncke, H.J., Alpert, B.S., & Gordon, L. (1986b). Preparing the amputated part for transfer. *Hospital Physician, 22*(3), 36-37, 40.

Hochbaum, S.R. (1986). Emergency airway management. *Emergency Medicine Clinics of North America, 4*, 411-425.

Huerta, C., Griffith, R., & Joyce, S.M. (1987). Cervical spine immobilization in pediatric patients: Evaluation of current techniques. *Annals of Emergency Medicine, 16*, 1121-1126.

Iversen, L.D., & Clawson, D.K. (1982). Manual of acute orthopedic therapeutics (2nd ed.). Boston: Little, Brown.

Jacobs, L.M., & Schwartz, R. (1986). Prospective analysis of acute cervical spine injury: A methodology to predict injury. *Annals of Emergency Medicine, 15,* 85-90.

Jaffe, D.M., Binns, H., Radkowski, M.A., Barthel, M.J., & Engelhard, H.H. (1987). Developing a clinical algorithm for early management of cervical spine injury in child trauma victims. *Annals of Emergency Medicine, 16,* 270-276.

Jehle, D., & Cottington, E. (1988). Effect of alcohol consumption on outcome of pedestrian victims. *Annals of Emergency Medicine, 17,* 953-956.

Kluger, J. (1988). The Miami project. *Discover, 9*(9), 60-66, 68, 70.

Knezevich, B.A. (1986). *Trauma nursing: Principles and practice.* Norwalk, CT: Appleton-Century-Crofts.

Kuska, B.M. (1982). Acute onset of compartment syndrome. *Journal of Emergency Nursing, 8*(2), 75-79.

Luce, J., Tyler, M., & Pierson, D. (1984). *Intensive respiratory care.* Philadelphia: W.B. Saunders.

Mace, S.E. (1985). Emergency evaluation of cervical spine injuries: CT versus plain radiographs. *Annals of Emergency Medicine, 14,* 973-975.

MacKenzie, E.J., Shapiro, S., & Siegel, J.H. (1988). The economic impact of traumatic injuries: One-year treatment-related expenditures. *Journal of the American Medical Association, 260,* 3290-3296.

Maher, A.B. (1986). Early assessment and management of musculoskeletal injuries. *Nursing Clinics of North America, 21,* 717-727.

Markison, R.E. (1984). Trauma to the extremities. In D.D. Trunkey & F.R. Lewis (Eds.), *Current therapy of trauma 1984-1985* (pp. 101-116). St. Louis: Mosby–Year Book, Inc.

Matsen, F.A. (1980). *Compartmental syndromes.* New York: Grune & Stratton.

Matsen, F.A., & Krugmire, R.B. (1978). Compartmental syndromes. *Surgery, Gynecology and Obstetrics, 147,* 943-948.

McCabe, J.B., & Nolan, D.J. (1986). Comparison of the effectiveness of different cervical immobilization collars. *Annals of Emergency Medicine, 15,* 93-96.

McSwain, N.E., Jr. (1980). Kinematics of orthopedic injury secondary to trauma. *Current Concepts in Trauma Care, 1,* 14-16.

Merritt, K. (1988). Factors increasing the risk of infection in patients with open fractures. *Journal of Trauma, 28,* 823-827.

Metcalf, J.A. (1986). Acute phase management of persons with spinal cord injury: A nursing diagnosis perspective. *Nursing Clinics of North America, 21,* 589-598.

Meyer, P.R., & Sullivan, D.E. (1984). Injuries to the spine. *Emergency Medicine Clinics of North America, 2,* 313-329.

Meyers, M.H. (1984). *The multiply injured patient with complex fractures.* Philadelphia: Lea & Febiger.

Myers, R.A. (1982). *Hyperbaric oxygen and the spinal cord.* Paper presented at the Seventh Annual Conference of the Clinical Application of Hyperbaric Oxygen, June 9-11, 1982, Anaheim, CA.

Nikas, D.L. (1986). Resuscitation of patients with central nervous system trauma. *Nursing Clinics of North America, 21,* 693-704.

O'Hara, M.M. (1987). Emergency care of the patient with a traumatic amputation. *Journal of Emergency Nursing, 13,* 272-277.

Pal, J.M., Mulder, D.S., Brown, R.S., & Fleiszer, D.M. (1988). Assessing multiple trauma: Is the cervical spine enough? *Journal of Trauma, 28,* 1282-1284.

Podolsky, S., Barraf, L.J., Simon, R.R., Hoffman, J.R., Larmon, B., & Ablon, W. (1983). Efficacy of cervical spine immobilization methods. *Journal of Trauma, 23,* 461-465.

Proehl, J.A. (1988). Compartment syndrome. *Journal of Emergency Nursing, 14,* 283-290.

Rea, R.E. (Ed.). (1991). *Trauma nursing core course (provider) manual* (3rd ed.). Chicago: Award Printing.

Rhee, K.J., Green, W., Holcroft, J.W., & Mangili, J.A. (1990). Oral intubation in the multiply injured patient: The risk of exacerbating spinal cord damage. *Annals of Emergency Medicine, 19,* 511-514.

Richmond, T.S. (1985). A critical care challenge: The patient with a cervical spinal cord injury. *Focus on Critical Care, 12*(2), 23-33.

Riggins, R.S., & Kraus, J.F. (1977). The risk of neurologic damage with fractures of the vertebrae. *Journal of Trauma, 17,* 126-133.

Ringenberg, B.J., Fisher, A.K., Urdaneta, L.F., & Midthun, M.A. (1988). Rational ordering of cervical spine radiographs following trauma. *Annals of Emergency Medicine, 17,* 792-796.

Rivara, F.P. (1990). Child pedestrian injuries in the United States: Current status of the problem, potential interventions, and future research needs. *American Journal of Diseases of Children, 144,* 692-696.

Roberge, R.J., Wears, R.C., Kelly, M., Evans, T.C., Kenny, M.A., Daffner, R.D., Kremen, R., Murray, K., & Cottington, E.C. (1988). Selective application of cervical spine radiography in alert victims of blunt trauma: A prospective study. *Journal of Trauma, 28,* 784-788.

Rosenthal, R.E. (1984). Emergency department evaluation of musculoskeletal injuries. *Emergency Medicine Clinics of North America, 2,* 219-244.

Schafermeyer, R.W., Ribbeck, B.M., Gaskins, J., Thomason, S., Harlan, M., & Atkisson, A. (1991). Respiratory effects of spinal immobilization in children. *Annals of Emergency Medicine, 20,* 1017-1019.

Skyhar, M.J., Hargens, A.R., Strauss, M.B., Gershuni, D.H., Hart, G.B., & Akeson, W.H. (1986). Hyperbaric oxygen reduces edema and necrosis of skeletal muscle in compartment syndromes associated with hemorrhagic hypotension. *Journal of Bone and Joint Surgery, 68-A,* 1218-1224.

Stauffer, E.S., & Mazur, J.M. (1982). Cervical spine injuries in children. *Pediatric Annals, 11,* 502-511.

Strange, J.M. (1987). *Shock trauma care plans.* Springhouse, PA: Springhouse.

Strauss, M.B., Hargens, A.R., Gershuni, D.H., Hart, G.B., & Akeson, W.H. (1986). Delayed use of hyperbaric oxygen for treatment of a model anterior compartment syndrome. *Journal of Orthopaedic Research, 4,* 108-111.

Strauss, M.B., & Hart, G.B. (1984). Compartment syndromes: Update and role of hyperbaric oxygen. *HBO Review, 5,* 164-182.

Sumchai, A.P., Sternbach, G.L., & Laufer, M. (1988). Cervical spine traction and immobilization. *Topics in Emergency Medicine, 10,* 9-22.

Teresi, L.M., Lufkin, R.L., & Hanafee, W.N. (1988). MRI of the cervical spine. *Applied Radiology*, *16*(8), 31-44, 49.

Trafton, P.G. (1984). Trauma to the extremities. In D.D. Trunkey & F.R. Lewis (Eds.), *Current therapy of trauma 1984-1985* (pp. 117-135). St. Louis: Mosby–Year Book, Inc.

Tyson, G.W., Rimel, R.W., Winn, H.R., Butler, A.B., & Jane, J.A. (1979). Acute care of the spinal-cord-injured patient. *Critical Care Quarterly*, *2*, 45-60.

Urbaniak, J.R., Roth, J.H., Nunley, J.A., Goldner, R.D., & Koman, A. (1985). The results of replantation after amputation of a single finger. *Journal of Bone and Joint Surgery*, *67-A*, 611-619.

Van Giesen, P.J., Seaber, A.V., & Urbaniak, J.R. (1983). Storage of amputated parts prior to replantation: An experimental study with rabbit ears. *Journal of Hand Surgery*, *8*, 60-65.

Walleck, C.A. (1988). Central nervous system II: Spinal cord injury. In Cardona, V.D., Hurn, P.D., Bastnagel Mason, P.J., Scanlon-Schilpp, A.M., & Veise-Berry, S.W. (Eds.), *Trauma nursing: From resuscitation through rehabilitation* (pp. 419-448). Philadelphia: W.B. Saunders Co.

Walt, A.J. (Ed.). (1982). *Early care of the injured patient* (3rd ed.). Philadelphia: W.B. Saunders.

Whitesides, T.E., Haney, T.C., Morimoto, K., & Harada, H. (1975). Tissue pressure measurements as a determinant for the need of fasciotomy. *Clinical Orthopaedics and Related Research*, *113*, 43-51.

Wohlstadter, T. (1979). Traumatic amputation: Management of the severed part. *Journal of Emergency Nursing*, *5*(4), 35-36.

Wojcik, J.B., & Morgan, A.S. (1988). Sternal fractures: The natural history. *Annals of Emergency Medicine*, *17*, 912-914.

Worsing, R.A., Jr. (1984). Principles of prehospital care of musculoskeletal injuries. *Emergency Medicine Clinics of North America*, *2*, 205-217.

Wright, J.G., Bogoch, B.A., & Hastings, D.E. (1989). The "occult" compartment syndrome. *Journal of Trauma*, *29*, 133-134.

Yeo, J.D., & Lowry, C. (1982). Treatment of spinal cord injured patients with hyperbaric oxygen: A series of 35 patients. Paper presented at the Seventh Annual Conference of the Clinical Application of Hyperbaric Oxygen, June 9-11, 1982, Anaheim, CA.

12 Elimination, Metabolism, and Sexuality

Gastrointestinal and genitourinary

■■

Diane M. Sklarov (Gastrointestinal trauma)
Pamela Stinson Kidd (Genitourinary trauma)

OBJECTIVES

❏ *Identify the mechanisms of injury responsible for blunt and penetrating trauma to the abdomen that impact elimination and metabolism.*

❏ *Discuss the pathophysiology of trauma to the abdomen, and discuss current treatment modalities.*

❏ *Analyze subjective and objective data to formulate appropriate nursing diagnoses for the patient who sustains abdominal trauma.*

❏ *Specify the nursing interventions indicated in care of the patient with abdominal trauma.*

❏ *Describe mechanisms of injury that result in a higher incidence of alterations in urinary elimination.*

❏ *Identify signs and symptoms and diagnostic data indicative of genitourinary (GU) injury.*

❏ *Relate appropriate nursing interventions for patients experiencing an alteration in urinary elimination and/or genital injury.*

❏ *Anticipate potential complications that arise from a GU injury.*

INTRODUCTION The gastrointestinal (GI) and genitourinary (GU) systems incorporate the processes of metabolism, elimination, and sexuality. Each organ functions individually but contributes to the overall physiologic processes of supplying energy substrates, eliminating and detoxifying waste products, and serving protective functions pertinent to the response to trauma.

Abdominal injuries account for nearly 10% of all trauma-related deaths occurring in the United States annually (Bresler, 1988). Both blunt and penetrating forces result in disruption of the phys-iologic integrity of the abdomen and its underlying structures. The etiologic mechanisms responsible for abdominal injury are blunt forces resulting most commonly from motor vehicle trauma, falls, and assault and penetrating forces resulting from acts of violence involving guns, missiles, and knives. Because these injuries are associated with the devastating sequelae of hemorrhage, shock, peritonitis, and ultimately death, rapid assessment and appropriate nursing interventions can significantly impact an individual's chance for survival.

The incidence of GU trauma in the civilian population is steadily increasing. This is probably related to the fact that accidents are the most common cause of death in people between 1 and 35 years of age (Baker, 1987). Previously, GU trauma was most prevalent in young men, because this segment of the population was more often involved in military combat, contact sports, and violent activities. The cultural transition whereby females now engage in more athletic competition and are employed in more diverse industrial occupations has increased the incidence of GU trauma in females.

GU trauma seldom occurs in isolation and is most often associated with abdominal injuries (McAninch, 1985a). However, anyone with trauma to the chest, flank, abdomen, pelvis, perineum, and genitalia should be suspected of having an associated GU injury. In the pediatric population, the kidney may be the most commonly injured organ by blunt trauma, exceeding brain, liver, and spleen (Peterson 1989).

GU injuries are often overlooked in the emergency department because initially, symptoms of this type of injury are not as dramatic or severe as other injuries and may not occur until several hours after injury. In one retrospective study, 214 deaths from external trauma with urologic injury were reviewed. Only 4 of the 214 deaths were attributed to urologic injury. Only 1 of the 4 deaths was related to an acute urologic injury: ruptured kidney with severe hemorrhage. The remaining 3 deaths were from sepsis secondary to a ruptured urethra or bladder (Cass, Luxemberg, Gleich, & Smith, 1987). Associated life-threatening injuries will take precedence during the resuscitation phase, the only exceptions being the rare renal artery avulsion injury and a ruptured renal pedicle. Both of these conditions are considered emergency situations requiring immediate surgery. Usually these patients will die of severe hemorrhage before reaching the emergency department. Fewer than 1% of trauma patients will have significant lower and upper urinary tract injury (Peterson, 1989).

Special needs of pregnant and pediatric trauma victims will be addressed only briefly, because these are discussed in depth in Chapters 16 and 17. Sexuality, a significant consideration when dealing with trauma patients, is intricately associated with the GU system and is discussed in that section. The gastrointestinal section is reviewed first.

CASE STUDY A 23-year-old woman is brought to the ED via a local fire rescue unit after being struck by a car. She is alert with initial vital signs as follows: BP, 90/60; AP, 112; R, 22. The only complaint is that of abdominal pain, and on physical examination the abdomen is markedly tender to palpation of the left upper quadrant, with a tire smudge mark visible in that area.

Based on anatomic location and mechanism of injury, what abdominal organ has the greatest potential for injury when blunt trauma occurs?

The spleen, located in the left upper quadrant of the abdomen, is the most commonly injured organ in blunt abdominal trauma.

In this type of injury, what diagnostic procedures are used to establish the necessity of laparotomy as a final surgical outcome?

Both diagnostic peritoneal lavage (DPL) and computerized tomography (CT) are used in the evaluation of splenic injury. Although DPL may be considered the procedure of choice, the hemodynamically stable patient suffering blunt trauma can benefit from noninvasive CT study. In the past, splenectomy was considered a relatively common resolution of injury; however, numerous studies indicating a significant incidence of postsplenectomy infection have led to more conservative, nonsurgical efforts to salvage tissue. This is supported by the capability of the spleen to heal with simple repair or careful monitoring in a select population.

What other structures lie within this quadrant and are at risk for injury?

The left upper quadrant contains the stomach, splenic flexure of the colon, tail of the pancreas, left kidney, and adrenal gland, in addition to the spleen.

What complications may result?

A high incidence of infection occurs in patients after removal of the spleen. In addition, abscess formation, pancreatitis, and recurrent hemorrhage can occur. Delayed splenic rupture can occur from 1 to 2 weeks after injury, resulting in hemorrhage into the peritoneum from a previously self-sealed laceration or hematoma to the spleen.

GASTROINTESTINAL TRAUMA
Mechanism of Injury
Blunt injuries

The initial evaluation of a patient presenting to the emergency department with abdominal trauma must include a thorough history of the precipitating event, with specific attention to the mechanism of injury. Trauma to the abdomen is attributable to blunt or penetrating forces. Blunt trauma sustained from a motor vehicle collision, fall, or physical assault produces two types of injuries: deceleration and compression. Deceleration injuries are directly related to Newton's law of motion, which states that a body at rest or in motion will maintain that state until interrupted by some force. In an automobile crash, the occupant's body stops its forward motion on impact with a seat belt or other fixed structure, whereas the abdominal organs continue to advance within their confined space until structural impact, tear, or rupture occurs (McSwain, 1984). The same principle applies whether the cause is a fall, physical attack, or sports injury.

Compression injuries occur when the abdominal contents are squeezed between the vertebral column and the impacting object itself. Specific organ systems at risk of injury include the pancreas, spleen, liver, and kidneys. The diaphragm is particularly vulnerable to compression injuries.

As many as 70% of trauma deaths are the result of blunt forces (Andrews, 1987). Both morbidity and mortality are increased in blunt trauma because of initially absent or equivocal physical findings. In addition, blunt trauma to the abdomen is rarely a singular event and may be seen with concurrent injuries to other body systems, especially the head and chest, in as many as 75% of patients (Cayten, 1984). Alcohol intoxication and drug usage can complicate the evaluation. The spleen and the liver are the organs most prone to injury, although the remainder of the abdominal organs may be involved (Gibson, 1987). Governmental regulation of mandatory use of seat belts and carseats has dramatically decreased the mortality associated with vehicular trauma, particularly in regard to occupants being thrown from the vehicle with subsequent lethal head injuries. Lap belts used without the adjacent shoulder harness can be responsible for abdominal injuries. In the same fashion, a "high-riding" lap belt causes the abdominal contents to bear the impact associated with deceleration (Cayten, 1984). If worn correctly, the combination seat belt allows the pelvis to absorb the shock of impact and to protect the abdominal contents (McSwain, 1984).

In an unrestrained pregnant woman, the uterus absorbs the impact of collision, offering no protection to the fetus. In blunt abdominal trauma in the pregnant woman, both the mother and the fetus are susceptible to injury. In addition to spleen and liver injuries resulting from blunt trauma to the abdomen, the pregnant woman can succumb to uterine rupture, although rare in occurrence, and abruptio placenta (see Chapter 16). The latter is more commonly seen and carries with it the likelihood of fetal demise. The extent of blunt abdominal injury and the trimester of pregnancy both affect the possibility of fetal injury, because the fetus may be alternately (1) protected by buoyancy and (2) exposed by virtue of the expanding uterus (Bremer & Cassata, 1986).

Knowledge of the mechanism of injury, physical assessment, and perhaps most important, a high index of suspicion are the nurse's tools to accurately identify and resolve potentially lethal injuries resulting from blunt abdominal trauma.

Penetrating injuries

Penetrating trauma to the abdomen is associated with acts of violence involving guns and knives, and patients with penetrating injuries are commonly seen in the emergency care setting. Although on the surface it is easier to identify an injury of this nature, an obvious and apparently localized wound may be accompanied by severely damaged underlying abdominal structures and viscera. Stab wounds to the abdomen are superficial in as many as 25% of the cases and fail to penetrate the peritoneal cavity (Frame, Timberlake, & McSwain, 1988). A surprisingly low mortality (1% to 2%) is associated with stab wounds (Gibson, 1987).

Obtaining a history of the type and size of weapon involved, as well as the direction and motion of the assault, is helpful but not always possible. The left upper and lower quadrants of the abdomen are especially prone to injury because of the prevalence of right-handed assailants (Briggs, Hendricks, & Flint, 1987). Female attackers are inclined to use a downward motion when wielding a knife, whereas men direct the angle upwards (Semonin-Holleran, 1988). Although reported, no conclusive research exists to substantiate this claim. Commonly injured organs involve the upper anterior abdomen, hence the spleen, liver, and diaphragm (Gibson, 1987).

Injuries resulting from bullets require consideration of velocity and weight of the missile. Missiles have the capacity to follow an erratic path and deflect from a bony structure, enhancing the potential for multisystem injury. The distance of the individual from the weapon fired and the trajectory and exploding properties of the bullet combine to affect mortality (Gibson, 1987). Furthermore, gunshot wounds to the abdomen penetrate the cavity in 80% of cases and cause intraabdominal injury in 92% to 98% (Gibson, 1987). The trajectory of the bullet to some extent determines the amount of tissue disruption. The presence or absence of both entrance and exit wounds should not be overlooked as information pertinent to the evaluation of extraabdominal derangement. The characteristics that differentiate an entrance from an exit wound lie ultimately within the realm of the ballistics expert or forensic pathologist to determine. However, the experienced trauma nurse can identify an entrance wound with a high degree of certainty, particularly if charring (the appearance of a powder burn) or tearing of the surrounding tissue occurs, which further suggests the firing occurred at close range. This information can aid in predicting the extent of injury, particularly if the bullet has completely traversed the abdominal cavity, but offers little substance to the overall clinical course of the patient and, further, does not alter nursing intervention. Virtually all abdominal organs are at risk from gunshot wounds, although the colon, liver, and small bowel are frequently injured (Gibson, 1987). The potential for hemorrhage is severe as a result of hollow organ perforation, visceral injury, and major vessel damage (Berman, Ricciardelli, & Savino, 1987).

In summary, the mechanism of injury involved in blunt and penetrating trauma supplies necessary information for the regulation and management of patients presenting with abdominal injury. Morbidity, mortality, and suggested treatment modalities differ for victims of blunt versus penetrating trauma.

Anatomic and Pathophysiologic Considerations

A review of normal anatomy and physiology of the abdomen is essential to understanding the impact of a traumatic event. A definition of terms commonly used in describing the abdomen is included to assist the reader. The *peritoneum* is a membranous sac that surrounds the *viscera* (hollow and solid organs). The peritoneum is divided into the *parietal* peritoneum (abdominal wall lining) and *visceral* peritoneum (organ lining). The *mesentery* is a double fold of peritoneum containing vessels and nerves attached to the *abdominal wall*, which encloses the abdominal organs. *Omentum* is comprised of peritoneum that connects the stomach and visceral organs. The *abdomen* is a portion of the body comprised of both hollow and solid organs with boundaries defined as extending from the diaphragm to pelvis.

Thoracic as well as abdominal trauma can contribute to injury of abdominal structures such as the liver, spleen, stomach, and diaphragm. The abdominal structures are classified as *intraperitoneal* or *retroperitoneal*. Those that are strictly intraperitoneal are the spleen, liver, stomach, bladder, uterus, ovaries, and fallopian tubes, whereas those that are solely retroperitoneal are the kidneys, ureters, rectum, and the major vascular structures of the vena cava, aorta, and portal vein. Some organs are comprised of both intraperitoneal and retroperitoneal portions and include the pancreas, duodenum, and colon. Retroperitoneal structures are afforded protection by the musculature of the back and the peritoneal cavity, whereas the remainder of the abdominal organs are protected, at least in part, by the thorax, spine, and pelvis.

To simplify the location of organs within the abdominal cavity, an imaginary line can be drawn through the umbilicus horizontally and vertically to divide the abdomen into four quadrants (Figure 12-1). The right upper quadrant houses the duodenum, gallbladder, liver, right kidney and adrenal gland, hepatic flexure of the colon, and head of the pancreas. The left upper quadrant contains the stomach, splenic flexure of the colon, spleen, tail of the pancreas, and left kidney and adrenal gland. The abdominal organs found in the right lower quadrant include the appendix, cecum, and right ovary and fallopian tube; the sigmoid colon and left ovary and fallopian tube are located in the left lower quadrant. The uterus and bladder are described as *midline organs* (Mansell, Stokes, Adler, & Rosensweig, 1974).

The anatomic changes that occur during pregnancy shift the contents of the abdomen and can render usual protective mechanisms ineffective. During the first trimester, the uterus is stationed deep within the pelvis and abdominal contents re-

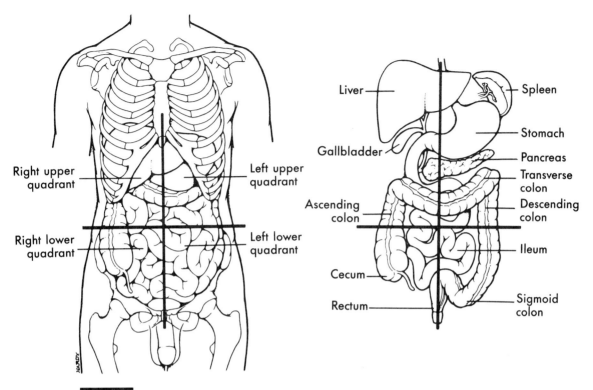

Figure 12-1   Abdominal contents. (From *The Practice of Emergency Care* (p. 386) by J.H. Cosgriff, Jr. and D.L. Anderson, 1984, Philadelphia: J.B. Lippincott.)

main essentially the same as in the nonpregnant female. As the pregnancy progresses, the gravid uterus provides protection to abdominal structures, although the stomach, liver, and spleen are compressed and displaced upward and the intestines posteriorly. With the onset of the third trimester, the bladder moves upward and assumes the position of an abdominal organ, away from its pelvic shelter (Bremer & Cassata, 1986).

Pediatric patients with abdominal injury present a unique challenge to practitioners because of the differences in anatomic proportions and growth patterns. Vital abdominal organs are relatively unprotected in the child—the kidneys, liver, spleen, and bladder are exposed to significant injury.

In summary, a knowledge of structural anatomy and physiology is a prerequisite to understanding the pathologic conditions that occur in trauma to the abdomen. Owing to its large size and vulnerable location, the abdomen is prone to

extensive damage and multiple system injuries are not uncommon.

General Assessment

The mechanism of injury and patient history form the basis of the subjective information in nursing assessment. This information is often not obtainable from the patient because of altered sensorium from a head injury or alcohol or drug ingestion, and the history must be pieced together from paramedic response teams, witnesses, and family members. A history of chronic illness, current medical problems, and medications is also useful but not always available.

Physical examination

A hands-on examination of the patient is necessary to provide additional information as to the extent of injury, as well as to determine basic physiologic defects. The assessment techniques of observation, auscultation, and palpation are fun-

Table 12-1 Special findings associated with abdominal trauma

Sign	Findings	Implications
Cullen's	Periumbilical ecchymoses	Peritoneal bleeding
Grey Turner's	Nontraumatic ecchymoses to lower abdomen/ flank	Retroperitoneal bleeding Possible hemorrhagic pancreatitis
Kehr's	Left upper quadrant pain radiating to left shoulder	Splenic rupture Diaphragmatic injury
Coopernail	Ecchymoses of perineum, scrotum, or labia	Pelvic fracture
Hematoma	Flank area	Renal injury

Note. From "Critical Nursing Care for Abdominal Trauma" by R. Semonin-Holleran, 1988, *Critical Care Nurse, 8*(3), p. 50.

damental to appraising bodily function. The physical appearance of the patient offers valuable clues to the underlying injury if an obvious insult such as stab or gunshot wound is not evidenced. Contusions, hematomas, lacerations, and even imprints (such as a tire tread mark) observed in given anatomic locations offer additional clues to injury. Distention of the abdomen or bladder can also be noted, as well as crepitus. Specific findings associated with abdominal trauma are listed in Table 12-1.

Auscultation to ascertain presence or absence of bowel sounds is vital for the patient experiencing abdominal trauma and should precede palpation in the physical examination. Signs and symptoms of peritoneal irritation from blood extravasation, as well as suspected organ damage, can be elicited by palpating the abdomen for rebound, guarding, referred pain, and rigidity (Semonin-Holleran, 1988). *Rebound tenderness* as an indicator of peritoneal irritation is described as pain that is elicited once pressure to the abdominal wall is removed. The patient contracting abdominal muscles in response to palpation of a sensitive area is called *guarding* (Lanros, 1988).

Pain *Referred pain* occurs in a location other than the point of palpation. An example of referred pain is Kehr's sign, where pain in the left upper quadrant of the abdomen radiating to the left shoulder is indicative of splenic disruption. The phenomenon of referred pain requires intensive neurologic research to understand the visceral and somatic pathways that transmit pain. Several hypotheses explain referred pain. One suggests the visceral and somatic fibers cross over at the same synapse site: the mind confuses the two sig-

nals, and the somatic sensation, which is more intense, produces pain in the region of innervation. For example, anterior and posterior pathways innervate the diaphragm at the level of C3 to C5. Anterior columns reflect sensation and pain; posterior columns reflect motor function (contraction) of the diaphragm. At the point where the pathways cross over, one hypothesis contends a "short circuit" develops where pain is referred to the shoulder region innervated by C3 to C5 (Romero-Sierra, 1986).

The term *rigid abdomen* is commonly used when the abdomen is exceptionally hard to the touch as a result of muscular contraction, often associated with hemoperitoneum. Voluntary rigidity is generally symmetrical, whereas involuntary rigidity is unilateral (DeGowin & DeGowin, 1976).

Diagnostic and Monitoring Procedures
Laboratory studies

Another parameter of objective assessment includes obtaining and interpreting laboratory data, both as a baseline and as an ongoing indicator of patient response. The basic studies elicited incorporate a hemoglobin (Hgb) and hematocrit (Hct) (complete blood count [CBC] if time allows), electrolyte profile, serum amylase, urinalysis, type and crossmatch, coagulation studies, and chest x-ray examination. The initial Hgb and Hct may be within normal range. Liver function tests such as serum glutamic oxaloacetic transaminase (SGOT), now known as *aspartate aminotransferase* (AST), and serum glutamic pyruvic transaminase (SGPT), now known as *alanine aminotransferase* (ALT), are often added to aid in diagnosis of hepatic or gallbladder injuries. A bilirubin level may be used also. These tests are useful adjuncts but rarely vital in the initial assessment of a trauma patient. An arterial blood gas is usually indicated to determine pH, oxygen saturation, and respiratory function.

Diagnostic peritoneal lavage

Reputable sources have published many studies regarding the efficacy of diagnostic peritoneal lavage (DPL) as a tool to determine the presence or absence of intraperitoneal blood in the abdomen indicative of organ perforation. Although this procedure is frequently used in the evaluation of blunt abdominal trauma, its use in penetrating trauma varies and will be discussed later in this section. The indications and contraindications for the use of DPL are listed in the box below.

Technique Three methods of peritoneal lavage are being used: closed, or percutaneous; semi open; and open, or cut-down (Burney, 1986). Advantages and disadvantages of each method exist; however, institutional guidelines dictate to some extent which method is ultimately employed.

Regardless of which method is used, proper preparation of the patient and equipment is necessary. The procedure should be explained to an alert patient, a step often overlooked in the sometimes hectic trauma area. If not already in place or otherwise contraindicated as discussed earlier,

a Foley catheter should be placed (to evacuate the bladder) and a nasogastric tube (to decompress the stomach) (Merlotti, Marcet, Sheaff, Dunn, & Barrett, 1985). This lessens the chance of perforation of the bladder or stomach during insertion of the lavage catheter. If the catheter is misplaced into an organ or peritoneal communication occurs, a sudden outflow of fluid may be noted, e.g., Foley output, nasogastric suction, or onset of diarrhea. The nurse should remember that DPL is a sterile invasive procedure.

The site chosen for DPL is the midline abdomen, a few centimeters below the umbilicus and superior to the pubis (Cayten, 1984). A supraumbilical site is recommended in the presence of a pelvic fracture to decrease the possibility of false positive results (Sherman et al., 1989). After a perpendicular insertion, the catheter is always directed toward the pelvis, since blood collects in this hollowed space (Burney, 1986). Evidence of previous abdominal incisions is a contraindication to DPL, since bowel perforation can occur secondary to adhesions; however, the site can be amended to an adjacent area (Cayten, 1984). Early pregnancy is treated in the same manner as the nongravid uterus. In the second and third trimester, the site is relocated to above the umbilicus, or culdocentesis may be substituted (Bremer & Cassata, 1986).

In the closed, or percutaneous, method of

Indications and contraindications for diagnostic peritoneal lavage

Indications	Relative contraindications	Absolute contraindications
Unidentified blood loss, hypotension	Morbid obesity	Laparotomy is clearly mandated
Indeterminate physical examination (alcohol, drugs, spinal cord trauma, head injury)	Gravid uterus or pelvic fracture (diversion of placement site)	Evisceration
Pelvic or rib fractures	Scarring indicative of previous abdominal surgeries (amended site)	
Patients requiring surgery with general anesthesia for other system injuries		
Equivocal physical findings with highly suspect mechanism of injury		
Stab wound with peritoneal penetration to rule out visceral injury		

DPL, a trocar catheter is inserted through a small abdominal incision into the fascia, peritoneum, and, finally, peritoneal cavity. This method is the quickest application of DPL, and it is performed without any visualization; therefore, risks exist of improper placement of the catheter with the possibility of visceral and organ damage upon entrance into the peritoneal cavity. The greatest percentage of false-positive results are present with this method because bleeding from the entry site is allowed to infiltrate the peritoneum. The use of lidocaine with epinephrine at the puncture site may decrease this occurrence (Burney, 1986). Sherman et al. (1989) advocate the use of the percutaneous method, finding accuracy rates of 98.8% and less time required to perform than the open method. The semiopen method involves a greater abdominal incision, such that the fascia can be exposed. The trocar is then advanced through an incision in the fascia more directly into the peritoneum with greater preservation of abdominal contents (Burney, 1986). The open technique has been highly regarded because of its safety but requires both additional time and skill on the part of the physician to complete. In this technique, the abdominal wall is excised in layers inclusive of the peritoneum, allowing direct visualization of the intraperitoneal space for placement of the trocar. It is the method of choice at most large trauma facilities.

Diagnostic criteria for DPL   Once the trocar is introduced, aspiration of gross blood, bile, or intestinal contents through the catheter is considered a positive result, indicating a need for laparotomy; therefore the procedure is terminated (Orban & Molitor, 1986). If blood is not found initially, 10 to 20 ml/kg or 1000 ml lactated Ringer's solution (normal saline or dialysis fluid may be used) is instilled into the abdominal cavity over 5 to 10 minutes. To allow for a mix of peritoneal fluid, manual pressure is applied to abdominal quadrants or the patient is turned side to side if not contraindicated. This is highly desirable, since laboratory analysis of lavage fluid is based on a standard dilution (Orban & Molitor, 1986). The fluid is then siphoned back into the original container via gravity. A return of 750 to 1000 ml is best for greater accuracy of cell counts; however, as little as 50 ml is adequate (Merlotti et al., 1985). Difficulty in obtaining return can be overcome by gentle palpation of the abdomen and careful manipulation of the catheter (catheter

may be lodged against tissue). The tubing must be patent to allow free backflow of fluid. The viscosity of the fluid is then interpreted initially, with clear fluid considered negative and any pink-tinged or cloudy return viewed as positive. The familiar method of the ability to read newspaper print through the fluid is still widely used as a gross indication of a negative result. The returned solution is routinely sent for stat analysis of red blood cells (RBCs), white blood cells (WBCs), Gram stain, and amylase for conclusive findings.

The standard criteria consider RBC counts of $100,000/mm^3$ or greater, WBC counts of $500/mm^3$ or greater, and the presence of bile to be positive findings. Results are considered equivocal if RBCs are between $50,000/mm^3$ and $100,000/mm^3$, and repeated DPL is indicated over time. Gomez et al. (1987) completed a literature review of 5715 patients who sustained blunt abdominal trauma and underwent subsequent DPL, comparing the findings against the "standard" criteria yielding an accuracy rate of 97.8%. Researchers who advocate decreasing the quantitative measures of RBCs to decrease false-positive results have found significant injury exists at levels between $20,000/mm^3$ to $100,000/mm^3$ (Gibson, 1987). The RBC count is a sensitive indicator of damage to the spleen and liver, both of which are highly susceptible to injury from blunt forces. If RBC counts are lowered, however, the same sensitivity principles that give DPL its merit in detecting intraperitoneal bleeding may warrant unnecessary laparotomy. Intestinal trauma without large extravasation into the peritoneal cavity will yield lower RBC counts; therefore WBC counts are more prognostic of small and large intestine disruption caused by inflammation and contamination (Bresler, 1988).

Amylase measurements in peritoneal lavage fluid appear to be predictors of visceral and pancreatic injury if greater than 100 international units per liter (IU/L.). Kusminsky, Tu, Brendemuehl, Tiley, and Boland (1982) report on 7 of 30 cases in which increased amylase levels were noted in peritoneal lavage fluid and amylase was increased in all retroperitoneal injuries. At the time of laparotomy, pancreatic and duodenal damage were found. It is of interest that the two duodenal injuries had a clear lavage return with insignificant RBC counts. Elevated amylase levels are indicative of pancreatic and small bowel injury but are not always immediately elevated, so the use of amylase values as absolute predictors is still being investigated.

Although DPL is widely used as a diagnostic tool in the evaluation of penetrating abdominal trauma, it is less definitive than when it is used in cases of blunt trauma. The incidence of peritoneal penetration from an anterior stab wound is relatively high (70%); however, subsequent visceral injury occurs in only 20% to 40% of cases (Gibson, 1987). Therefore high false-negative results from compulsory DPL can ensue. Cayten (1984), Gibson (1987), and Huizinga, Baker, and Mtshali (1987) advocate the conservative management of stab wounds to the abdomen, including local wound exploration if significant peritoneal signs are absent or if physical examination and the pathway of the object is indicative of a confined injury. After the wound is explored, if peritoneal penetration is confirmed, DPL is the next step in evaluation to determine if intraabdominal injury has occurred. Gunshot wounds to the abdomen, in contrast, are highly correlated to intraabdominal injury, and DPL is not routine. Determinants of positive lavage results differ when the mechanism of injury is a stab or gunshot wound. In penetrating trauma, researchers advocate the use of RBC count definitions of between $1000/mm^3$ and $10,000/mm^3$ as positive, because hollow viscera injuries (which do not bleed greatly) are associated with lower RBC counts, and this criteria would correlate with a lower percentage of missed injuries (Briggs et al., 1987; Gibson, 1987; Merlotti, Dillon, Lange, Robin, & Barrett, 1988).

Penetrating trauma to the back or flank area, which may represent retroperitoneal injury, is difficult to diagnose. If the peritoneal lining remains intact, damage to retroperitoneal structures and to the retroperitoneal portions of the pancreas, duodenum, and colon routinely will not be identified using DPL, since the fluid sampled is strictly intraperitoneal. However, seepage of RBCs from a retroperitoneal hematoma into the peritoneal cavity may provide a positive tap from an unexpected source. The box above right summarizes positive findings in DPL.

Radiographic studies

The chest x-ray study can identify concomitant pulmonary or cardiac injuries, as well as abdominal organ displacement. Because the physical examination usually identifies the need for laparot-

---

> ## Summary of positive findings in DPL
>
> Aspiration of ≥ 10 ml gross blood
> Aspiration of lavage return of feces, bile, intestine, or bacteria
> RBC $> 100,000/mm^3$ (blunt trauma)
> RBC $> 10,000/mm^3$ (penetrating trauma)
> WBC $> 500/mm^3$
> Lavage fluid return through chest tube or Foley catheter

---

omy, x-ray films of the abdomen are rarely useful in immediate assessment of the trauma patient except to identify free air or foreign bodies, such as bullet fragments. A retrospective study of 94 patients with stab wounds to the abdominal cavity suggests the limited value of abdominal films (Kester, Andrassy, & Aust, 1986). Abdominal films are equivocal at best as an indicator of intestinal injury, and more sophisticated technology, such as computed tomography (CT), is warranted.

Computerized tomography   In recent years advances in the use of CT in the evaluation of abdominal injuries have gained widespread approval. CT is used widely in the presence of blunt rather than penetrating trauma, since it is not as sensitive to hollow viscus injuries commonly seen with penetrating trauma (Briggs et al., 1987). However, peritoneal interruption by a penetrating force can be localized with its use.

A CT is advantageous in the hemodynamically stable patient and is recommended if a retroperitoneal injury is suspect. Retroperitoneal injuries can be missed using DPL and carry a high mortality (Bresler, 1988). Although a relatively uncommon injury, trauma to the pancreas can be evaluated best in conjunction with ultrasound, particularly in children and patients with low-density body fat (Jeffrey, Laing, & Wing, 1986).

CT can localize injury to the liver, spleen, and kidneys (commonly injured in blunt abdominal trauma), as well as indicate the amount of blood present. This is a valuable resource for evaluation of splenic and hepatic trauma that may be managed without laparotomy, a trend under significant study. Farnell et al. (1988) had notable success in nonoperative management of 22 patients with liver injury, based on CT localization of injury. The risks of surgical intervention and the possibility of postoperative infection encourage nonoperative management of these injuries in select situations. Hanna et al. (1987) advocate the use of DPL for blunt trauma, with CT reserved for stable patients who can be closely monitored. They further cite the need for qualified radiologic interpretation of CT findings and consider it a less accurate procedure than DPL. CT can be a useful adjunct in evaluation of the pediatric patient where conservative management may be recommended, since many liver lacerations heal without surgical intervention (Gibson, 1987). In children, where conservative management of splenic trauma has been more successful than in the adult population, CT is a means of evaluation (Gibson, 1987). Buntain, Gould, and Maull (1988) reported an accuracy rate of 97% using CT in evaluating 30 patients with blunt abdomen trauma resulting in splenic injury and further acknowledged the capability of CT to localize injury. In blunt abdominal trauma CT produces a relatively low incidence of false-positive results. DPL should not precede CT, since lavage fluid retained in the peritoneum can obscure findings and appear as intraperitoneal blood (Bresler, 1988; Federle, Crass, Jeffrey, & Trunkey, 1982). The postoperative risks of infection after splenectomy support the use of less radical methods of management. CT is costly, involves transfer to another department, and requires approximately 30 minutes to complete; however, it is a noninvasive procedure and carries no morbidity. As future research is available, CT will probably be more competitive in evaluating abdominal trauma of blunt origin.

Use of contrast   As discussed, CT is an excellent diagnostic tool to evaluate solid viscus injury (such as liver and spleen disruption), retroperitoneal injury, and intraperitoneal hemorrhage in the hemodynamically stable patient (Smedira & Schecter, 1989). GI contrast medium is a useful adjunct, generally reserved for the nonurgent evaluative examination. Barium is an inert, hypotonic product which is not absorbed. It allows for better detail and will not cause severe pulmonary disruption should it be aspirated. Barium is contraindicated if a perforation is suspected. Water-soluble contrast media, such as Gastrografin (diatrizoate meglumine) and Hypaque (diatrizoate meglumine and diatrizoate sodium solution) are absorbable, hypertonic solutions, which, if aspirated, can cause pulmonary edema or pneumonitis. Pancreatic and duodenal injuries can be well

diagnosed by CT using water-soluble media (Smedira & Schecter, 1989). Depending on the level of the organ being enhanced, media may take as long as 90 minutes to reach the level of the terminal small bowel.

The preferred route of contrast instillation in trauma is intravenous. Non-ionic products such as Omnipaque (iohexol), may be given by rapid injection (50 ml) or infusion (150 to 300 ml) in a matter of minutes. The use of IV contrast will show clear extravasation of media if visceral integrity has been disrupted, or enhance homogenicity if solid organs are intact. Allergic reactions to the IV media are limited, and few metabolic consequences occur.

Assessment and Interventions Related to Specific Injuries

Trauma to the abdomen can involve single-organ, multiple-organ, and vascular damage from a blunt or penetrating source. The major organ systems involved and relevant findings are discussed in the following section.

Diaphragmatic injuries

Because of the anatomic proximity of the thoracic cavity to the abdomen, penetrating or blunt trauma to the abdomen cannot be considered an isolated event, particularly if the area of involvement is between the fourth intercostal space and the tenth rib. Dual injuries are not uncommon and are termed *thoracoabdominal*. The most significant of these involves injury to the diaphragm, and both blunt and penetrating forces can be responsible. Although injury to the diaphragm itself may be minimal from penetrating trauma, damage to underlying structures of the chest or abdomen can result in hemothorax, pneumothorax, hemoperitoneum, and shock (Cowley & Dunham, 1982). Increased intraabdominal pressure as a result of blunt trauma to the lower chest or abdomen can lead to diaphragmatic rupture. Diaphragmatic injury is confined most commonly to the left side of the chest, since the liver protects the diaphragm on the right (Ramponi & Somerville, 1986). Generally, an upright chest film is sufficient to diagnose the presence of diaphragmatic injury. Findings on x-ray film may include an elevated hemidiaphragm, air-fluid levels above the left diaphragm, herniation of abdominal contents into the chest, and mediastinal shift (Symbas, Vlasis, & Hatcher, 1986). A previously placed nasogastric (NG) tube may be visible in the left chest, and if peritoneal lavage is performed, fluid may escape through a chest tube. More definitive studies include upper gastrointestinal (UGI) series and diagnostic pneumoperitoneum. Using fluoroscopy, air is injected into the peritoneum, and the path it follows through a diaphragmatic tear is observed. The patient is at significant risk for pneumothorax from the procedure (Ramponi & Somerville, 1986). DPL is considered a controversial means to diagnose thoracoabdominal trauma. Merlotti et al. (1988) disagree on the validity of chest films for diagnosis and support DPL for prediction of diaphragmatic injury with penetrating trauma.

Nursing interventions for the patient with a suspected or actual diaphragmatic injury are aimed primarily at ventilatory support with high-flow oxygen administration and meticulous attention to airway stability. The patient initially may be asymptomatic but may rapidly experience hypotension, respiratory distress, and tachycardia, particularly if herniation has occurred. On physical examination, the presence of bowel sounds in the chest, shoulder tip pain accelerated by deep breathing (Kehr's sign), or air sounds in the chest when testing NG tube placement is suggestive of diaphragmatic injury (Ramponi & Somerville, 1986). The first indication of diaphragmatic rupture may be intestinal obstruction, and formation of a paralytic ileus often results. Definitive management of a diaphragmatic rupture is surgical repair as soon as the patient's condition warrants so complications from herniation can be minimized (Symbas et al., 1986).

Esophageal injuries

Injury to the esophagus with resultant perforation is an uncommon finding in trauma. It is often an incidental occurrence associated with thoracic or peritoneal injury, but can be life-threatening. Penetrating injuries are more common than blunt trauma as a mechanism, since the esophagus is rather well protected. Cheadle and Richardson (1982) studied 19 patients with esophageal injuries over a 10-year period, with only one injury resulting from blunt trauma. All had associated injuries. A perforation may occur in any of three portions of the esophagus, and symptoms are related to location: cervicothoracic, midthoracic, and lower intraabdominal (Beal, Pottmeyer, & Spisso, 1988). Injuries may pro-

duce chest and abdominal pain, cervical crepitus, dysphagia, and dyspnea.

Lateral neck and chest films are indicated to rule out esophageal perforation, and findings include subcutaneous or mediastinal emphysema, mediastinal shift, and pneumothorax. These findings are not specific, however, for esophageal perforation. Diagnosis of esophageal perforation may be confirmed in the presence of pneumothorax or hydrothorax once a chest tube has been inserted for evacuation. If methylene blue is introduced into the esophagus, it will exit the chest tube if perforation is present (Cowley & Dunham, 1982).

Esophagography is a useful adjunct for determination of perforation. Controversy exists between using water-soluble and non-water-soluble contrast products when examining the esophagus. A negative Gastrografin swallow should be followed by a barium examination (Pass, LeNarz, Schreiber, & Estrera, 1987).

Endoscopy may be warranted for equivocal findings, provided associated injury does not preclude its use. Ideally, a nasogastric tube is placed to decompress the stomach. Because of its lack of flexibility, a Salem sump is more traumatic to the mucosa during insertion, but the air vent prevents mucosa from being irritated constantly during continuous suction. A Levin tube will also cause gastric irritation, and a smaller size may be used if only decompression is necessary.

Primary closure of the esophageal defect is the preferred method of management with most injuries occurring at the cervical region. Associated tracheal or abdominal injuries are handled as the area of injury is identified (Pass et al., 1987). Adequate airway maintenance and rapid evaluation are key, and nutrition via hyperalimentation or nasogastric tube must be maintained postoperatively. Antibiotic therapy is also an important treatment modality, since leakage of gastrointestinal contents can be injurious and lead to mediastinal infection (Ramponi & Somerville, 1986).

Splenic injuries

The spleen is the primary organ of injury from blunt forces applied to the abdomen (Gibson, 1987). Penetrating injuries resulting in splenic trauma are more uncommon, constituting only 6% of organ damage (Briggs et al., 1987). The spleen has a rich blood supply provided by the splenic artery and splenic vein, which accounts for the significant hemorrhage resulting from injury to this organ. The spleen as a solid organ is particularly susceptible to rupture, since it is protected only by the ribcage in the left upper quadrant. Associated injury is common, since the spleen is in proximity to the diaphragm, stomach, left kidney, a portion of the colon, and tail of the pancreas (Briggs et al., 1987).

Although DPL is widely used to confirm intrabdominal bleeding when blunt trauma occurs, CT is gaining wide support as a diagnostic tool. DPL carries an accuracy rate of nearly 98% for identification of splenic injury (Semonin-Holleran, 1988). However, CT is equally accurate in identifying specific areas of injury (subphrenic and subcapsular hematomas), as well as the amount of bleeding involved in splenic injury (Bresler, 1988). The hemodynamically unstable patient is probably better served by DPL than CT study.

In recent years the issue of splenic salvage rather than splenectomy as a surgical outcome has received considerable attention. This is at least in part due to the function of the spleen in controlling the body's immune response. Although an individual can live a normal life without the spleen, problems associated with postoperative infection have given rise to more conservative management regimens. Of course the degree of damage to the spleen will ultimately determine the preferred course of treatment. Kidd, Lui, Khoo, and Nixon (1987) reviewed 70 cases of splenic trauma, of which 17 were managed nonoperatively. Based on their findings, conservative management, which frequently has been documented as successful in children, can be applied to the adult population. Buntain et al. (1988) support the use of CT to determine splenic injury that can be managed nonsurgically. Sepsis of a pneumococcal origin is common after splenectomy in both the child and adult population and carries high morbidity and mortality. A current preventive strategy for patients with splenectomy, both adults and children, is administration of Pneumovax 23 (Semonin-Holleran, 1988). In addition, abscess formation, pancreatitis, and recurrent hemorrhage can occur postoperatively.

Patients with blunt and penetrating trauma to the abdomen that involves the spleen may present with findings ranging from left upper quadrant pain with radiation to the shoulder to frank hypovolemia. Diagnosis may be made by DPL, or CT

in the more stable patient, and nursing intervention is aimed toward treatment of shock.

The entity of delayed splenic rupture may occur in days or 1 to 2 weeks after injury to the spleen, resulting in hemorrhage into the peritoneum from a previously self-sealed laceration or hematoma to the splenic capsule (Cowley & Dunham, 1982). Careful monitoring of the patient being managed nonoperatively is therefore warranted. Nursing intervention is aimed at maintaining hemodynamic stability by intravenous therapy and attention to possibilities of rapid deterioration of the patient.

Hepatic injuries

Blunt and penetrating trauma to the abdomen accounts for damage to the liver in approximately 15% to 16% of cases (Briggs et al., 1987). Penetrating trauma from a stab wound can lacerate the liver and adjacent vessels but is generally more manageable than gunshot wounds, which can damage the parenchyma and carry a higher mortality from tissue destruction (Trunkey & Holcroft, 1983). Blunt trauma such as that found with deceleration injuries in vehicular trauma accounts for a high mortality, since isolated hepatic injury is uncommon.

The liver is a highly vascular organ, receiving its blood supply from the hepatic artery (25%) and the portal vein (75%) (Porth, 1982). When viewed on a plane, the liver is crossed by the inferior vena cava, branches of the hepatic artery, and the portal vein (Figure 12-2). Blood from the gastrointestinal system, spleen, and pancreas is delivered by the portal vein to the liver, which deposits outflow into the inferior vena cava and finally to the right atrium. In addition to this complex portal blood flow system, the liver itself houses approximately 200 to 400 ml of blood (Porth, 1982). Therefore damage to the liver or tearing of adjacent tributaries can result in profound hemorrhage. Indeed, control of hemorrhage both preoperatively and intraoperatively is the major management issue of liver trauma.

Clinical suspicion of liver trauma based on the mechanism of injury is the most reliable index from a diagnostic standpoint. To determine intraabdominal injury, DPL is certainly a procedure of choice for a patient with blunt trauma. Penetrating trauma, unless it can be determined by

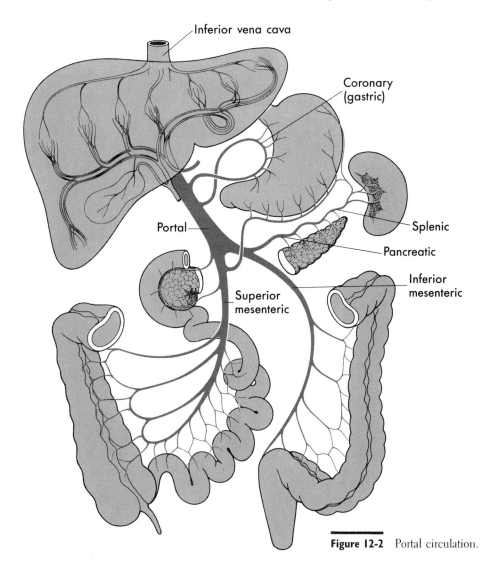

Figure 12-2 Portal circulation.

wound exploration to be superficial, is usually explored operatively and may be preceded by DPL to document hemoperitoneum (Briggs et al., 1987).

Abdominal films are considered to be of limited value to predict intestinal injury or perforation if clinical findings support significant injury (Kester et al., 1986). In the stable patient with questionable blunt injury, CT has proven to be a useful diagnostic mechanism. A current trend is to manage hemodynamically stable patients with equivocal physical examination by using CT initially and serially to pursue a nonoperative course

of management (Farnell et al., 1988). CT can elucidate specific areas of bleeding from damage to the liver, as well as the associated parenchymal injury (Bresler, 1988). Hanna et al. (1987) support the use of DPL in the evaluation of blunt trauma and view CT to be of limited diagnostic value in the unstable patient.

The liver has a unique hemostatic mechanism, and most minor lacerations will cease bleeding spontaneously. The right lobe is injured more frequently than the left. Hemorrhage from liver injury is generally pronounced and rapid so that an initial hematocrit determination may be of little value; hypovolemia and peritoneal signs are better indicators (Briggs et al., 1987).

The majority of nursing interventions are aimed at airway maintenance and treatment of shock. The patient's clinical presentation may be as simple as complaints of right upper quadrant abdominal pain or chest pain to profound hypovolemia. Commonly, the condition of patients with significant trauma appears somewhat benign and can deteriorate rapidly, before abdominal distention and loss of bowel sounds occur.

After surgical repair of the hepatic injury, infection, stress ulcers, and recurrent bleeding are common sequelae. Patients may develop hemobilia (bleeding from the biliary tree) or abscess formation, so external drainage via a T-tube is necessary. Because of the high incidence of postoperative infection, bleeding, and abscess formation, the use of packing to achieve hemostasis is used only for short term control during operative repair of the liver (Way, 1988). The liver has a regenerative capacity at the cellular level, so that as much as 80% to 85% can be removed with subsequent survival. This is important since, in addition to producing bile, the liver metabolizes drugs, carbohydrates, hormones, fats, and protein (Porth, 1982).

Gallbladder and biliary tract injuries

Gallbladder injury is uncommon as a result of trauma, but injury may occur to the gallbladder itself, the cystic or hepatic ducts, and the common bile or common hepatic ducts (Cowley & Dunham, 1982). Most injuries are diagnosed during laparotomy as an associated finding. Symptoms are related to the leakage of bile from the duct, which produces right upper quadrant pain and a small amount of bleeding provided no hepatic involvement exists. Penetrating wounds are responsible for duct injury and usually involve the portal vein or hepatic artery (Lucas & Ledgerwood, 1984). DPL with bile return is indicative of gallbladder involvement, and ultrasound can be used to identify gallbladder injury. Injury to the gallbladder is treated by cholecystectomy; injury to common bile ducts may necessitate anastomosis or primary closure.

Delayed rupture of the gallbladder can occur when an undiagnosed injury causes ongoing ischemia and necrosis of tissue. The interval between trauma and delayed rupture can be up to 6 months. The patient then presents with the same acute symptomatology and associated jaundice and/or ascites (Lucas & Ledgerwood, 1984).

Pancreatic injuries

Injury to the pancreas is rare; however, it can occur from both blunt and penetrating forces, with blunt injury of a crushing nature being more prevalent. Bicycle accidents with handlebar pressure to the abdomen, falls, and direct blows are common causes, and injury results from the compression of the pancreas against the vertebral column (Walker, 1986). The pancreas is somewhat protected by its primarily retroperitoneal location; however, elements situated in the retroperitoneal space, such as the duodenum, common bile duct, aorta, vena cava, and portal vein, allow for major disruption should blunt trauma occur (Maull, Rozycki, Vinsant, & Pedigo, 1987).

Trauma to the pancreas can produce subtle symptomatology, and it is well recognized that pancreatic trauma results in a high mortality by virtue of misdiagnosis, as well as associated injury (Jones, 1985). Hemorrhage from damage to the vasculature is a major consequence of retroperitoneal injury. If pancreatic trauma is an isolated injury, patients often have minimal complaints, such as upper abdominal pain or flank tenderness, particularly in the early diagnostic stages. These patients can deteriorate over time, with abdominal distention, peritoneal signs, and ensuing shock (Cowley & Dunham, 1982).

Many authors concur that serum amylase levels are a relatively poor predictor of pancreatic injury although, over time, serial elevations are diagnostic (Jones, 1985; Walker, 1986). DPL is used for abdominal trauma; however, CT is more conclusive for recognition of retroperitoneal injury (Bresler, 1988). Problems are associated with the accuracy of CT as a result of artifact and air or gas patterns, and DPL is not always positive with injury to the pancreas unless blood has escaped into the intraperitoneal space or unless the injury was to the relatively small portion of the pancreas (the tail) that is intraperitoneal. Maull et al. (1987) strongly support the use of CT, particularly when blunt abdominal injury is present, for diagnosis of retroperitoneal injury.

The pancreas consists of three portions: the head, the body, and the tail. The functions of the pancreas include enzyme production and storage, as well as insulin and glucagon production. Although hemorrhage is a problem with pancreatic injury, additional damage can be rendered by insult to the common bile duct (located near the head of the pancreas) and accessory pancreatic ducts, resulting in release of enzymes and subsequent pancreatitis, abscess, or fistula formation (Cowley & Dunham, 1982). Most pancreatic injuries necessitate drainage and can be managed by simple suturing. When more extensive damage occurs, particularly involving the body and tail, distal pancreatectomy is usually performed (Cowley & Dunham, 1982). Although insulin function may be preserved, enzyme secretion is often disrupted (Cowley & Dunham, 1982). Pancreatic fistula, abscess, and pseudocyst formation are late complications of pancreatic injury, made apparent when increased abdominal pain and/or fever occur. These complications are managed by drainage, either internal or external. For a stable patient, endoscopic retrograde cholangiopancreatography (ERCP) is useful in locating an injury site. During the acute phase of pancreatitis, NPO status prevails to avoid stimulation of pancreatic enzymes. The patient's nutritional state may be supplemented by total parenteral nutrition (TPN) or feeding catheter jejunostomy.

Because pancreatic injury may involve a subtle clinical presentation and many retroperitoneal injuries go undiagnosed, nursing intervention is guided by a high index of suspicion. Acknowledgment of clinical symptoms and mechanism of injury must be maintained, as well as anticipatory thinking regarding possible deterioration of the patient from an injury that lacks specificity.

Gastric and duodenal injuries

Trauma to the hollow organs of the GI or GU system can result in hemorrhage; however, damage is usually the result of leakage of organ contents and extravasation of fluids. Solid organs, such as the liver and spleen, bleed a great deal, and peritonitis is a late sign. On the other hand, hollow organs, such as the stomach and duodenum, demonstrate signs of peritoneal irritation early, followed by shock (Norton, 1984).

The stomach is injured more frequently by penetrating rather than blunt trauma (Cowley & Dunham, 1982). Nasogastric tube placement with resultant heme-positive return indicates gastric disruption. Because of its proximity to the liver, spleen, colon, kidney, and pancreas, blunt stomach trauma is rarely a solo entity. Provided the patient is hemodynamically stable, an upright chest or abdominal x-ray study may show free air in the peritoneum, suggestive of gastric damage, but this finding may be absent in as many as 50% of injuries (Norton, 1984). If gastric injury occurs singularly, repair and recovery are generally uncomplicated.

The stomach terminates in the duodenum, the beginning of the small intestine, where injury is more prevalent and more difficult to diagnose, since, with the exception of the superior portion, the duodenum is situated in the retroperitoneal space. The degree of injury to the duodenum from a penetrating source depends on the mechanism and the number of entry wounds, e.g., stab or gunshot wound, single or multiple. Blunt trauma to the duodenum can arise from a crush injury, deceleration, or compression, such as that associated with the lap portion of seat belts (Norton, 1984). If the injury occurs to the superior portion of the duodenum, the patient complains of abdominal pain and/or vomiting; if the injury is retroperitoneal, the patient initially may have an unimpressive clinical examination. Suspicion of a duodenal injury is paramount to its diagnosis because of conflicting signs and symptoms and equivocal findings on examination. Penetrating injuries are usually explored operatively if evidence of peritoneal penetration is found. DPL can render a false-negative result if the injury is in the retroperitoneum. CT and upper gastrointestinal studies are useful but must be reserved for a stable patient (Bresler, 1988). Water-soluble contrast studies will indicate duodenal injury if extravasation of the medium occurs (Cowley & Dunham, 1982). If no interruption of the duodenum exists, nonoperative observation is indicated. Repair of singular duodenal injuries involves debridement and closure. Tube decompression may be used, and a portion of the duodenum may be linked to the jejunum (duodenojejunostomy), if needed (Cowley & Dunham, 1982).

Nursing interventions involve stabilization of the patient via intravenous therapy, recognition of associated injuries, nasogastric decompression, and preparation of the patient for diagnostic procedures. Prophylactic antibiotic administration is indicated for any injury from which organ content leakage occurs.

Small bowel and colon injuries

The small intestine comprises the duodenum, jejunum, and ileum and is about 20 feet long.

Injuries to the duodenum were discussed separately. The small intestine's major function of water and nutrient absorption must be preserved for survival with at least 8 cm of terminal ileum and 30 cm of jejunum or products of digestion cannot be absorbed. Cholesterol and vitamin B_{12} are absorbed in the terminal ileum. Total parenteral nutrition is indicated for loss of small intestine function.

The small bowel is more resistant to injury than other abdominal organs, since it is not a fixed structure. Penetrating injury is more common than blunt trauma, and injury to this portion of the abdominal cavity is often associated with mesenteric and vascular disruption. The aorta, inferior vena cava, and superior mesenteric artery and vein traverse the small intestine, so associated hemorrhage secondary to injury can be evidenced (Briggs et al., 1987). Intraabdominal bleeding can be related to associated organ injury, such as the spleen or liver, but may involve leakage from the mesentery. Symptoms may include abdominal pain and/or peritoneal signs caused by irritation from leakage of blood or intestinal contents. As is found in other hollow organ injuries, the clinical examination may be equivocal (Feliciano & Mattox, 1984). Diagnostic adjuncts used to define small bowel injury include DPL and CT. As was discussed extensively, a minor injury, in this case of the mesentery or vasculature, can produce a positive lavage finding while CT can aid in localizing the amount and source of bleeding. Proponents for the use of CT in evaluation of small bowel trauma will argue that a DPL injury will result in unnecessary surgical exploration of minor injury because of its sensitivity (Bresler, 1988). The incidence of visceral injuries with trauma to the intestine is increased, so exploration for wounds of a penetrating source, particularly gunshots, is necessary (Feliciano & Mattox, 1984).

Colonic injury results from gunshot wounds and stabbings in 98% of cases (Briggs et al., 1987), and associated organ injury may be as high as 75% (Nelson & Walt, 1984). Mortality related to injury of the colon is highly related to contamination with bowel contents; therefore, early recognition and treatment is necessary. The function of the colon is water absorption and storage and propulsion of feces; the colon consists of the ascending, transverse, descending, and sigmoid colon (Schrock, 1988). The colon receives its blood supply from the superior and inferior mesenteric vessels originating from the aorta. Trauma to the transverse and sigmoid portions is more commonly caused by penetrating injury (Briggs et al., 1987).

Evisceration of the bowel and the membrane that encloses it (known as *omentum*) is a common finding with stab wounds and to a lesser degree with gunshot wounds. Evisceration is not always associated with disruption of visceral function; however, operative exploration and repair are the standard procedures (Huizinga, Baker, & Mtshali, 1987).

Radiologic studies to diagnose injury to the colon offer limited information, since free air or pneumoperitoneum may not exist. A paralytic ileus may develop from the nonmechanical obstruction that occurs from decreased peristalsis and peritoneal irritation. This finding often accompanies a postoperative course as well (Schrock, 1988).

DPL with a return of feces or vegetable matter is diagnostic for colon disruption, and blood and increased WBC counts are also found. The use of CT is controversial, and further study in this area is necessary (Bresler, 1988).

As in other injuries to abdominal organs, operative management depends on the extent and level of injury and, specific to the colon, the amount of contamination. Sepsis and fistula formation are common postoperative problems. Primary repair may be all that is necessary; however, the use of temporary or permanent colostomy is common. The types and sites of bowel diversion via colostomy include loop colostomy and end, or terminal, colostomy (Schrock, 1988). Whereas approximately 30 cm of the small intestine must be maintained for function, the colon may be removed and diverted through colostomy and allow for survival with only malabsorption problems occurring.

The importance of nutrition in the postoperative rehabilitation of the patient experiencing injury to the small or large intestine must be considered, since trauma increases the metabolic rate and impacts clinical progress. Tube feedings or intraoperative placements of adjuncts such as jejunostomy tubes are frequently used. Gastrostomy tubes carry a high incidence of reflux, so jejunostomy tubes may be better for feeding. Some disagree on whether to institute such feedings before bowel sounds return postoperatively.

The diagnosis of a mesenteric infarction is often presumptive and may accompany bowel trauma, particularly in the elderly population (Schrock, 1988). The thrombus formation may involve either the mesenteric arteries or veins and carries a high mortality. The symptomatology accompanying this finding may be obscure but the symptom that is *always* present is pain that is more profuse than the predisposing injury or condition should warrant. Essentially, damage to the mesenteric vasculature involves ischemia and leakage of bacteria into the circulation in a relatively short time—6 to 12 hours. The mucosal wall of the mesentery is involved, and the bowel infarcts secondary to the occlusion. Cardiogenic shock with peritonitis is the final outcome (Schrock, 1988). Once the diagnosis is confirmed, usually through angiography, the clinical course and ultimate survival of the patient depend on the degree of vessel involvement, whether the vessel is arterial or venous, and the ability to resect associated intestine to satisfactorily permit function of the organ. The prognosis is directly tied to the extent of damage and how quickly it is recognized.

Nursing care of the patient with real or suspected injury to the small and large intestines is related to assessment of hemodynamics and bowel sounds, and abdominal examination for observance of signs and symptoms of peritonitis. Gastric decompression is indicated via nasogastric tube, and early administration of intravenous antibiotics is necessary. When bowel contents protrude through the abdomen, the site should be covered with moist saline to preserve the mucosa. The patient, if awake, must be urged to avoid coughing or unnecessary movement that may result in increased evisceration. A posture of knee flexing may be useful (Semonin-Holleran, 1988).

Abdominal vascular injuries

The abdominal cavity receives the majority of its blood flow via the abdominal aorta and its channels. The circulatory flow throughout this system is complex, and the reader is urged to consult anatomic and physiologic references for specific circulation patterns. Some orientation is necessary to understand the impact of vascular injury in the abdomen. The portal venous system comprises the superior and inferior mesenteric, splenic, and gastric veins, which collect blood from the intestines, pancreas, and spleen.

This blood flow is directed through the hepatic veins. The portal vein and hepatic artery carry all blood to the liver and eventually terminate in the inferior vena cava. The combination of portal venous system and arterial flow through the liver is termed *splanchnic circulation*. The function of the inferior vena cava is to return blood from below the diaphragm. Its tributaries include the renal and hepatic veins. The superior and inferior mesenteric arteries arise from the aorta and supply portions of the colon and small intestine (Porth, 1982). The aorta bifurcates into the celiac axis, which gives rise to the gastric, hepatic, and splenic arteries. Hence every major organ within the abdomen is directly linked via a circulatory pathway to the aorta.

Trauma to the aorta or its branches is most commonly a result of penetrating injury and carries a high mortality from exsanguination. The vessels may be completely transected or lacerated or involve hematoma formation. Penetrating injuries that damage the aorta or vena cava are associated with injury to the surrounding organs as well (Briggs et al., 1987).

Blunt trauma is also a factor in vascular disruption. The vena cava may be torn as a result of deceleration injury, whereas the aorta is less frequently injured (Ward & Blaisdell, 1984). Collins et al. (1988) reported significant mortality associated with injury to the portal vein, hepatic artery, aorta, and vena cava, in descending order. Certainly the number of injuries and specific location contribute to overall survival. In addition, stab wounds are associated with lower mortality as compared with high-velocity gunshot wounds. An important consideration is that the liver has a rich blood supply from the inferior vena cava, hepatic artery, and portal vein and is the second most commonly injured organ in blunt trauma (Briggs et al., 1987).

Early recognition of vascular injury is associated with significant hypotension secondary to hemorrhage, peritoneal irritation, and abdominal distention. Exploration of such injuries is mandatory, and early laparotomy takes priority over diagnostic modalities. Management and survival of patients who sustain a vascular injury are related to rapid treatment of shock with volume replacement and blood products. The absence of femoral pulses on clinical examination is indicative of aortic dissection (Ward & Blaisdell, 1984).

Generally, although minor disruptions may be ligated during surgery, injury to the portal vein, superior mesenteric artery, and renal artery necessitate repair, or organ function can be lost.

Complications

Definitive treatment for organ disruption caused by abdominal trauma is often surgical intervention. In spite of meticulous attention to surgical procedure and to the preservation of a sterile environment, a number of postoperative complications can occur that have a deteminant effect on the patient outcome. These include wound infection, abscess and fistula formation, and stress ulcers.

Wound infection

Surgical infections share three common denominators: an agent, a host, and a defined space. The agents, or organisms capable of causing infection, are numerous. Some are easily treated (singular pathogens), whereas others (multiple organisms) are less amenable to therapy and can result in overwhelming sepsis, particularly if left untreated or unidentified. The host, in this case the trauma patient, offers an immunosupressed environment that the agent can easily access. In addition, the host may have medical conditions, such as diabetes or anemia, that impede otherwise normal healing processes. Some areas of the body are more prone to infection, particularly those characterized by decreased perfusion and/or limited nutrient and oxygen supply (Hunt & Jawetz, 1988).

Fever and leukocytosis are the hallmarks of the early development of postoperative wound infection. The suture line provides access for pathogens, and attention to the wound site, particularly if erythematous, alerts the practitioner to early treatable signs of infection (Hunt & Goodson, 1988.)

Abscess and fistula formation

Abscess formation associated with surgical intervention is an inflammatory process characterized by an accumulation of pus and fluid. Generally in a dependent, localized portion of the peritoneal cavity, abscess formation occurs as a result of environmental bacterial entry or as a consequence of a perforated viscus with the accumulation of necrotizing byproducts (Boey, 1988). Flu-

ids accumulate in response to gravity, so that the dependent portions of the abdomen, diaphragm, pelvis, and subhepatic spaces are generally affected (Boey, 1988). Any patient who experiences transient elevations in fever without a substantive origin and a unusually sluggish postoperative recovery should be suspect for abscess formation. Because a frank clinical picture may be absent, the practitioner's best tool is an index of suspicion, since the picture may be further clouded by antibiotic regimens, which may keep a virulent process temporarily at bay. Once the cause has been identified, the abscess must be quickly and completely drained, even if that process subjects the patient to another surgical procedure (Boey, 1988). Morbidity is compounded with delay, and multiple system compromise can ensue.

If left unchecked, the abscess can form an abnormal communication, a fistula, either between the cavity and the external environment or across organ paths. Fistulas are a common consequence of surgical procedures and are defined by the site where they develop, whether they are simple or complex in origin, and by the amount of fluid output (Schrock, 1988). Although a significant percentage of fistulas heal spontaneously, operative intervention with resection and end-to-end anastomosis may be indicated. Of paramount importance to fistula management is aggressive nutritional support (including TPN), maintenance of fluids and electrolytes, and control of sepsis resultant from a recurrent or incompletely drained abscess (Schrock, 1988). Furthermore, the caustic fluid drainage associated with fistula tracts must be both contained (to avoid skin breakdown) and measured and recorded (to facilitate adequate supplemental fluid intake) (Schrock, 1988).

Stress ulcers

The disruption of the body's hemostatic mechanisms as a result of trauma, sepsis, and shock can result in the development of acute ulcer formation in the stomach or duodenum (Way, 1988). Although the exact mechanism of action is unclear, stress ulcers develop as a result of both increased gastric secretion and an impaired mucosal layer secondary to ischemia (Way, 1988). Antacid therapy is instituted early in the postoperative period for the high-risk patient, because damage is clinically apparent only when hemorrhage occurs. Although hemorrhage can usually be contained by gastric lavage, in some cases operative intervention, specifically vagotomy or subtotal gastectomy, is indicated (Way, 1988).

Nursing Diagnosis

Clinical problems, such as those that exist in trauma, define the nursing role as that of anticipating the occurrence, assessing and monitoring the manifestations, and working with the medical discipline toward resolution of the patient care problem. It is difficult to label actual and high-risk diagnoses for the trauma patient because each clearly depends on an individual's presentation and severity of injury. A percentage of trauma patients present, for example, with splenic damage without the clinical manifestations of hypotension, hypovolemia, or respiratory compromise used to define the nursing diagnosis. Unless the patient situation dictates a problem to be actual, the patient will be at high risk for virtually all nursing diagnoses.

The nursing diagnoses presented here are based on the premise that patients are at risk for the complications of shock, respiratory compromise, sepsis, intraabdominal/retroperitoneal injury, and pain. The nursing diagnoses discussed are only a representative sample and by no means all inclusive. The nursing diagnoses most commonly used in abdominal trauma are presented in the table on pp. 384-385.

GENITOURINARY TRAUMA
Mechanism of Injury
Renal injuries

Blunt trauma produces 80% of all renal injuries. Of these injuries, 85% are the result of deceleration injuries from motor vehicle crashes. The remaining 15% are caused by falls and contact sports (McAninch, 1985b). Although the ratio is decreasing, 4 times as many men as women sustain renal injuries, with the majority being under 30 years old (Zoller, 1983). Penetrating injury to the kidney is related to gunshot or stab wounds. These injuries involve associated organ injury in 80% of the cases (McAninch, 1985b), usually affecting the liver, colon, spleen, and stomach. Children are more prone to renal injuries because their kidneys are proportionately larger and have a minimal layer of protective fat (Kearney & Finn, 1981).

Blunt trauma in the flank causes the twelfth rib to compress the kidney against the lumbar spine (Figure 12-3 illustrates the anatomic relationship among these three areas). This usually produces a contusion, but a fracture of the rib or the transverse process of the vertebrae can easily lacerate the kidney. Anterior renal injuries can occur when a patient receives a blow to the abdomen directly below the rib cage, such as that which occurs when a patient is involved in a motor vehicle crash and hits the steering column. This compresses the kidney between the object and the spine. This same mode of injury occurs when a patient is run over by an automobile. Rapid deceleration forces the kidney downward, placing a strain on the renal pedicle. This type of injury can result in the rupture of a major vessel or a stretching of the renal artery, producing a tear in the intima. This tear can produce a thrombus that occludes the vessel. These patients may present with fluid volume deficit and have additional injuries, clouding the diagnostic picture.

Ureteral injuries

The ureters are well protected by the spinal column, abdominal wall, colon, and pelvic organs. Blunt trauma is extremely rare. Most cases occur in persons less than 20 years old and are the result of severe abdominal compression, such as when a child is run over by an automobile. The ureter becomes crushed against the spinal column. The ureter is usually lacerated at the ureteropelvic junction (Salvatierra, 1984).

Penetrating ureteral trauma is twice as common as blunt ureteral trauma (Zoller, 1983). Associated injuries are common in these cases, especially gastrointestinal involvement. These patients tend to be severely injured and present in hypovolemic shock (Presti, Carroll, & McAninch, 1989). As a result, the ureteral injury is often overlooked until the patient goes to the operating room for repair of abdominal organs.

Bladder injuries

The majority of bladder injuries are the result of blunt trauma to a distended bladder. Figure 12-4 depicts this phenomenon. When distended, the bladder rises above the umbilicus, where there is less protection. Motor vehicle crashes, falls, direct blows, and sports injuries are the leading causes of trauma to the bladder (Hanno, 1985a).

Nursing diagnosis	Nursing intervention	Evaluative criteria
Fluid volume deficit Related to hypovolemia Secondary to hemorrhage As evidenced by poor skin turgor, altered vital signs, flank bruising, fluid accumulation on CT film	**Maintain fluid volume** Provide fluid resuscitation via two large-bore IVs. Prepare for use of colloids, type O neg. or type-specific blood as available. Monitor Hgb & Hct for decreases. Monitor BP, P, R, q15 min. Use MAST suit unless contraindicated to maintain BP >90 mm Hg; deflate slowly as BP stabilizes. Apply pressure to open wound; reinforce with pressure dressing. Monitor urine volume and specific gravity via urinary catheter and urinometer. Prepare patient for surgery or diagnostic procedures.	Patient will have the following: • palpable pulses, normal skin turgor, vital signs WNL; • unlabored respiratory rate of 14-20/min; • rate of hemorrhage slowed; • urinary output of 30 ml/hr.
Altered peripheral tissue perfusion Related to impaired blood supply to periphery As evidenced by decreased circulating blood volume, hypotension, peripheral vasoconstriction, pallor, cyanosis, cool temperature of extremities, capillary refill > 2 sec, hypothermia	**Promote perfusion** Monitor skin for color and temperature. Assess capillary refill and presence/absence of peripheral pulses. Assess mucous membranes. Maintain body warmth (blankets, warmed IV fluids). Remind patient to avoid crossing legs.	Patient will have the following: • extremities warm and pink; • capillary refill < 2 sec; • peripheral pulses present.

Ineffective breathing pattern
Related to shock and/or associated injury (e.g., diaphragm injury, esophageal tear) or aspiration
As evidenced by respirations shallow and slow or tachypneic;
ABGs: pH <7.35,
    pCO_2 >45,
    PO_2 <70,
    O_2 sat<90;
use of accessory muscles to breathe, use of involuntary splinting; decreased expansion of lungs caused by pain, concurrent injury to diaphragm; change in mental status secondary to hypoxia
	Promote ventilation
	Apply high-flow oxygen; adjust per ABG determinants.
	Monitor and interpret ABGs for fluctuations.
	Monitor airway patency, anticipate necessity for ventilatory support.
	Auscultate lung fluids for equality, presence of rales, or rhonchi wheezing.
	Monitor chest wall expansion.
	Monitor verbalization of chest discomfort.
	Assess breathing pattern, rate, and quality.
	Assess LOC q15 minutes; observe for changes in mentation, onset of confusion, restlessness.
		Patient will have the following:
		• respiratory rate maintained at 14-20 breaths/min;
		• ABGs within approximately normal limits;
		• equal bilateral chest movement (rise and fall); equal bilateral breath sounds;
		• no complaints of breathing difficulty;
		• stable Glasgow coma score.

Impaired skin integrity Related to tissue disruption by penetrating trauma As evidenced by disruption of skin surface/layers, evisceration of abdominal contents	**Promote tissue healing** Administer prescribed antibiotics to prevent overwhelming bacterial infection from open wound. Cleanse wound with antimicrobial solution if applicable; apply sterile dressing. Maintain body temperature via external warming (blankets) and internal warming (heated fluids).	Additional wound contamination and/or sepsis will be prevented by administration of antibiotics. Conservation of body temperatures will be maintained. Sterility will be maintained to degree possible. Patient will be immunized against tetanus if unprotected or of questionable status.

Nursing diagnosis	Nursing intervention	Evaluative criteria
	Maintain sterile field for diagnostic procedures to prevent infection. Administer tetanus prophylaxis as prescribed. Prepare for local wound exploration if deemed necessary. For eviscerated omentum, cover and protect abdominal contents with sterile wet dressing. Minimize movement of patient.	Strangulation, ischemia, and dehydration or eviscerated tissue will be avoided; evisceration will not extend.
High risk for injury As evidenced by retroperitoneal bleeding, peritoneal bleeding, colonic tears	**Detect additional injuries and complications** Determine and document mechanism of injury. Insert NG tube to decompress stomach; observe for blood. Observe and measure abdominal girth for distention. Auscultate and document presence or absence of bowel sounds. Palpate abdomen for signs of peritoneal irritation. Inspect and document areas of discoloration, contusion, or laceration. Prepare patient for diagnostic studies. Dipstick urine for presence of blood. Maintain adequate IV fluid intake. Monitor VS q15 minutes.	Intraabdominal injury will be ruled out or diagnosed. Abdominal distention and/or aspiration will be prevented. Changes in abdominal status will be noted. Abnormalities will be detected, documented, and reported.
Pain Related to tissue disruption As evidenced by communication of pain descriptions; nonverbal indicators (facial expression); moaning, crying, restlessness; autonomic responses (diaphore sis, BP, HR and respiration rate increase); abdominal guarding	**Promote comfort** Explain procedures, activities in calm, reassuring manner. Provide comfort measures as patient condition permits. Change position as appropriate (e.g., flex knees to relieve abdominal stress.) Provide diversional activity (e.g., conversation, focal point, concentration of breathing.) Limit abdominal palpation and rebound assessment to essential periods only.	Patient will relate increased comfort. VS will improve (e.g., HR decrease to normal range). Body tension will lessen. Restlessness will decrease.
High risk for infection As evidenced by ischemia, leakage of abdominal contents, abscess for mation	**Prevent infection** Recognize individuals at risk of abdominal content leakage (e.g., hollow organs injury). Anticipate need for administration of prophylactic antibiotic. Maintain sterile technique with dressing changes. Use aseptic technique and handwashing. Obtain blood and other tissue cultures when indicated.	Early changes will be detected. Patient will be afebrile. WBC count and differential will be WNL. Potential wound infection will be minimized. Clinical outcome will improve postoperatively.

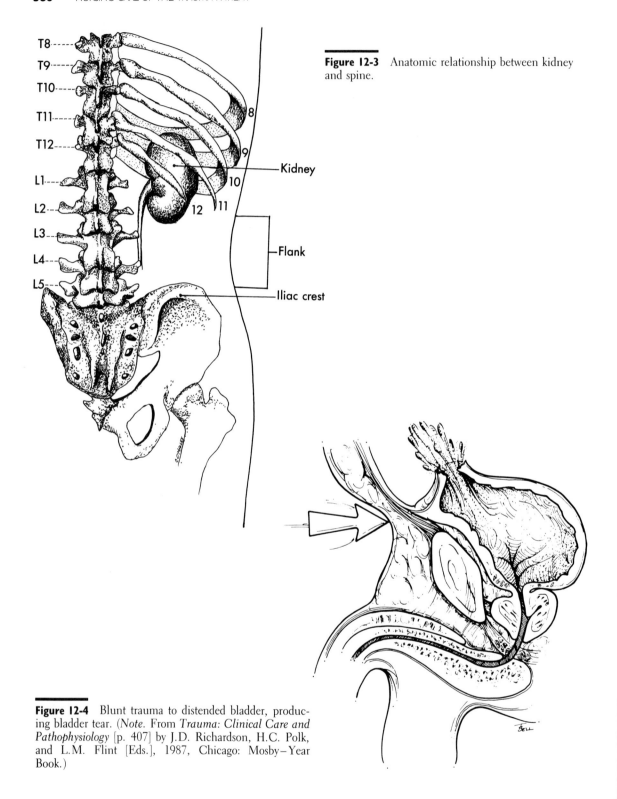

T8
T9
T10
T11
T12
L1
L2
L3
L4
L5

8
9
Kidney
10
11
12

Flank

Iliac crest

Figure 12-3 Anatomic relationship between kidney and spine.

Figure 12-4 Blunt trauma to distended bladder, producing bladder tear. (*Note.* From *Trauma: Clinical Care and Pathophysiology* [p. 407] by J.D. Richardson, H.C. Polk, and L.M. Flint [Eds.], 1987, Chicago: Mosby–Year Book.)

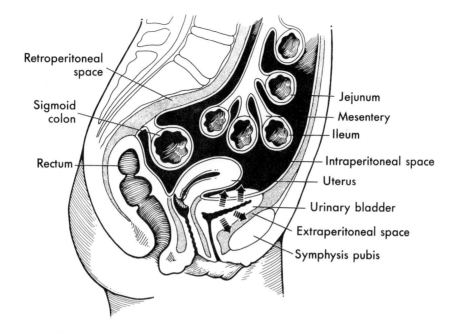

Figure 12-5   Anatomic relationship of bladder to peritoneal cavity. Bladder is partially covered by peritoneal membrane. Injury in this region produces intraperitoneal extravasation of urine.

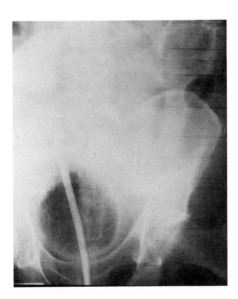

Figure 12-6   Bladder injury with both intraperitoneal and extraperitoneal extravasation of urine. (Courtesy Tucson Medical Center Radiology Department, Tucson, Ariz.)

Lacerations of the bladder can produce extraperitoneal or intraperitoneal (and in some cases both) extravasation of urine. Figure 12-5 illustrates how the bladder is partially covered by the peritoneal membranes. Extraperitoneal extravasation occurs in 80% of patients (Mitchell, 1984). This type of injury is the result of significant trauma and is associated with a pelvic fracture in 70% of all cases (Hanno, 1985a). In these situations, a fragment of pelvic bone is driven through the bladder or injury occurs contralateral to the site of the pelvic fracture because of compression (Carroll, Taylor, & McAninch, 1985b). Lacerations that produce intraperitoneal extravasation usually are in the area of the bladder fundus (Zoller, 1983). These injuries are frequently the result of a blow to the lower abdomen or compression secondary to a seat belt in a motor vehicle collision. In both instances the bladder usually is distended. A laceration with both intraperitoneal and extraperitoneal extravasation occurs most often in penetrating trauma (Figure 12-6). These patients have a higher mortality rate related to the presence of multiple associated injuries.

Urethral injuries

Urethral injuries vary in degree of occurrence and site of injury, depending on the age and sex of the patient. The urethra is about 5 times longer in males than in females and therefore is injured more often in males. In the male, the urogenital diaphragm divides the anterior and posterior urethra.

A urethral injury should be suspected when a patient has sustained perineal trauma, a straddle injury, or a pelvic fracture (Hanno, 1985b). The likelihood of urethral/bladder damage cannot be predicted with type and degree of pelvic fracture (Peterson, 1989). Blunt rectal trauma also has been associated with urethral disruption (Brunner & Shatney, 1987). Signs and symptoms of urethral injury include blood at the urethral meatus, inability to urinate, a high-riding prostate on rectal examination, and extravasation of blood or urine into the pelvic cavity or perineum.

Injury involving the anterior urethra, which includes the bulbous and penile urethra, usually occurs in isolation and does not involve other organs or sections of the urinary tract (Mitchell, 1984) (Figure 12-7). These injuries are often the result of a straddle fall where the urethra is crushed between the object fallen on and the pubic symphysis (Zoller, 1983). The anterior urethra can be damaged also by the use of foreign objects for sexual pleasure.

The posterior section of the urethra includes the junction point between the membranous and bulbous urethra (urogenital diaphragm) and the membranous and prostatic portions of the urethra. Injury to this section is most often the result of a motor vehicle crash where the pelvis is fractured (Harty, 1987; Zoller, 1983; Salvatierra, 1984). The posterior urethra can be damaged also by penetrating trauma.

Posterior urethral trauma is more common than bladder or anterior urethral injuries (Mitchell, 1984). It was previously thought that in cases of pelvic fractures, a bony fragment penetrated the urethra. This occurs infrequently, and usually the injury is the result of a shearing force applied to the membranous urethra above where it is anchored by the urogenital diaphragm. If the prostate is dislocated because of the force of impact, the injury may occur in the prostatic urethra. These injuries have a higher rate of complications.

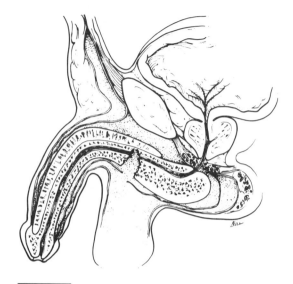

Figure 12-7 Depiction of anterior urethral injury.

The most common cause of urethral injury in the female is laceration by a spicule of bone from a fractured pelvis. This bone fragment may penetrate the anterior wall of the vagina. Therefore urethral injuries in the female are often regarded as open wounds (Mitchell, 1984).

Straddle injuries can damage the external urinary meatus, but usually the vulva is affected. Another source of urethral injuries in females are objects inserted into the vagina. These can cut through the vaginal wall and penetrate the urethra.

Genital injuries

Previously, genital trauma was most common in military personnel because of high-velocity missile injuries (Merrill & Palmer, 1985). The incidence of penetrating genital trauma is increasing in the general population, although most cases are the result of occupational accidents. A review of the literature did not reveal statistics comparing the incidence of blunt injuries with penetrating injuries, although blunt genital trauma is more common in patients less than 50 years of age (Brothers, 1985).

Many classifications of genital trauma exist. Avulsion injuries involve the skin from the penis or scrotum being ripped from the patient's body (Figure 12-8). This is commonly the result of an

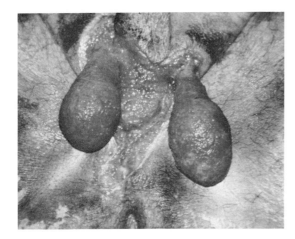

Figure 12-8 Scrotal avulsion injury. (Courtesy Tucson Medical Center Radiology Department, Tucson, Ariz.)

agricultural injury, where the patient's clothes become entrapped in a power takeoff of a farm tractor (Heeg, TenDuis, & Klasen, 1986). Penetrating genital injuries are generally the result of missile injury, so the salvage rate is lower. Penile amputation is frequently the result of self-mutilation. In 87% of these cases, the patient is believed to be psychotic (Jordan & Gilbert, 1989). Blunt genital trauma usually involves the scrotum and is the result of a straddle injury or a blow or kick to the area.

The incidence of genital trauma continues to rise in the female population. This is related to the increased participation of females in exercise programs, sports, and blue collar occupations. Blunt injuries are more common than penetrating injuries, with straddle accidents accounting for the greatest number.

Most vaginal injuries are lacerations produced by sexual assault. Sexual objects can lacerate the vagina as can consensual intercourse in women who are postmenopausal or who have experienced prolonged abstinence.

Anatomic and Physiologic Considerations
Kidneys

The kidneys lie in the retroperitoneum between the twelfth thoracic and second lumbar vertebrae. The adrenal glands lie on the superior medial aspect. The renal parenchyma is surrounded by a fibrous capsule. This capsule can promote hemostasis and prevent urinary extravasation after injury if it remains intact.

Twenty percent of cardiac output goes to the kidney. Massive hemorrhage can occur, since the renal artery arises from the aorta. The branches of the renal artery are end arteries. Very little collateral circulation exists; therefore thrombosed arteries must be repaired. The right renal vein drains directly into the inferior vena cava, so laceration of this vessel leaves the vena cava as a major bleeding site.

Ureter

The ureter is a tubular structure that connects the kidney to the bladder. It runs most of the length of the abdomen and pelvis and is located retroperitoneally. The ureter is a flexible structure and is firmly fixed only at the ureteropelvic junction, the site of most ureteral injuries. Flexibility prevents the ureter from sustaining injury in most cases of blunt trauma.

Bladder

The position and shape of the bladder vary with age, sex, and degree of distention with urine (Carroll, Taylor, & McAninch, 1985). In childhood and during pregnancy the bladder is an abdominal organ, predisposing it to a greater incidence of injury (Hanno, 1985a). The adult bladder is located in the pelvic region and ascends only when distended with urine. The superior surface, or dome, of the bladder is injured because it is not supported, is covered only by peritoneum, and is weak in structure. An injury here produces extravasation of urine peritoneally. The vesical neck of the bladder is the least movable part because it is supported by ligaments, fat, and fibrous tissue. Rupture here is common and results in extraperitoneal extravasation.

Urethra

The urethra is only 4 cm long in the female compared with 20 cm long in the male (Hanno, 1985b). Consequently, urethral injuries in females are rare. The urethra in males is divided into an anterior and posterior section by the urogenital diaphragm. The posterior urethra is in and above the urogenital diaphragm and includes the prostatic and membranous urethra. The prostatic urethra runs from the bladder neck to the prostate area. It is well supported and rarely injured. The membranous urethra passes through the urogenital diaphragm and attaches to the apex of the prostate. The posterior urethra is injured often as a result of shearing forces. The anterior section includes the bulbous and penile urethra. This section is located below the urogenital diaphragm and runs to the external meatus. Injury to the anterior section usually results from straddle injuries or external genital trauma.

In the male, the scrotum is covered by a thin layer of skin. It receives its blood supply from branches of the femoral and internal pudendal arteries. The testis and epididymis reside in each scrotal compartment and are suspended by the spermatic cord. The penis is covered by the corpus cavernosum. This dense fibrous sheath has a portion that is thinner and more susceptible to trauma, the tunica albuginea.

General Assessment

Assessment guidelines for the patient with GU injuries are presented in the box on the facing page. It is important to question the alert patient or the family, if the patient is unconscious, about preexisting renal disease. This may help to confirm that the uninjured kidney functions adequately, especially in cases where a nephrectomy may have to be considered. Additionally, polycystic, hydronephrotic, and horseshoe-shaped kidneys are highly susceptible to injury with very minor trauma.

Medications that the patient is taking at the time of injury should be documented. This may provide information that could alter the management of the injury. A small tear in the bladder with extraperitoneal extravasation of urine usually is managed conservatively. However, if the patient was taking co-trimoxazole (Septra) for a urinary tract infection, the extravasation of urine, especially when infected, could produce necrosis and septicemia. In this case it is favorable to surgically intervene and drain the retroperitoneal space. Likewise, if the patient has a history of chronic urinary tract infection or was experiencing hematuria before the injury, the interpretation of the urinalysis must be more suspect.

Assessment of the GU system begins after such priority measures as airway establishment and the initiation of IV fluids have been accomplished.

Certain mechanisms of injury result in a higher incidence of GU trauma. The trauma nurse should carefully evaluate any patient who has been struck by a motor vehicle. This type of injury often results in a renovascular problem (Zoller, 1983). A history of rapid deceleration injury, such as falls from heights, sledding accidents, and head-on automobile collisions, may produce blunt GU trauma. Penetrating injuries usually occur from knife and gunshot wounds to the abdomen, back, or lower chest wall. The right kidney is injured more frequently than the left because of its lower position in the abdomen and lack of skeletal protection (Odling-Smeed & Crockard, 1981).

Subjective data

Subjective data concentrate mainly on the patient's alteration in comfort. In kidney or ureteral injuries, pain is usually in the flank or upper abdominal area. It can mimic the pain experienced with the presence of renal calculi and may radiate to the groin or shoulder. Injuries to the lower urinary tract may result in suprapubic pain described as constant or boring. If the patient desires to void but is unable to or experiences severe pain on voiding, a lower urinary tract injury is suspected.

Extraperitoneal extravasation of urine will not produce much subjective data other than pain, as mentioned. Intraperitoneal extravasation can result in patient complaints of nausea, rebound tenderness, or tightness in the abdomen.

Objective data

Objective data are helpful in ascertaining GU injury. The patient should be undressed completely to facilitate assessment for ecchymoses and flank masses. Because of concommitant trauma, a patient may become agitated and require restraining. Sedation should be avoided if possible because pain is a major clue to GU injury. Adequate lighting is important because ecchymoses can indicate GU trauma. The lower rib area should be inspected for bruises because rib fractures occur from major force. Any force capable of fracturing ribs could compress the kidney. Blue discoloration of the flanks may indicate retroperitoneal bleeding, whereas discoloration of the perineal area may indicate a pelvic fracture and possible bladder or urethral injury. Any contusion of the abdomen could be symptomatic of GU injury, particularly renal injury, if the contusion is in the upper quadrant (McAninch, 1985).

The external meatus should be checked for bloody drainage, because this is a cardinal sign of anterior urethral injuries (McAninch, 1985a; Kidd, 1982; Salvatierra, 1984). Because of the speed with which trauma nurses must act, a catheter may be inserted without checking the meatus. Cleansing the area with povidone-iodine solution (Betadine) before examination may eliminate any sign of bleeding. Often patients with urethral injuries will present in hypovolemic shock secondary to blood loss from associated pelvic or abdominal injuries. Although it is essential to monitor urinary output in most cases of hypovolemic shock, when suspecting a urethral injury, it is better to depend on a central venous pressure measurement than to catheterize the patient and use urinary output for fluid titration.

After observing the patient, one should auscultate the abdomen for bowel sounds. A traumatic paralytic ileus can occur secondary to intraperitoneal urine extravasation or renal injuries. It is important to listen for the presence of bruits. A bruit can result from a renal vascular injury. Lack of breath sounds in the lower lung fields could indicate a pneumothorax from fractured ribs. As mentioned, fractured lower ribs, particularly the eleventh and twelfth ribs, can puncture the kidney, or the force producing the injury could have been strong enough to compress the kidney against the vertebrae.

Palpation of the abdomen should be performed gently. Palpation of the flanks may reveal a retroperitoneal mass, indicative of bleeding. Palpation can stimulate further bleeding and delay clot formation (Mitchell, 1984). If a mass is palpated, the areas should be marked and its measurement documented for a baseline assessment. Palpation of the bladder region can determine if distention is present, suggesting that bladder rupture has not occurred. If abdominal rigidity or guarding is noted, intraperitoneal extravasation may have occurred.

A rectal examination should be performed. A high-riding prostate or a boggy mass is indicative of a ruptured posterior urethra. Extravasated urine and blood dislocate the prostate. Figure 12-9 depicts dislocation of the prostate secondary to a rupture of the posterior urethra. Edema and hematoma formation within the pelvis can also dis-

GU trauma assessment guidelines

Initial actions

Initiate at least one IV line (large bore)
Remove all clothing
Obtain blood samples for complete blood cell count (CBC), BUN, creatinine, type and cross-match, electrolyte levels
Obtain vital signs
Obtain urine specimen for urinalysis, culture (unless urethral injury is suspected), dipstick (urine reagent strip, Chemstrip) measurement in the emergency department

History

When did the injury occur?
Where was the patient struck?
Where is the pain?
Is the pain increasing?
Was any tissue lost and recovered?
Was injury caused by motor vehicle crash, fall, machinery, blunt object, blow to abdomen, stab wound, or high- or low-velocity bullet?
Is there previous history of urologic disease or surgery?
Did patient urinate a short time before injury producing event?
Did patient void after injury? Was urine bloody? Was it a full amount?
What medications is the patient taking?
Does the patient have a history of hypertension, incontinence, infertility, or impotence?

Physical examination

Inspect ecchymoses on flank, over abdomen, or in perineum
Inspect external meatus for bleeding
Auscultate all abdominal quadrants for presence of bowel sounds before palpation and percussion
Auscultate for presence of bruit
Perform percussion of the bladder
Estimate flank and abdomen tenderness and rigidity
Measure abdominal circumference; check for distention
Palpate flank and abdomen for presence of mass and possible extravasation of urine or blood
Check for any shifting or dullness on percussion of abdomen
Perform rectal examination for position of prostate

Note. From "Genitourinary Trauma Patients" by P. Kidd, 1987, *Topics in Emergency Medicine, 9*(3), p. 74.

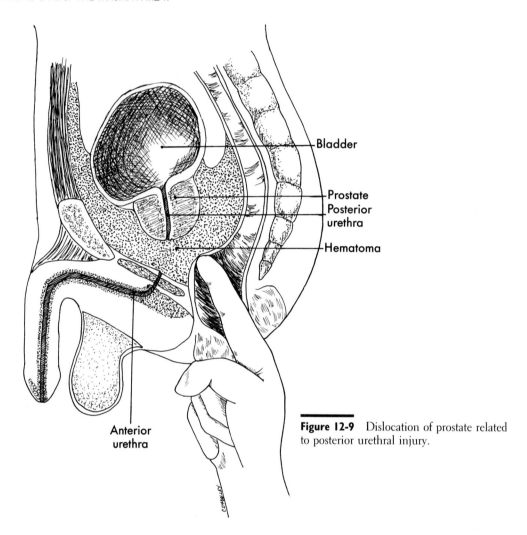

Figure 12-9 Dislocation of prostate related to posterior urethral injury.

place the prostate. If the prostate is palpable, a complete tear of the urethra is unlikely (Mitchell, 1984).

Percussion of the abdominal area may reveal dullness, indicative of extravasated urine or blood. If possible, the patient should be moved slightly to determine whether the dullness shifts, indicating fluid movement.

Diagnostic and Monitoring Procedures
Laboratory studies

Laboratory testing is not conclusive for patients with altered patterns in urinary elimination. Renal function tests must be obtained, so blood samples for BUN and creatinine levels should be drawn. The BUN may be elevated without an elevation in creatinine, secondary to dehydration. Therefore the creatinine level is a better indication of renal injury. When a renal vascular injury or a ruptured urethra associated with a pelvic fracture is suspected, a blood type and crossmatch is in order. The hemoglobin and hematocrit levels in a patient who was healthy before injury will be within normal limits unless the patient is severely hemodynamically compromised. Thus they are of little diagnostic value. The white blood cell count is usually mildly elevated in renal trauma, and polymorphonuclear leukocytes are increased (Zoller, 1983).

Much controversy exists about the clinical significance of hematuria. Hematuria is the single most common symptom of GU trauma and will occur in 90% of all cases (McAninch, 1985b). However, the degree of hematuria does not reflect the severity of the injury. The most severe GU injuries—renal vascular avulsion and main renal artery thrombosis—may not produce hematuria.

When catheterizing a patient, the trauma nurse *must* use strict sterile technique, lubricate generously, and not force the passage of the catheter. In some injuries, only microscopic hematuria will occur, and this finding can also result from careless or forceful catheterization. Hematuria may be transient, and the urine may clear by the second voiding. Therefore the first portion of the catheterized specimen should be sent for microscopic analysis (McAninch, 1989). Any patient with a positive dipstick test should have radiographic evaluation. These studies can be started while awaiting urinalysis results (Hanno & McAninch, 1985).

Radiographic studies

The box below includes common diagnostic testing used with suspected GU injury. Initially a flat plate abdominal film or kidneys, ureters, and bladder (KUB) film is obtained when GU trauma is suspected. KUB films can delineate size, shape, and position of the organs. Positive findings include scoliosis with the spine concaved toward the injured side, a unilateral enlarged kidney shadow, absence of psoas margin, and displaced bowel (Zoller, 1983). All of these signs could indicate hematoma or urine extravasation.

Preparing the patient for these films involves explaining why they are necessary. The emergency nurse should secure all IV tubings, lines, and monitoring devices. Tension is often placed

---

Common diagnostic tests for urologic trauma

KUB or abdominal flat plate film
Excretory urogram (EU), or intravenous
  pyelogram (IVP)
Renal arteriogram
Computed tomogram
Retrograde pyelogram
Cystogram
Retrograde urethrogram

---

on these items while the patient is being positioned. If an indwelling urinary catheter has been placed, it should be adequately taped so that unnecessary stress is not placed on the meatus. The catheter bag should be hung so it is always below the patient's abdomen. The catheter tubing should be checked for any kinkage to prevent retrograde urine drainage, which could compound the patient's initial injury.

Excretory urogram The excretory urogram (EU), otherwise referred to as the *intravenous pyelogram (IVP)*, is the diagnostic test of choice in upper urinary tract trauma. An iodine-based contrast medium is given IV, and x-ray films are obtained to determine dye passage. The dye flows first through the renal parenchyma and, in 3 to 5 minutes, through the renal calyces and pelvis. The ureters and bladder can be viewed 10 to 15 minutes after the dye is injected (Shetler, 1984). Hypotensive patients should be resuscitated before EU, since kidneys will not be well visualized without good perfusion (Neuwirth, Frasier, & Cochran, 1989).

Indications for the performance of an EU include patients who present with the following:
- Blunt abdominal trauma in all children
- Blunt abdominal trauma in adults with severe abdominal pain and hematuria (Neuwirth et al., 1989)
- Auto-pedestrian injury
- Falls from significant heights
- Penetrating abdominal wounds
- Fractures of lower ribs, vertebrae, or transverse processes
- Fractured pelvis
- Flank mass
- Paralytic ileus and abdominal pain after trauma (Zoller, 1983).

The EU cannot accurately diagnose bladder ruptures and urethral tears because of incomplete distention of the bladder. Incomplete distention could result in a small bladder tear being "missed." Therefore only the initial films of the kidney are usually obtained, expediting the procedure. The box on p. 394 summarizes abnormal findings on the EU.

The EU is a valuable diagnostic tool. It can provide information on both the damaged kidney and the uninjured one. If EU shows the patient to have preexisting renal disease, a nephrectomy will be used as a last resort. Figure 12-10 shows

Abnormal findings on excretory urogram

No dye excretion on one side   Indicative of a major vascular injury such as renal artery thrombosis or renal pedicle avulsion. This finding requires that an arteriogram be performed.

Dye extravasation   Indicative of a collecting system tear. This finding usually requires surgical repair.

Delayed excretion of dye   Indicative of a renal contusion or a minor laceration. This finding is managed conservatively.

Enlargement of renal outline   Indicative of an intrarenal hemorrhage. The size of the hematoma determines management *(to be discussed later in chapter).*

Reduction in renal size   Indicative of preexisting renal disease.

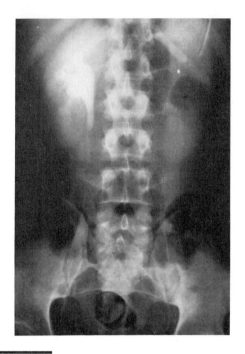

Figure 12-10   Excretory urogram showing poor excretion of dye from left kidney. (Courtesy Tucson Medical Center Radiology Department, Tucson, Ariz.)

poor excretion of dye from the left kidney.

Computed tomography   Computed tomography (CT) is used to provide additional information about renal function when the results of the EU are questionable. CT imaging has several advantages: it provides three-dimensional views; it is noninvasive; it provides excellent definition of lacerations, extravasation, and hematomas; and it can detect associated injuries (McAninch, 1985b). A disadvantage to CT is that it requires more patient cooperation than other radiographic studies.

CT allows more confidence in nonsurgical treatment. Two groups are evaluated better with CT than EU (Neuwirth et al., 1989):

- Individuals with stable vital signs but low hematocrit, with presence of rib fractures and substantial abdominal trauma
- Individuals with symptoms of abdominal trauma but in whom examination is unreliable because of altered mental status and/or spinal injury

Previously EU was the primary diagnostic tool for renal injury, but CT is being used with increasing frequency. Controversy exists over the ability of CT to detect renal vascular injury and minor renal injuries. In these cases, IVP may provide a more definitive diagnosis. The use of 1 to 2 cm sections on CT scanning can miss injuries. However, CT can provide determinate diagnoses of deep renal lacerations (extending into subcapsular cortex), ruptured kidney, and hematomas. In these circumstances, EU may indicate

an abnormality without providing anatomic detail as precisely as CT examination (Cass & Viera, 1987). Use of contrast enemas with CT scan improves retroperitoneal definition and may prevent unnecessary surgery (Peterson, 1989).

Renal arteriography   Renal arteriography is used when (1) the EU shows renal nonfunction, (2) clinical examination reveals bruit over the renal bed, or (3) the patient is clinically deteriorating. Arteriography can identify thrombosis of renal circulation (Figure 12-11). It is contraindicated in patients who cannot be stabilized (those patients go directly to the OR) and in patients with no patent femoral or axillary arteries for catheter placement (Zoller, 1983).

Retrograde pyelogram   Ureteral injuries can be detected by retrograde pyelogram, whereby a cystoscope is inserted through the urethra into the bladder and radiopaque catheters are threaded into the ureter, where contrast dye is injected. EU is unreliable in assessing injuries to the ureter. Patients who are hypersensitive to iodine-based dye often can tolerate this procedure better than an EU because the dye is not absorbed

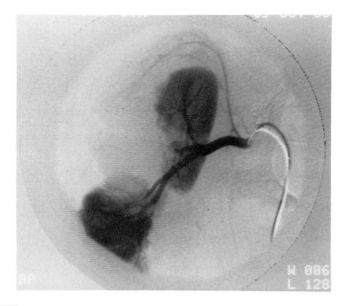

Figure 12-11   Renal arteriogram showing thrombosis of renal circulation. (Courtesy Tucson Medical Center Radiology Department, Tucson, Ariz.)

through the mucous membranes (Shetler, 1984). Yet a retrograde pyelogram cannot outline renal parenchyma, so major renal lacerations cannot be defined. Also, it is invasive and can introduce infection. Therefore retrograde pyelograms are not routinely performed. The ureters are seldom injured by blunt trauma. Penetrating trauma to the ureter may be explored surgically, negating the need for diagnostic testing, although the EU at times can show dye extravasation adjacent to the ureter.

Cystography   Cystography is used to diagnose bladder injuries. The EU does not effectively outline the bladder because of incomplete distention. Minor lacerations may go undetected. It has been reported to be 85% to 90% inaccurate in diagnosing bladder injuries (Kearney & Finn, 1981). Any patient with severe abdominal trauma with hematuria or a pelvic fracture should undergo cystography. Cystography is often completed in conjunction with retrograde urethrography, since it is necessary to pass a urinary catheter into the bladder. Previously it was thought if no urine was obtained by catheter, the bladder was ruptured (Mitchell, 1984). This is a false assumption because the patient may be anuric. Even if urine is withdrawn, a small puncture may still be present. Contrast medium, 30 to 50 ml, is injected

through the catheter. The patient will complain of pelvic and/or lower abdominal pain if extravasation is occurring. If contrast material outlines the bowel, an intraperitoneal tear is present. An extraperitoneal tear will demonstrate a starburst pattern where the dye accumulates in the extraperitoneal space. Small tears may go undetected unless after the initial contrast material is injected, an additional 50 ml is injected. This is sometimes referred to as *stress cystography*, and it can reveal minor lacerations. Contusions of the bladder can present as abnormalities in the outline, such as a teardrop appearance (Hanno, 1985a; Harty, 1987) (Figure 12-12). A teardrop configuration may be present also when a pelvic hematoma compresses the bladder (Carroll et al., 1985b).

Retrograde urethrography   Retrograde urethrography diagnoses urethral injuries. This test is indicated for any patient with pelvic fractures, blood at the urethral meatus, or perineal injury (Sandler & Burke, 1985). In the male, a urinary catheter is inserted into the penile meatus so that the balloon will be in the penile urethra. The balloon is filled with approximately 3 ml normal saline. Contrast medium is then injected and films obtained to determine if injury is present. The site of extravasation will determine if the injury is anterior or poste-

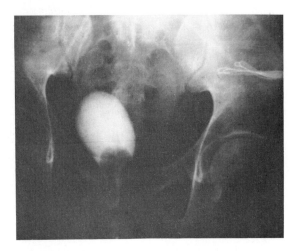

Figure 12-12 Cystogram showing "teardrop" bladder, indicating bladder contusion. (Courtesy Tucson Medical Center Radiology Department, Tucson, Ariz.)

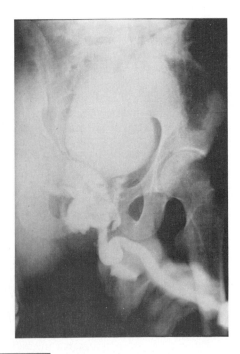

Figure 12-13 Retrograde urethrogram showing extravasation of dye from partial posterior urethral tear. (Courtesy Tucson Medical Center Radiology Department, Tucson, Ariz.)

rior. Figure 12-13 shows extravasation of dye from a partial posterior urethral tear.

Genital screening

Diagnostic testing provides vital information about the severity of injury in patients who have sustained genital trauma. Physical examination of the genitalia is not always helpful or possible because of the intense pain associated with this type of injury.

Transillumination of the scrotum is performed by passing a light through injured tissues. Non-transillumination can indicate testicular rupture. Testicular scanning and ultrasonography also can provide information about the integrity of the testicles and scrotal contents. Surgery is the only way to confirm rupture (Fournier, Laing, & McAninch, 1989).

Several of these diagnostic tests require full cooperation of the patient for adequate results to be obtained. The trauma nurse can explain briefly the rationale of the particular study to the patient to facilitate cooperation of the patient by alleviating anxiety. Questioning the alert patient about allergies to seafood can prevent a serious reaction to the dye. The patient should be observed closely for the development of hives or a sudden fall in blood pressure (Veise-Berry, 1983). These patients may receive blood transfusions and IV antibiotics concurrently, and either of these products can produce symptoms similar to those of a dye reaction.

Assessment and Interventions Related to Specific Injuries

Renal injuries Impaired tissue integrity
High risk for fluid volume deficit

It is difficult to detect a renal injury without completing radiographic studies, because the patient's signs and symptoms do not correlate well with the degree of injury. Hematuria is not a reliable indicator and will be absent with renal pedicle injury or renal vascular thrombosis (Zoller, 1983). Usually all patients with renal injuries will experience pain, ranging from mild, localized discomfort to generalized, severe pain. The presence of contusions or abrasions over the flank area or a flank or abdominal mass is also indicative of renal injury.

After radiographic studies, classification is per-

Stages of renal injury

Class I: Renal contusion

Findings   EU reveals enlarged renal outline. Patient has history of trauma and hematuria.

Management   Patient is admitted to hospital and placed on bedrest. Patient should be assessed often for presence or expansion of hematoma. Periodic urine specimens are obtained and compared for color change and number of RBCs.

Class II: Cortical laceration

Findings   EU reveals intravasation of dye through cortical laceration. Renal capsule is not usually torn, but perinephric hematoma can develop. Hematuria is present.

Management   Similar to class I. If capsule is torn and urine is extravasating, some urologists will administer antibiotics. Use of antibiotics is controversial, and they may be used only when patient has infected urine.

Class III: Calyceal laceration

Findings   Hematuria with flank trauma. EU will show intravasation of dye and disruption of pericalyceal system. Renal capsule is torn, and extravasation of urine will occur.

Management   Much controversy exists over best way to handle this injury. Conservative management is to monitor patient; transfuse as necessary. Those in favor of immediate surgery believe that complications are avoided (late bleeding, hypertension) and some of the kidney can be salvaged. Patients who underwent immediate surgery had shorter hospital stay in one study (Cass, Luxenberg, Gleich, & Smith, 1987a). Trauma nurse should be aware that surgical intervention may be possibility and be ready to prepare patient and family psychologically and the patient physically for such intervention.

Class IV: Complete renal tear or fracture

Findings   Patient experiences fluid volume deficit. Patient will have expanding flank mass. EU will show complete dye extravasation.

Management   Surgical intervention is indicated. Patients may be too unstable for radiographic evaluation, and this will be done in operating room. If patient is clinically stable and there is no chance of saving kidney, nephrectomy can be done on elective basis.

Class V: Vascular pedicle injury or renal artery thrombosis

Findings   EU shows nonvisualization of kidney. Arteriogram will reveal renal vascular damage or presence of thrombosis. Patient will be in shock, indicating severe fluid volume deficit, often with hematuria. This injury is rare, occurring in less than 2% of all renal trauma cases. Death may occur before reaching hospital.

Management   Early surgical intervention is necessary. After patency of airway is established, trauma nurse should concentrate on initiating at least two large-bore IV lines (14-gauge preferably) and obtaining blood for type and crossmatch. Uncrossmatched blood may be ordered. It has been estimated that the kidney can survive for 40 to 60 minutes without blood supply. Taking into consideration prehospital transport, stay in emergency department must be short. This patient should be in the operating room.

From "Genitourinary Trauma Patients" by P. Kidd, 1987, *Topics in Emergency Medicine, 9* (3), p. 77.

---

formed. This staging allows for basic management of the injury. The box above discusses the five stages in detail.

Management of major renal lacerations is controversial (class III). The majority of these lacerations result from blunt trauma. The presence of significant coexisting injuries does not necessarily indicate the severity of the renal injury (Yarbro &

Fowler, 1987). The latest research suggests that surgical repair may not be necessary. However, patients who were treated conservatively had a higher incidence of renal insufficiency and hypertension after trauma (Cass et al., 1987). Most sources agree on conditions that require surgical intervention in renal trauma. These conditions include expanding hematoma, pulsatile hematoma, penetrating trauma with urinary extravasation, vascular injury, and evidence of continued hemorrhage after the patient has received three units of blood (McAninch, 1985b; Salvatierra, 1984; Mitchell, 1984).

Ureteral injuries Altered patterns of urinary elimination
Pain

The physical examination is not always helpful in detecting ureteral injuries. Occasionally, urine may be present at the entrance or exit sites of the penetrating object. A retroperitoneal mass may form. Hematuria will be present when the ureter is partially torn or contused; however, if the ureter is completely transected, hematuria is absent (Zoller, 1983; Guerriero, 1985). An EU will detect a ureteral injury in 91% of the cases (Guerriero, 1985). If questions remain after the EU, a retrograde pyelogram will be performed.

Ureteral injuries are usually surgically repaired. Occasionally, a ureteral injury will be overlooked if the patient does not have an acute abdomen at time of injury or penetrating trauma. More than 50% of cases with delayed diagnoses result in a nephroureterectomy (Zoller, 1983). When a patient presents with fever, ileus, flank or abdominal discomfort, and hematuria, the trauma nurse should question the patient about any trauma he or she may have experienced within the past 3 weeks.

Bladder injuries Impaired tissue integrity
High risk for infection
Altered patterns of urinary elimination

The symptoms of bladder trauma are diverse and may differ according to whether intraperitoneal or extraperitoneal extravasation of urine has occurred. Generally, the patient will experience urinary retention; however, if the laceration is small enough, the patient may void 100 to 200 ml of urine (Mitchell, 1984). Hematuria is usually present, although it may be revealed only by microscopic examination. Suprapubic discomfort is present and will increase when the patient attempts to void.

Extravasation of urine Intraperitoneal extravasation will eventually produce symptoms of peritonitis. If the laceration goes undetected, a self-dialysis takes place, with the peritoneum serving as the dialyzing membrane. The patient will become hyponatremic, and the serum potassium and urea levels will increase (Mitchell, 1984). If the urine is uninfected, extravasation can be relatively harmless for 24 hours, producing only a chemical irritation (Mitchell, 1984). Associated injuries can interfere with the detection of symptoms. The abdomen will become distended, and an ileus will occur later. The patient will have elevated lactate dehydrogenase, BUN, and serum creatinine levels. These patients may present with decreased cardiac output, altered gastrointestinal tissue perfusion, and infection, depending on the severity of injury and delay in treatment (Harwood, 1983). Diagnostic peritoneal lavage is unreliable for intraperitoneal bladder rupture (Peterson, 1989).

Extraperitoneal extravasation initially will not produce changes in laboratory values. In these cases a suprapubic mass may be palpated. A bimanual examination may indicate a mass, which is the direct result of extravasated urine and blood. The suprapubic area may be indurated and red if treatment is delayed.

Treatment of bladder trauma depends on the severity of injury and location of extravasation. Contusions with gross hematuria and urinary retention are treated by the insertion of an indwelling urinary catheter until the hematuria clears. Drainage by catheter is not necessary if the patient can void. Intraperitoneal ruptures are usually treated with surgical exploration and suprapubic catheter drainage. Selected cases may be handled nonsurgically if coexisting intraperitoneal injury is not suspected (Peterson, 1989). Extraperitoneal rupture can be handled conservatively in some cases. These patients are placed in a semi-Fowler's position to facilitate urine flow. A cystogram is performed before removing the catheter to see if extravasation is still occurring. Complications can occur with this form of treatment, such as prolonged hematuria, infection, chronic alteration in renal tissue perfusion, and functional incontinence. Patients with large extraperitoneal tears or a fractured pelvis should have surgical exploration followed by suprapubic catheter drainage.

The trauma nurse should question the alert patient about the mechanism of injury when bladder trauma is suspected. The nurse should suspect bladder trauma in any patient who has a contusion in the lower abdominal area and has been involved in a motor vehicle crash while wearing a seat belt. It is necessary to determine if the patient has a history of participation in sporting activities. Patients should also be asked if they have had any difficulty voiding, if they have been voiding the usual amount, and if they have any preexisting GU problems.

On physical examination, the nurse should auscultate the abdomen and palpate for distention, rigidity, and the presence of a suprapubic mass. Obtaining a baseline abdominal girth measurement is desirable also. If the patient passes any urine while in the emergency department, the urine should be tested with a urine reagent stick (dipstick) before it is sent to the laboratory for analysis. In some settings, a urine reagent stick that tests for the presence of leukocytes may be used, which can indicate a preexisting infection when positive. Caution must be taken when interpreting these reagent sticks, since their sensitivity in identifying white blood cells (WBCs) decreases when the urine WBC is less than 50 (Propp, Weber, & Ciesla, 1989). Measuring baseline vital signs is important also, especially in cases of delayed treatment, because the patient's temperature may provide an additional diagnostic sign.

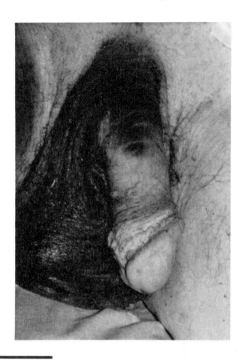

Figure 12-14   Urine collection in scrotal area from disruption of Colles' fascia. (Courtesy Tucson Medical Center Radiology Department, Tucson, Ariz.)

Urethral injuries	Altered patterns of urinary elimination
	High risk for functional incontinence
	High risk for sexual dysfunction

Anterior urethral injuries   Urinary extravasation will occur with anterior urethral injuries, the location depending on which fascial planes have been disrupted. If Buck's fascia has been damaged, blood and urine can travel from the thighs and anteriorly to the clavicular area (Hanno, 1985b). Colles' fascia is located in the perineum, and if it is disrupted, urine will collect in the scrotum and penis (Figure 12-14). This extravasation produces pain, swelling, and ecchymoses. A palpable mass may be present in the penile areas if the penile urethra has been lacerated or in the perineum if the bulbous urethra is damaged. Blood is usually present at the urinary meatus.

If the laceration is small and the patient can pass urine freely, treatment may be delayed. The patient may not present to the emergency department until the discomfort increases. When this delay occurs, necrosis of tissue results and infection may be present from the extravasated urine.

In any case of suspected urethral injury, a urinary catheter should not be passed except by a skilled practitioner or urologist. Retrograde urethrography will diagnose the site and extent of the injury. Passage of a catheter by an inexperienced person can convert a partial tear into a complete tear, increasing the likelihood of postinjury complications.

A contusion of the anterior urethra requires no treatment as long as the patient can pass urine. If the patient cannot urinate, a suprapubic cystostomy is performed to divert the urine from the site of injury. A partial tear can be treated by inserting a 14- or 16-French catheter for 5 to 7 days. A urethrogram is performed when the catheter is removed, and if extravasation continues, it is replaced (Harty, 1987; Zoller, 1983).

A complete tear should be surgically explored. Any hematoma is evacuated, and a suprapubic cystomy is performed. A primary reconstruction may be necessary if urethral tissue has been lost secondary to penetrating trauma.

Anterior urethral injuries often become infected, mostly with *Staphylococcus* or *Streptococcus*. These patients will generally receive aqueous penicillin and a broad spectrum antibiotic (Zoller, 1983). The major complications of these injuries are the formation of strictures and the loss of penile sensation (Mitchell, 1984).

Posterior urethral injuries The patient with a posterior urethral injury may have urinary retention with bladder distention. Blood may be present at the urinary meatus as seen in anterior injuries. Rectal examination may reveal a bogginess or dislocation of the prostate; however, this examination must be performed carefully because a partial rupture can be converted to a complete laceration.

Diagnosis of posterior urethral injuries is also accomplished by retrograde urethrography. A partial tear is suspected if periurethral extravasation occurs but some dye enters the bladder (Harty, 1987; Morehouse & MacKinnon, 1985). A partial tear will heal with fewer complications.

Management of posterior urethral injuries is controversial. Most physicians advocate the placement of a suprapubic cystostomy tube. A large risk of stricture formation exists with this method, which is then later repaired through urethroplasty. The alternative is to place a urethral catheter along with a suprapubic cystostomy tube. The urethra is allowed to heal over the urethral catheter (Harty, 1987). This method can convert a partial tear into a complete one and has a high risk of sexual dysfunction and functional urinary incontinence (Mitchell, 1984).

Female urethral injuries Diagnosis of female urethral injuries is made by retrograde urethrography. The patient will have urinary retention and may have a distended bladder and extravasation. Severe vaginal bleeding may be present if the vaginal wall has been penetrated.

Immediate repair of the urethra is preferred if the patient's condition permits (Mitchell, 1984). If a delayed repair is necessary, a higher risk of loss of urinary control and neurogenic damage exists. The female requires the full length of the urethra to be continent. Almost all lacerations of the urethra in females will result in some functional incontinence.

Urethral injuries in children The female child will present with the same symptoms and will be treated in the same manner as the female adult who has experienced a urethral injury. Therefore this discussion will be limited to the male child.

In the young male (before puberty), the prostate is not developed. The upper part of the posterior urethra is not supported. A shearing force to the urethra is received just below the bladder neck. This means that the injury is usually above the level of the external sphincter (the section of urethra with maximal urinary control) and above the level of the ejaculatory ducts. The future fertility of the child who experiences a posterior urethral injury is difficult to predict.

Diagnosis is made through retrograde urethrography. These patients will present with the same symptoms as the adult male (excluding bogginess of the prostate). An EU must be completed to ensure that no congenital anomaly of the kidneys exists that may have been aggravated by the injury.

Management of posterior urethral injuries is controversial, but most physicians favor delayed repair with initial placement of a suprapubic cystostomy tube. Patients managed in this manner have less sexual dysfunction after injury (Mitchell, 1984). Anterior urethral injuries in the young male are managed in the same manner as for those in the adult male.

Male genital injuries Pain
High risk for sexual dysfunction
High risk for body image disturbance
High risk for infection

Avulsion injuries Management of genital avulsions consists of removing injured skin from the penis, because the skin will become edematous if reapplied. However, scrotal skin is salvaged if it is still attached to the body by a pedicle (McAninch, 1989). If not enough scrotal skin is viable, the testicles are implanted in either inguinal or thigh pockets of skin. Thigh pockets typically are used in younger males because the pockets have a lower temperature, which promotes spermatogenesis.

The trauma nurse should cover open areas with moist saline packs. Any skin that is brought in by the patient or is removed is kept in a plastic bag or container and placed in ice slush in case it can be used in reconstruction. Tetanus toxoid and antibiotics are administered. The patient should be medicated for pain. These patients will go to surgery. The genital area is not cleansed until the patient receives general or spinal anesthesia in the operating room (Jordan & Gilbert, 1989). Closure should occur within 12 hours of injury.

Penetrating injuries, crush injuries, and burns Priorities in penetrating genital injuries are to control bleeding and prevent penile deformity. These injuries are sutured in the operating room unless curvature of the penis will result. In these cases the injury is packed with iodoform gauze and a compression dressing is applied. A urinary catheter is inserted for urinary drainage. Contaminated injuries may also be left open. Antibiotics and tetanus toxoid must be administered to these patients. The incidence of infection can be decreased by copious saline irrigation of the injured area. This may take place after the patient is medicated for pain.

Crush injuries to the genitalia are managed according to severity. In less severe injuries, the penis is elevated and ice packs are applied to reduce edema and decrease bleeding. Analgesics are given. If the injury is more severe and continues to bleed despite initial measures, a pressure dressing may be applied. If bleeding continues, surgical exploration is necessary because the testicle may be ruptured.

Burn injuries of the genitalia are treated like burns on other parts of the body. They are categorized as a critical burn. The area is flushed with sterile water or saline. Early surgical debridement is indicated, although it is almost impossible to immediately determine the extent of tissue damage. Early grafting is recommended (McAninch, 1989). Consequently, a second debridement after the patient is transferred from the emergency department may be necessary. In addition to irrigating the area, the nurse should administer tetanus toxoid and antibiotics. The patient's body should be assessed for the presence of other burned areas because chemicals and other agents can splash.

Amputations and fractures Amputations can be incomplete or complete. Incomplete amputation is managed by irrigating the area with saline, debriding devitalized tissue, and then realigning the portions of the penis. Formerly, complete amputations were treated by reanastomosing the urethra and fascia. No attempt was made to reestablish blood flow or neural function. After injury, these patients could ejaculate and have normal erections, but sensation was absent. Recently, microneurovascular repair has been conducted. The exact time frame for replantation is not known. The closer to the time of injury the better. Successful replantation has occurred later than 16 hours for normothermic ischemia and more than 24 hours for hypothermic ischemia. Penile tissue survives ischemia well (Jordan & Gilbert, 1989). Penile sensation usually returns within 3 months after injury (Merrill & Palmer, 1985).

The trauma nurse should place the amputated penis on a saline-soaked gauze pad inside a plastic bag and then pack the bag in ice slush (Jordan & Gilbert, 1989). The penile stump should be covered with a pressure dressing.

The penis can be fractured from direct trauma while it is erected. This may occur from having intercourse, masturbating, or being struck with an object. The patient will state that he heard a snapping sound and experienced severe pain and then a loss of erection. Swelling occurs quickly as a result of hemorrhage from the tear in the tunica albuginea. Coexisting urethral injury may be present. The penis may deviate to the opposite side of the injury secondary to hematoma formation (Orvis & McAninch, 1989). Management is controversial. Conservative treatment is catheterization, compression dressings, and application of ice packs. Antibiotics and enzymatic agents such as streptokinase may be administered, as well as diazepam to prevent erections (Peterson, 1989). The other method of treating this injury is to surgically evacuate the hematoma and close the tear. Recent research indicates that patients have less penile deformity and a shorter hospital stay when the injury is managed surgically (Harty, 1987; Merrill & Palmer, 1985; Elam & Ray, 1986; Orvis & McAninch, 1989).

The penis can be strangulated from objects placed around it as a result of sexual behavior or an attempt to stop incontinence. Treatment will depend on the length of time between when the object was placed and the patient sought health care. Most objects can be removed in the same manner as that used for an incarcerated finger ring. At times it is necessary to irrigate the penis (corpus cavernosum) distal to the object with heparinized saline to reduce the edema. Puncture wounds may be made in the penile skin to allow trapped blood to escape. As the trapped blood is removed, the penis will shrink to allow removal of the object (McAninch, 1985c). If the area must be opened, saline dressings are applied. Antibiotics and tetanus toxoid may be given, especially if the region appears infected.

Scrotal injuries   The patient with a scrotal injury may have acute pain, nausea, vomiting, faintness, and urinary retention. All patients with blunt trauma should be assessed for testicular rupture. Gonadal preservation requires early diagnosis of rupture. If the testicle cannot be palpated on examination, surgical exploration should be performed (Harty, 1987). The testicle can become dislocated by vector forces and may move beneath the abdominal wall (Brothers, 1985).

Closed reduction under general anesthesia is usually required. A reconstructed testicle can still usually produce hormones even if it cannot produce sperm. If the testicle can be palpated, the patient is initially treated with bedrest, scrotal elevation and support, ice packs, and antiinflammatory medication. Surgery may be necessary if the scrotum continues to swell.

A patient who experiences genital trauma has received not only a physiologic but also a psychologic trauma. In some cases, a psychologic problem may have initiated the genital injury. A psychologist may be included on the treatment team for these patients. A plastic surgeon is often necessary for cosmetic purposes. The trauma nurse should be supportive and explain why referrals are being made if the patient has questions. The patient's privacy should be respected. Careful documentation is necessary because sexual dysfunction may result.

> **Female genital injuries**   High risk for infection
> High risk for fluid volume deficit
> Pain
> High risk for rape-trauma syndrome

Vulva injuries   Injury to the vulva is often the result of straddle impact or assault where the tissue is kicked. Large blood vessels in the vulva rupture. The fascial sheets that cover the perineum are very strong and limit the depth of blood dispersion (Crombleholme, 1985). Large hematomas form that may require evacuation (Figure 12-15). Once evacuated, the cavity is packed and may require a Penrose drain. These patients may take sitz baths to relieve edema. If the wound is deep, antibiotics are administered. Minor hematomas are managed by applying ice, followed later by heat and analgesics. The trauma nurse should elicit in the history the approximate time of injury. This may provide information about the likelihood of the hematoma continuing to expand.

Penetrating vulva injuries may result from falling on a sharp object. The rectum, vagina, bladder, and intestine may be penetrated also because of their proximity and thin walls. The trauma nurse should try to obtain in the history an estimate of how long and how sharp the object was. This may help to determine the depth of penetration and the likelihood of performing peritoneal lavage. Because of the possibility of perforation, a careful and complete abdominal assessment is necessary.

Vaginal injuries   One case has been reported in the literature of a right hemidiaphragm laceration and pelvic viscera penetration from penetrating vaginal trauma (the patient reported she had fallen on a broom handle) (Gundlinger & Vester, 1987). Thus the trauma nurse must perform a complete assessment even when the injury "appears localized." Complications of penetrating vaginal wounds include pelvic abscess and vaginal strictures.

Blunt trauma to the vagina is rare. One case has been documented in the literature where a patient was waterskiing and a bolus of water produced a vaginal laceration (Crombleholme & Sweet, 1985). Treatment of lacerations depends on their location and the age and emotional status of the patient. Lacerations located in the fornix bleed heavily and require extensive retraction of the vaginal walls for repair. Patients usually receive general anesthesia for repair of these injuries. These lacerations have a higher rate of subsequent infection and intraperitoneal perforation (Crombleholme, 1985). Superficial lacerations are sutured after the patient receives local anesthesia.

Nursing Interventions

When dealing with patients who have a suspected urethral or renal injury, the trauma nurse must address fluid volume status first. Posterior urethral injuries in the male and urethral injuries in the female are often associated with pelvic fractures.

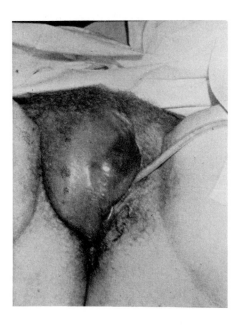

Figure 12-15 Vulva hematoma. (Courtesy Tucson Medical Center Radiology Department, Tucson, Ariz.)

The pelvis has a rich vascular supply, so these patients may have lost a great deal of blood. Priority measures will be starting two large-bore IV lines and infusing lactated Ringer's solution while obtaining a type and crossmatch.

While initially assessing the patient, the trauma nurse should remove all the patient's clothing. An area of extravasation of blood and urine may be missed if clothing remains on the patient. To determine sources of bleeding, it is crucial not to wash away any blood from the external meatus when cleaning the patient. This can be a helpful diagnostic sign that urethral injury has occurred. Although indwelling urinary catheters routinely are inserted in trauma patients to help ascertain fluid replacement needs, it is wise not to attempt to pass a urinary catheter. Central hemodynamic lines can be inserted for a reliable indicator of blood volume.

Documentation, although always important, should be thorough to avoid medicolegal problems. Information given to patients and parents should be documented. Exactly what procedures were done for the patient and any specialized services the patient obtained are important to discuss. These patients have the potential for disturbances in self-esteem, altered role performance,

and body image disturbance secondary to sexual dysfunction and alterated patterns of urinary elimination. To avoid litigation, it is helpful to document baseline data and the fact that proper care was administered.

These patients may need referral to psychiatric services or to a clinical nurse specialist so that they can discuss body image concerns. The trauma nurse should allow the patient to begin ventilating concerns, if any, and should honestly answer the patient's questions. A trusting relationship is necessary for the patient to adapt to a urethral injury and its high rate of complications. This should begin in the emergency department. The trauma nurse should request the services of community agencies that specialize in sexual assault cases, where available. It may be necessary to contact a counselor or clergy.

A child who has sustained a urethral or genital injury may be embarrassed to allow healthcare providers to assess the injury or to discuss symptoms. It is important to use terminology based on the cognitive level of the child. It may be helpful for the parents to be present during examination, because in today's society much emphasis is placed on not allowing another person to "look down there." In abuse cases, involvement of the

Table 12-2 Comparison of urologic injuries

Nursing diagnosis	Renal injuries	Ureteral injuries	Bladder injuries	Urethral injuries
Pain	Mild, localized tenderness to severe discomfort in groin, flank, upper abdomen. May radiate to groin or thigh of affected side	Flank, lower abdomen on affected side	Pelvic area, lower abdomen, suprapubic region. May radiate to shoulder	Suprapubic region
Altered patterns of urinary elimination	Hematuria may or may not be present (gross or microscopic)	Hematuria may or may not be present. Possible anuria	Small amount of bloody urine on catheterization. Strong urge to void but inability to do so	May be slight hematuria initially. Difficulty voiding. High incidence of functional incontinence with urethral injuries in females and with posterior urethral injuries in males after trauma
Fluid volume deficit	Possible	Possible	Possible	Unlikely
Altered genitourinary tissue perfusion related to infection	Possible	Possible	Unlikely	Unlikele
Infection as evidenced by N/V, abdominal distention and rigidity, absent bowel sounds, soft mass in flank	Possible	Possible	Possible with laceration of bladder fundus and penetrating trauma	Possible
High risk for alterated renal tissue perfusion	AV fistula; hydronephrosis, hypertension	Ureteral compression leading to hydronephrosis	Unlikely	Unlikely
Sexual dysfunction	Unlikely	Unlikely	Unlikely	Higher incidence of impotence and infertility with posterior urethral injuries in males

parents may prove to be a difficult situation. Children will require the presence of a strong, safe support system.

Appropriate nursing diagnoses for patients experiencing urologic tract trauma are included in Table 12-2. The diagnoses are compared in relation to the type of tissue disruption. Interventions and evaluative criteria, based on nursing diagnosis, are summarized in the table on p. 406 for urinary tract injuries and in the table on p. 407 for genital injuries.

Complications

Complications can occur after GU injury in spite of how meticulously the patient may have been managed. For example, renal injuries can result in hypertension. It is important to find out if the patient has a history of hypertension at the time of injury and if so how it is being managed. A later increase in diastolic pressure may be related to a preinjury condition and not a renin-angiotensin response. Urethral injuries can result in infertility, impotence, and incontinence. Documentation of any preexisting problems in these areas could reduce the chance of litigation later.

Regardless of the type of management, certain complications can occur after renal trauma. Early complications within the first month of injury are usually infection, secondary hemorrhage, and acute tubular necrosis with renal failure. These patients may experience altered patterns in urinary elimination, secondary to chronic infection, chronic alteration in renal tissue perfusion, and calculus formation. Hypertension is the most common of these later complications and occurs in 4% of renal injury patients (Zoller, 1983). Physiologically, this is related to scarring in the kidney, which decreases renal blood flow. Renin is released and converted eventually to angiotensin II, which produces vasoconstriction as a compensatory mechanism for increasing perfusion pressure. It is recommended that patients have a repeat EU 1 year after injury to detect complications. Blood pressure screening and urinalysis are again indicated at this visit.

Several complications can occur with posterior urethral injuries. Almost all patients will have some degree of stricture formation (Mitchell, 1984). Functional incontinence can result from neurologic damage. Sexual dysfunction may occur from psychogenic causes, thrombosis of vessels, damage to the penile artery, or neurologic

impairment. Damage to the internal sphincter in the bladder neck can result in failure of the sphincter to close during ejaculation. The seminal fluid will pass retrogradely into the bladder. The patient has the sensation of an ejaculation occurring but no external discharge. Infertility can result from damage to the ejaculatory ducts or seminal vesicles. In cases of retrograde ejaculation, sperm can be collected for artificial insemination.

SUMMARY In the team approach to care, particularly in the teaching hospital setting, interventions are usually shared among nurse and physician providers. A high index of suspicion associated with knowledge of the mechanism of injury provides valuable information to evaluate the extent of injury and the need for specific interventions. Blunt trauma to the abdomen is more difficult to evaluate because of the presence of normal physical findings on initial evaluation and stable patient presentation. However, the risk of significant intraabdominal injury is great. Injury resulting from penetrating trauma is generally more clearly defined. Special considerations must be given to the pregnant woman and pediatric patient who sustain injury.

Significant debate exists as to the efficacy of CT versus DPL in evaluating abdominal injury. The high mortality that exists as a consequence of abdominal trauma is related to hemorrhage, peritonitis, and sepsis and depends in part on the length of time from initial injury to arrival in the ED and the extent of associated injuries. In acute care, intervention is aimed at control of life-threatening disturbances measured against the element of time. Care of the patient with gastrointestinal trauma presents a unique challenge to nursing, since rapid and organized care can ultimately determine survival and return of the patient to a complete and productive life.

Care of a patient who has experienced GU trauma is likewise complex and challenging. It requires excellent assessment skills and the ability to detect subtle changes in a patient's condition. Although all patients should receive holistic care, these patients may require emotional assistance and psychologic or spiritual resources because of the nature and function of the GU organs. It is possible that astute care can prevent the occurrence of potentially devastating lifelong complications.

Nursing diagnosis	Nursing intervention	Evaluative criteria
Altered patterns of urinary elimination	**Restore normal pattern of urinary elimination** Insert urinary catheter unless urethral injury is suspected. Obtain blood for BUN and creatinine levels. Monitor urine output for amount and color. Test urine with dipstick for detection of hematuria. Percuss bladder for determination of distention. Percuss abdomen to detect dullness. Palpate skin over symphysis pubis to assess temperature. Assess urinary meatus for presence of blood. Assess perineum for ecchymoses and edema.	Urinary output will be at least 30 ml/hr. Hematuria, if present, will not increase.
Pain	**Promote comfort** Avoid sedation, because pain is a major clue to type of urologic injury. Administer non-narcotic analgesics. Use distraction techniques.	Patient will report a decrease in pain on a scale of 1 to 10.
High risk for fluid volume deficit	**Maintain adequate fluid volume** Obtain blood for type and cross-match, hemoglobin and hematocrit levels. Initiate two large-bore IV lines with normal saline or lactated Ringer's solution. Initiate oxygen therapy. Assess patient for diminishing LOC. Monitor vital signs. Anticipate surgical intervention; prepare patient for stat CT, IVP; complete operative permits and checklist (depending on institution). Assess flank region for expanding mass/hematoma, ecchymoses.	LOC will not deteriorate. Vital signs will stabilize with systolic BP of at least 90 mm Hg. Urine output will remain constant (preferably at least 30 ml/hr). Flank ecchymoses and masses will not extend.
High risk for infection	**Prevent infection** Administer broad spectrum IV antibiotic prophylactically. Obtain blood for CBC. Obtain urine specimen for culture and sensitivity. Obtain microscopic analysis of peritoneal fluid if lavage is performed. Administer tetanus toxoid. Monitor abdomen for dullness on percussion, distention. Assess bowel sounds. Monitor patient's temperature. Assess patient's description of pain location and intensity.	Patient's WBC will be WNL. Urine culture will be negative. Patient's abdomen will be nontender and nondistended, with bowel sounds present.

NURSING DIAGNOSES &
EVALUATIVE CRITERIA   *The patient with genital injury*

Nursing diagnosis	Nursing intervention	Evaluative criteria
Altered tissue perfusion	**Restore genital tissue perfusion** Initiate IV therapy. Obtain blood for CBC, type and crossmatch. Administer enzymatic agents as appropriate. Apply ice packs to area. Apply pressure dressings and/or packing to promote venostasis.	Blood flow will be maintained to genitalia as evidenced by pink skin color and warm tissue.
Pain	**Promote comfort** Administer narcotic analgesia. Use distraction techniques.	Patient will report decrease in pain on scale of *1* to *10*.
High risk for sexual dysfunction	**Prevent sexual dysfunction** Initiate referral to psychologist, urologist, and plastic surgeon as appropriate. Preserve all scrotal skin and penile sections by placing tissue in a plastic bag and place bag in a second container of iced saline slush solution. Cover open areas with moist sterile saline packs.	Avulsed tissue will remain viable for reimplantation.
High risk for infection	**Prevent infection** Administer IV antibiotics. Insert indwelling urinary catheter unless urethral injury is suspected. Administer tetanus toxoid. Assess patient's temperature. Monitor patient's abdomen for discomfort, distention, and absence of bowel sounds.	Patient's abdomen will remain supple and pain free. Urine will not communicate with avulsed, lacerated open tissue.

CASE STUDY A 35-year-old man presents to the ED via a local fire rescue unit, with an abdominal stab wound inflicted by a piece of glass. The patient is intoxicated and combative. Initial BP is 110/60; HR, 140; R, 22. The anterior portion of the abdomen is the site of injury, with intestine protruding from the entrance wound.

What are the priorities of care and assessment needs for a patient sustaining a stab wound with evisceration of abdominal contents?

Regardless of the mechanism of injury in abdominal trauma, the first priorities are is always airway, breathing, and circulation. Once a patent airway is established and circulation is ensured, physical assessment can proceed. Evaluation of the abdomen by auscultation to determine the presence or absence of bowel sounds is performed, followed by palpation to elicit pain, guarding, or rebound, with careful attention to the exposed intestine. Knowledge of the mechanism of injury is useful to determine the possibility of associated intraabdominal injury, and careful assessment of the body is necessary, since stab wounds often occur in multiples. Even with obvious peritoneal penetration, selective management is urged, which depends on the degree of evisceration, although most patients will undergo laparotomy. The wound and its contents must be protected from further injury and contamination; therefore, a sterile wet dressing is applied. Coughing, vomiting, or even movement carry the risk of further evisceration caused by increased intraabdominal pressure. Although the abdomen is the area with obvious injury, the chest must be assessed for equal lung sounds, bilateral movement, and respiratory exchange because of the abdomen's proximity to thoracic structures. Eviscerated contents, depending on the site, can herniate into the chest cavity and result in associated thoracic injury.

Ongoing monitoring of vital signs, mental status, and bodily functions is necessary. The patient with an altered sensorium caused by alcohol ingestion may impede evaluation efforts. If chronic alcohol consumption is a finding, inherent coagulation problems and underlying liver damage should be considered. Laboratory data must be secured and the patient readied for surgery if that is the treatment option. Fluid resuscitation must be carefully monitored because hemorrhage and shock may not be immediately present. Early administration of antibiotics is indicated to prevent infection.

What additional information regarding the mechanism of injury in the above scenario should be determined?

In the scenario, the mechanism of injury is defined as a stab wound to the abdomen from a piece of glass. It does not state how the glass arrived in the abdomen or how large the piece was. Additional information must be elicited and the following questions answered to adequately predict the extent of injury: Did the patient fall on the glass and, if so, from what height? This could indicate associated blunt trauma to the abdomen overlooked by the obvious wound presentation. Was the glass piece originally impaled and removed? The risk of intraabdominal injury is intensified if these situations exist, and selective management of a minor membrane disruption can be displaced in favor of laparotomy.

What complications may develop postoperatively from this type of injury?

A wide variety of postoperative complications, both short- and long-term, can ensue, including sepsis, abscess, and paralytic ileus formation. Ischemia to the bowel or its associated mesenteric circulation can result in lethal consequences if prompt recognition and management is not implemented. The patient also may need a temporary colostomy and nutritional support. The fact that the patient was intoxicated may reflect chronic alcohol abuse, which may lead to development of delirium tremens, difficulty with hemostasis, and inaccurate historical information.

RESEARCH QUESTIONS

- Is seat belt placement an indicator of specific organ system injury?
- Does patient teaching facilitate cooperation during diagnostic procedures in the trauma setting?
- Do patients who arrive in the emergency department with pneumatic anti-shock garments inflated achieve a better clinical outcome than those managed with only fluid resuscitation?
- What is the relationship between blood at the external meatus and the presence of urethral injury?
- What is the incidence of genitourinary injuries not detected in the emergency department?
- How often do emergency nurses initiate psychologic support services for patients with genital injuries not sustained by rape?

ANNOTATED BIBLIOGRAPHY

Briggs, E.E., Hendricks, D., & Flint, L.M. (1987). Penetrating abdominal trauma: Resuscitation, diagnostic evaluation, and definitive management. *Advances in Surgery, 20,* 1-46.
Comprehensive summary focused on penetrating abdominal trauma with a discussion of specific organ injuries, diagnostic intervention, and management strategies. This article offers the basics in an easily readable format.
Emergency Medicine 1985. 17 (Vol 11-16). Kidneys, ureters, bladder, urethra, female genitalia, male genitalia, respectively.)
Series that provides an excellent review (although dated) of genitourinary trauma. Each volume features a specific anatomic section of the genitourinary tract. Mechanisms of injury, pertinent objective data, diagnostic testing, and interventions are discussed as they relate to the specific section.

Federle, M.P., Crass, R.A., Jeffrey, R.B., & Trunkey, D.D. (1982). Computed tomography in blunt abdominal trauma. *Archives of Surgery, 117,* 645-650.
Retrospective study of 200 cases of blunt abdominal trauma that discusses the advantages of CT for diagnosis of intraperitoneal and retroperitoneal injuries.
Gibson, D.E. (1987). Abdominal trauma. *Trauma Quarterly,* 4(1), 11-25.
Thorough review of blunt and penetrating trauma to the abdomen, with special attention to individual organ damage. Advantages and disadvantages of the use of peritoneal lavage and CT are discussed.
Higie, S., Craven, K., & Neff, J. (1987). Standardized care plans: Blunt abdominal trauma. *Journal of Emergency Nursing, 13*(2), 114-117.
Accurate and functional plan of nursing assessment and intervention, using nursing diagnosis for the patient experiencing blunt trauma to the abdomen.
Neuwirth, H., Frazier, B., & Cochran, S. (1989). Genitourinary imaging and procedures by the emergency physician. *Emergency Medicine Clinics of North America, 7,* 1-28.
Comprehensive review of radiographic studies used in genitourinary trauma. Advantages and limitations of each procedure, as well as clinical controversies, are discussed.
Peterson, N. (1989). Complications of renal trauma. *Urologic Clinics of North America, 18,* 1111-1115.
Summary of the latest research in the area of complications of renal injury. Long-term management strategies are addressed.

REFERENCES

Andrews, J.F. (1987). Patterns in blunt trauma. *Trauma Quarterly, 3,* 1-5.

Baker, S. (1987). The neglected epidemic: Stone lecture, 1985. American Trauma Society Meeting. *Journal of Trauma, 27,* 343-348.

Beal, S.L., Pottmeyer, E.W., & Spisso, J.M. (1988). Esophageal perforation following external blunt trauma. *Journal of Trauma, 28,* 1425-1432.

Berman, H.L., Ricciardelli, C.A., & Savino, J.A. (1987). Abdominal trauma. *Patient Care, 21*(13), 105-123.

Boey, J.H. (1988). Peritoneal cavity. In L.W. Way (Ed.), *Current Surgical Diagnosis and Treatment* (pp. 404-420). Norwalk, CONN: Appleton & Lange.

Bremer, C., & Cassata, L. (1986). Trauma in pregnancy. *Nursing Clinics of North America, 21,* 705-716.

Bresler, M.J. (1988). Computed tomography v. peritoneal lavage in blunt abdominal trauma. *Topics in Emergency Medicine, 10,* 59-73.

Briggs, S.E., Hendricks, D., & Flint, L.M. (1987). Penetrating abdominal trauma: Resuscitation, diagnostic evaluation and definitive management. *Advances in Surgery, 20,* 1-46.

Brothers, L.R. (1985). Blunt scrotal trauma: A review. *Hospital Medicine, 21,* 61-80.

Brunner, R., & Shatney, C. (1987). Diagnostic and therapeutic aspects of rectal trauma: Blunt versus penetrating. *American Surgeon,* April, 215-219.

Buntain, W.L., Gould, H.R., & Maull, K.I. (1988). Predictability of splenic salvage by computed tomography. *Journal of Trauma, 28,* 24-32.

Burney, R.E. (1986). Peritoneal lavage and other diagnostic procedures in blunt abdominal trauma. *Emergency Medicine Clinics of North America, 4,* 513-526.

Carpenito, L.J. (Ed.) (1987). *Nursing diagnosis: Application to clinical practice.* Philadelphia: J.B. Lippincott.

Carroll, P., Lue, T., Schmidt, R., Trengrove-Jones, G., & McAninch, J. (1985a). Penile reimplantation: Current concepts. *Journal of Urology, 133,* 281.

Carroll, P., Taylor, S., & McAninch, J. (1985b). Major bladder trauma. In F.W. Blaisdell, D. Trunkey, & J. McAninch (Eds.), *Trauma management: Vol. II, Urogenital trauma* (pp. 69-75). New York: Thieme-Stratton.

Cass, A., Luxemberg, M., Gleich, P., & Smith, C. (1987a). Deaths from urologic injury due to external trauma. *Journal of Trauma, 27,* 319-321.

_____ (1987b). Long term results of conservative and surgical management of blunt renal lacerations. *British Journal of Urology, 59,* 17-20.

Cass, A., & Viera, J. (1987). Comparison of IVP and CT findings in patients with suspected renal injury. *Urology, 24,* 484-487.

Cayten, C.G. (1984). Abdominal trauma. *Emergency Medicine Clinics of North America, 2,* 799-821.

Cheadle, W., & Richardson, J.D. (1982). Options in management of trauma of the esophagus. *Surgery, Gynecology and Obstetrics, 155,* 380-384.

Collins, P.S., Maj, M.C., Golocovsky, M., Salander, J.M., Col, M.C., Champion, H., & Rich, N.M. (1988). Intraabdominal vascular injury secondary to penetrating trauma. *Journal of Trauma, 28,* S165-169.

Cowley, R.A., & Dunham, C.M. (Eds.) (1982). *Shock trauma/critical care manual: Initial assessment and management.* Baltimore: University Park Press.

Crombleholme, W.R. (1985). GU trauma inside and out: Female genitals. *Emergency Medicine, 17*(16), 15, 19-28.

Crombleholme, W.R., & Sweet, R.L. (1985). Female genital trauma. In F.W. Blaisdell, D. Trunkey, & J. McAninch (Eds.), *Trauma management: Vol. II, Urogenital trauma.* New York: Thieme-Stratton.

DeGowin, E.L., & DeGowin, R.L. (1976). *Bedside diagnostic examination.* New York: MacMillan Publishing.

Elam, A., & Ray, V. (1986). Sexually related trauma: A review. *Annals of Emergency Medicine, 15,* 576-584.

Farnell, M.B., Spencer, M.P., Thompson, E., Williams, H.J., Jr., Mucha, P., Jr., & Ilstrup, D.M. (1988). Nonoperative management of blunt hepatic trauma in adults. *Surgery, 104*(4), 748-754.

Federle, M.P., Crass, R.A., Jeffrey, R.B., & Trunkey, D.D. (1982). Computed tomography in blunt abdominal trauma. *Archives of Surgery, 117,* 645-650.

Feliciano, D.V., & Mattox, K.L. (1984). Small intestine injuries. In E.E. Moore, B. Eiseman, & C.W. VanWay III (Eds.), *Critical decisions in trauma* (pp. 206-208). St. Louis: Mosby–Year Book, Inc.

Fournier, G., Laing, F., & McAninch, J. (1989). Scrotal ultrasonography and the management of testicular trauma. *Urologic Clinics of North America, 16,* 377-385.

Frame, S.B., Timberlake, G.A., & McSwain, N.E. (1988). Trauma rounds. *Emergency Medicine, 20*(5), 59-60.

Gibson, D.E. (1987). Abdominal trauma. *Trauma Quarterly, 4,* 11-25.

Gomez, G.A., Alvarez, R., Plasencia, G., Echenique, M., Vopal, J.J., Byers, P., Dove, D.B., & Kreis, D.J., Jr. (1987). Diagnostic peritoneal lavage in the management of blunt abdominal trauma: A reassessment. *Journal of Trauma, 27,* 1-5.

Gundlinger, G., & Vester, S. (1987). Transvaginal injury of the duodenum, diaphragm and lung. *Journal of Trauma, 27,* 575-576.

Guerriero, G.W. (1985). Ureteral trauma. In F.W. Blaisdell, D. Trunkey, & J. McAninch (Eds.), *Trauma management: Vol. II, Urogenital trauma* (pp. 50-59). New York: Thieme-Stratton.

Hanna, S.S., Gorman, P.R., Harrison, A.W., Taylor, G., Miller, H.A.B., & Pagliarello, G. (1987). Blunt liver trauma at Sunnybrook Medical Center. *Journal of Trauma, 27,* 965-969.

Hanno, P.M. (1985a). GU trauma inside and out: The bladder. *Emergency Medicine, 17*(13), 21-31.

_____ (1985b). GU trauma inside and out: The urethra. *Emergency Medicine,* August 15, 161-168.

Hanno, P. & McAninch, J. (1985). GU trauma inside and out: The kidneys. *Emergency Medicine, 17*(15), 25-37.

Harty, P. (1987). Urologic trauma: Lower genitourinary tract. In J. Richardson, H. Polk, & L. Flint (Eds.), *Trauma: Clinical care and pathophysiology.* Chicago: Mosby–Year Book, Inc.

Harwood, A. (1983). Genitourinary trauma. *Emergency Medicine, 15*(6), 112-117, 120-121, 124-126.

Heeg, M., TenDuis, J., & Klasen, H. (1986). Power take-off injuries. *Injury, 17,* 28-30.

Huizinga, W.K.J., Baker, L.W., & Mtshali, Z.W. (1987). Selective management of abdominal and thoracic stab wounds with established peritoneal penetration: The eviscerated omentum. *American Journal of Surgery, 153,*(6) 564-568.

Hunt, T.K., & Goodson, W.H. III. (1988). Wound healing. In L.W. Way (Ed.), *Current surgical diagnosis and treatment* (pp. 86-98). Los Altos, CA: Lange Medical Books.

Hunt, T.K., & Jawetz, E. (1988). Inflammation, infection, and antibiotics. In L.W. Way (Ed.), *Current surgical diagnosis and treatment* (pp. 99-127). Norwalk, CONN: Appleton & Lange.

Jeffrey, R.B., Laing, F.C., & Wing, V.W. (1986). Ultrasound in acute pancreatic trauma. *Gastrointestinal Radiology, 11,* 44-46.

Jones, R.C. (1985). Management of pancreatic trauma. *American Journal of Surgery, 150,* 698-703.

Jordan, G., & Gilbert, D. (1989). Male genital trauma. *Clinics in Plastic Surgery, 15,* 431-442.

Kearney, G.P., & Finn, D.J. (1981). Trauma to the genitourinary tract. *Emergency Medicine, 13*(14), 69-77.

Kester, D.E., Andrassy, R.J., & Aust, J.B. (1986). The value and cost effectiveness of abdominal roentgenograms in the evaluation of stab wounds to the abdomen. *Surgery, Gynecology & Obstetrics, 162,* 337-339.

Kidd, P.S. (1987). Genitourinary trauma patients. *Topics in Emergency Medicine, 9,* 71-87.

Kidd, P.S. (1982). Trauma of the genitourinary system. *Journal of Emergency Nursing, 8*(5), 232-238.

Kidd, W.T., Lui, R.C.K., Khoo, R., & Nixon, J. (1987). The management of blunt splenic trauma. *Journal of Trauma, 27,* 977-979.

Kusminsky, R.E., Tu, K.K., Brendemuehl, J., Tiley, E., & Boland, J.P. (1982). The potential value of endotoxin-amylase detection in peritoneal lavage fluid. *American Surgeon, 48,* 359-362.

Lanros, N.E. (1988). *Assessment and intervention in emergency nursing.* East Norwalk, CT: Appleton & Lange.

Lucas, C.E., & Ledgerwood, A.M. (1984). Extra hepatic biliary tract injuries. In E.E. Moore, B. Eiseman, & C.W. VanWay III (Eds.), *Critical decisions in trauma* (pp. 194-196). St. Louis: Mosby–Year Book, Inc.

Mansell, E., Stokes, S., Adler, J., & Rosensweig, N. (1974). Patient assessment: Examination of the abdomen. *American Journal of Nursing, 74,* 1679-1702.

Maull, K.I., Rozycki, G.S., Vinsant, G.O., & Pedigo, R.E. (1987). Retroperitoneal injuries: Pitfalls in diagnosis and management. *Southern Medical Journal, 80,* 1111-1115.

McAninch, J.W. (1989). Management of genital skin loss. *Urologic Clinics of North America, 16,* 387-397.

McAninch, J.W. (1985a). Assessment and diagnosis of urinary and genital injuries. In F.W. Blaisdell, D. Trunkey, & J. McAninch (Eds.), *Trauma management: Vol. II, Urogenital trauma* (pp. 2-26). New York: Thieme-Stratton.

———— (1985b). Renal injuries. In F.W. Blaisdell, D. Trunkey, & J. McAninch (Eds.), *Trauma management: Vol. II, Urogenital trauma* (pp. 27-41). New York: Thieme-Stratton.

———— (1985c). GU trauma inside and out: Male genitals. *Emergency Medicine, 17*(17), 19-33.

McSwain, N. (1984). To manage multiple injury. *Emergency Medicine, 16*(4), 57-94.

Mee, S., & McAninch, J. (1989). Indications for radiographic assessment in suspected renal trauma. *Urologic Clinics of North America, 16,* 187-192.

Merlotti, G.J., Marcet, E., Sheaff, C.M., Dunn, R., & Barrett, J.A. (1985). Use of peritoneal lavage to evaluate abdominal penetration. *Journal of Trauma, 25,* 228-231.

Merlotti, G.J., Dillon, B.C., Lange, D.A., Robin, A.P., & Barrett, J.A. (1988). Peritoneal lavage in penetrating thoracoabdominal trauma. *Journal of Trauma, 28,* 17-22.

Merrill, D.C., & Palmer, J.M. (1985). Male genital trauma. In F.W. Blaisdell, D. Trunkey, & J. McAninch (Eds.), *Trauma management: Vol. II, Urogenital trauma.* New York: Thieme-Stratton.

Mitchell, J. (1984). The mechanism: Presentation of anterior urethral injuries. In J. Mitchell (Ed.), *Urinary tract trauma.* Bristol: Wright Press.

Morehouse, D.D., & MacKinnon, K.J. (1985). Urethral injuries. In F.W. Blaisdell, D. Trunkey, & J. McAninch (Eds.), *Trauma management: Vol. II, Urogenital trauma* (pp. 81-88). New York: Thieme-Stratton.

Nelson, R.M., & Walt, A.J. (1984). Colon injuries. In E.E. Moore, B. Eiseman, & C.W. VanWay III (Eds.), *Critical decisions in trauma* (pp. 210-212). St. Louis: Mosby–Year Book, Inc.

Neuwirth, H., Frasier, B., & Cochran, S. (1989). Genitourinary imaging and procedures by the emergency physician. *Emergency Medicine Clinics of North America, 7,* 1-28.

Norton, L.W. (1984). Stomach and duodenal injuries. In E.E. Moore, B. Eiseman, & C.W. VanWay III (Eds.), *Critical decisions in trauma* (pp. 198-200). St. Louis: Mosby–Year Book, Inc.

Odling-Smeed, W., & Crockard, A. (1981). *Trauma care.* New York: Grune & Stratton.

Orban, D.J., & Molitor, L. (1986). Abdominal trauma. In S. Cahill & M. Balshurs (Eds.), *Intervention in emergency nursing: The first 60 minutes* (pp. 203-224). Rockville, MD: Aspen Publishers.

Orvis, B., & McAninch, J. (1989). Penile rupture. *Urologic Clinics of North America, 16,* 369-375.

Pass, L.J., LeNarz, L.A., Schreiber, J.T., & Estrera, A.S. (1987). Management of esophageal gunshot wounds. *Annals of Thoracic Surgery, 44,* 253-256.

Peterson, N. (1989). Complications of renal trauma. *Urologic Clinics of North America, 18,* 1111-1115.

Porth, C. (1982). *Pathophysiology: Concepts of altered health states.* Philadelphia: J.B. Lippincott.

Presti, J., Carroll, P., & McAninch, J. (1989). Ureteral and renal pelvic injuries from external trauma: Diagnosis and management. *Journal of Trauma, 29,* 370-374.

Propp, D., Weber, D., & Ciesla, M. (1989). Reliability of a urine dipstick in emergency department patients. *Annals of Emergency Medicine, 18,* 560-563.

Ramponi, D.R., & Somerville, P. (1986). Chest trauma. In M.K. Fincke & N.E. Lanros (Eds.), *Emergency nursing: A comprehensive review* (pp. 229-230). Rockville, MD: Aspen Publishers.

Romero-Sierra, C. (1986). *Neuroanatomy: A conceptual approach.* New York: Churchill Livingstone.

Salvatierra, O., Jr. (1984). Genitourinary trauma. In J. Mills, M. Ho, P. Salher, & D. Trunkey (Eds.), *Current emergency diagnosis and treatment* (2nd ed.) (pp. 271-275). Los Altos, CA: Lange Medical Books.

Sandler, C.M., & Burke, J.T. (1985). Radiology of the urinary system in the emergency department. *Emergency Medicine Clinics of North America, 3*(3), 507-519.

Schrock, T.R. (1988). Large intestine. In L.W. Way (Ed.). *Current surgical diagnosis and treatment* (pp. 586-630). Los Altos, CA: Lange Medical Books.

Semonin-Holleran, R. (1988). Critical nursing care for abdominal trauma. *Critical Care Nurse, 8*(3), 48-56.

Sherman, J.C., DeLaurier, G.A., Hawkins, M.L., Brown, L.G., Treat, R.C., & Mansberger, A.R. (1989). Percutaneous peritoneal lavage in blunt trauma patients: A safe and accurate diagnostic method. *Journal of Trauma, 29,* 801-805.

Shetler, M. (1984). Excretory urogram and pyelogram. *RN,* June, 95-96.

Smedira, N., & Schecter, W.P. (1989). Blunt abdominal trauma. *Emergency Medicine Clinics of North America, 7*(3), 631-645.

Symbas, P.N., Vlasis, S.E., & Hatcher, C., Jr. (1986). Blunt and penetrating diaphragmatic injuries with or without herniation of organs into the chest. *Annals of Thoracic Surgery, 42,* 158-162.

Trunkey, D.D., & Holcroft, J.W. (1983). Abdominal injuries. In L.W. Way (Ed.). *Current surgical diagnosis and treatment* (pp. 224-225). Los Altos, CA: Lange Medical Books.

Veise-Berry, S.W. (1983). Nursing considerations during radiologic examination of the massively injured trauma patient. *Critical Care Quarterly, 6*(1), 55-65.

Walker, M.L. (1986). Management of pancreatic trauma: Concepts and controversy. *Journal of the National Medical Association, 78,* 1177-1182.

Ward, R.E., & Blaisdell, F.W. (1984). Abdominal aorta and vena cava injuries. In E.E. Moore, B. Eiseman, & C.W. VanWay III (Eds.), *Critical decisions in trauma* (pp. 218-220). St. Louis: Mosby–Year Book, Inc.

Way, L.W. (1988). Liver. In L.W. Way (Ed.). *Current surgical diagnosis and treatment* (pp. 459-470). Los Altos, CA: Lange Medical Books.

Yarbro, E., & Fowler, J. (1987). Renal trauma in rural Virginia. *Journal of Trauma, 27*, 940-942.

Zoller, G.W. (1983). Genitourinary trauma. In P. Rosen, F. Baker, G. Braen, R. Dailey, & R. Levy (Eds.), *Emergency medicine concepts and clinical practice, Vol. 1* (pp. 406-430). St Louis: Mosby–Year Book, Inc.

13

Tissue Integrity

Surface trauma

■■■■■■■■■■■■■■■■■■■■■■■■■■■■■■■■■■■■■■

Judy L. Larsen
Judie Wischman

OBJECTIVES

❑ Identify appropriate assessment of the following surface trauma: lacerations, abrasions, avulsions, contusions, puncture wounds, and mammalian bites.

❑ Discuss the appropriate management of the surface wounds just mentioned, including cleaning, closing, dressing, and tetanus prophylaxis.

❑ Select the appropriate wound care follow-up and patient instructions as indicated by the type of surface trauma.

❑ Understand the nursing diagnoses for patients with surface trauma, and apply these concepts to patient care situations.

INTRODUCTION Surface trauma occurs frequently and is often associated with other serious trauma. Because surface trauma is rarely life threatening, it is not the priority in trauma care. Yet surface trauma can have many serious implications for the patient. Complications such as bleeding, infection, scarring, or loss of function can mean significant long-term physical and psychologic changes for the patient. This area of trauma nursing provides rich opportunities for nursing assessment and intervention. Nurses become the experts in wound care and patient teaching for surface trauma. This chapter provides the trauma nurse with the basic knowledge needed to gain that expertise in the management of surface trauma.

CASE STUDY Mrs. Eve Johnson, a 75-year-old woman, was hit by a large truck while crossing the street. She fell on her left side and was dragged by the truck for a short distance. She did not lose consciousness. She was taken to the nearest hospital by ambulance, secured on a backboard and wearing a cervical collar.

In the ED she is alert and oriented. Her BP is 104/60; pulse, 120; and respiratory rate, 14. Her left arm and left upper thigh sustained large abrasions, embedded with dirt. A large laceration of the right knee is evident. Two moderate-size lacerations are present: one laceration is on her face, and one is in the occipital area of her scalp. A medical alert bracelet on Mrs. Johnson's right arm indicates that she has diabetes and has a history of high blood pressure.

In the initial assessment of Mrs. Johnson, what general considerations should be evaluated before beginning wound treatment?

Her BP is 104/60. Considering her history of hypertension, this BP could represent a hypotensive state. Mrs. Johnson should be evaluated for internal injuries and fractures.

Mrs. Johnson also has diabetes. Two areas must be considered because of this factor. It is important to determine if Mrs. Johnson is insulin dependent or if her blood sugar is controlled by oral agents. This information indicates the severity of the diabetes. Determining when she last took her medication and when she last ate is important to prevent either hypoglycemia or hyperglycemia. The vascular changes that occur with diabetes may decrease the blood supply to the wounds, slowing the healing process of Mrs. Johnson's injuries. She may require supervised dressing changes to allow monitoring of healing.

Should anesthesia be used before cleaning Mrs. Johnson's wounds?

Local anesthesia will provide the level of comfort needed for Mrs. Johnson to easily tolerate complete wound cleaning. The facial and scalp lacerations are anesthetized with an infiltration of lidocaine with epinephrine into the wound edge. Lidocaine with epinephrine is used because the vasoconstrictive properties of epinephrine will decrease bleeding in vascular areas, making repair easier. Within 10 minutes after injection, the lacerations can be cleaned without discomfort. The anesthetic effect will last 60 to 90 minutes. The knee laceration is infiltrated with plain lidocaine. Comfortable cleaning and repair can be completed after 10 minutes, and the effect will last 30 to 60 minutes. The abrasions are anesthetized with 4% lidocaine solution, which is applied by saturating gauze pads with the lidocaine solution and placing them directly over the abrasion. The anesthesia lasts only 20 minutes. Because Mrs. Johnson's abrasions are very large, it may be necessary to inject lidocaine around the abrasion edges to provide adequate anesthesia for cleaning.

Is there a difference in how these wounds should be cleaned?

Location and type of wound affect the cleaning method. Both the scalp and knee laceration will be irrigated with normal saline using a 35-ml syringe with an 18-gauge needle. The hair around the scalp laceration should be clipped, not shaved, before cleaning and repair. The facial laceration can be irrigated with a surfactant product like Shur Clens, because it is gentle and will not irritate the eyes if any solution gets near them. The abrasions should be scrubbed with a porous brush. All debris must be removed to prevent complications.

What complications can occur if the wounds are not cleaned completely?

All devitalized tissue and debris must be removed from the lacerations and the abrasions. This material becomes a foreign body in the wound and provides a medium for infection. The abrasions are considered tetanus-prone wounds because of the devitalized tissue present and the embedded

dirt. To prevent tetanus and other infections, all of the debris must be removed. Any dirt left in the abrasion can also cause permanent disfigurement. The epidermis heals over the dirt, resulting in a "tatooing" effect.

What are the important considerations for dressing Mrs. Johnson's wounds?

The lacerations all need a pressure dressing to eliminate dead space and reduce swelling. Excessive scarring can be prevented with a pressure dressing, because tension on the suture line is reduced by controlling edema. Special attention must be paid to the facial laceration. The knee must be immobilized to facilitate healing. This is of particular concern for Mrs. Johnson because of her decreased circulation. The knee will have a better chance of healing quickly if the process is not disturbed by motion. The abrasions should have an antibiotic ointment and a gauze dressing applied. Mrs. Johnson will need special assistance and instruction because the abrasions must be cleaned and redressed four times a day.

ANATOMIC AND PHYSIOLOGIC CONSIDERATIONS
Skin Layers

A fundamental knowledge of anatomy and physiology of the skin is necessary to understand anatomic relationships of injured tissue. Figure 13-1 shows the three layers of the skin: the epidermis, the dermis, and the subcutaneous tissue.

The outermost layer, the epidermis, contains stratified epithelial tissue. It is a protective surface and has no tensile strength. It contains rapidly reproducing cells that regenerate within 48 hours, a process called *epithelialization*.

The second layer of skin, the dermis, is referred to as the *true skin*. It is made up of connective tissue, elastic and collagen fibers. Hair follicles, sebaceous glands, sweat glands, and melanocytes are found in this layer. The dermal layer houses the blood vessels in the skin. A massive capillary network is located here, which contributes to significant edema in skin injuries. The dermis is characterized by good tensile strength, but has limited ability to regenerate to its original thickness.

The innermost skin layer is the subcutaneous layer. It consists primarily of fatty tissue. This layer has no tensile strength. The subcutaneous layer functions as an insulating cushion for heat

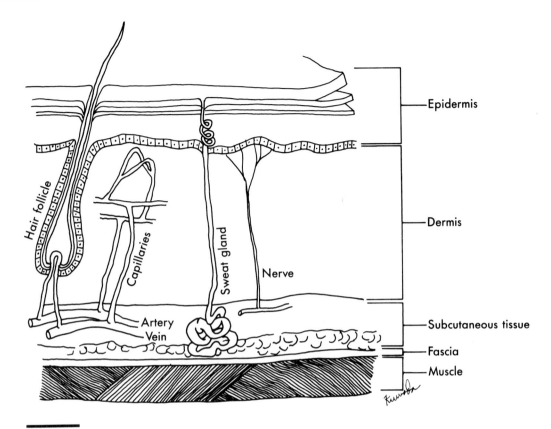

Figure 13-1 Skin layers.

retention and protection from trauma. Scar tissue is formed when collagen-forming fibroblasts from the subcutaneous layer are allowed to "migrate," or escape through the dermal and epidermal layers to the surface.

The box on p. 416 summarizes the structure and function of skin.

Wound Healing

Understanding the wound healing phenomenon is important to the nurse involved in wound care. Application of this knowledge can improve wound management techniques (Hunt, 1988) and provide a foundation for patient teaching.

Phases of wound healing

The process of wound healing occurs in three phases. The first phase, the inflammatory phase, lasts 3 to 5 days. It begins with the body's first defense, the intrinsic control of bleeding. Hemostasis usually occurs within 5 to 10 minutes after in-

jury. The vessels constrict, and a fibrin clot forms that unites the vascular wound edges. This vascular-cellular response disposes of bacteria, microorganisms, and dying tissue. Next, small vessels dilate, providing a fresh blood supply to the wound. Edema formation occurs in this phase (Fernandez & Finley, 1983). Release of histamine aids in cell membrane permeability, contributing to edema, but also allowing the defense cells to enter the wound site. As the white blood cells migrate into the wounded tissue, phagocytosis occurs. The final process in this phase is called *granulation*. A fibrin network clot forms a mechanical barrier and a physiologic filter against invading organisms.

The collagen or fibroplasia phase occurs next, lasting 2 to 3 weeks. Fibroblasts migrate to the wound, producing collagen. Collagen is a protein band that provides tensile strength to the wound as it heals.

The third phase is the maturation phase,

Structure and function of skin

Epidermis

Thickness of 0.04 mm
No blood supply
Composed of epithelium
Resident flora
No tensile strength

Dermis

Thickness of 0.5 mm
Main support structure
Contains nerve endings, lymphatics, vasculature, hair follicles, sebaceous glands, sweat glands, melanocytes
Normally moist
Good tensile strength

Subcutaneous tissue

Variable thickness
Reservoir for fat storage
Fibroblast formation
Temperature insulator
Shock absorber
Stores calories

Note. From "Wound Repair: A Review" by R. Bryant, 1987, *Journal of Enterostomal Therapy, 14,* p. 263.

---

which lasts from 3 months to several years. In this phase there is continuous collagen production and breakdown, resulting in constant changes in the appearance of the wound. These constant changes cause the injury site to become red, lumpy, dense, or sensitive. Gradually the injury site improves by becoming paler, thinner, and less tender. The maturation process is ongoing. Careful explanation to patients of wound maturation is important, because the poor cosmetic results that may be observed early in the healing process can cause them concern. Time can often be the best "plastic surgeon."

Types of wound healing

Wound healing occurs in one of three ways: primary, secondary, or tertiary intention. Primary intention, or primary closure, is the optimal method of wound healing. The best example is a sutured laceration where the wound edges are approximated. The underlying structures are aligned, eliminating dead space. This prevents the collection of fluid and formation of hematomas and

minimizes tissue defect and granulation formation (Dimick, 1988).

Healing by secondary intention occurs when extensive loss of tissue prevents wound edge approximation and closure. A common example of this is an avulsion, where portions of the skin and underlying tissue are missing. Granulation tissue forms to fill the gap between wound edges. There is a propensity toward scar formation and deformity (Trott, 1991).

Tertiary intention healing is the method of delaying primary wound closure. The wound is left open until edema has subsided, no infection is present, and all debris has been removed. The wound is then surgically closed. This leaves minimal tissue defect or scar formation. Wounds considered for delayed primary closure are those that are contaminated and infected or post-operative wounds in which massive swelling prevents safe or effective wound edge approximation (Dimick, 1988). Figure 13-2 shows the three types of wound healing.

Scar formation

The nurse must have basic understanding of how scars are formed to implement nursing interventions that foster the best cosmetic effect. The amount of scarring depends on the extent of injury to the skin layers.

Damage to the epidermis and the upper dermal layers can cause color changes. Often this is thought to be scarring when it is actually normal wound healing. The color change results from disruption of the melanocytes during injury. Redistribution of the melanocytes usually occurs as the epidermal layer heals.

Damage to the dermal layer can produce contour changes. Even though this "true skin" has good tensile strength, it has limited regenerative powers. Dermal injury with tissue loss is seen commonly as the acne pit, chicken pox mark, or a poorly repaired laceration.

"There is nothing in the true skin (dermis) that can scar" (G. Eade, personal communication, September, 1987). Scar tissue does not come from the dermal layer—it comes from the subcutaneous level. If the dermal layer cannot be closed, collagen-forming fibroblasts move freely from the subcutaneous layer to the top of the wound. These cells form the characteristic woody, lumpy, inelastic scar tissue. Figure 13-3

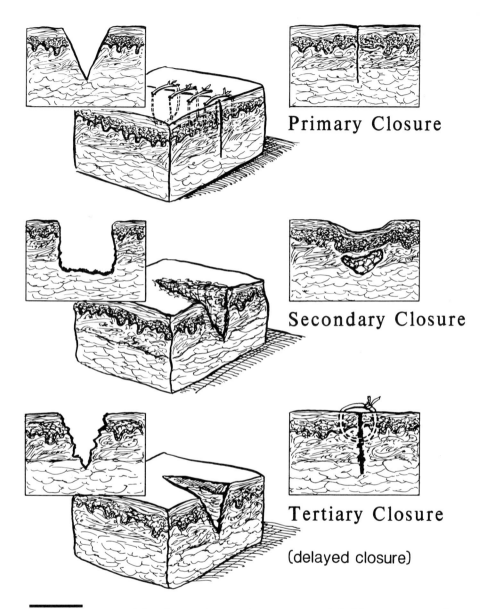

Primary Closure

Secondary Closure

Tertiary Closure

(delayed closure)

Figure 13-2   Types of skin closure. Primary closure is accomplished by suturing wound at time of initial patient presentation. Secondary closure occurs by allowing wound to heal by granulation. Tertiary closure, or delayed primary closure, is generally done 4 to 5 days after initial injury and allows any infectious process to be eliminated. (*Note.* From *Wounds and Lacerations: Emergency Care and Closure* [p. 82] by A. Trott, 1991, St. Louis: Mosby–Year Book, Inc.)

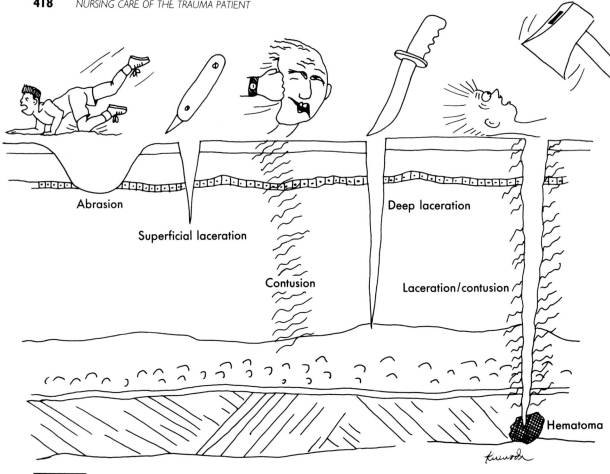

Figure 13-3 Damage to skin layers.

shows damage to the various skin layers.

Contused lacerations, full-thickness lacerations, and avulsions are types of wounds that may develop excessive (hypertrophic) scarring. Damage to all skin layers and interruption of the dermal approximation allow cells from the subcutaneous layer to migrate to the surface. Hypertrophic scarring is not a disturbance of the normal physiology of wound healing, but rather a "misdirection" of the collagen-forming cells from the subcutaneous layer and an over-production of collagen (Robson, 1988). An example of hypertrophic scarring is shown in Figure 13-4. Poor repair technique and excessive movement from inadequate immobilization of wounds over joints can contribute to excessive scarring. Hypertrophic scars generally fade and flatten over time.

Keloids are a different kind of excessive scarring. Keloid is a Greek word meaning "to grow beyond boundaries" (Robson, 1988). Collagen grows beyond the original wound boundaries to form the keloid. It is not the result of wound healing out of control. The collagen that forms keloids has a different composition from collagen of normal or hypertrophic scars. Certain areas of the body (the sternum, the mandible, the deltoid area) have a greater tendency to develop this disturbance. Plastic surgery cannot correct this condition because keloids return when removed. Treatment with steroids has had some success (Trott, 1991).

Impaired wound healing

Several conditions can impair wound healing. Many of the conditions outlined in the box on the facing page can be present in the trauma patient. Attention to the correction of these problems helps create an environment favoring maximal wound healing. The risk of scar formation can also be reduced when the conditions impair-

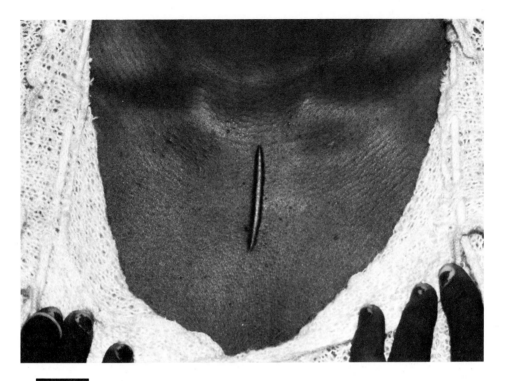

Figure 13-4   Example of hypertrophic scar. (*Note.* From *Wounds and Lacerations: Emergency Care and Closure* by A. Trott, 1991, St. Louis: Mosby–Year Book, Inc.)

ing wound healing are minimized. Attention to adequate approximation of all skin layers adds to a positive wound healing environment. This action prevents the subcutaneous tissue from migrating to the surface, thus preventing hypertrophic scarring. Dead space, with possible hematoma formation, is also eliminated.

Special Areas: Hand and Face

Surface trauma to the hand occurs frequently and has significant impact on our society. Approximately 16 million injuries occur each year, accounting for 90 million days of restricted activities and billions of salary dollars lost (Jupiter & Krushell, 1987). Nurses should understand the neuroanatomy of the hand to properly evaluate these injuries.

The three major nerves in the hand are the radial, ulnar, and median nerves, as shown in Figure 13-5. The acronym *RUM*, for *R*adial, *U*lnar, and *M*edian nerves, is a useful tool for remembering these nerves (Lampe, 1969). Table 13-1 outlines motor function, sensory distribution, and common nerve deficits.

Conditions that impair wound healing

Incomplete removal of devitalized tissue from initial injury, or subsequent rough handling

Foreign material—foreign bodies or residual infection

Shock—poor perfusion

Septicemia

Abnormal metabolic/electrolyte environment

Acidosis with or without hypoxia

Hepatic failure—leading to abnormal protein synthesis

Renal failure—uremia

Prolonged steroid administration—nitrogen and potassium depletion

Immune supression

Inadequate immobilization—damage to wound bed; stress on suture line

Malnutrition—lack of adequate caloric, protein, mineral, and vitamin intake

Delayed or incomplete eschar separation

Note. From *Pathology of Thermal Injury: A Practical Approach* (p. 23) by T.W. Panke and C.G. McLeod, 1985, Orlando, FL: Grune & Stratton.

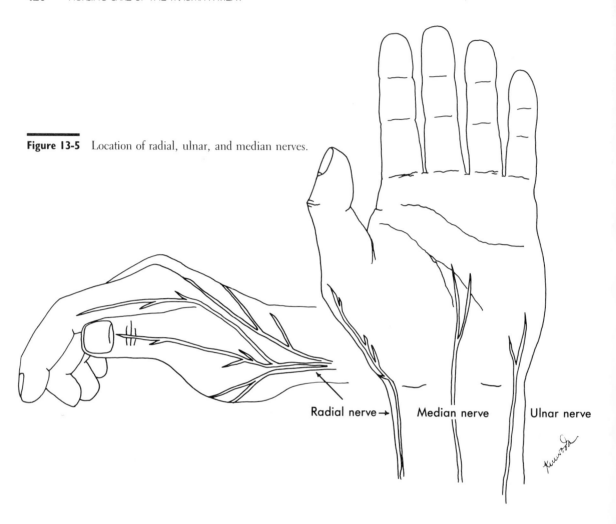

Figure 13-5 Location of radial, ulnar, and median nerves.

Table 13-1 Assessment criteria for nerves of the hand

	Radial nerve	**Ulnar nerve**	**Median nerve**
Motor assessment	Wrist extension Finger extension	Finger spreading/ approximation Paper between fingers	Flexion and pronation of thumb Thumb/fingertip approxi- mation
	Deficit: wrist drop	Deficit: "claw" hand and inability to hold paper between fingers	Deficit: inability to extend thumb
Sensory assessment	Dorsum of hand (1st, 2nd, 3rd, ½ of 4th digit) Over top of thumb	Palmar: ½ of 4th digit; all of 5th digit Dorsal: ½ of 4th digit; all of 5th digit	Palmar: thumb, 2nd, 3rd, ½ of 4th digit Dorsal: tips of 2nd, 3rd, 4th digit

The radial nerve's principle motor function involves wrist and finger extension. The most common deficit is wrist drop, where the patient cannot lift the wrist from a flat surface with the hand palmar side down.

The ulnar nerve's main motor function is finger spreading and approximation of the fourth and fifth fingers (ring and little fingers). The ability to hold paper between lateral and medial surfaces of these adjacent fingers demonstrates integrity of the nerve. The ulnar nerve controls extension of the fourth and fifth fingers through innervation of the interosseous muscles. The "claw" hand, or inability to extend the fourth and fifth fingers, is a common deficit of this nerve (Jupiter & Krushell, 1987).

The median nerve's motor function involves the ability to extend the thumb upward, palm side up, from a flat surface and thumb to fingertip approximation. Inability to perform the "thumbs up" movement indicates a deficit (Strange, 1987).

The fingers and toes can be described in several ways. The digits of the hand are referred to as follows: the thumb, pollex, or first finger; the index, or second finger; the middle, long, or third finger; the ring, or fourth finger; and the little, or fifth finger. The digits of the feet are referred to as follows: the hallux, big, or great toe; the long, or second toe; the middle, or third toe; the fourth toe; and the little, or fifth toe. A common terminology in the literature does not exist, and all of the terms just mentioned are correct.

Surface trauma to the face is a frequent occurrence. Because of the cosmetic implications of facial trauma, meticulous assessment and treatment are required. The facial nerve is divided into three major branches. The motor integrity of the nerve is demonstrated in facial expressions, such as smiling, kissing, grimacing, and raising of eyebrows (Dushoff, 1974). Sensory integrity is evaluated by the patients' ability to feel light pricking of the face with a needle.

GENERAL ASSESSMENT

The nurse's first priority is assessment of the total patient. The first step is evaluation of basic life functions, because most skin trauma injuries are not life threatening. Because some wounds are quite distracting or grotesque, the nurse's attention may be drawn from more subtle yet significant injuries. It should be remembered that circumstances creating surface trauma often impact other body systems.

The second step is to obtain additional data through elicitation of the history. General health factors affect healing and compliance with medical regimen. These include age, nutrition, and other illnesses or conditions, such as diabetes or immunosuppression. Gathering information about current medications and allergies is essential in this initial assessment phase because medications can affect the body's ability to heal and resist infection (Martinez & Burns, 1987). The therapeutic approach to wound care is directed by the cause and mechanism of injury, the duration of wound exposure, the degree of gross contamination, and the physical structures involved.

History

History relating to cause and mechanism of injury can provide information to guide individualized wound care (Trott, 1991). An accidental laceration by a clean knife demands different treatment than an avulsed laceration involving a lawn mower.

A key piece of historical data is the duration the wound was exposed to contaminants, because infection is correlated with exposure time (Edlich, Rodeheaver, Morgan, Berman, & Thacker, 1988). When the length of time is greater than 6 to 8 hours between the occurrence and treatment, suture repair may be questionable. Each situation must be evaluated individually, based on any prehospital treatment, history, and condition of the wound.

Physical Examination
Inspection

All wounds are considered to be contaminated (Dimick, 1988). It is important to determine if the wound is clean, dirty, or infected. The distinction between clean, dirty, and infected depends on the physical ability to remove contaminants. Dirty wounds can be made surgically clean by removing the contaminating agents, dirt, debris, and devitalized tissue. Infected wounds can not be made clean, because the contaminants are infectious organisms that have established a destructive cellular process, which cannot be altered by cleaning alone (Dimick, 1988).

The degree of contamination directly affects the incidence of infection (Edlich et al., 1988).

Some bacteria normally live on the skin, in saliva, and in the gastrointestinal tract. These organisms are unlikely to cause infection because they do not have access to serum. When these normal flora and the transient bacteria from the environment are introduced during injury to the skin, they come in direct contact with blood. This combination may produce infection, which can cause problems with wound healing. It is the amount of bacteria, not the type, that threatens the defense system, making the wound vulnerable to infection (Mancusi-Ungaro & Rappaport, 1986). Careful inspection and removal of foreign material supports the body's ability to resist infection and is key to the wound-healing process (Mancusi-Ungaro & Rappaport, 1986).

Vascular integrity

Vessels, bones, nerves, and tendons of the affected part should be examined to establish vascular integrity and motor and sensory function (Martinez & Burns, 1987). This part of the wound investigation is a relatively blind process and must be conducted carefully to prevent further tissue damage. Sites of injury should be inspected for continuous oozing, spurting (typical of arterial injury), and hematoma formation. Direct pressure is the best method to control bleeding. Its effectiveness requires pressure applied close to the source. A gauze roll or several gauze pads pressed against the bleeding site with force produces the best result. Applying several layers of reinforced dressing without manual force makes the pressure less direct and more dispersed. The excess gauze and reinforced dressing will simply absorb the blood, not stop the flow. The use of hemostats to clamp vessels can further damage vascular structures by crushing them. Blind grabs for bleeders may inadvertently injure nerves, which lie close to vascular structures (Trott, 1991). Distal pulses, skin color, and temperature should be evaluated if injury is near major vessels. The possibility of underlying structural damage must be evaluated carefully. Probing the wound is generally delayed until definitive wound treatment is started because of the possibility of inducing further tissue damage. Fracture of adjacent bony structures can occur from the impact of the injury; therefore radiologic studies may be required. Evaluation of the motor and sensory functions of the injured part will reveal muscle, nerve, or tendon damage.

Nerve function

A quick method to assess motor function of the three nerves is to have the patient grasp a pencil with all five fingers of the affected hand. The ability to perform this maneuver indicates the nerves are grossly intact (McGuire, 1982).

Sensory function of the hand nerves can be easily tested. A gentle pinprick to the web between the thumb and second (index) finger tests the radial nerve. The ulnar nerve is tested by pricking the tip of the fifth (little) finger. The median nerve's sensory function is tested at the tip of the index finger (Trott, 1991).

Tendon function

Early recognition of damage to tendons, because of their avascular nature, promotes healing and return of normal function. The extensor tendons, lying just beneath the dorsum of the hand, are injured most often. Figure 13-6 illustrates the most common extensor injury, the mallet finger. Damage to the distal interphalangeal portion of the tendon produces this injury (Jupiter & Krushell, 1987). Injury to the proximal interphalangeal and metacarpal phalangeal segments of the tendon results in inability to fully extend the digit (Lovett & McCalla, 1983).

Less often injured but critical to assess are the flexor tendons. These tendons, located on the palmar side of the hand, create an intricate pulley system. When these tendons are severed, inability to flex the involved finger and make a fist results. Flexor tendons retract when cut and are not easily visualized in the wound. Careful approximation can prevent adhesions and restriction of movement (Strickland, 1983). Elevation will also minimize adhesion and fibrous tissue formation, which may subsequently limit movement (Strange, 1987).

ASSESSMENT AND INTERVENTIONS RELATED TO SPECIFIC INJURIES

Lacerations Impaired skin or tissue integrity
High risk for fluid volume deficit
High risk for sensory/perceptual alterations

Lacerations are incised wounds. They result from injury with sharp or dull objects in conjunction with tearing or shearing that produces irregular tissue damage (Martinez & Burns, 1987). The nursing history should include three important components: duration of exposure, mechanism of

Mechanisms

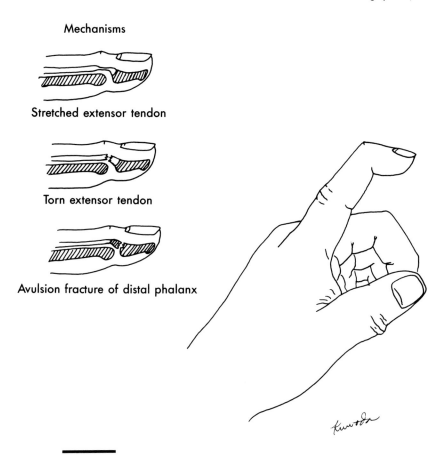

Stretched extensor tendon

Torn extensor tendon

Avulsion fracture of distal phalanx

Figure 13-6   Mallet finger—most common extensor tendon injury.

injury, and degree of contamination.

The time since occurence of the injury, in terms of length of environmental exposure, relates to the risk of infection. If this time exceeds 8 hours, primary closure may be questioned. The exception to this general concept is facial lacerations. Because of cosmetic implications, and the good vascular supply there is an extended time limit for closure of facial trauma (Dushoff, 1974).

Mechanism of injury, or how it occurred, indicates the extent of injury and the amount of contamination. A laceration occurring from a sharp knife is different from an injury from a fall against a large, dirty rock. The latter may result in a laceration with crushed edges and extensive tissue damage. This devitalized tissue creates a medium for infection (Phillips & Heggers, 1988). A wound heavily contaminated with dirt and gravel has greater chance of infection.

The treatment of lacerations is determined by

the type of wound healing appropriate for the injury. The decision for primary closure rests on a compromise between the likelihood of infection and the ability to provide favorable conditions for wound closure (Trott, 1991).

Wound preparation

Management of lacerations involves several steps: anesthesia, wound exploration, mechanical cleaning, and closure. After establishing adequate anesthesia, the laceration must be (1) inspected to rule out structural damage and (2) debrided conservatively. Any clearly nonviable tissue and foreign bodies must be removed. Further reconstruction of the wound shape may be necessary for the best plastic repair. Revision may include making jagged edges into straight ones. If a laceration is on the diagonal, or beveled, it may heal with a skin overhang. The dermis and epidermis should be trimmed to create a laceration that has edges perpendicular to the edge of the skin (Phillips & Heggers, 1988). These techniques provide better approximation of the wound edges.

After debridement and revision, copious irrigation under pressure is imperative to the mechanical cleaning of lacerations. This is accomplished with irrigation equipment and the appropriate wound cleaner.

Before wound closure, it is important to remove surface bacteria from the surrounding skin. This prevents inoculating the wound with skin flora. Wound edges can be cleaned with an antiseptic solution, like povidone-iodine. The solution should not enter the wound, because although iodine is bacteriocidal, it is also cytocidal, or lethal to cells.

Hair around the wound should be clipped, not shaved. Shaving can cause damage to hair follicles, resulting in bacterial proliferation (Martinez & Burns, 1987). Shaving has been associated with increased infection rates (Richless, 1985). Eyebrows should not be shaved because they are an important anatomic guide or landmark; their absence would make proper alignment difficult (Trott, 1991).

Wound closure

The wound is ready for closure once it is revised and cleaned. An important principle of wound closure is to match the skin layers (Dushoff, 1973). Closure is performed in layers to eliminate dead space, which prevents the formation of hematomas and fosters wound healing. The skin's greatest strength is in the dermal layer. The best repair is achieved when the the entire depth of the dermis is carefully approximated, which prevents the upward migration of cells from subcutaneous layer and minimizes scar formation. Careful alignment of skin layers eliminates uneven wound edges, which result in unsightly skin contours such as dermal override.

Wound edge eversion (skin's edges turned outward) is critical. This prevents the cut edges from rolling in (inverting) and continuing to bleed, forming hematomas. Also, inverted wound edges leave an uneven contour when they heal, which can be unsightly.

Laceration closure is accomplished by two methods: suturing and skin taping. The suturing technique should result in skin layer matching, wound edge approximation, and eversion. A commonly used technique is the square interrupted suture method. The suture is placed to form an elongated square, with the depth greater than the width. This bottle-shaped placement will evert the wound edges. If the width is greater than the depth, the edges will invert, or roll inward. Figure 13-7 demonstrates wound edge inversion and eversion.

Suture material Selection of the appropriate suture material is important because different types of suture have different functions. Absorbable sutures are generally used on the deeper layers. The materials used include plain and chromic catgut or synthetic polymers. These sutures support the wound during the critical healing phase and then dissolve (Bourne et al., 1988). Nonabsorbable sutures are used on the epidermis and the dermis. These sutures are made of silk or a variety of synthetic materials, such as nylon,

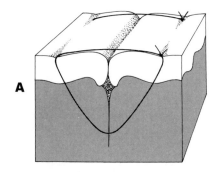 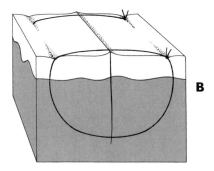

Figure 13-7 **A**, Incorrect placement of suture, causing wound edge inversion. **B**, Square interrupted suture method to ensure wound edge eversion.

polyethylene, and polypropylene. These sutures are removed when the healing process has closed the outer surface (Edlich et al., 1988).

All sutures potentially threaten the tissue defense systems and cause some inflammatory response. The trauma of needle insertion and the presence of the suture material itself increase the tissue susceptibility to infection. The extent of the tissue response depends on the chemical composition, the quantity, and the size of the suture and the individual's inherent tissue reaction (Edlich et al., 1988). Sutures made of natural fibers, such as silk or gut, produce the most tissue irritation. The smallest needle and suture for the task at hand should be used. Multiple-strand or braided sutures may be avoided because they can trap and hold bacteria. Monofilament or single-strand nylons or polypropylene are most often used for skin closure because they cause the least damage to the wound defenses (Edlich et al., 1988).

Reducing tension on the wound is the critical factor in suture placement. A wound under too much tension has the potential for increased local damage with tissue loss and possible infection (Trott, 1991). Permanent, conspicuous scarring in a railroad crosshatching fashion can result (Fernandez & Finley, 1983). Stitch hole scars also occur when pressure is on the suture line.

Wound tension can be reduced by closing the underlying layers first. Upper layer sutures must be placed at intervals to assure proper tension on the wound edges. A relationship exists between tension on the wound, the distance between stitches, and the distance of the stitch from the wound edge. The greater the tension on the wound, the closer the stitches should be to each other and to the wound edge (Dushoff, 1973). Large cuts require many small stitches to reduce the stress on the wound edge.

Sutures should be placed loosely. Traumatic wounds swell during the first few days of the inflammatory phase. As the wound swells, a snugly placed suture will quickly become too tight. Sutures should be placed loosely enough to approximate the wound edges, but not tight enough to cause tissue strangulation (Fernandez & Finley, 1983).

Wound tapes   Sterile wound tapes have advantages over sutures because they do not cause foreign body reaction and are less likely to produce infection (Martinez & Burns, 1987).

Wound tapes are used primarily in superficial, clean wounds where skin edges can be aligned easily. In deep, linear lacerations where underlying layers have been sutured, this alternative may be used to close the skin. Wound taping is also used to support the sutured wound after sutures are removed early to prevent the formation of needle puncture scars (Rodeheaver, Spengler, & Edlich, 1987). Wound tapes are popular for children because application does not require anesthesia or painful stimuli during wound closure (Richless, 1985).

Wound tapes are not indicated over joints or other body parts engaged in movement. In children and women with smooth skin, these closures provide excellent approximation of lacerations over the brow, under the chin, and across the cheek bones (Rodeheaver et al., 1987).

Before wound tapes are applied, the skin must be dry. Acetone, alcohol, or other skin preparation solvents are useful to remove skin secretions and moisture. An application of tincture of benzoin will enhance adherence of the strips to the skin. This adhesive adjunct can be toxic to tissue. Benzoin should be applied carefully as a thin film at the wound edge with a cotton-tipped applicator (Edlich et al., 1988).

Wound tapes are attached to one wound edge and then the other wound edge is pulled toward the taped edge before the remaining portion of the tape is applied to the skin. Application usually starts at one end of the wound, working toward the other end. If the wound has a slight amount of tension, a single strip should be placed at the center to reduce the tension, making even application from one end to the other easier. This anchoring strip can be replaced when working across the wound edge. Strips should be placed with caution to avoid wound edge inversion. The strips are placed along the wound so no gaping of skin occurs. The ends should be reinforced with tape to avoid rolling up of the edges. Figure 13-8 illustrates proper wound tape placement. Wound tapes are usually removed from the face in 2 to 3 days and in 5 to 10 days from other areas. When the tapes start to peel off, they are usually ready to come off.

Wound stapling   An alternative method for wound closure is the use of skin staples. Skin staples promote wound tensile strength equal to suturing (Roth & Windle, 1988). Ease of appli-

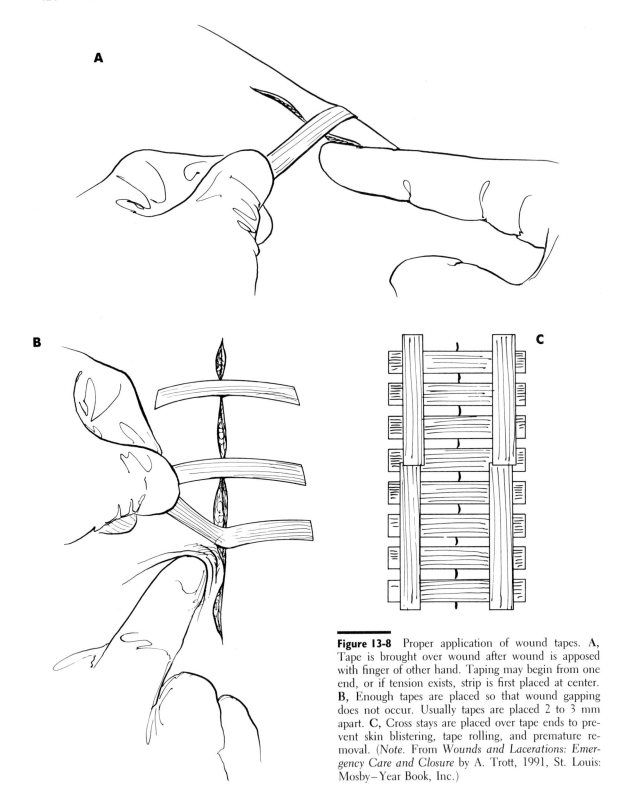

Figure 13-8 Proper application of wound tapes. **A,** Tape is brought over wound after wound is apposed with finger of other hand. Taping may begin from one end, or if tension exists, strip is first placed at center. **B,** Enough tapes are placed so that wound gapping does not occur. Usually tapes are placed 2 to 3 mm apart. **C,** Cross stays are placed over tape ends to prevent skin blistering, tape rolling, and premature removal. (*Note.* From *Wounds and Lacerations: Emergency Care and Closure* by A. Trott, 1991, St. Louis: Mosby–Year Book, Inc.)

cation with automatic stapling devices significantly decreases the time required for closure (Trott, 1991). Skin staples also cause less wound inflammatory response and have the same cosmetic effect when compared with standard suturing methods (Trott, 1991). Wound stapling can be used on linear lacerations of the scalp, trunk, and extremities. Stapling is usually avoided for hand or facial repair. Wound stapling has proven useful for temporary, quick closure of extensive wounds in trauma patients requiring immediate surgery (Trott, 1991).

Wound dressing

Most lacerations require a pressure dressing, which not only serves as a barrier to bacteria, but also compresses underlying tissue to minimize accumulation of fluids and limit dead space (Edlich et al., 1988). The pressure dressing is simply a primary dressing with the addition of a layer that provides compression. This can be done by adding a second layer of fluffed sterile gauze pads and an outer layer of conforming gauze. A pressure dressing reduces the chance of swelling. Maximal swelling occurs in 24 to 36 hours after injury, so the pressure dressing should be in place for this length of time. The pressure dressing, by the nature of its bulk, will immobilize the site of injury. Elastic wraps should be avoided, since they can exert excessive pressure on the wound site and cause circulatory complications.

Special considerations

Several frequently encountered special types of lacerations should be addressed. These lacerations are ones of the mouth, tongue, lips, nose, and ears.

Lacerations inside the mouth usually occur from crush injuries from a fall or an object jammed into the mouth. It is recommended that they be debrided and sutured (Dushoff, 1974). Mouth injuries heal rapidly. If the injury is unsutured, granulation tissue forms, leaving an uncomfortable lump. Salt water gargles (½ teaspoon salt to 8 oz. water) four times a day help keep the healing laceration clean.

The tongue is a vascular organ that heals rapidly. If lacerated and left open, it can be a source of bleeding. The tongue laceration is closed with large, absorbable sutures. Securing the tongue for repair may be difficult. A towel clip or single suture placed at the tip of the tongue after the patient is anesthetized can help to restrain this muscular organ.

Lip lacerations require careful anatomic approximation because of their cosmetic importance. The vermillion borders should be aligned exactly, because any deficit is noticeable. Local injection of an anesthetic can distort the form of the lip; therefore regional blocks are recommended for plastic repair (Richless, 1985).

If the nose is sutured, sutures must be removed early or suture tracks will remain because of the high concentration of sebaceous glands in the nasal area (Phillips & Heggers, 1988).

Ear lacerations need special attention because the skin is thin and cartilage is often exposed. Cartilage is poorly vascularized and does not hold stitches well. Careful and gentle approximation of wound edges is important because chondritis is a dreaded complication of external ear trauma. Field block anesthetic is used most often because of the limited space and unusual configuration of the ear (Trott, 1991). The dressing for the ear should serve as a splint yet not apply pressure to the area. Placement of a folded gauze pad behind the pinna next to the mastoid area supports the ear and relieves undue pressure on the cartilage when the over dressing is in place.

Patient teaching

Instructions for the patient with a laceration center around dressings and suture care. Circulation and sensation should be checked every 3 to 4 hours when a pressure dressing is in place. The dressing should stay in place for 24 to 36 hours, until maximal swelling has resolved. Patients may shower after the dressings have been removed, providing the suture line is carefully dried afterwards. Sutures are best kept dry and clean. The patient must understand the need for timely suture removal. If sutures are left in place too long, suture marks will occur. Sutures are removed early from the face, because this area is well vascularized and heals quickly. Other regions of the body heal more slowly and require sutures to be in place longer. Table 13-2 lists the normal suture removal times. Sutures are removed sooner in children, because children heal faster than adults and form suture marks sooner (Zukin & Simon, 1987). Sutures over joints should be removed later, because wounds in these areas present a greater chance of wound dehiscence secondary to movement.

Table 13-2 Suture removal timelines (in days)

Location	Adults	Children
Face	4-5	3-4
Scalp	6-7	5-6
Trunk	7-10	6-8
Arm (not joints)	7-10	5-9
Leg (not joints)	8-10	6-8
Joint		
Extensor surface	8-14	7-12
Flexor surface	8-10	6-8
Dorsum of the hand	7-9	5-7
Palm	7-12	7-10
Sole of the foot	7-12	7-10

Early suture removal (3 to 7 days) should be followed by skin tape for 7 to 10 days. The same is true for lacerations over the extensor surfaces of joints.

Note. From *Emergency Wound Care* (p. 130) by D. Zukin and R. Simon, 1987, Rockville, MD: Aspen Publishers.

Abrasions

Impaired skin integrity
Pain

Abrasions, "brush burns," or "road rashes" are the result of shearing forces that cause removal of the epidermis and the upper layers of the dermis. The nature of this injury embeds dirt and debris into the superficial layers of the dermis. Failure to remove all of this dirt and debris will result in traumatic tattooing, which is similar to a commercial tattoo (Trott, 1991). This permanent disfigurement is avoided with complete cleaning of all abrasions.

Wound preparation

Before meticulous cleaning, all abrasions require anesthesia. These wounds are painful to clean because nerve endings are exposed. For small wounds, topical anesthesia is usually sufficient. Larger wounds may require local infiltration of anesthetic to facilitate cleaning. Anesthetic is injected around the involved area in a fanning motion (Agris, 1976). For very large wounds, topical anesthetic may need to be applied in the center of the wound, a location difficult to infiltrate.

Scrubbing is the most effective method for mechanical removal of the embedded debris. Scrubbing should be done in a circular motion, using a sterile, soft-bristle toothbrush moistened with saline (King, 1984). Scrubbing should con-

tinue until all the debris is removed and slight capillary oozing occurs. Complete removal of embedded material, while avoiding further damage to injured tissues, is the key to preventing tattooing.

Wound dressing

Abrasions can be protected with a light covering of topical antibiotic ointment. This is applied four times a day after carefully removing the residual ointment from the previous application (King, 1984). The antibiotic ointment can be covered with a dry, sterile dressing if desired. The ointment keeps the wound moist, which prevents crusting. Reepithelialization occurs faster in this moist environment because the cells can move across the wound without interference from crusted wound exudate (Martinez & Burns, 1987).

Patient teaching

Patient teaching for abrasions includes dressing technique as just described and a warning about exposure to the sun. Exposure to direct sunlight must be avoided for the next 6 months (King, 1984), to prevent pigment changes in the area from over-stimulation of the melanocytes.

Avulsions

Impaired skin or tissue integrity
Pain
High risk for infection
High risk for self-care deficit
Impaired physical mobility
High risk for altered tissue perfusion
High risk for body image disturbance

Avulsions are injuries caused by a shearing force that creates a loss of tissue and prevents approximation of the wound edges. The four types of avulsions are "gouge" wounds, degloving injuries, pulping wounds, and amputations.

Gouge wounds

Gouge wounds involve removal of a section of epidermis and dermis. The missing tissue leaves a gap that must heal by secondary intention. The cardinal rule here is to "leave well enough alone" (Dushoff, 1974). This translates into meticulous cleaning with careful removal of all devitalized tissue so granulation can occur. Primary dressings are applied and left intact for long periods, allowing granulation to progress undisturbed.

Degloving injuries

Degloving injuries result from the stripping away of soft tissue from the bone by a shearing force. The most common injury site is the finger, as when a ring gets caught in machinery. Scalp and facial degloving can occur from the force of a fall, and extremity degloving can result from clothing caught in power machinery. Regardless of the mechanism of injury, the specific treatment for the wound itself is careful debridement and irrigation to create the best possible environment for good primary closure (Dula, Leicht, & Moothart, 1984). This can be accomplished only after adequate anesthesia. Large degloving injuries will require treatment in surgery with the patient under general anesthesia. The repair of a digital degloving injury can be accomplished with a regional nerve block (Richless, 1985). While the patient is effectively anesthetized, the wound and skin flap are irrigated and debrided. The skin flap is replaced and primarily closed. A compression dressing is applied to reduce swelling (Dula et al., 1984).

Pulping wounds

Pulping wounds are seen frequently after auto accidents when a patient's forehead hits the windshield with strong force. Removing all of the glass fragments is tedious but essential or the wound will "spit" glass for months after the injury. A hand vacuum is useful in removing loose glass fragments from the hair and surrounding area. Moistened cotton-tipped swabs are useful in the slow cleaning process. After the wound is thoroughly cleaned, single stitches can be used to tie down skin flaps (Trott, 1991). Overstitching must be avoided; the wounds will heal by granulation (Dushoff, 1974).

Amputations

The definitive treatment for most amputations occurs in the surgical suite. Presurgical care is focused on hemostasis of the stump and care of the amputated part. Hemostasis can be created with direct pressure and elevation of the injured part. The amputated part must be protected from dehydration and maceration. It should be placed in a container and the container surrounded with cool solution. The solution should not come in direct contact with the tissue. Keeping the part sealed from the air in a cool environment will prevent evaporation of fluid from the tissue. Refrigeration is appropriate, but *extreme* cold can destroy delicate tissue (Koszuta, 1984).

Skin grafting

Some avulsions with extensive tissue loss may require skin grafting. Some important points must be remembered about grafting. The donor site must not be a hair-bearing area unless the area to be grafted is hair-bearing. When transplanted, the hair follicles in the skin will continue to function (Cosgriff & Anderson, 1984). Grafts should be taken from areas with similar skin tones for a better cosmetic result. Selection of a donor site in an area with minimal exposure to the sun will reduce the risk of skin color change from sunlight-induced melanocyte stimulation.

Patient teaching

Patient teaching for avulsions is focused on the systemic signs of infections. Avulsion dressings are frequently left in place for as long as 10 days to avoid disruption of healing, making the observation of local response to infection impossible.

Contusions   Impaired skin and tissue integrity
High risk for fluid volume deficit
High risk for altered tissue perfusion
High risk for pain

Contusions are caused by blunt trauma to skin and underlying soft tissues. The epidermis and dermis remain intact. Crushed tissues disrupt small blood vessels in the dermis, causing bleeding. This creates the discoloration known as *ecchymosis*. Swelling from interstitial edema can occur also. Edema may damage underlying soft tissue because the pressure from increased amounts of interstitial fluid can be significant (Connolly, 1988). Treatment is aimed at comfort as well as detection and prevention of complications. Ice, elevation, and immobilization will generally control pain and swelling at the site of the injury.

Associated tissue injury

Crushing of tissue, even in the smallest contusion, can create a dimpling effect. As healing occurs, the upper layers of skin may adhere to muscle, creating an indentation. The "dimple" requires plastic surgery to correct.

Hematomas can form from bleeding into the

soft tissue. These are commonly reabsorbed without consequence and are treated with elevation and a pressure dressing to limit further bleeding (Martinez & Burns, 1987). Hematomas can become encapsulated and result in permanent subcutaneous deformity (Edlich et al., 1988). Treatment for encapsulated hematomas is incision and drainage.

The possibility of damage to underlying structures must always be considered. Fractures can easily be ruled out by x-ray study, but the underlying fascia can also be injured. In some cases this can develop into necrotizing fasciitis, a condition characterized by a rapid destruction of the subcutaneous tissue and deep fascia. Death is a common outcome (Svensson, Brookstone, & Wellsted, 1985). The development of the contusion into necrotizing fasciitis is associated with a distant area of sepsis, frequently a laceration injury sustained at the same time as the contusion. The devastating effects of an infected laceration in this case emphasize the benefits of meticulous wound care.

Another complication of contusion is compartment syndrome. This serious condition is the result of a crush injury in an area where there are tight fascial compartments (Hayden, 1983). Common locations include the anterior tibial and the deep posterior tibial compartments of the leg, the volar compartment of the forearm, and the interosseous compartments of the hand. Compartment syndrome is discussed in detail in Chapter 11.

Patient teaching

Patient teaching for contusions includes discussion about prevention of swelling and pain. The patient should receive a careful explanation of the importance of ice, elevation, and immobilization to reduce swelling and control pain. The patient must be familiar with the signs and symptoms of continued bleeding (enlarging ecchymotic area), the signs and symptoms of wound infection if other injuries are involved, and the signs and symptoms and significance of compartment syndrome.

Puncture Wounds

Impaired skin or tissue integrity
High risk for infection

Puncture wounds are penetrating wounds caused by a sharp, narrow, pointed object forced through the skin. The important issues in the assessment and treatment of puncture wounds are the presence of foreign bodies and infection. Also, a potential exists for underlying structural damage, depending on the location and depth of the puncture wound. The organ damage from an ice pick to the chest would certainly be the greatest concern from this puncture wound.

Most puncture wounds occur to extremities, with the largest percentage occurring to the feet (Edlich & Rodeheaver, 1984). The most common injury is a puncture wound from a dirty nail through a tennis shoe. In this case, bits of cloth, rubber plugs from the shoe sole, and rust can be impacted deep into the wound (Lammers, 1988). In one study of 887 patients, 8% to 15% of the puncture wounds of the foot progressed to cellulitis or localized abscess (Riley, 1984). Retained foreign bodies are frequently found in infected puncture wounds (Lammers, 1988). It is also known that a foreign body at the puncture site can increase the risk of osteomyelitis (Edlich & Rodeheaver, 1984). Given the association of retained foreign bodies and significant infection rates, it is prudent to rule out retained foreign bodies in all puncture wounds.

Assessment

The mechanism of injury is the first clue used to decide if the puncture wound is concealing a foreign body. The wound created by stepping on a dirty nail while wearing tennis shoes is more suspect than a simple puncture wound in the hand from a sewing needle. The nail, most likely found outdoors, will be forced into the foot by the weight of the body, bringing along bits of sock, shoe, and rust or dirt from the nail. In contrast, a needle creates a small wound, probably used in a much cleaner environment. This is a simple wound if the needle is intact, but becomes complex if the needle breaks off or is completely embedded.

Sharp pain with deep palpation over a puncture wound and pain associated with a mass are useful signs indicative of a hidden foreign body (Lammers, 1988). X-ray studies can sometimes assist in identifying the presence of retained foreign bodies, but frequently the objects are not radiopaque. Almost all glass can be seen on plain films because it contains lead, which is radiopaque (De Flaviis, Scaglione, Del Bo, & Nessi, 1988). Wood is not radiopaque unless it has been painted with paint containing lead, and even this does not ensure visualization. Rubber and metal can usually be viewed also (Lammers, 1988). Computed tomography, xeroradiography, and ultrasonography are used also as resources to identify and locate foreign bodies (De Flaviis et al., 1988).

Wound care

For simple, clean puncture wounds where retained foreign bodies have been ruled out, cleaning, dressing, and attention to tetanus status constitute complete wound care. Debridement and exploration are the only definitive actions when foreign bodies are suspected. A regional block is done to allow painless cleaning of the wound (Edlich & Rodeheaver, 1984). The wound is excised with a scalpel blade, punch biopsy, or cuticle clippers. Through this larger opening the wound is explored and foreign bodies and other contaminants are removed with irrigation and debridement (Lammers, 1988). The wound can be packed with fine mesh gauze and a bulky dressing applied for protection and drainage. The packing is changed daily until the wound heals (Edlich & Rodeheaver, 1984). Prophylactic antibiotics are recommended by some studies (Riley, 1984). All puncture wounds are classified as "tetanus prone" because of the chance of deep inoculation of contaminants, creating an anaerobic environment suitable to clostridium.

Special consideration: high-pressure injection injury

An uncommon yet very serious puncture wound is the high-pressure injection injury of the hand. These injuries present as small, innocuous puncture wounds. If they are left untreated, extensive tissue destruction results from the injection of the toxic substances used with these high-pressure guns. Substances such as paint, solvent, and grease are forced into the tissue at pressures as high as 12,000 pounds per square inch (psi) (Lammers, 1988). Regardless of the material injected, tissue devitalization is almost immediate and necrosis with gangrene from edema and ischemia can occur after 48 hours (Bucklew, Horner, & Diamond, 1985). Aggressive treatment with immediate, extensive decompression and debridement is necessary to prevent further damage (Schoo, Scott, & Boswick, 1980). The use of parenteral antibiotics and steroids as an adjunct to decompression and debridement therapy has proven somewhat beneficial for the treatment of this injury (Lammers, 1988).

Mammalian Bites

Impaired skin and tissue integrity
High risk for infection
High risk for body image disturbance

Mammalian bites account for 1% of all ED visits (Connolly, 1988). Dogs, cats, humans, and rodents account for about 98% of the bites. The remaining 2% result from all other species combined, including lagomorphs (rabbits), large herbivores (cows and horses), bats, and raccoons (Connolly, 1988). Dog bites constitute about 80% of these emergency visits, followed by cat bites, approximately 10%; human bites, about 5% to 10%; and rodents and other species, 2% to 5% (Kizer & Callaham 1984).

Assessment

The nurse must assess the same criteria for every type of mammalian bite. Of greatest concern is the potential for infection. All bites are inoculated with several different kinds of bacteria. The dog's mouth alone harbors more than 64 species of pathogens (Halverson, 1986). The risk of exposure to rabies is of concern in all nonhuman bites, whereas the transmission of blood-borne diseases must be evaluated for human bites. Tetanus status is vital to determine for all bite victims. The extent of damage to tissue is also an important assessment criterion. In many cases, the cosmetic implications of this injury are the greatest concern of the patient. The usual sites of animal bites, listed in order of frequency of occurrence, are the hands, arms, lower limbs, and face (Goldstein & Richwald, 1987).

Table 13-3 outlines the important characteristics of the common types of mammalian bites.

The circumstances of the bite play an important role in evaluating the risk of infection and the possibility of rabies. The time elapsed since the bite occurred is essential information in the history of all bite wounds—the longer the wound is exposed to the environment, the greater the chance of infection (Edlich et al., 1988). Because bite wounds are heavily contaminated wounds, time between injury and treatment becomes even more important. The history must also include the following information about the animal: type,

Table 13-3 Characteristics and treatment of mammalian bites

Factors	Cat	Dog	Human	Other (rodents/herbivores)
Organism	*Pasteurella multocida:* Virulent—often fulminant infection within 24 hours *Staphylococcus aureus:* usually responsible for infection after 24 hours (Goldstein & Richwald, 1987)	*S. aureus* *P. multocida:* 64 species found in a dog's mouth (Ordog, 1986)	*Eikenella corrodens:* human analog of *P. multocida* 40 species of aerobic and anaerobic streptococci and staphylococci common (Connolly, 1988)	Variety of organisms
Associated injury	Puncture wounds from needle-sharp teeth. Bone and joint penetration—possible osteomyelitis Cat scratches also introduce *P. multocida;* must be treated as bite	Crush injuries—avulsions and jagged lacerations	Occlusional—bite of assailant Self-inflicted—bite of own tongue or lip Closed-fist injury—bite of fist of an assailant, the most complicated human bite (Earley & Bardsley, 1984)	Herbivores cause crush injuries—rarely break skin
Risk of infection	20%-50% infection rate (Kizer & Callaham, 1984) Deep inoculation of bacteria	5% infection rate (Halverson, 1986)	15%-20% infection rate (Earley & Bardsley, 1984) Human mouth is a "microbial incubator" Closed-fist injury—highest risk for infection (Callaham, 1988)	Herbivores—crush injury: cannot be debrided—high risk (Callaham, 1988) Rodents seldom cause infection (Ordog et al., 1985)
Antibiotic coverage	High-dose penicillin covers *P. multocida* If *S. aureus,* add first generation cephalosporin or penicillinase-resistant penicillin	First generation cephalosporin or penicillinase-resistant penicillin (e.g., dicloxacillin) (Ordog, 1986)	Dual coverage needed: penicillin for *E. corrodens* and penicillinase-resistant penicillin for other organisms Combination drug—amoxicillin/clavulanate—covers most organisms (Goldstein, Reinhardt, Murry, & Finegold, 1984)	Each wound must be individually evaluated

relationship to the victim, current whereabouts, vaccination history, and general health. These factors can help determine the likelihood of the animal having rabies. It is also important to discover if the animal was provoked. Animals rarely bite without provocation (Kizer & Callaham,

1984). Rabid animals are the exception—they will attack without being provoked.

Infection risk

Several factors make bites at high risk for infection, as summarized in Table 13-4. Several kinds

Table 13-4 High risk factors for infection in bite wounds

Location	Type of wound	Patient population
Hand	Puncture	Age greater than 50 years
Wrist	Crush	Altered immune state
Foot		▪ asplenic
Over a joint		▪ chronic steroid use
Infant face/scalp		▪ chronic alcohol use
		▪ diabetic
		Poor nutrition
		Vascular impairment
		▪ diabetic
		▪ atherosclerosis
		Prosthetic or diseased heart valve or joint

of infection are possible from bite wounds. Localized cellulitis and abscess formation are most common (Kizer & Callaham, 1984). Lymphadenitis and lymphangitis can occur as infection spreads. Bacteremia and sepsis have been reported from mammalian bites (Callaham, 1988). Bites can also seed infection to distant parts of the body, such as prosthetic joints or valves (Kizer & Callaham, 1984). Scalp bites in infants have caused meningitis and intracranial abscess (Halverson, 1986).

Wounds that are at low risk for developing infection include bites on the face, scalp, lip, large clean lacerations, and bites from rodents (Ordog, Balasubramanium, & Wasserberger, 1985). These wounds will all do well if properly treated with meticulous wound care (Callaham, 1988).

Diagnostic tests

Laboratory studies such as Gram stain and culture are not necessary in fresh bites because the results rarely change the therapy. Infected wounds should be cultured if the antibiotic therapy fails or if the bite falls into the high-risk group, especially human bites of the hand (Kizer & Callaham, 1984). The culture should come from deep within the wound because contamination with many other organisms will occur from superficial specimens. Both aerobic and anaerobic cultures should be requested because anaerobes are present in about 70% of infected wounds (Callaham, 1991). It is helpful to list the type of wound

on the laboratory requisition (Halverson, 1986). This is especially true for human bites because *Eikenella corrodens*, the common organism isolated in human bites, is slow growing and requires a special medium (Callaham, 1988).

Whenever bony involvement is suspected, an X-ray examination is mandatory. The greatest incidence of underlying fracture is seen with craniofacial dog bites in small children and severe bite injuries of an extremity (Kizer & Callaham, 1984). The long, needle-like teeth of cats also penetrate bone (Halverson, 1986). Closed-fist injuries should be studied radiographically to look for foreign bodies, air in the joint, or osteomyelitis. As many as 70% of patients radiographed may have positive findings (Patzakis, Wilkins, & Bassett, 1987). Infection, joint penetration, and foreign bodies are all indications for hospital admission (Callaham, 1991).

Wound care

Meticulous mechanical cleaning of bite wounds is the most effective measure to reduce the chance of infection (Hurley, 1988). Irrigation is the first step. Bite wounds are irrigated with several hundred milliliters of 1% povidone-iodine solution. This solution is made by diluting the stock 10% povidone-iodine solution, using 10 parts of normal saline to 1 part of povidone-iodine (Kizer & Callaham, 1984). Although this breaks a rule of never using anything to irrigate a wound that cannot be used in the eye, the risk of infection outweighs the risk of damage to the cells. This irrigation is followed by irrigation with normal saline. Debridement is the second step of mechanical cleaning. This eliminates all crushed and devitalized tissue, as well as provides a straight wound edge. Removing this material will reduce the chance of infection approximately thirtyfold (Callaham, 1991).

There is no straight forward approach to the issue of suturing mammalian bites. Several studies have shown that properly irrigated and debrided wounds that are closed have a lower infection rate than those left open. (Kizer & Callaham, 1984). There is also a school of thought that dog bites can usually be closed and cat and human bites should never be closed (Phillips & Heggers, 1988). The definitive decision to close can be made only after evaluating each individual bite wound. High-risk wounds, such as bites to the hands or feet, bites inflicted by a cat, or bites to an immunosuppressed patient, are best left to heal by secondary intention or closed by delayed primary closure. The low-risk wounds of the face and scalp and large wounds that can be thoroughly cleaned are likely to do well with primary closure. Common sense plays an important part in balancing the need for closure against such factors as cosmetic concerns, use of the body part, and the risk of infection.

A bulky dressing is needed for every bite wound. This dressing serves three functions. First, it promotes removal of drainage from the wound because of the added layers of absorbent material. Bite wounds, particularly if not primarily closed, will form serous exudate. Second, a bulky dressing provides pressure, to obliterate dead space. The third purpose of a bulky dressing is immobilization. This is critical for all hand wounds, where movement can spread bacteria through the tissue planes (Kizer & Callaham, 1984). Infected extremities benefit from immobilization to prevent the infection from invading surrounding tissue.

Antibiotic administration

Not all victims of bite wounds need antibiotics. The practice of giving prophylactic antibiotics to every bite victim is outdated. Studies indicate that use of prophylactic antibiotics may benefit patients with high-risk wounds, but use of prophylactic antibiotics in low-risk bites is not indicated (Callaham, 1988). Irrigation and debridement are the most important factors in decreasing infection (Trott, 1991).

Frequently, patients do not receive medical attention for a few hours after inoculation of the bacteria. Oral administration of antibiotics requires several hours to demonstrate a useful blood level. Regardless of the type of bite or the antibiotic used, if antibiotics are given prophylactically to high-risk cases, the antibiotic must reach the site of inoculation rapidly (Callaham, 1988). Parenteral administration, preferably intravenous, is necessary to establish effective serum levels of the drug (Hurley, 1988). The beginning parenteral doses should be followed with a complete oral course of the antibiotic.

The decision regarding which antibiotic to administer for high-risk bites or established infections is difficult. No single agent is consistently active against all the potential bite wound pathogens (Goldstein & Richwald, 1987). The most likely infecting organism for the type of bite must be considered in choosing an antibiotic. Refer to Table 13-3 for treatment options.

Immunization

Tetanus prophylaxis   All mammalian bites are tetanus-prone wounds because they are contaminated with saliva (Halverson, 1986). The population of patients over 50 years of age account for the most tetanus cases related to bites (Callaham, 1991). Inadequate antibody levels in this group result because they have not had the required 10-year booster or were never vaccinated at all. For this group and for all bite cases, careful determination of tetanus immunization status is essential. Refer to Table 13-6, p. 442, for immunization recommendations.

Hepatitis B and HIV   For patients with human bites, the possibility of hepatitis B and HIV transmission must be evaluated. Patients bitten by known carriers of hepatitis B should receive appropriate prophylaxis. This consists of passive immunity with hepatitis B immunoglobulin (HBIG) 0.06 ml/kg as soon as possible and repeat in 3 months if active immunity has not been established with the hepatitis B vaccine. The protocol for hepatitis B vaccine is 1 ml IM on day 0, at 1 month and 6 months (Immunization Practices Advisory Committee, 1989). Bites received from HIV-infected or high-risk persons are considered low risk for HIV transmission by the Centers for Disease Control (Callaham, 1991) These wounds should be vigorously irrigated with 1% povidone-iodine, using precautions pertaining to body fluids, such as gloves and goggles (Callaham, 1991). A baseline HIV blood test with a 6 month follow-up can be obtained for patient reassurance.

Rabies prophylaxis   Rabies is a concern after every animal bite. Rabies is an acute, severe, viral infection of the central nervous system. It is nearly always fatal (Kizer & Callaham, 1984). Only three cases of recovery from rabies have been documented (Warrell & Warrell, 1988). Only one or two cases of human rabies occur in the United States annually (Callaham, 1991). Generally these cases originate outside of the country, especially in people visiting tropical countries, where rabies continues to be rampant (Fangtao et al., 1988).

At least 79% of confirmed animal rabies cases in the United States occur in wildlife (Connolly, 1988). High-risk animals include skunks, bats, raccoons, coyotes, and bobcats (Callaham, 1991). Domestic cat and dog bites are at low risk for developing rabies (Kizer & Callaham, 1984). The number of rabid dogs in the United States decreased from 8384 in 1946 to 95 in 1986 (Fishbein & Arcangeli, 1987). This reduction is primarily the result of mass vaccination.

The best defense against rabies is prevention. This is accomplished three ways: preexposure prophylaxis, postexposure treatment, and animal control.

Preexposure immunization is recommended for people engaged in high-risk activities or occupations (Kizer & Callaham, 1984). Veterinarians, animal control workers, postal workers, and spelunkers (cave explorers) have an increased risk of acquiring animal bites. Preexposure prophylaxis is usually given as a reduced regimen. The local public health department should be contacted for current area recommendations.

Postexposure treatment is extremely important. The rabies virus is fragile—it is easily destroyed by sunlight, drying, soap, and immunoglobulin (Callaham, 1991). Complete wound irrigation is an effective measure against rabies. Irrigation will reduce the concentration of rabies virus in exposed areas (Fangtao et al., 1988). The 1% povidone-iodine solution used for all bite wounds is appropriate for wounds where a low risk of rabies inoculation exists (Callaham, 1991). In situations where the risk of rabies inoculation is high, the wound should be irrigated with 1% benzalkonium chloride. This solution has been proven to kill the rabies virus (Kizer & Callaham, 1984).

Immunoprophylaxis should be considered for all animal bites deemed at high risk for rabies inoculation. Immunoprophylaxis generally consists of passive and active immunization. Passive immunization is established by injection of human rabies immunoglobulin (HRIG), 20 I.U./kg (Fishbein & Arcangeli, 1987). One half of the dose is given intramuscularly, and the remaining half is infiltrated in and around the wound for local viricidal effect (Fangtao et al., 1988). Active immunization consists of 1 ml of human diploid cell vaccine (HDCV) administered IM on days 0, 3, 7, 14, and 28 (Callaham, 1991). HDCV is known to have some side effects. Approximately

25% of patients have tenderness and itching at the injection site. Another 20% experience headache, myalgia, or nausea (Callaham, 1991). The public health department that has jurisdiction for the locality where the bite was sustained should be contacted for current area-specific recommendations (Callaham, 1991). Although serious side effects are rare, true allergic reactions have occurred and two cases of Guillain-Barré syndrome associated with HDCV immunization have been reported (Warrell & Warrell, 1988).

The most effective animal control is capture of the attacking animal. Domestic animals should be quarantined for 10 days. A vaccination history should be obtained. The animal is observed for signs of the disease. If signs develop, the animal should be sacrificed and the brain examined for the rabies virus. This is done using a fluorescent rabies antibody technique (FRA), which reveals the presence of rabies virus in the brain (Callaham, 1991). Wild animals should be destroyed and the brain examined by the FRA technique. Patient immunoprophylaxis should be started immediately after high-risk bites. If the FRA is negative, no further injections are necessary (Kizer & Callaham, 1984).

Patient teaching

Patient teaching for bite wound victims must center on the signs and symptoms of infection. The patient must have a firm understanding so in the event infection should occur, early treatment can be initiated. If an infection is established, the use of antibiotics and the expected healing course should be explained to the patient or family member. To help prevent the onset or spread of an infectious process, the importance of immobilization must be stressed. Immobilization can interfere with activities of daily living, so alternative methods of accomplishing these activities should be explored. If a threat of rabies exists, the patient or family member must understand the rabies injection schedule, the signs and symptoms of rabies, and the process of animal reporting. Local health departments are good resources for patients and nursing personnel.

GENERAL INTERVENTIONS
Patient Preparation

Fear and anxiety can create a less cooperative patient, decreasing the chance of maximal repair outcome. The psychologic considerations, such as providing reassurance, establishing rapport, assuring patient understanding, and using appropriate language, enhance cooperation and comfort the patient.

Appropriate positioning of the patient and adequate attention to the patient's physical comforts (e.g., empty bladder, warmth) are necessary to consider before initiating wound care. When dealing with children, the use of restraints may be necessary for patient protection.

Staff Preparation

The nurse should wear gloves, goggles, and a mask while examining the wound. This protects the patient from further wound contamination, such as droplet contamination from the examiner's mouth or introduction of new organisms from the hands (Edlich et al., 1988). Adhering to these wound precaution techniques protects the nurse from contracting bloodborne diseases. Gowns or aprons should be worn by the nurse during wound cleaning and whenever proximate to a draining wound. The appearance of some wounds is quite shocking, and staff should prepare themselves, support one another, and avoid alarming the patient.

Wound Preparation—Anesthesia

Anesthetizing the wound before treatment creates patient comfort, which is necessary to accomplish optimal cleaning. Trauma nurses should ensure that anesthesia is considered before cleaning. General anesthesia may sometimes be required to repair large, complicated wounds. If the maximal dose of local anesthetic is needed to do the repair, the concern for toxicity dictates the patient be transferred to the operating room.

Nitrous oxide

Nitrous oxide, delivered as 50% N_2O and 50% O_2, is a rapidly acting, patient-administered, safe alternative for pain control (Proehl, 1985; Stewart, 1985). This gas is a potent analgesic with weak anesthesia properties. It has been shown to be an effective agent for adults and children over 7 years of age undergoing laceration repair (Gamis, Knapp, & Glenski, 1989). Nitrous oxide is self-administered with a face mask or mouthpiece. As sedation increases, the seal between the mask and face or mouthpiece and lips is broken because the patient cannot hold the mask or

mouthpiece in place. The negative inspiratory demand valve that regulates the delivery of the gas cannot be triggered; therefore the patient controls the dose. The delivery system should never be anchored to the patient's face. It should be used only for patients who can hold the mask independently (Proehl, 1985).

Local anesthetic agents

A variety of local anesthetic agents are used in the treatment of surface trauma. The most common are lidocaine and bupivacaine, which can be administered topically or by injection.

Topical preparations   Frequently used external preparations are topical lidocaine solution, 2% to 4%; lidocaine jelly, 2.5%; and TEC solution (tetracaine, epinephrine, and cocaine). These products provide rapid, complete anesthesia without injection. Topicals work best on small abrasions and avulsions before cleaning. Depending on the extent of the abrasion or avulsion, the effect of external agents may create total anesthesia or at least make cleaning bearable. They are not absorbed through intact skin. Topical solutions are applied by pouring onto sterile gauze, which is placed directly over the wound and left in place for 5 to 10 minutes to take effect. If not enough time is allowed to induce anesthesia effect, unnecessary pain and fear can be created. Topical solution can sting when applied. Jelly can be used as a vehicle to remove dirt painlessly. It is water soluble and easily removable. The length of action for most topicals is 20 to 30 minutes.

TEC solution   TEC solution, also known as TAC (tetracaine, adrenaline, and cocaine), has become a popular agent because of good anesthesia properties and vasoconstrictive actions. There is some concern that the vasoconstrictive characteristics of TEC may increase susceptibility to infection by limiting access of defense cells to the wound (Barker, Rodeheaver, Edgerton, & Edlich, 1982). A recent study has shown that TEC does not increase bacterial proliferation; thus the concern about increased susceptibility to infection from TEC is questionable (Martin, Doezema, Tandberg, & Umland, 1990). TEC has advantages for children because a painful injection can be avoided and adequate anesthesia is reported (Anderson, Colecchi, Baronoski, & DeWitt, 1990). TEC is best used in small amounts to prevent systemic absorption. Careful monitoring of the vital signs is warranted to detect any signs of systemic effect, such as tachycardia or hypertension, although these side effects do not occur often (Fitzmaurice et al., 1990). Caution should be used when explaining the application of TEC to patients and families, especially when the patient is a child. The antidrug programs taught at many schools often emphasize the dangers of cocaine use; consequently, thoughtful explanation is needed to prevent anxiety for the patient and family (Weiss, 1989). Statistically, equivalent levels of anesthesia can be achieved with the deletion of cocaine, an increased concentration of tetracaine, and a decreased concentration of epinephrine (Trott, 1991). The deletion of cocaine from the solution eliminates the concern about the use of a controlled substance, making the choice of this variation of anesthetic solution even more attractive.

Injectable preparations   The solutions most frequently used for injection are lidocaine and bupivacaine. Injectables are used for large area abrasions, lacerations, deep puncture wounds, and avulsions. Table 13-5 summarizes the properties of these injectable agents.

Lidocaine with epinephrine   Epinephrine prolongs the duration of the effects of lidocaine by vasoconstriction, which delays absorption. This vasoconstriction reduces bleeding in vascular areas such as the face and scalp. It should be used with caution in places with low vascularity (fingers, toes, ears), because of the vasoconstrictive action. Lidocaine with epinephrine also diminishes the risk of systemic anesthetic toxicity because of the slower absorption rate of the drug. (Larrabee, Lanier, & Miekle, 1987). The epinephrine may delay wound healing, increase infection rates, and promote tissue necrosis by lim-

iting circulation to the injected area (Larrabee et al., 1987).

Bupivacaine   Bupivacaine (Marcaine) is used for extensive repairs because it is long acting (Spivey, McNamara, MacKenzia, Bhat, & Burdick, 1987). It is often used for regional blocks, which are useful in digit and facial injuries. These areas have limited space for expansion, and anesthesia injected directly into the wound can distort wound edges or create a tight compartment.

Administration   Anesthetics are usually injected into the dermal layer through the wound edge, as illustrated in Figure 13-9. Another method is to inject through the intact skin around the injury. This may be prudent for grossly contaminated wounds to prevent deep inoculation of bacteria (Richless, 1985). Injection through the wound edge produces less pain (Zukin & Simon, 1987). Injecting the solution slowly into the tissue, using a small-gauge needle (25- to 30-gauge), also reduces the pain of infiltration.

The acidic nature of local anesthetic solutions contributes to the discomfort of administration. A way to further reduce painful infiltration is to add sodium bicarbonate ($NaHCO_3$) to anesthetic solutions (Bartifield, Gennis, Barbera, Breuer, & Gallagher, 1990). By buffering the acidic pH, the injection is virtually pain free. The ratio of local anesthetic to $NaHCO_3$ is 10 parts anesthetic to 1 part $NaHCO_3$ solution. It is recommended that the mixture be prepared immediately before use. This eliminates concern regarding shortened shelf life of anesthetics caused by buffering (Christoph, Buchanan, Begalla, & Schwartz, 1988).

Local anesthetics can be administrated by us-

Table 13-5 Commonly used injectable anesthetics

Drug	Maximum dose	Onset of action	Length of action
Lidocaine (plain): 0.25%-2%	4.5 mg/kg	5-10 min	30-60 min
Lidocaine with epinephrine	7 mg/kg	5-10 min	60-90 min
Bupivacaine: 0.25%-0.5%	175 mg	5-10 min	3-6 hr

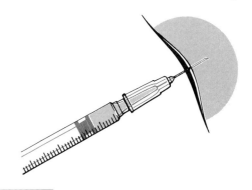

Figure 13-9   Local infiltration. Anesthetic is injected into wound edge, causing less pain than injecting through intact skin.

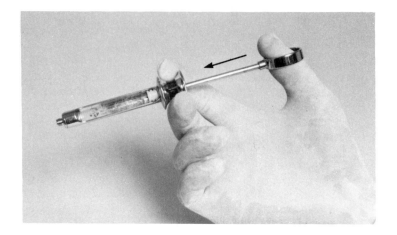

Figure 13-10 Spring-loaded cartridge for local anesthetic administration. (*Note.* From *Handbook of Local Anesthesia* [3rd ed.] by S.F. Malamed, 1990, St. Louis: Mosby–Year Book, Inc.)

ing a spring-loaded cartridge, as shown in Figure 13-10. Before treatment is begun, the effectiveness of anesthesia should be tested by gently pricking the area with a sterile needle.

Allergic reactions to local anesthetics are rare (Chandler, Grammer, & Patterson, 1987). A dilemma occurs when a patient states an allergy to local anesthetics. Pure lidocaine is rarely the offending agent. The allergy is usually (1) a reaction to the epinephrine in anesthetic agents, manifested as rapid heart rate and flushing; or (2) an allergic reaction (e.g., hives, flushing, mild respiratory distress) to the preservatives in the anesthetic agent (Swanson, 1983). Regular doses of lidocaine may be administered 30 minutes after giving a small (0.1 ml) intradermal test dose, providing no reaction occurs (Swanson, 1983).

The use of local injectable anesthetics involves precautions that must be observed which are summarized as follows:

1. Use the weakest effective solution to minimize the incidence of reactions.
2. Be familiar with the characteristics of the drug, and be aware of the total amount infiltrated. Do not exceed the maximum dose to avoid toxicity. Signs and symptoms of "caine" toxicity are shivers, shakes, tremors, euphoria or lethargy, convulsions, and cardiac arrest.
3. Be aware of the properties of lidocaine with epinephrine, as just described. Store lido-

caine with epinephrine in a different location from lidocaine, to prevent errors.
4. The use of one standard concentration of lidocaine reduces the possibility of dosage errors.
5. Avoid injecting excessive amounts of the anesthetic at the wound site. It can distort landmarks and tissue edges, resulting in scar formation or improper alignment (Martinez & Burns, 1987). Here a higher concentration anesthetic is useful, because less volume is required to produce anesthesia.

Wound Preparation—Cleaning

The primary objective of wound cleaning is to support the power of healing inherent in the tissue itself. This can be accomplished by using the appropriate wound cleaning agent and complete mechanical cleaning.

Agents

An appropriate wound cleaner is nontoxic, does not damage cells, has a high level of cleaning ability, is painless, and does not potentiate infection. The rule of thumb in choosing a wound cleaner is "never to use an agent to irrigate the wound that could not be used to irrigate the eye" (Martinez & Burns, 1987). A physiologic solution such as sterile normal saline can be used to dislodge foreign material without causing further injury to traumatized tissue. Another suitable cleaning agent is a nontoxic surfactant, poloxamer 188 (Shur Clens). The lubricating quality of this product reduces surface tension, facilitating the removal of debris (Rodeheaver, Kurtz, Kircher, & Edlich, 1980). It is particularly useful in the removal of tar and grease. Its painless application lends itself to pediatric and facial cases (Edlich et al., 1988).

Examples of inappropriate wound cleaners are povidone-iodine (Betadine), hexachlorophene (pHisoHex), and chlorhexidine gluconate (Hibiclens). Although they contain chemicals that effectively kill bacteria, these agents damage tissue defenses by causing inflammation, invite infection by destroying white and red blood cells, and cause considerable pain (Edlich et al., 1988). Other agents such as alcohol and hydrogen peroxide are also contraindicated as wound cleaners because of their caustic effects on tissue (Zukin & Simon, 1987). The box below outlines the toxicity of these solutions.

Several studies indicate that povidone-iodine antiseptic solution offers no therapeutic benefit in contaminated wounds (Edlich et al., 1988; Rodeheaver et al., 1982; Faddis, Daniel, & Boyer, 1977). One study reported a reduced infection rate in lacerations after a 60-second scrub with a dilute 1% povidone-iodine solution: 1 part 10% povidone-iodine solution to 10 parts saline (Gravett, Sterner, Clinton, & Ruiz, 1987). These wounds were also irrigated with large amounts of saline and debrided, both of which are measures that decrease the chance of infection in lacerations without the use of 1% povidone-iodine solution. Another study, comparing saline, Shur Clens, and 1% povidone-iodine solution as wound irrigation solutions, found no significant difference in infection rates (Dire, Hood, & Welsh, 1990). Povidone-iodine, because of its antimicrobial effect, reduces the number of bacteria on intact skin. It continues to be an ideal agent for preoperative disinfection of *intact* skin (Richless, 1985).

Methods

The key to proper wound cleaning is mechanical action (Trott, 1991; Dire et al., 1990). This is effectively accomplished by high-pressure irrigation, scrubbing, and debridement. These techniques can remove up to 90% of the contaminating bacteria in the wound (Richless, 1985). It must be remembered that the wound environment is the major concern. Bacteria will not grow where the conditions are not favorable. Mechanical cleaning alters the environment. The critical factor is the amount of bacteria removed, not the type of bacteria present.

High-pressure irrigation removes particulate matter from the wound. The preferred method is fluid delivered through an 18- or 19-gauge needle or plastic catheter with a 35-ml syringe (Rogness, 1985; Stevenson et al., 1976; Trott, 1991). This simple and practical system delivers the adequate hydraulic force, which is reported to be about 7 to 8 pounds per square inch (psi) when maximal amount of pressure is applied to the plunger (Edlich et al., 1988; Rogness, 1985; Stotts, 1983). Smaller syringes are clinically impractical because they can not provide the sustained stream or the large volume required to remove debris (Edlich et al., 1988). At least 200 ml of pressurized fluid is recommended. The tip of the needle or catheter should be placed as close to the surface of the wound as possible. This proximity will contribute to increased force of the irrigation. There are commercially available irrigation systems, such as Irrijet, with a spring-activated syringe for rapid refilling. These are easy to use and save time. The pulsing lavage devices, sold commercially for home oral care, are effective for irrigation when used with caution. Careful regulation of low pressure is required to prevent further damage to fragile tissue.

Toxicity of topical solutions

Saline = 0
Poloxamer 188 = 0
Povidone-iodine solution = 1+
Hydrogen peroxide = 6+
Povidone-iodine and detergent = 8+ (Betadine surgical scrub)
Hexachlorophene and detergent = 8+ (pHisoHex)
Chlorhexidine gluconate = 8+ (Hibiclens)
Isopropyl alcohol = 10+

Saline (0) is the standard. The higher the number, the more caustic the solution.

Note. From *Emergency Wound Care* (p. 30) by D. Zukin and R. Simon, 1987, Rockville, MD: Aspen Publishers.

Scrubbing a contaminated wound with a sponge has proven to be an effective means of removing bacteria (Edlich et al., 1988). Highly abrasive surgical brushes and sponges can traumatize tissue and impair the wound's ability to resist infection. The optimal sponge is soft and porous. In the case of deeply embedded debris, a stiffer brush, forcep, or scalpel may be needed to remove all foreign material, thus preventing the tattooing effect discussed earlier.

Debridement, a term coined by Napoleon's surgeon general, is the mechanical removal of devitalized tissue and foreign bodies (Martinez & Burns, 1987). Any material left in the wound will potentiate infection. Removal of tissue is done using forceps and scalpel to limit further trauma.

Wound soaking is not recommended. This technique is used as a temporizing measure until contaminated wounds can be completely cleaned and debrided. A recent study found that soaking wounds in 1% povidone-iodine solution did not reduce infection rates and saline soaks actually increased the wound bacterial counts (Lammers, Fourré, Callaham, & Boone, 1990).

Wound Closure

Specific wound closure is governed by the individual type of soft tissue injury. Definitive treatment for each type of surface trauma was discussed earlier in this chapter.

Dressings

After the wound has been treated, a functional dressing should be applied. A wound dressing protects the wound from external contaminants and compresses underlying tissues, minimizing accumulation of fluids and limiting dead space. It also immobilizes the area and keeps the wound moist, providing a "physiologic environment conducive to epithelial migration from wound edges across surface of the fresh wound" (Edlich et al., 1988).

Most wounds require a primary dressing. A primary gauze dressing consists of two parts. The first layer is a sterile, nonadhering layer that is in direct contact with the skin. The second is the sterile, absorbing layer. Synthetic dressings also may be employed as a primary dressing.

Gauze dressings The nonadhering quality of the first layer is important, to avoid disruption of healing and minimize pain. Fine mesh and pe-troleum jelly–impregnated gauze are commonly used because of their nonadhering qualities. If coarse mesh gauze is used directly against the wound, the gauze can become enmeshed in the dried exudate from the wound. This can cause both pain to the patient and the risk of premature removal of newly regenerated epidermis when the dressing is changed (May & Still, 1987). Coarse gauze dressings also have the disadvantage of shedding small particles and fibers into the wound, risking a foreign body reaction. The commercial dressings that are impregnated with antimicrobial agents such as scarlet red have shown no advantage in wound healing (May & Still, 1987; Gemberling, 1976). The significant quality for the first layer of the primary dressing is the fine gauge of the material. This covering also prevents dehydration. If wounds are kept moist, epithelialization proceeds more rapidly (Hunt, 1988).

The second layer of the primary dressing absorbs drainage and provides additional protection. The absorbing layer gains particular importance for complicated or contaminated wounds with the potential for infection. These wounds, compared with minor wounds and lacerations, are more likely to ooze exudate (Trott, 1991). The second layer of the primary dressing absorbs excess exudate, but still allows the wound to remain moist. The use of 4×4 sponges and large gauze pads as the absorbent layer can further support and immobilize the wound.

Synthetic dressings Transparent film dressings are widely used to maintain the microenvironment of the wound (Katz, McGinley, & Leyden, 1986). These occlusive wound dressings (Tegaderm, Op-site, Bioclusive) are water-vapor permeable, transparent, and easy to apply. External oxygen can penetrate the dressing to maintain an aerobic environment. The trapped wound exudate fluid provides nutrients and maintains relatively normal biochemistry for reepithelialization (May & Still, 1987). The accumulation of excessive moist exudate creates a culture medium for microorganisms to grow. It may be difficult to distinguish between normal wound exudate and infection. Accumulated fluid may be removed manually with a syringe and a fine-gauge needle. Although these dressings are an ideal primary covering, excessive exudate accumulation makes it difficult to keep the dressing in place (Edlich et al., 1988). A border of intact, uninjured skin around the wound is required for adhesion.

Recent research has shown that optimal wound healing occurs in an environment that reduces scar formation, prevents dehydration, maintains near physiologic temperature, and prevents bacterial contamination (Wayne, 1985). Semiocclusive, semipermeable dressings, such as Epi-Lock, maintain a 37° C temperature, which keeps the epithelial cell mitotic rate high for faster reepithelialization and maintains an environment that maximizes the phagocytosis of bacteria and wound debris (May & Still, 1987). These dressings offer significant benefits in the quality and rate of wound healing because of the environment they create. Epi-Lock is placed over the wound using surgical tapes, elastic net, or gauze wraps.

Another synthetic dressing used for short-term healing of partial-thickness wounds is Biobrane. This semiocclusive dressing is translucent, which facilitates wound visualization. It is made of nylon and silcone, which allows it to be flexible in all directions for full range of motion and patient comfort. Biobrane creates an environment similar to Epi-Lock, with the advantage of strong adherence to the wound (May & Still, 1987).

Nonadherent primary dressings can be held in place by a variety of attachments. Expandable mesh gauze rolls secure the dressing and conform to the patient's anatomy. Digit dressings can be secured with tube gauze creatively applied to allow visualization of capillary refill. Tape is often necessary to fasten the dressing to the skin. Hypoallergenic tapes are preferred and should be applied *around* the wound, not over. Taping over the dressing with nonporous tape traps excessive moisture, providing a medium for bacteria. Tape should never be applied completely around an extremity, because this may impede circulation from circumferential pressure as edema evolves.

Wound immobilization   Immobilization of the wound is needed to avoid disruption of the healing process. This is easily accomplished with complete dressing and splinting when the wound is over a joint. Of special concern is the hand. The hand must be dressed in the position of function, as shown in Figure 13-11. This position allows the metacarpophalangeal joint ligaments to be immobilized at their maximum length. When immobilized, ligaments tighten. Consequently, if they are immobilized in the shortened position, hand movement may be restricted when the dressing is removed (Connolly, 1988).

Averting Complications
Antibiotics

Antibiotic treatment is sometimes recommended for traumatic soft tissue wounds that have a high probability of infection (Trott, 1991). Sev-

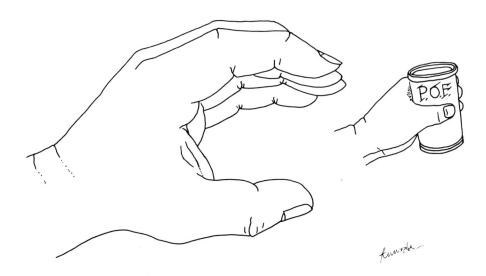

Figure 13-11   Correct hand position to maintain function.

eral types of wounds should be considered for antibiotic therapy. Wounds that have been open to the environment for extended or unknown periods of time are always suspect. Wounds of the hands and feet are prone to infection because of their distal anatomic location and exposure to greater environmental hazards. Facial wounds are less likely to become infected because of the vascular location. Wounds that are dirty or contaminated exhibit a higher incidence of infection, especially if contaminated with saliva, feces, or vaginal secretions. Wounds with extensive tissue damage are susceptible to infection because local tissue defenses are weakened.

Antibiotics should be administered as soon as possible after the traumatic event, while bacterial colony counts are low (Trott, 1991). Clinical studies show that antibiotics given preoperatively are more effective (Edlich et al., 1988). The objective of antibiotic therapy is to reach an effective blood concentration before or at the time of wound closure. Administration by the intravenous route results in the highest concentration and is frequently used in place of oral antibiotic administration (Edlich et al., 1988). Wound irrigation with antibiotic solutions is sometimes used to get early, high wound fluid concentrations of antimicrobials (Callaham, 1988).

Tetanus prophylaxis

Tetanus is a devastating neurologic disease with a 40% to 60% mortality. Approximately 50 deaths per year are reported in the United States (Giangrasso & Smith, 1985). Two thirds of the recent cases in the United States have followed surface trauma (Edlich et al., 1988). Meticulous wound care and proper immunization are the critical components in prophylaxis against tetanus.

Tetanus prophylaxis, when indicated, should occur within 72 hours from the time of injury. The tetanus bacillus *Clostridium tetani* is usually inoculated as a spore found in dirt, saliva, and feces (Knezevich, 1986). After this 72-hour "window of opportunity," the toxin from the spore may not be destroyed by the tetanus toxoid.

The decision to give tetanus immunization at the time of treatment depends on the patient's immunization history and the condition of the wound. Table 13-6 outlines the recommendations for tetanus prophylaxis.

The condition of the wound is evaluated to determine if it is tetanus prone. The box below lists the criteria for tetanus-prone wounds. A wound with any one of these clinical findings is considered dirty and more prone to infection. These tetanus-prone wounds dictate the recommendations for "All other wounds" outlined in Table 13-6.

The immunization history is essential to assure proper treatment. Patients older than 7 years require a booster of tetanus and diphtheria toxoid (Td) every 10 years, providing there is a history of primary immunization. Primary immunization, which provides active immunity, is a series of three doses of Td, the first two given 4 weeks apart and the third dose given 6 months after the second. If there is no history of primary immunization, passive immunity with tetanus immuno-

Table 13-6 Recommendations for tetanus prophylaxis

History of tetanus immunization (doses)	Clean and minor wounds		All other wounds	
	Td (a)	TIG (b)	Td	TIG
Uncertain	Yes	No	Yes	Yes
0-1	Yes	No	Yes	Yes
2	Yes	No	Yes	No (e)
3 or more	No (c)	No	No (d)	No

a Tetanus and diphtheria toxoid (Td)
b Tetanus immunoglobulin (TIG)
c Unless more than 10 years since last dose
d Unless wound is more than 24 hours old
e Unless more than 5 years since last dose

Note. From "ACIP Guidelines: Diphtheria, Tetanus, and Pertussis. Guidelines for Vaccine Prophylaxis and Other Preventive Measures,"—US 1985. *MMWR* 34, pp. 405-426, 1985.

Tetanus-prone wounds

- Exposed more than 6 hours
- Irregular configuration
- Puncture wounds
- Crush, burn, or frostbite injury
- Any sign of infection
- Devitalized tissue present
- Contaminated with saliva, feces, or soil

globulin (TIG) must be considered (American College of Emergency Physicians, 1986).

Immunization recommendations for children younger than 7 years are different. Primary immunization for children usually includes four doses spaced over the first 18 months and a booster in the fourth to sixth year. These immunizing doses include tetanus, diphtheria, and pertussis. The incidence and severity of pertussis is much greater in children age 7 and younger. Boosters after age 7 do not need to include the pertussis vaccine. Children younger than 7 years may also require passive tetanus immunity at the time of injury if the primary series is incomplete (American College of Emergency Physicians, 1987).

The National Vaccine Injury Act of 1986 requires healthcare providers to record the provider's name, address, and title; the type of tetanus vaccine given; the manufacturer; the lot number; and the date of administration for every tetanus immunization given. This information must be recorded on the patient's permanent medical record or in a permanent office log or file (Immunization Practices Advisory Committee, 1989).

The adverse reactions from the immunization are generally minor. Local erythema and induration are common, as well as mild fever and malaise. The only contraindication to tetanus immunization is a history of a severe hypersensitivity or neurologic response to a previous dose (Edlich at el., 1988).

Overimmunization creates a potential for increased adverse reactions to tetanus immunization. Td boosters are most often inappropriately administered to patients who have clean wounds and have been immunized within the past 10 years (Giangrasso & Smith, 1985). A complete history and strict attention to recommended tetanus prophylaxis standards can prevent this problem. The 72-hour "window of opportunity" allows the time to check immunization history, which is especially important for repeat patients or patients with altered consciousness.

Patient Teaching

Patient teaching is an essential ingredient in the wound treatment plan, since patient understanding is the basis for compliance. Several general concepts about wounds can be taught by the nurse to the patient.

Before patient discharge, specific instruction about when to change the dressing and how long to leave the dressing in place should be given. The use of ice, elevation, and immobilization should be encouraged to prevent swelling and reduce pain. The nurse should explain any application of medication to be used directly on the wound and should describe the signs and symptoms of infection, local and systemic, including advice for follow-up care if these occur.

Disfigurement is frequently a concern after injuries. An explanation about wound healing and scar maturation can lessen the anxious patient's apprehension. Because minor reactions to tetanus immunization are not uncommon, a brief explanation about reactions can be reassuring. Analgesics may be prescribed for wound pain. The nurse should explain their use to the patient. When over-the-counter analgesics are recommended and bleeding is a concern, the patient should be advised not to take aspirin. Wound-specific information should be included in patient instructions. Special considerations for common types of surface trauma are detailed earlier in this chapter.

Patient teaching is best followed with written instructions (Dames, 1991). The instructions should outline major points and include a list of supplies and directions for follow-up care (Trott, 1991).

SUMMARY   Numerous specialists assess the patient during ED care, and dressings and splints are often removed or displaced. An alert nurse can assure that optimal wound care is maintained during resuscitation, diagnostic testing, and definitive treatment.

It is important, if possible, for the initial treatment of surface trauma to occur before the patient is admitted to the intensive care unit. If wounds are not cleaned, they may be hidden under dressings and not noticed in time to prevent complications. Ideally, wounds should be cleaned and dressed in the ED or the operating room. Tetanus prophylaxis must be addressed early in the treatment plan. If this initial treatment is not completed, that fact must be clearly conveyed to the receiving staff.

The table on p. 444 outlines the nursing diagnoses and evaluative criteria for the patient with surface trauma.

Nursing diagnosis	Nursing intervention	Evaluative criteria
Impaired tissue integrity Related to structural defect As manifested by open wound, mottling of tissue	**Promote tissue healing** Assist with wound closure. Control bleeding with pressure. Apply sterile dressing to exposed tissue.	Hemostasis of wound will occur. Skin integrity will be re-established.
High risk for infection Related to disruption of skin barrier	**Prevent infection** Administer antibiotics as indicated. Administer tetanus toxoid and/or tetanus immunoglobulin (TIG). Assess wound for degree of contamination, mechanism of injury, and length of exposure. Administer meticulous mechanical cleaning. Apply protective dressing.	Wound cultures will be negative. No redness, swelling, or drainage will be present. Patient will be afebrile.
High risk for pain Related to edema, neural stimulation	**Promote comfort** Administer local anesthesia. Administer analgesia. Apply ice, and elevate. Provide immobilization with splints and dressings. Use distraction techniques.	Patient's self-rating score of pain on scale of 1 to 10 will decrease.
Impaired physical mobility Related to tissue impairment, pain, need for stablization As evidenced by guarding of injured body part, presence of splint	**Promote self-care** Administer analgesics. Apply appliances as needed (splints, slings, etc.). Refer to physical therapy. Teach alternative ADL techniques to patient and family.	Patient's impaired mobility will have minimal effect on activities of daily living.
Body image disturbance Related to edema, disfigurement As evidenced by verbal comments, social withdrawal	**Promote adjustment** Initiate referral to plastic surgeon if indicated. Teach patient and family about wound healing and scar behavior. Spend time listening.	Patient will understand. Patient will verbalize concerns.
High risk for altered tissue perfusion Related to edema, bleeding	**Promote perfusion to injured area** Encourage avoidance of clamps, tourniquets, and blind probing, unless essential to hemostasis. Apply ice and elevate injured part after insult, to minimize edema. Avoid circumferential, tight dressings.	Skin color will be normal. Capillary refill will be less than 2 seconds. Distal temperature will be normal.
High risk for sensory/perceptual alterations Related to disruption of sensory nerves	**Prevent sensory loss** Assess sensory distribution. Teach patient regarding numbness, which can occur secondary to edema versus serious nerve damage.	Patient will be able to feel sharp and dull sensations, temperature changes. Patient will report changes in sensation.

CASE STUDY   Robert Smith, an 18-year-old, was injured while trying to get out of a construction site guarded by dogs. As he was scrambling up a fence, one of the dogs bit his left leg and he lacerated his right cheek on the wire fencing. Going over the top of the fence, he fell to the ground, landing on his left side in the dirt. He sustained an abrasion over his forehead and left cheek, as well as a large contusion involving his left shoulder. Robert waited until Monday morning to seek medical care. On presentation, he was febrile and the bite wound was draining purulent exudate. Cellulitis involving the distal half of the lower leg was present. The cheek laceration was covered with dried blood and inflamed at the wound edges. The abrasion was embedded with debris and covered with purulent exudate. A large ecchymotic area was present around the left shoulder and upper arm.

What method of mechanical cleaning would be used for the bite wound?

Irrigation with 1% povidone-iodine, using a 35-ml syringe and 18-gauge needle, followed by irrigation with normal saline. It is important to remove all of the exudate from this wound and kill the present bacteria. This, in conjunction with antibiotic therapy, will treat the infection. When infection is not present in bite wounds, the treatment still includes irrigation with 1% providone-iodine solution. Bite wounds are heavily contaminated with many organisms. The bactericidal effect of this antiseptic solution is necessary to reduce the numbers of bacteria, despite the cytocidal effect on tissue. It also has viricidal properties, important when rabies is considered.

What special treatment modalities are required for the bite wound?

Intravenous antibiotics followed by a course of oral antibiotics are indicated because of the obvious wound infection. A wide-spectrum antibiotic is needed.

Evaluation of the need for rabies vaccination is indicated. In this case the location and history of the dog can be easily investigated.

Evaluation of tetanus status is required. This bite wound is considered to be tetanus prone because of the contamination by saliva, which can be the vehicle of transmission. The other wounds are tetanus prone because treatment was delayed and infection is present. Robert presented himself for treatment within the 72-hour limit, making tetanus prophylaxis warranted. If Robert is unsure of his immunization status, he will require Td and TIG.

Explain the desired method of closure for the bite wound and the cheek laceration.

The bite wound will be allowed to heal by secondary intention. Because of the obvious infection, suturing this wound is contraindicated. A cosmetic result is not of primary concern because of the location of this wound.

Delayed primary closure is indicated for the cheek laceration. This will done as soon as the possibility of infection is eliminated—3 to 5 days into the course of antibiotics. For the best cosmetic result, wounds should be closed before much granulation tissue has formed.

Describe the important patient instruction Robert will need to receive about his abrasion to avoid long-term complications.

Robert must avoid exposure of the abraded area to the sun for approximately 6 months. The sun can stimulate the melanocytes and cause uneven color changes.

What serious complication involving the shoulder contusion must be considered?

Because areas distant from the contusion are infected, necrotizing fasciitis is a possibility. The contused area should be carefully evaluated for increased pain or inflammation.

RESEARCH QUESTIONS

- Is there a difference in cosmetic result, perception of pain, and infection rate when abrasions are initially cleaned during immersion in a fluid medium "tank" versus at the bedside without immersion?
- What techniques are effective in diminishing the perception of pain during wound cleaning/irrigation?
- What meaning do physical scars of trauma have to patients posttrauma?
- Do dressings remain in place until the ordered date for recheck or dressing change? If not, why?
- Do patients report self-knowledge or nurse instruction for redressing their wound in the event that the dressing does not stay clean and dry until the date for recheck or dressing change?
- When is the added expense of a plastic surgeon's skill justified in repair of traumatic wounds? What criteria aid in the decision?
- What factors contribute to animal bites in children and adults? Can education decrease the risk?

RESOURCES

American Society of Plastic and Reconstructive Surgical Nurses
Box 56
North Woodbury Rd.
Pitman, NJ 08071
(609) 589-6247

International Association for Enterostomal Therapy
2081 Business Center Dr., Suite 290
Irvine, CA 92715
(714) 476-0268

ANNOTATED BIBLIOGRAPHY

Dushoff, I. (1973). A stitch in time. *Emergency Medicine, 2* (1), 1-16.
Article that presents the basic principles of suturing in a timeless, fundamental format, although somewhat dated. Several helpful "tricks of the trade," threaded throughout, make this interesting reading.

Dushoff, I. (1974). About face. *Emergency Medicine, 3* (11), 26-77.
Classic manuscript that details the management of surface trauma to the face. Many general wound treatment concepts are incorporated into the engaging text.

Edlich, R., Rodeheaver, G., Morgan, R., Berman, D., & Thacker, J. (1988). Principles of emergency wound management. *Annals of Emergency Medicine, 17* (12), 1284-1302.
Comprehensive review of wound management, focusing on scientific rationale with complete descriptions for clinical application.

Martinez, J., & Burns, C. (1987) Wound management. *Current Concepts in Wound Care, 10* (8), 9-16.
Excellent summary and discussion of the management of surface trauma, with emphasis on abrasions and lacerations. Several general wound treatment techniques are presented in an easily readable format.

Trott, A. (1991). *Wounds and lacerations: Emergency care and closure.* St. Louis: Mosby–Year Book, Inc.
Practical guide for the treatment of acute wounds. This book offers a step-by-step approach to wound care, augmented by several excellent, helpful illustrations.

REFERENCES

Agris, J. (1976). Traumatic tattooing. *Journal of Trauma, 16* (10), 798-802.

American College of Emergency Physicians (1986). Tetanus immunization recommendations for persons 7 years of age and older. *Annals of Emergency Medicine, 15* (9), 1111-1112.

American College of Emergency Physicians (1987). Tetanus immunization recommendations for persons less than 7 years old. *Annals of Emergency Medicine, 16* (10), 1181-1183.

Anderson, A., Colecchi, C., Baronoski, R., & DeWitt, T. (1990). Local anesthesia in pediatric patients: Topical TAC versus lidocaine. *Annals of Emergency Medicine, 19* (5), 519-522.

Barker, W., Rodeheaver, G., Edgerton, M., & Edlich, R. (1982). Damage to tissue defenses by a topical anesthetic agent. *Annals of Emergency Medicine, 11* (6), 307-310.

Bartfield, J., Gennis, P., Barbera, J., Breuer, B., & Gallagher, E. (1990). Buffered versus plain lidocaine as a local anesthetic for simple laceration repair. *Annals of Emergency Medicine, 19,* (12), 1387-1389.

Bourne, R., Bitar, H., Andreae, P., Martin, L., Finlay, J., & Marquis, F. (1988). In-vivo comparison of four absorbable sutures: Vicryl, Dexon Plus, Maxon, and PDS. *Canadian Journal of Surgery, 31* (1), 43-45.

Bryant, R. (1987). Wound repair: A review. *Journal of Enterostomal Therapy, 14* (6), 263.

Bucklew, P., Horner, W., & Diamond, D. (1985). High-pressure acid injection: Case report with recommended initial management and treatment. *Journal of Trauma, 25*(6), 552-556.

Callaham, M. (1988). Controversies in antibiotic choices for bite wounds. *Annals of Emergency Medicine, 17* (12), 1321-1330.

Callaham, M. (1991). When an animal bites. *Emergency Medicine, 20* (8), 105-113.

Chandler, M., Grammer, L., & Patterson, R. (1987). Provocative challenge with local anesthetics in patients with a prior history of reaction. *Journal of Allergy and Clinical Immunology, 79,* (6). 883-886.

Christoph, R., Buchanan, L., Begalla, K., & Schwartz, S. (1988). Pain reduction in local anesthetic administration through pH buffering. *Annals of Emergency Medicine, 17* (2), 117-120.

Connolly, J. (1988). Managing cuts and bruises. *Emergency Medicine, 17* (11), 78-100.

Cosgriff, J., & Anderson, D. (1984). *The practice of emergency care.* New York: J.B. Lippincott.

Dames, S. (1991). Initial wound management in the emergency department. *Focus on Critical Care, 2* (1), 1-3.

De Flaviis, L., Scaglione, P., Del Bo, P., & Nessi, R. (1988). Detection of foreign bodies in soft tissue: Experimental comparison of ultrasonography and xeroradiography. *Journal of Trauma*, 28 (3), 400-404.

Dimick, A. (1988). Delayed wound closure: Indications and techniques. *Annals of Emergency Medicine*, 17 (12), 1303-1304.

Dire, D., Hood, F., & Welsh, A. (1990). A comparison of wound irrigation solutions used in the emergency department. *Annals of Emergency Medicine*, 19 (6), 704-708.

Dula, D., Leicht, M., & Moothart, W. (1984). Degloving injury of the mandible. *Annals of Emergency Medicine*, 13 (8), 630-632.

Dushoff, I. (1973). A stitch in time. *Emergency Medicine*, 2 (1), 1-16.

Dushoff, I. (1974). About face. *Emergency Medicine*, 3 (11), 26-77.

Earley, M., & Bardsley, A. (1984). Human bites: A review. *British Journal of Plastic Surgery*, 37, 458-462.

Edlich, R., & Rodeheaver, G. (1984). Puncture wounds. *Comprehensive Therapy*, 10 (6), 41-49.

Edlich, R., Rodeheaver, G., Morgan, R., Berman, D., & Thacker, J. (1988). Principles of emergency wound management. *Annals of Emergency Medicine*, 17 (12), 1284-1302.

Faddis, D., Daniel, D., & Boyer, J. (1977). Tissue toxicity of antiseptic solutions. *Journal of Trauma*, 17 (12), 895-897.

Fangtao, L., Shubeng, C., Wang, Y., Chenzhe, S., Fanzhen, Z., & Guanfu, W. (1988). Use of serum and vaccine in combination for prophylaxis following exposure to rabies. *Reviews of Infectious Diseases*, 10 (4), 766-769.

Fernandez, A., & Finley, J. (1983). Wound healing: Helping a natural process. *Postgraduate Medicine*, 74 (4), 311-317.

Fishbein, D., & Arcangeli, S. (1987). Rabies prevention in primary care: a four step approach. *Postgraduate Medicine*, 82, (3), 83-95.

Fitzmaurice, L., Wasserman, G., Knapp, J., Roberts, DK, Waeckerie, J., & Fox, M. (1990). TAC use and absorption of cocaine in a pediatric emergency department. *Annals of Emergency Medicine*, 19 (5), 515-518.

Gamis, A., Knapp, J., & Glenski, J. (1989). Nitrous oxide analgesia in a pediatric emergency department. *Annals of Emergency Medicine*, 18 (2), 177-181.

Gemberling, R. (1976). Dressing comparison in healing donor sites. *Journal of Trauma*, 16 (10), 812-814.

Giangrasso, J., & Smith, R. (1985). Misuse of tetanus immunoprophylaxis in wound care. *Annals of Emergency Medicine*, 14 (6), 573-579.

Goldstein, E., Reinhardt, J., Murry, P., & Finegold, S. (1984). Animal and human bite wounds: A comparative study, Augmentin vs penicillin +/− dicloxacillin. *Postgraduate Medicine*, 56 (1), 105-110.

Goldstein, E., & Richwald, G. (1987). Human and animal bite wounds. *American Family Physician*, 36 (1), 101-108.

Gravett, A., Sterner, S., Clinton, J., & Ruiz, E. (1987). A trial of povidone-iodine in the prevention of infection in sutured lacerations. *Annals of Emergency Medicine*, 16 (2), 176-171.

Halverson, D. (1986, February). *Mammalian Bites*. Paper presented at the Emergency Medicine Conference, Seattle, Wash.

Hayden, J. (1983). Compartment syndromes. *Postgraduate Medicine*, 74 (1), 191-202.

Hunt, T. (1988). The physiology of wound healing. *Annals of Emergency Medicine*, 17 (12), 1265-1273.

Hunt, T. (1990). Basic principles of wound healing. *Journal of Trauma*, 30 (12), 122-128.

Hurley, D. (speaker). (1988). *Antibiotics in the treatment of human, cat, and dog bites*. Audio Digest Emergency Medicine. (cassette recording vol. 5, number 9, side A)

Immunization Practices Advisory Committee. (1989). Recommendations of the Immunization Practices Advisory Committee. *Morbidity and Mortality Weekly Report*, 38 (13), 226. Massachusetts: Massachusetts Medical Society.

Jupiter, J., & Krushell, R. (1987). Evaluating hand injuries. *Emergency Medicine*, 16 (11), 59-77.

Katz, S., McGinley, K., & Leyden, J. (1986). Semipermeable occlusive dressings. *Archives of Dermatology*, 122, 58-62.

King, C. (1984). Dealing with abrasions and lacerations. *RN*, 6, 53-56.

Kizer, K., & Callaham, M. (1984). A new look at managing mammalian bites. *Emergency Medicine Reports*, 5 (8), 53-58.

Knezevich, B. (1986). *Trauma nursing; Principles and practice* (pp. 153-175). Norwalk, Conn: Appleton-Century-Crofts.

Koszuta, L. (1984). Hand injuries. *Emergency*, 6 (6), 29-50.

Lammers, R. (1988). Soft tissue foreign bodies. *Annals of Emergency Medicine*, 17 (12), 1336-1347.

Lammers, R., Fourré, M., Callaham, M., & Boone, T. (1990). Effect of povidone-iodine and saline soaking on bacterial counts in acute, traumatic, contaminated wounds. *Annals of Emergency Medicine*, 19, (6), 709-714.

Lampe, E. (1969). Surgical anatomy of the hand. *CIBA Clinical Symposia*, 21 (3), 3-46.

Larrabee, W., Lanier, B., & Miekle, D. (1987). Effect of epinephrine on local cutaneous blood flow. *Head & Neck Surgery*, 9 (3), 287-289.

Lovett, W., & McCalla, M. (1983). Management and rehabilitation of extensor tendon injuries. *Orthopedic Clinics of North America*, 14 (4), 811-826.

Mancusi-Ungaro, H., & Rappaport, N. (1986). Preventing wound Infections. *Postgraduate Medicine*, 33 (4), 147-152.

Martin, J., Doezema, D., Tandberg, D., & Umland, E. (1990). The effect of local anesthetics on bacterial proliferation: TAC versus lidocaine. *Annals of Emergency Medicine*, 19 (9), 987-990.

Martinez, J., & Burns, C. (1987). Wound management. *Current Concepts in Wound Care*, 10 (3), 9-16.

May, S., & Still, J. (1987). Contemporary wound management with natural and synthetic dressings. *Ostomy and Wound Management*, 2 (3), 14-22.

McGuire, M. (1982). A "minor" hand injury? *RN*, 1, 28-32.

Ordog, G. (1986). The bacteriology of dog bite wounds on initial presentation. *Annals of Emergency Medicine*, 15 (11), 1324-1329.

Ordog, G., Balasubramanium, S., & Wasserberger, J. (1985). Rat bites: Fifty cases. *Annals of Emergency Medicine*, 14 (2), 126-130.

Panke, T.W., & McLeod, C.G. (1985). *Pathology of thermal injury: A practical approach*. Orlando, FL: Grune & Stratton.

Patzakis, M., Wilkins, J., & Bassett, R. (1987). Surgical findings in clenched-fist injuries. *Clinical Orthopaedics and Related Research*, 220 (7), 237-239.

Phillips, L., & Heggers, J. (1988). Layered closure of lacerations. *Postgraduate Medicine, 83* (8), 142-148.

Proehl, J. (1985). Nitrous oxide for pain control in the emergency department. *Journal of Emergency Nursing, 11* (4), 191-194.

Richless, L., (1985). Acute wound management. *Family Practice Recertification, 7* (3), 39-63.

Riley, H. (1984). Puncture wounds of the foot: Their importance and potential for complications. *Oklahoma State Medical Association Journal, 1* (77), 3-6.

Robson, M. (1988). Disturbances of wound healing. *Annals of Emergency Medicine, 17* (12), 1274-1278.

Rodeheaver, G., Bellamy, W., Kody, M., Spatafora, G., Fitton, L., Leyden, K., & Edlich, R. (1982). Bactericidal activity and toxicity of iodine-containing solutions in wounds. *Archives of Surgery, 117,* 181-186.

Rodeheaver, G., Kurtz, L., Kircher, B., & Edlich, R. (1980). Pluronic F-68: A promising new skin wound cleanser. *Annals of Emergency Medicine, 9* (11), 572-576.

Rodeheaver, G., Spengler, M., & Edlich, R. (1987). Performance of new wound closure tapes. *Journal of Emergency Medicine, 6* (5), 451-462.

Rogness, H. (1985). High-pressure wound irrigation. *Journal of Enterostomal Therapy, 12* (6), 27-28.

Roth, J., & Windle, B. (1988). Staple versus suture closure of skin incisions in a pig model. *Canadian Journal of Surgery, 31* (1), 19-20.

Schoo, M., Scott, F., & Boswick, J. (1980). High-pressure injection injuries of the hand. *Journal of Trauma, 20* (3), 229-238.

Spivey, W., McNamara, R., MacKenzie, R., Bhat, S., & Burdick, W. (1987). A clinical comparison of lidocaine and bupivacaine. *Annals of Emergency Medicine, 16,* 752-757.

Stevenson, T., Thacker, J., Rodeheaver, G., Bacchetta, C., Edgerton, M., & Edlich, R. (1976). Cleansing the traumatic wound by high-pressure syringe irrigation. *Journal of the American College of Emergency Physicians, 5* (1), 17-21.

Stewart, R. (1985). Nitrous oxide sedation/analgesia in emergency medicine. *Annals of Emergency Medicine, 14* (2), 139-147.

Svensson, L., Brookstone, A., & Wellsted, M. (1985). Necrotizing fasciitis in contused areas. *Journal of Trauma, 25* (3), 260-262.

Stotts, N. (1983). The most effective method of wound irrigation. *Focus on Critical Care, 10* (5), 45-48.

Strange, J. (1987). *Shock trauma care plans.* Springhouse, PA: Springhouse.

Strickland, J. (1983). Management of acute flexor tendon injuries. *Orthopedic Clinics of North America, 14* (4), 827-846.

Swanson, J. (1983). Assessment of allergy to local anesthetic. *Annals of Emergency Medicine, 12* (5), 316-318.

Trott, A. (1988). Mechanisms of soft tissue trauma. *Annals of Emergency Medicine, 17* (12), 1279-1283.

Trott, A. (1991). *Wounds and lacerations: Emergency care and closure.* St. Louis: Mosby–Year Book, Inc.

Warrell, D., & Warrell, M. (1988). Human rabies and its prevention: An overview. *Reviews of Infectious Diseases, 10* (4), 726-731.

Wayne, M., (1985). Clinical evaluation of Epi-Lock: A semi-occlusive dressing. *Annals of Emergency Medicine, 14* (1), 20-24.

Weiss, B. (1989). Children's antidrug program is working. *Journal of Emergency Nursing, 15* (2) 73-74.

Zukin, D.D., & Simon, R.R. (1987). *Emergency wound care* Rockville, MD: Aspen Publishers.

14 *Tissue Integrity*

Burns

■■■

Susan Engman Lazear

OBJECTIVES

❏ *Assess the depth and extent of injury for a given burn.*

❏ *Calculate the estimated fluid requirements for patients sustaining various types of burn injuries.*

❏ *Identify the special requirements of an electrically injured patient.*

❏ *Recognize the signs and symptoms of a suspected inhalation injury.*

❏ *List, in order of priority, the steps in the initial management of the major burn victim.*

❏ *Identify which patients are classified as major burn victims.*

❏ *Identify the typical burn injuries seen as child abuse injuries.*

INTRODUCTION   Burn injuries account for a significant proportion of the traumatic injuries sustained in the United States each year. Although the numbers are beginning to decline, approximately 2 million Americans are injured by fire annually, 75,000 are hospitalized for prolonged periods, and 12,000 die (Boswick, 1987a). Of these deaths, 50% are related to carbon monoxide poisoning and 30% of the patients admitted have sustained smoke and/or thermal damage to their ventilatory system.

Improved education and legislative efforts have begun to ameliorate these staggering statistics. The American Burn Association, through the work of its members, firefighters, and volunteers, has developed educational programs for all ages. School children are now learning fire safety and developing fire escape plans for their homes. The requirements of smoke alarms and sprinkler systems in public buildings, hotels, apartments, and other facilities have been enacted through state legislation. Federal regulations limiting the use of combustible, flammable products have

reduced the number of deaths. These regulations have specifically affected children, who had previously sustained mortal injuries when their clothing ignited, and airline crash victims, who were exposed to toxic by-products of burning plastic.

CASE STUDY   Ms. Anderson is a 43-year-old woman who fell asleep on her couch while smoking and subsequently sustained approximately 45% TBSA deep, partial-thickness burns. She is admitted to the ED unresponsive. Her BP is 140/72; P, 120; and RR, 24. Oxygen is being delivered by face mask.

What history is important to obtain from the prehospital care providers, family members, and others? What complications are suspected based on this history?

It is important to determine if Ms. Anderson was found in the house and in an enclosed space. The risk of smoke inhalation injury dramatically increases with the higher concentration of smoke in the room. The length of exposure to the heat, flame, and smoke will also impact the severity of Ms. Anderson's injuries. With a history of smoking and the associated pulmonary changes in her lungs, she is at risk for pulmonary sequelae, including adult respiratory distress syndrome (ARDS). In addition, it is important to ascertain the causes of Ms. Anderson's unresponsiveness, which could be secondary to either smoke inhalation or alcohol intoxication, or both. As with all burn patients, it is necessary to obtain information regarding the time that the injury was sustained, all circumstances surrounding the injury, past medical problems, allergies, current medications, as well as the patient's status on arrival of the prehospital care providers and any subsequent change in the patient's condition before arrival in the ED.

Based on the injuries sustained and the history obtained, what is the appropriate disposition of Ms. Anderson on completion of stabilization in the ED? What interventions are necessary to prepare for her disposition?

Ms. Anderson requires the facilities that are available at a burn center as outlined by the American Burn Association. Because of the extent of her injuries (greater than 45% total body surface area [TBSA], deep, partial-thickness burns), her possible smoke inhalation, and history of smoking, the patient is considered to be at high risk for mortality. Arrangements for transfer should be made by telephone with the nearest burn center. The referring and receiving physicians should discuss the patient's status, as well as requirements and arrangements for transport. During transfer, Ms. A. requires continuous fluid resuscitation, oxygen therapy, cardiac monitoring, a patent foley catheter, and maintenance of body heat. Prophylactic intubation before leaving the referring hospital will prevent loss of her anatomic airway secondary to swelling induced by heat and smoke inhalation. (A carboxyhemoglobin level drawn before her departure will allow for estimation of the degree of carbon monoxide poisoning she has sustained.)

CASE STUDY Jennifer is a 20-month-old toddler who is brought to the ED by her mother. She has sustained circumferential, full-thickness burns of her feet and hands. The mother states that the child was unattended in the bathtub with the older sibling, who turned on the hot water faucet, causing Jennifer's burns. On examination, Jennifer is whimpering in her mother's arms and withdrawing from the nurse. Her BP is 84 systolic; HR, 130; RR, 35.

What are the priorities in providing immediate aid for Jennifer?

Airway, breathing, and circulation are always first priority for all burn patients regardless of the extent of their burn injuries. The child should be removed from her mother's arms and placed on the examining table. Because of the questionable nature of these burns (the burns are typical of abusive burn injuries), the child may be separated from the parent. Fluid resuscitation may be accomplished by intravenous fluid administration. Although Jennifer may be able to meet her needs with oral fluids, full-thickness burns of the feet and hands are major injuries requiring admission to a burn center and IV placement is recommended. Pain control measures may be initiated. Debridement of the wounds can be delayed until after admission.

What special interventions are required for this pediatric burn victim?

The pediatric burn victim can become hypoglycemic very quickly in response to the stress reaction and the associated lack of glucose stores. The child under 8 years of age requires additional fluids containing dextrose to supplement the estimated fluid requirements calculated according to weight and TBSA injured (i.e., Baxter formula). Also, children have a different distribution of body surface area from the adult and, based on age, the TBSA percentages will vary. Disposition of the pediatric burn victim depends not only on the American Burn Association's recommended criteria but also on the parent's willingness to participate in the child's care and the child's compliance with medical restrictions. In this case as with many others, the child may need protection if abusive injuries are identified.

MECHANISM OF INJURY

Burns can be caused by a number of means. Not all burn injuries are caused by fire—chemicals, tar, electrical voltage, and lightning can cause burn wounds. Location, length of exposure, and mechanisms of injury will all impact outcome.

Of all burns, 60% are thermal injuries (Artz, Moncrief, & Pruitt, 1979). Exposure to flame, flash, steam, or scald causes tissue destruction. The nature of the injury sustained depends on the intensity of the heat, the size of the flame, the duration of the exposure, and the tissue injured.

Chemical Burns

Chemicals cause burns by denaturing protein within the tissues or by desiccating (dehydrating) the cells. The concentration of the agent and the duration of the exposure will impact the extent of injury. Alkali products cause deeper burns with more severe damage than acid agents. Powder burns are generally more ominous in outcome because the agent enters the pores and is therefore more difficult to remove. Prehospital professionals or lay people should begin removal of the agent. Once the chemical has been thoroughly removed, which must be done immediately on arrival of the patient to the ED, the wound is managed in the same manner as the thermal burn.

Electrical Burns

Electrical injuries are caused by an electrical force passing through the body. The type and voltage of the circuit, the pathway through the body, the duration, and the resistance of the body will determine the severity of damage. The electrical current enters the body through the skin, causing a localized external burn at the entry and exit sites and extensive damage internally between these two sites. The immediate damage is to the heart, lungs, and brain. Nerves, blood vessels, and muscle, being less resistant, are more easily injured, compared with bone and fat. The electrical current can cause tetanic contractions leading to respiratory paralysis and death, as well as fractures of the long bones. If the current passes through or near the heart, the cardiac electrical conduction system can be damaged, causing spontaneous ventricular fibrillation or other life-threatening dysrhythmias. Additionally, 20% of patients experiencing electrical injuries from sources of 1000 volts or greater require major amputation (Monafo, 1987).

The majority of lightning strike victims experience injury from the flashover phenomenon, in which most of the electrical energy does not transverse the body but flows around it. This is caused by the discharge of a static charge, which is repelled by accumulated like forces on the body, producing a shock wave (so-called *sledge hammer blow*) capable of causing such injuries as fractures and dislocations (Fontanarosa, 1988). Of patients surviving a lightning strike, 70% or more complain of paresthesias and/or paralysis, but both conditions are temporary (Monafo, 1987).

Tar Burns

Tar burns are often sustained by roofers, construction workers, and persons who repair roads. Hot tar comes in contact with the skin and cools, causing the tar to harden. The underlying burn depends on the temperature of the tar at the time of contact with the body. Determination of extent and depth of body surface injury can be accomplished only after the tar is removed with special agents.

Inhalation Burns

Inhalation burns cause two types of injuries. Above the glottis, the upper airway can be burned by the inhalation of hot air or smoke. This causes mucosal burns of the mouth, pharynx, and larynx, exhibited by blistering, edema, and potential loss of the anatomic airway. True thermal damage to the lower airway is rare (except with the inhalation of steam or explosive gases) because the body's protective mechanism is to cool the air that is inhaled.

A chemical tracheobronchitis develops in the lower airway as a result of the inhalation of chemical by-products of combustion found in smoke. Regardless of the type of offending chemical, the end organ response is the same. A loss of bronchial ciliary action (ciliary paralysis) occurs, as well as a decrease in surfactant production, progressive inflammation, and mucosal edema, leading to small airway closure and atelectasis. The tracheal and bronchial epithelia eventually slough, leading to hemorrhagic tracheobronchitis (Heimbach, 1983).

ANATOMIC AND PHYSIOLOGIC CONSIDERATIONS

Three zones of tissue damage occur at a burn site (Figure 14-1). The central "zone of coagulation" represents irreversible damage. Concentrically surrounding the zone of coagulation is the "zone of stasis," in which capillary blood flow is compromised. Edema formation and prolonged compromise of blood flow in this zone of stasis will cause a deeper and more extensive burn wound. For this reason, the depth and severity of burn wounds are not known for 3 to 5 days after the injury. The final zone of tissue damage is the "zone of hyperemia," signifying the area of superficial, peripheral damage, which will heal quickly on its own.

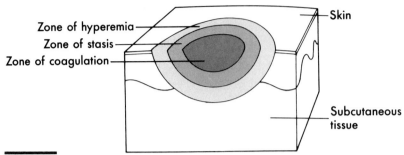

Figure 14-1 Zones of injury.

Depth of Injury

Controversy exists regarding the terminology of depth of injury (Cardona, Hurn, Mason, Scanlon-Schilpp, & Veise-Berry, 1988; Haynes, 1983; Monafo, 1987). Epidermal burns (in the past referred to as *first degree*) involve the superficial layers of the epidermis (Table 14-1 and Figure 14-2). These wounds blanch with pressure, and capillary refill is prompt. The injured area is reddened, is painful to touch, and will heal within 3 to 4 days without scarring. Because this layer rapidly regenerates, epidermal burns are not included in TBSA calculations.

Partial-thickness burns (second degree) can be superficial or deep. (see Table 14-1 and Figure 14-3). These wounds involve the entire epidermal layer and the superficial dermal layers. The portion of the epidermis that extends into the dermal layer through skin appendages (hair follicles, sebaceous glands, and sweat glands) remains viable in partial-thickness burns (Heimbach, 1986). Superficial partial-thickness wounds are identified by a mottled, moist, pink-red appearance and by the formation of thick-walled blisters. The wound is extremely painful because the pain sensors remain intact but exposed. Healing is accomplished by overgrowth of the epithelial cells from the skin appendages.

The deep, partial-thickness (DPT) burn extends into the lower reticular layer of the dermis and less skin appendages and epithelial cells are available for wound healing. The vast capillary network within the dermal layer accounts for the extensive edema formation associated with partial-thickness burns. These DPT wounds are sensitive to pressure but insensitive to pinprick and light touch. The wound will heal within 4 to 6 weeks but with unstable epithelium, hypertrophic scar-

ring, and contracture (Monafo, 1987). For this reason, many DPT burns are grafted within a week of injury.

All layers of the dermis and epidermis protruding into the underlying subcutaneous fat are damaged in full-thickness burns (third degree). The dermis has no regenerative capacity, and these wounds will heal by scar formation if not grafted. The burned area appears white, black, cherry red (because of interstitial hemorrhage), dry, leathery, and with thrombosed vessels (Figure 14-4). The pain sensors are destroyed, and, by definition, full-thickness burns are not painful. (However, it is imperative to remember the tremendous psychologic pain that accompanies a burn injury; also, rarely does a patient have only a full-thickness burn—the surrounding partial-thickness wound is extremely painful). However, as healing occurs and pain sensors regenerate, the pain increases.

Survivors with burns of bone and muscle (deep, full-thickness or fourth- or fifth-degree burns) are rare. These injuries require prompt debridement and possible amputation to prevent development of overwhelming metabolic acidosis from tissue destruction. These burns, depending on the extent and area involved, are not always considered fatal (Artz, Moncrief, & Pruitt, 1979).

The body's response to heat injury includes the following:
- thrombosis of the vasculature
- increased capillary permeability with an increased extravascular colloid oncotic pressure, resulting in translocation of fluid throughout the body
- loss of protein into the extravascular space.

The obstruction of blood flow caused by thrombosis is relieved within 24 to 48 hours in partial-

Table 14-1 Depth of injury

Characteristic	First degree	Second degree		Third degree
	Epidermal	Superficial, partial thickness	Deep, partial thickness	Full thickness
Morphology	Destruction of epidermis only	Destruction of epidermis and some dermis	Destruction of epidermis and dermis, leaving only some viable appendages	Destruction of epidermis, dermis, and underlying subcutaneous tissue
Skin function	Intact	Absent	Absent	Absent
Tactile and pain sensors	Intact	Intact	Intact, but diminished	Absent
Blisters	Present only after first 24 hours	Present within minutes; fluid-filled	May or may not appear as fluid-filled blisters; often is layer of flat, dehydrated "tissue paper" that lifts off in sheets	Blisters rare; usually there is layer of flat, dehydrated "tissue paper" that lifts off easily
Appearance of wound after initial debridement	Skin peels at 24 to 48 hours; normal or slightly red underneath	Red to pale ivory; moist surface	Mottled with areas of waxy, white, dry surface	White, cherry red, or black; may contain visible thrombosed veins; dry, hard, leathery surface
Healing time	3 to 5 days	21 to 28 days	30 days to many months	Will not heal; may close from edges as secondary healing if wound is small
Scarring	None	Present; influenced by genetic predisposition	Highest, because slow healing rate increases scar tissue development; influenced by genetic predisposition	Skin graft scarring is minimized by early excision and grafting; influenced by genetic predisposition

Note. Modified from *Trauma Nursing: From Resuscitation Through Rehabilitation* (p. 709) by V. Cardona, P. Hurn, P. Mason, A. Scanlon-Schilpp, and S. Veise-Berry, 1988, Philadelphia: W.B. Saunders.

Depth of burn

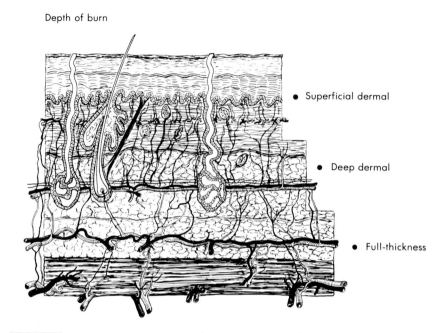

- Superficial dermal

- Deep dermal

- Full-thickness

Figure 14-2 Schematic of normal skin showing burn depth. (*Note.* From *Thermal Injuries* by D.P. Dressler, J.L. Hozid, and P. Nathan, 1988, St. Louis: Mosby–Year Book, Inc.)

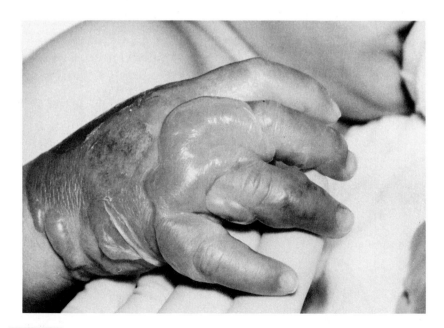

Figure 14-3 Partial-thickness burn with large bullae of dorsum of hand of child, caused by hot water. (*Note.* From *Thermal Injuries* by D.P. Dressler, J.L. Hozid, and P. Nathan, 1988, St. Louis: Mosby–Year Book.)

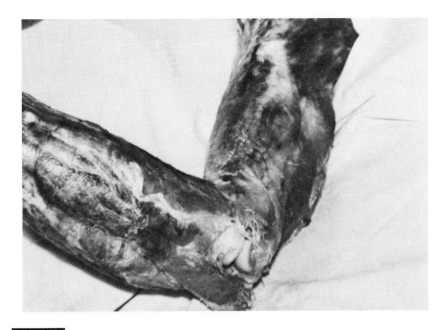

Figure 14-4   Full-thickness burn exposing elbow joint. (*Note.* From *Thermal Injuries* by D.P. Dressler, J.L. Hozid, and P. Nathan, 1988, St. Louis: Mosby–Year Book.)

thickness wounds but is prolonged for 3 to 4 weeks in the full-thickness injury (Artz et al., 1979). Although some experimental studies reported thrombosis of the arterioles, the venous system is now being implicated. Venules are susceptible to thermal damage because they are thin walled and this could hinder capillary outflow (Parke & McLeod, 1985). If infection or wound desiccation occurs, the thrombosis continues and circulation is not reestablished.

Vascular Changes

Capillary permeability increases for 2 to 3 weeks after injury; however, the most marked changes occur within the first 24 to 36 hours (Figure 14-5). Edema develops secondary to the loss of capillary integrity and occurs at the burn site in burns of 30% or less TBSA. Edema occurs throughout the body (although most pronounced at the burn site) in burns involving more than 30% TBSA (Artz et al., 1979).

Initially, blood viscosity increases after thermal injury secondary to a rise in the hematocrit as a result of vascular fluid shift into the interstitium. As aggressive fluid resuscitation is instituted, the hematocrit drops. An immediate hemolysis of the

red cells occurs, and the red blood cell has a reduced life span, in the range of 30% of normal (Artz et al., 1979). White blood cell count rises, with an increase in polymorphonuclear leukocytes. Platelet count and platelet survival time drop drastically during the first 5 days after injury, followed by an increase, which sustains for several weeks (Artz et al., 1979).

GENERAL ASSESSMENT

Regardless of the mechanisms of injury, additional history of the injury is important to ascertain, including length of exposure, location (open or enclosed), events preceding the injury, and time of the injury. These parameters are important prognosticators of severity and mortality. It is important to examine the patient for the smell of smoke, burns of the intraoral cavity, hoarseness, expiratory wheezes, and carbonaceous sputum. Carboxyhemoglobin (COHb) levels and arterial blood gas values should be determined as early clues for inhalation injuries.

All burn patients should be evaluated for life-threatening injuries causing airway, breathing, or circulatory compromise. Additional parameters to assess include vital signs, level of consciousness,

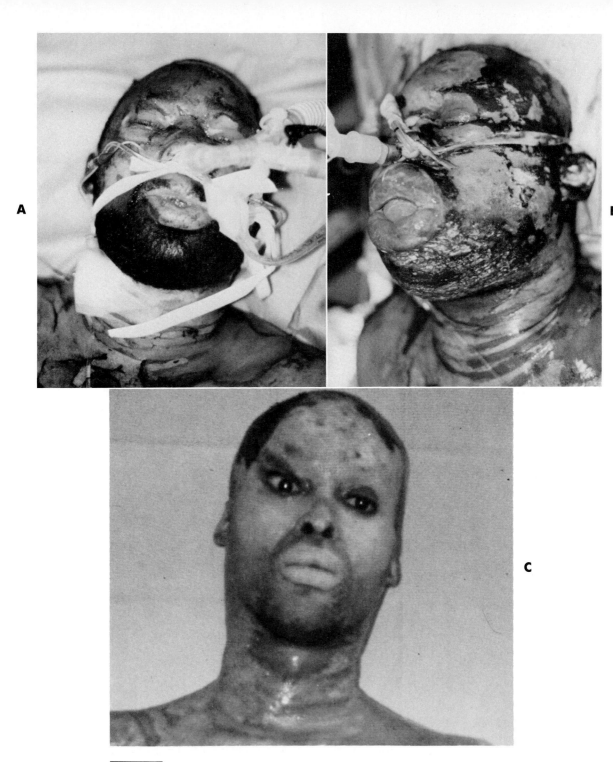

Figure 14-5 Facial edema. Patient was in a house fire and suffered 67% TBSA burns, including deep, partial-thickness and full-thickness burns to face. Photographs show progression of edema caused by direct injury, as well as the effects of fluid resuscitation for the major burn. **A,** 4 to 5 hours after-burn. **B,** 30 hours after-burn, showing distortion of facial features and necessity of intubation before the full extent of burn edema development. **C,** Facial contour 3 months after burn. (Note. Courtesy Anne E. Missavage, M.D., U.C. Davis Regional Burn Center, Sacramento, CA.)

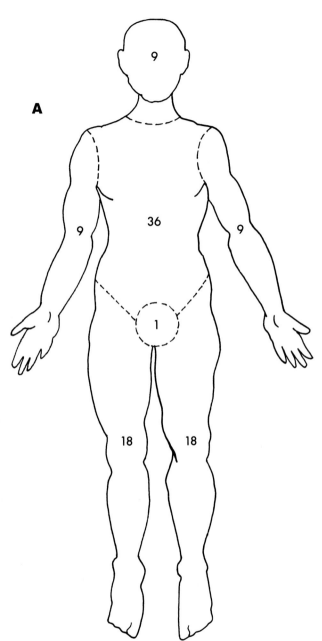

A

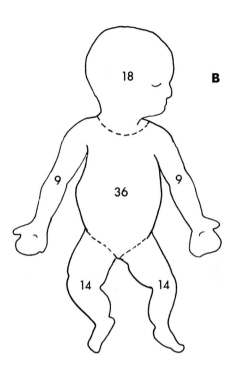

B

Figure 14-6   Rule of nines. **A,** Adult head and neck, extremities, and torso are labeled relative to their percent of total body surface area (TBSA) in multiples of nine. **B,** Infant/child diagram is slightly modified. Thorax is often misunderstood: chest + abdomen = 18%; back + buttocks = 18%.

core temperature, skin vital signs (including peripheral temperature and pulses), edema formation, depth and extent of injury, as well as the presence of compounding traumatic injuries (e.g., fractures, internal hemorrhage).

Extent of Injury

Fluid resuscitation requirements and disposition of the patient are two of the reasons that the amount of TBSA injury is calculated. The "rule of nines" was developed for ED and prehospital care providers to make quick estimation of the extent of injury. For example, a patient sustaining burns of the left forearm, lower portion of the abdomen, and left anterior and posterior thigh has sustained approximately a 22% to 24% burn. Corrections for age-related body surface area variations are easily made from modified charts based on the victim's age (Figure 14-6).

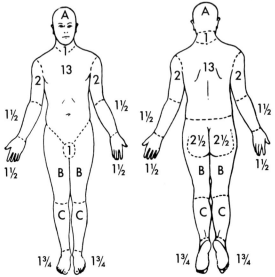

Relative percentage of areas affected by growth

	Age in years					
	0	1	5	10	15	Adult
A—½ of head	9½	8½	6½	5½	4½	3½
B—½ of one thigh	2¾	3¼	4	4¼	4½	4¾
C—½ of one leg	2½	2½	2¾	3	3¼	3½

Figure 14-7   Lund and Browder chart. (*Note.* From *Burns: A Team Approach.* [p. 160] by C. Artz, J. Moncrief, and B. Pruitt [Eds.], 1979, Philadelphia: W.B. Saunders.)

Lund and Browder developed an age-related chart that provides a more refined estimation of TBSA (Figure 14-7). To provide a more accurate calculation of the extent of injury, this chart can be used in conjunction with the palmar surface estimation (the patient's palm size is approximate to 1% of his TBSA). Computerized burn area measurement is also being developed to assist with accurate TBSA measurement (Scott-Conner, Clarke, & Conner, 1988).

Patients with preexisting illnesses should be managed with attention to their limitations. Patients with cardiac conditions may not be able to tolerate rapid, massive fluid replacement. Patients with diabetes have an increased need for insulin in response to the elevated serum glucose levels associated with the stress response. Patients with asthma and with chronic lung disease are at risk for severe respiratory compromise. Patients with a history of long-term use of immunosuppressive

agents have an increased risk of infection. Malnourished patients cannot meet the increased caloric needs associated with the increase in basal metabolic rate.

Triage

The American Burn Association has defined specific criteria for classifying severity of burns (Dimick, 1983). Admission to a burn center or community hospital for treatment as an out-patient is based on these criteria (Table 14-2). Burn centers deliver advanced, state-of-the-art burn care provided by a multidisciplinary team. Community hospitals may be able to care for burn victims if adequately trained staff and equipment are available.

Triage of burn patients from the field depends on the length of time in transport. If the patient requires the facilities of a burn center and transport time is 30 minutes or less, the patient should

Table 14-2 American Burn Association classification of severity of injury

Classification	Characteristics	Treatment facility
Minor	SPT* DPT† <15% TBSA adult DPT <10% TBSA child FT‡ <3% TBSA adult, child (not involving face, hands, feet, or perineum)	Out-patient or in-patient (for 24 hrs.)
Moderate	DPT 15%-25% TBSA adult DPT 10%-20% TBSA child FT 3%-10% TBSA adult, child (not involving face, hands, feet, or perineum)	Community hospital
Major	DPT >25% TBSA adult DPT >20% child FT >10% TBSA adult, child Burns of face, hands, feet, and perineum Burns complicated by: • inhalation injury • major associated trauma • preexisting illness • all major electrical injuries	Burn center

Note. From American Burn Association, 1983, Miami.
*Superficial, partial-thickness burns
†Deep, partial-thickness burns
‡Full-thickness burns

be admitted directly to the burn center. If transport times exceed 30 minutes, the patient should be transported to the closest facility for stabilization and IV fluid resuscitation (Trunkey, 1983) (see section on transport of burn patients).

GENERAL INTERVENTIONS
Stabilization

The goals of care of the burn victim are to minimize exposure to the causative agent, institute ABCs, assess for compounding injuries, and

transport the patient to the appropriate facility. Prehospital care providers must remember to protect themselves from injury while treating the patient. If the patient's clothing is on fire, the flame should be extinguished and the skin cooled with cool water (if burn is minor) or gelatinous impregnated dressings, which cause the transfer of heat from the wound to the dressing (Boswick, 1987c). Chemical burns should be flushed continuously; time should not be wasted searching for a specific neutralizing agent. Electrically injured patients should be monitored for cardiac dysrhythmias.

Suspected smoke inhalation injuries should be treated with application of a face mask or nasotracheal intubation and subsequent oxygen delivery at 100%. The patient should be protected from further contamination with a sterile or clean sheet covering. No ointment should be applied, because this may cause delay in evaluating the burn injury and may increase pain when it is removed. All jewelry and constricting clothing should be removed to prevent circulatory compromise. The patient should be transported with oxygen and intravenous (IV) fluids. Maintenance of body heat is another important goal during transport.

ED management of the burn victim should be expeditious—no longer than 30 to 45 minutes. The patient should be transferred and admitted to the appropriate level facility and definitive care begun as quickly as possible.

Burn victims should be evaluated as multiple trauma patients. Airway, breathing, and circulation receive immediate priority. A head-to-toe assessment for concomitant traumatic injuries (e.g., cervical spine injury sustained in a fall while escaping a burning building) relegates the burn wound to secondary priority. The patient should have admission blood work done, to include CBC, BUN, electrolytes, glucose, type and crossmatch, and a COHb level. Arterial blood gas studies, chest x-ray examination, and a urinalysis should be performed. Placing an IV line, foley catheter, and nasogastric tube, as well as initiating cardiac monitoring, should receive priority. Diphtheria tetanus (DT) (0.5 ml) should be administered and tetanus immunoglobulin (TIG) may be necessary, depending on the patient's immunization status. The staff should wear gowns, gloves, and masks during the ED stabilization to protect the patient from further contamination.

Ventilation

Burns of the face, head, and neck predispose the patient to airway compromise. Airway management, ventilatory support, and oxygenation are necessary. Prophylactic intubation using the nasotracheal route is indicated if the patient exhibits shortness of breath, decreasing level of consciousness, falling PaO_2, hoarseness, or swelling of the face and neck. Tracheostomy and cricothyroidotomy are contraindicated during the first 72 hours after injury because of the massive swelling that can occur, hindering anchoring and proper placement of the tube and further impairing skin integrity. Bronchoscopy may be performed to evaluate the extent of inhalation injury.

Smoke inhalation and/or carbon monoxide (CO) poisoning doubles the mortality rate for a burn of a given size. Carbon monoxide is a colorless, odorless, tasteless gas that is found in smoke. It has an affinity for hemoglobin that is more than 200 times greater than that of the oxygen molecule (Heimbach, 1983). This causes a shift of the oxygen dissociation curve to the left, resulting in tissue hypoxia. The half-life of CO on room air is 4 to 5 hours; on 100% oxygen, 80 minutes, and using hyperbaric flow at 3 atmospheres, 20 to 25 minutes (Davic & Hunt, 1977). Levels less than 10% usually produce no symptoms; at 20%, the patient complains of a headache and nausea and vomiting and exhibits a loss of manual dexterity (Mosley, 1988). A level of 30% causes confusion, lethargy, and ST segment depression on ECG; 40% to 60% produces coma; and levels greater than 60% are usually fatal (Heimbach, 1983).

Transcutaneous PO_2 analyzers have been found to be accurate in monitoring the oxygen delivery to tissues in the presence of carbon monoxide; however, pulse oximetry may be inaccurate during the first few hours after burn (Barillo, Mostropieri, Cohen, & Okunski, 1990; Barker & Tremper, 1987). During initial resuscitation, arterial blood gas measurements may be more advantageous in that information concerning adequacy of resuscitation (blood pH) and ventilation (PCO_2), as well as oxygenation (PO_2), is provided. Also, during the initial peripheral vasocontriction that occurs after burn injury, the use of oximetry may be limited. Therefore pulse oximetry is found to be most useful during the subacute phase of management (Barillo et al., 1990).

Any patient who has sustained CO poisoning (COHb level > 10%) or is exhibiting neurologic signs and symptoms should be placed on 100% oxygen therapy using a tight-fitting, nonrebreathing mask or endotracheal tube (although smokers and residents of urban centers may have a chronic COHb level of up to 10% [Desai, 1984]). Hyperbaric oxygen has been found to be beneficial in reducing the serum COHb level by forcing the CO molecule off the hemoglobin. However, the disadvantage of delaying resuscitation and stabilization and the hazards of barotrauma may contraindicate its use (Heimbach, 1986).

Several protocols exist for using hyperbaric oxygen (HBO) therapy (Heimbach, 1983, 1986). Generally, if the patient is admitted exhibiting signs and symptoms of CO poisoning, if the CO level is greater than 25%, if the burn is less than 40% TBSA, and if no associated medical problems or other injury will complicate care, hyperbaric oxygen treatment may be initiated (Heimbach, 1986).

Long-term sequelae of carbon monoxide poisoning include neurologic signs of impaired memory and neuropsychiatric disorders. Delayed consequences of severe hypoxic brain injury are documented (Heimbach, 1983). Cerebral hypoxia and hypoxic capillary leak may lead to cerebral edema, causing further neurologic complications (Desai, 1984). Carbon monoxide has also been found to be toxic at the cellular level. Use of HBO therapy will reduce the incidence of latent encephalopathy (Martindale, 1989).

Circumferential, full-thickness burns of the chest wall may cause ineffective gas exchange secondary to ineffective breathing patterns. Increased shortness of breath, decreased tidal volumes, and increased ventilatory pressures indicate worsening ventilatory status. Escharotomy (surgical release of contracted collagen) may be required to release the collagen fibers and underlying edema to promote full chest expansion.

Perfusion

Perfusion in the burn victim is compromised from the time of injury. The patient experiences a generalized increase in capillary permeability, causing loss of colloid, water, and electrolytes into the interstitial space, as previously discussed. In addition, sodium enters and potassium exits the cell, leading to a shift in the osmotic gradient,

Table 14-3 Fluid replacement formulas

Formula	Electrolyte solution	Colloid	Water	Rate	Example: 70 kg/45% TBSA (per 24 hours)
Evans	1 ml/kg/% TBSA normal saline (NS)*	1 ml/kg/%	2000 ml	½, 1st 8 hrs; ½, next 16 hrs	3150 ml NS 3150 ml colloid 2000 ml water 8300 ml TOTAL
Brooke	1.5 ml/kg/% TBSA lactated Ringer's solution (LR)	0.5 ml/kg/%	2000 ml	½, 1st 8 hrs; ½, next 16 hrs	4725 ml LR 1575 ml colloid 2000 ml water 8300 ml TOTAL
Modified Brooke	2-3 ml/kg/% TBSA lactated Ringer's solution	None	None	½, 1st 8 hrs; ½, next 16 hrs.	6300-9450 ml LR
Parkland (Baxter)	4 ml/kg/% TBSA lactated Ringer's solution.	None	None	½, 1st 8 hrs; ½, next 16 hrs	12,600 ml LR
Hypertonic formula	Rate based on urine output of 30 ml/hr with hypertonic LR (sodium, 250 mEq/L)	None	None	To maintain urine output	Unknown

which causes interstitial water to enter the cell. This fluid shift occurs rapidly during the first 8 hours after injury and tapers off after 18 to 24 hours (Artz et al., 1979).

The patient develops a severe intravascular fluid volume deficit in the form of burn shock, which, if untreated, can lead to cellular destruction and death. Controversies exist regarding the amount of fluid required to counteract these effects (Cardona et al., 1988; O'Neill, 1982; Robertson, Cross, & Terry, 1985). Ideally, the type, rate, and amount of fluid administered should be sufficient to maintain vital organ function (e.g., adequate cardiac output) without producing immediate or delayed deleterious effects (e.g., excessive edema).

Fluid replacement

Intravenous fluid replacement is suggested for deep, partial-thickness or full-thickness burns in excess of 15% to 25% TBSA in adults and 10% TBSA in children. Elderly patients are more prone to the effects of burn shock, and a smaller percentage of burned tissue (15% TBSA) is used as a guideline for fluid replacement. Fluid requirements are increased in patients with respiratory injuries resulting from smoke inhalation (Heimbach, 1983).

Table 14-3 lists guidelines for calculating fluid requirements. Generally, the amount varies between 2 and 4 ml/kg/% TBSA burned. O'Neill (1982) demonstrated that burns in excess of 35% TBSA require 4 ml/kg/% TBSA because of the greater basal metabolic rate and insensible water loss that these patients experience. Evaporative heat loss increases 4 to 20 times during the first 8 hours after injury. A second controversy exists between using crystalloid (i.e., lactated Ringer's solution) and/or colloids (e.g., plasma, albumin) during the first 24 hours after the burn. Some believe that the increased capillary permeability that exists may prohibit the use of colloids, because these agents would cross into the interstitial space, without providing vascular support (Wachtel, Frank, Fortune, & Inancsi, 1983). Finally, the use of dextrose-containing fluids remains unresolved. Dextrose is believed to create an osmotic diuresis, which is harmful to the hypovolemic patient early in the resuscitation.

The majority of these formulas (Table 14-3) suggest administering one half of the calculated fluid required within the first 8 hours and the second one half over the next 16 hours. Because the most significant fluid shifts occur in the first 8 hours after injury, this will provide vascular support to meet anticipated losses. Most formulas then suggest that the calculated fluid requirements be reduced by one third to one half for the second 24-hour period after-burn, and that dextran or colloid be administered (Cardona, Hurn, Mason, Scanlon-Schilpp, & Veise-Berry, 1988).

Circulation is also compromised secondary to the release of myocardial depressant factor. Immediately after injury, cardiac output drops precipitously, so that in burns of greater than 50% TBSA, the cardiac output is approximately 30% of the preburn value (Artz et al., 1979). In burns less than 40% TBSA, this factor has no consequence, but in burns over 60% TBSA, it is considered the primary cause of resuscitative failure. In addition, blood flow to the liver, bowel, and kidneys is altered. Adequate resuscitation can restore cardiac output and regional blood flow if initiated early in the postburn period (Artz et al., 1979).

Perfusion is also compromised in circumferential, full-thickness burns. Heat-induced shortening of dermal collagen and edema formation cause reduced capillary flow and subsequent tissue hypoxia. Loss of peripheral pulses (as determined by Doppler) indicates compromised circulation; an escharotomy can release the pressure within the intravascular space (using skin temperature and color as parameters for assessing perfusion will be inaccurate secondary to tissue destruction). Monitors are available to measure the intracompartmental pressure (see Chapter 11). A linear incision along the medial or lateral surface of the extremity should be only deep enough to cut through the eschar and reestablish blood flow to the affected area.

Sensory Perception

Alteration in the level of consciousness (LOC) of the burn victim may be secondary to any number of causes: hypoxia, CO poisoning, inadequate cerebral perfusion caused by burn shock, depression, associated head trauma, alcohol use, or drug use. History of the injury may be insufficient to rule out associated injuries and drug or alcohol use; therefore in-depth evaluation is required. Improved circulatory status with fluid resuscitation should demonstrate an improvement in the patient's LOC. Oxygen therapy and ventilatory support will help diminish hypoxia and effects of CO poisoning.

Burns of the eye are ophthalmologic emergencies. Corneal burns are suspected with the presence of blistering, singed eyelashes, and swelling, and are confirmed with fluorescein stain. Chemicals in the eye should be flushed continuously with saline. It may be necessary to use the Morgan therapeutic lens for prolonged irrigation. These patients should be examined by an ophthalmologist as soon as possible. (More in-depth discussion can be found in Chapter 10).

Pain

Dosage of analgesic is increased in the burn patient. The increased metabolic rate metabolizes drugs rapidly; thus the patient's requirements are greater (Cardona et al., 1988). Intravenous morphine sulfate, 2 to 4 mg every 20 to 30 minutes, is the drug of choice. Intramuscular medications are not absorbed uniformly secondary to decreased peripheral blood flow and therefore are contraindicated. In addition, medications given intramuscularly may cause a precipitous fall in blood pressure once peripheral circulation is reestablished.

Patient-controlled analgesia (PCA) is frequently used for the management of pain in burn patients. The use of inhaled 50% nitrous oxide/50% oxygen mixture during wound care in both the ED and the ICU has been found to be beneficial in controlling patients' pain during these procedures, while preventing oversedation. A study of the pain of burns demonstrated that pain is highly variable among patients, although the greatest pain is reported during therapeutic procedures (Choiniere, Melzack, Rondeau, Girard, & Paquin, 1989). Other techniques in use include distraction (imagery, music) and relaxation (massage, music, touch). The addition of antianxiety agents to the regimen of narcotic administration has been found to decrease the amount of opioid required to control pain.

Mobility

Associated trauma complicates care of the burn victim. Closed fractures may be overlooked and can cause internal, ongoing blood loss, increasing fluid requirements beyond expected needs. Closed compartment syndrome (see Chapter 11) may develop, which will necessitate performance of a fasciotomy. Application of splints or casts may be deleterious if swelling continues and may cause a tourniquet effect on the limb. In the event that immobilization is required for fracture management, external or internal fixation devices are the treatment of choice in the burned victim.

Improper wound management can lead to contracture formation with scarring. Contracture and subsequent loss of range of motion can be avoided with proper physical therapy and the application of pressure garments as soon as appropriate after injury.

Wound Care

Impaired tissue integrity is inherent in burn injuries. Although wound care does not receive immediate priority, institution of suggested protocols will prevent avoidable scarring and wound complications.

Wound care for major burns before transfer from the ED consists of superficial cleaning of the wound with soap, detergents, and water (removing rocks, dirt, and other debris); shaving or trimming surrounding hair (except eyebrows); and covering the wound with a topical antibiotic agent and a dry dressing. (Application of a topical antibiotic will depend on the protocols of the burn center to which the patient will be admitted; however, a survey of centers demonstrated that most centers do apply a topical agent, most commonly silver sulfadiazine (Taddonio, Thomson, Smith, & Prasad, 1990). Choice of topical agents includes silver sulfadiazine (Silvadene), which has the benefits of being a broad-spectrum antimicrobial agent that is not absorbed systemically, and is not painful on application. The disadvantages of the use of Silvadene are that its use may modestly delay wound healing, and approximately one third of patients become leukopenic during the first week of use (Zschoche, 1986). An alternative agent is mafenide acetate (Sulfamylon), which has better eschar penetration capabilities, is more effective against enterococci, and is the agent of choice in infected wounds. Disadvantages are that it is painful to apply and may cause an overwhelming systemic metabolic acidosis. Covering the wound with a thin layer of Kerlix will prevent staining of the patient's clothes and will protect tissue generation and graft adherence. Wounds may also be left undressed, and current research is ongoing to determine the optimal method (Warden, 1987.) However, if a wound is managed without a covering, application of additional

topical agent may be necessary as the patient moves in bed.

Dry dressings should be applied to prevent hypothermia and the risk of infection associated with moist dressing use. Application of cold water to stop the burning process 10 minutes after the injury has been reported to be ineffective because the tissues have already cooled by evaporative heat loss (Mikhail, 1988). Removal of blister covering is controversial (Boswick, 1987c; Rockwell & Ehrlich, 1990). Some believe that the blister covering will prevent further bacterial contamination; others believe that the devitalized tissue becomes a growth medium for infecting organisms (Boswick, 1987c). The burn blister fluid has been found to have several deleterious effects on healing of burn wounds, and it is recommended that this fluid be evacuated at the time of initial wound management (Rockwell & Ehrlich, 1990).

Grafting

Long-term care of major burns includes debridement and grafting of deep, partial-thickness and full-thickness wounds. Grafting generally occurs 4 to 5 days after resolution of tissue edema. Grafting has been used for wound protection to prevent bacterial contamination, to cover excised wounds, to reduce fluid and heat losses, to decrease pain, and to decrease the metabolic rate. Autograft (graft composed of the patient's own skin) provides the best match and acceptance. Not all wounds can receive autograft immediately, in which case human allograft (graft composed of cadaver or donated skin) or xenograft (graft retrieved from other species (e.g., pigskin) is placed over the wound to stimulate tissue growth and help prevent infection.

Other recent developments include manufactured wound coverings, including artificial skin and Biobrane (Table 14-4). These skin coverings are generally used when the burn covers more than 50% of the body surface and no available donor sites exist (Stern, McPherson, & Longaker, 1990). Artificial skin consists of a bilayer membrane, with one layer as an external barrier—the epidermal component, and a second layer as an internal environment—the dermal layer. The artificial skin (e.g., Integra) is applied to the burn wound and acts as a base for dermal growth. After time, the top layer of the artificial skin is removed

Table 14-4 Burn wound coverings

Type	Source	Purpose
Autograft	Patient's own skin or cell replication	Permanent replacement
Allograft (homograft)	Human cadaver	Temporary covering (3 to 5 days)
Xenograft (heterograft)	Pigskin	Temporary covering (3 to 7 days)
Artificial skin	Manufactured skin	Temporary covering (7 to 14 days) (part of membrane remains integrated in new skin; remainder is removed)
Biologic or biosynthetic dressings (e.g., Biobrane)	Manufactured membrane	Temporary covering that may act as base substance for dermal growth (complete removal once epithelization occurs)

intraoperatively and the wound is covered with meshed autografts. One-stage procedures and cultured skin substitutes are being developed (Burke, 1990; Hansbrough, 1990).

Biobrane is a temporary biosynthetic wound covering that acts also as a base substance for dermal growth. A patient with small, partial-thickness or full-thickness burns that need coverage can have Biobrane placed over the wound and be discharged, with a significant cost savings and reduced pain associated with typical dressing changes. Meshed Biobrane has been applied to areas of difficult topography (e.g., neck, axilla, elbow, buttocks) with good results (Phillips et al., 1990). Other biologic dressings that have been used in grafting include amnionic membranes and bovine and canine skin (Boswick, 1987c; Hansbrough, 1990).

An intensified effort should be made to harvest cadaver skin. Advances in cryopreservation techniques and storage have made allograft the wound covering of choice for most wounds (Boswick, 1987c). Regionalization of tissue banks and procurement networks and improved harvest and storage techniques for cadaver skin at tissue banks have increased availability of this precious resource (May, 1990). Meshing of grafts to achieve greater coverage allows the use of smaller donor grafts but may alter the cosmetic results.

Minor burns comprise approximately 95% of all burns treated in the United States, and many can be treated on an out-patient basis (Warden, 1987). Success depends on the patient's ability to change dressings, clean wounds, and recognize complications. Initial cleaning and debridement is done in the ED while the patient observes and

is taught the procedure. The wound can be covered with a single layer of saline-moistened gauze, gauze compresses, and, finally, an absorbent dressing. The patient should be instructed to (1) elevate the part to prevent swelling and (2) repeat wound care twice a day. Signs and symptoms of infection should be included in the patient teaching protocol, and the patient should be instructed to return immediately on recognition of any of these signs and symptoms. Out-patient topical antibiotic use is controversial because of various reports on effectiveness. Maintenance of a moist environment to stimulate epithelization is standard (Boswick, 1987c). Generally, the patient is instructed to return to the ED or clinic within 5 days for further evaluation and wound care (Haynes, 1983).

Elimination

Genital burn wounds complicate care because of the contaminated environment, as well as the difficulty in placing dressings over the folds of the groin area. For this reason, genital burns are classified as major burns and should be treated in a burn center.

Foley catheter placement is necessary for all patients with moderate or major burns and can be placed through a burned orifice. Urine output is an important parameter in the measurement of the adequacy of fluid resuscitation and should average, over 3 hours, 30 to 50 ml/hr in the adult and 0.5 to 1.0 ml/kg/hr in the child.

Myoglobinuria occurs as a result of muscle destruction. In deep, full-thickness burns and electrical burns, the release of myoglobin can potentiate the risk of developing renal failure. Inadequate urine output and pink-tinged urine are the hallmarks of myoglobinuria; however, confirmation is done by urinalysis. Increasing fluid intake may resolve the problem, but in severe cases, mannitol (12.5 g) IV will be required to help clear the renal tubules of myoglobin.

A nasogastric tube should be inserted in all burn patients with greater than 20% to 25% TBSA injured, because of ileus formation and subsequent nausea and vomiting, which may last as long as 5 days after injury. Any burn patient requiring long-distance transport may have a Salem sump tube placed and attached to continuous suction to prevent the risks of motion sickness and to allow for equilibration of pressure variances that occur with changes in altitude.

Adaptation

Burn injuries require long-term care and follow-up. Patients admitted to burn centers may have hospital stays longer than 3 to 6 months, and may experience multiple surgeries, possible loss of limb, disfigurement, and staggering hospital bills. The pain, fear, and loss of self-esteem are immeasurable (Ragiel, 1984; Shenkman & Stechmiller, 1987). Multidisciplinary teams, including physicians, nurses, physical and occupational therapists, respiratory therapists, nutritionists, social workers, and psychologists, can provide the patient with the comprehensive care required (Cardona et al., 1988).

Remarkable improvements in burn care during the past 3 decades have increased the survival rates in patients with large burns, as well as older patients. Overall mortality has declined from 24% in 1974 to 7% in 1984. Survival has also been accompanied by (1) an improvement in patients' satisfaction with their body image and (2) patients' ability to live more satisfied, happy, and productive lives (Burke, 1990). However, for this decreased mortality trend to continue, burn patients must be treated in facilities that are capable of providing state-of-the-art burn care in which aggressive intervention is undertaken. Special focus is needed on the inflammatory reaction and multiple organ failure and on inhalation injuries.

Transport Preparation

Transport of burn victims should follow American Burn Association guidelines for definitive care and may occur on two levels (Moylan, 1987): first, from the scene of the accident to the local hospital for stabilization; second, from the local facility to a treatment center specializing in burn care. In transport, it is important to provide for the physiologic needs of the patient and minimize contamination of the burn wounds.

Airway patency must be established before transporting the burn victim. Loss of airway patency and respiratory failure can occur in a patient sustaining smoke inhalation or burns of the face, head, or neck. Oxygen administration will reduce the half-life of carbon monoxide and minimize hypoxia. Intravenous fluid administration should be continued; therefore adequate fluids must be available to meet the patient's potential requirements. (See the box below for a list of transport equipment.) Continuous cardiac monitoring is important and should be considered a requirement for electrical burns. Maintenance of body heat can be accomplished with rescue blankets, which reflect heat loss back to the patient.

With the advent of sophisticated air ambulances, burn victims can be rapidly evacuated from outlying areas to major burn centers. The American College of Surgeons has guidelines for air ambulance operations, defining team configurations, equipment, and training of personnel (see Chapter 20). Helicopter transports are generally

---

Transport equipment for burn patients

Oxygen cylinders with regulators
Intubation equipment: laryngoscope, endotracheal tubes
Bag-mask resuscitator
Portable suction with suction catheters
Non-rebreather face mask of appropriate size
Lactated Ringer's solution (amount to meet calculated needs + ½)
IV infusion sets (with warming devices, if available)
Cardiac monitor with defibrillator
Foley catheter with drainage set
Nasogastric tube
Scalpel and dressings (escharotomy tray)
CODE (cardiac or cardiopulmonary arrest) medications
Clean, dry sheets
Rescue blanket
Vital sign flow sheet with input and output record
Patient's medical record

used within a 150 mile radius, whereas fixed-wing aircraft are used for longer distance. Air transport of patients requires the same planning and care as ground transport, with the additional concern for altitude effects on patient status.

ASSESSMENT AND INTERVENTIONS RELATED TO SPECIFIC INJURIES AND POPULATIONS
Pediatric Burn Injury

Pediatric burn victims have unique anatomic and physiologic needs. The incidence of burns as a form of child abuse has increased from 10% to 30% of all cases of reported abuse and are most prevalent in children younger than 3 years (Kelley, 1988). Burn patterns that may be indicative of abuse include full-thickness, circumferential burns of the feet, hands, or buttocks as a result of the child being forcibly held under scalding water; dry, linear burns resulting from a curling iron, stove burner, or radiator; small, circular burns from a lit cigarette being extinguished on the skin (Kelley, 1988). (Figures 14-8 and Figure 14-9). Accidental burns tend to leave irregular, erratic patterns, usually of more superficial depth (Gordon, 1979).

Ineffective gas exchange develops rapidly in the child with burns of the face, head, or neck. Because children have fewer collateral ventilatory pathways, airway maintenance, ventilatory support, and oxygenation must be initiated promptly in these children.

Circulatory support of the child is controversial. Estimation of fluid requirements based solely on the child's weight in kilograms and the TBSA burned may result in significant underresuscitation of the child (Carvajal & Parks, 1988). In addition, because children younger than 8 years have poor glycogen stores, which results in hypoglycemia, children will need additional glucose-containing maintenance fluids to supplement their calculated lactated Ringer's solution needs (see box on right). Assessing for the signs of adequate resuscitation (e.g., blood pressure, pulse rate, urine output) will ensure that the child is neither underresuscitated or overresuscitated. Close monitoring of the child's serum glucose using bedside blood glucose reagent strips (Chemstrip) will protect the child from a precipitous fall in serum glucose level.

Young children may not be able to express their physical and psychologic needs. Pain may be expressed in the form of crying; however, many other stimuli may cause the child to cry. Expression of needs through games and pictures may help establish a communication pattern with these children (see Chapter 17.)

Children with burns should be under constant supervision. The young child will not understand instructions to minimize contamination of the wound. Bumps, scrapes, and other injuries to the wound or graft may delay wound healing and lead to scar formation. Communication and expression of needs are difficult in the early developmental years of life. These children cannot express the severity of their pain and may be undermedicated. Involving parents and family members in the child's care is beneficial throughout the hospital stay.

Fluid requirements for pediatric burn patients

Lactated Ringer's solution for burn shock

2 to 4 ml/kg/% TBSA burned
 ½ in first 8 hours, starting from time of injury
 ¼ in second 8 hours
 ¼ in third 8 hours

D$_5$ ¼ Normal saline for maintenance

100 jt for first 10 kg
50 jt for second 10 kg   } Divided equally
20 jt for each remaining kg   } over 24 hours

Example: 25 kg child with a 40% TBSA deep, partial-thickness burn

Lactated Ringer's solution:
 2 to 4 ml/25 kg/40% = 2000 to 4000 ml/24 hours
 125 to 250 ml/hr during first 8 hours
 63 to 125 ml/hr during remaining 16 hours
D$_5$ ¼ normal saline
 1000 ml for first 10 kg   } 1600 ml/24 hrs =
 500 ml for second 10 kg   } 67 ml/hr
 100 ml for remaining 5 kg }
Total requirements: (including lactated Ringer's solution and D$_5$ ¼ NS)
 192 to 317 ml/hr during first 8 hours
 130 to 192 ml/hr during remaining 16 hours

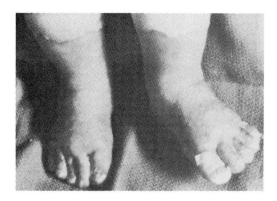

Figure 14-8 Bilateral forced immersion burns of feet and lower portions of legs of young child. "Stocking" configuration reflects uniform degree of involvement throughout burned areas and sharp, circumferential demarcation line proximally, which separates burned areas from proximal uninvolved skin. (*Note.* From "Inflicted Burns in Children" by J. Schanberger, 1981, *Topics in Emergency Medicine*, 3, p. 88.)

Nonthermal Burns

Chemical, electrical, and tar burns, as well as burns complicated by compounding traumatic injuries or preexisting illness, require special interventions.

Chemical

Chemical burns require immediate and continuous flushing with saline. The reaction caused by using the specific neutralizing agent often is exothermic (heat producing) and therefore can actually increase the severity of the injury. Of special note are hydrofluoric acid burns, in which a transcutaneous absorption of the fluoride ions into the subcutaneous tissue occurs, where the ions bind with calcium and cause severe, burning pain (Monafo, 1987). Treatment consists of copious water lavage and the application of magnesium hydroxide paste to bind the fluoride. If burning persists, calcium gluconate can be injected into the subcutaneous tissue after lavage and neutralization (Monafo, 1987). Once chemicals have been removed, the wound is treated as a thermal burn.

Electrical

Electrical injuries are considered to be like icebergs—only the tip of the damage can be visualized. As the voltage passes into the skin, a small burn occurs at the skin surface, while the majority of the damage occurs at the underlying mus-

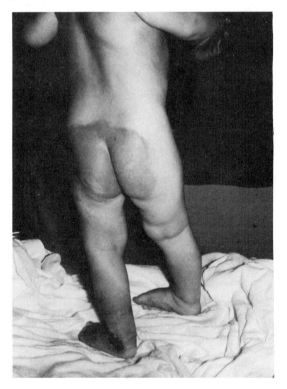

Figure 14-9 Partial-thickness hot water burns of child's buttocks and feet, caused by abuse. Note that buttocks would not be burned if child had stepped into water voluntarily. (*Note.* From *Thermal Injuries* by D.P. Dressler, J.L. Hozid, and P. Nathan, 1988, St. Louis: Mosby–Year Book.)

cular and vascular level. The damage that occurs depends on the density of the tissue through which the voltage passes. At very low currents, no adverse effects occur; increasing current can cause severe muscular contraction and paralysis of the respiratory muscles, leading to death by asphyxia. Energy and heat are dissipated through tissues— the larger the surface area of contact, the greater the dissipation. As an electrical current will do less harm if the area of contact is large (because of dissipation of energy and heat), the same current will do extensive damage if applied in a small area.

Extensive damage to muscle causes release of myoglobin, causing myoglobinuria. Voltage passing through the heart can damage the conduction system and can cause ventricular dysrhythmias. Necrotic tissue releases lactic acid, causing a severe, systemic, metabolic acidosis.

Many electrical burns occur from 120 volt AC household appliances (e.g., hair dryers, wall sockets, hot water heaters). These injuries are minor unless the time of contact with live wires is prolonged. Deep, extensive electrical injuries occur from high-voltage source (e.g., electrical transmission lines). However, with both types of injury, extent of damage is not easily ascertained. Long-term sequelae include amputation and cataract formation subsequent to extensive tissue damage.

The Lund and Browder chart for calculating body surface area injured provides an inaccurately low calculated fluid requirement when used for electrical burns. Patients with major electrical burns require fluids at 1 to 2 liters per hour or an adequate amount to maintain blood pressure and a urine output of at least 100 ml/hour. Mannitol (12.5 g) may be given judiciously to assist with the clearing of myoglobin, recognizing the osmotic effect on blood pressure. Sodium bicarbonate may be necessary to treat a low serum pH.

Tar

Tar burns may or may not cause extensive injury, depending on the temperature of the tar when it comes in contact with the skin. Once the tar has been cooled with cold water, ointment (Medisol, mineral oil, bacitracin, Neosporin) is applied to dissolve the tar. Tar should *never* be peeled off, because the depth and extent of burn will increase if attached, viable tissue is peeled

away. A dressing is then applied; it is removed after 18 to 24 hours, at which time most of the tar will have dissolved. During this interval, pain can be controlled for the thermally injured patient with small, frequent doses of morphine sulfate. After complete removal of the tar, the TBSA injured may be calculated. This percentage may be less than the percentage calculated on admission to the ED, and the patient may have been fluid overresuscitated. As with all burns, estimations of fluid requirements are merely guidelines and each patient must be followed individually for response to resuscitative efforts.

Associated Injury Risk

Simultaneous traumatic injuries may occur with the burn injury. Patients admitted with suspected or confirmed closed head injuries will require close monitoring of fluid status. Care must be taken to prevent overhydration of these patients and subsequent elevation of intracranial pressure. Blunt abdominal trauma can cause undetected hemorrhage that requires increased fluids and blood replacement—more than the calculated fluid required for burn shock resuscitation. In addition, the patient with a burned abdomen may give a false-positive examination on palpation, because touching the burned tissue may cause pain and the patient will withdraw. Diagnostic peritoneal lavage (DPL) may be done through burned tissue using aseptic technique to reduce the risk of infection.

EVALUATION

Signs of adequate resuscitative efforts include urine output of 30 to 50 ml/hr in the adult patient and 0.5 to 1.0 ml/kg/hr in the child, with the exception of the electrically injured patient, who requires a urine output of 100 to 200 ml/hr to prevent acute renal failure. The patient's level of consciousness will improve with improved cerebral blood flow and cardiac output and normal HbCO. Central venous pressure (CVP) measurements are beneficial in evaluating fluid status; however, most recommendations are placement of a CVP or Swan Ganz catheter only in patients with burns greater than 40% to 45% TBSA (Heimbach, 1986).

Vitals signs must be recorded in all burn patients and can be obtained over burned tissue. (To protect the patient and the blood pressure cuff, the patient's arm can be wrapped with a thin layer of gauze and the blood pressure cuff placed on top of the gauze.) Blood pressure is an indicator of fluid status; however, readings may be inaccurate if obtained in an area with severe edema (Rauscher & Ochs, 1983). Heart rate will be elevated initially and should return to within normal limits with adequate fluid administration and reduction in hypermetabolism.

Initial blood work will show an elevated hematocrit as a consequence of hemoconcentration. This should return to normal and may even drop to 30% to 35% within a few days after injury. Severe muscle damage can cause a dangerously low pH, which should be corrected with intravenous sodium bicarbonate. Patients with inhalation injuries will have a significant drop in PaO_2.

COMPLICATIONS
Inappropriate Fluid Resuscitation

Fluid overresuscitation and underresuscitation can be harmful to the burn patient. Continued signs of hypovolemic shock and sequelae are indicative of underresuscitation, which is the most common error of resuscitation. The pediatric and elderly patient are at risk for complications of overresuscitation. The elderly patient with a history of cardiac disease may be unable to tolerate rapid fluid administration, which can lead to congestive heart failure and pulmonary edema, increasing the mortality rate in this group of patients.

Infection

Systemic antibiotics are rarely indicated prophylactically in the burn victim (Boswick, 1987b). In the past, overwhelming resistant organisms developed from the liberal use of systemic antibiotics and caused a large number of deaths. Vigilant observation of culture and sensitivity reports, wound biopsies (usually performed at least twice weekly [Taddonio, Thomson, Smith, & Prasad, 1990]), as well as signs and symptoms of infection are imperative. Identification of an infecting organism is done using a punch biopsy or swab culture, and subsequently intravenous antibiotics are initiated. Exceptions to this recommendation are burn victims with open fracture sites; they should receive broad-spectrum antibiotics on admission. Topical antibiotics are used in large burns and may or may not be used for minor burns if meticulous wound care is performed.

The number of deaths from sepsis after burn injury is declining (Burke, 1990; Merrell, Saffle, Larson, & Sullivan, 1989). Burn size, presence of inhalation injury, and the extent of full-thickness injury are predictors for subsequent development of fatal sepsis. Improvement in fluid resuscitation, the practice of early excision, and improved medical care have greatly increased this decline in the number of deaths caused by sepsis (Merrell et al., 1989). Future development of new antimicrobial agents and the use of artifical wound coverings may further reduce this complication.

Infections in burn patients are often hospital-acquired, and although many methods of isolation are being used, the incidence of infection remains the leading cause of death among seriously burned patients (Lee, Marvin, Heimbach, Grube, & Engrav, 1990). A study to evaluate the effectiveness of a simplified barrier technique (handwashing, glove use, and plastic aprons) demonstrated a reduced incidence of cross contamination and proved to be cost-effective (Lee, Marvin, Heimbach, Grube, & Engrav, 1990). Astute awareness of the problem, as well as methods to prevent infection, should be foremost in the minds of all providers of health care for the burned patient.

SUMMARY Burns account for a significant portion of traumatic injuries. Regardless of the burn injury, airway, breathing, and circulatory requirements must remain as first priority. Assessment of the wound includes depth, extent, and a history of the injury. Resuscitation includes intravenous replacement of the large associated fluid losses. Wound care, protection from contamination, maintenance of body temperature, and pain control are subsequent priorities. Nursing diagnoses and evaluative criteria for the burned patient are presented in the table on pp. 470-471. Disposition of the victim to the appropriate facility will enhance the chance of survival and improve long-term outcomes. Burns in the elderly and children, as well as chemical and electrical burns, offer additional challenges to the ED healthcare provider. Thermal injuries are truly multisystem injuries and certainly impact the psychosocial realm in the acute, as well as the chronic, phases of care. A multidisciplinary approach to burn care will reduce mortality and morbidity of these injuries.

The patient with thermal injury

Nursing diagnosis	Nursing intervention	Evaluative criteria
Fluid volume deficit Related to capillary permeability, fluid extravasation As evidenced by systemic edema, decreased urine output, low PWCP, CVP	**Maintain adequate fluid volume** Monitor fluid replacement (see Table 13-3).	BP will be >90 systolic. Urine output will be 30-50 ml/hr (100 ml/hr for electrical burns). LOC will improve. CVP will return to WNL (2-6 mm H_2O).
Impaired gas exchange Related to decreased hemoglobin, alveolar damage, fluid shifts As evidenced by singed nasal hairs, carbonaceous sputum, upper airway edema	**Maintain oxygenation and ventilation** Adjust oxygen according to Pao_2. Anticipate escharotomy for full-thickness burns. Anticipate intubation for significant facial, neck, chest burns, and increasing SOB. Elevate HOB to promote full chest expansion.	Pao_2 will be 80-100 mm Hg. Chest excursion will improve. ABGs will improve. COHb will decrease.
High risk for hypothermia Related to loss of body heat through exposed skin	**Maintain body temperature** Administer warm, humidified oxygen. Administer warm IV fluids. Apply dry dressings. Use warming lights. Monitor core temperature. Avoid patient exposure to cold. Avoid use of wet saline soaks. Cover patient with rescue (e.g., Mylar) blanket.	Core temperature will be $\geq 37°$ C.
High risk for infection Related to damaged skin barrier, cellular destruction, presence of necrotic tissue, eschar	**Prevent infection** Apply topical antibiotics as indicated. Use aseptic technique. Wear apron/gown, glove, mask during interventions.	Cultures and sensitivities will show no growth.

Nursing diagnosis	Nursing intervention	Evaluative criteria
	Cover wounds for transport. Promote pulmonary hygiene and early mobilization.	
Pain Related to irritation of nerve endings, edema As evidenced by verbal complaints of pain, grimacing, change in vital signs	**Maximize comfort** Administer narcotics and/or sedation for moderate and major burns. Use imagery and relaxation techniques. Avoid IM injections.	Self-related pain score will decrease. Patient will comply with wound care.
Body image disturbance Related to disfigurement, edema, undesired change in functional abilities and role As evidenced by social withdrawal, verbal comments, anger	**Promote adaptation to change in image** Promote interaction with psychiatrist, psychologist. Promote interaction with family members. Encourage verbalization. Support interaction with other patients. Arrange interaction with previously burned patients as appropriate. Refer to PT/OT as appropriate.	Patient will verbalize feelings. Patient will be able to confront image in mirror.
Altered tissue perfusion Related to edema, coagulopathy, constrictive tissue and materials As evidenced by diminished pulses, cool distal extremities	**Enhance circulation** Perform Doppler checks. Evaluate circulation. Remove jewelry, constricting clothing. Ensure proper wrapping of wounds. Assist with peripheral escharotomy or fasciotomy. Explain need, procedure, alleviation of pain, and process of healing.	Peripheral circulation will improve. Capillary refill will occur within 2 seconds. Peripheral edema will decrease. Dressings will not constrict, and burned surfaces will not be in contact with one another.

CASE STUDY Mr. Roberts is a 37-year-old farmer who was thrown from his tractor when the engine exploded and ignited. He was brought to the ED at 3:15 PM by EMTs. On arrival he is unconscious and covered with soot. His BP is 96 by palpation; P, 136; and RR, 36 and shallow. He has burns of his head, back, abdomen, upper portion of chest, and distal portion of his right leg. His estimated weight is 75 kg. He is on a backboard with a cervical collar in place, and oxygen is being administered by face mask. The EMTs can relate little history as to the time and nature of the injury because the patient was found by his wife after an undetermined amount of time when he did not return to the house for lunch. However, the prehospital care report does include the following information: Mr. Roberts' clothes had been burned and were removed by the EMTs, the field surrounding the tractor had burned, and the smell of gasoline was present at the site.

In the order of priority, what are the appropriate steps in stabilizing Mr. Roberts?

Airway, breathing, and circulation receive first priority. Because the patient has burns of his head and upper portion of his chest with a poor respiratory effort, he should be prophylactically intubated and 100% oxygen should be provided. His unconsciousness may be caused by his decreased blood pressure, a closed head injury, or hypoxia and hypercarbia. Two large-bore intravenous lines should be established, with infusion of a crystalloid solution at 300 to 500 ml/hr. The rate should be increased or decreased, based on his vital signs and response to therapy.

Because no time of injury can be ascertained, it is possible that Mr. Roberts is experiencing at least a 3- to 4-liter fluid deficit. The details of the partial history should be considered: Mrs. Roberts states that her husband did not return for lunch and she then went looking for him. Therefore it can be assumed that his injury occurred during the morning, before his normal lunch break. (It is now 3:15 PM, at least 3 hours after he was to return to the house.) After intubation and establishment of intravenous access, a thorough head-to-toe assessment for compounding traumatic injuries must be instituted. Blood samples should be sent to the laboratory for electrolytes values, type and crossmatch, and glucose, hematocrit, hemoglobin, and carboxyhemoglobin levels. An arterial blood sample should be drawn for ABG studies. A Foley catheter and NG tube should be inserted. Mr. Roberts should receive 0.5 ml of diphtheria toxoid (or tetanus toxoid) IM. Subsequently, if no other injuries are found, wound care can be instituted.

After initial evaluation, it is determined that Mr. Roberts has sustained the following injuries: approximately 48% deep, partial-thickness burn, an open tibia/fibula fracture of his right leg, possible smoke inhalation, and a suspected lacerated spleen (based on mechanism of injury and ecchymosis over the left upper quadrant of his abdomen). Based on this additional information, what therapies should be instituted for Mr. Roberts?

Specific fluid requirements can be calculated using one of the accepted formulas. Based on his weight and percentage of TBSA burned, the patient requires between 450 and 900 ml/hr for the first 8 hours. However, his resuscitation has already been delayed at least 3 hours and to administer the calculated fluid required (3600 to 7200 ml) requires an infusion rate of between 700 and 1400 ml/hr for the first 5 hours. Also, both the smoke inhalation injury and the splenic hematoma require additional IV fluids, including packed red cells. Mr. Roberts will continue to have a low blood pressure until adequate fluid resuscitation to meet his ongoing losses is achieved. Also, because initiating intravenous fluid resuscitation was delayed (fluids are calculated from time of injury), he is probably extremely hypovolemic. Increasing fluids over and above the calculated needs may be necessary, but close monitoring of the signs of adequate resuscitation is imperative.

The physician must decide if Mr. Roberts should go to the operating room for an exploratory laporatomy. An abdominal CT scan or diagnostic peritoneal lavage can help determine the extent and seriousness of his injury. The open tibia/fibula fracture will require intervention by an orthopedic surgeon; again, the urgency of such treatment will depend on the patient's condition. However, because of the open fracture, broad-spectrum intravenous antibiotics should be initiated soon after admission to the ED. Obtaining a core temperature will demonstrate the extent of existing hypothermia.

Because of the extent of his burn, as well as the compounding traumatic injuries, Mr. Roberts requires admission to a burn center. Transport arrangements should be initiated soon after his admission to the ED. Determination of the extent of stabilization required can be discussed with the receiving physician in the burn center. Mr. Roberts' wounds can be cleaned and covered with sterile gauze. He should remain on the backboard with the cervical collar in place until his cervical spine has been cleared of injury by x-ray examination. Before transport, maintenance of body heat and prevention of further contamination must be initiated. Mr. Roberts should remain in the ED no longer that 45 to 60 minutes, unless awaiting the arrival of the transporting team.

RESEARCH QUESTIONS

- What are the effects of nursing interventions on hypothermic states in the massively burned individual?
- How can ED care of the burn victim be improved?
- What is the best approach to be used with the next-of-kin in requesting harvesting of donor skin?

- Is it possible to successfully manage a patient on an out-patient basis after minor skin grafting?
- How do patients manage the pain of wound dressing changes at home?
- Is there a way to quantify sequential Doppler results in the assessment of peripheral vascular compromise secondary to burn edema?
- What depth and percentage of TBSA burn should serve as the criterion to avoid use of cool saline towels in an effort to avoid hypothermia, yet maximize comfort?
- What nursing interventions reduce anxiety and pain during dressing changes and other painful procedures (Marvin et al., 1991*)?
- What community-based follow-up would best meet the physical and emotional needs of the patient with burns and his or her family (Marvin et al., 1991*)?
- What nursing interventions promote healing of donor sites and skin grafts (Marvin et al., 1991*)?

RESOURCES

American Association of Tissue Banks (AATB)
1350 Beverly Rd., Suite 220-A
McLean, VA 22101
(703) 827-9582

American Burn Association
Department of Surgery, R310
University of Miami
Box 016310
Miami, FL 33101
(305) 547-6187

International Society for Burn Injuries
2005 Franklin St. #660
Denver, CO 80205
(303) 839-1694

National Fire Protection Association (NFPA)
Batterymarch Park
Quincy, MA 02269
(617) 770-3000

National Institute for Burn Medicine
909 E. Ann St.
Ann Arbor, MI 48104
(313) 769-9000

Phoenix Society (Burn Rehabilitation)
11 Rust Hill Rd.
Levittstown, PA 19056
(215) 946-4788

---

*The reader is directed to this reference for an in-depth discussion of research priorities in burn nursing.

Radiation Emergency Assistance Center and Training Site (REAC/TAS)
General Information: Oak Ridge Associated Universities
Box 117
Oak Ridge TN 37831
(615) 576-3131
24 hour Hotline: (615) 482-2441, Beeper, #241

ANNOTATED BIBLIOGRAPHY

Boswick, J. (1987). *The art and science of burn care*. Rockville, MD: Aspen Publishers.

One of the most recent textbooks on burn care. This manual covers all aspects of burn care from the prehospital phase through rehabilitation. Each chapter is concise and to the point. Chapters highlighting wound care are especially good, including many photographs.

Robertson, K., Cross, P., & Terry, J. (1985). CE burn care: The crucial first days. *American Journal of Nursing*, 85(1), 30-45.

First of a series of articles regarding burn care. The information is easy to read and very complete. Although continuing education credit is no longer available for this course, the self-examination is most beneficial. The same journal issue also reviews nutritional needs and rehabilitation of patients with thermal injury.

McLaughlin, E.G. (1990). *Critical care of the burn patient: A case study approach*. Rockville, MD: Aspen Publishers.

Book with a unique format for presenting information regarding nursing care of burn patients. Each chapter begins with a brief description of the topic at hand and is followed by one or more case studies. Subsequently the information is brief but quite thorough. Further in-depth information is included in the discussion of the case studies. Each chapter ends with a good reference list.

REFERENCES

Artz, C., Moncrief, J., & Pruitt, B. (Eds.) (1979). *Burns: A team approach*. Philadelphia: W.B. Saunders.

Barillo, D., Mostropieri, C., Cohen, M., & Okunski, W. (1990). How accurate is pulse oximetry in patients with burn injuries? *Journal of Burn Care and Rehabilitation*, 11 (2), 162-166.

Barker, S. & Tremper, K. (1987). The effect of carbon monoxide inhalation on pulse oximetry and transcutaneous PO_2. *Anesthesiology*, 66 (5), 677-679.

Baxter, C. (1990). Future prospectives in trauma and burn care. *Journal of Trauma*, 30 (12) Suppl., S208-209.

Boswick, J. (Ed.) (1987a). *The art and science of burn care*. Rockville, MD: Aspen Publishers.

Boswick, J. (1987b). Initial care of burn wounds. In J. Boswick (Ed.), *The art and science of burn care* (pp 37-39). Rockville, MD: Aspen Publishers.

Boswick, J. (1987c). The role of dressings in treating burn wounds. In J. Boswick (Ed.), *The art and science of burn care* (pp 53-63). Rockville, MD: Aspen Publishers.

Burke, J. (1990). From desperation to skin regeneration: Progress in burn treatment. *Journal of Trauma*, 30 (12), S36-40.

Cardona, V., Hurn, P., Mason, P., Scanlon-Schilpp, A., & Veise-Berry, S. (1988). *Trauma nursing: From resuscitation through rehabilitation*. Philadelphia: W.B. Saunders.

Carvajal, H., & Parks, D. (1988). *Pediatric burn management*. Chicago: Mosby–Year Book, Inc.

Choiniere, M., Melzack, R., Rondeau, J., Girard, N., & Paquin, M. (1989). The pain of burns: Characteristics and correlates. *Journal of Trauma*, 29 (11), 1531-1539.

Davic, J.C., & Hunt, T.K. (Eds.) (1977). *Hyperbaric oxygen therapy*. Bethesda, MD: Undersea Medical Society.

Desai, M. (1984). Inhalation injuries in burn victims. *Critical Care Quarterly*, 7 (3), 1-6.

Dimick, A. (1983). Triage of burn patients. In T. Wachtel, V. Kahn, & T. Frank (Eds.), *Current topics in burn care* (pp 15-18). Rockville, MD: Aspen Publishers.

Fontanarosa, P. (1988). Lightning and related injuries. *Journal of Emergency Medical Services*, 13 (7), 37-43.

Gordon, M. (1979). Nursing care of the burned child. In C. Artz, J. Moncrief, & B. Pruitt (Eds.), *Burns: A team approach* (pp 390-410). Philadelphia: W.B. Saunders.

Hansborough, J. (1990). Current status of skin replacements for coverage of extensive burn wounds. *Journal of Trauma*, 30 (12) Suppl. S155-162.

Haynes, B.W. (1983). Emergency department management of minor burns. In T. Wachtel, V. Kahn, & H. Frank (Eds.), *Current topics in burn care* (pp 19-24). Rockville, MD: Aspen Publishers.

Heimbach, D. (1983). Smoke inhalation: Current concepts. In T. Wachtel, V. Kahn, & H. Frank (Eds.), *Current topics in burn care* (pp 31-39). Rockville, MD: Aspen Publishers.

Heimbach, D. (1986). *Pearls from the top*. Unpublished protocol, University of Washington, Seattle.

Kelley, S. (1988). Physical abuse of children: Recognition and reporting. *Journal of Emergency Nursing*, 17 (2), 82-90.

Lee, J., Marvin, J., Heimbach, D., Grube, B., & Engrav, L.H. (1990) Infection control in a burn center. *Journal of Burn Care and Rehabilitation*, 11 (6), 575-580.

Martindale, L. (1989). Carbon monoxide poisoning: The rest of the story. *Journal of Emergency Nursing*, 15 (2), 101-104.

Marvin, J.A., Carrougher, G., Bayley, B., Weber, B., Kinghton, J., & Rutan, R. (1991). Burn nursing delphi study. *Journal of Burn Care and Rehabilitation*, 12 (2), 190-197.

May, S. (1990). The future of skin banking. *Journal of Burn Care and rehabilitation*, 11 (5), 484-486.

McLaughlin, E.G. (1990). *Critical care of the burn patient: A case study approach*. Rockville, MD: Aspen Publishers.

Merrell, S., Saffle, J., Larson, C., & Sullivan, J. (1989). The declining incidence of fatal sepsis following thermal injury. *Journal of Trauma*, 29 (10), 1362-1366.

Mikhail, J. (1988). Acute burn care. *Journal of Emergency Nursing*, 14 (1), 9-18.

Monafo, W. (1987). Thermal injuries. In R. Stine & R. Marcus (Eds.), *A practical approach to emergency medicine* (pp 411-421). Boston: Little, Brown.

Mosley, S. (1988). Inhalation injury: A review of the literature. *Heart and Lung*, 17 (1), 3-9.

Moylan, J. (1987). First aid and transportation of burn patients. In J. Boswick (Ed.), *The art and science of burn care* (pp 41-44). Rockville, MD: Aspen Publishers.

O'Neill, J. (1982). Fluid resuscitation in the burned child: A reappraisal. *Journal of Pediatric Surgery*, 17 (5), 604-607.

Parke, T.W., & McLeod, C.G., Jr. (1985). *Pathophysiology of thermal injury: A practical approach*. Orlando, FL: Grune & Stratton.

Phillips, L., Jarlsburg, C., Mathoney, K., Gracia, W., Meltzer, T., Smither, D., & Robson, M. (1990). Meshed Biobrane: A dressing for difficult topography. *Journal of Burn Care and Rehabilitation, 11* (4), p 347-351.

Ragiel, C. (1984). The impact of critical injury on patient, family and clinical systems. *Critical Care Quarterly, 7* (4), 73-78.

Rauscher, L.A., & Ochs, G.M. (1983). Prehospital care of the seriously burned patient. In T. Wachtel, V. Kahn, & H. Frank (Eds.), *Current topics in burn care*. Rockville, MD: Aspen Publishers.

Robertson, K., Cross, P., & Terry, J. (1985). The crucial first days. *American Journal of Nursing, 85* (1), 30-45.

Rockwell, W., & Ehrilich, H. (1990). Should burn blister fluid be evacuated? *Journal of Burn Care and Rehabilitation, 11* (1), 93-95.

Scott-Conner, C., Clarke, K., & Conner, H. (1988). Burn area measurement by computerized planimetry. *Journal of Trauma, 28* (5), 638-641.

Shenkman, B., & Stechmiller, J. (1987). Patient and family perception of projected functioning after discharge from a burn unit. *Heart and Lung, 16* (5), 490-496.

Stern, R., McPherson, M., & Longaker, M. (1990). Histologic study of artificial skin used in the treatment of full-thickness thermal injury. *Journal of Burn Care and Rehabilitation, 11* (1), 7-13.

Taddonio, T., Thomson, P., Smith, D., & Prasad, J. (1990). A survey of wound monitoring and topical antimicrobial therapy practices in the treatment of burn injury. *Journal of Burn Care and Rehabilitation, 11* (5), 423-427.

Trunkey, D. (1983). Transporting the critically burned patient. In T. Wachtel, V. Kahn, & H. Frank (Eds.), *Current topics in burn care* (pp 11-14). Rockville, MD: Aspen Publishers.

Wachtel, T., & Fortune, J. (1983). Fluid resuscitation for burn shock. In T. Wachtel, V. Kahn, & H. Frank (Eds.), *Current topics in burn care* (pp 41-52). Rockville, MD: Aspen Publishers.

Wachtel, T., Frank, H., Fortune, J., & Inancsi, W. (1983). Initial management of major burns. In T. Wachtel, V. Kahn, & H. Frank (Eds.), *Current topics in burn care* (pp 25-28). Rockville, MD: Aspen Publishers.

Wachtel, T., Kahn, V., & Frank, H. (1983). *Current topics in burn care*. Rockville, MD: Aspen Publishers.

Warden, G. (1987). Outpatient management of thermal injuries. In J. Boswick (Ed.), *The Art and Science of Burn Care* (pp 45-51). Rockville, MD: Aspen Publishers.

Zschoche, D. (1986). *Mosby's comprehensive review of critical care* (3rd ed.). St Louis: Mosby–Year Book, Inc.

15 Adaptation

Psychosocial and spiritual

■■

Karen Kidd Lovett

OBJECTIVES
- ❏ Incorporate the concept of holism into trauma nursing practice.
- ❏ Develop an awareness of the emotional and spiritual responses of the trauma patient.
- ❏ Gain an understanding of the nurse's own emotional, mental, and spiritual responses in given trauma situations.
- ❏ Address the challenge of relating to the trauma patient as a human being.

INTRODUCTION The impact of trauma on peoples' lives is analogous to the ripple effect demonstrated when a rock is tossed into a pool of water. Trauma disrupts and agitates, sending out its effects in ever-widening circles.

Whether patients arrive at an emergency department (ED) or trauma center by way of ambulance with sirens, by helicopter from a remote area, or by private car speeding through traffic, the effect is traumatic, unsettling, and a continuity of the momentum that began with the traumatic event. Patients experience inner turmoil and desperately seek an internal balance. They may feel their boundaries closing in or breaking down. They may feel vulnerable or exposed, out-of-balance, uncertain, out-of-control; in short, they feel threatened and, as a result, experience intense anxiety and loss of control.

This chapter examines the center of the "pool" (the patient, both psychologic and spiritual aspects) and the "ripples" (family, friends, medical personnel), all of whom are affected by the action of the "rock" (the trauma-producing event).

ANXIETY

Anxiety is a physiologic reaction to a threat. We become anxious when we feel threatened. The response to that threat is a "call to arms" involving the physical, mental, and emotional capacities needed to either defend or to escape the danger. Although adaptation in the face of trauma is needed, it can also be detrimental if these adaptive reactions are either extreme or persistent.

Anxiety incorporates the basic emotions of anger and fear. Anxiety serves as a signal that we think we are threatened or in some kind of danger (Lester, 1983). This anger and fear is referred to as the "fight or flight" response (Figure 15-1), which results from the body's attempt to mobilize against the threat. In today's world there is little to actually fight and almost no place to flee. As a result, people experience anxiety. In a nontraumatic situation, people will probably begin to deal effectively with the threat. However, as the terms *emergency*, *crisis*, and *trauma* indicate, this is a time when cognition and emotional responses may be skewed. The following section deals briefly with anxiety's inherent emotions: anger and fear.

Anger

Anger is an aggressive response to a conscious or unconscious threat. Anger itself can be threatening or unacceptable to the person, and so it may

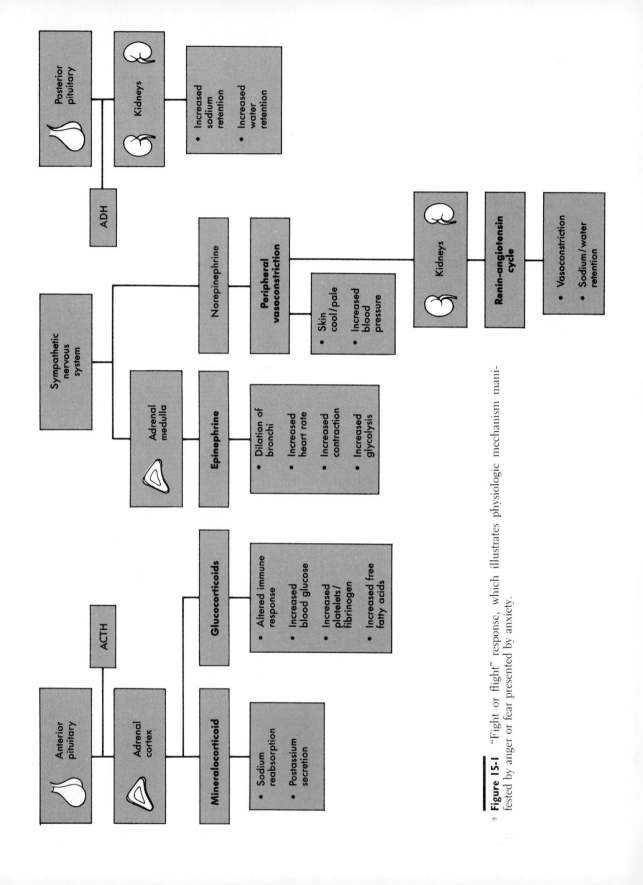

Figure 15-1 "Fight or flight" response, which illustrates physiologic mechanism manifested by anger or fear presented by anxiety.

find expression in forms other than those commonly recognized as anger. One of the more subtle forms anger takes is humor, particularly humor that has a bite or sting. Derogatory remarks aimed at either patients or the medical profession can be a telltale sign of passive anger.

Passive aggression is a form of anger that springs from the person's subconscious and is often so subtle that neither nursing staff nor patients connect the actions with anger. Passive aggression in patients may take many shapes, of which two are common: dragging things out, which might be expressed as lack of cooperation during bathing, and "forgetting" something, necessitating staff making additional trips to the patient's room. Nurses are also susceptible to passive aggressiveness in that professional conduct often imposes behaviorial guidelines that limit the expression of anger or frustration often produced by "uncooperative" patients.

The threats to which persons respond are many and varied. These are perceived as threats because they "endanger" that to which the person is attached or has invested himself or herself.

Self-directed anger

Perhaps the most obvious and the most pertinent component of this discussion is the threat to the physical self. When our bodies are endangered, our very lives are in jeopardy. The following illustrates how the anger reaction may present.

CASE STUDY The ICU nurses complained about Mr. B., a 27-year-old whom they described as "hateful, obnoxious, and uncooperative." He made hurtful, sarcastic remarks, with the result that the nurses were beginning to avoid him. He was obviously angry and directing the anger toward the care team. Mr. B. had been in an auto accident, made a good recovery, and was discharged. Two months later he experienced a rupture of an undetected dissecting aortic aneurysm. Complications after recovery resulted in permanent renal failure.

Mr. B. was embittered and antagonistic. In short, he was angry. He was angry because life, as he had known it, had been disrupted. He was angry because he could no longer work, his expected life span had been greatly reduced, he was dependent on a "machine" for life maintenance, his relationships with his wife and his 3-year-old daughter were adversely affected, and his self-image had been mutilated.

The ICU nurses, dialysis technicians, and physicians became the target of this anger. He believed that they should have been able to "do something" to heal him, to restore his life to the way it was before the auto accident and the renal failure. Because they could not "heal him" and had not been able to detect the aortic aneurysm, he angrily lashed out at them in hurtful and inappropriate ways.

Nursing intervention The nurses were hurt (threatened) by his remarks concerning their ability to care for him and responded by distancing themselves from him (flight) when possible. Others responded in a retaliatory manner by directing ill-natured remarks toward Mr. B. and by delaying response to his call (examples of passive aggression and the flight response).

Mr. B.'s response should be understood as a reaction to his life-threatening situation and not as a personal attack on the staff. With that understanding, it is easier to deal with the patient in a more responsible way. A basic technique is to name his behavior and that of the care team. For example:

> Well, Mr. B., you've surely had a rough time of it haven't you? I think I would be angry and scared if it had happened to me. I'm wondering if that is how you are feeling?

It is vital for the staff to know if what they are assuming about the patient is correct. If he replies that he is feeling scared and/or angry, they could continue talking with him in this manner:

> Let's see if we can work together to find a way to help the situation. When you make hurtful comments to the staff, we no longer look forward to coming in to see you. And then we both lose something.

The patient may or may not respond in a cooperative manner, but he has been treated in a responsible way and as a person capable of making decisions. In addition, he now knows the response his behavior causes among the staff and has heard the consequences of continuing the same behaviors. It is helpful for the concerns of the nurses and their response to the patient to be vented in a constructive way and for the staff to realize the attacks made by Mr. B. were the result of his personal struggle.

Danger to the extended self

People are not just self-contained physical entities—they have emotional involvements and investments in other people. They possess things, ideas, and beliefs; thus they are also threatened and subsequently angered when extended parts of their self are endangered.

> For example, when my son was a toddler at play in the back yard, I happened to notice a small snake raising its head out of its hole in the ground. It was too close to my child! I ran to my son, picked him up, and carried him into the house. Shaking with anger, I got a hoe and went back to the area where the snake had been sighted. By this time it had crawled out of its hole. I began to attack the snake with an intensity I had not known I possessed. I was literally shaking with rage.

My physical self had been in no danger but I perceived danger to my extended self that was heavily invested in my child.

As anyone who works in hospitals is aware, tension is present in patients, their families, and their friends. It may be just beneath the surface or may be easily visible. In either case, hospital personnel must be aware of its presence and be prepared to deal with it in a therapeutic manner. Often anger is more obvious from the family than from patients themselves. Family and friends are sometimes more able to fight the threatening situation than the patient, whose reaction may be that of shock, denial, grief, or fear.

The reverse of this reaction is demonstrated when families and friends find it "too much" (threat) to deal with the illness of their loved one. (This is particularly true in the event of sudden or unexpected death.) Some of the more common adaptive responses are as follows:

- Denial: Often this is the first stage in the process of coming to terms with the trauma. Denial is a way of avoiding a harsh or painful reality. In this phase family members may trivialize symptoms and resist treatment. When families and patients remain in this stage—clinging to unrealistic expectations and refusing to accept the truth of the situation—they must be viewed as being in crisis. Support, empathy, and quiet presence of the nurse and other staff members is greatly needed. If the nurse perceives that the family is involved in the denial process,

the situation should be carefully monitored. Should they seem to be "stuck," the attending physician or nurse educator may need to schedule a conference to help answer questions and facilitate acceptance and understanding of the patient's condition. However, the family should be given some time to come to terms with the situation; denial is usually part of the adjustment process.

- Disorganization: Once the family and patient accept the situation, they may react in negative ways, insulting nurses and physicians, or each other. They may demand special attention, make irrational statements, and display irrational behavior. Their world is in chaos. They need their situation and feelings acknowledged by the staff. They need support and "concrete" assistance. Perhaps the nurse could offer them suggestions on coping with routine matters such as household duties, which continue to need attention even during hospitalization. The nurse can refer them to social service agencies that can provide support and aid during times of trauma. They should be reminded to eat and to rest and to share the visitation times. All of these suggestions help give shape and boundaries to their world, which has lost its familiar shape and its comfortingly familiar boundaries.

- Hyperorganization: Another form of adaptation, hyperorganization is easily recognized in the tremendous business observed in the family. They become concerned with details and procedures to the extent that they may actually neglect the patient's needs, as well as their own. They need encouragement to sit and talk with one another about what has happened and how they feel about it (Bluhm, 1987).

Perceived threat to objects

Although it may sound strange, people develop "relationships" with objects and places. Anyone whose new car was dented or whose new carpet received a red fruit juice spill will have an immediate understanding of what is meant by "relationship" with a thing. People also invest meaning in communities, institutions, and sports. When something happens to threaten one of these, the people too may be threatened, anxious, and angry.

A patient was brought into the trauma unit after an automobile accident in which he was moderately injured and the driver of the other car was critically injured. The patient's concern, however, was for his new red sports car, which was damaged, and not for the other driver. Members of the staff became angry with the patient for his lack of concern. The staff was angry even though they were under no physical threat from the attitude of the patient. However, their value system was attacked, and therefore their reaction was one of anger.

Threat to one's ideas or beliefs

Philosophies, culture, community values, and religious doctrines are primary foundations on which people build approaches to and ways of life. Therefore when the ideas and beliefs we consider to be important are threatened, ignored, ridiculed, made legal (e.g., the legalization of marijuana) or illegal, or disagreed with, we are threatened and become anxious, which may present itself as anger (Lester, 1983). Figure 15-2 demonstrates the relationships between things, ideas, and people.

Mr. T. is a Jehovah's Witness. The trauma team insists that he need a blood transfusion because his blood pressure remains 80 systolic and he is going to the OR for an exploratory laparotomy. When his family is told of his need for a blood transfusion, they become defensive and angry. During the discussion, the family becomes so angry they yell at the trauma team, insisting that Mr. T. not be transfused. Some members of the trauma team also become very agitated and respond in anger to the patient's family. The value system of the trauma team and the belief system of the patient and his family are in intense conflict. To not do everything possible to save the patient is a severe threat to the integrity of the health profession, but to allow the blood transfusion strikes at a fundamental belief of the patient. The threats to both belief systems result in anger, confrontation, fear, and frustration.

Misplaced anger

Feelings of helplessness, rage, and frustration are likely to be projected onto the care team by patients and families. Our society has elevated science to an almost "god-like" status. Health pro-

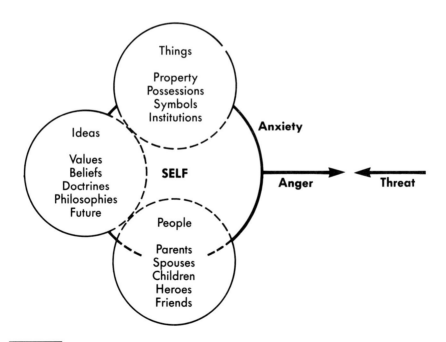

Figure 15-2 Ripple effect as illustrated by conjoining circles showing patient and patient's extended self. (*Note.* From *Coping with your Anger: A Christian Guide* [p. 30] by A.D. Lester, 1985, Philadelphia: Westminster Press.

Interventions for misplaced anger

- Remember that the feelings are misdirected. Whether they are projected feelings or not, nasty comments hurt. It is important to have someone you can talk with about the reaction that such remarks engender within you.
- State what you observe in a nonthreatening way.
- Follow with an offer to listen or to refer to chaplain or counseling consult team.
- Touch the patient. Of course you touch the patient a great deal while delivering care, but take a few seconds to pat an arm or smooth the hair back away from the patient's face. In general, touch, however brief, breaks down the feelings of isolation that develop during illness. However, regional and ethnic differences must be considered. For example, to Navahos, touch by an "outsider" is not welcomed—it is considered an invasion of the soul and is literally "off limits." (Orgue, Blech, & Monrroy, 1983.)
- Should a patient recoil or "freeze," be aware that such a reaction may signal the possibility of previous abuse. Sensitivity to the patient (i.e., the patient reaches for you or touches you) and common sense must be your guide.

fessionals are expected to "fix-it," and when that "security" fails, if the person or persons are threatened, anger will result. The caregiver may be unjustly criticized or verbally abused. Strategies to handle the situation may assist the caregiver. The suggestions in the box above have proven successful in many situations where anger is misplaced.

Fear

The Hebrew word for fear is *yahrah*, which also means honor, revere, and respect. In Greek, *phobos* means fear, respect, reverence, stand in awe. Fear is both affective and volitional. It is not just felt; it is also decided on, thought about. Both psychologically and theologically, fear is neutral, it is not good or bad, not right or wrong, it just is. It does, however, have acute physical manifestations, as does anger, that the nurse, as caregiver, can see. Fear becomes right or wrong, normal or pathologic, on the basis of its context or object. Fear acknowledges the power or authority of an entity. A fear object may be a creature, a person, an idea or thought, such as dying, failure, loss of control, embarrassment, or grief. Fear objects must have two characteristics: *omnipotence*—the power that gives the ability to hurt or destroy, create, make, confirm, or affirm; and *access*—one must be vulnerable to the fear. We do not fear that which does not have power. We do fear our own helplessness, because suddenly we have no power.

To become part of the trauma team, the nurse must become totally familiar with the world of the trauma unit. After that familiarity is achieved, the dials and hoses and machines no longer are frightening and the sights and sounds and smells are accepted. This is probably not the case for the patient or the family. If conscious, the patient is confronted by a massive sensory assault, which only adds to the disorientation already present. The bright lights, the metallic sounds, the conversations, the blood, and the pain all take on new and heightened importance in the world of the patient. Even the silences after the general overabundance of noise and activity are suddenly freighted with meaning. When the regular beep of the heart monitor stops in the cubicle next to the patient, he or she may wonder, "Why did that stop?" "Did the patient die?" "Did the machine stop or malfunction?" "Could it be me next?" (Figure 15-3 shows a patient's view.)

Because the staff is familiar with this environment, they may forget how strange and frightening it is to the patient. As part of the team the nurse will be asked the same questions over and over and will give the same answers over and over. As a result, the answers may grow short, and explanations may be filled with acronyms and jargon or, even worse, explanations may be omitted altogether in the rush of delivering care.

People who work in emergency situations daily can become calloused and distant. The apparent callousness or remoteness may mask the pain, fear, and feelings of vulnerability these situations engender. Nurses do not have time to feel the fear and the pain of each patient, nor do they have time to *be conscious* of their own fears. But they *do experience* the fear and the pain. Nurses are aware that they too are finite human beings and that they are vulnerable to the same injuries and assaults as those being experienced by the patient.

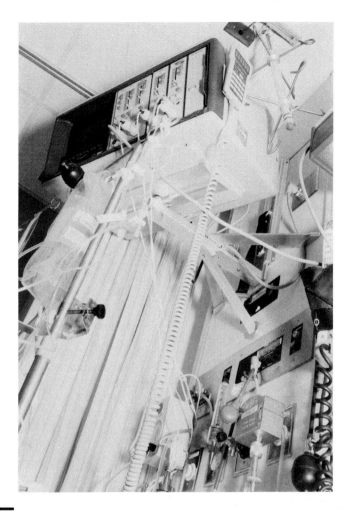

Figure 15-3   View from patient's perspective in intensive care unit. (*Note.* From *Principles and Practice of Adult Health Nursing* [1st ed.] by P.G. Beare and J.L. Myers, 1990, St Louis: Mosby–Year Book, Inc.)

Theologically, an aspect of a fear object is that it may also be a faith object. Particular people, places, ideas, and objects that are feared are also likely to be worshiped. What one fears assumes a central place in one's life. Thus it is possible to view God as a fear object. To believe that God is powerful and to believe that God loves are acknowledgments of omnipotence and are also acknowledgments of honor and reverence. Many believe that the fear object can and will use power for good. Others may believe that power is also used for bad or evil and thus see their illness as punishment or as an effort by the fear object to teach them something or to get their attention.

CASE STUDY   Sarah, a college student, was hit by a truck while riding her bicycle. She is Catholic and a fairly active member of her parish. She had missed mass the past three Sundays because of pressures of school work and home life. She expressed her guilt and fear to the nurse stating, "I knew I would be punished for my sin."

An ideation such as this is not uncommon and is not indigenous to any particular denomination.

People need desperately to "make some sense" of their situation, in other words, to make meaning or to find a reason for. One way of assigning meaning or answering the "why" is to assign the action to God. To say it was God's will or purpose makes more sense to some than to say it was "just chance" or "dumb luck" that they were hit by a truck. However, many will also assign their situation to just that—"bad luck" and nothing more.

Nursing intervention

The nursing response to such statements or questions might be the following:
- To invite patients to explain why they feel they are being punished
- To offer to call a chaplain or to contact the patients' own clergy. If none is available, it might be helpful to ask what they think God wanted them to learn. Are they learning it? Is life going to be different? (Cox-Gedmark, 1980)
- To encourage patients to talk, to explore ideas, and to search for meaning in their life situation as pertains to the crisis event (Clark, 1987)

Coping behaviors

Crises interrupt the everyday routine of life. They throw people out of balance. Yet some individuals handle crisis situations very well, coping successfully, whereas others experience maladaptive coping. Coping behaviors begin once the perception of threat occurs. It must be remembered that even what is seen as pathologic or unsuccessful coping is a coping response (Clark, 1987).

Patients may react in one or a combination of several ways or they may use all of the behaviors at different stages of their anxiety. For example, patients may do one of the following:
- Attempt to change one of the characteristics of the anxiety-producing factor—either decide that it is not all-powerful or deny it access (fight). This may be seen in the patient who responds by kicking and screaming.
- Retreat or escape—shock or denial, repression or suppression (flight). Patients may deny they need a physician, or they may refuse treatment in their effort to keep the reality of their situation "at bay." When this occurs, they should be gently and calmly confronted with all the facts available. This should include a calm statement of their injury, their current status, and treatment plans. The nurse must take time to tell the patient what is going on and what is going to happen. Because of the disorientation resulting from pain, shock, or medications, this will probably need to be done more than once. It may be appropriate to call in the hospital psychologist, social worker, or chaplain, if available.
- Submit or surrender—let the fear object (person, place, thing, or event) be the boss.

Why do some cope better than others, and what can the health care professional do to aid successful coping? Recalling the "rock in the pool" imagery (the rock disturbs the water at a specific site but also affects the whole of the pool), the nurse must consider the multidimensional history of the person experiencing the crisis (just as no part of the person is unaffected by the trauma, so too no one particular event is experienced in isolation from the preceding event of that life). Meninger refers to the concept of homeostasis. He proposes that all behavior, whether of cells, organs, emotions, or cognition, is a continuous attempt to preserve or regain "organismic integrity." This is done through some degree of adjustment or adaptation of the physiologic or emotional system. People seek constancy and balance. Changes in the balance (homeostasis) of any system signal involvement throughout the whole and "may sometimes grossly affect the steadiness of other partial systems" (Meninger, Mayman, & Pruyser, 1963).

The following provides several illustrations of what has been discussed thus far.

CASE STUDY Dr. W., a 43-year-old man, was working late in the laboratory of his dental office when two intruders entered and demanded drugs and money. In the ensuing scuffle, Dr. W. received a bullet wound to the left lower quadrant of his abdomen. The .22 caliber bullet perforated the sigmoid colon, necessitating an emergency laparotomy with a resection of the injured colon ending with a Hartmann pouch. He is conscious at the time of arrival and when told he will need surgery, he vehemently denies that this is true. He says, "Surgery is just not necessary. Take out the bullet and let me go home. I've got to go to the police station and see if I can identify the guys that broke into the office and shot me!" The surgeon explains that the bullet has lodged harmlessly in the paraspinous muscles and will not need to be removed. Dr. W. requests that his fiancée be notified. When she arrives, he says, "Please don't let them cut me; I don't need surgery." "Just take the bullet out and send me home," and later, "I'm sorry, I'm so sorry to put you through all of this."

His early reaction of denial is beginning to be outweighed by fear and guilt. It should be remembered that more than one aspect of a person's life is impacted by traumatic situations and more than one emotion is present also. However, one of the emotions will be predominant at any given time.

An appropriate nursing intervention is for the nurse to state what he or she observes and then ask some exploratory questions, For example, "Dr. W., you seem to be very anxious about the possibility of surgery. Have you had an operation or an experience with surgery in the past?" He does indeed have a history of medical experiences that is contributing to his reactions.

At the age of 9 he was diagnosed as having polio. A fascia lata graft to the anterior abdominal wall was done to repair damage secondary to denervation after the polio. This surgery was done to postpone a spinal fusion, which he would have at age 12. He also had several surgeries on his foot and leg to repair damage and to facilitate movement. He made a successful recovery from these surgeries and dedicated himself to an extremely healthy life-style. He ate a carefully balanced diet, exercised, and in general developed a philosophy of life and health that stated, "One can determine whether one is sick or well; one can prevent illness through thought and practice of a healthy life-style." Until this time in his life, his philosophy has held true, but suddenly he is in the hospital, through no fault of his own and in spite of his precautions, and is once again facing surgery. Now Dr. W. becomes conscious of all the experiences of his childhood illness, subsequent painful surgeries, and prolonged rehabilitation. The memories are painful and frightening and threaten Dr. W. in several areas, including the following:

- Acute awareness of his finitude: He is confronted with his limitations.

- Loss of control: Work, marriage plans, physical intrusion, and lack of ability to prevent injury are all out of his hands.
- Jeopardized body image: Once again he is faced with this issue.
- Shaken philosophy of life and health: He has been true to his philosophy; nonetheless, he is injured, hospitalized, and facing surgery.
- Guilt: Pertaining to his patients, employees, and especially his fiancée, he feels guilty because his patients will be inconvenienced; his employees will not be able to work full time during his hospitalization and subsequent recovery time; and postponement of the wedding is a real possibility.
- Grief: (See pp. 486-487 for a more detailed discussion of grief.)

Because of the complex nature of Dr. W.'s past, referral to a mental health professional for counseling may be appropriate. Nonetheless, several interventions can successfully be performed by both the ED and ICU nurses that will lessen the patient's anxiety. All patients have a great need to feel trust in those giving them care. Interventions are as follows:

- One of the easiest and most effective ways of doing this is through mutuality; affirmation of personhood, that of the nurse and the patient. This may be done by making good, steady eye contact, introducing oneself, and calling the patient by name. This simple, basic human touch adds dignity and humanity to what is often, of necessity, a less than dignified experience (Drew, 1986,).
- Lessen the sense of isolation by explaining as much as possible what is going on and why. This is important even for patients who seem to be comatose and is invaluable for any family who may be present. Information concerning future treatment plans and expected results is also helpful and affirming to the patient (Bourdon, 1986).
- Lessen the sense of loss of control: where possible, give the patient some choices in care. Choice, no matter how small, is associated with personhood. Patients who are threatened by their experience of loss of control are reassured when they understand the temporary nature of the experience (Cox-Gedmark, 1980; Bourdon, 1986).

- Help the patient identify and define his or her feelings: "I wonder if this is frightening for you?" "All the machines may seem dehumanizing, but they are for the purpose of . . . ."
- Express genuine empathy and concern: "I'm sorry you are so uncomfortable; may I rearrange your pillows?"
- Convey hope.
- Encourage additional supportive resources: chaplain, social worker, clergy, friends.
- Encourage questions: "Is there anything that I can explain to you?"
- Confront denial: "Dr. W., you have been shot, and the bullet has perforated the sigmoid colon; you need to have surgery."
- Listen to what the patient says. The effective nurse learns to listen with not only the ears but also the eyes, the touch, and, indeed, all the senses.

Grief as a coping behavior

Grief is a reaction to loss. When persons become physically ill, perhaps suffering paralysis or loss of body parts or function, their natural reaction is one of grief. These losses are much like the death of a loved one. The patients must move through the mourning process just as bereaved persons move through the process of mourning. If balance and some measure of health are to be regained, adjustment, adaptation, and acceptance of the changes must occur (Oates, 1982). Patients and their families often react to a period of hospitalization with grief. One reason for this is that hospitalization reaches into so many areas of life, affecting not only functioning as individuals, but also relationships (family, friends, employers/employees, and community). Hospitalization affects the following:

- The ability to work. Whether a temporary interruption or a permanent disability, this factor has a significant bearing on the grief reaction. So much self-worth and respect of others are based on work or profession. Hospitalization puts this in jeopardy.
- Relationships with family and friends. Hospitalization often causes significant role reversals, increasing stress and the need for grief work. It can also open old wounds in relationships and family patterns. On the other hand, hospitalization may generate positive responses: reconciliations occur; people express care and concern; people realize for the first time how really important the other person is to them.
- Self-esteem. This is more often an issue when significant physical change is associated with the trauma. Although many patients will go through a period of lessened self-esteem, it is generally more of a problem in traumas that produce prolonged life-style changes, for example, heart attacks, severe burns, injuries resulting in paralysis, loss of limb, and loss of sight or any of the senses. (Nurses should be aware of the emotional state of children and adolescents—even traumas that will be of a relatively short duration may cause great distress in younger patients.) Self-esteem also can be a problem with persons whose self-esteem rests on their work or profession.
- Independence. See a discussion of this in the section on control.

The grief reaction process may be divided into three major phases (Bowlby, 1980):

- The first phase is a protest or refusal to believe that what has occurred is real. (Note Dr. W.'s denial of the need for surgery.) Shock, which is nature's anesthetic, is often a part of this phase of grief and, at this point, is actually helpful because it cushions the initial blow of a traumatic event and allows time for the person to come to grips with the reality of the situation.
- The second phase is disorganization, characterized by despair and helplessness.
- The third phase is reorganization. This is usually a time of gradual adjustment in which the patient begins to reorganize and regain control of his or her life. It may be a time of acknowledging limitations (temporary or permanent) yet also can be a time of discovery and focusing on strengths.

Most patients are helped by the realization that grief is a natural and temporary process, which most people overcome. However, it is also important to remember that no two persons experience grief in exactly the same way. Periods of returning to earlier phases of grieving—taking one step forward and two steps back—may occur. The patient may be thrown back into more intense grieving after having moved far down the road toward healing. For example, the anniversary of an accident or surgery or hearing of a situation that is similar to his or her own can cause a reversal in the grieving process. Even revisiting the hospital can adversely affect the person. Also, the caregiver must be aware of the effects grief can have on bodily functioning, as well as these emotional and cognitive effects. Patients should be made aware of these facts about grief. The nurse should tell the patients, their families, and their friends (who are subject to the same griefs and coping behaviors as the patient) that grief is a process and is a part of their trauma from which they will recover. Many books are available on this subject and often social services, chaplain services, or other psychologic support services will have materials that can be given to the patients and their families.

Physical pain

The primary awareness of patients may center around the actual physical pain they experience. Oates states the following (Oates, 1982):

> We are talking about primary pain caused by real irritation of nerve endings such as the pinching of central nerves by shattered vertebrae. The cycle of pain needs careful attention from the point of view of the patient's reaction. The cycle of pain begins with the stimulation or irritation of the nerve endings themselves. This is followed by shock: pain hits the patient. It carries with it a stunning, blunting, shocking effect. Shock is followed by fear. The response of the patient is a fear reaction amounting to panic. Muscles tense up, increasing the pain. This reaction differs according to immediacy, amount of control, and the degree of pain tolerance. The fear or panic reaction calls for a muscular tonicity of bracing against additional thrusts of pain. This tension predisposes the organism to more pain, finishing or closing the cycle: pain-fear-muscle spasm-tension-more pain. The need for relaxation as a means of slowing down and eventually breaking the vicious circle is evident.

CASE STUDY   Ms. G., a 52-year-old woman, an R.N., and a former ED supervisor, was brought to the ED after involvement in a multiple car accident. She feels frightened and lonely. Additionally, she realizes for the first time how impersonal a trauma care situation can be. She is in intense pain from multiple injuries, including a broken back, ankle, collar bone, and several ribs. She is trembling from shock and fear. She feels isolated, yet because of her professional experience, she understands and even anticipates the care procedures, which increases her anxiety. Her respiration and pulse rates are elevated. One of the nurses takes her hand and begins to gently stroke her arm. The nurse calls her name, makes eye contact, and says, "Ms. G., my name is Nancy. I imagine all this must be pretty scary for you right now. We know you are in a lot of pain, and we are going to help you. Your husband and daughters have arrived, and we will let them come back to see you in just a little while." Ms. G. begins to calm down somewhat, and her breathing becomes more regular and her muscles relaxed.

Several things happened during the very few moments of the nursing intervention:

- Ms. G. was recognized as a person. By identifying herself and calling Ms. G. by name, the nurse recognized the patient as an individual. She gave her the gift of personhood and dignity.
- The current life situation of the patient was recognized. By naming the fearful situation in an empathetic manner, the nurse reassured the patient that her feelings and perceptions were accurate and that the care team recognized and understood them.
- Hope was conveyed. The nurse quietly reassured the patient of the care being given and that care would continue.
- Additional support was provided. Giving the patient the information that her family had arrived and that she would soon be able to see them provided additional emotional support for Ms. G.

Ms. G. later stated that she felt the nurse's personal attention to her was a turning point. She then felt that she was no longer "the broken back in room 2," but was once again a person. She also felt she had a contact: someone who cared about her and not just her injuries, although she stressed that the high level of competent care was also reassuring.

Post traumatic stress disorder   The nurses noticed very specific patterns of speech and behavior as Ms. G. began to be conscious for longer and longer periods. She showed signs of increased anxiety and talked repeatedly about her brush with death and the fear that "it could happen again anytime." She described herself as helpless and expressed a strong doubt that she would ever be able to drive again. At one point she even expressed a doubt that she could ever work in a hospital again.

What Ms. G. was experiencing is not an uncommon result of traumatic occurrences. The impact of trauma has been known and studied for many years. It is known by many names, including *shell shock*, *Viet Nam Vet's disease*, *stress response syndrome*, and most recently *post traumatic stress disorder* (American Psychiatric Association, 1987). The posttrauma response is most often found in cases of bereavement, disaster (natural or caused by humans), transportation accident, violent crime, accidental personal injury, or the witnessing of any of these. Signs and symptoms of the response for the caretaker to be alert for are the following (American Psychiatric Association, 1987):

- Reexperiencing of the traumatic event. This may occur through recurring and intrusive remembrances of the event, recurring "bad" dreams of the event, reliving the experience in sudden and intrusive ways, flashbacks, hallucinations, and high psychologic distress when in situations reminiscent of the traumatic event.
- A numbing of response or an avoidance of stimuli that might be associated with the trauma. Efforts are made to avoid thoughts, feelings, activities, or situations that could cause remembrance of the trauma, forgetting important aspects of the trauma, loss (or lessening) of interest in important activities, feeling detached or estranged, and a sense of a shortened life span.
- Arousal increase. This is demonstrated as sleep disturbances, increased irritability or anger, difficulty maintaining concentration, hypervigilance, increased startle response, and physical response to events that resemble the trauma.

These signs and symptoms must last for at least one month to be diagnosed as Post Traumatic Stress Disorder but may not show up for several months after the trauma actually occurs.

Many life events are stressful. Even positive occurrences, such as the birth of a child, marriage, a new job, and a wage increase, are stressors and require adjustment. The psyche must as-similate the new data; it must incorporate the new reality into the old. In short, an "adjustment" period is required. In most cases this is done with only mild disruption of life processes. However, in the case of the intensely traumatic event, the process is not so simple, requiring much emotional work and reshaping of cognition and cognitive processes (Alvarez, Horowitz, Kaltreider, & Wilner, 1980; Mechanic, 1977; Kirby, Kuch, & Swinson, 1985; Mendelson, 1987; Welch, 1987; Horowitz & Krupnick, 1981)

Role of the family in the trauma or emergency department What was happening to Ms. G.'s family as they gathered in the trauma unit waiting area? What was their response to the information about Ms. G.'s injuries? Indeed, what dynamics are active in the days after the accident as Ms. G. is moved into the ICU and later transferred to a rehabilitation center? The following are some possible reactions:

- Stress must be considered as a possibility. No family or patient will react in a predictable manner. Therefore the nurse must be familiar with the many reactions persons may have to stress.
- Shock and denial function much the same way in the family as in the patient, as a bumper or cushion that allows time for the "sorting through" of the event or events.
- Disorganization occurs as the family unit is thrown out of balance. Their normal structure of daily life (even if that life has involved home care of a chronically ill patient) is disrupted. This in itself is a stressor and contributes to the confusion and disorganization of the family system.

BODY IMAGE

Each person has a picture or image of his or her own body—the physical self. It is an image that is very difficult, and often traumatic, to change. For example, persons who have been overweight, especially as children, who then lose weight often have problems adjusting to their new image and in fact carry the mental picture of themselves as overweight for a long time. The same holds true for people who have been thin and then gain weight. In their mind's eye, they are still slender, and so accepting and dealing with a weight problem becomes more difficult because of the mental image of their physical being.

Trauma victims may have a sudden, dramatic

bodily change with which they must deal. The impact of this lasts far beyond the period of hospitalization. Whether the injury is that of a gunshot wound, a burn, loss of a limb, paralysis, or a temporary colostomy, the patient's world is disrupted and will never be exactly the same again.

In a traumatic school bus accident where the gas tank exploded on impact with another vehicle, dozens of children suffered second- and third-degree burns. The immediate and intense pain was accompanied by the threat of scars and disfigurement. The children soon began to ask how they were going to look when they got well, whether they could be fixed, and if they were going to need an operation. Dealing with the reality of altered physical appearances is painful and frightening. Grief reactions and adjustment are not quickly accomplished. Most patients will have moments of reliving the traumatic event. They will often have nightmares and flashbacks, as well as conscious replaying of the event or events. The ability to talk about the feelings and memories will lessen the pain of those memories and feelings.

For some patients the only way to begin to understand a change in body image is to begin to struggle for meaning and for a more complete understanding of who they really are. This includes discovering what about them is still the same. The assessment process addresses not only physical appearances but other parts of their selves that may have grown during the traumatic events that have changed their lives—such things as their abilities to love, think, listen, discern, and even laugh. Supportive families, communities, nurses, and doctors are integral components of the regaining of balance and health. Additionally, introduction of the patient to resources such as support or therapy groups and/or professional counseling is desirable (Cox-Gedmark, 1980).

SPIRITUAL ADAPTATION

I prayed all the way to the hospital. I was so scared, and I prayed so hard!

What did you pray?

Well, you know it's sort of funny, I was praying for God to help Frank be O.K. and that I wouldn't wreck or anything, but I was also sort of angry with God. Do you know what I mean? It just seemed so unfair . . . after all, Frank's doing God's work . . doing ministry and all . . . it just didn't seem fair. God was being unfair!

This verbatim reflects much of the duality of the spiritual problems invoked by trauma. On one hand, the faith of the minister's wife sustained her and provided hope; on the other hand, her sense of "fair play" had been violated. Her husband, a young minister, had fallen from the roof of a parishioner's barn while helping with repairs. He had landed on a pile of rocks and was unconscious and bleeding from the mouth. The farm, in a remote area, had no phone service, so she brought him to the hospital in her car. Her belief in the basic ground rules had been shaken. That she felt free to express her frustration and questions indicates a sound belief system and willingness toward growth and maturity of her religious ideation.

Crises of faith are common during times of trauma. The shape and cause of the crises are as diverse as the people themselves, yet common themes and factors are present, which, when identified, assist the care team in deciding on a therapeutic approach.

Obviously, hospital personnel have neither the time nor the training to do a spiritual inventory. However, it is a simple thing to ask the patient and accompanying family and friends if they want to see a chaplain or to have a minister, priest, or rabbi called. Willis (1977) notes that some people resist the introduction of clergy and cast them in a negative role of death messenger, harbinger of God's wrath, or a somber-faced person who imposes Bible reading or prayer on them instead of drying their tears and comforting and encouraging them. However, many others find comfort and support in the presence of clergy or chaplain. Indeed, many view clergy as representing God (Oates, 1982) and possessing God's wisdom. Similarly, even people who are not particularly religious find comfort, strength, and inspiration in sacred scriptures and prayers during times of trauma. The caregiver has little way of knowing the belief system of the patient or the family and so must simply ask them. An offer to call the patient's clergy or to notify the hospital chaplain is always correct and shows concern for the whole person.

Questions of faith arise in times of trauma because the person's understanding or beliefs in the nature of God have been tested and have been found either lacking or shaken, and thus threatened.

Who God is and how God acts are topics that

consume much time and energy for theologians, scholars, and clergy, which is to be expected. Yet whenever people think about God and shape beliefs about God's actions, they are thinking theologically. All persons of faith, whether that faith is great or small, have a theology. These foundations of belief are tested in times of emergency and trauma. A discussion of some common themes that are frequently encountered in crisis situations follows.

Themes of Belief

A major theme of belief that often surfaces is that of a wrathful God. This is a difficult concept and can be distorted into thoughts of God as an angry, vengeful puppeteer. This faith model is often the springboard for such questions and statements as "What have I done to deserve this?" "Am I being punished?" "I guess God wanted to get my attention." "I guess God wanted to teach me something." Well-meaning family members, relatives, or clergy may make statements or quote bits of scripture that indicate God's responsibility for an illness or an accident, never realizing the devastating effects these quotes may have on the patient. When persons' whole faith systems are built on systems of rewards and punishments, it is likely that excessive guilt, questions, and fear will accompany illness and accidents. Persons with this belief may have a difficult time expressing their fears, anger, resentment, and questions. It is helpful to acknowledge that although many are taught that to question God or to express anger toward God implies a lack of faith, the Hebrew and Christian traditions record such questions and expressions frequently. In the Old Testament of the Bible, Job was devastated by loss of his land, his crops, his children, and his physical health. He also had to endure the persistent interrogation of his friends, who would have him search his life for some sin that would cause his afflicted state. Yet Job protested his innocence, and not only questioned God, but shouted:

> No wonder then if I cannot keep silence; in the anguish of my spirit I must speak, lament in the bitterness of my soul (Job 7:11 [Jerusalem Bible, 1968]).
>
> Suppose I have sinned, what have I done to you, you tireless watcher of mankind? Why do you choose me as your target? Why should I be a burden to you? (Job 7:20 [Jerusalem Bible, 1968]).

In Habakkuk also is found cries of complaint and outrage:

> How long, Yahweh, am I to cry for help while you will not listen; to cry 'Oppression!' in your ear and will not save? (Habakkuk 1:2 [Jerusalem Bible, 1968]).

The patient needs reassurance that the questions and emotions being expressed are normal; everyone feels them. Indeed, such questions and feelings may be understood as one of the ways God gives to help people understand and deal with what has happened to them.

Religious faith or the lack of it can be a highly emotional and sensitive area. Incidents of illness and trauma are not times for teaching but are rather, times for reassurance and comfort. The caregiver must be aware, though, of the impact of the faith structure on the healing process of the patient. The patient is working within that structure. Therefore the caregiver is called on to recognize the faith dynamics that are present.

SUDDEN DEATH

Despite all that modern health care can do, sudden, unexpected death is a reality. Once again the pool imagery is a reminder that the ripples caused by the impact of the trauma (death) reach to all parts of the pool and in this manner impact the lives of others.

Members of the family may or may not be present at the time of death. Nonetheless, they will eventually need attention. How this is done can have tremendous impact on their grief process (Dubin & Sarnoff, 1986; Fanslow, 1983).

If the family is present before the time of death, they must be kept aware of the current status of the patient. They must also be told if and when death is imminent and be given a chance to say good-bye (Fanslow, 1983). The family should have information about the care procedures being followed, as well as facts about the injury or trauma itself. It is recommended to arrange for additional support (e.g., chaplain, social worker, psychiatric nurse, clergy, friends).

In some hospitals, family members are given the option of being present during resuscitation attempts. This is a highly controversial subject that requires more study. However, the preliminary evidence indicates more beneficial results from the family members' presence than from their exclusion (Fanslow, 1983; Post, 1986; Post & Rhee, 1985).

If the family is not present at the time of death, they must be notified. It is a shocking experience to be called by hospital ED personnel and told that a loved one is either gravely ill or has died. Generally it is best to tell the family that the person is in the ED and request that they come as soon as possible, rather than to notify of the death by phone. The caller should suggest that the family member(s) have someone come with them. The nurse should ensure that the family knows which hospital is calling and the location. If possible, a phone number should be given to them so that they can call to verify the information. When the family lives a long distance from the hospital, they should probably be told of the death. It is important that they have someone with them. If necessary, a hospital staff member should notify the Red Cross or police department and request their assistance.

When the family arrives, they should be met by a staff member and taken to a quiet room (Dubin & Sarnoff, 1986; Justice, 1982). Staff should postpone requesting signature or preference in funeral homes. The physician in charge should tell the family as candidly as possible what has happened. A variety of responses can be anticipated. The most common first response is one of shock and denial. They may cry or begin to deny, saying, "No, I don't believe it" or "I was just with her!" Sometimes family members will react in anger and begin to blame the medical personnel, the hospital, or each other. This is not the appropriate time to try and reason with them or to justify medical techmiques, but is rather a time to present a calm, quiet attitude of acceptance and understanding (Dubin & Sarnoff, 1986). The staff member's presence is important. The family may or may not remember what the staff says (although that is important too), but they will remember whether someone was there. Although these people may not be rude or inconsiderate in normal circumstances, sudden, unexpected death is not normal and their reaction may not be either.

The medical staff will need to answer questions posed by the family and reassure them that every effort was made to resuscitate their loved one. If at all possible, the family should be taken to a private place. A phone should be made available for their use (Dubin & Sarnoff, 1986; Justice, 1982).

Staff should ask if the family would like to see "Mr. _____" or "Jane." The nurse should never refer to the deceased person as "the body." If the cause of death was violent, the family may need to be prepared. The body should be cleaned, unnecessary machines removed, and clean coverings arranged before the family is brought into the room. Most families want to see the loved one, and indeed this is an aid to the grief process, which confronts them with the reality of the death. Some last words may be spoken or prayers said. The family must not be rushed during this last private time together. It is not uncommon for the spouse to kiss or hold the patient in an effort to revive him or her. When there is no response, hysteria may set in. This, however, is not an indication for sedation. In fact, sedation at this point seems to prolong the initial grief stage (Dubin & Sarnoff, 1986; Fanslow, 1983; Huff, 1989). It is better to offer physical support, a glass of water or cup of coffee, and encouragement to breathe slowly and deeply.

Because sudden, unexpected death is difficult at best, the staff may have a tendency to remain withdrawn and coldly professional, distancing themselves from the grief. This is a form of coping and denial and should be carefully attended. It is acceptable for the nurse to share emotions in a genuine and sensitive way, rather than hurrying to the next duty. However, the nurse must not burden the family with a recitation of his or her own woes, but should express sympathy and understanding. For example, "This is really hard; you must be reeling" is a better response than "I know just how you feel; my Aunt Jeannie died just like that." The nurse's open response may encourage their tears, rage, or recollections. The family should be given an opportunity to speak. They may talk of the loved one or of themselves. What is most important is that the nurse encourage the first faltering steps on the way to grief.

After the family has had time with the loved one, it may be necessary to begin the paperwork. Should an autopsy be needed, the nurse should explain that this does not mean mutilation or disfigurement. Also, the nurse should explain the method of transporting the deceased to the medical examiner or to the funeral home and how the family may obtain a copy of the medical examiner's report (Dubin & Sarnoff, 1986) It is helpful if the information and procedures can be written down.

No one feels adequate to help in such grief situations. The feelings are not incorrect; no one *is* adequate. The staff must, however, make an effort to touch one another, to keep the almost overwhelmingly impersonal atmosphere of EDs from being the norm. The staff cannot heal, but they can help bind the wounds with genuine empathy and quiet, comforting presence.

CONTROL

I have put this section last because I believe this issue to be a current that flows throughout each of the cases and topics discussed previously. My favorite part of a roller coaster ride is where it comes to an end. What was a childhood delight has become a time of stress, panic, and extreme anxiety. Why? What has caused such a complete turnabout in my enjoyment of a popular amusement park ride? It is very simple: I cannot tolerate such extreme feelings of loss of control that are produced by the hurtling and whirling action of the roller coaster.

I know a man who has a difficult time riding in a car if someone other than he is driving. Why? He needs to be in control.

Existential psychology tells us that the root of the fear of being "out of control" or, conversely, the need to be "in control" arises from death anxiety. We ward off our fear of death, which we cannot control, by attempting to control that which we can (Yalom, 1980).

Everyone has a degree of anxiety about death; that is only natural. We have not as yet personally experienced death and whether there is a belief in an afterlife and whether one anticipates the afterlife to be malicious or benign, there is still some anxiety concerning death's occurrence. One of the ways we deal with this anxiety is through manipulation of our lives and sometimes the lives of others. A sense of mastery is gained through the ordering of our days, and if we have a feeling of control, we have a feeling that death can be kept at bay if only we can remain in control.

The emotional component that keeps our systems on track, running smoothly, and in order is control. We fear loss of control, not only in ourselves but also in those around us. We are extremely uncomfortable when someone "loses it" in our presence. It threatens our sense of "self-control." After all, if this person could lose control, then perhaps we could also! That is a major reason why it is so important for the caregiver to remain calm and steady. The world of the patient is already tilting and whirling, and he or she looks to you to steady the world, to bring back some measure of control to life. Self-direction is one of the foundations on which authentic personhood is built. When we lose that ability or capacity for self-determination, for ordering our world, a part of the self is lost. This is a threat to the self and produces the emotional reactions that have been discussed.

When a patient is admitted to the trauma center, one of the first questions he or she may have, whether spoken or unspoken, is "Am I going to die?" When something unexpected happens, there is a great awareness of loss of control, and death anxiety (often unrecognized as such) comes washing over the patient. These life situations initiate a powerful rush of death anxiety so that the patient is overwhelmed and displaces or represses the death anxiety. Instead of being fearful of an experience of "not being" (at least in the same state of life as is currently known), the patient becomes fearful about something specific, an object or a situation (Yalom, 1980). Because the fear or anxiety is then "located," it can be managed and provides a way of once again gaining mastery over the death anxiety. A measure of control is regained.

One of the tasks of the caregiver is to reduce anxiety to tolerable levels. Therefore it is easy to see how important the element of choice becomes in treatment. As mentioned, the ability to make some choices, "to have a say" in one's care, provides a sense of control and helps restore equilibrium to the patient's world. The reality of intense resuscitation may make "patient choice" seem ridiculous, but an effort should be made by the nurse to allow some semblance of control. This could be achieved, for example, by asking the patient which visitor to allow in first, or ask the patient if he or she would like an extra warm blanket.

The theme of control runs like a stream throughout the topics discussed in this chapter. It is present in every case and life situation. It is vitally important to the sense of well-being and worth. The nurse should remember it while caring for patients. To tend to the needs of the deepest part of their selfhood is to reach where no medicine and no technology can reach.

SUMMARY   The purpose for the inclusion of this chapter on psychologic and spiritual adaptation to trauma in a nursing text is to reaffirm a truth. The truth is simply this: we are whole beings. We are body, mind, and spirit. Impact on one of these aspects of the self impacts the whole, just as the rock in the pond sends out ripples affecting the entire surface of the water.

The nurse should approach each patient as a whole, complex, living, changing personality. If that is done, the patient will receive nursing care that the best health insurance plan in the world cannot buy. The table below summarizes psychosocial nursing interventions for the trauma patient.

NURSING DIAGNOSES & EVALUATIVE CRITERIA   *The patient requiring psychosocial adaptation*

Nursing diagnosis	Nursing intervention	Evaluative criteria
High risk for fear Related to uncertain prognosis, unexpected injury	**Promote trust** Answer questions in clear, understandable terms and in a caring manner. Encourage patient to acknowledge fears, and assure patient that fear is a normal response.	Patient will state that fear is decreased.
High risk for anxiety Related to physiologic threat	**Relieve anxiety** Treat patient as a person capable of making decisions if physical condition allows. Anticipate passive aggression by patient toward health care providers. Do not react with aggression toward patient or withdraw from patient.	Patient will participate in decision-making as physical condition allows. Patient will state that anxiety is decreased.
Ineffective patient coping Related to inexperience in coping with a stressful event the magnitude of traumatic injury	**Promote effective coping** Help patient to identify previously used helpful coping strategies. Obtain psychosocial and spiritual resources for patient. Permit presence of patient's social support network (e.g., family, friends).	Patient will use effective coping strategies.

COMPETENCIES
The following clinical competencies pertain to **caring for the trauma patient with psychosocial and spiritual needs.**

☑ *Demonstrate assessment of patient's psychosocial and spiritual needs.*

☑ *Make referrals to the chaplain and other social service staff, based on assessment.*

☑ *Allow patient to participate in decision-making when appropriate.*

RESEARCH QUESTIONS

- Does the patient's sense of "loss of control" adversely affect the healing process? Conversely, does the patient's sense of "being in control" or "managing" the illness aid recovery?

- What type of educational process would best prepare the nursing staff for successful interaction with death and dying issues? This would include the patient and the family, as well as the personal reaction of the nurse.

- Much emotional distancing by the staff frequently occurs when dealing with the patient who is hospitalized because of a suicide attempt. However, these patients often need personal interaction very much. What can be done to facilitate more personalized care of the patient who has attempted suicide?

RESOURCE

The Society for Traumatic Stress Studies
Box 1564
Lancaster, PA 17603-1564
(717) 396-8877

ANNOTATED BIBLIOGRAPHY

Good, W.V., Nelson, J.E. (1968, revised). *Psychiatry Made Ridiculously Simple.* Miami: Medmaster.
Various psychiatric problems, treatment, and medications highlighted in an interesting and understandable manner. Authors' straightforward explanations are done with a minimum of "medicalese," and are interwoven with humor and illustrations. An excellent addition to the library of both medical and lay persons.

Lester, A.D. (1983). *Coping with your anger: A Christian guide.* Philadelphia: Westminster Press.
Insight by way of theology and psychology for persons to deal creatively with anger. The author writes in an appealing and empathetic style. To understand reactions that are out of proportion with the situation, this is a "must" to read.

Oates, W.E., & Oates, C.E. (1985). *People in pain: Guidelines for pastoral care.* Philadelphia: Westminster Press.
A fine volume that interweaves the knowledge and expertise of one of America's foremost pastoral counselors and his son, a well-known and highly respected neurologist. Together they explore the physiologic, psychologic, and spiritual dimensions of pain. This should be a required text for all of the "helping" professions.

REFERENCES

American Psychiatric Association (1987). *Diagnostic and statistical manual* of mental disorders (3rd ed.). Washington, DC: Author.

Bluhm, J. (1987). Helping families in crisis hold on. *Nursing,* Oct., 44-46.

Bourdon, S.E. (1986). Psychological impact of neurotrauma in the acute care setting. *Nursing Clinics of North America, 21,* 629-639.

Bowlby, J. (1980). *Loss: Sadness and depression: Vol. 3.* New York: Basic Books.

Clark, S. (1987). Nursing diagnosis: Ineffective coping. I. A theoretical framework. *Heart and Lung, 16,* 670-676.

Clark, S. (1987). Nursing diagnosis: Ineffective coping. II. Planning care. *Heart and Lung, 16,* 677-683.

Cox-Gedmark, J. (1980). *Coping with physical disability.* Philadelphia: Westminster Press.

Drew, N. (1986). Exclusion and confirmation: A phenomenology of patients' experience with caregivers. *Image, 18,* (2), 39-43.

Dubin, W.R., & Sarnoff, J.R. (1986). Sudden unexpected death: Intervention with the survivors. *Annals of Emergency Medicine, 15* (1), 54-57.

Fanslow, J. (1983). Needs of grieving spouses in sudden death situations: A pilot study. *Journal of Emergency Nursing, 9,* (4), 213-216.

Horowitz, M.J., Wilner, N., Kaltreider, N., & Alvarez, W. (1980). Signs and symptoms of posttraumatic stress disorder. *Archives of General Psychiatry, 37,* 85-92.

Huff, L.A. (1989). *People in crisis* (3rd ed.). Reading, MA: Addison-Wesley Publishing.

Ingram, T.L., Hurley, E.C., & Riley, M.T. (1985). Grief-resolution therapy in a pastoral context. *Journal of Pastoral Care*, 39 (1), 69-72.

Justice, W.G. (1982). *When death comes*. Nashville: Broadman Press.

Krupnick, J.I., & Horowite, M. (1981). Stress response syndromes: Recurrent themes. *Archives of General Psychiatry*, 38, 428-435.

Kuch, K., Swinson, R.P., and Kirby, M. (1985) Posttraumatic stress disorder after car accidents. *Canadian Journal of Psychiatry*, 30, 426-427.

Lester, A.D. (1983). *Coping with your anger: A Christian guide*. Philadelphia: Westminster Press.

Mechanic, D. (1977). Illness behavior, social adaptation, and management of illness: A comparison of educational and medical models. *Journal of Nervous and Mental Disease*, 165, 79-87.

Mendelson, G. (1987). The concept of posttraumatic stress disorder: A review. *International Journal of Law and Psychiatry*, 10, 45-62.

Meninger, K., Mayman, M., & Pruyser, P. (1963). *The vital balance* (p. 106). New York: Viking Press.

Minnick, A. (1983). Locked-in syndrome. *Journal of Neurosurgical Nursing*, 15, 77-79.

Oates, W.E. (1982). *The Christian pastor* (3rd ed.) (pp. 48-55). Philadelphia: Westminster Press.

Oates, W.E. (1987). *Behind the masks: Personality disorders in religious behavior* (pp. 70-81). Philadelphia: Westminster Press.

Oates, W.E., & Oates, C.E. (1985). *People in pain: Guidelines for pastoral care*. Philadelphia: Westminster Press.

Orgue, M., Blech, B., & Monrroy, L. (1983). *Ethnic nursing care: A multicultural approach*. St. Louis: Mosby–Year Book, Inc.

Post, H. (1986). *Sudden death in the emergency department: Survivors speak of their presence during resuscitation*. A report to the College of Chaplains. Also, published: Richardson, Tex: *Christian Medical Society Journal*, Summer 1985.

Post, H., & Rhee, K. (1985). Sudden death in the emergency room: What does compassion mean to the survivors? *Christian Medical Society*, 16 (3), 9-11.

Rodgers, C.D. (1983). Needs of relatives of cardiac surgery patients during the critical care phase. *Focus on Critical Care Oct.*, 50-55.

Swizer, D.K. (1974). *The minister as crisis counselor*. Nashville: Abingdon Press.

Welch, M. (1987). Trauma recovery: An ethnography (An unpublished *thesis prospectus* from University of Connecticut, Department of Anthropology, Spring 1987.)

Willis, W. (1977). Bereavement management in the emergency department. *Journal of Emergency Nursing*, 3, 35-39.

Yalom, I.D. (1980), *Existential psychotherapy* (pp. 262-268). New York: Basic Books.

IV

TRAUMA THROUGHOUT THE LIFESPAN

16 Trauma in Pregnancy

Linda K. Manley

OBJECTIVES

❑ Identify common mechanisms of injury and injury patterns in the gravid trauma patient.

❑ Recognize injuries that may have been the result of a pathologic condition peculiar to the pregnancy itself (e.g., eclampsia, abruptio placenta).

❑ Describe normal anatomic and physiologic changes that occur during pregnancy.

❑ Describe how the initial resuscitation of the gravid trauma patient must be modified to accommodate and preserve normal changes.

❑ Explain how the secondary survey differs in the pregnant trauma patient, and explain the importance of assessing fetal status.

INTRODUCTION Innovative technology and the opportunity for early prenatal care have dramatically reduced perinatal mortality during the past two decades. When perinatal deaths are trauma-related, however, a similar decrease has not been observed. Trauma during pregnancy is currently the leading cause of death and disability in the obstetric patient and fetus.

Injuries are estimated to occur in 6% to 7% of all pregnancies, although most are minor in nature (Baker, 1982; Buchsbaum, 1979a). In a 5-year retrospective review of trauma admissions to a level I facility, Drost et al. evaluated a total of 318 pregnant trauma patients, admitting 25 (8%), which was 0.3% of the overall trauma admissions (Drost et al., 1990). Level I trauma center orientation and continuing education efforts are often directed toward the adult trauma victim, with less emphasis placed on the pediatric, geriatric, and obstetric trauma patient (Zuspan, 1990).

Motor vehicle crashes are the leading cause of maternal death, followed by violent assault and suicide (Baker, 1982). Pregnancy can aggravate preexisting family stress and increase domestic violence (Hillard, 1985). Anatomic changes throughout pregnancy alter the woman's center of gravity, predisposing her to falls. With each succeeding trimester, the likelihood of an accident increases (Jackson, 1979). By the third trimester, minor trauma occurs more frequently than at any other time during female adulthood (Neufeld, Moore, Marx, & Rosen, 1987).

This chapter addresses issues for the practitioner faced with the complex problem of managing two victims. Optimal maternal and fetal outcome requires a thorough understanding of injury patterns, recognizing normal anatomic and physiologic changes, and modifying the initial resuscitation. Maternal resuscitation is the only means of fetal resuscitation.

CASE STUDY Lori, 28 years old and 32 weeks pregnant, was involved in a head-on collision. Although not ejected, Lori was found unrestrained with head, chest, and possible abdominal injuries. Prehospital care providers state Lori was "stable" en route to the hospital. On arrival to the emergency department (ED), she has a nasal cannula, cervical spine immobilization, and one 20-gauge IV in place. Initial BP is 100/60; pulse, 104; and respirations, 20.

What are three changes that occur in the cardiovascular system during pregnancy?

Circulating blood volume increases approximately 40%. The major components of the blood, the plasma, and erythrocyte volume, however, rise at a disproportionate rate, with plasma volume increasing more than erythrocyte volume. The results are a decrease in the hemoglobin, to 11 g, and a "physiologic anemia" of pregnancy.

Heart rate increases 10 to 15 beats per minute (bpm). Tachycardia, though, is still considered a pulse greater than 100 bpm.

Blood pressure decreases 5 to 15 mm Hg during the second trimester.

What is the most accurate way to assess an **early** *(<20%) blood volume deficit in the gravid patient?*

Maternal hypervolemia offers the gravid patient a 30% to 35% cushion before classic signs of hypovolemic shock in the mother become evident. Uteroplacental blood flow, though, is shunted from the fetal circulation to the maternal circulation much earlier. An excellent indicator of maternal hypovolemia is the presence of hypoxia in the fetus, which can be assessed by determining the fetal heart rate (FHR). A 20% volume deficit, then, may have no effect on the mother, but a dramatic effect on the fetus.

Initial arterial blood gases (ABGs) reveal pH, 7.31; Pao$_2$, 88 torr; and Paco$_2$, 42 torr. What do these values indicate?

Pregnancy is associated with an increase in the tidal volume, but no change in the respiratory rate, which results in a physiologic "hyperventilation" and a resultant decrease in the Paco$_2$ to approximately 30 torr. Thus a Paco$_2$ of 42 torr may be abnormal and require further evaluation.

MECHANISM OF INJURY
Motor Vehicle Crashes

Motor vehicle crashes occur nearly 10 times more frequently than other accidents for women in their reproductive years (Jackson, 1979; Crosby, 1983). Traffic accidents are responsible for the majority of maternal deaths, with fetal death most often resulting from maternal death. More than 48,700 deaths and 1,800,000 disabling injuries were attributed to motor vehicle accidents in 1987, at a national cost of $64.7 billion (National Safety Council, 1988). Unfortunately, statistics regarding the obstetric trauma patient are not available.

During a motor vehicle crash, the gravid uterus receives not only the impact of the steering wheel or dashboard, but the inertial forces of mass versus momentum (Baker, 1982). All moving bodies have kinetic energy that must be dissipated before they are able to stop. Kinetic energy in a moving automobile is imparted by the engine and dissipated by the tire friction and brakes; occupants are slowed with the car because of their friction against the seats. If the vehicle and occupant are uniformly decelerated and slowed, nothing happens. If the vehicle and occupant decelerate at different rates, however, a massive amount of force is delivered to the occupant in a brief amount of time. The human body can tolerate extreme impact forces if applied over an extremely short period of time, but individual organs and tissues have widely varying tolerances to impact. Injury is usually the result of organ displacement and subsequent hemorrhage. In a motor vehicle crash, the pregnant woman is at risk for premature labor or a uterine injury (i.e., abruptio placenta, uterine rupture).

During the early 1960s, the use of the lap-belt restraint system by pregnant women was closely scrutinized. Rubovits (1964) reported a case of uterine rupture in a woman wearing a lap belt alone. He suggested that lap belts increased the risk for fetal and maternal injury by focusing the force directly over the uterus. Crosby and Costiloe (1971), however, found that the greatest risk to the gravid woman was ejection from the car if unrestrained. Unrestrained pregnant women ejected from a vehicle had a 33% death rate, which dropped to 5% when not ejected. Fetal death rate was highest (47%) when the mother was ejected, versus 11% when not ejected.

Of interest, the benefit of the lap belt appears to be greatest for the mother. Crosby and Costiloe (1971) found the fetal death rate of lap-belted survivors was actually slightly higher (2%) than that of the unbelted survivors. This may be due to the fact that during a crash the uterus remains in motion until checked by an outside force, which, in this case, is the lap belt. Forward flexion over the belt results in uterine distortion, which may result in shearing at the placental attachment site, especially with an advanced pregnancy (Crosby & Costiloe, 1971). Uterine pressure, normally 50 mm Hg during labor, has been shown to rise to as high as 550 mm Hg, 10 times greater, during a collision (Crosby, 1979). It is unlikely, though, that the fetus would be killed solely by this short-lasting, extreme pressure gradient.

The most ideal restraint system at present is a three-point restraint—lap belt and shoulder harness. Crosby, King, and Stoute (1972) found that when properly used, this system reduced fetal death from 50% to 8.3% in primate studies. The shoulder harness prevents forward flexion over the belt and diffuses impact force sustained by the placenta, uterus, and fetal structures. Correct positioning of the three-point restraint system is essential. The lap belt is worn low, below the uterus, and tight across the pelvis; the position of the shoulder harness is unchanged. Some advocate placement of a cushion between the seat belt and abdominal wall, which may further help to distribute the deceleration force (Mathews, 1975). Mathews (1975) describes a case of uterine rupture in a woman, 25 weeks pregnant, involved in a head-on collision, who was wearing a loosely fitted lap-shoulder safety harness. Laparotomy revealed a fetus and placenta lying free in the abdominal cavity with 3500 ml of blood. The mother survived, but the fetus did not. However, uterine rupture is extremely rare.

In general, the following are common injury patterns found in pregnant women involved in severe motor vehicle crashes (Crosby, 1979):

- The severity of injury to the pregnant woman closely parallels the severity of physical damage to the vehicle.
- Severe life-threatening injuries are usually multiple; however, the leading cause of maternal death is from a head injury.
- Internal injuries are usually accompanied by intraperitoneal hemorrhage and hypovolemic shock.
- The likelihood of fetal death is proportional to the severity of maternal injury.
- Women with multiple injuries are likely to lose the fetus as a result of an abruptio placenta and/or maternal shock.
- Pelvic fractures are associated with a high incidence of placental separation and fetal injury.

Use of seat belts and prevention should be, at least initially, a primary concern for public health and medical professionals. The position of the woman in the car and whether a restraint system was used must be ascertained and reported by emergency medical services (EMS) personnel at the scene.

Penetrating Trauma

The most common penetrating injury to the abdomen during pregnancy is a gunshot wound (Buchsbaum, 1979b). To a lesser extent, penetrating injuries also result from any number of objects, including swords, files, wooden stakes, knives, animal horns, and barbeque forks. Maternal and fetal outcome in penetrating trauma is related to the number of maternal organs injured. In general, the more organs injured, the worse the prognosis.

As the uterus occupies an increasingly larger portion of the abdominal cavity, the likelihood of uterine injury increases. The gravid uterus acts as a shield for the mother and protects the more vital maternal structures (i.e., intestines, liver, spleen).

Gunshot wounds

The actual incidence of gunshot wounds during pregnancy is not known, but probably exceeds the reported rate, with most occurring in urban areas. A gunshot wound to the nonpregnant uterus is rare, because the normal uterus is shielded by the bony pelvis (Buchsbaum, 1979b). During pregnancy, however, it is the organ most likely to be injured. The uterus is not considered a vital organ, and maternal mortality resulting from an abdominal gunshot wound is surprisingly low (Buchsbaum, 1975). This may be due, in part, to the shielding effect of the uterus, as well as the transfer of energy directly into the dense uterine musculature.

It is assumed that organs in the path of the bullet may be injured. Detecting the course of the bullet once it has entered the body is extremely difficult; thus surgical exploration is required. Usually, a bullet that enters the gravid uterus is likely to come to rest there.

Fetal outcome is far worse than maternal outcome with an abdominal gunshot wound, with mortality rates ranging from 41% to 71% (Bushsbaum, 1979b). Direct injuries to the fetus can cause injury and death in utero; indirect injury to the cord, placenta, or membranes can also cause fetal death. Furthermore, alterations in maternal homeostasis (i.e., hypovolemic or neurogenic

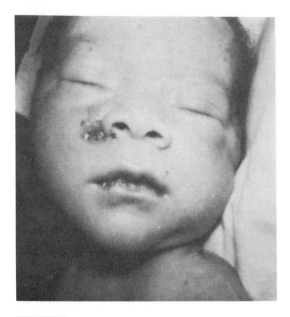

Figure 16-1 Puncture wound to right nasolabial fold resulting from small-caliber bullet. (*Note.* From "Gunshot Wound of the Pregnant Uterus: Case Report of Fetal Injury, Deglutination of Missile, and Survival," by H.J. Buchsbaum and P.A. Caruso, 1969, *Obstetrics and Gynecology*, 33, p. 673.)

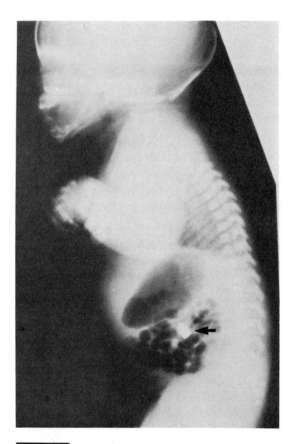

Figure 16-2 Bullet found in fetal abdomen on x-ray examination. (*Note.* From "Gunshot Wound of the Pregnant Uterus: Case Report of Fetal Injury, Deglutination of Missile, and Survival" by H.J. Buchsbaum and P.A. Caruso, 1969, *Obstetrics and Gynecology*, 33, p. 673.)

shock) can adversely affect the fetus and negatively impact on outcome.

Case review The mother at 34 to 36 weeks gestation was struck in the abdomen by a low-velocity, small-caliber bullet. X-ray examination revealed the bullet lodged in the uterus. Surgical exploration revealed an entrance wound on the anterior surface of the uterus with no other organ injury identified. A live infant with an Apgar score of 9 was delivered by cesarean section. Examination of the infant failed to reveal any wounds to the abdomen or thorax, and the bullet was not located in the uterine cavity. Examination of the infant found a puncture wound to the right nasolabial fold (Figure 16-1) with no injury to the palate or tongue. A whole body x-ray examination of the newborn revealed the bullet in the abdominal cavity (Figure 16-2). Apparently, after penetrating the cheek, the bullet was subsequently swallowed and later retrieved when the infant passed it per rectum (Buchsbaum, 1979b).

Case review A 23-year-old mother at 36 weeks gestation was shot in the abdomen with a low-velocity, .38-caliber bullet. X-ray examination of the maternal abdomen revealed the bullet to be in the uterus, lodged in the arm of the fetus. A live, 1700 g, infant was delivered by cesarean section; the mother sustained no associated injuries. The infant had an entrance wound posteriorly in the right flank and an exit wound in the right anterior chest wall, with the bullet resting in the right arm. The infant sustained a right tension pneumothorax (Figure 16-3), which was managed with tube thoracostomy and intubation. When the baby was 12 hours of age, meconium was oozing from the entrance wound, and subsequent surgical exploration revealed kidney, colon,

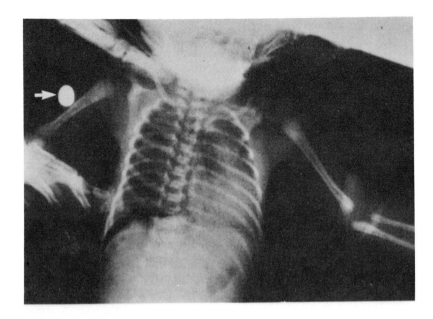

Figure 16-3   Thoracoabdominal gunshot wound with fetal survival of 36-week fetus with tension pneumothorax. (*Note.* From K. Brown, R. Bhat, O. Jonasson, and V. Dharmapuri, 1979, *Journal of the American Medical Association*, 237, pp. 2409-2410.)

liver, and diaphragm injuries, which were repaired. The infant was discharged on day 34 (Buchsbaum, 1979b).

Stab wounds

Stab wounds to the abdomen are less common than gunshot wounds and have a more optimistic prognosis for both the mother and fetus (Buchsbaum, 1979b). With stab wounds, an organ may be able to slide away from the advancing blade, with ultimately fewer organs being injured.

Abdominal stab wounds can be divided into those occurring in either the upper quadrant or the lower quadrant. Two thirds of abdominal stab wounds occur in the upper abdomen above the umbilicus (Neufeld et al., 1987). Overlying loops of bowel, displaced upwards by the expanding uterus, are easily injured. If local exploration reveals the penetration of the peritoneal cavity, surgical exploration is frequently indicated. Stab wounds to the lower abdomen are more likely to injure the uterus, with the other organs shielded to some degree. If serious maternal and fetal injury is ruled out by local wound exploration, diagnostic peritoneal lavage, urologic studies, and

serial hematocrit values, lower abdominal injuries can be managed without laparotomy (Gatrell, 1987).

Thermal Injuries

Most burn units nationwide admit women who are pregnant, yet literature on this subject is scarce. Burns can be the result of a direct thermal or electrical injury.

Burns

Between 1951 and 1974, the burn unit of the U.S. Army Institute of Surgical Research admitted 19 pregnant women between the ages of 16 and 37 years (Taylor, 1979). All burns were caused by flames or explosions. Of the 19 admitted, 11 were burned by flammable liquids, 5 by clothing, 2 by house fires, and 1 by an aircraft accident. Of interest, 2 of the patients burned by flammable liquids used gasoline as a means of committing suicide. The extent of the burns ranged from 6% to 92% of the total body surface area (BSA), with the third-degree component ranging from no BSA to 83.5% BSA. The duration of the pregnancy varied from 5 to 36 weeks, with the majority occurring during the first two trimesters.

The most striking finding by the Institute of Surgical Research team was that the outcome of the pregnancy was primarily determined by the extent of the mother's burn injury and ultimate fate of the mother. Seven women had burns of greater than 60% BSA, and all seven died. Six of the seven pregnancies terminated before the mothers' death, with two stillborns and four live births of infants weighing from 680 to 2500 g; only the 2500 g infant survived.

Twelve women survived their burns, and of these, 10 were discharged with their wounds healed and the pregnancy intact. Only one fetus died, and this coincided with a severe burn wound cellulitis. The study suggests that maternal survival is usually accompanied by fetal survival. If the mother's burns are lethal (>50% BSA), the pregnancy will usually terminate spontaneously before her death.

Several factors contribute to, and frequently coexist with, the loss of a pregnancy in the burn victim—namely, hypotension, hypoxia, sepsis, and electrolyte imbalance (Taylor, 1979). Hypotension, secondary to hypovolemia, results in uteroplacental constriction and is a complication easily remedied by close monitoring and early, aggressive fluid replacement. Hypoxia, another frequent complication accompanying burn injuries, further decreases uterine blood flow and fetal oxygenation. Gravid patients with major burns are at risk for overwhelming systemic infection and septic shock, frequently the terminal event. Electrolyte balance, particularly the serum sodium level, must be closely followed in burn patients. The U.S. Army series was associated with a fairly high incidence of dilutional hyponatremia, which may contribute to the onset of premature labor.

Finally, burn victims are frequently at risk for both carbon monoxide and cyanide toxicity as a result of the combustion of plastic materials found in homes. Carbon monoxide poisoning in pregnancy can result in fetal and infant death or severe neurologic impairment in the offspring (Zalstein & Koren, 1990). Carboxyhemoglobin and cyanide levels should be obtained during the initial evaluation of the burned obstetric patient. Regional poison control centers can be instrumental in assisting with the patient's management.

Electrical injuries

Although electrical injuries occur infrequently, all pregnant women sustaining even a minor electrical shock should immediately notify their attending physician, because this injury is associated with an extremely high fetal mortality. Leiberman et al. (1986) followed six women, 21 to 40 weeks pregnant, who received minor household electrical shocks from a lamp, iron, wall outlet, oven, and washing machine. The current path was from the hand to the foot. None of the women were burned or appeared otherwise injured. Despite the lack of obvious injuries, three stillbirths occurred among the six women. Of the three fetuses who survived, two were observed to have oligohydramnios, a complication where an abnormally small amount of amniotic fluid is produced. Most injuries occurred on standard household circuits, not on bathroom circuits, which are protected by ground fault interrupter circuits (GFIC). It was suggested that even if a GFIC had been activated, the current may still have been high enough to injure the fetus. A current considered safe for children and adults may not be safe for a fetus.

In an electrical accident, the fetus is a potential victim in an otherwise harmless event (Leiberman et al., 1986). The low resistance of the vascular uterus and abundancy of the amniotic fluid may funnel the current directly through the uterus, predisposing the fetus to injury (Gatrell, 1987). Fetal damage may also result from changes in fetal heart conduction or lesions in the uteroplacental bed (Leiberman et al., 1986). Burn marks have been noted on infants who survived the initial electrical injury (Rees, 1965).

Of interest, electrical currents used for therapeutic reasons during pregnancy have not been found to have a detrimental effect on fetal outcome. For example, electroconvulsive therapy applied to the head of psychiatric patients, for depression, did not impact negatively on fetal outcome (Repke & Berger, 1984). Pregnant women requiring elective or emergent countershock, with energy currents up to 300 watt/seconds, have also had excellent fetal outcomes (Neufeld et al., 1987). This may be because with both procedures, the current path did not directly cross the uterus and the fetus was closely monitored.

Lightning injuries In 1983, 93 people were struck by lightning in the United States (National

Safety Council, 1988). Although this occurrence is extremely rare in the pregnant patient, it has been documented (Pierce, Henderson, & Mitchell, 1986). With rapid advanced life support, women who are in cardiopulmonary arrest and who appear dead can be successfully resuscitated and resume a normal life. Intrauterine fetal death, however, occurs 50% of the time, and, as with other electrical injuries, the fetus is at an increased risk. Rare cases of intrauterine survival have occurred after exposure to lightning, and long-term follow-up of the infant has been normal (Flannery & Wiles, 1982).

Sports Injuries

Pregnant women may be at a greater risk for an athletic injury because of the anatomic and physiologic changes associated with pregnancy. Although physiologic performance factors are important, the body movements required by each sport also must be considered. Locomotion may be slowed because of an increasing mass, altered upright posture, and increased fluid retention (Nicholas, 1979).

Six main types of motion are used during most sporting activities: walking, running, jumping, kicking, throwing, and stance. During the first and second trimester, running and stance usually pose no significant problem. During the third trimester, however, the same motions may result in severe fatigue or strain (Nicholas, 1979). Injuries are much more likely in sports where running, kicking, throwing, and jumping are essential components.

Participation in contact sports, such as softball and hockey, beyond the first trimester carries a strong risk of receiving high-velocity blows to the uterus (Haycock, 1982). Pregnancy, though, does not preclude participation in many other sports, including jogging, tennis, bicycling, and paddleball, and is frequently encouraged for cardiovascular fitness. The fetus is well cushioned in the amniotic sac, and the likelihood of injury is small.

Most injuries incurred during pregnancy affect the musculoskeletal system, although they can also affect the nervous system, viscera, chest, head, and face. The most disconcerting injuries to the musculoskeletal system during pregnancy are sprains, strains, dislocations, and fractures.

Sprains and strains

Sprains are defined as injuries to the joints in which ligaments binding the joint are torn or stretched. If sprains are not treated properly during pregnancy, a residual disability can follow postpartum. Strains are defined as muscle-tendon tears. The most serious and difficult strain to treat during pregnancy is a back strain, usually caused by excessive twisting motions or fatigue. Women who play contact and endurance sports are predisposed to back strain. Pregnancy causes ligament laxity and muscle stretching and changes the mechanics of posture. During prolonged sports activities, further stretching or tearing of the supporting spinal and pelvic muscles can occur. It can be difficult to differentiate a fracture and nerve root irritation from disk protrusion or a simple strain.

Dislocations and fractures

For the most part, diagnosis and treatment of dislocations and fractures of the pregnant woman parallel those of her nonpregnant counterpart. A few sports injuries have a particular importance, especially those involving the pelvis. During pregnancy, hormonal influences cause a softening of most joints, including the sacroiliac joint. Falls occurring with the legs wide apart can separate the pelvis, injure the coccyx, or tear the adductor tendons and result in a serious and painful disability (Nicholas, 1979). Prevention of such injuries is extremely important.

Pelvic fractures are more common in certain sports, such as hiking, mountain climbing, or riding a horse, motorcycle, or bicycle. The hazard with pelvic fractures is excessive callus formation, which will malalign the pelvic canal. X-ray studies are permissible and should be used if the woman has crepitus, severe swelling or ecchymosis, spasm, gait disturbance, or weakness of a lower extremity. When possible, the abdomen should be shielded from unnecessary x-rays.

Although not specifically injured, the fetus can be adversely affected when the mother engages in vigorous sports activities. Maternal exercise influences the fetal heart rate and breathing patterns (Gorski, 1985). Pregnant women with uteroplacental insufficiency are more likely to have more significant fetal changes during exercise and should be closely monitored. Severe hyperthermia, induced by extremely strenuous exercise or environment, should be avoided, because it can affect fetal development, especially in early pregnancy.

ANATOMIC AND PHYSIOLOGIC CONSIDERATIONS

Nearly every organ system undergoes major changes during pregnancy, and, in some instances, it may be this change that initiates the injury.

Ventilation

The major anatomic change in the respiratory system occurs primarily with the diaphragm, which is elevated approximately 4 cm and increases in excursion 1.0 to 1.5 cm (Cruikshank, 1979). The respiratory rate does not change. During pregnancy, tidal volume increases 40% with a subsequent decrease in residual volume (Cruikshank, 1979). Progesterone, known to be a potent respiratory stimulant, may be responsible for the increased tidal volume (Brooks, 1983). It is important to note that this "hyperventilation of pregnancy" results in a decreased arterial $Paco_2$ level, falling to approximately 30 torr during the second trimester, a level which is maintained throughout the pregnancy (Cruikshank, 1979). The gravid patient compensates for a respiratory alkalosis with a reduction in serum bicarbonate to approximately 22 mEq/L (normal, 26 mEq/L); thus, the pH is maintained within normal limits (Brooks, 1983). During pregnancy, the respiratory center becomes much more sensitive to minute changes in the $Paco_2$ level. For example, a 1-torr increase in arterial CO_2 in the nonpregnant woman increases minute ventilation 1.5 liters per minute (lpm). A similar increase in the gravid patient increases minute ventilation 6.0 lpm, a 400% increase (Cruikshank, 1979). Another significant change is a marked (43%) increase in oxygen consumption (Brinkman & Woods, 1979). The gravid woman has a significantly reduced oxygen reserve compared with her nonpregnant counterpart, and hypoxemia can easily result (Neufeld et al., 1987) (Table 16-1).

Relatively short periods of severe hypoxia may have detrimental effects on the developing fetus, although this is controversial. One interesting study examined the possible effects of hypoxia on mice during early gestation (Clemmer and Telford, 1966). Shortly after fertilization, several mice were placed in a low-oxygen environment (<6% FIo_2) for 6 hours. The animals were sacri-

Table 16-1 Maternal hemoglobin, blood gases, and oxygen consumption during pregnancy

	Gestational weeks			
	12	24	32	38
Hgb (g/dl)	12.5	11.5	10.8	11.1
Pao_2 (mm Hg)	107.6	104.1	102.5	101.3
$Paco_2$ (mm Hg)	29.7	28.0	30.2	31.1
V_E (L/min)	8.4	10.3	10.4	11.1
Vo_2 (ml/min)	160	200	230	280

(*Note.* From Effects of Hypovolemia and Hypoxia on the Conceptus by C.R. Brinkman and J.R. Woods, Jr. In H.J. Buchsbaum [Ed.], 1979, *Trauma in Pregnancy,* Philadelphia: W.B. Saunders.) V_E, Minute ventilation; Vo_2, oxygen consumption.

ficed at term and the fetuses delivered alive; the newborns were sacrificed one day later and examined. The most striking finding was that 28% of the baby mice were found to have cardiac defects, compared with 7.5% of the controls. Of the cardiac anomalies, 71% were septal defects; the second most common anomaly was an intraventricular defect.

The fetus may be able to tolerate brief periods of hypoxia (i.e., <10 minutes) without detrimental effects. Several physiologic adaptive mechanisms provide some degree of protection (Seldon & Burke, 1988). First, the oxygen-hemoglobin dissociation curve for fetal hemoglobin lies to the left of the maternal curve, which results in greater oxygen saturation at any given partial pressure of oxygen. Second, the fetus survives with a normal hypercarbia (12 to 15 mm Hg higher than maternal) and decreased level of carbonic anhydrase. And last, the reflex fetal response to hypoxia results in selective vasoconstriction, which shunts blood to critical fetal organs—the brain, heart, adrenals, and placenta.

Perfusion

Dramatic alterations occur in the cardiovascular and hematologic system early in pregnancy. During the first 10 weeks, cardiac output rises to 6 to 7 lpm and remains at this level for the duration of the pregnancy. Circulating blood volume (CBV) increases, on the average, 40%, with individual variations ranging from 20% to 100% (Cruikshank, 1979).

Vital sign assessment

Changes in the cardiovascular system affect vital signs. Heart rate increases 10 to 15 beats per minute (bpm) throughout pregnancy, reaching a maximum during the third trimester (Cruikshank, 1979). During both the sleeping and waking state, the pulse ranges from 80 to 95 bpm. Tachycardia, defined as a pulse rate greater than 100 bpm, is still considered a sign of hypovolemic shock, but can result also from fear and anxiety.

Cardiac monitoring may reflect changes in the electrocardiogram. During pregnancy, the heart is pushed upward and rotated forward by the elevated diaphragm, with the electrical axis deviating about 15 degrees to the left (Cruikshank, 1979). Lead III may reveal flattened or inverted T waves, and Q waves may appear in lead III and aV_F. Ectopic beats, usually supraventricular, are more common during pregnancy.

Pregnancy is associated with a vasodilated state caused by hormonal influences. Systolic blood pressure typically falls 5 to 15 mm Hg during the second trimester, rising to nonpregnant levels near term. A blood pressure greater than that of nonpregnant levels is *never* normal during pregnancy and may signify a dangerous obstetrical complication—preeclampsia, or pregnancy-induced hypertension (PIH).

Supine hypotensive syndrome

Supine hypotensive syndrome, also known as the inferior vena cava syndrome, is a common complication of late pregnancy. Supine hypotension is defined as a mean blood pressure decrease of 15 mm Hg and a sustained increase in pulse of 20 bpm. Supine hypotension results when the heavy gravid uterus compresses the major pelvic veins, inferior vena cava, and abdominal aorta, reducing venous return to the heart. This syndrome can result in a marked reduction in uterine blood flow. Unrecognized supine hypotension can sequester as much as 30% of the circulating blood volume and pool it into the venous system (Brinkman & Woods, 1979). Noninvasive monitoring has shown oxygen saturation to decrease in a small percentage of pregnant women in the supine position (Calvin, Jones, Knieriem, & Weinstein, 1988); this study, however, terminated at 5 minutes and did not evaluate prolonged use of the supine position, as would occur with the anesthetized woman or one immobilized on a backboard for a prolonged period. It must

be assumed that all women who are more than 20 weeks pregnant are at risk for supine hypotension, reduced uterine blood flow, and decreased oxygen saturation. The inferior vena cava is located on the right side of the body; thus, positioning the pregnant woman on the left side can reduce caval compression and increase cardiac output by 25% (Brinkman & Woods, 1979). Proper positioning is critical! The position of choice is the left lateral recumbent position at a 15- to 30-degree angle. If this is not possible, manually displacing the uterus off to the left side can be equally effective. Information on immobilizing the gravid trauma patient is discussed under Primary Survey in this chapter.

Fluid volume deficit: hypovolemia

Pregnancy-induced **hyper**volemia offers a protective, cushioning effect for the mother, allowing for a loss of 30% to 35% of the CBV before "classic" signs (i.e., tachycardia, poor peripheral perfusion, hypotension) of hypovolemic shock occur. Early signs of maternal **hypo**volemia are extremely difficult to identify and are best assessed by determining the fetal status (i.e., fetal heart rate (FHR), fetal movement [Table 16-2]). The fetus initially demonstrates hypoxia with an elevation in the FHR (normally FHR is 120 to 160/minute), followed by bradycardia. A 10% to 20% maternal CBV deficit will have minimal effects on the mother, but profound effects on the fetus. Animal studies have shown that when blood volume is rapidly depleted, uterine blood flow is markedly reduced before any change is noted in the maternal blood pressure (Brinkman and Woods, 1979). Unlike the kidney, brain, myocardium, and skeletal muscles, the uterus is incapable of increasing blood flow in the face of decreasing perfusion (Brinkman and Woods, 1979). Catecholamines, released during times of stress (i.e., acute blood loss, anxiety, fear) have potent alpha-adrenergic properties, which result in vasoconstriction. The uterine vascular bed is richly endowed with alpha-adrenergic receptors (Brinkman and Woods, 1979). An early response of maternal hemorrhage is marked uteroplacental constriction, caused by catecholomine release, resulting in a decreased oxygen supply to the fetus. It has been suggested that the fetus may be better able to tolerate maternal shock early in the pregnancy, although literature on this subject is scarce (Buchsbaum, 1975).

Table 16-2 Signs of hypovolemic shock in pregnancy

Circulating blood volume deficit	Early (20%)	Late (25%)
Pulse	<100 beats per minute	>100 beats per minute
Respiratory rate	12-20 per minute	>20 per minute
Blood pressure	Normal	Hypotensive
Skin perfusion	Warm, dry skin	Cool, ashen skin
Capillary refill	<2 seconds	>2 seconds
Level of consciousness	Alert	Agitated, lethargic
Urine output	>30-50 ml/hr	<30-50 ml/hr
Fetal heart rate*	High; low, with late decelerations	High, low, absent, late decelerations

*Fetal heart rate normally 120-160 beats per minute

The stress response in the nonpregnant patient is, as mentioned, vasoconstriction, resulting from catecholamine release. The stress response in the gravid patient, with the exception of uterine vascular bed, is one of vasodilation, possibly resulting from hormonal changes (Gatrell, 1987). Progesterone may blunt the angiotensin response, whereas estrogens depress sympathetic activity and locally dilate blood vessels. Maternal vasodilation response occurs mostly in the first two trimesters, with vasoconstriction predominant in the last trimester.

Late shock, loss of 30% to 35% of the CBV, is associated with the more "classic signs" of hypovolemic shock, that is, a weak, thready pulse; pale skin; lethargy; decreased urine output (<30 to 50 ml/hr); and possibly hypotension. At this stage, the fetal heart rate may be severely abnormal or absent. Cyanosis may not be noted in the cardiovascular assessment because this finding may be absent with advanced hemorrhagic shock and anemia. Cyanosis may not occur in the patient with a hemoglobin level below 5.9 g.

Central venous pressure (CVP) can be helpful in assessing maternal cardiovascular status and the woman's response to fluid resuscitation. Much confusion exists concerning what normal CVP values are during pregnancy. The Committee on Trauma, American College of Surgeons (1988) notes that the resting CVP is variable, and regardless of the initial reading, it is serial CVP measurements that are helpful. The gravid woman responds to fluid resuscitation as does her nonpregnant counterpart. For example, in the nonpregnant patient, rapid infusion of 250 ml of an isotonic fluid should elevate the CVP 2 to 4 cm H$_2$O (Gatrell, 1987).

Maternal bleeding may be associated with fetal bleeding into the maternal circulation, resulting in isoimmunization (Resnik, 1985). If the gravid woman has Rh-negative blood, an Rh-positive fetus may sensitize her and cause hemolytic disease for that or a later pregnancy (Gatrell, 1987). As little as 0.01 to 0.03 ml of fetal blood will sensitize 70% of Rh-negative patients (Mollison, 1973). Rh-immune globulin should be administered in appropriate doses. Testing for maternal-fetal hemorrhage will be reviewed in more depth under Sexuality: Reproductive Changes in this chapter.

Hematopoiesis

Alterations also occur in the major blood components. Both plasma and red blood cell volume rise, but at a disproportionate rate. Plasma volume increases by 50%, whereas erythrocyte volume increases by 30% to 35%. This results in a fall in the hemoglobin to 10.5 to 11.0 g during the last trimester and what is more commonly known as a "physiologic anemia" of pregnancy. This should be considered when reviewing complete blood count (CBC) results. Also, when reviewing the CBC, the white blood cell (WBC) count increases during pregnancy and can reach values as high as 18,000/mm^3, rising even higher during labor (Vander Veer, 1984). This may be an important factor to consider because the WBC count can be a diagnostic aid in the evaluation of abdominal trauma.

Hematologic changes that accompany pregnancy result in a hypercoagulable state. Fibrinogen levels double, clotting factors VII, VIII, and IX increase, and circulating plasminogen activator decreases. This may protect against maternal hemorrhage, but spontaneous thrombosis is a hazard (Gatrell, 1987). It has been suggested that the decreased viscosity of the blood, resulting from the falling hemoglobin level, may help protect against this complication to some extent. Bleeding, clotting, and prothrombin times remain unchanged.

Obstetric complications, such as eclampsia, abruptio placenta, intrauterine death, and missed abortion, are associated with a greater propensity for disseminated intravascular coagulation (DIC) (Gatrell, 1987). The placenta contains a large amount of thromboplastin, and the uterus is a major source of plasminogen activator. Injury to either the placenta or uterus can produce a consumptive coagulopathy and fibrinolysis.

It has been suggested that the risk of a spontaneous aortic dissection increases with pregnancy (Neufeld et al., 1987). Of dissecting aneurysms in women younger than 40 years, 50% occur during pregnancy. Predisposing factors may include an increased cardiac output, hypervolemia, and hypertension associated with eclampsia.

Abdominal System

Throughout pregnancy, gastric motility is reduced and emptying time is increased. Hormonal influences have a relaxing effect on the gastroesphageal sphincter and may limit its ability to prevent regurgitation (Brooks, 1983). Thus the pregnant woman is much more susceptible to vomiting and subsequent aspiration. It must always be assumed that the gravid patient has a full stomach.

Anatomic changes in the abdominal organs complicate diagnosis. Uterine enlargement leads to passive and active stretching of the abdominal wall and alters the woman's response to peritoneal irritation from blood or intestinal contents. Guarding and rigidity may be diminished or absent, making the physical examination far less rewarding than in the nonpregnant patient (Cruikshank, 1979). The initial abdominal examination includes assessment of bowel sounds and rebound tenderness while observing for contusions or abrasions to the abdominal wall, which could indicate the direction from which the injury occurred (Crosby, 1979).

Organs besides the uterus injured in abdominal trauma include the liver, pancreas, and spleen. The frequency and outcome from liver injuries is not statistically different between the pregnant and nonpregnant patient. Liver function

tests (LFT) do not reveal a change in the serum aspartate aminotransferase (AST) or lactic dehydrogenase (LDH) levels; the alkaline phophatase value, though, increases progressively throughout pregnancy and is 3 to 4 times higher at term (Cruikshank, 1979).

Spontaneous splenic rupture can be fatal during pregnancy and may or may not be related to a traumatic injury. It has been suggested preexisting congenital anomalies triggered by the "hypervolemic" state may predispose the gravid woman to a splenic rupture (Neufeld et al., 1987). Currently, evidence to support this theory is lacking.

Mobility: Musculoskeletal Changes

During pregnancy, the hormone *relaxin* causes the ligaments of the symphysis pubis and sacroiliac joints to loosen. This facilitates vaginal delivery by making the rigid pelvis more flexible (Cruikshank, 1979). Marked widening of the symphysis pubis occurs by the seventh month of gestation. The pelvis is actually less susceptible to fracture during pregnancy as a result of this increased mobility. It is this mobility, though, coupled with a protuberant abdomen, that leads to an unsteady gait. Falls are much more common during pregnancy than at any other time during adulthood (Cruikshank, 1979).

The skeletal system is well maintained during pregnancy despite a drop in calcium metabolism and a rise in the maternal parathyroid hormone (PTH). The fall in total calcium is nearly identical to the fall in serum albumin; thus the concentration of ionized calcium remains fairly constant (Cruikshank, 1979). A state of "physiologic hyperparathyroidism" occurs as levels of PTH rise during pregnancy (Cruikshank, 1979).

Responsiveness: Preeclampsia and Eclampsia

Physiologic changes occurring in the central nervous system (CNS) are unclear. A dangerous complication of pregnancy greatly affecting CNS functioning is preeclampsia, or toxemia, of pregnancy. Preeclampsia is a poorly understood, complex, multisystem disorder, which presents after the twentieth week of pregnancy. It is characterized by hypertension—defined as an increase in the systolic blood pressure of 30 mm Hg and an increase in the diastolic blood pressure of 15 mm Hg, or greater than 90 mm Hg—and proteinuria. Generalized edema and hyperreflexia help support the diagnosis but need not be present

(Brooks, 1983). It has been postulated that the cause of this disorder is genetic or immunologic, although this is controversial (Jagoda & Riggio, 1991).

Preeclampsia can progress to the convulsive phase, eclampsia. Eclampsia is associated with a high perinatal mortality rate, possibly as high as 30% to 35% worldwide (Cavanagh, Knuppel, & O'Connor, 1982). Eclampsia is reported to be present in .05% to .2% of all deliveries and is most common in primigravidas, older multigravidas, women with diabetes, and women with preexisting chronic hypertension (Neufeld et al., 1987).

Seizure activity resulting from eclampsia can easily be mistaken for a head injury in the traumatized obstetric patient. Although the pregnant trauma patient presenting with coma or seizure activity may have a trauma-induced intracerebral bleed, it must be assumed that the seizure activity has an eclamptic etiology (Cruikshank, 1979; Neufeld et al., 1987). Seizure activity and apnea result in marked maternal and fetal hypoxia. It can have a lethal outcome for both the mother and fetus if not aggressively treated.

Case review

A 28-year-old woman, 41 weeks gestation, was found unconcious in a cattle feed lot, presumably attacked by a bull. En route to the hospital, she developed grand mal seizure activity and was hypertensive (BP, 170/100). She has 3+ proteinuria on admission. The assumption of a severe head injury is made and an extensive neurologic examination is done, including computerized tomography of the brain, which is negative. At this point, the correct diagnosis of eclampsia is recognized. In the interval before diagnosis, however, irreversible damage has been sustained, and both the mother and fetus subsequently die (Cruikshank, 1979).

Elimination: Genitourinary

Several anatomic changes occur in the renal system. Marked dilation of the renal pelves and ureters occurs at 10 weeks gestation and persists until 6 weeks postpartum (Cruikshank, 1979). The right side is usually more dilated than the left, and dilation does not occur below the pelvic brim (Cruikshank, 1979). The bladder is displaced anteriorly and superiorly by the the expanding uterus and is considered an abdominal organ. As an abdominal organ, it is more susceptible to injury.

Hypervolemia increases renal plasma flow (RPF). Nonpregnant RPF is about 475 ml/minute, which increases to 750 ml/minute by 16 weeks gestation and is maintained at this level throughout the pregnancy (Cruikshank, 1979). The glomerular filtration rate (GFR) increases by 67% (Cruikshank, 1979). As a result of the increased RPF and GFR, serum creatinine and blood urea nitrogen levels fall below nonpregnant levels. Elevation of these values may indicate preeclampsia.

During the first two trimesters, the pregnant woman has a greatly enhanced diuretic response to a water load (Cruikshank, 1979). Large amounts of fluid necessary for resuscitation during this time usually pose no significant problem for the kidneys. During the third trimester, however, the ability of the kidney to excrete a similar water load dimishes; this is most pronounced in the patient with preeclampsia. Aggressive fluid resuscitation necessary for circulatory support is not contraindicated, but demands close monitoring.

The urinalysis during pregnancy may reveal glycosuria, which is not particularly alarming, because most pregnant patients have an increased amount of glucose in the urine (Cruikshank, 1979). Likewise, a small number of leukocytes may be noted, but their presence is not a reliable sign of renal disease or injury. The presence of erythrocytes, however, is never normal and may indicate renal disease or a urinary tract injury.

Metabolic: Hormonal Changes

Changes occurring in the endocrine system during pregnancy are complex. The most significant change is with the pituitary gland. During pregnancy, the pituitary gland doubles in size and requires a much greater blood flow than usual. Hypotension can lead to ischemic necrosis of the anterior pituitary, followed by hemorrhage into the gland when the circulation is restored (Cruikshank, 1979). Sheehan's syndrome, a long-term complication of pituitary necrosis, can result and is the most common nonneoplastic cause of hypopituitarism. Sensitive hormones, such as the gonadotropins, growth hormone, thyrotropin, ACTH, and prolactin, are then lost.

Sexuality: Reproductive Changes

Certainly the most obvious changes during pregnancy occur in the reproductive system. Uterine size increases from 7 to 36 cm in length, uterine weight from 70 to approximately 1000 g (Cruikshank, 1979), and uterine blood flow, normally less than 2% of the cardiac output, to 25% during pregnancy (Brinkman & Woods, 1979). At term, the CBV flows through the uterus every 8 to 11 minutes. Uterine blood flow is increased by several mechanisms: an increase in cardiac output, hypervolemia, and, most important, low uteroplacental vascular resistance (Brinkman & Woods, 1979). As noted, uterine blood flow is extremely sensitive to catecholamine release and hypoxia, with marked vasoconstriction resulting.

Estimating gestational age can be difficult in the unresponsive woman (Figure 16-4). An easy method involves measuring in centimeters (cm), from the top of the symphysis pubis to the top of the uterus (fundus). The duration of pregnancy is approximated by the height of the uterus. For example, by 20 weeks, fundal height is approxi-

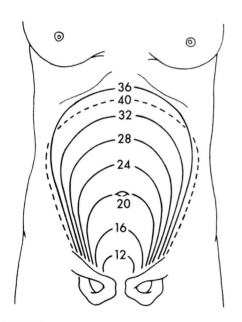

Figure 16-4 Size of uterus at various weeks' gestation. (*Note*. From Anatomic and Physiologic Alterations in Pregnancy that Modify the Response to Trauma [p. 29] by D.P. Cruikshank. In H.J. Buchsbaum [Ed.], 1979, *Trauma in Pregnancy*, Philadelphia: W.B. Saunders.)

mately 20 cm, roughly at the level of the umbilicus. At 28 weeks, the beginning of the third trimester and fetal viability, fundal height is between the umbilicus and costal margin (approximately 28 cm). And at term, fundal height is at the level of the costal margin.

During the first trimester, the uterus is seldom subjected to direct trauma, and the fetus is well protected within the bony confines of the pelvis. Although the issue is controversial, many believe that injuries occurring during this time are not usually associated with a higher rate of miscarriage (Baker, 1982). A causal relationship in any posttraumatic abortion is extremely difficult to determine because 10% to 20% of *all* pregnancies terminate in a spontaneous abortion.

Beyond the first trimester, the protuberant uterus is much more vunerable and is the most common organ injured with severe abdominal trauma. To some extent, the uterus and its contents are cushioned in the front by the bowel, bladder, and anterior abdominal wall and in the back by the spine and strong back muscles (Crosby, 1979). The amniotic fluid further cushions the fetus and offers some degree of protection.

As noted, the pregnant woman is at an increased risk for an abruptio placenta or uterine rupture. Although the exact mechanism of an abruptio placenta, or placental separation, is unclear, it is thought that the elastic nature of the myometrium (smooth muscle of the uterus) allows for significant distortion of the uterus (Kettel, Branch, & Scott, 1988). The placenta, however, is a relatively fixed and inelastic structure. Thus a shearing force is created, which predisposes the placenta to separation, bleeding, fetal distress, and, if severe, fetal death. Placental abruption has been estimated to occur in 6.6% to 66% of traumatized patients (Kettel et al., 1988). Abruption must be considered in every case of maternal abdominal trauma. Most occur immediately, and almost all within 48 hours (Gatrell, 1987).

Typically, the patient with an abruption presents with abdominal pain and uterine tetany, which may or may not be accompanied by vaginal bleeding. With 20% of the cases, the pain may be unimpressive and the bleeding sequestered behind the placenta, making the diagnosis difficult (Gatrell, 1987). Minor placental separations, less than 10%, will produce a decidual hematoma and a placental infarct may be noted at term delivery. Involvement of 10% to 25% of the placenta often initiates labor, whereas more extensive separations, greater than 25% to 30%, cause fetal distress, threatening fetal survival, and require immediate delivery (Vander Veer, 1984; Gatrell, 1987). Fetal mortality is almost a certainty if more than half of the placental surface is involved. Severe abruptio placenta is characterized by uterine hypertonus, with baseline intrauterine pressures of 20 mm Hg or more (Resnik, 1985). Usually an abruption large enough to terminate a pregnancy will do so within 48 hours of the traumatic event (Neufeld et al., 1987). Abruptio placenta is the most common cause of DIC in obstetrics, but does not usually occur when the fetus is still alive (Resnik, 1985).

As noted, fetal-maternal hemorrhage can result from blunt or penetrating abdominal trauma. A large fetal hemorrhage poses a great threat to the fetus but may not be apparent until shortly before the fetus's death. Some authors suggest pregnant victims sustaining significant blunt

trauma have a Kleihauer-Betke (KB) test done, which detects fetal hemoglobin (Hg-F) (Gatrell, 1985). Fetal-maternal hemorrhage detection is based on the resistance of fetal cells to alkali (Neufeld et al., 1987). The KB test mixes a maternal blood sample with alkali, and the ratio of fetal cells and lysed maternal material is recorded, enabling prediction of the volume of fetal blood leaked into the maternal circulation. The KB test is indicated for all Rh-negative mothers and those with the potential for an abruptio placenta. A recent study, however, revealed that the KB test was correct in only 27% of patients; the authors felt the test was of no value in predicting adverse obstetric outcome (Towery, English, Wisner, 1991).

Case review

A 28-year-old woman, approximately 24 weeks pregnant, was involved in a head-on collision (Figure 16-5). The patient, an unrestrained driver, sustained head and abdominal injuries. En route to a level I facility, she was alert and oriented with stable vital signs; fetal assessment re-

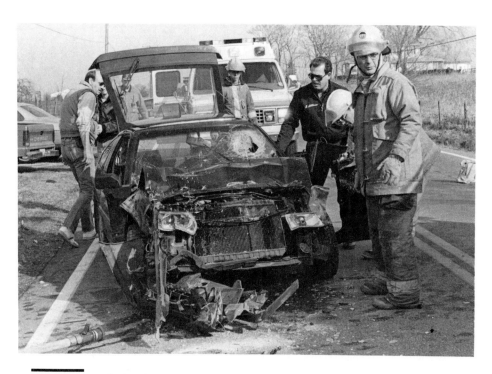

Figure 16-5 Vehicle of woman, 24 weeks pregnant, who sustained late abruptio placenta and subsequent fetal demise. (Courtesy Gary Johnson.)

vealed regular FHTs (140 bpm). In the ED, the patient has signs of a cardiac contusion and is admitted for cardiac monitoring. Frequent fetal evaluation reveals a normal FHR up until 4 hours after injury, when it suddenly disappears. Ultrasound reveals fetal demise and a placental abruption with fetal-maternal hemorrhage.

Uterine rupture is uncommon, with the incidence estimated at approximately 1% (Rothenberger, Quattlebaum, Perry, Zabel, & Fischer, 1978). The rupture most commonly occurs at the fundus after the twentieth week of pregnancy (Gatrell, 1987). Previous uterine surgery may be a predisposing factor, but not always. Hemorrhage is minimized if the placenta detaches and the uterus contracts. Fetal survival is exceedingly rare, but known to occur. Uterine repair should be attempted because subsequent childbearing may be desired.

Case review

A 17-year-old, approximately 18 weeks pregnant, was the unrestrained front seat passenger ejected 35 feet from the car. She presented to the local ED with head, chest, abdominal, and lower extremity injuries. In the ED, she is tachycardic (110 bpm) and pale; BP is 100/60; and initial Hgb is 9 g. Fundal height is estimated at the umbilicus, but FHTs are absent; there is no significant abdominal tenderness. The patient is transferred to a level I trauma center, where she is taken immediately to surgery after a DPL is positive. Laparotomy reveals an 18-week-old fetus, with placenta attached, in the peritoneal cavity (Figure 16-6). Other injuries include a lacerated spleen, which requires a splenectomy, mesenteric artery lacerations, a lumbar fracture, and extremity fractures. The uterus is repaired with primary suture, and the patient is discharged home 2 weeks later.

Recent evidence suggests that even with what appears to be a minor collision, prolonged continuous fetal monitoring (for a minimum of 24 hours) is indicated (Agran, Dunkle, Winn, & Kent, 1987). Towery et al. (1991) found that external fetal monitoring and ultrasound evaluation detected most obstetric complications within the

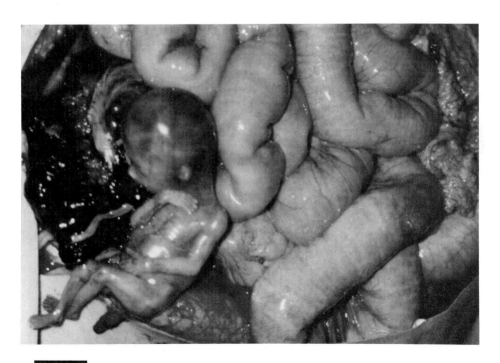

Figure 16-6   Uterine rupture with subsequent fetal demise of 18-week fetus. (Courtesy Steve Santanello, D.O.)

first 6 hours of a trauma admission. On occasion, though, a prolonged delay can occur in some cases. A multidisciplinary approach is essential.

GENERAL ASSESSMENT AND INTERVENTIONS

The physiologic response of the mother is self-preservation at the expense of the fetus. Initially, resuscitative efforts are directed primarily to the mother, because maternal resuscitation is the only means of fetal resuscitation. A systematic approach is necessary in the care of **all** trauma patients, regardless of the pregnancy status. Initial resuscitation priorities for the gravid patient are not different; however, the management must be modified to preserve and accommodate normal anatomic and physiologic changes.

Primary Survey

The primary survey, as described in Chapter 7, is directed at identifying and correcting life-threatening injuries. The primary survey addresses the ABCs (airway, breathing, circulation) and deficit, an abbreviated neurologic examination.

Airway and cervical spine control

Without a doubt, the number one priority for every trauma patient is establishing and maintaining a patent airway. This is done simultaneously while providing cervical spine control. The cervical spine is the most mobile and weakest portion of the spine. Disruption is relatively easy, but repair difficult (Albright et al., 1979). As mentioned numerous times throughout this text, all trauma patients must be considered to have a cervical spine fracture until proven otherwise by a complete set of x-ray films (anteroposterior, lateral, odontoid views). Prehospital and ED management includes immobilization of the entire spine on a backboard, with the addition of a cervical immobilizing device and hard collar. Of particular importance in the pregnant patient over 20 weeks gestation is tilting the backboard to the left side 15 to 20 degrees to offset the potential problem of supine hypotension. Tilting is done **after** the woman has been rapidly secured to the backboard with a minimum of three straps.

Airway management, discussed in Chapter 8, can be done by several methods, including the chin lift or jaw thrust, bag-valve-mask device, intubation, or cricothryoidotomy. Initial maneuvers to open the airway do not differ in the pregnant patient. Intubation should be given early consideration in the woman with a decreased level of consciousness (not responding to voice), significant facial, neck or chest injuries, or signs of advanced hypovolemic shock. Nasal intubation is the method of choice in the gravid woman with spontaneous respiratory effort but without evidence of maxillofacial trauma. If an airway cannot be obtained by any other means, a surgical cricothyrotomy should be done with placement of a 7.0 cuffed endotracheal tube in the trachea. Early intubation and hyperventilation will maximize maternal oxygen delivery.

While assuring a patent airway, the caregiver must remember that pregnant women are at a greater risk for vomiting and subsequent aspiration. A nasogastric tube should be placed during this phase to reduce this risk, and the patient should be observed for gastric bleeding.

Breathing

After a patent airway has been secured, attention is directed toward maximizing oxygenation. Major life-threatening thoracic injuries (i.e., tension pneumothorax, sucking chest wound, massive hemothorax, flail segment), are rapidly evaluated and corrected. Signs of a tension pneumothorax are similar to those that occur in the nonpregnant patient and are described in detail in Chapter 8. With the gravid patient, diaphragmatic elevation requires that tube thoracostomy, if required, be performed one or two interspaces above the normal site (Neufeld et al., 1987). Some advocate more aggressive use of chest tubes in the pregnant patient with thoracic trauma to minimize the adverse effects of hypoxia on the fetus (Gatrell, 1987).

Supplemental, high-flow oxygen via a nonrebreather mask is mandatory for every injured pregnant woman, regardless of how minor the injury may appear. As noted, pregnancy is associated with a marked increase in oxygen consumption and reduced maternal oxygen reserves (Neufeld et al., 1987). Hypoxic tissue damage occurs rapidly when the pulmonary system is compromised by injury (Neufeld et al., 1987). It must be remembered that the fetus is very sensitive to maternal hypoxia. There is never any reason to withhold oxygen from a pregnant trauma patient.

It is interesting to note that supplemental oxygen alone will not reverse fetal hypoxia in the presence of maternal hypovolemic shock (Brinkman & Woods, 1979). Maternal shock results in uteroplacental constriction, thereby decreasing fetal perfusion and oxygenation. Supplemental oxygen is beneficial to the fetus only when uteroplacental perfusion is restored, which totally depends on maternal volume replacement. Supplemental oxygen given to normovolemic mothers does improve fetal oxygenation. (Brinkman & Woods, 1979).

Baseline ABGs should be drawn on arrival to the ED and reevaluated at frequent intervals. It must be remembered that normal "hyperventilation" during pregnancy results in a decrease in the $Paco_2$ level to approximately 30 torr; thus arterial $Paco_2$ levels above this may be a subtle sign of respiratory compromise.

Circulation

After meticulous attention is given to airway and ventilation, the injured woman's hemodynamic status is evaluated. Active external blood loss is halted, venous access obtained, and aggressive fluid resuscitation implemented.

A common question involves use of the military anti-shock trousers (MAST) or pneumatic anti-shock garment (PASG) during pregnancy. Unfortunately, no prospective studies have been done concerning use of the MAST/PASG during pregnancy, and the issue remains a controversial one. The general belief is that the leg compartments but not the abdominal compartment can be safely inflated. Inflation of the abdominal compartment can induce supine hypotension by compressing the inferior vena cava and further impede uterine blood flow. The patient's abdominal girth during the the last trimester would probably preclude use of the abdominal compartment.

Venous access includes placement of two, if not three, large-bore (i.e., 16-gauge or greater) peripheral intravenous lines for fluid and blood replacement. Early venous access and aggressive fluid resuscitation are of extreme importance. As discussed, maternal shock and the concomitant catecholamine release reduce uterine blood flow long before clinical signs are apparent in the mother. Fetal hypoxia occurs early. Fluid resuscitation with a crystalloid solution should be started in volumes estimated at 3 times blood loss

(Vander Veer, 1984; Committee on Trauma, American College of Surgeons, 1988). Both lactated Ringer's solution and dextran, a synthetic plasma volume expander, have been successful at restoring circulating maternal volume (Buchsbaum, 1979c). Lactated Ringer's solution is superior to dextran in that it can return the fetal heart rate to normal in the clinical setting of hypovolemic shock. Dextran has not been shown to affect the fetal heart rate and fetal circulation because it has a fairly high molecular weight and does not leave the intravascular compartment and replace interstitial fluid losses as does lactated Ringer's solution. Interstitial fluid translocation is necessary for metabolic exchange at the cellular level (Buchsbaum, 1979c). Albumin, also a volume expander, can be given, but it is expensive and may result in a deterioration of the pulmonary function by worsening pleural effusions.

The most satisfactory response is obtained when both the volume and red blood cells are replaced together, as in whole blood transfusion (Buchsbaum, 1979c). In the acute setting, type O-negative blood can be used with type-specific blood administered when it becomes available. Ideally, large amounts of fluid and blood rapidly administered should be warmed to body temperature before infusing. Rafferty, Keefer, and Barash (1983) recommend maintaining a hematocrit of at least 30% as a goal in the acutely hemorrhaging pregnant women.

Finally, circulatory assessment includes ascertaining cardiac function. Generally, all pregnant women with multiple injuries should have a 12-lead ECG during the stabilization phase and should be closely observed for a cardiac contusion. Ventricular ectopy and runs of ventricular tachycardia can occur with chest trauma (Selden & Burke, 1988).

Disability

As described in Chapter 10, a rapid neurologic evaluation is undertaken for assessment of increased intracranial pressure (ICP). The gravid woman presenting with seizure activity must be assumed to be eclamptic. Treatment in this case consists of securing the airway, halting seizure activity, controlling blood pressure, and delivering the baby as soon as possible (Jagoda & Riggio, 1991). Seizure activity can be controlled with several drugs, including an intravenous barbiturate such as thiopental (75 to 100 mg) or diazepam (5 to 10 mg) (Brooks, 1983). This will decrease cerebral lactate production by decreasing cerebral metabolism (Brooks, 1983); both drugs add to postictal depression.

The most common drug given to preeclamptic or eclamptic patients in the United States is a 20% solution of magnesium sulfate ($MgSO_4$). Clinical evidence suggests that magnesium sulfate can control and even prevent eclamptic convulsions by decreasing acetylcholine release from the prejunctional motor neuron, thereby depressing muscle membrane excitability (Brooks, 1983). The loading dose is 4 g IV, followed by 2 to 3 g IV per hour. An alternative approach is to follow the 4 g loading dose with 5 g IM and repeat this every 4 hours (Neufeld et al., 1987). The therapeutic range is 4 to 6 mEq/L (4 to 7 mg/ml). Magnesium sulfate can cause transient hypotension possibly secondary to relaxation of skeletal muscles. Signs of toxicity include loss of deep tendon reflexes (DTRs), cardiac conduction defects (i.e., P-Q interval prolonged, widened QRS complex), bradycardia, respiratory depression, and cardiac arrest (Brooks, 1983). Loss of DTRs precede respiratory depression, and close monitoring of the patellar reflex should help prevent an overdose (Brooks, 1983). The patellar reflex is a valuable bioassay that is immediate, reliable, and free (Stubbs & Heins, 1985). When magnesium sulfate is given to the gravid woman who initially had DTRs but subsequently loses patellar reflex, it usually indicates levels of magnesium of 8 to 10 mEq/L (8 to 10 mg/ml) above the therapeutic range. Maternal overdose can be managed with calcium gluconate, 1 g IV push over 3 minutes. Calcium increases the release of acetylcholine from the prejunctional motor neuron and may be beneficial in reversing the effects of magnesium sulfate (Brooks, 1983). Magnesium sulfate crosses the placenta; therefore, after delivery, the neonate may also display decreased muscle tone, respiratory depression, or apnea, as toxic effects of maternal therapy. IV calcium gluconate is effective also for the neonate.

The gravid woman presenting with eclampsia and seizure activity should be considered for an immediate cesarean section because eclampsia is associated with high fetal mortality and morbidity.

Secondary Survey

The secondary survey is a thorough head-to-toe examination designed to identify and treat non–life-threatening injuries (i.e., fractures, abrasions). Essentially, this examination does not differ from the examination of the nonpregnant patient as discussed in Chapter 7. In the pregnant woman, though, special consideration must be given to abdominal, uterine, and fetal evaluation.

Abdominal assessment

Delays in diagnosis of intraperitoneal hemorrhage can have a catastrophic outcome; thus definitive diagnostic evaluation must be undertaken quickly. Use of abdominal paracentesis, a peritoneal needle tap, is a controversial issue during pregnancy. Buchsbaum (1979c) believed that this procedure is more hazardous in the pregnant patient because uterine enlargement and compression of the small bowel pose an increased risk of injury to intraabdominal organs. Also, a fairly high rate of a false-negative tests occurs when blood loss is concealed; only the positive tap is valid (Baker, 1982). Diagnositic peritoneal lavage (DPL) may be a safer route. Rothenberger et al. (1978) report a 100% success rate, devoid of complications, when DPL was done in a series of 12 pregnant women. Currently ultrasound is the preferred imaging technique used to ascertain intraabdominal injury (Haycock, 1984).

Uterine assessment

Uterine assessment includes measuring fundal height, tenderness, and irritability. Measuring fundal height is a quick way to estimate gestational age and is usually accurate within 2 to 4 weeks. Serial measurement may indicate a concealed uterine hemorrhage (Gatrell, 1987). Also, the shape and contour of the uterus should be frequently evaluated, because a change may indicate a uterine rupture (Gatrell, 1987). The uterus is further assessed for tenderness and irritability. Uterine tetany, irritability, contractions, and abdominal pain can be warning signs of both maternal and fetal danger. Complications (i.e., abruptio placenta, uterine rupture) can result in massive hemorrhage and place the mother and the fetus in jeopardy.

Evaluation of the perineum should include a formal pelvic examination if vaginal bleeding is

not present. Vaginal bleeding during the third trimester warrants immediate consultation by an obstetrician. The presence of amniotic fluid in the
vagina, as evidenced by a pH of 7 to 7.5, should
be noted, because this suggests ruptured chorio-
amniotic membranes (Committee on Trauma,
American College of Surgeons, 1988). Cervical
effacement and dilation, fetal presentation, and
the relationship of the fetal presenting part to the
ischial spines should be documented also.

At this time, information related to the patient's medical and obstetric history should be obtained. This includes pregnancy status (i.e., grav-
ida, para), date of the last menstrual period
(LMP), expected date of confinement (EDC), or
due date, current medications, allergies, events
before the injury, and last meal.

Fetal assessment

Fetal assessment includes checking for fetal
movement and the FHR. In general, any fetal
movement felt is a positive sign. The FHR is usually obtainable by Doppler scan at 10 to 14 weeks
of age, and by stethoscope at 20 weeks of age, although this is difficult in a noisy environment
(Franaszek, 1985) (Figure 16-7). Early signs of fetal distress and hypoxia include changes in the
FHR (i.e., bradycardia, defined as a pulse of less
than 110 bpm, and late fetal decelerations) (Neufeld et al., 1987). The FHR should be continually monitored, and the team caring for the injured woman must be versed in the interpretation
of various fetal heart rate patterns (Gatrell, 1987).
Collaboration with the obstetric nursing staff is
ideal. Fetal heart rate evaluation and uterine ultrasonography are integral components of the
evaluation (Drost et al., 1990).

Definitive Therapy

Definitive care, simply defined, is getting the
right patient to the right facility at the right time.
With the pregnant trauma patient, this allows for
definitive obstetric and neonatal consultation. A
specialized team should be immediately available
and able to intervene on behalf of both the
mother and the fetus.

Definitive care may be in part determined by
the mechanism of injury. For example, surgical
exploration is preferred in the management of all
gunshot wounds to the abdomen, including those

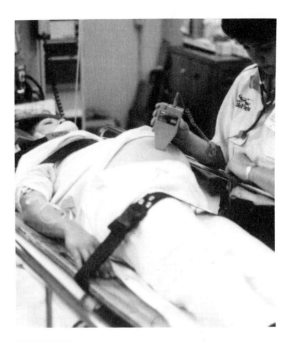

Figure 16-7 Fetal heart tones obtained by determining
flow using Doppler scanning.

that occur during pregnancy. When the issue of
definitive care is considered, the ideal scenario is
that both the mother and fetus do well. Severe
maternal injury, however, may result in maternal
survival and fetal death. Severe maternal hemorrhage often necessitates surgery and anesthesia,
both of which require special considerations. Another difficult scenario is the pregnant woman in
full cardiopulmonary arrest. Postmortem cesear-
ean section may be necessary to salvage the fetus.
Each of these situations will be discussed briefly.

Anesthesia considerations

Physiologic alterations during pregnancy have
important anesthetic implications for the critically
injured obstetric patient. On the positive side, the
hypervolemic and vasodilated state accompanying
normal pregnancy provides the mother with a
cushion against precipitous blood pressure falls
after regional anesthesia and sympathetic nervous system blockade (Brooks, 1983). Functional
changes in ventilatory parameters, however, can
result in dramatic falls in venous and arterial oxygenation during periods of apnea; supine hypo-

tension further decreases cardiac output and oxygenation (Brooks, 1983). Oxygenation before intubation, as with all patients, is essential. The concentration of inhalation agents required to produce anesthesia in a pregnant woman may be decreased, which results in a more rapid induction (Brooks, 1983).

Gastric slowing, as noted, poses a special problem for anesthesiologists and obstetricians, because pulmonary aspiration is a leading cause of anesthesia-related deaths. Mask-delivered analgesic (i.e., nitrous oxide) may precipitate an unwanted loss of conciousness and predispose the woman to vomiting and aspiration in an unprotected airway. Once again, placement of a nasogastric tube is also essential.

Preparation for anesthesia often includes administration of an oral antacid, placement of two large-bore intravenous lines, and access to four units of whole blood and blood warmers. In the setting of hemorrhagic shock, volume replacement may be difficult, if not impossible, until the cause is disclosed. If the patient becomes hypotensive with a falling CVP, ketamine, 1 mg/kg, may help support maternal circulation because of its sympathomimetic properties, with only a minimal increase in uterine tone (Brooks, 1983; Gatrell, 1987). With severe hypotension (systolic BP < 70 mm Hg), succinylcholine alone, 1.0 to 1.5 mg/kg, may be a better agent. Potent alpha-adrenergic agents may be used to treat life-threatening maternal hypotension until intravascular volume can be restored. However, these agents markedly diminish uterine blood flow. Adverse effects, though, must be disregarded when maternal safety is jeopardized. Most likely, maternal hypotension will correlate with neonatal asphxia, and the neonate will require aggressive resuscitative measures including blood replacement.

General principles of anesthesia for the critically ill or injured pregnant woman include obtaining a careful history, current medications, drug allergies, and past anesthesia experiences. Family members, when possible, should be consulted about any familial problems related to anesthesia. A history of neurologic disease or deficit should be elicited if regional anesthesia is being contemplated.

Cardiopulmonary resuscitation

The pregnant woman in cardiopulmonary arrest poses an extremely difficult challenge because

anatomic and physiologic changes require a different approach to resuscitation. Compression of the abdominal aorta by the heavy gravid uterus in late pregnancy markedly reduces venous return and uteroplacental blood flow. Manually displacing the uterus to the left side while CPR is in progress is of utmost importance. Oxygen and vasopressors alone will not improve fetal perfusion in hypovolemic shock, mandating that aggressive fluid resuscitation is implemented. Vasopressors further impair fetal oxygenation by increasing uteroplacental resistance. Close monitoring of arterial blood gases is also important, because maternal acidosis constricts uteroplacental vasculature. Lee et al. (1986) recommend more frequent use of sodium bicarbonate during resuscitation; however, a note of caution: a combined metabolic and respiratory alkalosis is also deleterious. Frequent ABG determinations assist with guiding bicarbonate replacement, as well as assessing oxygenation.

In the nonpregnant patient, open heart massage, when rapidly performed, has been found superior to closed chest massage because it can generate improved coronary, carotid, and aortic blood flow and increase cardiac output and arterial pressure (Sanders, Kern, & Ewy, 1983). Lee et al. (1986) suggest that open heart massage be implemented in the gravid woman if external chest compression is ineffective after 10 to 15 minutes, despite ventilation, positioning, fluid challenges, and acid-base management. However, Bocka et al. (1988) believe the best chance of maternal and fetal salvage is when open-chest cardiac massage is implemented sooner, that is, within 5 minutes. Further actions, especially clamping the descending aorta, may restore circulation to the mother but impair blood flow to the placenta (Brocka et al., 1988).

Perimortem (postmortem) cesarean section

Weber (1971) describes the postmortem cesarean section as a procedure shrouded in mystique and antiquity and overshadowed by fear, religion, and law. Certainly it is one of the rarest procedures ever performed. Postmortem cesarean sections date back to Greek mythology when Apollo delivered Aesculapius from the dead Coronis (Weber, 1971). The earliest recorded reference to a successful postmortem cesarean section was in 237 BC (Weber, 1971). On record, about 200 infants have been rescued from certain death by a cesarean section performed on a dead or dying mother (Gatrell, 1987). Strong and Lowe (1989) state that this procedure is underemphasized on the skills list of the emergency physician. They theorize that postmortem cesarean sections may result in at least a 15% infant success rate. Furthermore, an emergency cesarean section may alter maternal hemodynamics, restoring a pulse in clinically dead women.

In 1971 Weber reviewed approximately 150 cases and noted factors related to a successful outcome. The most important factor was fetal maturity. At 28 weeks gestation, the beginning of the third trimester, fetal weight is approximately 1000 g and fetal viability 50%. Circumstances surrounding the mother's death also affect fetal outcome. If the mother's death approaches slowly, as with infections, systemic diseases, and malignancies, the fetus is subjected to long-term hypoxia and outcome is poor. When the mother's death is abrupt, however, fetal outcome is markedly improved, because the fetus can tolerate approximately 10 minutes of anoxia without severe subsequent cerebral or neuromusculature damage (Weber, 1971). After 15 minutes, success is rare. Thus Weber (1971) proposed a grading system for immediate postmortem cesarean section that can be used in the event of a sudden arrest in a woman 28 or more weeks pregnant:

Time from maternal arrest to cesarean section	Outcome
5 minutes	Excellent
5 to 10 minutes	Good
10 to 15 minutes	Fair
15 to 20 minutes	Poor
20 to 25 minutes	Unlikely

As mentioned, an immediate cesarean section may be lifesaving for both the fetus and mother. The procedure for a cesarean section is relatively easy and clear-cut once the difficult decision has been made. Higgins (1987) suggests the following actions be done:

1. Continue chest compressions and ventilation with the uterus manually displaced to the left side.
2. Obtain any sharp instrument, preferably a scalpel.
3. Use sterile technique within reason.
4. Use a vertical midline incision through the abdominal cavity to the uterus; incise the uterus and remove the fetus.

5. Have a separate team, neonatal if possible, resuscitate infant.
6. Remove the placenta.
7. Continue CPR, and re-evaluate.

Neonatal resuscitation

During the perinatal period, asphyxia, resulting in hypoxemic-ischemic encephalopathy, is a major cause of death and disability. A rapid, aggressive approach, focusing on oxygenation, improving perfusion, and maintaining the core temperature, is essential for an optimal outcome (Figure 16-8).

Initial assessessment of the neonate often uses the Apgar scoring method (Table 16-3), which evaluates several parameters including heart rate, respiratory effort, muscle tone, reflex irritability, and color. A score is calculated usually at the end of the first minute and then again at 5 minutes. If the infant is not responding well, the Apgar score is repeated at 5 minute intervals, up to 20 minutes, until a score of 8 or better is noted on two successive evaluations (Benitz & Sunshine, 1985). The Apgar score can help assess the degree of asphyxia and response to treatment and, to a lesser extent, predict survival or possible neurologic sequelae (Benitz & Sunshine, 1985). Immediate intervention is not delayed until the score is ascertained. Every ED should be equipped with an easily accessible neonatal resuscitation tray (see the box on p. 521).

After delivery, the neonate is dried with prewarmed towels while the mouth and nose are gently suctioned with a bulb syringe or DeLee suction catheter (American Heart Association, American Academy of Pediatrics, 1988). The infant is placed supine, with the head dependent to facilitate drainage of secretions, on a warming table or crib with a radiant warmer. Initial assessment begins with the infant's response to these measures.

A lusty cry, pulse greater than 120 bpm, and good muscle tone usually correlates with an Apgar score of 8 or greater. Little intervention is needed other than suctioning and maintaining the infant's core temperature. All infants have difficulty tolerating a cold environment. If a warmer is not available, use of warm towels may help.

Poor respiratory effort and air exchange and pale or cyanotic skin correlates with an Apgar score of 4 to 7. Interventions include supplemental oxygen by mask or brief bag-valve-mask venti-

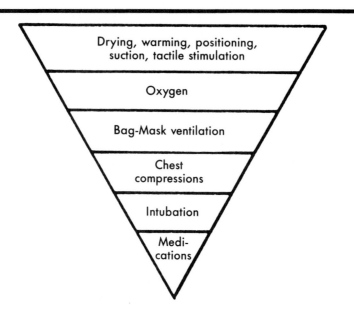

Figure 16-8 Inverted pyramid reflecting approximate relative frequencies of neonatal resuscitative efforts. (*Note.* From *Textbook of Advanced Pediatric Life Support* by American Heart Association, 1988, Dallas: Author.)

Table 16-3 Apgar scoring method

Sign	0	1	2
A ppearance (color)	Blue, pale	Cyanotic hands and feet, pink body	Completely pink
P ulse	Absent	<100 beats per minute	>100 beats per minute
G rimace (reflex irritability or response to suction catheter)	No response	Grimace or minimal avoidance	Cry, cough, or sneeze
A ctivity (muscle tone)	Flaccid, limp	Some flexion	Well flexed, active
R espiratory effort	Absent	Gasping, weak cry	Strong, lusty cry

Resuscitation equipment for the emergency room

Items that should be readily accessible

Radiant warmer
Suction with manometer
Resuscitation bag (250-500 ml)
Face masks (newborn and premature size)
Laryngoscope
Laryngoscope blades (straight 0 and 1)
Medications
    Epinephrine (1 : 10,000)
    Sodium bicarbonate (4.2%)*
    Volume expander

Items that should be on newborn resuscitation tray

Bulb syringe
DeLee suction trap
Endotracheal tubes (2.5, 3.0, 3.5)
Suction catheters (one 5F and two 8F taped to the
    appropriate ET tube)
Endotracheal tube stylet
Umbilical catheter (5F)
Syringe (10 and 20 ml)
Three-way stopcock
Feeding tube (5F and 8F)
Towels
OB kit/cord-cutting materials

Note. From *Textbook of Pediatric Advanced Life Support*
(p. 70) by American Heart Association, Dallas: Author
*If the adult 8.4% solution is the only one available, it
should be diluted 1 : 1 with sterile water.

lation, gentle airway suctioning, and close observation for improvement in the respiratory status. The majority of neonates respond extremely well to a high-oxygen environment.

An Apgar score of 3 or less is given to an apneic or gasping infant with flaccid muscle tone and cyanosis. Aggressive measures must be implemented immediately, beginning with bag-valve-mask ventilation with 100% oxygen and intubation within the next 15 to 30 seconds if no improvement. Again, in the vast majority of cases, the heart rate will respond well to ventilation. A pulse of 60 to 80 requires external cardiac massage using either the two-finger method over the midsternum, or encircling the infant's chest with both hands and applying compression with the thumbs. The depth of compression is ½ to ¾ inch, at a rate of 120 bpm. The quality of the compressions is assessed by palpating a femoral or brachial pulse. A pulse that slows after intubation could indicate improper tube placement, a unilateral or bilateral pneumothorax, or a severe congenital anomaly (i.e., diaphragmatic hernia, tracheal or laryngeal stenosis, congenital heart block).

The pregnant trauma patient

Nursing diagnosis	Nursing intervention	Evaluative criteria
Altered tissue perfusion Related to increase in erthyrocyte and plasma volume	**Maintain circulation** Obtain blood for CBC, type and crossmatch.	Hct will maintain at 30%.
	Monitor for early, subtle signs of hypovolemic shock.	FHR will maintain at 120-160 bpm. Maternal pulse will be less than 100 bpm. Respiratory rate will be less than 20 per minute. Skin will be warm and dry with capillary refill ≤2 seconds. LOC will be alert and oriented.
	Insert urinary catheter if no urethral or pelvic injury. Obtain urine for red blood cell detection.	Urinary output will be maintained at 30-50 ml/hr. Blood in urine will not increase.
	Position patient on left side if 20 weeks or more pregnant, by tilting backboard 15-20 degrees, or manually displace uterus to left side.	Blood pressure will remain within normal limits; the potential for supine hypotension will be minimized.
	Provide for means of rapid fluid resuscitation.	Two, or large-bore IVs (16-gauge or greater) will be established. Isotonic solutions will be used. Fluids will be warmed when possible.
	Minimize blood loss by: • direct pressure • MAST/PASG inflation of legs only	Ongoing hemorrhage will be minimized.
High risk for impaired gas exchange Related to increased oxygen consumption, decreased residual tidal volume	**Promote ventilation** Assess for adequate gas exchange by obtaining an arterial blood gas.	$Paco_2$ will be maintained at 30.
	Maximize oxygenation by providing supplemental oxygen.	Oxygen will be administered by a nonrebreather mask if breathing spontaneously or 100% if assisted.

Nursing diagnosis	Nursing intervention	Evaluative criteria
	Assess both maternal and fetal oxygenation.	The following will be maintained: • maternal pulse ≤100 bpm • respiratory rate ≤20 per minute • LOC alert • FHR and movement within normal limits
High risk for aspiration Secondary to decreased gastric motility	**Maintain airway patency** Place nasogastric tube to minimize vomiting and aspiration. Place endotracheal tube if patient has a decreased LOC. Maintain patient NPO status.	Patient will not vomit or aspirate. Intake and output will be closely monitored.
High risk for altered cerebral perfusion Secondary to preeclampsia or pregnancy-induced hypertension	**Promote cerebral blood flow** Assess for signs of PIH: • diastolic pressure > 90 mm Hg; • decreased LOC; • proteinuria; • hyperreflexia.	Blood pressure will remain within normal limits. Patellar reflex will remain normal. Protein will not be excreted in the urine. Level of consciousness will remain normal with no complaints of headache, blurred vision, or dizziness.
	If signs of preeclampsia, anticipate the need for: • supplemental oxygenation; • $MgSO_4$ (4 g loading dose; followed by 2-3 g per hour); • Valium. If $MgSO_4$ administered, observe closely for signs of toxicity: • loss of DTRs; • cardiac conduction defects; • hypotension; • fetal depression.	Patient will not experience seizure activity. If administered, dose of $MgSO_4$ will be maintained within the therapeutic range.

COMPETENCIES The following clinical competencies pertain to **caring for the pregnant trauma patient.**	☑ Demonstrate knowledge of anatomic and physiologic changes during pregnancy.
	☑ Demonstrate knowledge of altered lab values during pregnancy.
	☑ Apply cervical spine immobization device correctly; demonstrate correct method of tilting a backboard when supine hypotensive syndrome is of concern.
	☑ Demonstrate techniques to minimize maternal hemorrhage (i.e., direct pressure, MAST/PASG inflation).
	☑ Correctly perform a fetal assessment using a Doppler stethoscope to obtain the fetal heart rate.
	☑ Correctly perform a uterine assessment to estimate gestational age through fundal height measurement.

SUMMARY Crosby (1983) describes a state of "diagnostic and therapeutic paralysis" when the trauma patient is discovered to be pregnant. With education and cooperation among the critical care team providers, this need not be the case. The key to both maternal and fetal survival is a knowledge of common injury patterns, recognition of normal anatomic and physiologic changes, and an aggressive approach to resuscitation with meticulous attention given to the ABCs. The table on pp. 522-523 presents a summary of nursing diagnoses and evaluative criteria for the pregnant trauma patient.

RESEARCH QUESTIONS

- What is the knowledge base of ED and prehospital personnel regarding anatomic and physiologic changes in the obstetric patient?
- What is the relationship between prehospital and ED fluid resuscitation and maternal and fetal outcomes?
- Devise a triage scoring tool that will identify the obstetric trauma patient at risk in the field setting.

REFERENCES

Agran, P.F., Dunkle, D.E., Winn, D.G., & Kent, D. (1987). Fetal death in motor vehicle accidents. *Annals of Emergency Medicine, 16*, 1355-1358.

Albright, J., Sprague, B., El-Khoury, G., & Brand, R. (1979). Fractures in pregnancy. In H.J. Buchsbaum (Ed.), *Trauma in pregnancy* (pp. 142-166). Philadelphia: W.B. Saunders.

American Heart Association, American Academy of Pediatrics. (1988). *Textbook of pediatric advanced life support.* Dallas, Author.

Baker, D.P. (1982). Trauma in the pregnant patient. *Surgical Clinics of North America, 62*, 275-289.

Benitz, W.E., & Sunshine, P. (1985). Neonatal resuscitation. In N.M. Nelson, *Current therapy in neonatal-perinatal medicine 1985-1986.* (pp. 360-368). Philadelphia: B.C. Decker.

Bocka, J., Courtney, J., Pearlman, M., Tintinalli, J., Lorenz, R., Swor, R., Krome, R., & Glover, J. (1988). Trauma in pregnancy. *Annals of Emergency Medicine, 17*, 829-834.

Brinkman, C.R., & Woods, J.R. (1979). Effects of hypovolemia and hypoxia upon the conceptus. In H.J. Buchsbaum (Ed.), *Trauma in pregnancy* (pp. 52-81). Philadelphia: W.B. Saunders.

Brooks, G.Z. (1983). Anesthesia for the critical-care obstetric patient. In R.L. Berkowitz, *Critical care of the obstetric patient* (pp. 73-131). New York: Churchill Livingstone.

Buchsbaum, H.J. (1975). Diagnosis and management of abdominal gunshot wounds during pregnancy. *Journal of Trauma, 15*, 425-429.

Buchsbaum, H.J. (1979a). In H.J. Buchsbaum (Ed.), *Trauma in pregnancy* (pp. vii-viii). Philadelphia: W.B. Saunders.

Buchsbaum, H.J. (1979b). Penetrating injury of the abdomen. In H.J. Buchsbaum, (Ed.), *Trauma in pregnancy* (pp. 82-100). Philadelphia: W.B. Saunders.

Buchsbaum, H.J. (1979c). Diagnosis and early management. In H.J. Buchsbaum (Ed.), *Trauma in pregnancy* (pp. 40-51). Philadelphia: W.B. Saunders.

Calvin, S., Jones, O.W., Knieriem, K., & Weinstein, L. (1988). Oxygen saturation in the supine hypotensive syndrome. *Obstetrics and Gynecology, 71*, 872-877.

Cavanagh, D., Knuppel, R.A., & O'Connor, T.C. (1982). Preeclampsia and eclampsia. In D. Cavanagh, R.E. Woods, T.C. O'Connor, & R.A. Knuppel, (Eds.), *Obstetric emergencies* (pp. 107-132). Philadelphia: Harper & Row.

Clemmer, T.P., & Telford, I.R. (1966). Abnormal development of the rat heart during prenatal hypoxic stress. *Proceedings of the Society for Experimental Biology and Medicine, 121*, 800.

Committee on Trauma, American College of Surgeons. (1988), *Advanced trauma life support*, Chicago: Author.

Crosby, W.M. (1979). Automobile injuries and blunt abdominal trauma. In H.J. Buchsbaum, (Ed.), *Trauma in pregnancy* (pp. 101-127). Philadelphia: W.B. Saunders.

Crosby, W.M. (1983). Traumatic injuries during pregnancy. *Clinical Obstetrics and Gynecology, 28,* 902-912.

Crosby, W.M., & Costiloe, J.P. (1971). Safety of lap-belted restraint for pregnant victims of automobile collisions. *New England Journal of Medicine, 284,* 632-636.

Crosby, W.M., King, A.I., & Stout, L.C. (1972). Fetal survival following impact: Improvement with shoulder harness restraint. *American Journal of Obstetrics and Gynecology, 112,* 1101-1106.

Cruikshank, D.P. (1979). Anatomic and physiologic alterations of pregnancy that modify the response to trauma. In H.J. Buchsbaum (Ed.), *Trauma in pregnancy* (pp. 21-39). Philadelphia: W.B. Saunders.

Drost, T.F., Rosemurgy, A.S., Sherman, H.F., Scott, L.M., and Williams, J.K. (1990). Major trauma in pregnant women: Maternal fetal outcome. *Journal of Trauma, 30,* 574-578.

Flannery, D.B., & Wiles, M. (1982). Follow-up of a survivor of intrauterine lightning exposure. *American Journal of Obstetrics and Gynecology, 142,* 238-239.

Franaszek, J.B. (1985). Trauma in pregnancy. *Topics in Emergency Medicine, 5,* 51-56.

Gatrell, C.B. (1987). Trauma and pregnancy. *Trauma Quarterly, 4,* 67-85.

Gorski, J. (1985). Exercise during pregnancy: Maternal and fetal response. *Medicine and Science in Sports and Exercise, 17,* 407-416.

Haycock, C.E. (1982). Injury during pregnancy: Saving both the mother and fetus. *Consultant, 22,* 269-274.

Haycock, C.E. (1984). Emergency care of the pregnant traumatized patient. *Emergency Medicine Clinics of North America, 2,* 843-851.

Higgins, S.D. (1987). Emergency delivery: Prehospital care, emergency department delivery, perimortem salvage. *Emergency Medicine Clinics of North America, 5,* 529-539.

Hillard, P.J.A. (1985). Physical abuse in pregnancy. *Obstetrics and Gynecology, 66,* 185-190.

Jackson, F.C. (1979). Accidental injury: The problem and the initiatives. In H.J. Buchsbaum, (Ed.), *Trauma in pregnancy* (pp. 1-21). Philadelphia: W.B. Saunders.

Jagoda, A., & Riggio, S. (1991). Emergency department approach to managing seizures in pregnancy. *Annals of Emergency Medicine, 20,* 80-85.

Katz, M. (1984). Maternal trauma during pregnancy. In R.K. Creasy, & R.R. Resnik, *Maternal fetal medicine: Principles and practice* (pp. 772-780). Philadelphia: W.B. Saunders.

Kettel, L.M., Branch, D.W., & Scott, J.R. (1988). Occult placental abruption after maternal trauma. *Obstetrics and Gynecology, 71,* 449-453.

Lee, R.V., Rodgers, B.D., White, L.M., & Harvey, R.C. (1986). Cardiopulmonary resuscitation of pregnant women. *American Journal of Medicine, 81,* 311-318.

Leiberman, J.R., Mazor, M., Molcho, J., Haiam, E., Maor, E., & Insler, V. (1986). Electrical accidents during pregnancy. *Obstetrics and Gynecology, 67,* 861-863.

Matthews, C.D. (1975). Incorrectly used seat belt associated with uterine rupture following vehicular collision. *American Journal of Obstetrics and Gynecology, 115,* 1115-1116.

Mollison, P.L. (1973). Clinical aspects of Rh immunization. *American Journal of Clinical Pathology, 60,* 287.

National Safety Council. (1988). *Accident facts.* Chicago: Author.

Neufeld, J.D.G., Moore, E.E., Marx, J.A., & Rosen, P. (1987). Trauma in pregnancy. *Emergency Medicine Clinics of North America, 5,* 623-640.

Nicholas, J.A. (1979). Sports injuries. In H.J. Buchsbaum (Ed.), *Trauma in pregnancy* (pp. 189-203). Philadelphia: W.B. Saunders.

Pierce, M.R., Henderson, R.A., & Mitchell, J.M. (1986). Cardiopulmonary arrest secondary to lightning injury in a pregnant woman. *Annals of Emergency Medicine, 15,* 597-599.

Rafferty, D.T., Keefer, J.R., & Barash, P.G. (1983). Fluid management in the massively bleeding obstetric patient. In R.L. Berkowitz, *Critical care of the obstetric patient* (pp. 47-61). New York: Churchill Livingstone.

Rees, W.D. (1965). Pregnant woman struck by lightning. *British Medical Journal, 1,* 103.

Repke, J.T., & Berger, N. (1984). Electroconvulsive therapy in pregnancy. *Obstetrics and Gynecology, 63,* 395.

Resnik, R. (1985). Third trimester bleeding. In N.M. Nelson, *Current therapy in neonatal-perinatal medicine* (pp. 71-73). Philadelphia: B.C. Decker.

Rothenberger, D., Quattlebaum, F.W., Perry, J.F., Zabel, J., & Fischer, R.P. (1978). Blunt maternal trauma: A review of 103 cases. *Journal of Trauma, 18,* 173-178.

Rubovits, F.E. (1964). Traumatic rupture of the pregnant uterus from seat belt injury. *American Journal of Obstetrics and Gynecology, 90,* 828-829.

Sanders, A.B., Kern, K.B., & Ewy, G.A. (1983). Improved survival from cardiac arrest with open chest massage. *Annals of Emergency Medicine, 12,* 138 (abstract).

Seldon, B.S., & Burke, T.J. (1988). Complete maternal and fetal recovery after prolonged cardiac arrest. *Annals of Emergency Medicine, 17,* 346-349.

Strong, T.H., & Lowe, R.A. (1989). Perimortem cesarean section. *American Journal of Emergency Medicine. 7,* 489-494.

Stubbs, T.M., & Heins, H.C. (1985). Elampsia. In N.M. Nelson, *Current therapy in neonatal-perinatal medicine.* Philadelphia: B.C. Decker.

Taylor, J.W. (1979). Thermal injuries. In H.J. Buchsbaum, *Trauma in pregnancy* (pp. 128-141). Philadelphia: W.B. Saunders.

Towery, R., English, P., & Wisner, D.H. (1991). Kleihauer-Betke tests, uterine ultrasound, and external fetal monitoring in pregnant women after blunt trauma. *Journal of Trauma, 31,* 1032 (abstract).

Vander Veer, J.B. (1984). Trauma during pregnancy. *Topics in Emergency Medicine, 5,* 72-77.

Weber, C.E. (1971). Postmortem cesarean section: Review of the literature and case reports. *American Journal of Obstetrics and Gynecology, 110,* 158-165.

Zalstein, E., & Koren, G. (1990). Occupational exposure to chemicals in pregnancy. In G. Koren, *Maternal-Fetal toxicity: A clinician's guide* (p. 194). New York: Marcel Dekker.

Zuspan, S.J. (1990). Essential trauma nursing knowledge included in level I trauma center orientation and continuing education programs. *Journal of Emergency Nursing, 16,* 141-144.

17 Trauma in Childhood

■■■

Renee Semonin-Holleran

OBJECTIVES

❑ Discuss the problems and prevention of pediatric trauma.

❑ Identify the sources of pediatric trauma by age group.

❑ Describe the specific assessment and interventions required to care for the pediatric trauma patient.

❑ Identify differences between the adult and pediatric trauma patient related to specific traumas, such as head, chest, and abdomen.

❑ Discuss when and how to transport the pediatric trauma patient.

INTRODUCTION Trauma is the leading cause of death until the fourth decade of life in the United States. It has been estimated that 20,000 children die and 100,000 are disabled each year because of trauma-related injuries (Zorludemir, Ergoren, Yucesan, & Olcay 1988). In 1986, according to the National Safety Council (1987) figures, 16,000 children under the age of 15 died from accidental injuries. Included in these statistics were 3400 deaths from motor vehicle accidents; 1208 from fires or burns; and 1200 from drowning.

Regardless of what statistics are quoted, it seems certain that trauma is a major cause of death and disability in the pediatric population. However, in spite of the abundance of medical and nursing resources available in this country, little has been done to organize the care of the pediatric trauma patient.

CASE STUDY Sara is a 24-month-old patient brought to the emergency department (ED) after having been crushed between two cars. She is moaning, pale, and cyanotic. Her blood pressure is 60 by palpation; heart rate, 180; and respirations, 10.

What would normal vital signs be for Sara?
Sara is 24 months old. A quick and simple formula to calculate her normal blood pressure is:

$$80 + (2 \times [\text{age of the child in years}]).$$

Therefore her normal blood pressure is 84. The Pediatric Advanced Trauma Course from the American Heart Association (Chameides, 1988) recommends that if a 10 mm Hg fall in systolic blood pressure occurs, careful assessment for shock is required. Her respiratory rate should be between 20 to 30.

What is the most likely type of trauma that Sara may have incurred?
The most common pediatric trauma seen in the ED is head trauma. Gilmore (1987) and Peclet et al. (1990) noted that head trauma accounts for some 250,000 pediatric admissions and 4000 childhood deaths annually in the United States.

PEDIATRIC TRAUMA SYSTEMS

Results of a survey (Listing of Children's Hospitals with Emergency Departments in the United States, 1988) reported that approximately 50 EDs in the United States have pediatric emergency departments. Unfortunately, these are not evenly distributed throughout the country. Therefore a significant number of pediatric trauma resuscitations are done in EDs that are not dedicated specifically to the pediatric patient, much less the pediatric trauma patient.

Research continues to demonstrate that the care of the pediatric trauma patient is different from that for the adult and inappropriate care

527

contributes to higher mortality and morbidity (Mayer, 1985). In a recent study, Mueller, Rivara and Mayer (1988) found that children and young adolescent pedestrians who were struck by motor vehicles were at greater risk of death when injured in rural areas than in urban areas. Some of the reasons suggested by the authors were distance from the hospital and amount of experience with the care of these patients.

Henderson (1988) noted that several research studies have shown evidence that children suffer a higher mortality and morbidity than adult trauma patients. Although critically injured pediatric trauma patients make up a small percentage of the emergency medical services (EMS) population, their outcomes are less than optimal when they are not cared for in an organized and systematic manner consistent with their special needs.

Several solutions have been proposed to decrease the mortality and morbidity that is associated with pediatric trauma. Harris, Latchaw, Murphey, and Schwaitzberg (1989), Henderson (1988), Mayer (1985), and Seidel and Henderson (1991) have all noted the need for an organized, systematic approach to the care of the pediatric trauma patient. Included in these systems would be (1) education of the prehospital care provider; (2) well-developed prehospital emergency medical transport systems, including the use of both ground and air transport; (3) emergency departments approved for pediatric care; and (4) pediatric trauma centers or pediatric critical care centers that have immediate access to computed tomography and pediatric intensive care units, rehabilitation resources, community support, and prevention programs.

Between 1985 and 1990, 20 states received funding from the government through the Emergency Medical Services for Children (EMSC) grants. The goals of the EMSC development continue to be that all ill or injured children will receive state-of-the-art emergency medical care; pediatric services will be integrated into an EMS system that is provided with optimal resources; and the EMSC component of the EMS system will include a spectrum of services ranging from primary prevention of illness and injury to problem identification, acute care, and rehabilitation (Seidel and Henderson, 1991).

The American Academy of Pediatrics has developed a position paper that describes the pediatrician's role in the emergency care of children. Among the important roles of the pediatrician are the provision of education to parents to prevent illness and injury; referral to appropriate care centers; and formation of networks with emergency medical services to provide the highest level of care to the critically injured child (Bushore, 1988). In addition, a pediatric committee has been formed within the Emergency Nurses' Association. One of the goals of this group is to address the issues that arise in the care of the pediatric trauma patient in the ED, as well as offer methods to prevent pediatric trauma.

TRAUMA SUSCEPTIBILITY

The sources and patterns of pediatric trauma vary by age and are related to different causes. Sources of trauma are associated with growth and developmental skills. Specific growth and developmental information for each age group is listed later in this chapter.

The pediatric patient can suffer trauma from both blunt and penetrating origins. Blunt trauma is a more common mechanism of injury seen in the pediatric patient (Peclet, et al., 1990). However, the incidence of penetrating trauma sustained by the pediatric patient has increased. About 4500 children die annually from gunshot wounds (Beaver et al., 1990).

More boys than girls are injured in all age groups. This is particularly true for older children. At present there is no one particular explanation for this (Schwaitzberg & Harris, 1987).

Infants

During the first year of life, the infant (birth to 12 months) develops from a state of complete dependence to one of vigorous exploration of his or her person and environment. Initially the infant is at risk from injury related to the improper use of equipment, such as cribs or child restraints. As children grow and explore their environment, crawling, standing, and the ability to grasp and manipulate objects can place them at risk for injury.

Motor vehicle crashes are the most common cause of trauma deaths in infants. The majority of these deaths occur because the infant is unrestrained or improperly restrained while in a moving vehicle (Schwaitzberg & Harris, 1987).

Infants are also at risk for burn injuries, particularly scald injuries. The emergency nurse must be alert to the possibility of child abuse as the cause.

Orlowski (1989) noted that about 3000 children younger than 5 years are treated annually in hospital emergency departments for submersion accidents. These accidents occur in residential pools. It has been estimated that pediatric submersion accidents would be decreased by 60% to 80% if proper barriers were used.

Toddlers and Preschoolers

Toddlers and preschoolers are children from 1 to 6 years of age. As children mature, they are left alone more often, and in the process of exploring their environment, they are at greater risk of becoming injured. Toys, open spaces, and newfound independence contribute to the possibility of toddlers and preschoolers being injured. They can climb to amazing heights, open drawers and closets, have limited reading ability, and are still clumsy in many skills.

Children younger than 5 years are also very susceptible to injuries from cars, vans, and trucks. Because of their increased mobility and small size, younger children are at considerable risk of sustaining significant injury from motorized vehicles while they play on driveways, parking lots, and sidewalks (Winn, Agran, & Castillo, 1991).

Schwaitzberg and Harris (1987) noted that toddlers and preschoolers are most likely to be injured in a fall. Falls usually occur while in the home and occur particularly from furniture and stairs. Falls that occur outside of the home generally involve playground equipment.

School-Age Children

School-age children (6 to 12 years of age) continue to develop increasing independence. They are now away from the home and spend much of their time in school. School-age children become active independently outside of the home. Because of this, school-age children are at greater risk of being involved in pedestrian accidents. Bicycles and other wheeled vehicles, such as mopeds and all-terrain vehicles, become a source of injury and death.

Because children spend a significant amount of time in school, playgrounds and sports also can be a source of trauma. Safe use of equipment and the proper attire for each sport can help reduce the risk of injury.

Adolescents

Adolescents (13 to 18 years of age) provide a unique challenge to emergency nursing. Adolescents have access to cars, alcohol, and drugs. They are mobile and tend to take unnecessary risks. Peer groups are important. Sports activities are intense.

Paulson (1988), in completing a comprehensive assessment of the sources of adolescent injuries, noted that the road posed the greatest source of trauma for the adolescent. Included are injuries from motor vehicle crashes, bicycles, and motorcycles. To illustrate, in 1985, 12,460 deaths occurred of people 15 to 24 years old, as a result of motor vehicle crashes (Paulson, 1988).

Greensher (1988a) found that persons 15 years and older accounted for almost two thirds of bicycle-related deaths in 1985. Such behaviors as wrong-way riding, not obeying traffic laws, and nighttime riding increased the risk of being injured.

Other wheeled devices, such as skateboards, minibikes, minicycles, trailbikes, mopeds, and all-terrain vehicles (ATVs), provide additional sources of trauma. Greensher (1988a) noted that particularly the ATV has been increasingly posing a risk to adolescents. Injuries related to ATVs that were treated in EDs rose from 63,900 in 1984 to 85,900 in 1985 (Greensher, 1988a). Many consumer, medical, and nursing organizations, including the Emergency Nurses' Association, have begun to take an active role through state and federal legislation to regulate the sale and safe use of wheeled vehicles to decrease the number of lives lost.

Unfortunately, alcohol frequently is involved in adolescent deaths and injuries caused by trauma. Of adolescent drivers involved in fatal multivehicle crashes, 25% have blood alcohol content greater than 0.1%, and 75% of the adolescent drivers involved in fatal nighttime single-vehicle crashes have a significant (greater than 0.1%) blood alcohol content (Paulson, 1988).

Alcohol is a factor not only related to motor vehicle crashes, but also present in other injuries. Orlowski (1988) stated that more than 50% of adolescents who were involved in drowning or near-drowning were using alcohol.

An important concern for the emergency nurse when caring for the injured female adolescent is the possibility of pregnancy. The patient may not volunteer this information, and the trauma team may unsuspectingly be caring for two victims.

As discussed, multiple sources can contribute to pediatric injuries and their resultant mortality and morbidity. Nurses who care for the pediatric trauma victim need an understanding about human growth and development, both physically and psychosocially, to be aware of these sources. Specific differences between the adult and pediatric trauma patient are discussed in the next section.

PREVENTION OF TRAUMA IN CHILDHOOD

One of the major focuses of the care of the pediatric trauma patient should be on prevention of injury. Currently several methods are being applied for the prevention of injury. These include using safety devices, such as child restraint systems and helmets; instituting educational programs, such as the National Safe Kids Campaign; and providing a safe environment, such as the building of fences around swimming pools.

A survey conducted by the Children's Hospital Medical Center in Washington (Staff, 1988) found that most parents needed more information about the major causes of injury and death to their children. Parents expressed more concern about drug abuse and kidnapping than about motor vehicle crashes, burns, or drowning.

The survey also suggested that parents believed they were least prepared to cope with victims of auto crashes and near-drowning, which comprised about three fifths of accidental childhood deaths in 1986. However, more than 70% of the parents surveyed expressed an intense interest in learning how to use safety equipment and prevent injuries and deaths. The majority of parents also believed that the responsibility to prevent these accidents rested with the children's families.

Vehicular Safety

Education and protective devices may offer some hope. Yet if preventive measures are not used appropriately, they can cause further damage. An example of improper use of safety equipment is cited by Bull, Stroup, and Gerhart (1988). They present a case study of a 3-month-old infant inappropriately restrained in a car seat. Consequently, the infant died of a severe liver injury after being involved in a motor vehicle crash.

In addition, the authors conducted a survey of the use and misuse of car seats. They discovered that car seats were not always properly secured in cars and sometimes not secured at all, harness straps were not used, infants were incorrectly positioned in the seats, and protective shields were not placed over the child.

Greensher (1988b) noted that three kinds of car seats are presently in use in this country. These are rear-facing infant safety seats for infants who weigh 20 pounds; convertible seats for both infants and toddlers who weigh 40 pounds (forward-facing for toddlers and rear-facing for infants); and booster seats for children weighing between 30 and 60 pounds. Children who are 4 to 5 years of age or who weigh more than 40 pounds can use lap belts. For these devices to be effective, the child must sit straight up against the seat. In addition, recent safety recommendations made by consumer protection agencies have indicated the need for shoulder harnesses as well as lap belts for passengers (including older children) who ride in the back seat of cars (Greensher, 1988b).

Helmet Use

The use of helmets for bicycle riders has been offered as another solution to decrease the mortality and morbidity related to head trauma. O'Malley, Born, Delong, Shaikh, and Schwab (1987) found that bicyclists and infant or child passengers were at a greater risk of fatal head injury than motorcyclists. In the study the age range of those injured was from birth to 24 years.

Thompson, Frederick, Rivara, and Thompson (1989) found that bicyclists who wore a helmet had a 85% reduction in risk of head injury and an 88% reduction in risk of injury to the brain. The researchers evaluated 235 patients who had suffered a head injury related to a bicycle crash. More than 60% of the bicyclists with head injuries were children under 14 years of age. Only about 2% of children under 15 years of age who suffered a head injury were wearing a helmet.

More research is needed to learn the best

methods to prevent or decrease injuries. The proper use of safety devices, children and parental education, and provision of a safe environment will make a difference. Teaching injury prevention is an extremely important responsibility of all nurses who care for victims of trauma.

ANATOMIC AND PHYSIOLOGIC CONSIDERATIONS
Growth and Development

A basic understanding of human growth and psychosocial development can help in the initial assessment of the pediatric trauma patient. Table 17-1 offers information on specific weight, height, and psychosocial skills for the pediatric patient (Wong and Whaley 1986; Hazinski 1984).

Numerous authors have pointed out that children are not "little adults." However, just as for the adult trauma patient, initial assessment and management of children's airways, ventilation, and circulation are mandatory to decrease mortality and morbidity. Specific differences should be addressed when caring for the pediatric trauma patient. The box on p. 533 lists some of the specific differences between the pediatric and adult trauma patient. The following discussion offers the assessment and intervention skills that may be useful for the trauma nurse when caring for the pediatric trauma patient.

Airway

The young child's airway differs from the adult's in several ways. Small children and infants have a large tongue relative to the size of their oropharynx. The tongue is more likely to block the airway of an unresponsive child. Also, infants younger than 6 months of age are nose breathers, and obstructions in this area can cause airway compromise.

Other anatomic differences between the child and the adult include the proximity of the child's tongue, hyoid bone, and epiglottis, which may make visualization of the glottis more difficult. The child's epiglottis is soft and floppy and may be difficult to pick up with the laryngoscope, making intubation more complex.

The vocal cords of a young child are more pliable than those of the adult and are easier to damage. The larynx lies more anteriorly, leading to more frequent intubation of the esophagus.

The child's airway is narrowest at the cricoid ring. This narrowed area can be damaged, causing edema and possibly stenosis. For this reason it is recommended that uncuffed tubes be used in children younger than 8 years (Eichelberger & Pratsch, 1988). Table 17-2 contains information from the Pediatric Advanced Life Support Course (Chameides, 1988), which suggests the appropriate size of laryngoscope blade, endotracheal tube, and suction catheter that should be used based on the child's age.

Ventilation

The respiratory rate of children is faster than that of the adult. Table 17-3 gives some parameters of normal respirations for the pediatric patient.

Perfusion

The circulatory status of the child is assessed in conjunction with airway and breathing. Differences in heart rates exist between the adult and the child. It is essential to consider this when caring for the pediatric trauma patient. For example, a heart rate of 88 in an infant indicates an emergency, whereas in an older child or adult that rate would be considered normal. Table 17-3 shows normal ranges in heart rate. The box on p. 533 presents a simple formula to quickly calculate the pediatric systolic and diastolic blood pressure. According to the *Textbook of Pediatric Advanced Life Support* (Chameides, 1988), the lower limits of the pediatric blood pressure can be calculated using the formula 70 + (2 × [the child's age in years]). The upper limits of the child's blood pressure can be calculated using the formula 90 + (2 × [the child's age in years]). These three formulas provide the trauma nurse with parameters to monitor the blood pressure of the injured child. In addition, an appropriately fitting pediatric cuff is important in determining an accurate blood pressure.

Mobility

Specific differences exist between the adult and pediatric musculoskeletal and cervical spine. The child's periosteum is thicker, and this can lead to more rapid healing. This can be a problem if the fracture has not been properly reduced. The injury may heal improperly and contribute to loss of function (Barkin & Rosen, 1987; Karlin, 1987; Marcus, 1986; Mayer, 1985).

The child's bones are more pliable and porous

Table 17-1 Comparison of growth and development skills

Age	Weight	Height	Physical development	Psychosocial	Major fear	Pain
Infant (Birth-12 months)	Gaining weight	At 1 year, height should be 50% greater than at birth	Initially has primitive reflexes, such as Babinski; progresses to rolling over, crawling, grasping objects, to walking	Should be interacting with environment	Separation from parents	Feels pain.
Toddler (1-3 years)	Average weight: 26-28 pounds; after 3 years, gains about 3-5 pounds per year	Increases in height about 2-2½ inches per year	Begins to have bowel and bladder control; very active—climbing, running, riding three-wheeled vehicles	Very curious and loves to explore; can solve simple problems; helps undress self; has limited vocabulary and increased attention span	Separation from parent(s); has high security need	Will meet pain with intense emotional distress
Preschool-age child (3-5 years)	Average weight: 50 pounds	Average height: 46 inches	Jumps rope; rides a bicycle; ties shoelaces; draws a person with six parts; can open doors and windows; goes up and down stairs	Has 2100-word vocabulary; begins questioning parents' beliefs; honesty important; identifies with parent of same sex; relies on parent(s) for security	Separation; loss of control; mutilation; the unknown; and the dark	Needs to express pain
School-age child (6-12 years)	Average weight: 60-100 pounds	Increases in height 2-2½ inches per year	Has increased physical skills; involved in organized sports; rides a bicycle and other wheeled vehicles, such as skateboards, mopeds	Begins some logical thinking; peer group important; cares for pets; can understand about illness and its effects	Mutilation and death	May attempt to be stoic about pain
Adolescent (13-20 years)	Adult size	Adult size	Menses begins; nocturnal emission; becomes sexually active; obtains driver's license	May experiment with drugs, alcohol; performs abstract thinking; peer group important	Loss of control; altered body image; separation from peers	May be hyperresponsive to pain

Table 17-2 Sizes for pediatric airway equipment

Age	Laryngoscope	Endotracheal tube size	Suction catheter (French)
Infant (Birth-12 months)	Miller 0-1	2.5-4.5 (uncuffed)	5-8
Toddler (1-3 years)	Miller 2 Flagg 2	4.5 (uncuffed)	8
Preschool-age child (4-5 years)	Miller 2 Flagg 2	5.0 (uncuffed)	10
School-age child (6-12 years)	Miller 2 MacIntosh 2	5.5-7.0 (uncuffed to the age of 8)	10-12
Adolescent (13-20 years)	MacIntosh 3 Miller 3	7.0-8.0 (cuffed)	12

Note. Adapted from *Textbook of Pediatric Advanced Life Support* (p. 26) by L. Chameides (Ed.), 1988, Dallas: American Heart Association.

Specific differences between the adult and pediatric trauma patient

- Growth, development, and psychological skills vary with age.
- Children have smaller airways with more soft tissue and a narrowing of the cricoid cartilage. The openings of the trachea and esophagus are closer together, which can make intubation more difficult.
- Children have faster respiratory rates and become hypoxic more quickly.
- The temperature control mechanism is immature in infants and small children.
- Children are easily dehydrated.
- Children have faster heart rates.
- Young children's extremities are likely to appear mottled. This may be a response to cold. Capillary refill may be a better indicator of circulatory status in the child.

Estimating blood pressure for the pediatric patient

Systolic BP (mm Hg) = (2 × Age in years) + 80

Diastolic BP (mm Hg) = ⅔ systolic

Table 17-3 Normal respiration and heart rates for the pediatric patient

Age	Respiration (breaths/minute)	Heart (beats/minute)
Infant (birth-12 months)	30-60	120-160
Toddler (1-3 years)	25-40	90-140
Preschool-age child (4-6 years)	22-34	80-110
School-age child (6-12 years)	18-30	75-100
Adolescent (13-18 years)	12-20	60-100

than the adult's. As a result, they may not completely break and when they do, a specific fracture pattern is produced. The types of fracture patterns produced include buckle fractures, plastic bends, and greenstick fractures (Karlin, 1987).

The epiphyseal (growth) plate, which acts as a shock absorber, is still developing in the child. The bone is divided into four parts. These parts are the diaphysis (the shaft of the bone), the metaphysis, the epiphysis, and the epiphyseal plate. The epiphysis is at the end of the bone near the joint and is separated from the metaphysis by the epiphyseal plate (Barkin & Rosen, 1987). Damage to the growth plate can be devastating, leading to

Table 17-4 Salter classification of epiphyseal injuries

Type	Description	Mechanism of injury
1	Complete separation of epiphyseal plate without a fracture. Growth problems are rare.	Side-to-side force
2	Most common type of injury. Epiphysis is separated with a fracture of the metaphysis. Growth problems are rare.	Shearing and bending force
3	Intra-articular fracture from joint surface to growth plate. Appropriate reduction necessary for adequate blood supply to decrease damage.	
4	Occurs across growth plate, extending from joint surface to a portion of the metaphysis. Surgical open reduction and internal fixation is necessary. The prognosis is guarded.	
5	Occurs through epiphyseal plate. Because of crushing injury, will generally result in growth problems.	Crushing force

Note. Adapted from *Pediatric Trauma Care* (p. 103) by M. Eichelberger and G. Pratsch, 1988, Rockville, MD: Aspen Publishers.

cessation of growth and a shortening of the extremity.

Injuries to the epiphyseal plate have been classified traditionally by Salter and Harris (1965). The classification consists of the mechanism of injury, the type of treatment needed to treat the injury, and the prognosis for recovery from the specific injury. Table 17-4 contains the Salter classification adapted from Eichelberger and Pratsch (1988).

The cervical spine of the pediatric patient differs from the adult's until around the age of 10 years. Several distinct differences between the adult and pediatric spine must be considered by the trauma nurse. The pediatric patient has incomplete ossification with increased cartilage, presence of epiphyseal lines, and increased mobility of the cervical spine (Marcus, 1986). The increase of cartilage to bone in the young child appears on x-ray film as a wider space between the vertebrae. Multiple epiphyseal lines are present on the first two cervical vertebrae of the young child. These appear as smooth lines in predictable places. They may be mistaken for fractures. However, fractures are generally irregular in shape and in unpredictable places. The mobility of the child's cervical spine produces subluxation, which is demonstrated on x-ray examination, that makes it difficult to determine whether it is normal or abnormal. An example is the subluxation of C2 on C3 of up to 4 mm seen on lateral flexion in 40% of children between the ages of 1 to 7 years (Marcus, 1986).

GENERAL ASSESSMENT AND INTERVENTIONS
Airway

As with the adult trauma patient, initial airway management for the child should always be performed with cervical spine immobilization. A hard cervical spine collar or specific pediatric backboard should be used to protect the child's cervical spine. Cervical collars are now available for the infant and smaller child, which provide immobilization without interfering with the airway (see Chapter 11).

If the child is in respiratory distress or exhibits signs and symptoms of poor oxygenation, such as altered mental status and poor capillary refill, oxygen should be initiated. Awake and semicomatose children offer a challenge in maintaining proper position of oxygen delivery devices, such as nasal cannulas and masks. Many children are fearful of having something in their nose or wrapped around their face. A useful technique the trauma nurse may employ is holding an oxygen mask close to the child's face (parent may do this as well) to allow the oxygen to blow by the child, while keeping the child from becoming fearful or agitated, as may occur by placing the device directly on the child.

The child's trachea is shorter than the adult's. The average length of the newborn's trachea is 4 to 5 cm and grows to about 7 cm in the 18-month-old (Eichelberger & Pratsch, 1988). Thus intubation of the right main stem bronchus or perforation of the trachea could occur.

As stated, initial airway management in the pediatric trauma patient requires close attention to the cervical spine. If the child is breathing, the chin-lift or jaw-thrust maneuver may be employed. The mouth should be checked for any foreign material and the material, if visualized, should be quickly removed. Children may be found with such material as blood, vomitus, toys, or gum obstructing their airway. The appropriate size of suction catheter should be available for clearing the airway. A bulb syringe and Delee catheter are needed for the infant, and catheters ranging in size from 8 to 14 French will be useful for other pediatric patients.

If initial repositioning of the airway is unsuccessful, mechanical adjuncts may be required. These include oral and nasopharyngeal airways, esophageal airways, tracheal intubation, and cricothyrotomy.

Oral and nasopharyngeal airways must be available in smaller sizes for the pediatric patient. Oral airways range in size from 4 to 10 cm in length (Guedel sizes 000 to 4). The appropriate size is determined by placing the oral airway next to the child's face with the flange at the level of the central incisors and the bite block parallel to the hard palate. The tip of the airway should reach the angle of the jaw (Chameides, 1988). This airway can be used only in the patient without a gag reflex. The nasopharyngeal airway is available in sizes from 12 to 36 French. The appropriate length is estimated by measuring from the tip of the nose to the tragus of the ear (Chameides, 1988). These airway adjuncts can serve only as temporary airways and will not protect the child from aspiration.

The esophageal airway is not recommended in the child. Because the child's face and esophageal length varies, determining the appropriate size of tube can be difficult. In addition, the complication of intubating the trachea combined with failure to recognize this could be fatal to the pediatric patient (Chameides, 1988). Breath sound assessment can be more difficult in the child than in the adult because of the size of the child's chest and transmission of sound. The endotracheal tube may be in the stomach, and sound transmission may suggest that it is in the trachea.

Orotracheal intubation is the recommended approach for the infant and young child in the presence of respiratory failure. Nasotracheal intu-

bation in children can cause nosebleeds or obstruction of the tube by adenoidal tissue (Eichelberger & Pratsch, 1988). However, some physicians do prefer its use for long-term intubation. The oral tube may be changed after stabilization (Cardona, Hurn, Mason, Scanlon-Schipp, & Veise-Berry, 1988).

Table 17-2 (p. 533) illustrates the child's age and recommended tube size, but other "formulas" may be used to estimate tube size. These include (1) using the diameter of the child's little finger; (2) measuring the tube to the child's external nares; and (3) using the following formula to calculate the tube size in millimeters:

$$\frac{16 \ + \ age \ in \ years}{4}$$

Tube placement should be confirmed with a chest X-ray examination, and the tube should be secured with tape. Tincture of benzoin will help to keep the tape in place on the child's face and help to keep the tube from moving. Tracheostomy tape should not be tied around the tube, since it could kink the tube or compress it decreasing the size of its lumen. It is important to assess the child's breath sounds for tube location every time the child is moved.

Another useful technique that can be used to assess tube placement is to measure the length of tube from the gum line to the adaptor part of the endotracheal tube. This length is then recorded on a tongue blade and used as a baseline. This tool can be used repeatedly (Morrow, 1988).

Sedation and paralyzing agents

Medication may be required to facilitate safely intubating the child when the child is still awake, combative because of head injury, clenching his or her jaw, or coughing or gagging. In addition, medication will decrease the possibility of causing an increase in intracranial pressure during intubation, particularly for the patient with head trauma.

Suggested drugs that might be used include Pentothal (2 to 4 mg/kg); vecuronium (0.1 mg/kg); fentanyl (Sublimaze) (1.7 to 3.3 mcg/kg for children 2 to 12 yr.—it is not recommended for children under 2 years of age); and succinylcholine (Anectine) (1.5 mg/kg) (Karb, Queener, & Freeman, 1989). When succinylcholine is used for children, they should be premedicated with atro-

---

Intubation protocol for the pediatric trauma patient

1. Assist the child's ventilation with bag-valve-mask or anesthesia bag with 100% oxygen.
2. Assemble all needed equipment, including emergency equipment. Be sure it is all functioning.
3. Connect a cardiac monitor to the child. Be sure that the IV line is functioning. (Note that succinylcholine can be given through an intraosseous needle.)
4. Premedicate the child with atropine sulfate 0.01 mg/kg if using succinylcholine. Be sure to document a pupil assessment before administering the atropine sulfate.
5. Before paralyzing or sedating the child, perform and document a brief neurologic assessment.
6. Premedicate the child with suspected head injury with lidocaine 1.5 mg/kg intravenously.
7. If the child is alert, consider the use of diazepam 0.1 to 0.2 mg/kg or lorazepam 0.05 mg/kg; this will help make the child amnesiac to the event.
8. Administer paralyzing or sedating agent, and assist ventilation until intubation completed.
9. Assist with intubation by immobilization of cervical spine and applying cricothyroid pressure.
10. **Always** talk to and touch the child. Remember the child may be sedated or paralyzed, but the child can still experience pain and may require medication.

---

pine sulfate (0.01 mg/kg) to decrease the possibility of bradyrhythmias. It is important to emphasize that if the child is alert at all, providing amnesia with diazepam (Valium) (0.1 to 0.2 mg/kg) or lorazepam (Ativan) (0.05 mg/kg) can help make the procedure less anxiety provoking (Eichelberger & Pratsch, 1988; Karb et al., 1989; Syverud et al., 1988). The box above contains a suggested protocol to follow when medicating the child for intubation.

Before intubating the patient who has suffered a head injury, lidocaine (1.5 mg/kg) may be given intravenously. Lidocaine has demonstrated the ability to decrease the acute rise in intracranial pressure that may come with the intubation procedure (Barkin & Rosen, 1987).

An alternative method for airway management is the cricothyrotomy. This procedure can be performed by either using a needle or actually making a surgical incision and then inserting an endotracheal tube or tracheostomy tube. Indications for cricothyrotomy include massive maxillofacial trauma, unusual patient anatomy, foreign body obstruction, and known cervical spine fracture.

This type of airway intervention is useful in the older child and adolescent, but in children younger than 8 years the cricothyroid membrane forms the narrowest segment of the airway and the cricothyrotomy may not be effective. However, if no other airway intervention has been successful, a cricothyrotomy may be indicated (Chameides, 1988).

Breathing

The bag-valve device with a face mask can be used to assist ventilation when there is respiratory difficulty or apnea. Two types of bags are available to assist pediatric breathing: self-inflating devices and anesthesia ventilation systems. The self-inflating bag is available in both a pediatric and infant size. It does not require an oxygen source to fill because of its recoil. This device will deliver 21% oxygen unless attached to an oxygen source (Chameides, 1988). Most of these bags are equipped with a pressure-limited pop-off valve that is set between 35 and 45 cm H_2O. This helps decrease the chances of injuring the child's pulmonary system (Chameides, 1988).

The anesthesia bag requires more experience for proper use. This bag requires a gas flow for it to inflate. In addition, an overflow valve must be adjusted so that barotrauma does not occur to the patient's pulmonary system. Many of these bags are attached to a pressure meter to monitor pressure during ventilation of children. A pressure of 35 mm Hg is generally adequate and safe (Chameides, 1988).

No matter what type of resuscitation bag is used, a mask of appropriate size must be used if bag-valve-mask ventilation is to be effective. The mask should extend from the bridge of the nose to the cleft of the chin, covering the nose and mouth. Pressure to the eyes should be avoided. The mask should be transparent so that any material that may be obstructing the airway can be visualized (Chameides, 1988).

If any difficulty in ventilating the child occurs,

a thorough assessment of the chest is imperative. Injuries that require immediate treatment include tension pneumothorax, a sucking chest wound, massive hemothorax, and flail chest.

Because young children are aerophagic (swallow air) and use abdominal muscles in ventilation, a nasogastric tube should be inserted to decompress the abdomen. This will also prevent the possibility of aspiration.

If the child is placed on a ventilator, the settings are usually as follows: the normal tidal volume is 10 to 15 ml/kg; inspiratory time is generally ≥ 0.5 seconds; peak inspiratory pressure is 20 to 30 cm H_2O; rate is based on the child's age; and positive end expiratory pressure (PEEP) is 3 to 5 cm H_2O (Chameides, 1988). The effectiveness of ventilation must always be continuously assessed by observing the rise and fall of the child's chest; the color and capillary refill; changes in mental status; and oxygenation (ABGs).

Perfusion

The child's general appearance, color, and mental status provide important parameters of circulatory status. An adequately perfused child responds to the environment and recognizes the parent.

The child's color should be pink. Because the pediatric heart rate is normally fast and can easily increase with stimulation, such as agitation, capillary refill is a better indicator of peripheral perfusion. Brisk capillary refill (less than 2 seconds) is a normal response (Chameides, 1988).

If the child has suffered a cardiac arrest, both basic and advanced cardiac life support must be initiated, using the standards that were developed by the American Heart Association and published in the *Textbook of Pediatric Advanced Life Support* (Chameides, 1988). An infant has been defined as an individual ranging in age from birth to 1 year; a child is from 1 to 8 years of age. After 8 years of age, the patient may be managed with adult CPR techniques. Table 17-5 contains a summary of basic cardiac life support for the infant and child.

Establishing intravenous access

Establishing an intravenous (IV) access, particularly in the smaller child, can sometimes be a difficult and time-consuming process. Mayer (1985) suggests that the simplest and safest way to obtain venous access in the child is by percutaneous peripheral vein cannulation. Suggested sites include dorsum of the hand, the antecubital fossa, the saphenous vein at the ankle, and the external jugular vein in the neck. Catheter size varies from 24- to 22-gauge in the infant to 20- to 18-gauge in the older child.

Mayer (1985) notes that the central venous lines via the subclavian, internal jugular, and femoral route that are often used in the adult trauma patient may not be as useful and could be potentially dangerous to the pediatric patient. The stress of an emergency situation could make the procedure even more difficult for the inexperienced practitioner. Complications include pneumothorax, tension pneumothorax, infiltration into the thoracic cavity, cardiac tamponade, and hematoma formation.

Cannulation of the femoral vein has been associated with specific serious complications. These include avascular necrosis of the femoral head, femoral vein thrombosis, and femoral ar-

Table 17-5 Basic cardiac life support for the pediatric patient

	Age of the child	
	Birth to 1 yr	**1 to 8 yr**
Compression		
Site	Midsternum	Lower third of sternum
Mechanism	Two fingers encircling the child's chest	Heel of the hand
Depth of the Compression	½-1 inch	1-1½ inches
Rate	100/min	80-100/min
Compression/breath ratio	5:1 (pause for ventilation)	5:1 (pause for ventilation)

Note. Adapted from *Textbook of Pediatric Advanced Life Support* (p. 16) by L. Chameides (Ed.), 1988, Dallas: American Heart Association.

tery thrombosis. Any of these complications can interfere with the growth and development of the child's extremity (Mayer, 1985). Mayer (1985) recommends the use of peripheral venous cutdowns and intraosseous infusions as alternatives when percutaneous venous access cannot be obtained rapidly. It is interesting to note, however, that in the *Pediatric Advanced Life Support Course* (Chameides, 1988), percutaneous cannulization of the femoral vein is recommended.

An important point that must be emphasized is that the pediatric trauma patient, just as the adult trauma patient, may require fluid resuscitation and an intravenous access is necessary to accomplish this. Several techniques are available, and the trauma nurse should be aware of these to assure that the pediatric patient does not suffer unnecessary complications. The following discussion presents another technique to gain vascular access in the pediatric patient.

Intraosseous infusions

Rosetti, Thompson, Aprahamian, Darin, and Mateer (1984) found that even at pediatric centers, venous access was not always rapid or achieved. They conducted a 3-year retrospective study of 66 pediatric arrests that were treated in the ED. In 24% of the patients, it took 10 minutes or longer to establish intravenous access, and in 6% of the patients, no access was ever obtained. It took an average of 24 minutes to perform a cutdown.

Tsai & Kallsen (1987) discovered that attempting IV access contributed to longer scene time for prehospital care providers. The authors suggest that because of (1) low success rate in obtaining IV access in children under 13, (2) prolonged scene times when IV access is attempted, and (3) lack of opportunities to maintain pediatric IV skills, other routes of infusion, such as intraosseous, may be more useful.

Intraosseous infusion has been reported in the literature since 1922. Tocantins (1940) reported the use of this method for infusing such fluids as blood through the bone marrow. The development of specific intraosseous needles (Jamshidi and Cook) has reintroduced the use of this method, particularly in the prehospital and ED setting.

An intraosseous infusion uses the vascular network of long bones to transport fluids and drugs

---

Drugs and fluids that may be administered by an intraosseous route	
Drugs	**Fluids**
Epinephrine	Colloids
Lidocaine	Crystalloids
Naloxone	Blood
Atropine	
Sodium bicarbonate	
Bretylium tosylate	
Calcium chloride	
Dopamine	
Dobutamine	
Antibiotics	
Succinylcholine	
Diazepam	
Lorazepam	

---

from the venous sinusoid, to the central venous canal, to the nutrient emissary veins, and finally to the systemic venous circulation. Because the medullary cavities are encased in a noncollapsible bony cortex, they do not collapse in shock.

Intraosseous infusions may be used when IV access cannot be obtained, to assure patient survival. Kanter, Zimmerman, and Straus (1986) suggest that if after 5 minutes no IV access has been established, an intraosseous infusion should be attempted.

The box above contains a list of drugs and fluids that have been safely infused through an intraosseous needle. The ideal site for intraosseous infusion in the child younger than 3 years is the proximal tibia, 1 to 2 cm below the tibial tuberosity on the flat medial surface. This site is usually easily accessible during resuscitation and can be secured. For the older child, the distal tibia, 2 cm proximal to the medial malleolus with needle directed slightly cephalad, can be used. The sternum has been recommended for adults, but may be difficult to use when CPR is being performed. The box above contains a summary of the procedure for the insertion of intraosseous needles, and Figure 17-1 is an illustration of the procedure.

Complications that have been observed with the use of intraosseous needles are extravasation of fluid and osteomyelitis. Osteomyelitis has been reported, but its incidence is very low and possi-

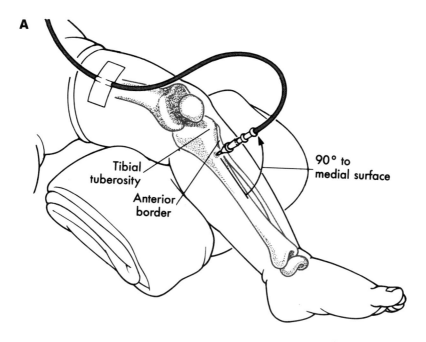

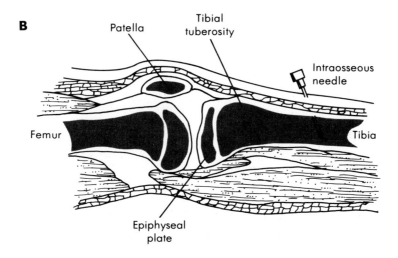

Figure 17-1   **A,** Intraosseous infusion technique. **B,** Insertion. (*Note.* **A,** Redrawn from *Pediatric Advanced Life Support* [p. 44] by L. Chameides [Ed.], 1988, Dallas: American Heart Association. **B,** From *Emergency Pediatrics: A Guide to Ambulatory Care* [3rd ed.] by R.M. Barkin and P. Rosen, 1990, St. Louis: Mosby–Year Book, Inc.)

Intraosseous insertion procedure

1. Select appropriate size needle:
   - infants younger than 18 months: 18- or 20-gauge needle
   - children older than 18 months: 13- or 16-gauge needle
2. Prepare the site with antiseptic solution.
3. Anesthetize the area if the child is alert.
4. Select desired site. A gentle twisting motion is required for insertion.
5. Direct the needle away from epiphyseal plate.
6. Needle placement can be verified by:
   - needle standing up without support
   - aspiration of blood
7. Flush needle with fluid to remove any clots on tip of needle.
8. Secure needle with gauze pads or tracheostomy tape.
9. Observe for complications associated with use of central lines, such as infiltration, localized irritation, and embolus.
10. Remember, this is a temporary line. When able, alternative venous access should be obtained.

---

bly could be related to prolonged use of the needle or use of hypertonic and strongly alkaline solutions (Manley, Haley, & Dick, 1988).

Theoretic complications include damage to the growth plate and pulmonary emboli. To date, neither of these complications has been reported in the literature.

Estimating blood loss

The normal circulating blood volume in the pediatric patient makes up about 7% to 8% of the child's body weight. A child's blood volume can be estimated at 85 ml/kg. An example is a 10-kg child whose circulating blood volume is 850 ml and who loses 160 ml of blood because of trauma. Practitioners familiar only with the adult trauma patient may not consider the 160 ml blood loss to be excessive, but it represents about 20% of the child's circulating blood volume. Children also tend to have lower hemoglobin and hematocrit levels than adults. The range of hemoglobin is 11 to 12 g for those 14 years of age and younger. The hematocrit values range from 33% to 36% for the same age group (Eichelberger & Pratsch, 1988).

Hypovolemia

As with the adult trauma patient, there is much controversy about the treatment of hypovolemia related to trauma in children. The colloid versus crystalloid debate has research to support both sides. However, regardless of which treatment is selected, certain parameters should be observed in the fluid resuscitation of the pediatric patient.

Eichelberger and Pratsch (1988) and Mayer (1985) advocate the use of lactated Ringer's solution in the initial resuscitation of shock. When shock has been identified, a fluid bolus of 20 ml/kg should be initiated. If the child's weight is unknown, a table of weights corresponding to age of the child should be consulted. According to the *Textbook of Pediatric Advanced Life Support* guidelines (Chameides, 1988), the fluid bolus can be repeated up to 60-100 ml/kg for the child in profound shock. To assure the appropriate fluid bolus is given, the trauma nurse should use a method to control the infusion, such as a Buretrol or a stopcock on the IV tubing.

The child should be closely monitored for a response, including increase in blood pressure, slowing of heart rate, and improvement in color. The normal blood pressure and heart rate for the age of the child must be used as a baseline when evaluating the child's present vital signs. If no change occurs, a repeat fluid bolus should be given. A urinary output of 1 ml/kg/hr should be maintained and closely monitored. If the child does not exhibit any signs of circulatory improvement, blood should be administered at 10 ml/kg of packed red cells or 20 ml/kg of whole blood (Eichelberger & Pratsch, 1988).

Pneumatic anti-shock garments (PASG) and military anti-shock trousers (MAST) are available and one of these may be used, especially during transport of the child. These devices should be used with caution. If the abdominal compartment is inflated, it may interfere with the child's ventilatory ability, because young children are abdominal breathers.

Neurologic Assessment

The neurologic assessment of the pediatric patient is related to the child's growth and development. The trauma nurse must be aware of the cognitive stages of pediatric development to make an appropriate neurologic assessment. Because the child may be afraid, crying, separated from the parent, and, for certain ages, unable to comprehend or follow instructions, neurologic assessment may be difficult. As with the adult trauma patient, neurologic assessment of children consists of five components: level of consciousness; pupillary response; motor assessment; sensory assessment; and vital signs.

Two useful tools are available to perform and document a brief pediatric neurologic assessment and a gross measure of responsiveness. The box on the left presents the AVPU method, which is a gross measurement of responsiveness, and the box below presents the pediatric-modified Glasgow coma scale, which can be used for children 5 years and younger.

Exposure

Young children, because of their large body surface area/mass ratio, are very susceptible to increased heat loss and are less able to regulate their body temperature. Hypothermia may result. Hypothermia can cause pulmonary hypertension, increased hypoxia, and metabolic acidosis (Eichelberger & Pratsch, 1988).

The child needs to be especially protected from temperature stress during trauma resuscita-

---

AVPU method for pediatric neurologic assessment

A Alert

V Responds to verbal stimuli

P Responds to painful stimuli

U Unresponsive

Pediatric-modified Glasgow coma scale

Eyes opening

Score	>1 Year	<1 Year
4	Spontaneously	Spontaneously
3	To verbal command	To shout
2	To pain	To pain
1	No response	No response

Best motor response

Score		
6	Obeys	Spontaneous
5	Localizes pain	Localizes pain
4	Flexion-withdrawal	Flexion-withdrawal
3	Flexion-abnormal (decorticate)	Flexion-abnormal (decorticate)
2	Extension (decerebrate)	Extension (decerebrate)
1	No response	No response

Best verbal response

Score	>5 Years	2-5 Years	Birth-23 Months
5	Oriented and converses	Appropriate words and phrases	Smiles, coos, appropriately
4	Disoriented and converses	Inappropriate words	Cries; consolable
3	Inappropriate words	Persistent cries or screams	Persistent, inappropriate crying and/or screaming
2	Incomprehensible sounds	Grunts	Grunts; agitated/restless
1	No response	No response	No response

Note. From *Severe Head Trauma* (p. 5) by J. Simon, 1988. Presented at Pediatric Emergencies, Williamsburg: Resource Applications.

Table 17-6 Pediatric trauma score

Component	Severity category		
	+2	+1	-1
Size	>20 Kg	10-20 Kg	<10 Kg
Airway	Normal	Maintainable	Unmaintainable
CNS	Awake	Obtunded	Comatose
Systolic BP	>90 mm Hg	90-50 mm Hg	<50 mm Hg
Open wounds	None	Closed fracture	Open/multiple fractures
Cutaneous	None	Minor	Major/penetrating

TOTAL (POINTS) _____

Note. From "The Pediatric Trauma Score as a Predictor of Injury Severity in the Injured Child by J. Tepas, D. Mollitt, and J. Talbert, 1987, *Journal of Trauma, 27*, p. 14.

tion. Heating lights, warm blankets, and warm intravenous fluids will help prevent the complications of hypothermia. In addition, the child's temperature should be monitored frequently during trauma resuscitation.

Trauma Scoring

As with the adult trauma patient, it is important to determine quickly the severity of the child's trauma and the potential for mortality and morbidity. A pediatric trauma score (PTS) has been developed and is being evaluated. Ramenofsky et al., (1988) and Tepas, Mollitt, and Talbert (1987) have considered the use of the PTS for determining the severity of injury and the need for advanced care. Table 17-6 presents the pediatric trauma score. Each item in the instrument receives a score ranging from +2 to -1. The points are then totaled. Ramenofsky et al., (1988) found that the PTS offers the potential to help prehospital care providers and ED personnel decide when a child should be transferred for more definitive care, such as to a pediatric trauma center. The scores on the scale range from +12 (no injury) to -6 (fatal injury). The researchers found, after evaluating 469 pediatric trauma cases, that a prehospital PTS score of 8 or less indicated a severely injured child—one who should be transferred to a facility with the most advanced level of care.

Family Considerations
Death and dying

The family is an interdependent system. When a child is traumatically injured or dies, the entire family is affected. Because trauma is the leading

cause of death for the pediatric population, it is likely that many of these sudden deaths may occur or conclude in the ED. Death of a child affects the family unlike any other stress.

The manner in which the sudden illness, injury, or death is communicated to the family is extremely important. Dubin and Sarnoff (1986) noted that

> the initial contact that emergency department caregivers have with the survivors [family] has a significant impact on their grief response. Inadvertent inhibition of the grief process can result in a pathologic response with an increased risk of morbidity or mortality [for those left behind].

In addition, the greatest fear most young children experience is separation from their parents. Many times this is a necessity, particularly during initial resuscitation. It is important for the trauma nurse to involve the family as much as possible. Perhaps one of the most critical things the trauma nurse can do for the family is to provide them with information. Controversy has always existed about how to communicate to the family what is being done for the child. Many argue that verbal communication is not enough.

A study was conducted by Doyle et al. (1987) regarding allowing families to remain with their members during resuscitation. The family member was seated within touching distance of the individual when possible. A survey was used to collect data. The survey was given to the families who participated in the study. All the family members who responded stated that they believed that everything that could be done was done for their family member. Of the people who answered, 76% believed that their adjustment to the patient's death was made easier by being with the patient at the moment of death. Many family members stated that they had a chance to say good-bye.

The family unit is the system that responds to the stress of a sudden or untimely death. Nurses, physicians, and others in the ED make up a subsystem with whom the family will interact. The effects of this interaction will have long-term consequences on the family as a whole. Therefore communicating and allowing family participation are two meaningful nursing interventions that are provided by the trauma nurse.

Child abuse

About one million cases of child abuse occur in the United States annually; of these, approximately 2000 to 4000 children die. It has been estimated that 10% of the children younger than 5 years who are treated in the ED have been abused (Kelley, 1988).

Injuries that have been associated with child abuse include head injuries; burns; injuries to the ears, nose, and mouth; abdominal trauma; and fractures. A detailed history of the injury, including physical findings, a subjective report, previous injury history, laboratory and radiographic studies, and assessment of family functioning, will help determine if the injury is accidental or intentional.

It is the responsibility of ED physicians and nurses in all 50 states to report suspected child abuse. The agency who receives and acts on the report varies from state to state. It is critical that the trauma nurse realize that reporting suspected abuse may save the child's life.

Family education

If the injury is one that is treatable in the ED and the child and family will be sent home, the trauma nurse has an opportunity to teach the family about prevention. Providing information about growth and development and the sources of injury to the child may contribute to decreasing further injury and accidental deaths.

Pain Management

The pain management of the patient with multiple trauma has only recently been evaluated by trauma team members. Concern of contributing to the patient's altered mental status and interfering with the patient's blood pressure, pulse, and respirations has resulted in many multiple-trauma patients—both adult and children—being undermedicated for pain during the initial management of trauma.

Broome and Lillis (1989) and Hazinski (1984) noted that the child's stage of growth and development and his or her previous experience with painful or perceived painful events influence the child's response to pain. Table 16-2 contains a summary of how the child may respond to pain related to age.

Broome and Lillis (1989) and McCaffery and Beebe (1989) describe several nursing interventions that may be used by the trauma nurse in the management of pediatric pain. These include understanding how the child perceives the painful experience based on the child's level of growth and development; using techniques that help distract the child from the pain, such as the child's favorite toy, color, or music; and allowing the parent to support the child when possible.

Cutaneous stimulation has been found to be of use in reducing the pain related to particular procedures such as infiltration of anesthesic, IV insertion, and drawing blood. McCaffery and Beebe (1989) suggest massage/pressure, vibration, heat/cold, and topical anesthetics may make pain more bearable.

One topical anesthetic that has been used in the pediatric patient is TAC (Trott, 1985). TAC is an equal-parts mixture of tetracaine, 0.5%; epinephrine, 1:2000 concentration; and cocaine, 11.8%. This mixture is applied to the wound by saturating a piece of gauze. It should not be used on the ear, tip of the nose, penis, or any other easily compromised vascular site (Trott, 1985).

A critical point that the trauma nurse must remember when caring for the injured child is that no matter what the age, the child can feel pain. Both narcotics and nonnarcotic analgesics can be used in the pediatric patient, though the dosages and effects of the drugs may vary because of the growth and development of the child. Pain assessment and intervention are essential components in the evaluation and care of the injured.

ASSESSMENT AND INTERVENTIONS RELATED TO SPECIFIC INJURY
Head Injury

Altered responsiveness

The most common type of pediatric trauma seen in the ED is head trauma. It has been estimated that in the United States about 500,000 head injuries occur in children annually. About 25,000 of these children will die or are permanently disabled because of injury (Eichelberger & Pratsch, 1988).

The initial management of pediatric head injury is focused on maintenance of an airway with concurrent cervical spine immobilization, breathing, and circulation. When the child is hemodynamically stable, a CT scan should be performed. Only about 15% of children with head injuries require surgery (Eichelberger & Pratsch, 1988).

Pediatric head injuries have been classified as minor, moderate, and severe. Children with a Glasgow coma scale score of 14 or 15 are in the minor head injury category. These children generally have suffered localized trauma to the head, such as a scalp laceration or a concussion with a transient loss of consciousness. Children with a minor head injury should be observed and their family given clear and understandable instructions about how to continue this observation at home.

A child with a moderate head injury has a Glasgow coma scale score of 9 to 12. Using the modified coma scale for the pediatric patient, this includes the young child who is crying and cannot be comforted, as well as the older child who is combative. These children should be admitted and a head CT scan performed.

The CT results will dictate the treatment. Nursing care of these patients requires continuous assessment. Protecting the child from injury and providing a safe environment in the ED is needed to decrease the possibility of further injury.

Severe head injury is suspected when the Glasgow coma scale score is less than 8. The major focus of treatment is rapid evaluation of the cause by CT and prevention and management of increased intracranial pressure. The box (upper right) presents a summary of care for the pediatric patient with severe head trauma.

Thoracic Injury

Ineffective breathing pattern
Impaired gas exchange

Only about 25% of all trauma to children involves the chest. Twice as many boys as girls suffer thoracic trauma (Mayer, 1985). Even though this is not a common type of trauma in children, some specific differences exist between the adult

---

Summary of care for the child with severe head injury

1. Intubate child for hyperventilation and prevention of aspiration. Maintain P_{CO_2} between 20% and 25% (Gilmore, 1987).
2. Perform CT scan and cervical spine evaluation. Maintain cervical spine immobilization until injury possibility has been ruled out.
3. Administer medications that may be used to control intracranial pressure (ICP) in the pediatric patient:
   Mannitol 0.25 to 1 g/kg IV (15% or 20% solution)
   Furosemide 0.5 to 1.0 mg/kg IV
   Dexamethasone 0.25 mg/kg IV
   Fentanyl 0.02-0.03 mg/kg IV
4. Monitor ICP.
5. Pentobarbital coma may be used to control ICP: 3 to 20 mg/kg initially; blood levels are then maintained between 25 and 40 mcg/ml.
6. Hypothermia may be used to decrease increased ICP.
7. Elevate head 10 to 30 degrees when cervical spine has been cleared.
8. Administer anticonvulsant therapy if seizures occur.
9. Assess neurologic status continuously.
10. Talk with, touch, perform range of motion, turn, and position the child as tolerated. Involve family in the child's care. Use familiar sounds and environment when possible for the child.

---

and pediatric patient in its initial recognition and management.

The child's chest is very compliant. Because of this, the child may suffer severe injury to the chest and have little external evidence. Children are also aerophagic and may swallow enough air to decrease effective ventilation.

Traumatic asphyxia

Perhaps one of the most dramatic injuries that occurs to children is traumatic asphyxia. Traumatic asphyxia was first described in 1837 as the "masque ecchymotique." Traumatic asphyxia occurs because of direct compression to a compliant thoracic cage against a closed glottis. This causes a sudden and dramatic increase in intratracheal and intrapulmonary pressure and temporary vena caval obstruction (Mayer, 1985). The signs and symptoms include a bluish discoloration of the skin of the face and neck; petechiae of the face, neck, and chest; and subconjunctival hemorrhage. Because of the sudden increase in pressure, the child needs to be evaluated for abdominal, pulmonary, and intracranial injuries that may have occurred.

The management of thoracic trauma in the pediatric patient is based on maintenance of airway, breathing, and circulation and early recognition of the extent of the traumatic injuries to prevent mortality and morbidity. Chest tubes should be the appropriate size and should be placed carefully to avoid damage to the developing breast buds in young females. Table 17-7 contains chest tube sizes based on age.

Abdominal Injury

Altered urinary and bowel elimination
High risk for altered nutrition: less than body requirements

Abdominal trauma accounts for only a very small number of trauma-related deaths in the pediatric population (Mayer, 1985). Kane, Cronian, Dorfman, and DeLuca (1988) noted that abdominal injuries account for 10% of trauma-related deaths. It should be remembered that the abdominal cavity is a large potential space and children have less circulating blood volume and can exsanguinate much more quickly than the adult patient.

The most frequently injured abdominal organs in the child are the liver and spleen. These organs are injured more frequently as the result of blunt abdominal trauma from motor vehicle accidents, falls, and blows to the upper quadrant. The management differences between the adult and pediatric trauma patient are based on the diagnosis and treatment of abdominal trauma. To

---

> ### Indications for peritoneal lavage for the pediatric trauma patient
>
> - Altered response to painful stimuli because of:
>   — head trauma
>   — alcohol or drug ingestion
> - Fractures of the lower ribs, pelvis, lumbar spine
> - Positive abdominal findings
> - Hemodynamic instability

preserve organ tissue and in the case of the spleen to maintain immune competence, the trend is to avoid operative intervention in the pediatric patient (Haftel, Mahour, & Senac 1988; Kane, Cronian, Dorfman, & De Luca 1988; Pearl et al., 1989).

The CT scan has emerged as an effective method to evaluate for abdominal injuries in the hemodynamically stable child who has suffered blunt abdominal trauma. If the child has suffered penetrating trauma, such as a gunshot wound, laparotomy is still recommended (Eichelberger & Pratsch, 1988; Kane et al., 1988; Mayer, 1985). The box above shows indications for peritoneal lavage in the pediatric trauma patient. If a diagnostic peritoneal lavage is to be performed on the pediatric trauma patient, 10 to 20 ml/kg of 1.5% of dialysis solution or buffered lactated Ringer's solution is instilled (Mayer, 1985).

If the child remains hemodynamically stable and the CT scan does not reveal other intraabdominal injuries, the child may be managed nonoperatively. It has been observed that many injuries to the liver and spleen resolve spontaneously (Eichelberger & Pratsch, 1988; Kane et al., 1988).

Musculoskeletal or Spinal Injury

Impaired physical mobility

The incidence of cervical spine trauma in the young child has been noted at 2% to 3% (Marcus, 1986). However, the cervical spine of the child should always be immobilized and protected just as for the adult trauma patient. Dietrich, Ginn-Pease, Bartkowski, and King (1991) conducted a study that found that children did sustain significant spinal trauma and many times this was not very obvious. The immobilization of the

---

Table 17-7   Chest tube sizes for the pediatric patient

Age of the child	Tube size (French)
Newborn	8 to 12
Infant	14 to 20
Child	20 to 28
Adolescent	28 to 42

Table 17-8 Common pediatric musculoskeletal injuries

Type of fracture	Mechanism of injury
Clavicle fracture	Falls from heights, such as from the top bunk bed, trees
Midshaft fracture of the humerus (spiral)	Possible child abuse; direct blow to the humerus
Supracondylar fracture	Fall on extended arm
Distal radius and ulna fracture	Fall on outstretched arm
Crush injury of distal phalanx	Door closed on digits, such as car door
Nursemaid's elbow (dislocation of elbow)	Child is pulled or lifted by one arm
Femur fracture	Child struck by a car, bicycle; other wheeled-vehicle crashes
Tibia fracture	Rotational injury

cervical spine was discussed previously in this chapter.

Musculoskeletal injuries are managed after major injuries have been stabilized. Extremity pain is a cardinal symptom of injury in the pediatric patient. Fractures of vascular long bones, such as the femur, can be a significant emergency for the child because of potential blood volume loss. Table 17-8 presents a list of some common musculoskeletal injuries and their mechanisms of injury.

A history about the possible mechanism of injury should be taken. A physical examination of the injured area should include evaluation for swelling, open wounds with bone protruding, deformity, color changes in the limb, presence of pulse, diminished or absent capillary refill, loss of motion, decreased sensation, and any pain or tenderness. If the ED physicians and nurses are not experienced in evaluating pediatric x-ray films, comparison views between the injured and uninjured extremities may be helpful.

Any open fractures should be cultured for aerobic and anaerobic organisms. The wound should be covered with a moist, sterile dressing, and antibiotic therapy should be initiated. An orthopedic consult is necessary.

The specific treatment of the injury depends on the type of injury and its location. Children's sizes are available for traction devices, such as the Hare or Thomas traction splints. Splints can be composed of boards or some type of firm surface, slings, and tape. Also, air splints are available in a children's size. Regardless of what splinting device is used, it must be assessed for proper placement and fit. Included in the assessment should be neuromotor, sensory, and vascular status of the affected extremity. Barkin and Rosen (1987) note that casts are not usually applied to pediatric fractures until 48 hours after the injury. This allows for swelling to decrease; however, when neurovascular compromise exists, intervention should be immediate.

Recognition of potentially vulnerable musculoskeletal injuries should be accomplished quickly by the trauma nurse. In addition, such musculoskeletal injuries as spiral fractures or injuries that do not correspond to the child's current growth and development skills should be more closely evaluated for potential child abuse. The failure to identify and properly treat a musculoskeletal injury in the injured child could lead to long-term, devastating consequences.

TRANSPORT OF THE INJURED CHILD

Trunkey (1988) asserts that an organized or regionalized approach to trauma care will definitively improve trauma mortality and morbidity. For the pediatric trauma patient, this could make the difference between life and death.

Because only a limited number of centers are specifically dedicated to pediatric trauma care, centers with the capability and resources to care for the pediatric trauma patient should be identified and used in a timely manner. The advent of sophisticated prehospital care and ground and helicopter transport can contribute to the use of these centers.

The Children's Hospital National Medical Center in Washington, D.C. recommends that a child be transferred under the following conditions: if there is no pediatric expertise available; if the child needs a diagnostic procedure not available; if the child's condition may deteriorate and require more specific care; and if the family requests the child be transferred.

Hart, Haynes, Schwaitzberg, and Harris (1987) provide precise reasons to transfer the pediatric patient. These guidelines are presented in the box below.

In 1989 the American Academy of Pediatrics formed a multidisciplinary interest group that developed recommendations for the interhospital transport of the critically ill or injured pediatric patient (Day et al.,1991). Among their recommendations were the following:

1. Pediatric patients should be transported by those who are skilled in the care of the pediatric patient and who maintain those skills.
2. Standards should be developed that address the type of education and training that is needed for pediatric transport.
3. Quality assurance should be an integral part of any pediatric transport system.

4. Some type of pediatric transport data base should be developed.
5. Multicenter research should be conducted related to the transport of the critically ill or injured patient.

If the child is to be transferred, a decision must be made concerning the best method of transport to use of those transport methods available. Chapter 20 discusses the advantages and disadvantages of particular transport methods.

After the method of transport has been selected, the child will need to be stabilized as much as possible for transfer. The box below presents measures that should be addressed before transport.

Recommendations for transport of the pediatric trauma patient

- Serious injury to one or more organ systems
- Hypovolemic shock requiring more than one blood transfusion
- Orthopedic injuries, such as two or more long bone fractures, fractures of the thoracic cage, compromised neurovascular status, fractures of the axial skeleton
- Spinal cord injuries
- Blunt abdominal trauma with hemodynamic instability
- Patients requiring ventilatory support
- Extremity reimplantation
- Head injuries with cerebral spinal fluid leak, altered mental status, deteriorating neurologic status, increased ICP, and GCS less than 9
- Burns involving more than 15% TBSA
- Falls from heights
- Motor vehicle crashes involving associated fatalities, extrication time longer than 15 minutes, speeds more than 55 miles per hour, and pedestrians who have been struck
- Trauma score less than 13

Note. From "Air Transport of the Pediatric Patient" by M. Hart, D. Haynes, S. Schwaitzberg, and B. Harris, 1987, *Emergency Care Quarterly, 3,* p. 23.

Stabilization of the injured child for transport

1. Stabilize the airway.
2. Immobilize the cervical spine.
3. Perform brief assessment for injury identification.
4. Obtain baseline vital signs.
5. Connect cardiac monitor to patient.
6. Insert nasogastric tube.
7. Place two intravenous lines.
8. Dress open wounds.
9. Obtain a history of mechanism of injury.
10. Draw blood specimens for laboratory studies, and bring along any results that have been obtained.
11. Splint fractures.
12. Insert Foley catheter.
13. Insert temperature probe.
14. Obtain paperwork.
15. Be sure the family knows about the transfer, has directions to the receiving facility, and has an opportunity to see the child before leaving. If the child is critical, the family should wait until the transport team leaves before they leave.

The pediatric trauma patient

Nursing diagnosis	Nursing intervention	Evaluative criteria
High risk for altered cerebral tissue perfusion Related to cerebral edema, decreased blood volume	**Promote cerebral blood flow** Stabilize ABCs. Administer drugs to decrease ICP. Monitor neurologic status, including: • Glasgow coma scale; • motor/sensory; • pupils; • vital signs. Touch and talk to the child, and provide care based on developmental phase. Decrease excessive sensory stimulation.	Child will have: • adequate airway; • Po_2 and Pco_2 within desired limits for type of injury and desired outcome; • GCS score above 12. Child will respond to the environment.
High risk for ineffective breathing pattern and impaired gas exchange Related to abdominal breathing, obligatory nasal breathing	**Promote ventilation** Recognize need for intubation (uncuffed tubes to age 8). Ventilate the child, using the appropriate calculated tidal volume, device, and rate. Insert nasogastric tube to decompress the stomach, facilitate ventilation, and prevent aspiration. Monitor respiratory response.	Tracheal trauma and barotrauma will not occur. Abdomen will be decompressed. Aspiration will be prevented. Equal breath sounds will be present. Capillary refill will be within normal limits.
High risk for fluid volume deficit Related to circulating blood volume (see Estimating Blood Loss)	**Promote adequate perfusion** Calculate appropriate fluid bolus. Administer 20 ml/kg of normal saline or lactated Ringer's solution.	

**NURSING DIAGNOSES &
EVALUATIVE CRITERIA**   *The pediatric trauma patient—cont'd*

Nursing diagnosis	Nursing intervention	Evaluative criteria
	Monitor results of fluid bolus.	Normal blood pressure and pulse for age of the child will be maintained.
	Monitor child for the following signs and symptoms of shock: • altered mental status; • sluggish or absent capillary refill; • inadequate urinary output. Evaluate child for sources of blood loss by: • measuring abdominal girth; • assessing extremities for injuries.	Capillary refill will be <2 secs. Urinary output will be 1-2 ml/kg.
High risk for pain Related to destruction of tissue, stimulation of nerve endings	**Promote comfort** Administer pain medication based on mg/kg.	Child will be able to express pain (use subjective measures).
High risk for fear Related to unfamiliar surroundings, separation from family	**Promote calm** Talk to and explain procedures to child based on developmental stage. Distract child with toys, colors, or sound. Allow parent with child as much as possible. Recognize major fear of the child based on growth and development. Use restraints for safety and not for punishment.	Child will cooperate. Family will be involved as much as possible. Consult Table 17-1, p. 532. No injury will occur from restraints.

COMPETENCIES
The following clinical competencies pertain to **caring for the pediatric trauma patient.**

☑ Perform assessment in relation to anatomic and physiologic considerations.

☑ Document assessment using developmentally appropriate scales (e.g., pediatric-modified Glasgow coma scale).

☑ Calculate appropriate dose of medications/intravenous fluids for the pediatric trauma patient.

☑ Demonstrate appropriate interventions for maintaining airway patency in the pediatric patient.

☑ Establish or assist in the establishment of intravenous access (e.g., intraosseous infusion) in the pediatric trauma patient.

☑ Perform baseline psychologic assessment of family and child to determine if response is developmentally appropriate and if a counseling referral is necessary.

☑ Report suspected cases of child abuse to appropriate authorities.

SUMMARY The care of the pediatric trauma patient requires a skilled and organized approach. The table pp. 548-549 contains a summary of the care of the injured child. At present resources devoted specifically to the pediatric patient are limited. When prevention and education have failed, early identification of injuries, prompt and appropriate interventions, and transferring of the child, if indicated, should be accomplished. Harris (1987) states:

> Pediatric trauma care is becoming an art form best practiced by pediatric surgeons who regard it as their field of special interest. The concept of dedicated pediatric trauma units and teams is not new. Both are apt to meet well-intentioned resistance from some traditionalists, but emotional and physiologic differences of the young patients and the need to cope with pediatric trauma as a syndrome require special techniques and organization best provided by pediatric trauma centers.
>
> If 10 more years are spent adapting for children this progress made in adult trauma centers, lives needlessly will be lost and the momentum of medical progress is impeded. As a society, as parents, we must not waste any more time or any more children.

This is a challenge that trauma nurses must face. Trauma nurses are in a position to provide the best care and vital information about prevention of pediatric trauma. Nursing as a profession and community must decrease the mortality and morbidity that robs society of its children.

CASE STUDY Erin is a 7-year-old patient brought to the ED by helicopter after being involved as a passenger in a motor vehicle accident. The car was hit on the side where she was sitting. She was wearing her shoulder harness and seat belt.

Erin is alert and oriented with no obvious injuries to her head. Her strongest complaint is pain on the left side of her "stomach." She has significant bruising over the upper portion of her abdomen.

Her blood pressure is 70/50; pulse, 140; and respirations, 30. Erin weighs 30 kg.

What are normal vital signs for Erin?

Erin, a 7-year-old, is considered a school-age child. The formula of 80 + (2 × [child's age in years—in this case, 7]) would calculate a normal systolic pressure of 94. Erin's normal diastolic would be two thirds of the systolic, or approximately 60. According to the *Textbook of Pediatric Advanced Life Support* (Chameides, 1988), the lower limit of the pediatric systolic blood pressure is calculated by using the formula 70 + (2 × the child's age in years) or in Erin's case, 84. Erin's normal pulse rate should be around 100, and her respirations 18 to 30. Erin's vital signs indicate that she is in shock. In addition, because her mental status is appropriate, she is probably in compensated shock, but is at risk of deteriorating because of fluid volume deficit.

Based on mechanism of injury and the initial physical findings, what organ may Erin have injured?

The mechanism of injury to Erin's abdomen was

blunt trauma to the upper quadrant, probably related to the seat belt. Based on her complaint and the physical finding of bruising, she probably has sustained a splenic injury.

How would fluid resuscitation be accomplished for Erin?

The amount of fluid Erin will need is based on calculating 20 ml/kg. The fluid of choice is either normal saline or lactated Ringer's solution. Based on her weight of 30 kg, Erin's initial fluid bolus will be 600 ml. After this bolus, improvement in her blood pressure and decrease in her pulse would indicate a positive response to the fluid. If response is not adequate, the initial fluid bolus may be repeated. If response is still not adequate, infusion of 10 ml/kg of packed red blood cells may be needed, particularly since blood loss has probably occurred from the potential splenic injury.

What type of behavior could the trauma nurse expect from Erin?

Because Erin is 7 years old, she possesses the ability to understand what is happening to her. It will be important for the trauma nurse to talk to Erin and not around or "through" her. Erin will probably be cooperative if procedures are explained to her.

What types of fears may Erin experience based on her age?

Erin's fears are based on the unknown. This is probably a new experience for her, and since she was transported without her parents, no one is there for her to rely on. Erin is old enough to have some knowledge about death and may be afraid that she may die or that her family has died.

RESEARCH QUESTIONS

- Is the pediatric trauma score a useful predictor of the extent of injury?
- Does a pediatric trauma center decrease mortality and morbidity related to pediatric trauma?
- What preventive strategies work best to decrease injury in the pediatric trauma patient?
- What is the best way to communicate sudden death of a child to a family?
- What are effective nursing interventions that can be used to decrease the perception of pain in the injured child?

RESOURCES
General information

American Academy of Pediatrics
Publications Department
141 NW Point Blvd.
Elk Grove Village, IL 60009
(312) 228-5005

Clearinghouse on Child Abuse and Neglect Information
PO Box 1182
Washington, DC 20013
(703) 821-2086

Emergency Medical Services for Children (EMSC)
A Report to the Nation
Published by National Center for Education in Maternal and
     Child Health
Washington, DC 20057

Emergency Nurses' Association
Pediatric Committee
230 East Ohio St., Suite 600
Chicago, IL 60611
(312) 649-0297

National Maternal and Child Health Clearinghouse
38 and R St. NW
Washington, DC 20057

National SAFE KIDS Campaign
Resource Catalog
111 Michigan Ave.
Washington, DC 20010-2970
(202) 939-4993

Pediatric Interhospital Critical Care Transport: Consensus of
     a National Leadership Conference
The Children's Hospital of Alabama
1600 7th Ave. South
Birmingham, AL 35233

Bereaved parents

Bereaved Parent Support Group Pediatric Project
PO Box 1880
Santa Monica, CA 90406
(213) 828-8963

Compassionate Friends
PO Box 1347
Oak Brooks, Il 60521
(312) 990-0010

Drug education

National Federation of Parents for Drug Free Youth
8730 Georgia Ave. # 200
Silver Springs, MD 20910
800-554-KIDS

Parents Reaching Out Service
D.C. General Hospital Department of Pediatrics
1900 Massachusetts Ave. SE
Washington, DC 20057
(202) 727-3866

Pediatric resuscitation equipment

Armstrong Medical Industries
Broselow Pediatric Resuscitation Measuring Tape
PO Box 700
Lincolnshire, Il 60069-0700
(800) 323-4220

Maxishare Corporation
The First 5 Minutes
763 18th St.
PO Box 2041
Milwaukee, WI 53201

Mosby–Year Book, Inc.
Pediatric Emergidose Cards
11830 Westline Industrial Dr.
St. Louis, MO 63146
(800) 325-4177

ANNOTATED BIBLIOGRAPHY

Eichelberger, R., & Pratsch, G. (1988). *Pediatric Trauma Care.* Rockville MD: Aspen Publishers.
   Recently published textbook authored by both a physician and a nurse. It contains not only the pathophysiology associated with pediatric trauma, but an overview of the entire pediatric trauma resuscitation process.
Mayer, T. (1985). *Emergency management of pediatric trauma.* Philadelphia: W.B. Saunders.
   Textbook that contains an in-depth discussion of the pediatric trauma patient. In addition, the text contains detailed suggestions of pediatric management, including equipment suggestions.
Tsai, A., & Kallsen, G. (1987). Epidemiology of pediatric prehospital care. *Annals of Emergency Medicine, 16*(3), 284-292.
   Article that evaluated 3184 prehospital care forms that reflected treatment and transportation of pediatric patients. The authors then identified some of the factors that contributed to the need for prehospital care by the pediatric patient. These factors included the time of day; on-scene time required for pediatric stabilization; and outcome of pediatric resuscitation in the field.

REFERENCES

Barkin, R.M., & Rosen, P. (1990). *Emergency pediatrics: A guide to ambulatory care* (3rd ed.). St. Louis: Mosby–Year Book, Inc.
Beaver, B., Moore, V., Peclet, M., Haller, J., Smialek, J., & Hill, J. (1990). Characteristics of pediatric firearm fatalities. *Journal of Pediatric Surgery, 25*, 97-100.
Broome, M., & Lillis, P. (1989). A descriptive analysis of pediatric pain management research. *Applied Nursing Research, 2* (2), 74-81.
Bull, M., Stroup, K., & Gerhart, S. (1988). Misuse of car safety seats. *Pediatrics, 81* (1), 98-101.
Bushore, M. (1988). Children with multiple injuries. *Pediatrics in Review, 10* (2), 49-57.
Campbell, J. (1988). *Basic trauma life support.* Englewood Cliffs, NJ: Brady Book.
Cardona, V., Hurn, P., Mason, P., Scanlon-Schipp, A., & Veise-Berry, S. (1988). *Trauma nursing: From resuscitation through rehabilitation.* Philadelphia: W.B. Saunders.
Chameides, L. (Ed.) (1988). *Textbook of pediatric advanced life support.* Dallas: American Heart Association.
Day, S., McCloskey, K., Orr, R., Bolte, R., Notterman, D., & Hackel, A. (1991). Pediatric interhospital critical care transport: Consensus of a national leadership conference. *Pediatrics, 88* (4), 696-704.
Dietrich, A., Ginn-Pease, M., Bartkowski, H., & King, D. (1991). Pediatric cervical spine fractures: Predominantly subtle presentations. *Journal of Pediatric Surgery, 26* (8), 995-1000.
Doyle, C., Post, H., Burney, R., Maino, J., Keefe, M., & Rhee, K. (1987). Family participation during resuscitation: An option. *Annals of Emergency Medicine, 16* (6), 673-675.

Dubin, W., & Sarnoff, J. (1986). Sudden unexpected death: Interventions with survivors. *Annals of Emergency Medicine, 15* (1), 54-57.
Eichelberger, M., & Pratsch, G., (1988). *Pediatric trauma.* Rockville, MD: Aspen Publishers.
Gilmore, H. (1987). Emergency management of head trauma in children. *Emergency Care Quarterly, 3* (1), 37-46.
Greensher, J. (1988a). Non-automotive vehicle injuries in adolescents. *Pediatric Annals, 17* (2), 114-121.
Greensher, J. (1988b). Recent advances in injury prevention. *Pediatrics in Review, 10* (6), 171-177.
Haftel, A., Mahour, G., & Senac, S. (1988). Abdominal CT scanning in pediatric blunt trauma. *Annals of Emergency Medicine, 17* (7), 684-689.
Harris, B., Latchaw, L., Murphey, R., & Schwaitzberg, S. (1989). A protocol for pediatric trauma receiving units. *Journal of Pediatric Surgery, 24* (5), 419-422.
Harris, B. (1987). Recommendations for pediatric trauma care in hospitals. *Emergency Care Quarterly, 3* (1), 65-75.
Hart, M., Haynes, D., Schwaitzberg, S., & Harris, B. (1987). Air transport of the pediatric trauma patient. *Emergency Care Quarterly, 3* (1), 21-26.
Hazinski, M. (1992). *Nursing care of the critically ill child* (2nd ed.). St. Louis: Mosby–Year Book, Inc.
Henderson, D. (1988). The Los Angeles pediatric emergency care system. *Journal of Emergency Nursing, 14* (2), 96-100.
Kane, N., Cronian, J., Dorfman, G., & De Luca, F. (1988). Pediatric abdominal trauma: Evaluation by CT. *Pediatrics, 1*, 11-15.
Kanter, R., Zimmerman, J., & Straus, R. (1986). Pediatric emergency access: Evaluation of a protocol. *American Journal of Diseases of Children, 140*, 132.
Karb, V., Queener, S., & Freeman, J. (1989). *Handbook of drugs for nursing practice.* St. Louis: Mosby–Year Book, Inc.
Karlin, L. (1987). Musculoskeletal trauma. *Emergency Care Quarterly, 3* (1), 57-60.
Kelley, S. (1988). Physical abuse of children: Recognition and reporting. *Journal of Emergency Nursing, 14* (2), 82-90.
Listing of children's hospitals with emergency departments in the United States. (1988). *Journal of Emergency Nursing, 14* (2), 130-131.
Manley, L., Haley, K., & Dick, M. (1988). Intraosseous infusion: Rapid vascular access for critically ill or injured infants and children. *Journal of Emergency Nursing, 14* (2), 63-69.
Marcus, R. (1986). *Trauma in children.* Rockville MD: Aspen Publishers.
Mayer, T. (1985). *Emergency management of pediatric trauma.* Philadelphia: W.B. Saunders.
McCaffery, M., & Beebe, A. (1989). *Pain: Clinical manual for nursing practice.* St. Louis: Mosby–Year Book, Inc.
Morrow, J. (1988). Simplifying nursing management of pediatric airways and intravenous infusions. *Journal of Emergency Nursing, 14* (2), 103-106.
Mueller, B., Rivara, F., & Mayer, T. (1988). Urban-rural location and the risk of dying in a pedestrian-vehicle collision. *Journal of Trauma, 28* (1), 91-94.
Narkewicz, R. (1988). The epidemiology of injuries in adolescents. *Pediatric Annals, 17* (2), 84-96.
National Safety Council. (1987). *Accident facts* (NSC Publication No. ISBN: 0-87912-137-8). Chicago: Author.

O'Malley, K., Born, C., Delong, W., Shaikh, K., & Schwab, C. (1987). A triage tool for trauma center transfer. *Topics in Emergency Medicine*, 9 (1), 71-78.

Orlowski, J. (1989). It's time for pediatricians to "rally 'round the pool fence." *Pediatrics*, 83 (6), 1065-1066.

Orlowski, J. (1988). Adolescent drowning. *Pediatric Annals*, 17 (2), 125-132.

Paulson, J. (1988). The epidemiology of injuries in adolescents. *Pediatric Annals*, 17 (2), 85-96.

Pearl, R., Wesson, D., Spence, L., Filler, R., Sigmund, E., Shandling, B., & Superina, R. (1989). Splenic injury: A 5-year update with improved results and changing criteria for conservative management. *Journal of Pediatric Surgery*, 24 (5), 428-431.

Peclet, M., Newman, K., Eichelberger, M., Gotschall, S., Guzzetta, P., Anderson, V., Randolph, J., & Bowman, L. (1990). Patterns of injury in children. *Journal of Pediatric Surgery*, 25 (3), 85-91.

Ramenofsky, M., Ramenofsky, M., Jurkovich, G., Threadgill, D., Dierking, B., & Powell, R. (1988). The predictive validity of the pediatric trauma score. *Journal of Trauma*, 28 (7), 1038-1042.

Rivara, F. (1988). Motor vehicles injuries during adolescence. *Pediatric Annals*, 17 (2), 107-113.

Rosetti, V., Thompson, B., Aprahamian, C., Darin, J., & Mateer, J. (1984). Difficulty and delay in intravascular access in pediatric arrests (UAEM Abstracts). *Annals of Emergency Medicine*, 13, 406.

Schwaitzberg, S., & Harris, B. (1987). The epidemiology of pediatric trauma. *Emergency Care Quarterly*, 3 (1), 1-6.

Seidel, J., Hornbeim, K., Kuznets, D., Finklestein, J., & St. Geme, J. (1984). Emergency medical services and the pediatric patient: Are their needs being met? *Pediatrics*, 73 (6), 769-772.

Seidel, S., & Henderson, D. (Eds.). (1991). Emergency medical services for children. Washington: National Center for Education in Maternal and Child Health.

Simon, J. (1988, June). *Severe head injury.* Paper presented at the meeting for Pediatric Emergencies, Williamsburg, VA.

Staff, (1988, July). Parents underestimate dangers of preventable childhood injuries. *Emergency Medicine and Ambulatory Care News*, p. 12.

Syverud, S., Borron, S., Storer, D., Hedges, J., Dronen, S., Braunstein, L., & Hubbard, B. (1988). Prehospital use of neuromuscular blocking agents in a helicopter ambulance program. *Annals of Emergency Medicine*, 17 (3), 236-242.

Tepas, J., Mollitt, D., & Talbert, J. (1987). The pediatric trauma score as a predictor of injury severity in the injured child. *Journal of Trauma*, 22, 14-18.

Thompson, R., Frederick, T., Rivara, F., & Thompson, D. (1989). A case-control study of the effectiveness of bicycle safety helmets. *New England Journal of Medicine*, 320 (21), 1361-1367.

Tocantins, L. (1940). Rapid absorption of substances into the bone marrow. *Proceedings of the Society for Experimental Biology and Medicine*, 45, 292-296.

Trott, A. (1985). *Minor wound care.* New York: Medical Examination Publishing Co.

Trunkey, D. (1988). Trauma care at mid-passage: A personal viewpoint. *Journal of Trauma*, 28 (7), 889-895.

Tsai, A., & Kallsen, G. (1987). Epidemiology of pediatric prehospital care. *Annals of Emergency Medicine*, 3, 284-292.

Walker, M., Storr, B., & Mayer, T. (1984). Factors affecting outcome in the pediatric patient with multiple trauma. *Child's Brain*, 11, 387-397.

Wilson, M. (1983-1985). Childhood injury control. *Pediatrician*, 12, 20-27.

Winn, D., Agran, P., & Castillo, D. (1991). Pedestrian injuries to children younger than 5 years of age. *Pediatrics*, 88 (4), 776-782.

Wong, D., & Whaley, L. (1990). *Clinical manual of pediatric nursing (3rd ed.).* St. Louis: Mosby–Year Book, Inc.

Zorludemir, U., Ergoren, Y., Yucesan, S., & Olcay, I. (1988). Mortality due to trauma in childhood. *Journal of Trauma*, 28 (5), 669-671.

18 *Trauma in the Elderly*

Rodney Newman

OBJECTIVES

❑ Discuss the significant impact that trauma in the elderly patient has on healthcare resources.

❑ Identify the physiologic changes that occur in aging patients that may affect their survival after trauma.

❑ Recognize the need of aggressive care for the elderly trauma patient in the prehospital setting, the emergency department, and the intensive care unit.

❑ Describe the pathophysiology of multisystems organ failure that may occur in the elderly trauma patient.

❑ Develop a systematic assessment for identifying complications and the complex response the elderly patient may have to trauma.

INTRODUCTION Trauma is a major catastrophic event in the elderly population. This segment of the community, those over 60 years of age, currently represents 11% of the U.S. population (Horst, Farouck, Sorensen, & Bivins, 1986). It is estimated that the elderly population will increase more than 18% by 1996 (Fisher & Miles, 1986) and 50% by the year 2025 (U.S. Bureau of the Census, 1976). Trauma is the fourth leading cause of death in people older than 55 years and the fifth leading cause in people older than 75 years (Cancer Statistics, 1984).

CASE STUDY A 68-year-old woman fell down a flight of stairs in her home. She had severe right hip pain and lay on the floor for approximately 16 hours before a neighbor found her. Her skin was cool, clammy, & pale, and she responded only slightly to stimuli. In the emergency department (ED), the patient is quickly evaluated and found to be hypotensive. The ED nurse auscultates a blood pressure of 80/65, palpates a heart rate of 116, and observes a respiratory rate of 36. Capillary refill is prolonged, temperature is 35.4° C, and the lower extremities are mottled. Marked skin tenting is demonstrated, and the patient's mucous membranes are dry. Her level of consciousness (LOC) is diminished, and she responds

only when the trauma nurse manipulates the patient's right leg. The right leg is shortened and externally rotated.

Oxygen is quickly started by mask at 8 L/minute. Multiple large-bore intravenous catheters are placed, and warm fluid resuscitation begins with lactated Ringer's solution. Gradually the patient's LOC and vital signs improve. Arterial blood gas values and other laboratory data are within acceptable ranges. X-ray films demonstrate a comminuted fracture of the right hip. The patient is taken to the operating room for internal fixation of the fracture. During the procedure, three units of packed red blood cells are given. After surgery she is taken to the intensive care unit (ICU). She recovers uneventfully until the third postoperative day, at which time she develops a low-grade fever, confusion, tachycardia, and dyspnea. Bilateral infiltrates are demonstrated on her chest x-ray film. The dyspnea is accompanied by hypoxemia, demonstrated by a Pao_2 of 50 mm Hg. The patient requires intubation and mechanical ventilation. A pulmonary artery catheter is placed, and the readings indicate that the patient is hemodynamically stable.

Laboratory data reveal a rising creatinine level with decreased urinary output, indicating renal failure. On the eighth day, the bilirubin increases, demonstrating liver dysfunction. The cardiac output and blood pressure begin to fluctuate, requiring pharmacologic support. The surgical incision fails to heal, and skin over the bony prominences breaks down as a result of protein wasting despite total parenteral nutrition (TPN). Even with aggressive medical and nursing care, the patient deteriorates into a comatose state with increasing hemodynamic instability. She dies 21 days after injury.

Does the time delay in receiving care in this case play a major role in the outcome? If so, why?

Time is of the utmost importance when dealing with any trauma patient, especially an elderly patient. Studies have shown that the longer the time lapse from injury to treatment, the higher the incidence of complications (Wilson, 1982). In this case, several major concerns exist. First, a fractured hip results in the loss of 1.5 to 2.5 liters of blood from the fracture (Peltier, 1984). This blood loss may result in hypovolemic shock, yet general dehydration may mask a drop in hematocrit and the tachycardic response may be limited by the aging process or medications.

Second, 16 hours without fluid intake secondary to immobility contributes further to hypovolemia, hypoxemia, inadequate tissue perfusion, and decreased LOC. Because this patient experienced muscle injury, rhabdomyolysis, a breakdown of the muscle myoglobin, may develop, which can affect renal and hepatic function. Time, therefore, was a major determinant to the outcome in this patient.

What is the pathophysiology of this progressive multisystems organ failure (MOF)?

Multisystems organ failure (MOF) is a syndrome that results from an inciting event (e.g., trauma, sepsis, hypotension), followed by a sequential failure of lungs, liver, kidneys, and heart (Cerra, 1988). The pathophysiology is complex and will be discussed in more detail later in this chapter. However, the common factor in MOF seems to be hypoxia. Hypoxia begins a vicious cycle of several mediator systems leading to organ failure. Mediators of the complement system and by-products thromboxane A_2, and by-products of phospholipase result in endothelial injury, increased capillary permeability, third spacing (interstitial edema), and cellular dysfunction. Significant cellular dysfunction results in dysfunctional organs, and death of the patient is the result. The current therapy of MOF is aimed at prevention,

reversal of hypoxia with early and aggressive care, and multisystems support.

What are the primary goals in the initial treatment and care of this patient?

As with other trauma patients, the ABCs (**a**irway, **b**reathing, **c**irculation) apply in the care of the elderly trauma patient, with some important considerations. The airway and breathing must be protected and supported. The respiratory system in the elderly is fragile and requires additional assessment and laboratory data to ensure its proper care (i.e., frequent arterial blood gas (ABG) determinations, an adequate hemoglobin, and oxygen support to maintain the Pao_2 between 60 and 80 mm Hg). Proper pulmonary toilet will help the older patient's lung clear during the trauma crisis. Support of circulation may be difficult because of preexisting diseases, such as congestive heart failure, renal dysfunction, and chronic lung disease. Additional therapeutic guidance with hemodynamic monitoring is essential to ensure optimal filling pressures and to prevent increased workload on the cardiovascular system. Therefore the *sine qua non* of trauma care in the elderly is to (1) optimize all vital functions quickly and accurately and (2) be prepared for rapid, unexpected changes.

TRAUMA SUSCEPTIBILITY

Many researchers have demonstrated that injuries in the elderly are less common than in any other segment of the population. However, the mortality and morbidity are higher than for any other age group with similar injuries (Hogue, 1982; Iskrant & Joliet, 1968; Oreskovich, Howard, & Copass, 1984). Functional limitation status before injury seems to be the primary predictor of mortality. Patients with preexisting functional limitations had a sixfold increase in mortality versus the same-aged patients without limitations (Hansen & Davis, 1991). The Major Trauma Outcome Study (MTOS) reviewed 46,613 major trauma patients and demonstrated that when patients were grouped together by the injury severity scale score and correlated to age, elderly patients had a significantly higher mortality rate than younger patients (Finelli, Jonsson, Champion, Morelli, & Fouty, 1989; Hansen & Davis, 1991) (Table 18-1).

The elderly patient seems to be more prone to injury because of the physiologic changes that oc-

Table 18-1 Relationship of ISS* to mortality

	% Mortality	
ISS range	**Over 65 years**	**Under 65 years**
1-15	3.1	0.4
16-24	15.4	5.5
25-34	48	17.5
35-44	61.1	25.8
45-54	66.7	41.7
over 54	100	88

Note. From "A Control Study for Major Trauma in Geriatric Patients" by F.C. Finelli, J. Jonsson, H.R. Champion, S. Morelli, and W.J. Fouty, 1989, *Journal of Trauma, 29,* p. 545.
*ISS represents the injury severity scale score: the higher the score, the greater the severity of injury.

Table 18-2 Conditions associated with or predisposing to accidents in the elderly

Medical conditions	**Neurologic conditions**
Orthostatic hypotension	Transient ischemic attacks
Osteoarthritis	Seizures
Rheumatoid arthritis	Syncope
Peripheral vascular disease	Parkinson's disease
Cardiac dysrhythmias	Subdural hematoma
Aortic stenosis	Tremors
Hypothyroidism	Neuropathy
Diabetes mellitus	Myelopathy
Nutritional deficiencies	
Generalized debility	

Note. Modified from "Typical Geriatric Accidents and How to Prevent Them" by J.E. Escher, C. O'Dell, & S.R. Gambert, 1989, *Geriatrics, 44*(5), pp. 55 & 66.

cur with age. Decreased visual acuity, hearing loss, slower reaction time, and problems with balance and mobility all play a major role in the elderly sustaining trauma (Escher, O'Dell, & Gambert, 1989) (Table 18-2). Physiologic changes in the elderly will be discussed in more detail later in this chapter.

There seem to be many reasons for the increased mortality. A controversial reason is that of preexisting (before injury) diseases. However, studies have not found a significant correlation between preexisting disease and mortality in the elderly trauma patient (Allen & Schwab, 1985; Oreskovich et al., 1984; Trunkey, Siegel, & Baker, 1983). Shock after trauma has been shown to be a major determinant of survival in all age groups (Linn, 1983). The physiologic changes that occur in the elderly patient may prevent an appropriate response to shock or trauma, thus contributing to a higher mortality. Of elderly patients, 43% develop cardiac and pulmonary complications after shock compared with an insignificant number of complications in younger patients (DeMaria, Pardon, Merriam, Casanova, & Gann, 1987).

Ethics and Finance

Another contributing factor for increased mortality of the elderly trauma patient is age. Age may be inappropriately used as a triage criterion, leading to delays in medical care, thus resulting in increased mortality. Overestimation of surgical risk and underestimation of remaining functional lifespan can result in decisions that the patient is "too old" or at too high a risk for surgery (Keating & Lubin, 1990). Age, in and of itself without regard to functional capacity, has not been shown to be a significant determinant of survival (Bobb, 1987). Each trauma case must be reviewed individually. The practice of denying care strictly because of age is of questionable ethics. Because of today's resource conservation and concern with healthcare dollars, judicious care must be considered in all patients. Many elderly patients contribute much to society and to deny them care based on some predetermined age limit denies society many blessings.

Aside from the higher mortality and morbidity, the increased financial costs of care for the elderly trauma patient as compared with the younger trauma patient must be considered. The elderly patient consumes one third of all healthcare resources expended on trauma care (Finelli et al., 1989; Mueller & Gigson, 1983). This is primarily the result of prolonged hospitalization, treatment of complications, and prolonged rehabilitation and home health care.

It is clear that the care of the elderly trauma patient will be a common need in the future, considering the current growing geriatric population. This will affect the initial resuscitation in the prehospital setting and the ED. The long-term care provided in the intensive care unit (ICU), on the general floor, and in the rehabilitation unit, as well as the care provided by home healthcare agencies, will also be impacted. The nurse must be able to understand the complex needs of the elderly patient created by traumatic injuries to provide the care required to improve patient outcome.

ANATOMIC AND PHYSIOLOGIC CONSIDERATIONS

The human body is capable of growth, movement, repair, maintenance, and reproduction. Far beyond these physical abilities are the mental and psychologic powers that endow each human with its unique personality. As life progresses, the body and mind undergo many changes. These changes can be subtle and may not be recognized except by faltering steps or lapses of memory. The aging of all body systems plays a major role in the survival and recovery of the geriatric trauma patient.

General Appearance

The aging process produces changes that are visually obvious, such as changing body composition, posture, and skin appearance. The proportion of body fat to muscle mass increases. By the age of 75, body fat increases by 16%. This additional fat is stored in the abdomen and hips. The fat content of the arms and legs decreases. Dehydration may be reflected by skin tenting when skin is pinched or elevated over the hands and forearms. Because fat contains less water than muscle, an increase in body fat results in a decrease of total body water by approximately 8% (Jessup, 1984).

Increase in body fat has a profound effect on drug distribution. Drugs may accumulate in fat tissue at concentrations equal to plasma, thus leading to unpredictable drug responses (Matteson, 1988a; Schwertz & Buschmann, 1989). A complicated orchestration of variables, such as body size, body composition, protein content, and fat distribution, leads to the effect drugs have on an elderly patient (see box, upper right).

Caution must be used in administering drugs, especially those with renal or hepatic clearance. Drugs with short elimination half-lives should take precedence or the time between doses prolonged with careful monitoring of effect.

Weight loss in the elderly occurs and results from decreases in nutritional intake caused by decreased appetite and limited resources. Nutritional deficiencies are common in the elderly and may contribute to elderly patients not surviving

---

Changes in drug absorption and distribution associated with aging

- Slower absorption of oral and parenteral drugs
- Slower absorption of suppositories because of decreased blood supply to the rectum
- Slower drug distribution because of the reduction of active and passive transport systems
- Higher drug levels because of:
  —fewer plasma proteins to bind
  —decreased metabolism in the liver
  —decreased body mass and surface area
- Less drug excretion because of decreased renal function

Note. Modified from "Common Pathological Conditions in Elderly Persons: Nursing Assessment and Interventions" by P.A. Kidd & M. Murakami, 1987, *Journal of Emergency Nursing, 13,* p. 334-341.

---

trauma (Dougherty, 1988). Nutritional deficiencies will be discussed later in the chapter.

Posture in the elderly begins to change as calcium is lost from the bone. Spinal osteoporosis is responsible for changes in height and posture. The trunk shortens as the intervertebral spaces narrow. This results in a body position that is stooped forward, with flexion of the knees, hips, and elbows, and a backward-tilting head (Figure 18-1). Such a posture shifts the center of gravity from the hips to the upper torso, affecting balance (Jessup, 1984; Snell, 1980). This contributes to the high incidence of falls in the elderly population (Waller, 1974). Geriatric falls at home account for 48% of blunt injuries and 72% of all fatal falls (DeMaria et al., 1987; Escher et al., 1989). Falls at home have been attributed to deteriorating health before the accident (Bobb, 1987). Thoracic and lumbar vertebral body collapse plus kyphosis of the spine and the accompanying "dowager's hump" can drastically alter posture, safe mobility and patient comfort (see Figure 18-1).

Repeated falls or unexplained injuries may occur in the elderly patient. The nurse must have a high index of suspicion in this type of patient for neglect or abuse (see box, p. 560).

The skin becomes thin and less elastic as a person grows older. Atherosclerosis and other vascular changes result in decreased blood supply to the skin. This leads to retarded cell replacement, and thus healing is reduced. This reduction in

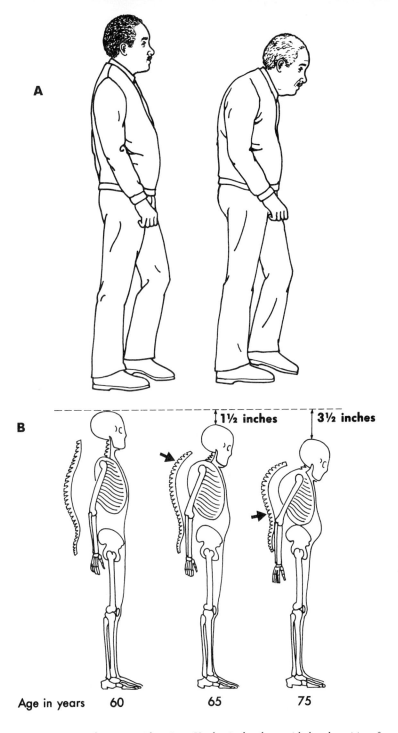

A

B

1½ inches   3½ inches

Age in years   60   65   75

Figure 18-1   **A,** Changes in posture and stance with aging. Kyphosis develops with head position forward of vertical axis, compensatory extension of neck, and forward displacement of scapulae; compression of vertebrae with loss of height; lessening of lordotic lumbar curve; and slight flexion at hips and knees. This shifts center of gravity from hips to thorax, contributing to falls. **B,** Natural history of spinal osteoporosis over time. In early stages of disease, asymptomatic loss of height (1 to 1½ inches) occurs as result of changes in upper thoracic vertebrae *(arrow)*. Later stages of disease are characterized by painful collapse of lower thoracic and lumbar vertebrae, which may account for loss of 2 to 2½ inches per episode. Body height remains stable between collapse fractures. Significant loss of height ceases when costal margins come to rest on iliac crests. (*Note.* **B** redrawn from Long-term observations on aged women with pathologic osteoporosis [p. 20] by M.R. Urist, M.S. Gurvey, and D.O. Fareed. In U.S. Barzel [Ed.], 1970, *Osteoporosis*, New York: Grune & Stratton.)

healing may lead to the formation of decubitus ulcers in the bedridden patient. Friable skin is often evidenced by open abrasions or avulsions from minimal friction during repositioning or even simple tape removal. Retarded cell replacement may impede the healing of surgical incisions, providing an entrance for bacteria and increasing the risk of wound disruption. Increased vascular fragility may produce ecchymosis and blood loss even with minor trauma. The sweat glands decrease in size, number, and function, which leads to dry, fragile skin, decreased perspiration, and a diminished ability to regulate body temperature. Aging not only produces wrinkles, but inhibits the skin's ability to protect the body.

Activity and Mobility

Fractures are common in the older population and take longer to heal because of osteoporosis. When an individual reaches about the age of 40, bone loss begins. Diet, hormonal changes, and physical activity effect this bone loss. Women have a higher percentage of osteoporosis (25%) than men (12%), as a result of hormonal changes during menopause (Jessup, 1984). Osteoporosis is an important yet minimally investigated problem for men. Hypogonadal elderly white men may be at increased risk for low impact hip fractures (Standley, Schmitt, Poses, & Deiss, 1991).

Orthopedic trauma constitutes a large part of the injuries seen in an ED. This is true in the el-

derly patient because of osteoporosis, which results in brittle bones that are easily fractured (Figure 18-2). The outer shell of bones, or cortex, is responsible for support, while the inner, spongy, bone-containing trabeculae serve as sites for bone formation (Matteson, 1988). Trabecular bone loss begins earlier than cortical bone loss. The vertebral bodies, wrists, and hips, have a large amount of trabecular bone; therefore these areas are at greatest risk of fracture with aging (Jowsey, 1977).

The elderly frequently suffer from arthritis, which decreases flexibility of all joints, especially the cervical spine, and may decrease reaction time. The combination of osteoporosis and arthritis can contribute significantly to the likelihood of elderly persons sustaining skeletal trauma. Inability of elderly persons to move out of the way of danger, to look in all directions to see an oncoming vehicle, or to brace themselves from a fall directly contribute to their sustaining fractures, which results in prolonged immobility.

Muscle weakness results from loss of muscle cell mass, a 10% to 20% decrease in motor unit size, and a prolonged conduction time through the motor unit (Jessup, 1984). This decreases strength of the individual, causes fatigue of all muscle groups, and provides little protection to the skeletal frame against trauma. An elderly person is less likely to be able to avoid injury and more likely to fatigue under the stress of trauma. Fatigue results in immobility and subsequent respiratory failure related to the immobility. These changes are not universal for all elderly patients. There is some suggestion that many of these changes may be secondary to a sedentary life-style and not primarily due to the aging process (Phipps, Long, Woods, & Cassmeyer, 1991).

As described, functional status is an important determinant of postinjury outcome. Rating scales to assess functional status have been developed, such as the PULSES profile, which measures general functional performance including **p**hysical condition, **u**pper limb functions, **l**ower limb functions, **s**ensory components, **e**xcretory functions, and **s**upport factors (Granger, Albrecht, & Hamilton, 1979).

Immobility caused by traumatic injuries of the musculoskeletal system and the prolonged recovery from other injuries has many hazards. Each physiologic system becomes stressed. The musculoskeletal system has an accelerated rate of muscle atrophy, loss of strength, contractures, skin break-

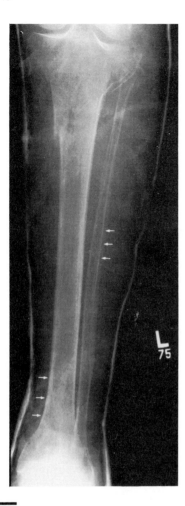

Figure 18-2 Complex proximal tibia-fibula fracture in 78-year-old man struck by car. Note thinning of cortex (*arrows*) and extensive demineralization of bone. (*Note.* From Comorbidity in Geriatric Patients [p. 224] by D.R. Kauder and C.W. Schwab. In K.I. Maull, H.C. Cleveland, G.O. Strauch, and C.C. Wolferth [Eds.], 1990, *Advances in Trauma* [Vol. 5], St. Louis: Mosby-Year Book, Inc.)

down, and osteoporosis. The urinary system suffers because of stasis associated with immobility, which creates such complications as urinary tract stones and infections, imposing additional stress to the kidney. The cardiovascular system may be compromised by venous thrombosis, orthostatic hypotension, and tachycardias. The lungs may develop atelectasis and pneumonia. Furthermore, because of inactivity and isolation, the geriatric patient may experience psychologic deterioration.

Ventilation

Acute respiratory failure is a major complication after trauma in any age group. The physiologic changes that occur in the elderly patient increase susceptibility for the development of respiratory insufficiency. Muscle weakening and rigidity in the thoracic cage result in restricted ventilation and decreased vital capacity. The older patient must expend about 10% more energy on breathing than a younger person because of these changes. An ineffective cough mechanism related to muscle weakness may lead to the retention of pulmonary secretions, resulting in infections. After individuals reach the age of 70, respiratory fluids decrease by 30%, producing tenacious secretions, mucous plugging, and an increased rate of infection (Jessup, 1984). Airway clearance and gas exchange are challenged by the aging process.

A greater risk for aspiration and pneumonia exists because of delayed gastric emptying, decreased lower esophageal sphincter tone, and decreased laryngeal reflexes (Katz & Fagraeus, 1990). Diaphragmatic support of breathing has greater importance in the elderly, which can be aided by positioning, avoiding large meals, and reducing postoperative intraabdominal pressure by special techniques in abdominal cavity closure.

Elderly patients experience changes in the elastin and collagen components of the lung. This causes a decrease in tensile strength, decreased recoil during expiration, smaller alveoli, and thickening of the capillary basement membrane. Apical ventilation increases, and basilar ventilation decreases, resulting in a ventilation/perfusion mismatch (areas of lung being perfused but not ventilated) and a decreasing oxygen tension. An acceptable value of PaO_2 changes dramatically with age, as depicted in Table 18-3 (Shapiro, Harrison, & Walton, 1979). Trauma or surgical stress may impact the pulmonary reserves enough to become a significant problem, resulting in acute respiratory failure.

Perfusion

Physiologic changes that occur with normal aging may be detrimental to the heart during the severe or prolonged stress of trauma. The left ventricle thickens by 25% because of fibrosis, sclerosis, and fatty infiltration of the endocardium and myocardium, resulting in a heart that contracts less forcefully. This is a direct result of decreased left ventricular compliance and a delay in the normal

Table 18-3 Acceptable arterial oxygen tensions at sea level for the elderly breathing room air

Age (years)	Pao$_2$ (mm Hg)
< 60	> 80 (normal 95-97)
60	80
70	70
80	60
90	50

Note. Modified from *Clinical Applications of Blood Gases* (4th ed.) (p. 82) by B.A. Shapiro, R.A. Harrison, R.D. Cane, and R. Kozlowkski-Templin, 1989, Chicago: Mosby–Year Book, Inc.

filling time (Lakatta, 1983; Zamfirescu, 1982). The resting heart rate may not change with age; however, maximal heart rate, stroke volume, and O$_2$ consumption decrease about 1% per year after the age of 20 (Goldman, 1979; Hassock & Bruce, 1982; Kennedy & Caird, 1981). The ejection fraction (the amount of blood pumped by the heart with each contraction) also decreases to less than 60% (Port, 1980). A summary of cardiovascular changes can be seen in Table 18-4.

Aging, therefore, results in a decreased ability to increase heart rate and cardiac output with stress. Coronary blood flow decreases 16% to 35% by the age of 70 years (Lakatta, 1983). The elderly patient may be more prone to myocardial ischemia, infarction, shock, and intraoperative complications. A significant number of elderly patients will have myocardial infarctions without the typical accompanying symptoms (Gottlieb & Gerstenblith, 1988). Often the elderly patient in shock will develop cardiac failure precipitated by a silent myocardial infarction during or shortly after a traumatic event.

"Silent" myocardial infarctions may occur when a person is under anesthesia or awake. Although chest pain usually does accompany myocardial infarction and ischemia in the elderly, it has been shown to be reported less frequently with increasing old age (Bayer et al., 1986; Bell, Dixon, & Sehy, 1991). "Anginal equivalents" (breathlessness, faintness, or extreme fatigue) may be the evidence of myocardial ischemia rather than chest pain, since an increased tolerance to pain exists in many elderly people (Harrel, 1988).

Electrophysiologic changes occur in the heart that delay myocardial repolarization. An increased recovery period may lead to increased irritability and ectopy, which in turn may cause fatal dysrhythmias. The electrocardiogram may display increased wave intervals, amplitude, and a leftward shift in the QRS axis (Bachman, Sparrow, & Smith, 1981). These electrical changes indicate myocardial hypertrophy and a decreased automaticity.

Vascular changes

Arterial elasticity decreases as a result of sclerosis and an increased deposition of calcium in the walls of major arteries. This results in increased peripheral resistance and altered organ blood flow. Systolic blood pressure rises, causing an increased cardiac workload. All vessels become fibrotic and tortuous. The capillary membrane thickens, leading to decreased diffusion of substances between the capillaries and cells (Goldman, 1979).

Blood pressure control may be greatly affected because of the aging process and/or medications. Baroreceptors become less sensitive, and the vascular changes discussed earlier can result in hypertension or orthostatic hypotension. The National High Blood Pressure Education Program (NHBPEP, 1980) reported that 40% of white people and 50% of black people older than 65 years have hypertension. This places the elderly hypertensive patient at high risk for cardiovascular disease and sudden death (Kannel, 1981). Elderly patients are more difficult to assess and treat than younger hypertensive patients.

Orthostatic hypotension may result from chronic diseases, prolonged bedrest, medications, volume depletion, and acute injury (Rowe, 1987). It has also been noted that there is a 50% prevalence of vasovagal reactions causing syncope in the elderly patient. Elderly patients with syncope have decreased norepinephrine levels at the time of the syncopal episode (Hackel, Linzer, Anderson, & Williams, 1991). With advancing age the arterial and cardiac muscles become less responsive to beta-adrenergic stimulation. These changes may blunt the elderly patient's response to exercise, stress, and shock (Yin, 1980).

Hemopoietic system

Hemopoietic activity of the bone marrow decreases by 50% in patients over 60 years of age, as demonstrated in Table 18-5. It was recently noted

Table 18-4 Heart rate, cardiac output, and blood volume changes in the elderly

Parameter	Age (years)						
	20	**30**	**40**	**50**	**60**	**70**	**80**
Maximal heart rate		190	182	174	164	155	146
Resting heart rate		76	72	68	66	62	59
Cardiac index ($l/min/m^2$)	3.5–3.7	3.5	3.0	2.8–3.1	2.6–3.7	2.4–3.6	2.4
blood volume (l/m^2)	2.7			2.6	2.6	2.5	

Note. Modified from "Physiology of Aging of the Heart" by R.D. Kennedy and F.I. Caird, 1981, *Cardiovascular Clinics, 12,* p. 3.
Note. Values include several studies and are means for groups.

Table 18-5 Changes in blood components with age

Component	Change	Implication
Erythrocytes	Reduced	Fatigue
Hemoglobin	Reduced	Fatigue
Hematocrit	Reduced	Fatigue
Leukocytes	Same counts but decreased function	Decreased resistance to infection
Lymphocytes	Reduced	Decreased resistance to infection
Platelets	Increased aggregation	Clotting problems

Note. Modified from *Gerontological Nursing: Concepts and Practices* (p. 195) by M.A. Matteson and E.S. McConnell, 1988, Philadelphia: W.B. Saunders.

that lower erythropoietin (EPO) levels may not be as significant as once thought. When compared with those of younger patients, the EPO levels were not lower if controlled for hematocrit (Powers, Krantz, Collins, & Meurer, 1991). Red blood cell (RBC) mass decreases and the RBCs become less flexible and may not survive as long in the vascular system.

Mild anemia in the elderly is relatively common but has not been shown to be the direct result of the aging process. Rather, it is linked to the effects of chronic disease, dementia, depression, and nutritional deficits. The incidence of anemia is highest in the institutionalized elderly (Clark & Delafuente, 1988). Iron-deficiency anemia is most problematic for the elderly when compared with other anemias with similar hemo-

globin levels, since oxygen transfer to tissues is impacted.

Coagulation abnormalities may become apparent in the elderly patient. Aging increases platelet aggregation and decreases fibrinolytic activity, which may result in deep venous thrombosis (DVT) or cerebral vascular accident (CVA). The potential for bleeding tendencies is greater in the elderly patient because of the many medications taken, including aspirin, ibuprofen, and warfarin (DeNicola & Casale, 1983).

The normal compensatory response to shock is to increase cardiac output by increasing heart rate and stroke volume. The majority of elderly patients cannot compensate, and cardiac output may decrease. There are fewer red blood cells to carry O_2 to the cells, which may precipitate angina, myocardial infarction, stroke, and other organ dysfunction. The normal signs of shock, such as tachycardia, may not be present if the patient is taking beta blocker medications. Shock is also more difficult to treat in the elderly because their response to such treatment measures as vasopressors is less predictable (Cerra, 1988).

Several studies support the benefits of exercise in the elderly patient to improve or delay the effects of aging on the cardiovascular system (Bortz, 1982; Harris, 1983; Larson, 1984). Consistent prior exercise may have a profound positive effect in the elderly patient involved in trauma. Further study is needed.

Sensory and Perception

The elderly brain decreases in size (atrophies) by approximately 7% without a resulting loss of intellectual function. A decrease in cerebral blood flow and oxygen utilization causes loss of cerebral cortex neurons. These structural changes may result in a diminished emotional response, confusion, and a narrowing of interests that were previously pursued, such as hobbies or professional endeavors. Increased levels of monoamine oxidase and serotonin and decreased levels of norepinephrine may be associated with depression in the elderly. Attempted suicide in the elderly population may be associated with depression or lingering illness. The elderly give fewer indications that they are contemplating suicide and tend to be more successful in their attempts than younger patients (Cutter, 1983).

In the elderly patient, injury to the head is common because of elderly patients' loss of balance and slower reaction time to protect themselves during a fall. Subdural hematomas may result from a fall or motor vehicle accident or may occur spontaneously. Health care providers may attribute the typical signs and symptoms of increased intracranial pressure to the process of senility or dementia and an actual injury may be overlooked. Any elderly patient presenting with increased drowsiness, confusion, and cognitive impairment should be assessed for a subdural hematoma or other neurosurgical emergencies. Delays in surgical intervention to remove the hematoma may have disastrous results.

In the shock state with an insufficient mean arterial pressure (MAP), less blood is delivered to the brain, which may cause an increase in cerebral dysfunction and anoxic encephalopathy. Assessment of the patient's level of consciousness (considering possible preexisting senility, dementia, or Alzheimer's disease) becomes very difficult. The MAP must be within normal limits to adequately perfuse the brain and prevent cerebral dysfunction, especially in the presence of arteriosclerosis.

Psychologic changes also occur that may affect the geriatric patient's recovery from trauma. Posttraumatic stress disorder (PTSD) may occur with any trauma patient. The PTSD is characterized by recurrent nightmares, intrusive thoughts, or flashbacks of the traumatic event. After an acute phase that includes anxiety symptoms, the patient will tend to become depressed and somatic symptoms may appear. Unfortunately PTSD may affect the elderly patient more severely because of limited social support systems. Many older patients are widowed and "don't want to be a burden" on their children and do not seek their family's help (Figley, Scrignar, & Smith, 1988).

Mental status in the elderly is a complex issue. Terminology is variable, such as dementia, ICU psychosis, "sundowner's" syndrome, and acute confusion, but specific definitions can be found in the *Diagnostic and Statistical Manual III* (APA, 1987), which is used routinely by psychiatric health professionals. Of most importance is to focus on helping to determine whether the disturbance or change in behavior is acute or progressive in onset and whether it is organic or psychologic in nature. A person can be oriented to person, place, and time and yet be acutely confused, thus requiring a more detailed mental status examination (Kroeger, 1991). Attention, speech, mood and affect, thought processes and content, judgment, insight, and memory should be evaluated. Trends in findings are most helpful, and any organic cause must be identified and treated. Arranging activities of daily living on a schedule similar to the patient's home schedule, allowing visitation and personal items, providing activity during waking hours, reviewing medication lists with pharmacy, frequently checking and interacting with patients, and using restraint only as needed should help to minimize negative consequences of confusion.

Thermoregulation

The older person's ability to regulate body heat production and heat loss is altered. The actual role of the hypothalamus and hormonal action of thermal regulation is not fully known. The first factor in heat production is glucose metabolism in the muscle, which produces heat. An elderly person with less body muscle mass cannot produce adequate amounts of heat from the metabolic processes within the muscle. Even though the elderly patient may have an increased amount of body fat, conservation of heat is inadequate. This may also be caused by hypothyroidism and a decreased metabolic rate, as described in the endocrine section of this chapter. Second, the body normally regulates heat through the vasoconstriction or dilation of blood vessels within the subcutaneous fat and skin. Because the elderly patient has significant changes in the blood vessels and how they respond to stimuli, heat regulation may become a problem.

This may explain why the elderly patient responds to infection with hypothermia instead of hyperthermia. Temperatures may vary from standard normals as much as 3° F in the elderly population. Therefore the most appropriate action is to establish a norm for each patient and assess the trend (Castle, Norman, Yeh, Miller, & Yoshikawa, 1991; Darowski, Najim, Weingerg, & Guz, 1991; Thatcher, 1983).

Nutrition

The gastrointestinal tract rarely deteriorates in the elderly patient and even in diseased conditions can still sustain life. However, elderly patients may have many variables affecting their nutritional intake. Appetite, economic status, proximity to the grocery store, and an inability to prepare the food all play a role in patients' nutritional status (Matteson, 1988a).

Gastrointestinal (GI) motility and secretion of digestive juices decrease. The mucosa of the GI tract also begins to atrophy. Because of atrophy of the gastric mucosa, the lack of hydrochloric acid, and a diminished supply of the intrinsic factor for vitamin B_{12} absorption, pernicious anemia may develop, leading to anemia and a decreased O_2-carrying capacity. When these problems occur, they may complicate the recovery of the elderly patient from trauma.

Upper gastrointestinal (UGI) bleeding is a growing problem in elderly patients. They have a higher complication rate with UGI bleeding than their younger counterparts. Relapse bleeding is higher—about 60% to 90% rebleeding in the first year. The main risk factors for the elderly developing UGI bleeds are high use of non-steroid antiinflammatory drugs, genetic disposition, smoking, and Heliobacter pylori infections of the stomach. Several studies are now in progress to control H. pylori infections to reduce UGI bleeding in the elderly (Miller, Burton, Burton, & Ireland, 1991; O'Riordin, Tobin, & O'Murain, 1991).

Also, a direct correlation exists between dysfunction in protein synthesis, enzyme production, and hormone synthesis and a poor nutritional status (Cerra, 1987). Poor ventilation can result from poor nutrition, leading to further complications (Arora, Dudley, & Rochester, 1982; Hunter, Carey, & Lash, 1981). This results from inadequate substrate delivery to the muscles of respiration. Diminished respiratory muscle contraction and muscle fatigue develop, and respira-

tory failure is the end result (Ingersol, 1989). Malnutrition also retards wound healing as a result of diminished or altered protein synthesis and a negative nitrogen balance. In the elderly this has greater meaning because of general reduction in cell generation.

In the adult patient the glycogen reserve is approximately 1200 to 1600 calories. The glycogen reserve is usually the body's energy source for 2 to 6 hours after eating and is depleted within 12 to 24 hours (Dougherty, 1988). If a person does not eat after a 12- to 24-hour fast, the body will switch to fat metabolism to produce glucose, or gluconeogenesis. The by-products of lipolysis are ketones and other acids, which may stress renal function. In-patient "fasts" must be avoided or limited by early institution of nutritional support.

Diverticulitis may be a devastating complication of the high stress of trauma in the elderly. Inflammation of one or more diverticuli occurs in 20% to 40% of nonstressed patients with diverticulosis. Diverticulosis, an endemic and virtually epidemic condition in aging America, may be exacerbated by the stress of trauma. Complications of diverticulitis may include bowel obstruction, hemorrhage, fistula formation, and sepsis. A sequel to diverticulitis is perforation and intraabdominal sepsis (Counselman, 1988).

Fluid Volume and Electrolyte Status

Function of the aging kidney declines steadily. Between the ages of 40 and 90, 50% of the renal function is lost (Hollenberg, Adams, & Solomon, 1974). This progressive loss of functional nephrons and decreased renal cell growth is the result of several factors: a 53% loss of renal blood flow, a falling glomerular filtration rate, and increased hyalinization of the tubules. This may lead to a "washout phenomenon" that contributes to the inability of the aged to concentrate urine. This is demonstrated by a decreased urine specific gravity and osmolality (Rowe, Shock, & DeFronzo, 1976). Older patients, presumably because of excess secretion of antidiuretic hormone (ADH), may experience a 20% decrease in free water clearance and may develop hyponatremia with intravenous hydration (Sunderam & Mankikar, 1983). Impaired renal responsiveness to ADH levels places the patient at risk for hypernatremia when water deprived (Beck, 1990).

Potassium abnormalities may also develop in

the elderly because of decreased renin/angiotensin levels (Lonergan, 1988). During the stress of trauma, low mean arterial pressure (MAP) causes the kidney to release large amounts of renin. Renin is converted in several steps to angiotensin, a powerful vasoconstrictor and a stimulator of aldosterone. Aldosterone affects the kidney's ability to excrete potassium. Because the renin response in the elderly is blunted, potassium levels may elevate to lethal extremes.

The renal excretion of drugs is also impacted by the changes in kidney function. Although glomerular filtration rate declines with age, the serum creatinine concentration remains normal, since lean muscle mass decreases with age. Use of this serum value to determine renal function or to gauge medication dosages is erroneous. For clinical management, calculation of the creatinine clearance is important. A common formula is (Cockcroft & Gault, 1976; Yurick, Spier, Robb, Ebert, & Magnussen, 1989):

$$\frac{(140 - \text{age}) \times \text{lean body weight in kg}}{72 \times \text{serum creatinine level}}$$

Acid-base problems take longer to correct secondary to impaired renal function and the decreased clearance of many drugs. Subsequently, drug reactions are more common among the elderly. The renal function of older patients is also more vulnerable to insults by such pharmacologic therapies as dopamine, epinephrine, and nephrotoxic antibiotics (Ouslander, 1981; Tinetti, 1983). Evaluation of new drugs such as the monobactam antibiotic *aztreonam* as an alternative to aminoglycosides is indicated in the elderly at higher risk for toxicity (Beam, 1989).

Endocrine and Immunocompetence

Many changes in the endocrine system occur with aging. These changes are related to the amount or rate of secretion of the hormone and the response of the target organ. The pituitary gland, called the *master gland*, suffers a decreased blood supply and fibrosis develops. However, no documented changes in the concentrations of adrenocorticotropic hormone, thyroid-stimulating hormone, growth hormone, or the luteinizing hormone have been published.

The thyroid gland undergoes fibrosis. The triiodothyronine (T_3) levels decrease 25% to 40%

but thyroxine (T_4) levels are unchanged. A corresponding decrease occurs in the basal metabolic rate. The pancreas becomes less sensitive to glucose levels, resulting in glucose intolerance and hyperglycemia. This is extenuated in the shock state, caused by catecholamines released with stress or infused during treatment.

Little research has been done to study the changes in the endocrine system in trauma and even less in the elderly patient involved in trauma. Many studies are beginning to show the effects of shock on the cell, but the role of the endocrine system is still a mystery (Chernow et al., 1986; Cleamons, Chaudry, & Daigneau, 1984). This area needs further study. The endocrine system controls many body functions. Considering that all other systems in the elderly patient are at less than optimal function, it is logical to think that endocrine dysfunction in the elderly trauma patient may have detrimental effects.

The defensive, homeostatic system of the body undergoes progressive degeneration, resulting in an inability to fight infections. White blood cell numbers do not change except for a decrease in the total percentage of lymphocytes and their overall function. This may lead to a decreased resistance to infections (DeNicola & Casale, 1983). An older patient has a decreased concentration of natural antibodies to fight common infections. Yet, an increase in autoantibodies may cause a higher incidence of autoimmune problems. The immune system does not respond to antigens and other mediators as readily because of cellular and hormonal immunosuppression. The occurrence of sepsis has been reported as high as 41%. Sepsis has been associated with a 50% mortality in elderly trauma patients (Horst et al., 1986). Sepsis results from lymphocyte/macrophage dysfunction occurring several days after traumatic insult (see box on p. 567).

The elderly patient may also exhibit atypical symptoms of infections, such as hypothermia, confusion, immobility, or other organ dysfunction not directly associated with the infection. Infections are common in the older patient and sometimes difficult to diagnose and treat. Therefore care must be taken to prevent the entrance of bacteria into the body by using meticulous sterile technique in the elderly trauma patient. Table 18-6 reviews the primary changes that occur in the body systems with the aging process.

Conditions that may predispose elderly persons to infections

Underlying chronic diseases
Impaired organ function
Acute illness
Nutritional deficiencies
- vitamin
- mineral
- protein
- caloric
Dehydration
Use of certain medications
- steroids
- non-steroid antiinflammatories
Stress
Immobility
Environmental exposure to pathogens
Urinary retention

Incontinence
- urinary
- fecal
Invasive procedures
Skin thinning and slow healing
Decreased pulmonary clearance
Increased microbial colonization
Diminished saliva production
Reduced esophageal motility
Impaired febrile response
Circulatory insufficiency
Depression
Impaired mentation
Impaired immunity
Decreased gag reflex, decreased gastric emptying, lower esophageal sphincter tone and laryngeal reflexes

Note. Adapted from "Immunologic Impairment, Infection, and AIDS in the Aging Patient" by F.L. Cohen, 1989, *Critical Care Nursing Quarterly, 12*(1), p. 41.

Table 18-6 Primary physiologic changes in the elderly

Body system	Change	Body system	Change
Skin	Loss of subcutaneous tissue Decreased sebaceous secretions Thinning hair	Liver	Decreased drug metabolism Decreased protein synthesis
Muscular	Increased fat substitution for muscle Muscle atrophy	Gastrointestinal	Decreased digestive enzymes Decreased absorption and mobility
Skeletal	Loss of calcium from bones Shrinkage of vertebral disks Deterioration of cartilage	Endocrine	Decreased utilization of insulin Cessation of progesterone Decline of estrogen Decline in testosterone
Pulmonary	Reduced chest wall compliance Decreased vital capacity Increased residual volume Reduced cough reflex Reduced ciliary action Decreased lung recoil Decreased diffusion capacity	Vision	Decreased ability to focus Loss of color sensitivity Decreased dark adaptation Decreased peripheral vision Increased sensitivity to glare Increased incidence of retinal detachment
Cardiac	Endocardial thickening Decreased cardiac output Increased atherosclerosis Orthostatic hypotension	Hearing	Difficulty in speech discrimination Degeneration of auditory pathways
Renal	Decreased renal blood flow Decreased glomerular filtration rate Decreased creatinine clearance	Immunological	Decreased resistance to infection More susceptible to autoimmune disease

Note. Modified from *Clinical Geriatrics* by I. Rossman, 1972, Philadelphia: J.B. Lippincott.

The physiologic changes of old age slowly begin to upset the homeostatic integration of all systems in the body. These changes are usually tolerated because of a corresponding decrease in an older person's activity level. The insult of trauma pushes the compensatory mechanisms of all patients to the limit. A young patient has multiple reserves to meet the metabolic demands of trauma, but the adaptive mechanisms of the elderly often are pushed beyond their reserves. The result is that with minimal trauma the elderly patient may develop multiple organ failure leading to death.

GENERAL ASSESSMENT

The assessment of the elderly trauma patient is not unlike the normal trauma assessment. The differences will reflect the limited reserves of the elderly patient to compensate for the increased stress of the traumatic insult. The primary survey must assess and identify life-threatening problems.

Airway

The airway must be managed. The oral airway must be cleared and dentures removed. Many elderly patients have dentures, which may obstruct the airway if they fall out of place. Frequent assessment for equal bilateral breath sounds is mandatory. It should be remembered that fractures of the spinal column are common with the elderly trauma patient (Bryson, Warren, Schedhlem, Mumford, & Lenaghan 1987). The spine must be stabilized until spinal fractures are ruled out by radiologic examination. Radiographic clearance is often more difficult in the elderly because of degenerative changes. Care must be taken during cervical spine immobilization with regard to postural changes of aging. Excessive hyperextension has contributed to problems with airway management.

Breathing

The adequacy of ventilation must be assessed. A normal tidal volume (V_T) is approximately 5 ml/kg. During stress the respiratory rate increases, and V_T increases to 10 to 15 ml/kg. The elderly patient with a decreased functional residual capacity (FRC) and weaker respiratory muscles may not be able to move air in and out of the lungs. This leads to hypoventilation and eventually respiratory failure. Breath sounds, chest excursion, and respiratory effort must be assessed frequently.

Crackles and wheezes are important to assess because they may indicate (1) early fluid overload during fluid resuscitation or (2) congestive heart failure. Diminished breath sounds in the bases may be common. Chest wall integrity must be assessed for injury, which may cause a decrease in respiratory function. Rib fractures are seen frequently in the older trauma patient even with minimal chest injuries. Fractured ribs may increase the risk of pneumothorax and are often associated with underlying contusion.

The angle of the ribs should be examined. Chronic lung disease may first present itself by the ribs becoming horizontal as lung volumes increase and the anterior/posterior ratio of the chest becomes 1:1. Oxygen support is extremely important to ensure proper oxygenation. ABGs should be obtained frequently to check PaO_2, O_2 saturation, and O_2 content. Pulse oximetry has been used successfully in many critically ill patients to monitor oxygenation. Several studies have used the oximeter in an elderly population with good correlation with arterial blood gases (Palve & Vuori, 1989).

Circulation

Circulation must be assessed and red cell mass restored to ensure optimal O_2 carrying abilities. Blood pressure and mean arterial pressure must be monitored. The MAP should be kept above 70 mm Hg to ensure perfusion of the kidney. A BP of 120/64 may be significantly low for a patient with atherosclerosis and hypertensive disease. Assessment of urinary output is a good indicator of perfusion. Normal urine output in the elderly should be maintained at approximately 0.3-0.5 ml/kg/hr. Attempting to maintain a greater urine output may result in fluid overload and the start of a cyclic need for diuretics followed by volume expansion. Fluid boluses rather than hourly intravenous rate increases are encouraged (Cohen, 1990).

The elderly patient cannot tolerate a prolonged shock state. With the higher incidence of atherosclerosis in the older patient, acute myocardial infarction can occur. The ECG must be monitored to enable prompt treatment of dysrhythmias. Knowledge of patients' baseline rhythm from past medical history may be helpful. During fluid resuscitation, a central intravenous line provides the ability to obtain central venous pressure (CVP) readings, which should be maintained between 6 to 8 cm H_2O to ensure adequate fluid resuscitation.

The CVP may be elevated if a patient has pulmonary hypertension or chronic pulmonary disease, which is common in the elderly population. Congestive heart failure must also be aggressively assessed for, prevented, and treated. Auscultation for crackles and wheezes and an S_3 heart sound is important. A pulmonary artery catheter if often necessary to assess the older patient correctly.

Disability

A rapid neurologic examination is now conducted. The level of consciousness (LOC) is a very sensitive indicator of cerebral blood flow. A decrease in the LOC may indicate poor brain perfusion, increasing intracranial pressure, or occurrence of a cerebral vascular accident in the elderly patient. An arterial line should be inserted to monitor MAP to ensure adequate perfusion pressure to the brain. A baseline neurologic history is invaluable and should be obtained from the family. Spinal cord function can be assessed quickly if the patient can move all extremities. The spinal cord must be protected until all vertebrae are x-rayed. Confusion and depressed cognitive abilities should alert the trauma nurse of the possibility of a subdural hematoma. Because of brain atrophy and the fragility of cerebral blood vessels, bleeding may occur with minimal trauma. An early computerized tomography (CT) scan may decrease the 70% mortality associated with elderly patients with subdural hematomas. In the process of exposing the patient to assess and institute therapy, special attention is required to prevent heat loss.

Secondary Survey

After the primary survey and initial resuscitation is conducted, a detailed head-to-toe assessment and history can be completed. A history can reveal useful information, such as previous medical problems, medications being taken, and significant events occuring before the accident. For example, a patient may have been experiencing chest pain before losing control of his or her car and crashing into a tree. This will alter therapy considerably. Attention should be paid to finding medical information cards or bracelets.

Additional laboratory work is indicated in the elderly trauma patient that may not be done initially on a younger patient. Electrolytes, especially potassium, magnesium, calcium, and phosphate levels, should be obtained. These electrolytes have been associated with cardiac dysrhythmias and sudden death. Creatinine and blood urea nitrogen (BUN) levels will help to assess renal function, which may already be compromised because of the aging process. Serial liver and cardiac enzymes may be important to follow in the elderly patient after trauma.

Tissue integrity

The development of pressure sores is a complication in the care of a trauma patient. The elderly are at high risk because of skin, subcutaneous tissue, and muscle changes with age. Both extrinsic factors (e.g., friction, moisture, pressure) and intrinsic factors (limited mobility, suboptimal nutrition, use of traction for fractures, altered mental status, incontinence) contribute to the potential for decubiti (Stone, 1991). Pressure points vary, depending on the patient's position—supine, lateral, or sitting. Direct compression of bone, muscle, subcutaneous fat, and the dermal layer of the skin eventually destroys tissue in all these layers, creating a cone-shaped pressure gradient that is widest within the fat and muscle and narrow at the skin surface initially. Shearing forces cause the loose superficial fascia to slide against the firmly attached deep fascia, damaging vessels within. Tissue necrosis develops with a wide base.

Prevention starts with identifying patients at risk and assuring consistent, careful examination of the skin for evidence of compressive or shearing forces. It is especially important to document all abrasions and wounds after the traumatic injury and monitor their healing, as well as common pressure points. Special assessment tools (such as the Norton scale, which assesses physical condition, mental state, activity, mobility, incontinence, and a list of high-risk medical diagnoses and laboratory abnormalities) allow identification of high-risk patients who would benefit from high-risk prevention measures. These include air support/kinetic beds, special boots, and prominent bone protectors and extensive use of mobility aids with the assistance of physical and occupational therapy.

GENERAL INTERVENTIONS

The existing research and treatment modalities for traumatic injuries are based on a younger patient population. It is conceivable that what is effective for the young may not be effective for the old (Bobb, 1987).

Support of Ventilation and Perfusion

Basic resuscitative efforts apply. Establishment of an airway, proper ventilation, and maintenance of circulation and vascular pressure are still extremely important. However, the degree of aggressiveness, especially in the use of invasive techniques, may vary. It is better to be aggressive with therapy and monitoring too soon than to do too little too late. Care can always be reduced but may not be beneficial late in the course of therapy. Little data is available on the treatment of the elderly trauma patient. The elderly may benefit by aggressive restoration of red blood cell mass, maintaining a higher hematocrit than that tolerated for young patients (Horst et al., 1986). This is logical when considering that hypoxemia may be the key factor in multiple organ failure (Shoemaker, 1987) and that the normal physiologic changes of aging may cause any degree of hypoxia to be detrimental. By increasing the red blood cell mass during times of traumatic shock, it is theorized that more oxygen will be transported to the cell, thus preventing tissue hypoxia.

The resuscitative therapies outlined in other chapters of this book apply and should be followed. Research must be conducted to optimize the care delivered to the elderly patient who has sustained trauma. The care must be directed toward the normalization of physiologic parameters, and aggressive monitoring should be used to follow therapy in the elderly patient to prevent complications of resuscitation, such as congestive heart failure (CHF).

Supporting and maintaining oxygen transport has been discussed in other sections of this book. An optimized cardiac preload, a maximized cardiac output, and an adequate hemoglobin level will ensure oxygen transportation to the cell. Vascular compliance may need to be manipulated with vasodilators or vasopressors to maximize tissue perfusion.

Prevention of Infection

Multisystems organ failure resulting from trauma must be treated in an aggressive manner. Decreased perfusion caused by hypovolemic, cardiogenic, or septic complications must be corrected. Hemodynamic monitoring is essential in preventing hypervolemia and in assessing adequate restoration of fluids. Infection must be treated with judicial use of antibiotics and surgical drainage whenever possible. Prevention of infection must be foremost in the nurse's mind. Sterile care of intravascular catheters, sterile suctioning, implementing skin care, and monitoring for infection are all critical interventions.

Early mobilization has been demonstrated to reduce many complications of trauma and should be accomplished as soon as the patient is hemodynamically and neurologically stable (Border, 1988). This may include taking patients to surgery earlier, immobilizing fractures, and using tilt tables, cardiac chairs, or any other device that maintains stability yet gets the patient out of the supine position.

Nutritional Support

Metabolic support with nutrition is essential. Nutritional problems occur because of the body's inability to either obtain or utilize the substrates of glucose, free fatty acids, or amino acids. Nutrition will improve healing, supply energy, and improve the immunologic defenses of the body. Careful monitoring at the bedside to prevent hyperglycemia or hypoglycemia will prevent many problems for the critically ill elderly patient (Newman, 1988). Abnormal glucose metabolism can alter healing, metabolic function, and neurologic status. This is important when dealing with an older patient who may already be malnourished.

The actual caloric needs of the elderly trauma or critically ill patient are not known. Research is underway to establish the nutritional requirements of the elderly patient. It is important to follow weight changes in the elderly patient. A change of 5% in the past month or 10% in the past 6 months may indicate nutritional risk. Low protein is also a significant risk factor; serum albumin of less than 3.5 g suggests visceral protein depletion. Nutritional support should be started early and aggressively maintained to establish a 3

Types of abuse

Physical abuse
This type of abuse is mandated by law to be reported:

- direct physical harm, including shoving, pushing, hitting, shaking, and hair-pulling
- lack of medical care or overmedication
- sexual exploitation
- unreasonable physical constraint
- prolonged deprivation of food or water

Financial abuse

- theft
- misuse of funds or property
- extortion
- duress
- fraud

Emotional (psychologic) abuse

- verbal assaults
- threats
- creating fear
- isolation
- withholding emotional support

Violation of rights

- coercion
- locking up
- abandonment
- forced removal from home or forced entry into a nursing home (excluding clients viewed by the court or mental health law to be gravely disabled and in need of such placement)

Neglect (denial of basic needs)

- failure to provide food
- failure to provide clothing
- failure to provide shelter
- failure to provide for health and safety
- failure to provide for medical care

Self-neglect

Note. From Elder Abuse Task Force of Santa Clara County. (1987). *Elder Abuse: Guidelines for Professional Assessment and Reporting* (pp. 1-18). Author.

---

to 5 g/dl positive nitrogen balance (Champagne & Ashley, 1989).

Potential for Abuse or Neglect

Elder abuse has been estimated to occur annually in 4% of the U.S. elderly population (U.S. House of Representatives Select Committee on Aging, 1981). One million cases is astounding, yet only one in six cases is believed to be reported to authorities. It is important that the various types of elder abuse are understood. The box above lists examples of physical, financial, and emotional abuse, as well as violation of rights, neglect, and self-neglect. Also, specific indicators are listed in the box on pp. 572-574 to assist in identifying possible incidents of abuse, neglect, mistreatment, and exploitation. Physicians should also be encouraged to list elder abuse or "other adult abuse" as the primary etiologic diagnosis at discharge to spur proper investigation and interven-

tion and to develop a base to determine occurrence rates (Appleton, 1988). Awareness of local adult protective statutes should assure that health professionals have the appropriate forms and are aware of referral/reporting policies. One study found that a majority of patients presenting to an ED and diagnosed with abuse did not initially complain of abuse (Jones, Dougherty, Schelble, & Cunningham, 1988). A hospital-based screening protocol to assist in detection of elder abuse may be extremely useful. Figure 18-3 shows one example, which includes sections for medical and psychosocial history, physical assessment, and diagnostics.

Many significant and specific nursing problems must be considered to assess, monitor, and care for the older patient with traumatic injuries. These problems will be outlined by each physiologic system, addressing the important nursing diagnoses and nursing interventions in the table on pp. 579-583.

Indicators for determining abuse

The following are indicators that should be considered to determine whether each type of abuse may be present. These are warning signs to alert you to the possibility of abuse. Further assessment and documentation are necessary to determine whether there is actual abuse, as some indicators may be present without the existence of abuse. See the following section for assistance with assessment and documentation.

Indicators provided for these areas:
1. Quality of family/caregiver involvement indicators
2. Physical abuse indicators
3. Financial abuse indicators
4. Emotional (psychologic) abuse
5. Rights violations indicators
6. Neglect indicators

1. Quality of family and caregiver involvement as an indicator

There are many behavioral responses that the caregiver (suspected abuser) may exhibit. These responses may give you significant information as to the possibility of abuse.

- The older person may not be given the opportunity to speak for him or herself, or to see others without the presence of the caregiver (who may be a suspected abuser).
- Caregiver may appear under stress, may look pressured, show frustration, anger, or sadness.
- The family member or caregiver "blames" the elderly person (e.g., accusation that incontinence is a deliberate act).
- There is a problem with alcohol, drugs, or medications.
- Flirtations, coyness, etc., indicate the possibility of an inappropriate sexual relationship.
- There is aggressive behavior (threats, insults, harassment or threatening gestures).
- There is previous history of abuse to others (e.g., children, spouse).
- Caregiver was abused as a child, or accepts violence as a way of life.

- Caregiver exhibits tendency toward unpredictable behavior.
- There may be unrealistic beliefs based on promises made previously (e.g., that at all costs they should keep the elder at home).
- There is social isolation of family, or isolation or restriction of activity of the older person within the family unit (e.g., denying the need for social interaction).
- Lack of close family ties are evident.
- Security and affection is withheld or is nonexistent.
- There may be an obvious absence of assistance, questionable attitude, indifference or anger towards the dependent person.
- The caregiver appears unable to understand care needs or shows poor judgment.
- There are conflicting accounts of incidents by the family, neighbors, or person interviewed.
- There is an unwillingness or reluctance to comply with service providers in planning for care and implementation.

2. Physical abuse indicators

The following indicators do not signify physical abuse or neglect per se. They can be clues, however, and thus helpful in assessing the client's situation. The physical assessment of abuse should be done by a physician or other trained professional.

- Any injury incompatible with explanation
- Injury that is not being cared for properly
- Cuts, pinch marks, scratches, lacerations, or puncture marks
- Bruises, welts, or discolorations
  - bilaterally on upper arms
  - clustered on trunk, but may be evident over any area of body
  - presence of old and new bruises at the same time

  - unexplained bruises/welts in various stages of healing
  - injury reflects shape of article used to inflict injury (electric cord, belt buckle)
  - injuries are sometimes hidden under the breasts or on other areas of the body normally covered by clothing
- Dehydration and/or malnourishment without illness-related cause; loss of weight
- Pallor
- Sunken eyes, cheeks
- Evidence of inadequate or inappropriate administration of medication
- Eye injury
- Torn, stained, bloody underclothing

Note. Modified from Elder Abuse Task Force of Santa Clara County. (1987). *Elder Abuse: Guidelines for Professional Assessment and Reporting* (pp. 1-18). Author. Adapted in part from San Francisco Elder Abuse Prevention Task Force and the Monterey County Departments of Health and Social Services.

2. Physical abuse indicators—cont'd

- Bruises, swelling or bleeding in external genitalia, vaginal, or anal areas
- Poor skin hygiene.
- Absence of hair and/or hemorrhaging beneath the scalp
- Soiled clothing or bed
- Burns that may be caused by cigarettes, caustics, acids, friction from ropes or chains, or contact with other objects
- Signs of confinement (tied to furniture, bathroom fixtures, locked in room)
- Lack of bandages on injuries or stitches when indicated, or evidence of unset bones

3. Financial abuse indicators

This list is not intended to be exhaustive, but is intended to convey possible abuse. Great care must be taken before making accusations.

- Unusual activity in bank accounts
- Activity in bank accounts that is inappropriate to the older adult, e.g., withdrawals from automated banking machines when the person cannot walk or get to the bank
- Power of attorney or deeds to real property obtained when person is unable to comprehend the financial situation and/or to give a valid power of attorney or deed
- Unusual interest in the amount of money being spent for the care of the older person; concern that too much money is being spent
- Refusal to spend money on the care of the conservatee; numerous unpaid bills, overdue rent, when someone is supposed to be paying the bills
- Recent acquaintances expressing affection for a wealthy older person with assets
- Recent change of title of house in favor of a "friend" when the older person is incapable of understanding the nature of the transaction or does not even realize the transfer took place
- Caregiver asks only financial questions of the worker; does not ask questions related to care
- Caregiver has no obvious means of support

Repeated skin or other bodily injuries should be fully described and careful attention paid to their location and treatment. Frequent use of the emergency room and/or hospital or health care "shopping" may also indicate physical abuse. The lack of necessary appliances such as walkers, canes, bedside commodes; lack of necessities such as heat, food, water; and unsafe conditions in the home (no railings on stairs, etc.) may indicate abuse or neglect. Abuse may also occur if the elderly person's level of care is beyond the capacity of the caregiver or lack of appropriate supervision is given.

- Recent will has been drawn
  —when the person is clearly incapable of making a will
  —when the person does not fully realize there are changes in beneficiaries
  —friends or relatives urging the person to make a new will and elder does not clearly indicate she/he wants one
- Placement not commensurate with alleged size of the estate
- Lack of amenities, i.e., TV, personal grooming items, appropriate clothing when the estate can afford them
- Personal belongings such as art, silverware, jewelry are missing
- Caregiver tries to isolate older adult from old friends and family; tells older person no one wants to see him/her, and older person then becomes isolated and alienated from those who care for her/him; comes to rely on caregiver alone who then has total control of finances
  —promises of life-long care in exchange for willing or deeding of all property/bank accounts to caretaker
  —Signatures on checks, etc., that do not resemble older person's signature
  —Checks and other documents signed when older person cannot write
  —Absence of admission agreement for cost of care in residential care homes

Continued.

Indicators for determining abuse—cont'd

4. Emotional (psychologic) abuse indicators

The person may exhibit these behaviors, but of themselves they do not indicate psychologic abuse or neglect. If these behaviors are present, the evaluator needs to also consider the items listed under "Quality of Family/Caregiver Involvement" and evaluate further for abuse. If no indication of abuse, make a referral for evaluation of health status including mental health, if appropriate.

- Ambivalence
- Deference
- Passivity
- Fear of caregiver or healthcare provider
- Fearfulness expressed in the eyes; may look away from caregiver or health care provider
- Withdrawal
- Depression
- Helplessness
- Hopelessness
- Resignation

5. Rights violations indicators

- Coercion has been used to force person into convalescent hospital or other care facility
- Person has been locked in home, in car, in room, or out of home
- Visitors, phone calls, access to phone, or reception of mail has been prevented
- Denied appropriate clothing
- Denied food/water, or health care (exceptions may occur due to changing issues in "right to die;" seek legal consultation or contact Adult Protective Services (APS)
- Sensory deprivation including withholding the following necessary items:
  —hearing aid
  —dentures
  —eyeglasses
  —assistive devices (walker, cane, wheelchair, prosthesis)
- Restricted access to personal hygiene including bladder/bowel routine.

6. Neglect indicators

Failure by care provider to:
  —assist with personal hygiene or provide food, clothing, or shelter
  —provide for medical care for physical and mental health needs
  —protect from health and safety hazards
  —prevent malnutrition

AKRON GENERAL MEDICAL CENTER
GERIATRIC ABUSE PROTOCOL

Account No.	EMD No.
Full Name of Patient	Date

MEDICAL & PSYCHOSOCIAL HISTORY: (Quote Where Possible)

1. **History of present illness/injury.** If patient, caregiver, or other informants (EMS, police) give different histories, document what is said by each.

   _____

   _____

   _____

2. **Past medical history.** Other current problems, severe cognitive and/or physical impairment requiring extended care, history of abuse or neglect, repetitive admissions because of injuries or poor health. _____

   _____

   _____

3. **Dependence on caregiver.** Financial, physical, and or emotional support. Social isolation.

   _____

   _____

   _____

4. **Recent household crises or conflicts.** Inadequate housing, financial difficulties, dysfunctional relationships. _____

   _____

   _____

5. **Can the patient relate to instances of:**
   - rough handling
   - sexual abuse
   - alcohol or drug abuse by family
   - verbal or emotional abuse
   - isolation and/or confinement
   - misuse of property or theft
   - threatened
   - gross neglect (fluids, food, hygiene)

   _____

   _____

   _____

6. **Interview with caregiver:**
   - recent household conflicts
   - knowledge of patient's medical condition; care and medicine required
   - mental health of caregiver - abuse as a child, poor self-image, history of violent behavior
   - willingness and ability to meet elder needs
   - commission of any threatening or abusive acts
   - demonstration of poor self-control - blaming the patient for being old or ill, denial, exaggerated defensiveness

   _____

   _____

   _____

Figure 18-3 Geriatric abuse protocol and screening tool. (*Note.* From *Geriatric Emergency Medicine* [pp. 536-539] by G. Bosker, G.R. Schwartz, J.S. Jones, and M. Sequeira [Eds.], 1990, St. Louis: Mosby–Year Book, Inc.)   *Continued.*

AKRON GENERAL MEDICAL CENTER
GERIATRIC ABUSE PROTOCOL

Account No.	EMD No.
Full Name of Patient	Date

PHYSICAL ASSESSMENT:

Temp_____ Pulse _____ Resp _____ B.P. _____ Weight _____

1. **General appearance** (include condition of clothing).
   _____
   _____

2. **Current mental/emotional status.** Mental status exam; behavior during exam - extremely fearful or agitated, overly quiet and passive, depressed. _____
   _____

3. **Physical neglect.** Dehydration and/or malnutrition, inappropriate or soiled clothing, poor hygiene, injury that has not received proper care, evidence of inappropriate care (eg, neglected gross decubiti).
   _____
   _____

4. **Evidence of sexual abuse.** Torn, stained, or bloody underclothing; bruises or bleeding of genitalia, anal areas; signs of STD. _____
   _____

5. **Physical abuse findings** (also mark on pictures below):
   _____
   _____

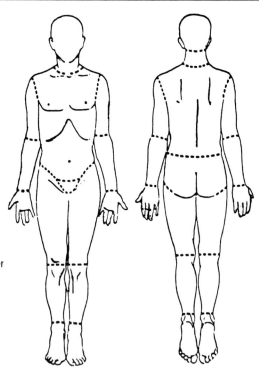

Indicators

Head injuries
  Absence of hair
  Hemorrhaging below scalp
  Broken teeth
  Eye injuries
Unexplained bruises:
  Face, lips, mouth
  Torso, back, buttocks
  Bilaterally on upper arms
  Clustered, forming patterns
  Morphologically similiar to
    striking object
  In various stages of healing
Unexplained burns:
  Cigar or cigarette burns
  Immersion burns
  Friction from ropes or chains
  Patterned like electric iron, burner
Sprains/dislocations
Lacerations or abrasions:
  Mouth, lips, gums
  Bite marks

Figure 18-3—cont'd   Geriatric abuse protocol and screening tool. (*Note.* From *Geriatric Emergency Medicine* [pp. 536-539] by G. Bosker, G.R. Schwartz, J.S. Jones, and M. Sequeira [Eds.], 1990, St. Louis: Mosby–Year Book, Inc.)

AKRON GENERAL MEDICAL CENTER
GERIATRIC ABUSE PROTOCOL

Account No.		EMD No.
Full Name of Patient		Date

DIAGNOSTICS

1. **Color photos** - labeled with name of patient, date, photographer, witness. Include picture with ruler in plane or lesions and picture of patient's face.

2. **Laboratory confirmation** (depending on type of injury/neglect present):
   - complete blood count
   - Partial thromboplastin time, prothrombin time, platelet count (easy bleeding)
   - Urinalysis, electrolyte panel (dehydration)
   - GC and chlamydia cultures, wet mount, VDRL (sexual abuse)
   - Radiologic screening for fractures
   - Metabolic screening for nutritional or endocrine abnormalities
   - Serum drug levels or toxicologic screens (over - or undermedication)

3. **Computerized axial tomogram** (CAT scan) - major changes in neurological status or head trauma that could result in subdural hematoma.

ASSESSMENT

1. No form of abuse is evident
2. Psychological abuse-verbal assault, threats, isolation
3. Material abuse or theft
4. Physical abuse - deliberate inappropriate care, direct beatings, sexual abuse
5. Physical neglect; determine causes:
   - age or frailty of caregiver
   - caregiver's lack of knowledge of patient's condition; care or medicine needed
   - physical or mental illness of caregiver
   - lack of support systems for the caregiver
   - financial difficulties

In my opinion, the medical findings are consistent with:

_____
_____
_____

FINAL DISPOSITION: _____
_____

SIGNED: _____

      Attending Physician   Date

_____

      Nurse   Date

_____

      House Officer   Date

Figure 18-3—cont'd   For legend see opposite page.

SUMMARY The elderly population is growing, and many attempts are being made to improve the quality of the "golden years." Increased physical activity programs, social stimulation programs, and better medical care are adding to this quality. As the elderly population grows, so does the incidence of trauma in this population group. The nurse involved with the care of the injured elderly patient must be astute regarding the special needs of the elderly. The understanding of the physiologic changes and the assessment differences and the monitoring of the elderly patient's response to trauma are basic skills the nurse must acquire.

Each system must be assessed, monitored, and supported to obtain optimal patient response. As this high technologic support and care is given, the nurse must not forget the patient's psychologic aspects and needs. Independence is linked to psychologic well-being and must be considered in discharge planning. A survey of American Association of Retired Persons members showed that more than 80% preferred an option of home health care to long-term stays in nursing homes (Lindsey, 1988). Community support groups, such as Community and Home Injury Prevention Project for Seniors (CHIPPS) in San Francisco, assist the elderly to prevent injury by providing home safety assessments, medication counseling, educational programs, and discounted installation of safety devices. Efforts must continue to provide for alternative living and healthcare arrangements for the elderly that benefit clinical, financial, and psychosocial needs.

A reverent respect should be given to the many years of service the elderly have given to society. Nurses are well prepared to extend this holistic approach to the care they provide. If they provide the "high tech care" and the psychologic support all patients deserve, nurses will demonstrate that nursing has developed and matured into a true profession.

NURSING DIAGNOSES &
EVALUATIVE CRITERIA   *The elderly trauma patient*

Nursing diagnosis	Nursing intervention	Evaluative criteria
High risk for impaired gas exchange and ineffective airway clearance Related to respiratory muscle weakness, decreased chest wall compliance, decreased vital capacity, thickened pulmonary mucosal bed	**Promote ventilation** Perform pulmonary assessment by: • assessing level of patient's dyspnea and its impact on activity. Maintain airway Monitor secretions. Place in semi-Fowler's position. Avoid increased intraabdominal pressure Suction prn and encourage cough: • presuction oxygenate; • suction less than 10 seconds; • postsuction oxygenate. Provide hydration by: • using humidified oxygen; • ensuring judicious fluid management; Administer O_2 therapy. Monitor for hypoventilation. Assist with intubation as necessary by: • assessing need; • maintaining airway.	Breathing patterns will improve. Respiratory rate will maintain at 16-18 breaths/min. Adventitious sounds will be absent. No respiratory fatigue will occur. Stridor will be absent. Denture will fit correctly. Bilateral breath sounds will be equal. Patient will maintain own airway or artificial airway will be stable. Secretions will be mobilized. Sputum will be clear in color and not frothy, as in pulmonary edema. Use of diaphragm will be unhindered. Breath sounds will improve. ABGs will be normal for age (see Table 18-3). Color will improve. O_2 desaturation will be minimal during suctioning and other therapies. Preload will equal 14-16 mm Hg. Mucous membranes will be moist. Urine output will equal 0.5 ml/kg/hr or greater. No abnormal skin tenting will be present. Mucous plugging will be avoided. IV fluids will be administered per orders. I & O and daily weights will be stable. ABGs will be normal for age. Cyanosis will be absent. Pulse oximeter O_2 saturation will be above 90%. Hypoventilation will be detected early. Pa_{CO_2} will be 40 mm Hg. Artificial airway will be maintained. Pa_{O_2} and Pa_{CO_2} will be within normal limits for age and previous history. Artificial airway will be maintained in correct position and confirmed by x-ray examination and breath sounds.

Continued.

Nursing diagnosis	Nursing intervention	Evaluative criteria
High risk for impaired gas exchange and ineffective airway clearance —cont'd	Monitor mechanical ventilation by: • monitoring ABGs • assessing for complications • monitoring V_T and VC, compliance, P/F ratio, negative inspiratory pressure (NIP); • following chest x-ray reports.	Respirations will be stable on ventilator. ABGs will be within normal limits. Patient will be free of ventilation-precipitated problems. V_T will equal 5 ml/kg; VC will equal 10 ml/kg. Compliance will increase; P/F ratio will be >250-300; NIP will be stronger. X-ray film will show resolving fluid and/or air. Tube placements will be reported as optimal (ETT, chest tubes, central lines, etc.)
High risk for altered tissue perfusion and fluid volume deficit Related to decreased RBC production, atherosclerosis, decreased compensatory mechanisms	Maintain circulation Perform perfusion assessment by: • determining the history of fluid loss; • observing skin color and turgor; • monitoring vital signs for the elderly; • monitoring hemodynamics; • monitoring laboratory data; • monitoring urine output. Provide aggressive pulmonary care. Establish IV lifeline. Provide fluid volume replacement by: • monitoring intake and output; • monitoring patient's weight. Treat perfusion problems.	 Precipitating cause will be corrected. Mucous membranes will be moist. No abnormal skin tenting will be present. BP will be consistent with past history. Systolic BP will be above 100 mm Hg or MAP will be greater than 65 mm Hg. No orthostatic hypotension present. Heart rate will be 60-100/min. Respiratory rate will be 16-18/min. LOC will be within norm for age. CVP will be normal (4-8 cm H_2O) (5-11 mm Hg). PWP will be normal (10-16 mm Hg). Hematocrit will be 35-40%. Hemoglobin will be 13-15 g. Partial thromboplastin time will be 25-40 sec. Prothrobin time will be 11-13 sec. Pao_2 will be normal (Table 18-3). $Paco_2$ will be normal (35-40 mmHg). Urine output will be ≥0.5 ml/kg/hr. Specific gravity will be 1.015-1.025 Breath sounds will be clear. Secretions will be mobilized. Physical activity will increase. Large-bore IV cannulae will be placed. Sterility will be maintained at sites. I & O and weight will be stable. Hemodynamics will be normalized. Blood/blood products will cause no reaction. Acidosis will be prevented.

Nursing diagnosis	Nursing intervention	Evaluative criteria
	Provide the following multisystem support: • nutritional support; • inotropic support;	TPN Glucose will be within normal limits. Albumin will be >3.5 g. MAP will be >65. Only the lowest dopamine dosage will be required. PWP will be optimized. Urine output will be normal.
	• ventilatory support.	ABGs will remain within normal limits. Adequate rest will be provided between sessions of ventilatory exercise during weaning.
	Prevent the following complications: • respiratory distress;	Patient will deny dyspnea. Respiratory rate will be within normal limits.
	• congestive heart failure;	Exercise tolerance will increase. JVD will be normal. S_3 heart sound will be absent. Lungs will be clear.
	• renal failure;	Urine output will be 0.5 ml/kg/hr. Blood urea nitrogen will be <20 mg. Creatinine clearance will be normal for age.
	• liver failure.	AST, LDH, and bilirubin will be normal. PT and PTT will be within normal limits.
High risk for sensory/perceptual alterations Related to decreased neurotransmitters and stimulation of sensory tracts, decreased pain perception, disrupted daily schedule because of hospitalization	**Promote environmental orientation** Decrease noise and light. Allow rest periods. Provide clock and calendar and personal effects. Explain procedures. Maintain privacy. Encourage visitors. Institute fall precautions.	Mental status will be unchanged. Patient will be oriented to person, place, and date/time. Patient will interact with others appropriately. No hallucinations will occur; sleep cycle will be maintained. Patient will maintain sense of dignity and some control over environment. Signs of depression will be absent. No falls or slips will occur.
High risk for pain Related to traumatic injury, disruption of tissue	**Promote comfort** Perform pain assessment, noting: • characteristics of the pain; • comparison of pain with past experiences. Provide pain control measures by: • changing position; • elevating body part; • providing range of motion; • providing heat or cold packs; • massaging area (except calf muscle).	Patient will verbalize pain appropriately. Patient will be free of pain or pain will be lessened. Measures will control pain; sedatives will not be required.

Continued.

Nursing diagnosis	Nursing intervention	Evaluative criteria
High risk for pain—cont'd	Use distraction techniques by: • talking with patient; • encouraging visitor interaction; • providing music, T.V., etc.	Patient will rank pain less with techniques.
	Administer pain medications effectively by: • providing prescribed dose at appropriate intervals; • using visual analog scale to determine intensity of pain.	Pain will be controlled without excessive sedation Patient will not be heavily sedated.
	Administer sedatives effectively by: • assessing for —pain —hypoxemia —comfort measures; • administering small doses of drugs with short half-lives; • monitoring effect (elderly very sensitive to sedatives).	
High risk for impaired tissue integrity Related to decreased mobility, altered peripheral perfusion, incontinence	**Maintain tissue perfusion** Assess risk factors, including: • altered nutrition; • decreased skin perfusion; • overly dry or wet skin; • prolonged bedrest; • mechanical forces.	Risk factors will be eliminated or reduced.
	Assess skin (especially pressure points) and use decubitus flow sheet to observe and document: • color, texture, sensation; • vascularity; • infections.	Color, texture, and sensation will be normal. Skin will be free of excoriation. Skin will be free of infections and decubiti.
	Implement pressure relief devices, such as: • sheepskin; • alternating air pad; • Egg crate pad; • kinetic beds.	Skin will be clean, dry, and free of reddened areas and decubiti.
	Keep skin clean and dry, including: • exposing skin to air; • limiting use of waterproof pads; • changing absorptive pads frequently when necessary to use. Turn frequently. Avoid shearing forces—use trapeze bar as possible. Institute continence training.	
	Improve circulation by: • maintaining normothermia; • treating shock;	Skin will be warm and pink

Nursing diagnosis	Nursing intervention	Evaluative criteria
	• massaging and moisturizing during skin care; applying protective skin care products to reddened areas; • performing range of motion. Facilitate early ambulation with PT/OT assist prn. Maintain proper fluid balance. Maintain nutrition, including: • evaluating fit and use of dentures; • consulting dietitian for special needs; • engaging family support for special treats and emotional support.	Use of adaptive aids will allow increasing mobility. I&O will be about equal. No tissue weeping will occur. Serum albumin will be stable and > 3.5 g. Dentures will fit and will be in place. Patient will voice meal preferences.
High risk for altered nutrition: less than body requirements Related to decreased GI function, intake	**Assess nutritional status** Weigh patient daily. Measure and record intake and output. Monitor laboratory data, including: • BUN; • serum albumin; • electrolytes; • calcium, magnesium. Encourage oral intake. Provide frequent, small meals with assistance as needed. Determine food preference. Monitor enteral/TPN feedings, including: • monitoring I & O; • maintaining infusion rate; • checking stomach residuals for enteral feedings; • monitoring blood glucoses; • assessing for complications.	Patient will maintain weight. Fluid status will be normal. BUN will be <20 mg. Albumin will be >3.5-4 g. Electrolyte values will be within normal range. Calcium and magnesium values will be within normal range. Normal caloric intake (45 cal/kg/24 hr) will be maintained. Patient will resume PO intake. If patient cannot maintain calorie intake orally, invasive feedings will be provided. Patient will be free of complications, such as: • infections; • hyperglycemia; • hypoglycemia; • hyperosmolality; • acid-base problems; • electrolyte problems; • aspiration; • ileus; • diarrhea.

CASE STUDY   A 68-year-old man was involved in a motor vehicle collision (MVC). The paramedic unit had a difficult time extricating the patient, and the primary survey revealed head and neck trauma, respiratory compromise, and shock. As the paramedic team started to treat the patient, he arrested as the result of ventricular fibrillation. Defibrillation was carried out with the return of a sinus rhythm with occasional ventricular ectopy. The patient was endotracheally intubated. Two IV lines of NS were started, and the patient was quickly transported to the E.D.

The trauma team has been notified by radio of the suspected injuries and is prepared as the patient enters the trauma room. The airway is secured, but the trauma nurse notes left chest lag, right tracheal deviation, and cyanosis. The ED physician places a 36-Fr. left chest tube, and the patient's color immediately improves. Blood samples are drawn for type and crossmatch, chemistries, liver and cardiac enzymes, and arterial blood gases. Notable bleeding is slight, except for minor abrasions and lacerations. The abdomen is distended, and no bowel sounds are present. Because of the decreased LOC (Glasgow coma scale score of 6) of this patient, a nasogastric tube and urinary catheter are inserted and a peritoneal lavage is performed with frank bloody fluid return. A large bruise over the left upper abdomen is noted. The patient is unresponsive, head and cervical spine x-ray films are within normal limits, and spinal safeguards are discontinued. Head CT scans demonstrate increased intracranial pressure with a 2 cm shift of midline structures but a nonoperative lesion.

The ECG reveals ventricular ectopy and ST wave changes, so a 12-lead ECG is obtained. In leads II, III, and aV_F, a Q wave, ST elevation, and T wave inversion are noted. Lidocaine is started with a 1 mg/kg bolus followed by a 2 mg/min continuous infusion. The patient is then taken to the OR for laparotomy and placement of an intracranial bolt.

How does airway management differ in the elderly trauma patient?

The airway must be the first priority in the care of the severely injured patient regardless of age. In the elderly patient it is even more important to lessen the risk of hypoxemia. Hypoxemia may result in death immediately or may precipitate MOF, as discussed earlier. Elderly patients normally have a lower Pao_2, and further decreases may not be tolerated. In addition to hypoxemia, the risk of hypercapnea exists, which results from hypoventilation. The elderly patient will not normally retain CO_2, although many elderly have preexisting obstructive airway disease. Those with weakened respiratory muscles and a rigid thoracic cage from arthritis may hypoventilate in response to the additional stress of trauma. An elevated CO_2 will cause respiratory acidosis, vasodilation, hypotension, dysrhythmias, and a left shift in the oxyhemoglobin dissociation curve—problems the elderly patient cannot tolerate. Hypotension may lead to decreased blood flow to the heart and brain. If atherosclerotic disease is present, an infarct of cardiac or cerebral tissue may occur. Dysrhythmias and poor O_2-carrying ability secondary to anemia may decrease the supply of O_2 to the cells and result in worsening hypoxia.

This patient also has a head injury, which puts him at high risk for a spinal cord injury; the patient must be treated as such until spinal cord injury is ruled out by x-ray examination. Because of the demineralization of the bone in osteoporosis, cervical fractures may be seen in the elderly patient involved in trauma although radiographic confirmation is more difficult. Deceleration injuries (e.g., whiplash, in particular) can easily injure the cervical spinal cord. The airway should always be supported, but care must be taken to prevent additional injury to the neck. Stabilization of the neck should be maintained in an aligned position and thoroughly supported. As the neck is supported and stabilized, intubation can be accomplished to secure the airway, if needed.

Why would this patient demonstrate ventricular ectopy and ECG changes?

There are three possible explanations for this occurrence. First, the patient with severe thoracic and abdominal trauma may have also sustained a cardiac contusion. Second, he may have had a myocardial infarction while driving, passed out or even arrested, and then crashed his car. Third, hypotension or the stress associated with injury may trigger arrhythmias in an aged heart with atherosclerosis and decreased compensatory ability. The answer may be found in the patient history. This patient is 68 years old, which places him in the high-risk category for heart disease. Does this patient have a history of coronary artery disease (CAD)? Does he have a medical alert bracelet or other emergency identification suggesting CAD? If a history is not known, the trauma nurse must rely on objective diagnostic data. The 12-lead ECG demonstrated ischemic changes seen in the inferior part of the heart, suggesting an acute myocardial infarction (AMI). If he had sustained a cardiac contusion, the changes would have been primarily anterior, and Q wave development is rare in a contusion unless trauma is very severe. Care will be the same initially (e.g., cardiac monitoring, lidocaine administration, assessment for failure), but additional testing with cardiac enzymes must be done in the critical care unit. If CAD is the problem, care should be undertaken to reduce the complications that can impede the elderly patient's recovery from trauma.

What type of monitoring would be expected?

The elderly patient who either sustains a cardiac contusion or has a myocardial infarction may develop congestive heart failure (CHF). A pulmonary artery catheter may be necessary to manage fluid status. If after chest trauma, the patient develops jugular venous distention, crackles in the lung bases, and S_3 or S_4 heart sounds, CHF should be suspected. The course of management should include a diuretic, digoxin, O_2 therapy, and rest. If symptoms do not abate, a pulmonary arterial catheter can be used to monitor pulmonary wedge pressure (PWP). The PWP indicates volume status of the patient. If the PWP is less than 6 mm Hg, IV fluids should be administered. If the

PWP is greater than 14 to 16 mm Hg, a diuretic or vasodilator may be used. This patient had a PWP of 24 mm Hg, cardiac index (CI) of 1.8 L/min/m², systemic vascular resistance (SVR) of 2300 dynes, O_2 delivery of 1000 ml/min, and a consumption of 150 ml/min.

This patient had severe cardiogenic shock. Furosemide, nitroglycerine, and dobutamine were started. The PWP decreased to 18 mm Hg, and the SVR decreased to 1600 dynes. This is the result of the diuretics and vasodilator therapy. By optimizing the PWP and SVR and the administration of dobutamine, the CI increased to 3.0 L/min/m². Oxygen delivery increased because of improved hemodynamics, and consumption greatly improved because of better capillary perfusion. In addition, the serum lactate level dropped from 6 to 2.5 mmol. This demonstrated an improvement in the tissue perfusion and oxygenation.

As with most drugs, however, care must be taken in elderly patients because of their inability to metabolize and excrete medications normally. As discussed earlier, physiologic changes that occur in the liver and kidneys may have further dysfunction in the elderly trauma patient.

RESEARCH QUESTIONS

- Do elderly patients require different fluid resuscitation techniques from the younger trauma patient?
- What are the differences in mortality and morbidity between younger and older age groups with the same posttraumatic resuscitative techniques?
- Should the elderly patient be intubated and mechanically ventilated sooner than the younger patient to prevent hypoxic complications after trauma?
- Do weaning procedures differ between the elderly and the younger trauma patient with respiratory failure?
- Is there a difference in the incidence of pulmonary infections in elderly trauma patients receiving aggressive nursing care and those placed on kinetic therapy beds?
- What are the cost/benefits (financial, emotional, ethical) of resuscitating the elderly trauma patient?
- What preventive measures are available to decrease the incidence of trauma in the elderly population?

- Why do elderly patients become septic sooner after trauma than younger patients?
- What techniques are most effective to accurately monitor LOC in the patient with dementia or Alzheimer's disease?
- Does blood administration to obtain higher hemoglobin levels in the elderly trauma patient improve survivability and prevent complications?

RESOURCES

American Association of Retired Persons (AARP)
601 E St. NW
Washington, DC 20045
(202) 434-2200
This association maintains a large selection of high-quality consumer publications ranging in topic from "Your Health" to "Managing Money and Choosing Health Care Services." Videotapes are also available on such subjects as home safety & elder abuse. The National Elder Care Institute on Health Promotion publishes "Perspectives" and serves as a clearinghouse as part of AARP.

Area Agencies on Aging
The Older Americans Act in the 1970s divided the United States and its territories into area agencies; approximately 700 exist today. They provide services to the aging themselves or contract to community agencies. The Federal Administration on Aging disburses money to state departments, which distribute money to the area agencies. Community services include legal assistance, meals, housing, and transportation, ombudsmen, and a senior information and referral service. To contact, call the operator for the area code in question and ask for the *Area Agency on Aging.*

Professional Organizations

American Society of Aging
833 Market St., Suite 512
San Francisco, CA 94130-1824
(415) 882-2910
National Council on Aging
600 Maryland Ave. SW, West Wing 100
Washington DC 20020
(202) 479-1200 or 1-800 424-9046

ANNOTATED BIBLIOGRAPHY

Bobb, J.K. (1987). Trauma in the elderly. *Journal of Gerontological Nursing, 13,* 28-31.
  Research article that reviews the past literature in geriatric trauma that demonstrates an increased mortality and morbidity of the elderly patient. It is a clear and concise study and addresses the significant problems that may affect the survival of the elderly trauma patient. An excellent point presented is that age is not always a determinant of survivability. More research is needed.
Border, J.R. (1988). Multiple organ system syndrome. In F.B. Cerra (Ed.), *Perspectives in Critical Care* (pp. 23-29). St. Louis: Quality Medical Publications.

Excellent review of the current research in multisystems organ failure. The article outlines the pathophysiology of MOF and its detrimental effects on all patients. It also suggests that the elderly patient is at higher risk for MOF than the younger trauma patient. Enforced supine position, broad-spectrum antibiotics, and invasive procedures all play a major role in the development of MOF. The elderly are more prone to these therapeutic interventions than the younger patient.

REFERENCES

Allen, J.E., & Schwab, C.W. (1985). Blunt chest trauma. *American Surgeon, 51,* 697-700.
American Psychiatric Association (APA) Task Force on Nomenclature and Statistics. (1987). *Diagnostic and statistical manual of mental disorders* (3rd ed.—revised), (DSM-III-R). Washington, DC: American Psychiatric Association.
Appleton, W. (1988). Elder abuse: Diagnose, treat, cure (letter to editor). *Annals of Emergency Medicine, 17* (10), 1104-1105.
Arora, N.S., Dudley, M., & Rochester, M. (1982). Respiratory muscle strength and maximal voluntary ventilation in undernourished patients. *American Review of Respiratory Disease, 126,* 5-8.
Bachman, S., Sparrow, D., and Smith, L.K. (1981). Effects of aging on the electrocardiogram. *American Journal of Cardiology, 48*(3), 513-516.
Bayer, A.J., Chadha, J.S., Farag, R.R., & Pathy, M.S. (1986). Changing presentation of myocardial infarction with increasing old age. *Journal of the American Geriatrics Society, 34,* 263-266.
Beam, T.R., Jr. (1989). The role of Aztreonam in treating infections in the elderly. *Infections in Medicine, 6*(2), 58-64.
Beck, L.H. (1990). Perioperative renal, fluid, and electrolyte management. In H.J. Keating III, (Ed.), *Clinics in geriatric medicine: Perioperative care of the older patient, 6* (3), 557-569. Philadelphia: W.B. Saunders.
Bell, J.E., Dixon, L., & Sehy, Y.A. (1991). Physical assessment: The breast and the pulmonary, CV, GI, and GU systems. In W.C. Chenitz, J.T. Stone, and S.A. Salisbury (Eds.), *Clinical gerontological nursing: A guide to advanced practice (pp. 51-69).* Philadelphia: W.B. Saunders.
Bobb, J.K. (1987). Trauma in the elderly. *Journal of Gerontological Nursing, 13,* 28-31.
Border, J.R. (1988). Multiple organ system syndrome. In F.B. Cerra (Ed.), *Perspectives in critical care* (pp. 23-29). St. Louis: Quality Medical Publications.
Bortz, W.M. (1982). Disuse and aging. *Journal of the American Medical Association, 248*(10), 1203-1208.
Bromley, H.R., Frei, L.W., Nelson, L.D., & Shoemaker, W.C. (1988). How much perfusion is enough? In F.B. Cerra (Ed.), *Perspectives in critical care* (pp. 31-44). St Louis: Quality Medical Publications.
Bryson, B.L., Warren, K., Schedhlem, M., Mumford, B., & Lenaghan, P. (1987). Trauma to the aging cervical spine. *Journal of Emergency Nursing, 13*(6), 334-341.
Cancer Statistics (1984). *Cancer, 34,* 51.
Castle, S.C., Norman, D.C., Yeh, M., Miller, D., & Yoshikawa, T.T. (1991). Fever in the elderly nursing home resident: Are the older truly colder? *Journal of the American Geriatrics Society, 39,* 853-857.

Cerra, F.B. (1987). Hypermetabolism, organ failure, and metabolic support. *Surgery*, 191, 1-14.

Cerra, F.B. (1988). Multiple organ failure syndrome. In F.B. Cerra (Ed.), *Perspectives in critical care* (pp. 1-22). St. Louis: Quality Medical Publications.

Champagne, M.T., & Ashley, M.L. (1989). Nutritional support in the critically ill elderly patient. *Critical Care Nursing Quarterly*, 12(1), 15-25.

Chernow, B., Reed, L., Geelhoed, G.W., Anderson, M., Teich, S., Meyerhoff, J., Beardsley, D., Lake, C.R., & Holaday, J.W. (1986). Glucagon: Endocrine effects and calcium involvement in cardiovascular actions in dogs. *Circulatory Shock*, 19, 393-407.

Clark, R.L. Jr., & Delafuente, J.C. (1988). Anemias. In J.C. Delafuente and R.B. Stewart (Eds.), *Therapeutics in the elderly* (pp. 157-166). Baltimore: Williams & Wilkins.

Cleamons, M.G., Chaudry, I.H., & Daigneau, N. (1984). Insulin resistance and depressed gluconeogenic capabilities during early hyperglycemic sepsis. *Journal of Trauma*, 24, 701-708.

Cockcroft, D.W., & Gault, M.H. (1976). Prediction of creatinine clearance from serum creatinine, *Nephron*, 16, 30-33.

Cohen, M.M. (1990). Perioperative responsibility of the surgeon. In H.J. Keating III (Ed.), *Clinics in Geriatric Medicine: Perioperative care of the older patient*, 6 (3), 557-569. Philadelphia: W.B. Saunders.

Counselman, F. (1988). Two sides of acute abdomen in the elderly. *Emergency Medicine*, 30, 56-74.

Cutter, F. (1983). *Art and the wish to die*. Chicago: Nelson-Hall.

Darowski, A., Najim, Z., Weingerg, J.R., Guz, A. (1991). Hypothermia and infections in elderly patients admitted to the hospital. *Age and Ageing*, 20, 100-106.

DeMaria, E.J., Pardon, R., Merriam, M.A., Casanova, L.A., & Gann, D.S. (1987). Survival after trauma in geriatric patients. *Annals of Surgery*, 206, 738-743.

DeNicola, P., & Casale, G. (1983). Blood in the aged. In D. Platt (Ed.). *Geriatrics* (pp. 252-292). New York: Springer-Verlag.

Dougherty, S. (1988). The malnourished patient. *Critical Care Nurse*, 8, 13-22.

Escher, J.E., O'Dell, C., & Gambert, S.R. (1989). Typical geriatric accidents and how to prevent them. *Geriatrics*, 44(5), 54-69.

Figley, C.R., Scrignar, C.B., & Smith, W.H. (1980). PTSD: The aftershock of trauma. *Patient Care*, May 15, 111-127.

Finelli, F.C., Jonsson, J., Champion, H.R., Morelli, S., & Fouty, W.J. (1989). A case control study for major trauma in geriatric patients. *Journal of Trauma*, 29(5), 541-547.

Fisher, R.P., & Miles, D.L. (1986). Trauma demographics in this decade. *Journal of Trauma*, 26, 673-676.

Goldman, R. (1979). Decline in organ function with aging. In I. Rossman (Ed.), *Clinical geriatrics (2nd ed.)* (pp. 23-59). Philadelphia: J.B. Lippincott.

Gottlieb, S.O., & Gerstenblith, G. (1988). Silent myocardial ischemia in the elderly: Current concepts. *Geriatrics*, 43(4), 29-34.

Granger, C.V., Albrecht, G.L., & Hamilton, B.B. (1979). Outcome of comprehensive medical rehabilitation: Measurement by PULSES profile and the Barthel index. *Archives of Physical Medicine and Rehabilitation*, 60, 145-154.

Hackel, A., Linzer, M., Anderson, N., Williams, R. (1991). Cardiovascular and catecholamine response to head up tilt in the diagnosis of recurrent unexplained syncope in elderly patients. *Journal of the American Geriatrics Society*, 39, 663-669.

Hansen, L.C., & Davis, M. (1991). Use of life-sustaining care for the elderly. *Journal of the American Geriatrics Society*, 39, 772-777.

Harrel, J.S. (1988). Age-related changes in the cardiovascular system. In M.S. Matteson and E.S. McConnell (Eds.), *Gerontological nursing: Concepts and practice* (pp. 193-217). Philadelphia: W.B. Saunders.

Harris, R. (1983). Cardiovascular disease in the elderly. *Medical Clinics of North America*, 67(2), 379-393.

Hassock, K.R., & Bruce, R.A. (1982). Maximal cardiac function in sedentary normal men and women: Comparison of age-related changes. *Journal of Applied Physiology*, 53(4), 799-804.

Hogue, C.C. (1982). Injury in late life: part I: Epidemiology. *Journal of the American Geriatrics Society*, 30, 183-190.

Hollenberg, A., Adams, D., & Soloman, H. (1974). Senescence and the renal vasculature in normal man. *Arch Res*, 34, 309-316.

Horst, H.M., Farouck, N.O., Sorensen, V.J., & Bivins, B.A. (1986). Factors influencing survival of elderly trauma patients. *Critical Care Medicine*, 14, 681-684.

Hunter, A., Carey, M., & Lash, H. (1981). The nutritional status of patients with COPD. *American Review of Respiratory Disease*, 124, 376-381.

Ingersol, G.L. (1989). Respiratory muscle fatigue research: Implications for clinical practice. *Applied Nursing Research*, 2, 6-14.

Iskrant, A.P., & Joliet, P.V. (1968). *Accident and homicide*. Cambridge: Harvard University Press.

Jessup, L.E. (1984). Physical changes and physical assessment of older individuals. In B.M. Steffi (Ed.), *Handbook of Gerontological Nursing*. New York: Van Nostrand Reinhold.

Jones, J., Dougherty, J., Schelble, D., and Cunningham, W. (1988). Emergency department protocol for diagnosis and evaluation of geriatric abuse, *Annals of Emergency Medicine*, 17 (10), 1006-1015.

Jowsey, J. (1977). *Metabolic diseases of bone*. Philadelphia: W.B. Saunders.

Kannel, W.B. (1981). Systolic blood pressure, arterial rigidity, and risk of stroke: The Framingham study. *Journal of the American Medical Association*, 245(12), 1225-1229.

Katz, S.M., & Fagraeus, L. (1990). Anesthetic considerations in geriatric patients. In H.J. Keating III (Ed.), *Clinics in Geriatric Medicine: Perioperative care of the older patient*, 6(3), 499-510. Philadelphia: W.B. Saunders.

Keating, H.J. III, & Lubin, M.F. (1990). Perioperative responsibility of the physician/geriatrician. In H.J. Keating III (Ed.), *Clinics in Geriatric Medicine: Perioperative care of the older patient*, 6(3), 459-467. Philadelphia: W.B. Saunders.

Kennedy, R.D., & Caird, F.I. (1981). Physiology of aging of the heart. *Cardiovascular Clinics*, 12(1), 1-8.

Kroeger, L.L. (1991). Critical care nurses' perceptions of the confused elderly patient. *Focus on critical care, 18*(5), 395-400.

Lakatta, E.G. (1983). Determinants of cardiovascular performance: Modification due to aging. *Journal of Chronic Disease, 36*(1), 15-30.

Larson, B. (1984). Health and aging characteristics of highly physically active 65-year-old men. *International Journal of Sports Medicine, 5*(6), 336-340.

Lindsey, L. (1988). Living arrangements for the elderly: Alternatives to institutionalization. In J.C. Delafuente and R.B. Stewart (Eds.), *Therapeutics in the elderly* (pp. 83-92). Baltimore: Williams & Wilkins.

Linn, B.S. (1983). Surgery and the elderly patient. In R.D.T. Cape & R.M. Coe, *Fundamentals of geriatric surgery* (pp. 68-87). New York: Raven Press.

Lonergan, E.T. (1988). Aging and the kidney: Adjusting treatment to physiological changes. *Geriatrics, 43*, 27-33.

Matteson, M.A. (1988a). Age-related changes in the gastrointestinal system. In M.A. Matteson & E.S. McConnell, *Gerontological nursing: Concepts and practices* (pp. 266-277). Philadelphia: W.B. Saunders.

Matteson, (1988b). Age-related changes in the musculoskeletal system. In M.A. Matteson & E.S. McConnell, *Gerontological nursing: Concepts and practice* (pp. 171-191). Philadelphia: W.B. Saunders.

Miller, D.K., Burton, F.R., Burton, M.S., & Ireland, G.A. (1991). Acute upper gastrointestinal bleeding in elderly persons. *Journal of the American Geriatrics Society, 39*, 409-419.

Mueller, M.S., & Gigson, R.M. (1983). Age differences in health care spending. *Social Security Bulletin, 36*, 18.

National High Blood Pressure Education Program Coordinating Committee (NHBPEP). (1980). *Statement on hypertension in the elderly* (pp. 2-7). Bethesda: National Institutes of Health.

Newman, R.H. (1988). Bedside blood sugar determinations in the critically ill. *Heart & Lung, 17*, 667-669.

Oreskovich, M.R., Howard, J.D., & Copass, M.K. (1984). Geriatric trauma: Injury patterns and outcome. *Journal of Trauma, 24*, 565-570.

O'Riordin, T.G., Tobin, A., & O'Murain, C. (1991). Heliobacter pylori infections in the elderly dyspeptic patients. *Age and Ageing, 20*, 189-192.

Ouslander, J.G. (1981). Drug therapy in the elderly. *Annals of Internal Medicine, 95*, 711-722.

Palve, H., & Vuori, A. (1989). Pulse oximetry during low flow cardiac output and hypothermia states immediately after open heart surgery. *Critical Care Medicine, 17*, 66-69.

Peltier, L.F. (1984). Program #13: Fat embolism. In *The Sound Slide Library Selection*. Chicago: American Academy of Orthopaedic Surgeons.

Phipps, W.J., Long, B.C., & Woods, N.F., & Cassmeyer, V.L. (Eds.) (1991). *Medical-Surgical nursing: Concepts and clinical practice*. (4th ed.). Ed.) St. Louis: Mosby–Year Book, Inc.

Port, S. (1980). Effects of age on the response of the left ventricle ejection fraction to exercise. *New England Journal of Medicine, 303*(20), 1133-1137.

Powers, J.S., Krantz, S.B., Collins, J.C., & Meurer, K. (1991). Erythropoietin response to anemias as a function of age. *Journal of the American Geriatrics Society, 39*, 30-32.

Rowe, J.W. (1987). Clinical consequences of age-related impairment in vascular compliance. *American Journal of Cardiology, 60* (12), 68-71.

Rowe, J., Shock, N., & DeFronzo, R. (1976). The influence of age on the renal response to water deprivation in man. *Nephron, 17*, 276-278.

Samuelson, B. (1983). Leukotrienes: Mediators of immediate hypersensitivity reactions and inflammation. *Science, 220*, 568-575.

Schwertz, D.W., & Buschmann, M.T. (1989). Pharmacogeriatrics. *Critical Care Nursing Quarterly, 12*(1), 26-37.

Shapiro, B.A., Harrison, R.A., Cane, R.D., & Kozlowski-Templin, R. (1989). *Clinical application of blood gases*. Chicago: Mosby–Year Book, Inc.

Shoemaker, W.C. (1987). Circulatory mechanisms of shock and their mediators. *Critical Care Medicine, 15*, 787-794.

Snell, R.S. (1980). *Clinical Neuroanatomy for Medical Students*. Boston: Little, Brown.

Standley, H.L., Schmitt, B.P., Poses, R.M., & Deiss, P. (1991). Does hypogonadal contribute to the occurrence of minimal trauma hip fractures in elderly men. *Journal of the American Geriatrics Society, 39*, 799-771.

Stone, J.T. (1991). Pressure sores. In W.C. Chenitz, J.T. Stone, & S.A. Salisbury (Eds.), *Clinical gerontological nursing: A guide to advanced practice* (pp. 247-265). Philadelphia: W.B. Saunders.

Sunderam, S., & Mankikar, G. (1983). Hyponatremia in the elderly. *Age and Ageing, 12*, 77-80.

Taylor, A.E., Matalon, S., & Ward, P. (Eds.). (1986). *Physiology of oxygen radicals*. Bethesda: American Physiological Society.

Thatcher, R.M. (1983). 98.6° F: What is normal? *Journal of Gerontological Nursing, 9*(1), 22-27.

Tinetti, M.E. (1983). Effects of stress on renal function in the elderly. *Journal of the American Geriatrics Society, 31*, 174-181.

Trunkey, D.D., Siegel, J., & Baker, S.P. (1983). Panel: Current status of trauma severity indices. *Journal of Trauma, 23*, 185-201.

U.S. Bureau of the Census. (1976). Current population reports. Washington, D.C.: Author.

U.S. House of Representatives Select Committee on Aging (1981). *An examination of a hidden problem*. 97th Congress (Committee publication No. 97-277). Washington, DC, Government Printing Office.

Waller, J.A. (1974). Injury in the aged. *New York State Journal of Medicine, 74*, 2200-2207.

Wilson, R.F. (1982). Future treatment of shock. In R.A. Cowley and B.F. Trump (Eds.), *Pathophysiology of shock, anoxia and ischemia* (pp. 500-506). Baltimore: Williams & Wilkins.

Yin, F.C.P. (1980). The aging vasculature and its effects on the heart. In M.L. Weisfeld (Ed.), *The aging heart: Its function and response to stress* (pp. 137-214). New York: Raven Press.

Yurick, A.G., Spier, B.E., Robb, S.S., Ebert, N.J., & Magnussen, M.H. (1989). *The aged person and the nursing process* (3rd ed.). Norwalk, Conn: Appleton & Lange.

Zamfirescu, N.R. (1982). Functional peculiarities of the heart in the aged. *Physiology, 19*(2), 73-79.

SELECTED
TRAUMA SEQUELAE

Relationships Between Physiologic Processes

Anticipating complications

■■

Kathleen B. McLeod
Wayne C. McLeod
Janet A. Neff

OBJECTIVES

❏ Identify the major complications that increase the morbidity and mortality of trauma patients.

❏ Recognize early signs and symptoms of complications, and anticipate appropriate nursing interventions.

❏ Recognize the factors that may increase the incidence of complications.

❏ Describe the physiologic interactions that contribute to the course of recovery for the trauma patient.

❏ Outline the metabolic changes and requirements of the trauma patient.

INTRODUCTION Many potential complications affect the morbidity and mortality of trauma patients. Resuscitative measures, though life and limb saving, may predispose the patient to a myriad of complications that are both iatrogenic and physiologic in nature. Careful attention to nursing technique will decrease the incidence of avoidable infection. In addition, a working knowledge of the potential complications that may arise within hours to weeks of admission will enhance safe nursing care and decrease the chances of damaging sequelae.

CASE STUDY Daniel, a 65-year-old man, was an unrestrained driver of a passenger car who was involved in a one-vehicle rollover at 55 miles per hour. He was ejected and found 20 feet from his car. Treatment initiated before the patient's arrival in the emergency department (ED) included full cervical spine immobilization on a backboard, placement of two large-bore IVs with infusion of normal saline, and 100% oxygen by endotracheal tube. The paramedics reported that he was unconscious initially and then became combative. Initial BP was 80/50; pulse, 140; and respirations, 30 and labored.

In the ED, the patient is examined and is found to have multiple abrasions on all extremities, diminished breath sounds in the right chest, several broken ribs, and a fractured pelvis. Immediate ED intervention includes insertion of a chest tube, rapid fluid resuscitation and blood replenishment, placement of an indwelling urinary catheter, and attainment of a standard panel of laboratory tests and radiologic studies.

The patient stabilizes after the resuscitative efforts, and BP is 130/70; pulse, 95; and respirations, 20 (unassisted). The admitting diagnoses for Daniel are right pneumothorax, multiple right rib fractures without a flail segment, closed head injury, right pubic rami fracture, and multiple abrasions.

List at least five factors that place this patient at risk for developing postinjury infection.

Multiple factors predispose Daniel to develop infection. The prehospital initiation of IV lines and endotracheal intubation under suboptimal conditions are two of the most common. Insertion of chest tubes, urinary catheter, and other invasive devices may introduce pathogens. Patients who experience shock may have translocation of bacteria from the intestinal tract to the circulatory system (Baker, Deitch, Li, Berg, & Specian, 1988). Multiple blood transfusions and use of steroids and antibiotics, in addition to the traumatic event itself, increase the likelihood for infectious sequelae. Immobility and impaired respiratory function are also contributory factors.

What physiologic changes can be assessed in this patient that may indicate the onset of sepsis?

The initial phase of sepsis is characterized by alterations in levels of consciousness indicative of hypoxia. These include disorientation, restlessness, and apprehension. Bounding tachycardia is often present, as is a warm, dry skin with a flushed appearance. Respirations tend to be shallow and rapid, and urine output diminishes. Because cardiac output levels remain elevated, the blood pressure will reflect normal to slightly low normal values even in the presence of vasodilation. Temperature is usually elevated but occasionally will be subnormal.

Is this patient at risk for developing disseminated intravascular coagulation (DIC)?

This patient has an increased risk for developing DIC related to several factors. Four main factors precipitate the onset of DIC: hypotension, hypoxemia, acidemia, and circulatory stasis. Daniel shows evidence of shock with tachycardia and a blood pressure of 80/50. He may become both hypoxic and acidotic related to his chest injuries, and will likely have circulatory stasis secondary to shock and immobility. Thus he is at risk for DIC, which may be caused by one or a combination of these factors.

MECHANISM OF INJURY

Infection leading to sepsis and ultimately multiple organ failure (MOF) are among the topics discussed in this chapter. DIC, whether a manifesta-

tion of sepsis, massive blood replacement, or other causative factors, may create an even more complex situation for the critically injured.

Factors that place trauma patients at risk for major complications include those with mechanisms creating sustained hypoperfusion, invasive microbial infections, unstabilized long bone fractures, undebrided wounds, and inflammatory foci, such as pancreatitis (Flint, 1991). Patients experiencing alterations in airway protection or clearance are at high risk for aspiration.

In the presence of complex injuries, compensatory mechanisms in stress may mimic apparent complications early in the patient's course. Therefore it is necessary for the trauma nurse to have a basic understanding of the physiologic responses to trauma.

ANATOMIC AND PHYSIOLOGIC CONSIDERATIONS
Physiologic Responses to Trauma

Severe trauma and prolonged resuscitative measures alter the normal physiology and trigger the stress response. After the initial restoration of circulatory volume, the body develops a hyperdynamic state that serves to enhance the healing process. Unless other events, such as perfusion deficits and uncontrolled infection, complicate the process, the peak of this response is generally seen 48 to 72 hours after injury and diminishes within 7 to 10 days (Mirtallo, 1988).

The response is directly proportional to the extent of injury, and energy expenditure will elevate with increases in cardiac output and oxygen consumption. Mobilization of the body's resources to meet the demands of healing are exhibited by muscle and visceral protein breakdown for energy and a negative nitrogen balance.

In a fasting, noninjury state, glycogen is broken down to glucose, but available glycogen is depleted within 24 hours. Fat is subsequently converted to fatty acids for energy. To sustain functioning, the brain, blood, and bone marrow must have glucose as an energy source. This is then generated from amino acids obtained by breaking down protein. In the injured state, protein is broken down at the same time as fat. Protein is not a deferred energy source, which is why early nutritional support is so necessary. Because the greatest protein stores are found in muscle, fasting will produce breakdown of these reserves.

The body eventually adapts by using ketone

Table 19-1 Summary of neuroendocrine stress responses and resulting effects

Neuroendocrine	Effects on metabolic processes	Net results
↑ Catecholamines ↑ Glucocorticoids ↑ Glucagon ↑ Growth hormone ↓ Insulin	Glycogenolysis Gluconeogenesis Lipolysis Proteolysis	Provision of substrate for energy
↑ Catecholamines ↑ Glucocorticoids ↑ Vasopressin (ADH) ↑ Aldosterone	Sodium and water retention	Defense of fluid volume

Reparative phase		Net results
↑ Insulin ↓ Glucagon ↑ Growth hormone and other growth factors ↑ Thyroid hormones		Protein synthesis Cell proliferation Restoration of fat deposits

Note. From Stress Response (p. 307) by A.M. Lindsey and V.K. Carrieri. In V.K. Carrieri, A.M. Lindsey, and C.M. West (Eds.), 1986, *Pathophysiological Phenomena in Nursing*, Philadelphia: W.B. Saunders.
↑, Increase; ↓, decrease.

bodies for energy in starvation. In the stress response to injury, glucose requirements are much higher and adaptation may not occur (Van Way, 1991). This stress response is initiated in the central nervous system and involves the sympathetic nervous system, multiple hormones, cytokines, and acute-phase proteins.

ADH

A complex cascade of hormonal releases complete the stress process. Antidiuretic hormone (ADH), also referred to as *arginine vasopressin*, is stimulated secondary to an increase in plasma osmolality and a decrease in the circulatory volume. Subsequently, free water absorption in the distal tubules and collecting ducts occurs, thereby increasing the specific gravity and diminishing urinary output. In addition, ADH stimulates glucose production in the liver through increased glycogenolysis and gluconeogenesis (Kenney, 1986). Table 19-1 summarizes stress responses.

The renin-angiotensin complex is then stimulated by diminished sodium levels reaching specific parts of the nephron. Catecholamines, ACTH, vasopressin, and glucagon are also responsible for the stimulation of renin, which in turn initiates angiotensin production. The major

role of angiotensin is aldosterone stimulation by the adrenal cortex. Aldosterone may also be stimulated by elevated potassium levels and is sometimes referred to as the *scavenger hormone*, because it promotes further improvement in the efficiency of sodium and water reabsorption (Kenney, 1986). Additionally, catabolism is stimulated with a loss of body cell mass, with increasing mobilization of fatty acids and utilization of amino acids necessary for gluconeogenesis (Bailey, 1991).

Cortisol and catecholamines

Another hormonal response seen is the production and release of cortisol, which is initiated by the secretion of ACTH. The net purpose of cortisol in the response to trauma and volume loss is to increase glucose production, which occurs by inhibiting hepatic enzymes that break down glucose. The overall effect is an increase in circulating blood glucose, accelerated muscle breakdown, and enhanced protein synthesis in the liver.

Principal mediators in the increases of metabolism and oxygen consumption are catecholamines, such as epinephrine. Their release functions to increase core glucose supply and enhance glucose utilization in the periphery. This occurs by promoting the breakdown of fat and protein for energy and glucose breakdown in peripheral tissues (Kenney, 1986). It is interesting to note that catecholamine secretion tends to be only 10% above normal after an uncomplicated surgery, but may increase more than 50% in patients with peritonitis and 100% in patients with extensive burns (Baue, 1991).

The secretion of insulin, which is basically inhibited by the release of catecholamines, is indirectly stimulated by cortisol and other hormones that promote hyperglycemia (Kenney, 1986). Insulin plays a major role in the metabolic response because it increases glucose and amino acid uptake and promotes protein synthesis, thereby boosting available energy. It inhibits the breakdown of fat and glycogen (Figure 19-1).

Electrolyte imbalances, particularly elevated potassium levels, related to infusions of blood and blood products, interstitial fluid shifts, and lysing of traumatized tissue may result from compensatory or resuscitative measures (Cardona, 1985).

Cytokines

Cytokines are low-molecular-weight proteins that regulate the differentiation, generation, and immunoregulatory function of various cells, including lymphocytes and macrophages (Priest, 1991). Prominent cytokines implicated in the development of the septic state include tumor necrosis factor (TNF) and interleukin-1 (IL-1). Also known as peptide regulatory factors, they are a family of proteins whose chief effects are seen on other cells (Van Way, 1991). These proteins have been associated with key roles in the pathogenesis of septic shock and as toxic secondary mediators of gram-negative sepsis; TNF, also known as *cachectin*, acts as the major mediator (Priest, 1991).

Studies have shown that the cellular physiologic response to TNF is nearly identical to that of endotoxins. Responses include fever or hypothermia, tachycardia, elevated cardiac output, decreased systemic vascular resistance, and decreased visceral blood flow. Higher concentrations are associated with hypotension, acidosis, and circulatory collapse with resulting MOF (Priest, 1991). TNF has been found to induce the production of IL-1, which produces the same responses as TNF. Thus it appears that TNF and IL-1 act synergistically in some circumstances.

Clinical studies are underway to evaluate the administration of monoclonal antibodies to TNF in septic patients. Research has supported monoclonal antibody addition to IL-6 in protecting mice against the lethal effects of both *Escherichia coli* and TNF (Sugerman, 1991).

Although the potential actions of IL-1 are numerous, purified preparations of IL-1 appear to have similar responses as plasma divalent cations, namely iron, zinc, and copper. Reductions in plasma iron and zinc and increases in copper levels have been known to occur in trauma and infection (Fry & Polk, 1987). Reductions in iron and zinc may actually retard bacterial growth, while copper deficiency states have been identified with increased frequencies of infection. Interleukin-1 appears to stimulate lactoferrin release from neutrophils, thus binding with circulating plasma iron. This is further removed from the system by reticuloendothelial cells (Fry & Polk, 1987).

Inflammatory indicators

The inflammatory response is a complex pathologic process of cellular and histologic reactions. It is often difficult to identify early infection in the trauma patient because the inflammatory response is triggered by the direct trauma, as well as foreign bodies, such as bullets, sutures, drains, catheters, and dirt. As a result, it is not uncommon for the white blood cell (WBC) count to elevate to 20,000-40,000/mm^3 immediately after severe trauma (Hoyt, 1988). The release of catecholamines can also trigger and increase white blood cell production.

Fever, which is clinically defined as 100.5° F (37.8° C) or higher, is activated by the formation of polymorphonuclear leukocytes (PMNs), monocytes, and macrophages, which stimulate the release of endogenous pyrogens. These pyrogens travel to thermosensitive neurons in the anterior hypothalamus, producing peripheral vasoconstriction. Thus body surface temperature is reduced, and shaking chills ensue as skeletal muscles contract in response to the activation of somatic motor nerves by thermal receptors of the skin. The net result is an increase in body heat and fever production.

Thermoregulatory mechanisms can be altered by several factors, which may inhibit the detection of fever by altering the normal temperature set point of the patient. The patient with a central nervous system injury that interferes with the

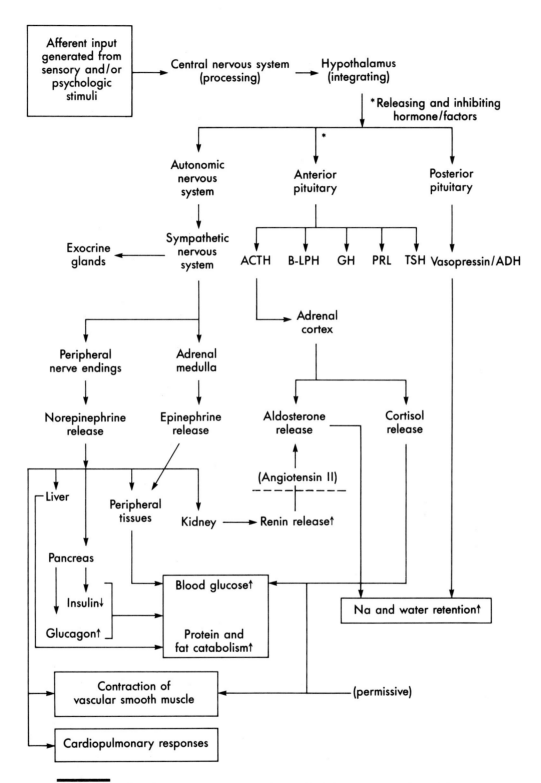

Figure 19-1 Physiologic responses in stress. (*Note.* From Stress Response [p. 305] by A.M. Lindsey and V.K. Carrieri. In V.K. Carrieri, A.M. Lindsey, and C.M. West (Eds.), 1986, *Pathophysiological Phenomena in Nursing*, Philadelphia: W.B. Saunders.)

skin's thermoregulatory functions could have a set point of 96° F (35.6° C). Thus an increase to 99° F (37.2° C) would be clinically indicative of a fever. Any patient with an injury to the hypothalamus, which is the primary regulator of the autonomic functions including thermoregulation, may exhibit hyperthermia or lack of control of body temperature and set point. This is especially true in young children. Elderly patients with deteriorating skin function may have lower than normal set points (Hoyt, 1988). On the other hand, the patient with an implanted mechanical device, such as a pacemaker, will have a higher thermal set point and appear to have a chronic low-grade fever, related to chronic stimulation of the inflammatory response.

It is difficult to diagnose infection. The normal inflammatory response after trauma to tissues alters body temperature (febrile) and white blood cell count and differential. Clinical manifestations indicative of infection, such as redness, swelling, heat, pain, and decreased function of the traumatized area, may be present secondary to the injury.

Other compensatory responses to injury include an increase in the left ventricular function with an increased cardiac index, increased pulse rate, stroke index, and left ventricular stroke work. Total systemic peripheral resistance (afterload) is diminished. Classically, the hypermetabolic state is demonstrated by increased oxygen consumption (Savino, 1987).

During the first 5 days after injury, the body enters a diuretic phase to mobilize and excrete fluids and electrolytes, which often results in hypovolemia accompanied by less than normal sodium and potassium levels. Urinary nitrogen loss occurs in proportion to the amount of skeletal muscle breakdown and the degradation of injured tissue (Mirtallo, 1988).

DIAGNOSTIC AND MONITORING PROCEDURES

The WBC count is useful to determine the presence of infection or sepsis. The WBC count may be elevated to 15,000/mm^3 and frequently exceeds 20,000/mm^3. In the presence of gram-negative sepsis, the WBC values may be normal, which is considered to be a grave indicator (Wilson, 1985). The differential will indicate a shift to the left, with 80% to 95% PMNs and an increase in bands, indicating the rapid production of im-

mature white cells. Lymphocyte counts less than 1500/mm^3 denote probable host defense impairments. In the presence of inflammation, monocytes (which become macrophages) rapidly multiply, to envelop foreign particles.

Chemistries

Chemistry values may be beneficial in detecting the development of impending organ failure from sepsis. Glucose levels increase despite insulin administration, and LDH levels tend to rise early, which is a nonspecific indicator of impending organ failure. As renal dysfunction ensues, the blood urea nitrogen (BUN) and creatinine values increase. Alkaline phosphatase elevation is seen with eventual hyperbilirubinemia as hepatic failure begins. Serum albumin may be reduced secondary to increased gluconeogenesis from protein sources. Albumin shifts into the interstitial space because of vascular permeability and is decreased in the presence of impaired liver function.

A standard progression of blood gas abnormalities is seen as shock and MOF worsen. The first stage encountered is respiratory alkalosis, with or without metabolic alkalosis, followed by metabolic acidosis. Uncompensated metabolic acidosis is seen next, culminating in a combined respiratory and metabolic acidosis (Roberts, 1985).

Enzymes such as serum glutamic-oxaloacetic transaminase (SGOT) and serum glutamate pyruvate transaminase (SGPT) (aspartate aminotransferase [AST] and alanine aminotransferase [ALT], respectively) may be abnormal from sepsis, shock, or the injury itself; thus they are not reliable indicators of liver failure in the absence of other symptoms (Flint, 1988).

Plasma proteins

Plasma proteins, namely albumin, transferrin, and prealbumin, are negative acute-phase reactants. They indicate more than just nutritional factors, and changes in their levels should be evaluated together, not separately. Interest is also growing in monitoring total protein by albumin and globulin levels.

Albumin Serum albumin concentration is the best single nutritional test for predicting patient outcome. Possessing a half-life of 18 days, it is the major protein synthesized by the liver. The primary functions are to preserve plasma oncotic pressure and transport other substances. The long half-life, however, limits the value for detecting acute nutritional changes. Albumin levels between 2.8 and 3.5 g/dl are thought to represent mild protein depletion, whereas levels less than 2.2 g/dl indicate severe depletion (Smith & Mullen, 1991).

Transferrin   Possessing a half-life of 8 days, serum transferrin is a beta-globulin that transports iron in plasma and may help prevent bacterial infection by actually binding iron. Reduced plasma iron levels have been associated with slowing of bacterial proliferation (Fry & Polk, 1987). The short half-life may provide an advantage over albumin as a nutritional indicator; however, clinical studies have not demonstrated significant value differences (Smith & Mullen, 1991). Levels less than 200 mg/dl are indicative of protein depletion.

Prealbumin   The half-life of prealbumin is 2 to 3 days, and measurable changes occur in prealbumin levels within 7 days of changes in nutrient intake (Smith & Mullen, 1991). Although these changes can be detected more rapidly than that of albumin, it has not been proven to predict poor outcome better than either albumin or transferrin (Smith & Mullen, 1991). As an index of nutritional progress, renal and hepatic function must be stable. Substantial patient risk and protein depletion are appreciated when prealbumin levels fall lower than 15 mg/dl.

ASSESSMENT AND INTERVENTIONS RELATED TO SPECIFIC CONDITIONS
Septic Syndrome and Septic Shock

Of patients who survive more than 2 days after trauma, the majority of subsequent deaths are attributed to infection (Dellinger, 1986). Infectious complications occur in more than half of the severely injured patients and account for 78% of the late deaths seen in trauma morbidity (Procter, 1987).

Confusion sometimes exists in the description and meaning of the term *sepsis*. For the purposes of this chapter, sepsis will be defined as a syndrome characterized by the signs and symptoms of severe infection. It may progress to the disseminated infectious state characterized by septic shock. Multiple organ failure (MOF) may ensue as a result of sepsis. It is important to realize, however, that the septic syndrome and MOF can occur in the absence of infection. In more than 30% of patients with trauma-related sepsis and

MOF, a specific focus cannot be identified (Meakins, 1991).

Predisposing factors

Multiple factors predispose trauma patients for development of infection. From the time the patient is injured on the scene, the inflammatory mechanisms are hard at work to inhibit the growth of bacteria via phagocytic mechanisms. The nurse must consider all the possibilities of contamination that are inherent to the prehospital environment, as well as the clinical setting.

When the patient is injured, breaks usually occur in the integumentary system, which is the largest protective organ the body has in the host defense system. Abrasions and lacerations may occur, as well as the collection of foreign matter in each of these. Trauma patients will usually present to EDs with many artifacts of the accident scene, including dirt, oil, gasoline, glass, rocks, bullets, and other foreign bodies.

In urgent, life-threatening situations, there is little time or opportunity to adequately prepare IV puncture sites, wash hands, and maintain aseptic technique. One study showed that IVs started in the field by EMTs and paramedics are likely to have a complication rate more than 4.5 times higher than those initiated within the hospital setting (Lawrence & Lauro, 1988). Any invasive procedure may introduce exogenous bacteria. Indwelling catheters, tubes, and monitoring devices provide a conduit for microbial invasion.

Studies have shown that a positive correlation exists between alcohol use and the incidence of trauma. According to the facts distributed by the American Trauma Society in 1987, 50% to 55% of the national traffic deaths were alcohol related. Trauma patients with a history of alcohol abuse have a high incidence of developing infection related to trauma for several reasons, including breakdown of protective barriers, exposure, and preexisting malnutrition.

The incidence and severity of infections among the alcohol abuse population have prompted researchers to study the direct effect of alcohol on the immune system. Acute intoxication inhibits the normal delivery of PMNs to sites of bacterial invasion (MacGregor, 1986). The ingestion of alcohol significantly interferes with antibody responses and suppresses macrophage function. Therefore the nurse must monitor carefully for the onset of infection in the patient with a history of alcohol ingestion. Patients with both episodic and chronic usage should be considered immunosuppressed.

High-risk sites of infection

The critically ill patient who requires intubation and ventilatory support has an increased susceptibility to infection. Of nosocomial pneumonias, 74% of cases are seen in surgical patients, and the risk is increased 21 times for those requiring continuous ventilatory support (Johanson, 1988). One study demonstrated that despite standard pulmonary toilet, 70% to 90% of ventilator patients in an ICU setting after 1 week were colonized with hospital-acquired bacteria in the oropharynx and digestive tract. The primary organisms were *Enterobacter* and *Pseudomonas*. More than 60% of these patients developed pulmonary infections (Kerver et al., 1988).

Injuries to soft tissues may be a potential source of infection secondary to the accumulation of blood or necrotic skin and tissue, which provide an excellent culture medium for bacterial growth (Rush, Kelly, & Nichols, 1988). Treatment should be aggressive in respect to surgical evacuation and debridement.

The presence of devitalized tissue from direct organ injury produces a catabolic response. Prolonged activation of the catabolic neuroendocrine system will ultimately cause large muscle atrophy, colonic and gastric stasis, lethargy, and capillary leaks secondary to prolonged complement release. This serves a prime role in the onset of organ failure (Babikian, 1989). Roth's studies (Rush et al., 1988) have demonstrated that the addition of povidone-iodine to the irrigating solution used to debride wounds may prevent postoperative wound infection when used concomitantly with parenteral antibiotics. The use of povidone-iodine remains controversial however. The reader is referred to Chapter 13 for more information.

The trauma nurse must also consider internal sources as the potential infectious site. Experimental studies in mice demonstrated that bacterial translocation from the gut is promoted when a disruption of intestinal microflora, impaired host immune defenses, and a physical disruption of the intestinal mucosa occur. Mice subjected to varying time frames of shock were documented to have ileal mucosal necrosis that became more profound the longer they were in shock (Baker et al., 1988).

This study suggests that the presence of extended periods of shock or possibly the severity of shock may predispose traumatized patients to the translocation of indigenous bacteria into the blood. Recent experimental studies showed that this phenomenon may be reversed with selective administration of vasodilators directly into the mesenteric circulation or systemic administration of thromboxane synthetase inhibitors (Herndon, 1991). Figure 19-2 summarizes these and other effects of critical factors on GI functioning.

The central nervous system (CNS) must be considered a possible source of infection, especially in the presence of intraventricular monitoring devices. Subarachnoid bolts are less commonly an infectious source than intraventricular pressure monitors that allow therapeutic drainage of cerebrospinal fluid (CSF) (Procter, 1987). One study documented subarachnoid bolts to be associated with no infection rate over 1 year, and subdural catheters to have a very low incidence of related infection. A 14% infection rate occurred over the same time period in patients with ventricular catheters (Smith, 1987). Patients with open skull fractures and basilar skull fractures also are at risk for CNS contamination. The trauma nurse must maintain a high index of suspicion with head-injured patients, since their levels of consciousness frequently are decreased. This complicates the assessment of meningeal infection.

Another potential source of infection leading to sepsis and MOF is the presence of occult intraabdominal abscesses. Frequently they do not produce bacteremia; therefore blood cultures may be negative. The process may be so insidious that it may not be recognized until organ failure occurs. Failure to recognize and treat the source of infection producing MOF results in 100% mortality (Procter, 1987).

Open fractures carry the potential for infection, related to wound contamination and devitalized soft tissue created by the fracture. Antibiotics are often initiated while the patient is still in the ED. Open fractures are cultured in some institutions before antibiotics are initiated, since a correlation exists between the eventual infecting organisms and those initially cultured. The most common ones are *Staphylococcus aureus* and *Escherichia coli*. Generally cephalosporins with gram-negative activity provide adequate prophylaxis (Procter, 1987).

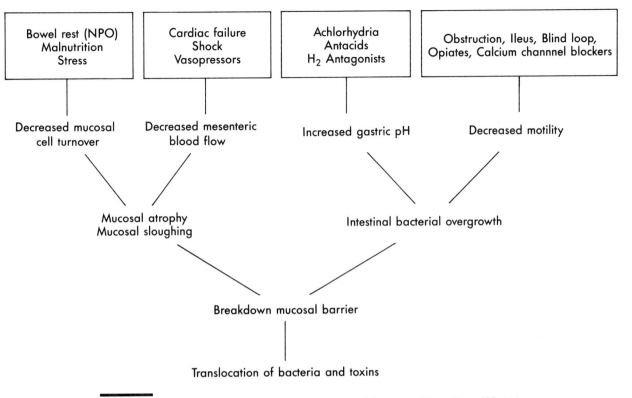

Figure 19-2 Effects of critical illness on gastrointestinal function. (*Note.* From "Nutrition and Trauma: Techniques of Nutritional Support" by R.H. Rolandelli and M.J. Koruda, 1991, *Trauma Quarterly*, 7(2), p. 34.)

Assessing for Signs and Symptoms of Sepsis

Nursing assessment of the trauma patient should be performed frequently, using a systematic and complete approach. During these ongoing evaluations of patient status, some indicators may be helpful in anticipating potential complications.

Most patients who have had major trauma to the chest or abdomen can be expected to develop some level of atelectasis or pneumonitis. This generally surfaces about 24 to 48 hours after surgery, presenting with signs and symptoms of fever, diminished bronchial breath sounds, and infiltrates on chest x-ray films (Wilson, 1985).

Wound infections will generally manifest themselves 5 to 7 days after injury. Exceptions to this are beta hemolytic streptococcal and clostridial infections, which may develop in 24 to 48 hours. It may take 2 weeks or longer for host defense-impaired persons and those on antibiotics to develop outward signs and symptoms of infection.

Nearly all patients with indwelling urinary cath-

eters will have bacteria in their urine after 5 days of catheter placement. Although this becomes a significant factor to nursing care, it is believed to be an infrequent cause of bacteremia and sepsis (Wilson, 1985). Caplan and Hoyt's study (Carpenter, 1987) demonstrated that although urinary infections account for 18% of all infections, UTIs account for only 3% of bacteremias.

Hyperdynamic phase

Sepsis can be broken down into two phases: the hyperdynamic stage and the hypodynamic stage (see box, p. 600). Initially the hyperdynamic phase is typically a normal or increased cardiac output state. Release of hormonal and chemical substances that are stimulated by microorganisms originally result in a peripheral vasodilation, producing warm, flushed skin.

Central nervous system alterations, such as restlessness, confusion, and increasing anxiety, may be the first observable manifestations of this

---

Comparison of phases in septic shock

Early septic shock
Hyperdynamic phase

- vasodilation (warm, pink skin)
- increased cardiac output
- increased stroke volume
- increased pulse pressure
- normal or elevated initial BP
- increasing signs and symptoms of shock:
  —increased respirations
  —urine < 25 ml/hr
  —metabolic acidosis

Advanced septic shock
Hypodynamic phase

- hypovolemia
- decreased cardiac output
- reduced oxygen transport
- increased capillary permeability
- increased vasoconstriction (cold, clammy skin, mottled or cyanotic)
- oliguria
- vasodilation in presence of gram-negative endotoxins

---

hyperdynamic state. In alcoholic patients, the cause of these symptoms may be misleading and difficult to differentiate from delirium tremens.

The blood pressure will remain normal or high at the onset of sepsis as long as the cardiac output remains elevated. The pulse is generally full and bounding secondary to increases in stroke volume and pulse pressure.

The respiratory rate characteristically increases with a reduced tidal volume and a minute volume of 1.5 to 2.0 times the normal level (Wilson, 1985). Septic patients tend to be air swallowers and may rapidly develop an ileus, even without abdominal infections. The skin tends to be warm, dry, and flushed during this hyperdynamic phase.

Failure to thrive, sometimes demonstrated by listlessness and lack of energy, may be one of the first indicators of impending or unsuspected sepsis, which may culminate in MOF. The elderly population is especially susceptible, secondary to impaired host defense systems and altered physiologic processes. Chapter 18 further explains immunosuppression in the elderly.

Fevers may be low grade and intermittent initially; white blood count may be slightly elevated with a left shift. Increased PMNs, especially bands, are present.

Hypodynamic phase

Continuation of the septic state is manifested by hypovolemia and low cardiac output as the compensatory mechanisms begin to fail. Increasing capillary permeability resulting in interstitial fluid and electrolyte shifts—particularly in the lungs—is the main cause of the decreased circulating volume creating the poor cardiac output. Increasing vasoconstriction causes cool, clammy skin, which may appear either mottled or cyanotic (Wilson, 1985) (see the box on the left). With progression in the hypodynamic phase, vasodilation will occur in the presence of gram-negative endotoxins.

Multiple Organ Failure

One definition of MOF in the trauma patient is the decompensated pathologic response to injury, which is initiated and enhanced by microbial invasion (Flint, 1988). It is the final stage of the postinjury response, with a 95% mortality rate, which begins days to weeks before clinical indicators surface (Cerra, 1991), and is said to be present when more than one system or organ cannot support their activities (Baue, 1991). It has been reported to be the cause of death in 80% to 85% of surgical intensive care unit deaths, with the cost of stay ranging between $21,763 and $294,568 (Bailey, 1991).

The development of organ failure has been described to occur secondary to inadequate perfusion from initial circulatory deficits, thus producing tissue hypoxia and limiting the functional capacity of some vital organs. This is especially true when the overall metabolic demands are increased (Shoemaker, Appel, & Kram, 1988).

Six common threads are observed in the development of MOF (Baue, 1991). The first is shock, ischemia, or circulatory instability after injury, with a subsequent increased cardiac output and hyperdynamic phase. Second is immobility with mechanical respiratory compromise. Third, tissue injury/inflammation creates the activation of cellular humoral mediators. Fourth, infections activate the systemic responses (interleukins, TNF, and others). Fifth is bacterial overgrowth with or-

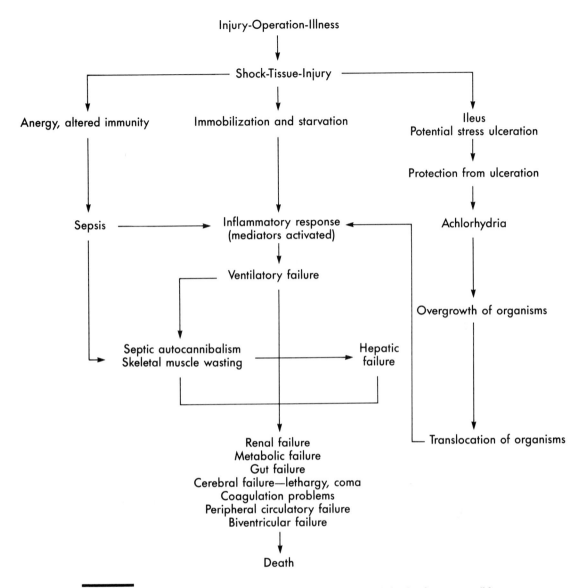

Figure 19-3 Contributing factors to multiple organ failure and death after injury. (*Note.* From "Nutrition and Metabolism in Sepsis and Multisystem Organ Failure" by A.E. Baue, 1991, *Surgical Clinics of North America, 71*(3), p. 550.)

ganism translocation into mesenteric lymph nodes, and inflammatory mediator stimulation (gut failure syndrome). Ultimately, the metabolic demands on skeletal muscle and the liver result in protein metabolic failure, namely septic autocanniabalism and hepatic failure, leading to death. Figure 19-3 summarizes contributory factors to MOF after injury.

The major organs affected in MOF are lungs, kidneys, liver, and the central nervous system, which ultimately create major abnormalities in glucose, protein, and fat metabolism. The severely injured will develop a respiratory failure requiring ventilatory support (Baue, 1991). An associated circulatory instability results, followed by renal insufficiency and rising bilirubin levels from hepatic dysfunction. This impacts greatly on the nutritional demands of the patient as well. Baue's research showed the mortality rate approaching 60% to 80% with three or more failed organs. Thus the best treatment for MOF is prospective support of organ function, adequate nutrition, and the prevention of failure.

It becomes difficult to initially segregate MOF from sepsis, because the onset of organ failure appears to coincide strongly with the onset of overt bacterial infection. Some evidence also supports the theory that tissue injury to organs may be caused by the release of bacterial products into the circulation from an injured or infected lung (Johanson, 1988). Patients suffering from peritoneal contamination caused by penetrating abdominal injuries are seen to have MOF onset in the second or third week after injury when associated with abdominal infections (Flint, 1988).

More recently it has been hypothesized that MOF is caused when the macrophage releases cytokine and oxygen-free radicals in response to shock followed by reperfusion. These radicals cause increased capillary permeability, vasodilation, decreased blood volume, and organ ischemia. Altered cell metabolism thereby disturbs the function of distant organs (Cerra, 1991).

Assessing for signs and symptoms of multiple organ failure

Assessment and detection of MOF is organ specific and often insidious. Tachypnea and cyanosis may indicate hypoxemia, which is usually the earliest specific manifestation of MOF. The onset of jaundice, a late sign, is indicative of liver failure.

The renal system, in comparison with pulmonary, immune, cardiovascular, and other systems, accounts for the highest mortality reported in trauma patients both young and old (Finelli, Johnsson, Champion, Morelli, & Fouty, 1989). The first signs of renal failure may be polyuria, azotemia, or abnormal free water clearance. Both transient oliguria and diuresis may occur, which are nonspecific indicators.

"Coffee ground" nasogastric aspirate may be the first sign of impending gastrointestinal failure characterized by varying degrees of ulceration and bleeding. Table 19-2 summarizes additional clinical manifestations of organ failure.

Table 19-2 Clinical manifestations of organ failure

Organ	Clinical manifestations
Lung	Hypoxemia, tachypnea, increased intrapulmonary shunt fraction, loss of compliance, pulmonary edema
Liver	Progressive hyperbilirubinemia, cholestatic jaundice, altered amino acid clearance
Kidney	Polyuria/oliguria, elevated BUN and creatinine
Gastrointestinal system	Bleeding, ileus, loss of mucosal barrier function, endoscopic evidence of mucosal erosions
Hematologic system	Disseminated intravascular coagulation, thrombocytopenia, bleeding, increased fibrin split products, decreased fibrinogen
Central nervous system	Lethargy, coma, EEG changes, hyporeflexia, confusion

Note. From Sepsis and Multiple Organ Failure (p. 996) by L.M. Flint. In E.E. Moore, K.L. Mattox, and D.V. Feliciano (Eds.), 1991, *Trauma* (2nd ed.), Norwalk, CT: Appleton & Lange.

Disseminated Intravascular Coagulation

Disseminated intravascular coagulation (DIC), also known as *consumption coagulopathy* and *defibrination syndrome*, appears to be partially causative of MOF. Activation of coagulation and fibrinolytic systems after trauma may be associated with the development of respiratory distress possibly related to thromboembolism (Riberg et al., 1986).

Predisposing factors

DIC is an acquired bleeding disorder, which occurs as a secondary phenomenon, not as a primary one. Obstetrical complications, neoplasms, hemolytic processes, hypotension, hypothermia, sepsis, and rattlesnake bites place the patient at risk for developing DIC. Regardless of the specific cause, four common factors are predisposing: (1) arterial hypotension, often associated with shock; (2) hypoxemia; (3) acidemia; and (4) stasis of capillary blood (Vogelpohl, 1981). Trauma can account for all four of these factors.

Multiply injured trauma patients may require

massive blood transfusions for hemodynamic stabilization, which may increase their susceptibility to DIC. *Massive blood transfusion* is defined as the administration within a 24-hour period of a volume of blood and blood components equal to or exceeding the patient's estimated blood volume (Kruskall et al., 1988). Although rapid transfusion of blood and blood components may be life-saving in the traumatized patient, it is associated with a special set of complications.

Blood stored at 4° C develops storage defects that may assume greater significance in massive transfusions than in low-volume elective transfusions. Factors V and VIII, the labile factors, decline during preservation in the liquid state (Rutledge & Sheldon, 1988). Occasionally this leads to a bleeding diathesis that is a predisposition to abnormal hemostasis during or after resuscitation.

This bleeding abnormality has been attributed to resuscitation with blood and fluid deficient in both coagulation factors and viable platelets, and is called a *dilutional coagulopathy* (Kruskall et al., 1988).

DIC is an inappropriate, accelerated, and systemic activation of the coagulation cascade, in which both thrombosis and hemorrhage may occur simultaneously (Griffin, 1986). To understand the pathophysiology of the disorder, the trauma nurse must review the normal clotting physiology.

Coagulation   Normal clotting mechanisms are a complex interaction of thrombotic and antithrombotic activity. Two pathways are involved in thrombin formation: the extrinsic pathway and the intrinsic pathway (Figure 19-4).

Normal intact endothelium interacts mini-

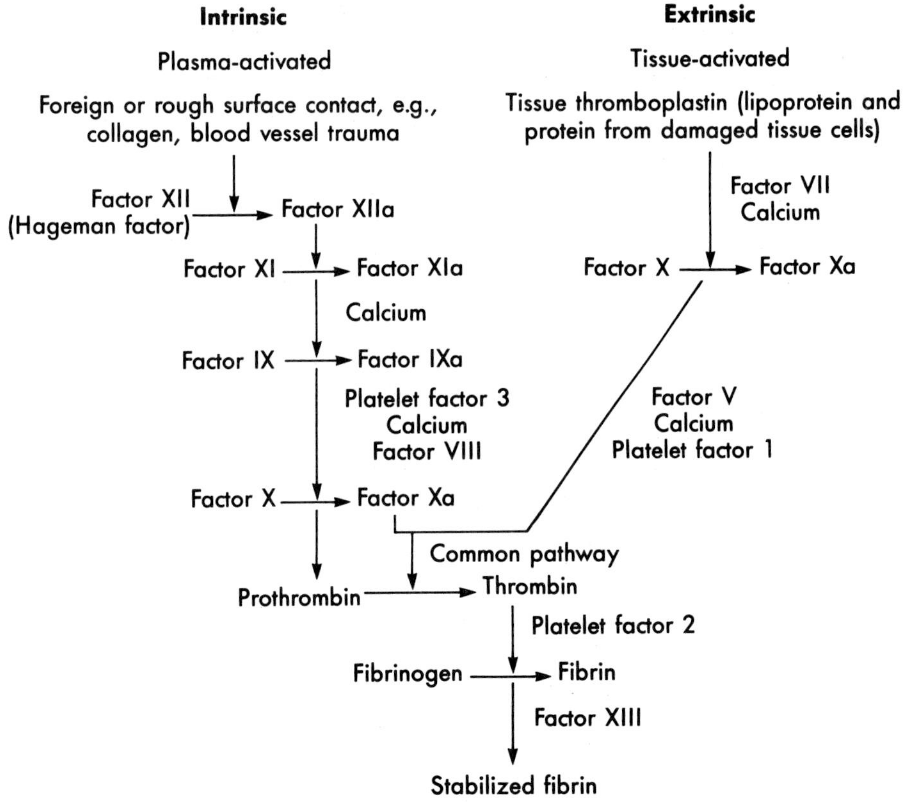

Figure 19-4   Pathways to coagulation. (*Note.* From "Disseminated Intravascular Coagulation: A Nursing Challenge" by B.A. Suchak and C.B. Barbon, 1989, *Orthopaedic Nursing*, 8(6), p. 63. Adapted from *Textbook of Medical Physiology* by A.C. Guyton, 1986, Philadelphia: W.B. Saunders; and *Guide to Diagnostic Procedures* by R.M. French, 1980, New York: McGraw-Hill.)

mally with circulating blood cells and maintains platelets in an inactive state by the synthesis and secretion of the potent antiaggregatory prostaglandin, *prostacyclin* (Stump & Mann, 1988). Under conditions of vascular trauma, the endothelium assumes a more prothrombotic state. The release of thromboplastin from the vascular injury stimulates the extrinsic pathway. The more complex intrinsic pathway is more difficult to activate and much harder to stop, since it self-perpetuates (Vogelpohl, 1981). Collagen under the endothelial cells of the intima of the vein is referred to as the *subendothelial matrix*. Exposure to this matrix leads to von Willebrand factor–mediated platelet adherence and collagen-induced platelet activation. The damaged endothelium also serves as a direct target for platelet adherence. These combined factors activate the intrinsic clotting mechanisms. Ultimately, the two converge and proceed to the same end: the production of fibrin thrombi and stable clots. Massive intravascular clotting is prevented because the body has a check and balance system using antithrombolytic agents to prevent systemic intravascular coagulation.

Antithrombins II and III, naturally occurring coagulation inhibitors, are found in the plasma. Antithrombin II (heparin) neutralizes free circulating thrombin. Antithrombin III neutralizes active clotting enzymes. Also, the endothelium can be a source of a key fibrinolytic enzyme, tissue plasminogen activator (TPA) (Stump & Mann, 1988). Factor XII activates plasminogen and stimulates its conversion into fibrinolysin. Fibrinolysin then digests fibrinogen and breaks down the fibrin thrombi.

The breaking down of the fibrin thrombi results in fibrin split products (FSPs), also known as *fibrin degradation products (FDPs)*, which are anticoagulants in nature. The FSPs interfere with the clot formation of platelets, thrombin, and fibrinogen as a compensatory mechanism. Thus no massive intravascular coagulation occurs.

Coagulopathy Why then does massive bleeding occur with DIC? Most patients with DIC have suffered an episode of prolonged hypotension. In arterial hypotension, arterial vasoconstriction combined with capillary dilation and the opening of preferential arteriovenous shunts lead to stagnation of blood in many capillaries. This blood rapidly becomes acidotic, which promotes coagulation. Also, thrombin liberated into the circulation by the intrinsic and extrinsic coagulation cascade catalyzes the activation of fibrinogen. This causes more fibrin to be produced and deposited into the microcirculation. In the capillaries, fibrin threads begin to form clots, which decreases flow of nutrients to the body cells, resulting in tissue ischemia. The most susceptible organs to tissue ischemia are the brain, kidneys, lungs, gastrointestinal (GI) tract, pancreas, adrenal glands, and the pituitary gland (Griffin, 1986). Failing organs may be further impaired by platelet clumping, another consequence of thrombin formation.

The average adult has approximately 100,000 miles of capillaries. The rapid acceleration of the clotting process in the microcirculation results in the rapid consumption of prothrombin, fibrinogen, platelets, factor V, and factor VIII. These cannot be replaced quickly enough to balance the dynamic equilibrium between clot formation and clot lysis (Vogelpohl, 1981). As a result of the decreased availability of coagulation factors and the increased amount of anticoagulants, the patient's blood cannot form stable clots in places where they are needed and bleeding occurs into the skin, from body orifices, and at sites of catheters and incisions (Figure 19-5).

Assessment and diagnosis

Although the clinical history is important, DIC is diagnosed primarily by laboratory studies. A battery of tests is used to verify DIC. Table 19-3 presents the laboratory findings.

The nursing assessment is critical in the detection and diagnosis of DIC. First, the nurse must always be alert for early signs of impaired tissue perfusion. These include subtle mental status changes, such as restlessness, confusion, and inappropriate behavior, as well as more overt physical signs and symptoms, such as hypotension, dyspnea, tachypnea, syncope, and even hemiplegia. All of these signs and symptoms may result from cerebral hypoxia. Impaired tissue perfusion may lead to organ necrosis and failure, such as acute renal tubular necrosis resulting in diminished urine output.

In the presence of DIC, blood may ooze from mucous membranes, needle puncture sites, incisions, or around catheters into body orifices. The nurse should inspect the patient's skin for purpura, hemorrhagic bullae, wound hematomas,

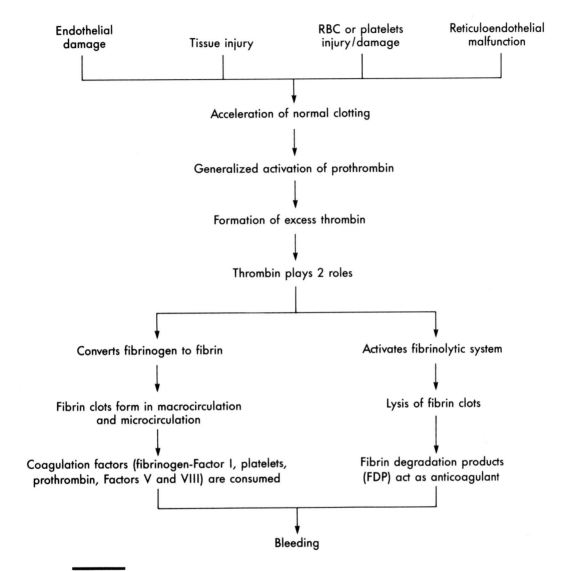

Figure 19-5 Coagulation process in DIC. (*Note.* From "Disseminated Intravascular Coagulation: A Nursing Challenge" by B.A. Suchak and C.B. Barbon, 1989, *Orthopaedic Nursing*, 8(6), p. 63. Adapted from *Textbook of Medical Physiology* by A.C. Guyton, 1986, Philadelphia: W.B. Saunders; and *Guide to Diagnostic Procedures* by R.M. French, 1980, New York: McGraw-Hill.)

Table 19-3 Laboratory data reflective of DIC

Test	Normal values	Values in DIC
Hemoglobin	♂ 14.0-16.5 g/dl	↓
	♀ 12.6-14.2 g/dl	↑ or ↓
Hematocrit	♂ 42%-52%	↓
	♀ 37%-47%	
Red blood cells	♂ 4.6-6.2 million/ml	↓
	♀ 4.5-5.4 million/ml	
White blood cells	4500-11,000/ml	↑
Platelet count	150,000-400,000/mm³	<100,000/mm³
Prothrombin time	12-14 seconds	Prolonged
Partial thromboplastin	45-65 seconds	Prolonged
Fibrinogen	195-356 mg/dl	<160 mg/dl
Fibrin split products	2-10 mg/ml	Elevated

♂, Male; ♀, female.

gangrene, widespread ecchymoses, and petechiae.

Occult bleeding may cause abdominal distention, guaiac-positive stool or emesis, hematuria, and changes in the color of the skin. Symptoms of occult bleeding that should be noted are malaise, weakness, altered sensorium, and headache. Acrocyanosis, characterized by sharply defined, irregularly shaped, cyanotic patches on the periphery of arms and legs, may result from fibrin deposited in the microcirculation (Griffin, 1986). Acrocyanosis may lead to gangrene.

Treatment of disseminated intravascular coagulation

The most controversial issue in DIC is treatment. Through the 1950s the recommended treatment was replacement with whole fresh blood, platelets, and clotting factors, such as fibrinogen and fresh frozen plasma. In the 1960s a new treatment was attempted using aminocaproic acid (Amicar), which acted by inhibiting profibrinolysis, the breakdown of fibrin by the proteolytic enzyme system. Initial results were promising; however, serious complications developed, with an 80% failure rate.

Also in the 1960s, treatment with heparin was instituted based on the reasoning that heparin would block the fundamental problem of enhanced clotting activity (Shoemaker, Ayres, Grenvik, Holbrook, & Thompson, 1989). Heparin's major action is to prevent the activation of thrombin. Heparin also neutralizes free-circulating thrombin, inhibits further progression of thrombi in capillaries, and prevents the activation of factor X. To this date, a controlled, prospective, clinical trial with heparin has never been performed to validate the effectiveness of heparin use in DIC. Controversy still exists as to the most effective activated partial thromboplastin time (APTT). APTTs from 1.5 to 3 times the control have been cited in the literature (Suchak & Barbon, 1989).

The one major and most important principle in the treatment of DIC agreed on by most is to treat the underlying cause. Nursing care priorities include rapid recognition, control of hemorrhage, and support of psychosocial needs for the patient and family.

GENERAL ASSESSMENT AND INTERVENTIONS
Nutrition

Survival of the trauma patient after the initial resuscitation depends on prevention of infection/sepsis, preservation of vital organs, and avoidance of malnutrition. Depending on the severity and the number of body systems involved, the total energy expenditure (TEE) can be elevated as much as 15% to 50% (Hurst, Koetting, & Lang, 1988). This impacts greatly on the immobilized, immunocompromised patient who may be ventilator dependent. Complete dependence on the medical and nursing team to provide life-sustaining support and meet nutritional demands becomes a requirement.

Previously in this chapter, the metabolic response to stress and injury was outlined. More specifically, the body undergoes a process of metabolic prioritization for the repair of tissue and system impairments. The hormonal cascade results in rapid lysis of protein, increased rate of fat utilization, and water and salt conservation. Gluconeogenesis and ureageneisis are accelerated and have a depleting effect on lean body mass. These processes, when sustained, will place the patient in a catabolic and malnourished state, predisposing them to complications of trauma.

The catabolic state that follows the shock phase of the injured patient generally occurs 3 to 10 days after the traumatic incident and is characterized by increased protein metabolism (Hassan & Danziger, 1988). This hypermetabolic state results in simultaneous mobilization of protein and fat in the face of elevated glucose levels that are present in response to stress. Patients with these responses consistently exhibit increases in protein degradation and increases in urinary nitrogen excretion. The accelerated loss of protein can be tolerated for a short period, but eventually will result in total body nitrogen loss, or negative nitrogen balance, if there is no intervention (Hassan & Danziger, 1988).

Two basic methods for estimating nonprotein caloric needs are used in the nutritional care of the trauma patient: (1) the Harris-Benedict equation and (2) calorimetry (Cerra, 1988). The Harris-Benedict method (see box below) is an equation that calculates the basal energy expenditure (BEE) based on height, weight, sex, and age, in the resting, nonstressed state.

For energy requirements in the injured patient, a stress factor is multiplied into the formula, thereby calculating the total daily expenditure (TDE) (Hsieh, 1988). Expired gas analysis applies principles of indirect calorimetry through the use of metabolic carts or ventilated-hood calorimeters to analyze expired gas. These devices measure expired carbon dioxide production and oxygen consumption as part of the equation to calculate the respiratory quotient and resting metabolic expenditure (RME). The RME is representative of the actual energy expenditure at the time of measurement; thus an added stress factor does not need to be calculated into the formula (Cerra, 1988). Resting energy expenditure can be calculated in patients with a thermodilution pulmonary artery catheter.

The RME, although quite accurate, is an expensive method and labor intensive. Conversely, the Harris-Benedict method is easy to use, requires no special technology, and can be rapidly calculated. Another quick estimate of nonprotein caloric need is to use ideal body weight for the formula 30 kcal/kg/day. Multiple methods are available for nutritional assessment as described in the box on p. 608 and are incorporated into screening tools (Figure 19-6).

Use of Energy Sources

In the traumatized patient, body protein can be catabolized at a rate of 75 to 150 g/day, which may ultimately result in a loss of 300 to 600 g of lean body mass daily (Hassan & Danziger, 1988). Therefore stressed patients may require between 2.5 to 3.5 g/kg/day of supplemental protein. There are no known storage mechanisms or sites for protein; therefore if it is used for energy and is not replenished, a deficiency will result. An interrelationship exists between caloric intake and protein requirements, providing for a proportional amount of nitrogen retention to the amount of caloric support.

Most tissues have the ability to utilize fat as an energy source; however the nervous system and wound tissues are excluded. Fat becomes a major source of energy for the body as free fatty acids (FFAs) are released into the circulation after an injury. Basically, glucose uptake diminishes in the periphery from several factors, creating an environment for fat to be the accessible energy source.

Although the reason is not clear, ketone production is not greatly increased in the response to trauma. It is hypothesized, however, that the rise of insulin in response to the initial surge of glucose seems to inhibit the triglyceride lipase activity. Thus serum-free fatty acid levels increase, but less than might be expected compared with energy requirements (Stanek, 1988).

Nitrogen balance

Comparison of urinary nitrogen output and nitrogen intake provides an estimate of lean body

---

Harris-Benedict equation for basal energy expenditure (BEE) calculation

Men

BEE = 66 + (13.7 × wt) + (5 × ht) − (6.8 × a)

Women

BEE = 665 + (9.6 × wt) + (1.7 × ht) − (4.7 × a)

wt, Weight in kilograms (kg = 2.2 pounds); *ht,* height in centimeters (cm = 2.54 inches); *a,* age in years. Total BEE is expressed in kilocalories.

Methods for nutritional assessment

1. Weight

   $$\% \text{ Ideal body weight} = \frac{\text{Actual wt} \times 100}{\text{Ideal wt}}$$

   $$\% \text{ Weight loss} = \frac{\text{Usual wt} - \text{actual wt} \times 100}{\text{Usual wt}}$$

2. Albumin (serum): 4 to 5 g/kg
3. Transferrin: $(0.8 \times \text{TIBC}) - 43$

   (In moderate to severe malnutrition, correlation with TIBC is not accurate; direct measurements should be done.)

4. TLC $= \dfrac{\% \text{ Lymphocytes} \times \text{WBC}}{100}$

5. Skin tests: *Candida,* streptokinase, and mumps tests are commonly used; malnourished patients will not respond to two or more antigens.

6. CHI: 24-hour urine collection; creatinine level compared with standard $\dfrac{\text{Actual excretion} \times 100}{\text{Standard excretion}}$

   affected by age, diet, and urine collection technique

7. TSF: Measurement of skin-fold thickness with calipers; comparison with norms.
8. MAC: Measurement of circumference at midpoint of distance from acromion to olecranon; comparison with norms.
9. MAMC $=$ MAC $- (3.14 \times \text{TSF})$

   (normal $=$ 25.3 cm in males; 23.2 cm in females)

Nutritional deficits	None	Mild	Moderate	Severe
% Ideal body weight	>90	80-90	70-79	<70
% Weight loss	0-5	5-15	15-25	>25
Serum albumin (g/dl)	>3.5	3-3.5	2.1-2.9	<2.1
TLC (thousands of cells/mm^3)	>2.0	1.2-2.0	0.8-1.2	<0.8
Transferrin (mg/dl)	>200	150-200	100-150	<100
CHI % standard	>90	81-90	71-80	70-60
TSF % standard MAC	>90	51-90	31-50	<30
MAMC % standard	>90	51-90	31-50	<30

Note. Data from Medical grand rounds lecture notes by R. Fisher, 1982, Yale-New Haven Hospital, New Haven, Conn.; and from *Pocket Manual of Surgical Nutrition* (p. 29) by F.B. Cerra, 1984, St. Louis: Mosby—Year Book, Inc.
wt, Weight; *TIBC,* total iron-binding capacity; *TLC,* total lymphocyte count; *WBC,* white blood cell count; *CHI,* creatinine-height index; *TSF,* triceps skin fold; *MAC,* midarm circumference; *MAMC,* midarm muscle circumference.

---

mass and protein status. Nitrogen output that exceeds the intake is indicative of continued protein catabolism (negative nitrogen balance). Nutritional support should be instituted before the development of severe and prolonged negative nitrogen balance. Essential amino acids in and of themselves do not provide a source of energy, but they allow for protein synthesis so that nitrogen is available.

The goal of therapy is to create a positive nitrogen balance while maintaining body weight and increasing hepatic protein synthesis (Mirtallo, 1988). Prevention of weight loss in excess of 10% of the preinjury weight is targeted (Martindale & McCarthy, 1988).

Glutamine

Translocation of bacteria has been attributed in part to bowel mucosal atrophy. Experimental models have shown that glutamine administration in both total parenteral nutrition (TPN) and enteral feedings demonstrated less small bowel mucosal atrophy than did control models (Priest, 1991). Thus glutamine administration in the gut may play a key role in maintaining a functional GI mucosal barrier.

STANFORD UNIVERSITY HOSPITAL
DEPARTMENT OF NUTRITION & FOOD SERVICES

**INITIAL NUTRITION
SCREENING**

ADDRESSOGRAPH STAMP - MEDICAL RECORD NUMBER, PATIENT NAME

ADM. DATE:	SCREEN DATE:	RISK FACTOR (RF)

S: Wt History 6 mos. PTA:　☐ Stable　☐ Gain *　☐ Loss *

　　　　　　*Explain _____

　　APPETITE:　☐ Stable　☐ < NL*　☐ > NL*　* Explain _____

　　GI PROBLEMS:　☐ None　☐ N　☐ V　☐ D　☐ Constipation　☐ Chew/Swallow Problem

　　　　　　☐ Other _____

　　SPECIAL DIET PTA:

　　FOOD ALLERGIES:

Risk factor column (S section):
YES　NO
WT HX　☐　☐
GI　☐　☐

O:　Ht _____ Wt _____ ☐ Actual ☐ Stated　Usual Wt _____　Desirable Body Wt _____

　　Age _____　% Usual Wt _____　Desirable % Body Wt _____

　　Date _____ Albumin _____ GM/DL ☐ WNL　☐ Marginal Depletion (2.9-3.2)　☐ Severe Depletion (< 2.9)

　　OTHER LABS _____

　　DIET ORDER _____

　　DIAGNOSIS _____

Risk factor column (O section):
HT/WT　☐　☐
LABS　☐　☐
DIET　☐　☐
DX　☐　☐

A:　NUTRITIONAL STATUS:　☐ High Risk (>3 RF)　☐ Moderate Risk (1-3 RF)　☐ Low Risk (0 RF)

TOTAL RF SCORE =

　　☐ Unable to determine nutritional status due to lack of sufficient screening data.

P:　☐ Dietetic Technician to provide Basic Nutrition Services
　　　Reevaluate in　3　5　7　10　14　days　　　　Next Follow-up Date: _____

　　☐ Referred to Registered Dietitian for Comprehensive Nutritional Assessment

　　☐ Refer to Progress Notes Dated _____ .

　　☐ _____
　　　_____
　　　_____
　　　_____
　　　_____
　　　_____

Signature/Title　　　　　　　　　　　　　　Date

15-661 (10/90)　　WHITE – MEDICAL RECORD COPY　CANARY – DIETITIAN COPY　PINK– DIETETIC TECHNICIAN COPY

Figure 19-6　Initial nutritional screening tool. (Courtesy Stanford University Hospital Department of Nutrition and Food Services.)

Nutritional Support
Enteral

Enteral routes of nutrition have proven to maintain the GI tract integrity, to be cost efficient, and to decrease the risk of sepsis. Therefore in many instances this method is preferred over parenteral techniques.

The GI mucosa normally is a sufficient barrier that prevents bacterial translocation into the systemic circulation. However, in the face of bacterial overgrowth and/or mucosal atrophy, this barrier is subject to breakdown. This gut dysfunction can be reversed or minimized by the administration of early enteral feedings (Rolandelli & Koruda, 1991) (see Figure 19-2).

Patients undergoing laparotomy may have a feeding gastrostomy or jejunostomy inserted at the time of surgery. Other patients without significant contraindications may have a nasogastric feeding tube inserted. In the presence of delayed gastric emptying secondary to anesthesia or postoperative shock, the feeding access will be placed distal to the stomach, either surgically, endoscopically, or by fluoroscopy.

Continuous, uniform feedings directly into the small bowel are more beneficial to the trauma patient than intermittent nutritional supplements (Guenter, 1985). These continuous feedings have been associated with less stool frequency, shorter times to achieve nutritional goals, and greater tolerance in patients with hemodynamic instability (Rolandelli & Koruda, 1991).

Common complications that may be seen when enteral feedings are used include (1) aspiration if gastric feedings are given and (2) diarrhea from the hyperosmolarity or bacterial overgrowth of the solutions. Prevention of complications depends on the following nursing techniques:
- ensuring proper tube placement
- ensuring proper patient position while receiving feeding: head of bed elevated 30 degrees if not contraindicated
- ensuring proper supplement dilution
- administering supplement at appropriate rate
- routinely checking residuals

Clogging of the feeding tube is sometimes unavoidable, but may be minimized by routine irrigations with tap water or saline and special care in flushing after medication administration. Some tubes are difficult to aspirate, thereby complicating checks of residual.

Studies have suggested that the small bowel is relatively resistant to postoperative and traumatic ileus and that the activity of the small bowel returns several hours after an insult (Rombeau & Caldwell, 1984). This is in contrast to colonic activity, which may not return for several days. Adynamic ileus occurs more commonly in the stomach and colon than in the ileum (Baue, 1991). These studies suggest that the stomach and colon may not tolerate enteral feedings in the first few days after injury, but the small bowel may.

Historically, bowel sounds have been used as criteria for determining the optimal time for instituting enteral feedings. According to Hull (1985), the small bowel retains its capacity to absorb fluids and nutrients in the presence of ileus. Nutritional efforts that bypass the stomach may be instituted earlier in the trauma patient than they have been in the past. This may decrease the complication rate, provide a more cost-effective method, and provide efficacy equal to total parenteral nutrition (Adams et al., 1986).

Preferably, feedings are started within 24 hours of injury. In the presence of abdominal injury, this may be difficult, related to an ileus caused from either direct injury or surgery. In these cases, a catheter jejunostomy has been advocated. Feedings can then be started within a few hours after surgery; starting with an isotonic solution at 30 to 50 ml/hr and taking about 5 days to advance the delivery to sufficient calories to meet the patient's metabolic requirements (Van Way, 1991). A residual amount that equals the past hour's feeding infusion plus 50 ml is considered high.

Several classifications of enteral diet formulations have been cited by Rolandelli & Korunda (1991), based on nutrient composition. They include the following:
- **Polymeric** These diets are considered complete and contain 100% of the recommended daily allowances (RDA) of vitamins and minerals when 2 liters are administered. They are lactose-free and of high molecular weight composition with low osmolarity. Most contain 1 to 3 kcal/ml. They are generally palatable and can be used for oral supplementation or tube feedings. They are the initial choice for oral or enteral feedings when GI digestion and absorption are intact. According to Rolandelli & Koruda (1991),

these diets are suitable for 90% of trauma patients.

- **Oligomeric** These diets are composed of elemental nutrients, which require minimal digestion and leave little residue in the colon after nearly complete absorption. They contain 1% to 30% fat and are considered complete with all essential minerals and vitamins. These diets are relatively hyperosmolar and can cause diarrhea if administered too rapidly. Oligomeric diets cost approximately 5 times that of polymerics and are basically unpalatable. They are easily delivered by fine-bore feeding tubes.
- **Modular** Modular feeding allows for alterations in the ratio of basic nutrients to meet special nutrient requirements in hepatic failure, electrolyte imbalances, and short bowel syndrome, to name a few. They require astute monitoring and advanced expertise to provide continued nutrition without deficiencies.

Table 19-4 illustrates the classification of current enteral formulas. Enteral nutrition is contraindicated in complete mechanical intestinal obstruction, high-output intestinal fistulae, shock, severe diarrhea, and with a prognosis not warranting aggressive nutritional support.

Parenteral

When a patient has lost normal gut function, parenteral nutrition can be utilized for meeting high caloric and metabolic requirements. When used aggressively, it can greatly improve the nitrogen balance status. Protein calories are generally not calculated for TPN usage because the goal is to use amino acids for protein synthesis and not as an energy source (Guenter, 1985). Carbohydrate supplied as highly concentrated dextrose provides the energy medium. Of the calculated caloric and nitrogen requirement, 50% to 75% should be infused during the first 24 hours to determine tolerance and electrolyte requirements, before the rate of TPN administration is advanced.

It is interesting to note that the use of TPN may have an effect on the development of sepsis and MOF. Animal studies have shown that a statistically significant increase in the cecal bacterial count and impairment of the intestinal defenses occurred when TPN was used (Alverdy, Aoys, &

Table 19-4 Classification of enteral formulas

Polymeric	Oligomeric	Modular
1 kcal/ml	**Elemental**	**Carbohydrate**
Ensure/HN	Vivonex TEN	Polycose
Renu	Travasorb STD	Medical
Osmolite/HN		Hycal
Sumacal	**Low residue**	Calplus
Isocal	Precision LR	
Sustacal	Precision HN	**Fat**
	Flexical	Microlipid
1.5 kcal/ml		Lipomul
Ensure Plus/HN	**Peptide based**	MCT
Sustacal HC	Peptamin	
	Vital HN	
3 kcal/ml	Criticare	**Protein**
Isocal HCN	Reabilan	Casec
Magnacal		Promix
	Special—hepatic	Propac
Fiber	**encephalopathy**	EMF
containing	Hepatic-aid	Aminess
Enrich	Travasorb-Hepatic	
Jevity		**Complete**
Compleat	**Special—renal**	**modular**
Ultracal	**failure**	Nutrisource
	Amin-Aid	
	Travasorb Renal	
	Special—stress/	
	trauma	
	Trauma-aid	
	Stresstein	
	Criticare	
	Impact	

Note. From "Nutrition and Trauma: Techniques of Nutritional Support" by R.H. Rolandelli and M.J. Korunda, 1991, *Trauma Quarterly, 7*(2), p. 40. (Reprinted by permission from "Enteral Nutrition in the Critically Ill" by M.J. Koruda, P. Geunter, and J. Rombeau, 1987, *Critical Care Clinics, 3,* pp. 133-153. Copyright 1987. W.B.Saunders).

Moss, 1988). This correlates with the study by Baker et al. (1988) regarding translocation of gut bacteria into the systemic circulation.

The subclavian site is the preferred route of administration for TPN, because other sites have proven to increase the risk of such complications as thrombophlebitis. Subclavian vein thrombosis may develop in approximately 5% to 15% of patients receiving TPN. It commonly occurs 1 to 2 weeks after the onset of therapy, demonstrated by unilateral swelling of the arm, shoulder, neck, or head. The use of catheters that are heparin-bonded, Silastic, or coated with water-activated lubricants, as well as the addition of 1000 to 2000 units of heparin per liter of parenteral solution, have reduced the incidence of thrombus formation (Grant, 1988).

The most common complication of TPN is infection at or around the insertion site. The presence of the catheter and hypertonic glucose solutions increases the risk of migration of bacteria along the catheter walls. Any hospital that routinely cares for critically ill and nutritionally supported patients should have stringent protocols for parenteral nutrition. These protocols should address the use of strict aseptic technique, specific instructions on vascular access, catheter management, solutions, and the management of complications.

The second most common complication of parenteral nutrition is hyperglycemia. Insulin may be added to the infusion, or fat may be used as a primary calorie rather than glucose.

Nursing considerations for patients with parenteral infusions should include routine TPN site dressing change per hospital protocol, continued assessment for changes in breath sounds, maintenance of blood return within the line, and assessment for leakage or visible change around the catheter site. Chest x-ray films should be obtained after the initial insertion for documentation of proper catheter placement.

Special Considerations

The trauma patient may have altered responses to injury related to direct trauma to organs, sepsis, organ failure, DIC, or a combination of factors that create disruptions in metabolism.

In patients who exhibit respiratory difficulties, caloric doses that meet the basal requirement are required, with special attention given to the amount of carbohydrates. Excessive carbohydrate infusions will increase carbon dioxide levels and lead to increased respiratory effort, which may lead to hypercarbia, respiratory acidosis, and increasing ventilator dependency (Grant, 1988). The administration of fat as an energy source will minimize the amount of carbon dioxide produced from fuel oxidation.

Renal impairment affects the body's ability to regulate electrolytes and nitrogen waste products, acid-base balance, and fluids. Tolerance to the usual nutritional load will be diminished, which may produce additional complicating factors, such as azotemia, acidosis, hyperkalemia, and hypermagnesemia. The recommended approach in renal failure is to dose nutrients to tolerance with a protein restriction, increased calorie-nitrogen ratio, and selected addition of electrolytes (Mirtallo, 1988).

Patients with hepatic failure must have careful consideration of protein, fat, and carbohydrate doses. Encephalopathies may develop or progress with intolerances to protein and accumulation of free fatty acids from IV administration of fat. A modest restriction of protein and careful use of lipids to prevent excessive fat accumulation are recommended when signs of increasing encephalopathy or increases in serum ammonia develop (Mirtallo, 1988). Excess calories are responsible for fatty infiltration of the liver; therefore the caloric dose necessary to achieve a positive nitrogen balance should not be exceeded.

SUMMARY Caring for the trauma patient can be complex because many variables exist that may complicate the patient's outcome. Coagulation abnormalities may ensue in the midst of treatment for infection or organ failure. Iatrogenic infections may complicate the patient's condition even more. Considering the multitude of problems that may arise, the trauma nurse must be astute in assessment and treatment of the multiply injured patient. Prevention and minimizing morbidity and mortality in the trauma patient should be of primary concern. The table on pp. 613-618 outlines pertinent nursing diagnoses and evaluative criteria for the multiply injured patient.

NURSING DIAGNOSES &
EVALUATIVE CRITERIA   *The multiply injured patient*

Nursing diagnosis	Nursing intervention	Evaluative criteria
Altered tissue perfusion Related to bleeding Secondary to changes in clotting cycle As evidenced by change in mental status, petechiae, cool skin	**Minimize perfusion deficit** Obtain arterial blood gases as appropriate. Obtain blood for laboratory studies to include prothrombin, partial thromboplastin time, hemoglobin, hematocrit, fibrinogen levels, and fibrin split products. Observe for bleeding at venipuncture sites, mucous membranes, catheter insertion sites, and incisions. Monitor for hematuria, hematemesis and occult blood in stool; report if present. Assess for increased bleeding or new sites of hemorrhage. Monitor arterial pressure, electrocardiogram, pulse, and respiration every 30 to 60 minutes. Assess level of responsiveness every 30 to 60 minutes. Auscultate heart and breath sounds. Monitor intake and output. Avoid intramuscular injections; minimize number of venipunctures by scheduling draws collectively. Monitor distal extremities for altered neurovascular status.	 Patient's coagulation profile will return to normal parameters (refer to Table 19-3). Patient will exhibit no evidence of bleeding. Vital signs will remain stable. Patient will show no deterioration in mentation. Lungs will remain clear. Peripheral pulses will be equal and present. No edema or pain to dorsiflexion of foot will be present.
Decreased cardiac output Related to hypovolemia, capillary permeability, failure of compensatory mechanisms Secondary to sepsis AND **Infection** Related to bacterial, fungal, or viral invasion, localized or systemic, actual or potential As evidenced by vasodilation, fever, drainage of pus from wound	**Promote blood flow distribution** Obtain cultures of fluids from IV sites, sinuses, surgical and nonsurgical wounds; also culture sputum, urine, blood, cerebrospinal fluid (if indicated). Draw blood specimens and monitor laboratory data, including hemoglobin and hematocrit, coagulation profile, and white blood count. Obtain computerized tomography scans, as ordered, to identify areas of potential abscesses. Obtain x-ray studies, as ordered, (chest x-ray and abdominal films) to detect fluid accumulation, free air, or abscesses.	 Cultures will be negative. White blood cell count will be within normal limits or decreasing to normal. Differential count will be without shift. Abscesses will be drained effectively with interventional radiology techniques or surgical intervention.

Continued.

NURSING DIAGNOSIS	NURSING INTERVENTIONS	EVALUATIVE CRITERIA
Decreased cardiac output AND **Infection—cont'd**	Administer antibiotics as indicated. Administer oxygen as indicated. Deliver appropriate fluid, blood, and/or blood products as ordered. Assess for shock. *Hyperdynamic* signs and symptoms are tachycardia; tachypnea; warm, pink skin; hyperthermia; restlessness, other changes in level of consciousness; respiratory alkalosis. *Hypodynamic* signs and symptoms are tachycardia; tachypnea; pallor; hypothermia; oliguria; unresponsiveness; disseminated intravascular coagulation; hypotension; decreased cardiac output. Assess for effects of pharmacologic therapy. Monitor vital signs every 15 minutes or as needed. Monitor pulmonary arterial pressure and pulmonary catheter wedge pressures every 1 to 2 hours as ordered. Monitor cardiac output as ordered. Monitor core temperature; keep patient warm and dry; avoid chills. Maintain intravenous lines (at least two large-bore); accurately measure intake and output. Wash hands frequently; maintain strict aseptic technique; adhere to institutional infection control measures. Assess for signs and symptoms of wound infection, to include redness, swelling, drainage, temperature changes, fever, pain. Monitor urine glucose (glucosuria may precede impending sepsis).	Therapeutic levels of antibiotics will be maintained, and physician's choice of antibiotic will reflect the results of culture and sensitivity studies. Patient will be alert and oriented to person, place, time. Early detection and management of the hyperdynamic phase will occur to prevent progression to hypodynamic stage. Vital signs will be within normal parameters. Pulmonary catheter wedge pressure will be 4-12 mm Hg. Pulmonary artery pressure will be 25/10 (15 mean pressure). Cardiac output will be 5L/min. (Cardiac index should be calculated.) Patient will be normothermic. Intake and output and weight changes will be thoroughly documented. Quality improvement audits will show adherence to invasive procedure policies. Signs and symptoms of wound infection will be absent. Glucosuria will be absent.
Impaired gas exchange Related to accumulation of fluid in alveoli and pulmonary interstitium As evidenced by oxygen desaturation with activity, difficulty weaning from ventilator	**Promote diffusion of gases** Draw blood for arterial blood gases and/or monitor pulse.oximetry. Administer oxygen as indicated. Administer bronchodilators as indicated. Provide chest physiotherapy and incentive spirometry as prescribed.	Patient will demonstrate improved ventilation as evidenced by nonlabored breathing, clear lungs, and arterial oxygen and carbon dioxide levels within normal parameters.

NURSING DIAGNOSIS	NURSING INTERVENTIONS	EVALUATIVE CRITERIA
	Assess patient's respiratory status, rate, rhythm, chest expansion, breath sounds, skin color. Assess for signs of bronchospasm. Suction frequently or as needed. Assist and teach patient to cough and deep breathe. Turn and/or reposition patient every 2 hours; Consider use of rotating beds for increased pulmonary toilet.	Respiratory rate will be 12-20/min; chest expansion will be equal and adequate. No retractions or wheezing will be present. Sputum will be of normal color and consistency.

Altered nutrition: less than body requirements
Related to hypermetabolic and hypercatabolic trauma responses and absent oral intake
As evidenced by delayed wound healing, weight loss, difficulty weaning from ventilator
	Maintain nutritional balance
	Perform serial measurements of skinfold thickness and midarm muscle circumference.
	Assist with caloric calculations, type, and amount of dietary supplements.
	Assist with insertion of feeding device as appropriate (i.e., central line for parenteral nutrition; gastric/duodenal tubes for enteral nutrition.)
	
	Recognize value of varied serum studies in interpretation of recent change in nutritional status.
	
	Monitor serum laboratory results—glucose, creatinine, blood urea nitrogen, electrolytes, liver enzymes, complete blood count, prothrombin time, magnesium, calcium, phosphorus, and osmolality.
		Patient will maintain nutritional status to meet body requirements and promote healing (see box, p. 608)
		
		Complications of nutritional therapy, such as the following, will be minimized:
		Enteral
		
		• aspiration;
		• altered bowel elimination—diarrhea.
		Parenteral
		
		• air embolus;
		• hydrothorax.
		Biologic half-lives of nutritional markers will be considered as patient's nutritional status is evaluated:
		• prealbumin 2.5-3 days;
		• transferrin 4-8 days;
		• albumin 14-20 days.
		Serum laboratory values will be within normal limits—desired adult values are listed below (significant differences for children are noted):
		• glucose: 70-100 mg/dl (generally treated if 180-200)
		  newborn: 20-60
		  1st yr.: 50-130;
		• osmolality: 275-295 mOsm/kg water;
		• magnesium: 1.6-2.5 mEq/L
		  newborn: 1.5-2.3
		  child to age 12: 1.2-1.9;
		• phosphorus: 2.5-4.5 mg/dl
		  newborn: 5.0-10.5
		  1 yr: 4.0-6.8
		  10 yrs: 3.4-6.0;

Continued.

NURSING DIAGNOSIS	NURSING INTERVENTIONS	EVALUATIVE CRITERIA
Altered nutrition: less than body requirements—cont'd		• calcium: 8.5-10.3 mg/dl or 4.5-5.6 mEq/L newborn: 7-12 mg/dl 2-16 yrs: 9-11 mg/dl; **Trace elements** • zinc: 50-150 mcg/dl; • copper male: 70-140 mcg/dl female: 85-155 mcg/dl child: 30-150 mcg/dl; • sodium: 135-145 mEq/L; • potassium: 3.5-5.5 mEq/L newborn: 5.0-7.7; • chloride: 98-108 mEq/L; • urea nitrogen (BUN): 9-20 mg/dl 1-2 yrs: 5-15; • creatinine: 0.4-1.3 mg/dl <5 yrs: 0.1-0.5; • iron: 50-150 mcg/dl newborn: 100-250 infant: 30-80 child: 40-120; • aspartate aminotransferase (AST): 10-35 IU/L; • alanine aminotransferase (ALT): 10-40 IU/L newborn: 2-3 times adult AST/ALT 1-5 yrs: 1½ -2 times adult AST/ALT.
	Administer appropriate nutrient. Administer insulin as directed. Obtain chest x-ray film after insertion of central line and flexible, small-bore feeding tube. Assess patient's nutritional status on admission; check for food allergies, preexisting diseases that affect nutrition, current medication, alcohol use, height, and weight.	Invasive lines will remain optimally positioned. Pneumothorax will not develop. Patient will maintain positive nitrogen balance (nitrogen intake [grams] minus urine urea nitrogen plus 4). During optimal support, a positive balance of 3-5 g is expected. Nutritional history will be documented. Patient's weight will compare with norms for age and height.
	Monitor weight, maintain strict intake and output measurement and recording, and assess for fluid overload or deficit.	Weight loss will be avoided. (Weight changes of 0.5 kg/day = fluid imbalances; a nutritionally induced weight gain of 1 kg is approximately equivalent to a positive caloric balance of 7000 cal/week.)

NURSING DIAGNOSIS	NURSING INTERVENTIONS	EVALUATIVE CRITERIA
	Obtain urine for routine monitoring.	Urine specific gravity, glucose, ketones, and protein will all be within normal limits.
	Monitor for signs and symptoms of hyperglycemia and hypoglycemia.	Abnormal assessment parameters will be avoided, or detected and reported.
	Assess for signs of fatty acid deficiency, including alopecia, decreased immunity, thrombocytopenia, and prolonged wound healing.	
	Assist with coping mechanisms to decrease fear and anxiety that may increase metabolic demands.	
High risk for injury Related to tube feeding and total parenteral nutrition (TPN): aspiration, altered bowel elimination, electrolyte imbalance, infection	**Maintain patency and sterility of tubes and lines as appropriate** <u>Tube feedings</u> Check tube placement by gastric air pop, aspiration, residual, and/or x-ray examination	
	Color the feeding with dye if aspiration possible.	Color of sputum will not reflect dye color added to feeding.
	Elevate head of bed while feeding and for 30 to 60 minutes after gastric feeding, unless contraindicated; For continuous feeding, check for excessive residual and use side-lying position and/or elevation of head.	
	Use special precaution when dealing with small-bore, flexible feeding tubes, which are mobile and easily displaced.	
	Assess breath sounds and changes in respiratory pattern during and after feeding.	Breath sounds will remain clear to auscultation, and x-ray findings will be negative.
	Consult with dietician regarding correct supplement for gastric vs. jejunal feeding.	
	Consult with pharmacy regarding correct administration of medications.	Maximal absorption and action of drugs will occur; tube will remain patent.
	Gradually increase rate and concentration of supplement, and monitor tolerance; report diarrhea.	Diarrhea will be controlled or prevented.
	Cleanse administration set per protocol, and place only a 4-hour infusion amount of solution in administration set at a time.	Enteritis induced by bacterial overgrowth will be avoided.

Continued.

....

NURSING DIAGNOSIS	NURSING INTERVENTIONS	EVALUATIVE CRITERIA
High risk for injury—cont'd	Total parenteral nutrition Assure aseptic technique during insertion and maintenance of site/tubing changes. Assess central lines for patency. Report abnormal laboratory values to physician and nutritional support team.	No leakage, redness or edema at site will occur. Blood will return on aspiration. Fingerstick glucose will be within normal limits. (See nursing diagnosis: *altered nutrition*).
High risk for altered oral mucous membrane Related to use of systemic antibiotics, nothing by mouth (NPO) status, altered coagulation status	Maintain integrity of mucous membranes Administer nystatin or other agents as appropriate for thrush. Assess mucous membranes, tongue, and gums every 4 to 8 hours. Brush teeth with soft toothbrush bid or prn. Apply lip balm or petroleum jelly for dry lips. Remove dentures and clean bid—assure proper fit. Report evidence of caries or tooth pain, especially if patient immunologically labile. Explain rationale for episodes of NPO status. Rinse mouth with dilute peroxide or dilute mouthwash solutions. Use dampened oral swabs to keep oral mucosa moist.	The patient's oral mucosa will remain clean, moist, and free from disruption. The patient will verbalize oral comfort and maintain appetite. Patient will comply with NPO status.
Anxiety and Fear Related to threat of death and loss of independence Secondary to long-term hospitalization and complications As evidenced by patient comments, nonverbal gestures	Facilitate patient adjustment to illness Assess level of patient fears and understanding of current condition. Maintain a nonstressful environment. Provide appropriate information about condition, procedures, and laboratory studies. Encourage questions. Maintain and assist with coping strategies. Be sensitive to needs, and observe nonverbal clues. Facilitate visiting by significant others. Decorate and organize room according to patient wishes.	Patient will exhibit decreased symptoms of anxiety/fear. Patient will display new coping strategies. Significant others will verbalize needs and concerns.

CASE STUDY Mr. W. is a 25-year-old man involved in a two-vehicle MVC on a rural stretch of highway. He was one of three occupants in a small compact car that was broadsided by a large sedan traveling at 55 to 60 mph. The car was extensively damaged and torn into three sections. Because the closest medical assistance was approximately 30 minutes away, dual response of an ambulance and an air rescue helicopter was initiated simultaneously.

When the first ground unit arrived, they found Mr. W. lying amidst the wreckage, conscious but confused, and moving all four extremities. The environmental Fahrenheit temperature was in the low 40s. He had no obvious external injuries. An initial patient survey was conducted, and BP was 150/80; HR, 110; and respirations, 24. Mr. W. was considered to be stable and was prepared for transport on a long spine board with a cervical collar in place. Two large-bore IVs were initiated with normal saline infusing at a keep-open rate, and PASG was applied, but not inflated.   The helicopter arrived several minutes later and initiated transport to the nearest trauma center. En route, Mr. W.'s vital signs remained unchanged; however, his level of consciousness diminished to the point of unresponsiveness. Nasotracheal intubation was performed for airway protection and to ensure adequate oxygenation, especially in light of his probable closed head injury.

What are the potential complications that may be anticipated for this patient?

Mr. W. has the potential for several severe and life-threatening complications as a result of his injuries. Sepsis may be anticipated based on invasive procedures performed under less than ideal con-

ditions. The patient was exposed to the elements for an extended time, increasing his risk of hypothermia and the chances of developing coagulation disorders. Without knowing the cause of his decreasing level of consciousness, caregivers must suspect that he has hypoxia, hypovolemia, and/or an intracranial bleed.

On arrival in the trauma/resuscitation room, Mr. W. is found to open his eyes only to pain. His blood pressure has dropped to 40 systolic with a pulse rate of 130. Total trauma score is 4, and core temperature, measured by urinary catheter probe, is 30° C (86° F). Several more intravenous lines are placed and about 2000 ml of warmed crystalloid and 4 units of packed red blood cells are infused in an effort to stabilize his condition within the first 35 minutes.

Urinary catheter and nasogastric tube returns are grossly positive for blood. A diagnostic peritoneal lavage is performed, the return of which is also grossly bloody. Arterial pressure of 70 is obtained per invasive monitoring, and Mr. W. is immediately taken to the operating room suite. Results from his initial blood draw reveal a hemoglobin of 8 g/dl and a hematocrit of 25%.

The operative management of Mr. W. includes the placement of bilateral chest tubes and a left thoracotomy for the evacuation of accumulated blood. A diaphragmatic herniation is present with abdominal contents in the chest cavity; this is appropriately repaired. Exploratory laparotomy reveals an avulsed spleen requiring splenectomy. A triple-lumen subclavian line, pulmonary artery catheter, and feeding jejunostomy tube are inserted intraoperatively.

Intraoperative blood loss is estimated at 12 units, with autotransfusion by cell saver reinfusing 5000 ml of autologous blood. An additional 14 units of packed red blood cells are transfused, along with 10 units of platelets, 4 units of fresh frozen plasma, and 20 liters of crystalloid solution.

Mr. W. survives surgery and is transferred to the trauma intensive care unit. Laboratory values reveal a platelet count of 107,000/mm^3; prothrombin time, 14.1 seconds; partial thromboplastin time, 40.1 seconds; fibrinogen, 195 mg/dl; and fibrin split products, 20-40 mg/ml.

After stabilization of the immediately life-threatening injuries, the following injuries are also identified:

- multiple rib fractures
- brain contusions with hemorrhage and coma
- fractures of C2 and C4
- multiple pelvic fractures
- massive retroperitoneal hematoma
- subdural hematoma
- coagulopathy
- left clavicle fracture

Based on the injuries that were sustained by Mr. W., he is a prime candidate for developing sepsis, MOF, and DIC. Awareness of the patient's predisposing factors and trends in laboratory data reveal a consumptive coagulopathy within the first 24 hours. Differentiation as to whether DIC was prompted by his hypothermia, shock, or blood replacement is less important than the nurse's knowledge of predisposing factors for early assessment and treatment.

Nutritional consultation determines a 3270 calorie and 82 g protein need daily. Both enteral and parenteral alimentation are initiated to meet metabolic demands. The initiation of invasive monitoring along with TPN are two more predisposing components for sepsis.

The white blood cell count over the first 4 days increases from 5800 to 17,300, and then to 24,000. Staphylococci sepsis is detected by blood culture, and Mr. W. continues to show signs of progressive multiple organ failure by increasing BUN (as high as 152 mg/dl), increasing creatinine (as high as 8.1 mg/dl), and oliguria. Dialysis is initiated and maintained for several weeks. Hepatic enzymes elevate progressively, indicating liver failure as well. After several weeks of struggling to overcome the injuries and profound complications, Mr. W. dies from multiple organ failure and irreversible brain injuries.

Trauma nurses and prehospital personnel must consider the potential for sequelae and the entire extent of injury that may be present. Recall that the initial prehospital care providers considered this patient to be "stable" in the field because he was moving all four extremities and had adequate vital signs. Mechanisms of injury are essential in elevating the index of suspicion for all health care providers.

Mr. W. was very much like most trauma patients who are seen nationally. He was a young, healthy, man, under the age of 39. It is very easy to underestimate the magnitude of injury based on initial assessment and vital signs. However, as seen, patients like Mr. W. may compensate for their injuries for some time after the incident. Complications are not easily managed, especially in the complex patient like Mr. W. Increased knowledge and anticipation of potential complications and injury control will decrease the morbidity and mortality seen in trauma care delivery today.

RESEARCH QUESTIONS

- What percent of planned caloric intake is lost in enteral feedings with fine-bore feeding tubes during delays to ensure tube placement after dislodgement, questioned aspiration, lack of ability to aspirate residual, and tube replacement because of obstruction?
- What methods of maintaining enteral tube patency are cost efficient and time efficient?
- What protocol will maximize early nutritional support in the patient with high risk of poor tolerance to enteral feedings as a result of the use of paralytic agents, sedatives, and opiates?
- What impact does frequency and intensity of patient activity/mobility have on tolerance of enteral feedings?
- What level of satiety do patients feel when receiving TPN?
- Do patients sense differences between supplement solutions administered at room temperature and those administered directly from a refrigerated source?
- Do patients accurately identify when they are ready for oral feedings?
- How frequently and how promptly are nutritional recommendations from dietician specialists instituted?

ANNOTATED BIBLIOGRAPHY

Cerra, F.B. (1988). Nutritional and metabolic support. In K.L. Mattox, E.E. Moore, & D.V. Feliciano (Eds.), *Trauma* (pp. 869-876). Norwalk, CT: Appleton & Lange.
Overview of the nutritional and metabolic needs of the trauma patient.

Griffin, J.P. (1986). Be prepared for the bleeding patient. *Nursing '86, 6,* 34-40.
Simple, easy-to-understand article describing bleeding disorders.

Rolandelli, R.H., & Koruda, M.J. (1991). Nutrition and trauma: Techniques of nutritional support. *Trauma Quarterly, 7*(2), 32-63.
Overview of the indications, methods, complications, and nutritional requirements for enteral and parenteral supplementation of the injured patient.

Rush, D.S., Kelly, J.P., & Nichols, R.L. (1988). Prevention and management of common infections after trauma. In K.L. Mattox, E.E. Moore, & D.V. Feliciano (Eds.), *Trauma* (pp. 223-234). Norwalk, CT: Appleton & Lange.
Overview of common infections and their prevention. Attention is given to infections originating from chest and abdominal trauma.

REFERENCES

Adams, S., Dellinger E.P., Wertz, M., Oreskovich M.R., Simonowitz, D., & Johansen, K. (1986). Enteral versus parenteral nutritional support following laparotomy for trauma: A randomized prospective trial. *Journal of Trauma, 26*(10), 882-891.

Alverdy, J.C., Aoys, E., & Moss, G.S. (1988). Total parenteral nutrition promotes bacterial translocation from the gut. *Surgery, 104,* 185-190.

Babikian, G.M. (1989). Physiologic response to the traumatic wound. *Trauma Quarterly, 5*(2), 1-5.

Bailey, P.M. (1991). The metabolic response to injury: Overview and introduction to multiple system organ failure. *Trauma Quarterly, 7*(2), 1-11.

Baker, J.W., Deitch, E.A., Li, M.A., Berg, R.D., & Specian, R.D. (1988). Hemorrhagic shock induces bacterial translocation from the gut. *Journal of Trauma, 28,* 896-904.

Baue, A.E. (1991). Nutrition and metabolism in sepsis and multisystem organ failure. *Surgical Clinics of North America, 71*(3), 549-565.

Cardona, V.D. (1985). Complications of trauma. In V.D. Cardona (Ed.), *Trauma nursing* (pp. 155-163). Oradell, NJ: Medical Economics.

Carpenter, R. (1987). Infections and head injury: A potentially lethal combination. *Critical Care Nursing Quarterly, 10*(3), 1-11.

Cerra, F.B. (1988). Nutritional and metabolic support. In K.L. Mattox, E.E. Moore, & D.V. Feliciano (Eds.), *Trauma* (pp. 869-876). Norwalk, CT: Appleton & Lange.

Cerra, F.B. (1991). The systemic septic response: Concepts of pathogenesis. *Journal of Trauma, 30*(12), S169-S174.

Dellinger, E.P. (1986). In D.D. Trunkey, & F.R. Lewis (Eds.). *Current therapy of trauma - 2.* (pp. 105-110). Philadelphia: B.C. Decker.

Finelli, F.C., Johnsson, J., Champion, H.R., Morelli, S., & Fouty, W.J. (1989). A case control study for major trauma in geriatric patients. *Journal of Trauma, 29*(5), 541-548.

Flint, L.M. (1988). Sepsis and multiple organ failure. In K.L. Mattox, E.E. Moore, & D.V. Feliciano (Eds.), *Trauma* (pp. 879-891). Norwalk, CT: Appleton & Lange.

Flint, L.M. (1991). Sepsis and multiple organ failure. In E.E. Moore, K.L. Mattox, & D.V. Feliciano (Eds.), *Trauma* (2nd ed.) (pp. 995-1006). Norwalk, CT: Appleton & Lange.

Fry, D.E., & Polk, H.C. (1987). Host defense and organ system failure. In J.D. Richardson, J.C. Polk, & L.M. Flint (Eds.), *Trauma: Clinical care and pathophysiology* (pp. 41-75). Chicago: Mosby–Year Book, Inc.

Grant, J.P. (1988). Nutrition in the trauma patient. In J.A. Moylan (Ed.), *Trauma surgery* (pp. 501-534). Philadelphia: J.B. Lippincott.

Griffin, J.P. (1986). Be prepared for the bleeding patient. *Nursing '86, 6,* 34-40.

Guenter, P. (1985). Nutritional care of the trauma patient. In V.D. Cardona (Ed.), *Trauma nursing* (pp. 195-202). Oradell, NJ: Medical Economics.

Hassan, E., & Danziger, L.H. (1988). Metabolic response to injury. *Trauma Quarterly, 4*(4), 1-7.

Herndon, D.N. (1991). What's new in surgery for 1991: trauma and burns. *American College of Surgeons Bulletin, 76*(1), 56-58.

Hoyt, N.J. (1988). Infection and infection control. In V.D. Cardona, P.D. Hurn, P.J. Mason, A.M. Scanlon-Schlipp, & S.W. Veise-Berry (Eds.), *Trauma nursing from resuscitation through rehabilitation* (pp 224-256). Philadelphia: W.B. Saunders.

Hsieh, N.L. (1988). Nutritional assessment for the critically ill adult. *Problems in Critical Care, 2* (4), 527-537.

Hull, S. (1985). Enteral versus parenteral nutrition support: Rationale for increased use of enteral feeding. *Zeitschrift fur Gastroenterologie, 23*(Suppl.), 55-63.

Hurst, J.M., Koetting, C.A., & Lang, C.E. (1988). Multiple trauma. *Trauma Quarterly, 4*(4), 67-76.

Johanson, W.G. (1988). Infection in acute respiratory failure. *Intensive and Critical Care Digest, 7*(1), 5-6.

Kenney, P.R. (1986). Neuroendocrine response to volume loss. *Trauma Quarterly, 2*(3), 18-27.

Kerver, A.J., Rommes, J.H., Mevissan-Verhage, E.A., Hulstaert, P.F., Vos, A., Verhoef, J., & Wittebol, P. (1988). Prevention of colonization and infection in the critically ill patient: A prospective randomized study. *Critical Care Medicine, 16,* 1087-1092.

Kruskall, M.S., Mintz, P.D., Bergin, J.J., Johnston M.F.M., Klein, H.G., Miller, J.D., Rutman, R., & Silberstein L. (1988). Transfusion therapy in emergency medicine. *Annals of Emergency Medicine, 3,* 327-335.

Lawrence, D.W., & Lauro, A.J. (1988). Complications from IV therapy: Results from field-started and emergency department–started IVs compared. *Annals of Emergency Medicine, 17*(4), 314-317.

MacGregor, R.R. (1986). Alcohol and immune defense. *Journal of American Medical Association, 256,* 1474-1478.

Martindale, R.G., & McCarthy, M.S. (1988). Enteral and parenteral nutrition in the trauma patient. *Trauma Quarterly, 4*(4), 47-58.

Meakins, J.L. (1991). Etiology of multiple organ failure. *Journal of Trauma, 30*(12), S165-S168.

Mirtallo, J.M. (1988). Nutrition in the critically ill patient. *Trauma Quarterly, 4*(4), 9-18.

Priest, B.P. (1991). Trauma and the septic state: Pathophysiological mechanisms and the role for parenteral nutrition. *Trauma Quarterly, 7*(2), 12-18.

Procter, C.D. (1987). Infection and trauma: An overview. *International Anesthesiology Clinics, 25*(1), 163-173.

Riberg, B., Medegard, A., Heideman, M., Gyzander, E., Bundsen, P., Oden, M., & Teger-Nilsson, A.C. (1986). Early activation of humoral proteolytic systems in patients with multiple trauma. *Critical Care Medicine, 14,* 917-925.

Roberts, S.L. (1985), *Physiological concepts and the critically ill patient.* Englewood Cliffs, NJ: Prentice-Hall.

Rolandelli, R.H., & Koruda, M.J. (1991). Nutrition and trauma: Techniques of nutritional support. *Trauma Quarterly, 7*(2), 32-63.

Rombeau, J.L., & Caldwell, M.D. (1984). *Enteral and tube feeding.* Philadelphia: W.B. Saunders.

Rush, D.S., Kelly, J.P., & Nichols, R.L. (1988). Prevention and management of common infections after trauma. In K.L. Mattox, E.E. Moore, & D.V. Feliciano (Eds.), *Trauma* (pp. 223-234). Norwalk, CT: Appleton & Lange.

Rutledge, R.G., & Sheldon, G.F., (1988). Bleeding and coagulation problems. In K.L. Mattox, E.E. Moore, & D.V. Feliciano (Eds.), *Trauma* (pp. 809-817). Norwalk, CT: Appleton & Lange.

Savino, J.A. (1987). Hemodynamic monitoring in trauma. *Trauma Quarterly, 3*(3), 13-29.

Shoemaker, W.C., Appel, P.L., & Kram, H.B. (1988). Tissue oxygen debt as a determinant of lethal and nonlethal postoperative organ failure. *Critical Care Medicine, 16,* 1117-1120.

Shoemaker, W.C., Ayres, S., Grenvik, A., Holbrook, P.R., & Thompson, W.L. (1989). *Textbook of critical care* (2nd ed.). Philadelphia: W.B. Saunders.

Smith, K.A. (1987). Head trauma: Comparison of infection rates for different methods of intracranial pressure monitoring. *Journal of Neuroscience Nursing, 19*(6), 310-314.

Smith, L.C., & Mullen, J.L. (1991). Nutritional assessment and indications for nutritional support. *Surgical Clinics of North America, 71*(3), 449-457.

Stanek, G.S. (1988). Metabolic and nutritional management of the trauma patient. In V.D. Cardona, P.D. Hurn, P.J. Mason, A.M. Scanlon Schlipp, & S.W. Veise-Berry (Eds.), *Trauma nursing from resuscitation through rehabilitation* (pp. 284-315). Philadelphia: W.B. Saunders.

Stump, D.C., & Mann, K.G. (1988). Mechanisms of thrombus formation and lysis. *Annals of Emergency Medicine, 17,* 1138-1145.

Suchak, B.A., & Barbon, C.B. (1989). Disseminated intravascular coagulation: A nursing challenge. *Orthopaedic Nursing, 8*(6), 61-69.

Sugerman, H.J. (1991). What's new in surgery for 1991: Critical care and metabolism. *American College of Surgeons Bulletin, 76*(1), 16-19.

Van Way, C.W. (1991). Nutritional support in the injured patient. *Surgical Clinics of North America, 71*(3), 537-548.

Vogelpohl, R.A. (1981). Disseminated intravascular coagulation. *Critical Care Nurse, 3,* 38-43.

Wilson, R.F. (1985). Special problems in the diagnosis and treatment of surgical sepsis. *Surgical Clinics of North America, 65,* 965-986.

VI

NURSING WITHIN THE TRAUMA CONTINUUM

20 *Air Transport of the Trauma Patient*

Renee Semonin-Holleran

OBJECTIVES

❏ Describe the history of helicopter transport and flight nursing in the United States.

❏ Outline the advantages and disadvantages of helicopter transport.

❏ Discuss the effects of flight on human physiology.

❏ Discuss the effects of flight on equipment used in patient care.

❏ Describe the specific assessment and interventions for patient transport by helicopters.

❏ Outline the safety issues involved in flight nursing.

❏ Summarize the ethical issues involved in flight nursing.

INTRODUCTION Hospital-based helicopter services have been developing rapidly over the past 20 years. Along with the development of flight programs has been the evolution of flight nursing. Nursing of the critically ill or injured can now be accomplished outside the confines of the emergency department (ED) and the intensive care unit (ICU). This nursing care is contributing to decreasing the mortality and morbidity of specific patient populations because patients are now afforded accessibility to care that was limited in the past (Baxt, 1986; Burney et al., 1988; Carraway et al., 1984; Harless, Morris, Cenzig, Holt, & Schmidt, 1978; Uhlhorn & Jacobs, 1982).

Trunkey (1988) stated that two vital ways trauma-related mortality and morbidity will be reduced are (1) effective prehospital care and (2) regionalization of trauma services. The use of hospital-based helicopter programs and flight nurses provides a mode to improve the care of the traumatically injured patient.

In 1987 the National Flight Nurses Association in collaboration with the American College of Surgeons developed a course that specifically addresses the care of the trauma patient by the flight nurse during transport. The Flight Nurse Advanced Trauma Course (FNATC) was first offered in 1988.

The primary goal of the course is to provide flight nurses with the skills and knowledge to give the highest level of care to the traumatically injured patient. The course is composed of both lectures and skills stations. The lecture material addresses flight physiology and its effects on the injured patient; safety; communications; mechanisms of injury; legal issues; transport considerations; and stress management. The skills stations include advanced airway management; fluid resuscitation; cervical spine and chest x-ray interpretation; invasive skills laboratory; and initial management, stabilization, and transport.

In 1991 the text *Flight Nursing: Principles and Practice* (Lee, 1991) was published. This was a landmark in the development of the practice and profession of flight nursing. Contained in this text arc the fundamentals of flight nursing. It serves as an additional resource that can be used for the care of the trauma patient being transported by air.

The focus of this chapter is to discuss the history of flight nursing, discuss the ethical issues related to the practice of flight nursing, and identify the advantages and disadvantages of air transport of the traumatically injured patient. In addition, the physiology of air transport, the stresses of flight, and specific assessment and interventions for transport will be addressed. Finally, the safety issues involved in the practice of flight nurses will be discussed.

FLIGHT NURSING
Historical Review

The first recorded transport of patients by air was in 1870. Wounded soldiers were transported by hot air balloon during the Prussian siege of Paris. In 1918 the United States Army had air ambulances based in Louisiana and Texas (Lee, 1987). Table 20-1 contains some historical milestones in the use of helicopters for patient transport.

Laurette M. Schimmoler has been credited with beginning a national movement for nurses' participation in air medical transport. In 1933 she and other interested flight nurses formed the Emergency Flight Corps. In 1936 the name of the organization was changed to the Aerial Nurse Corps of America (Lee, 1987). The goals of the organization were to provide physically qualified and technically trained registered nurses to transport patients by air and improve air ambulance service, particularly focusing on patient safety in flight (Lee, 1987).

Unfortunately, the Aerial Nurse Corps was not recognized by the military. However, in 1942 the military developed a training program for flight nurses that had requirements similar to those of the Aerial Nurse Corps. The military flight nursing course contained courses in aeromedical physiology, survival tactics, mental hygiene, and eventually combat readiness. Because of the military connection, the participation of flight nurses increased during WW II (Lee, 1987).

Finally, in 1966 Ms. Schimmoler was recognized by the military for her contributions to flight nursing. Her foresight laid the foundation for nurses to demonstrate the need for nursing care outside of the hospital.

The experience of using helicopters to trans-

Table 20-1 Historical milestones in the use of air transport for patient transport

Year	Event
1870	Injured soldiers were transported by hot air balloon.
1918	Two U.S. Army air ambulances were based in Louisiana.
1945	First helicopter rescue was conducted.
1950-1953	Korean conflict showed helicopters were useful in patient transport. By the end of the war, about 20,000 men had been transported by helicopter.
1965-1972	Helicopter transport was used the most in Vietnam. More than 800,000 individuals were transported.
1967-1971	Department of Transportation feasibility study for the use of helicopters in the civilian population was conducted. Seven states participated.
1970	Military Assistance to Traffic and Safety (MAST) was begun at Fort Sam Houston, Texas. MAST provided aeromedical assistance to civilian police and fire agencies for patient transport.
1972	First hospital-based helicopter program "Flight for Life" was begun at St. Anthony's Hospital in Denver
1973	Use of helicopters began in statewide trauma care systems in Maryland and Illinois.
1976	Second helicopter-based program was established at Hermann Hospital, Houston.
1991	A total of 253 air medical services were in operation.

port patients in both the Korean and Vietnam wars led the Department of Transportation to evaluate the use of helicopters in civilian care in 1967. The first hospital-based helicopter program was begun in 1972 at St. Anthony's Hospital in Denver, and the service was staffed by flight nurses. In 1976 Hermann Hospital in Houston introduced the first registered nurse and physician flight crew.

Table 20-2 Comparison of various aircraft used to transport patients

Fixed-wing aircraft model	Cruise speed (km/hr)	Range (km)
Lear 25	864	2240
Lear 35	864	3520
Lear 36	864	4160
Falcon 50	480	5280
MU-2	480	2290

Rotor-wing aircraft model	Cruise speed (mph)	Range (nautical miles)
ASTAR	130	410
Dauphin 2	162	550
A-109	140-150	440
Longranger	145	368
Bell 412 SP	140	400
BO-105	130	308
BK-117	155	308
S-76	167	400

Note. From "Aeromedical Transport" by J. Hodges, 1989, *Emergency Care Quarterly, 4*, pp. 8-10.
1 km = ⅝ mile; 1 mile = 1.609 km.

The American Society of Hospital Based Emergency Aeromedical Services (ASHBEAMS) was organized in 1980. It is now known as the Association of Air Medical Services (AAMS). The National Flight Nurses Association (NFNA) was formed in 1981. Both organizations are devoted to the development and implementation of standards that provide the highest level of care and safety for the air transport of patients.

The 1991 Program Directory published in the *Journal of Air Medical Transport* listed 253 programs that operate services that transport patients by air. These services include both helicopter and fixed-wing transport programs. The majority of these programs are supported by hospitals. The estimated cost of most programs range between 1.0 and 1.3 million dollars a year (Hodges, 1989). However, the amount could be higher or lower, depending on the size of the programs and the types of aircraft that are used. See Table 20-2 for a comparison of fixed-wing and rotary-wing aircraft.

Macione and Wilcox (1987) published a study that gave a general description of helicopter emergency services and how they are used in the United States. They found that programs in rural areas had larger patient volumes than those in urban and suburban areas. Single-aircraft programs averaged 40 flights per month; multiple-aircraft programs averaged 57 flights per month. Trauma patient transports made up about 50% of patient transports. About 15% to 25% of these patients were transported directly from the scene. Macione and Wilcox's data suggested that helicopter programs, however, tend to vary as much as the hospitals that support them.

Flight Team Composition

Since the beginning of helicopter use in the civilian arena, there has always been discussion about who should be members of the flight team and what education they should have. There is little argument about the pilot's role, but who should be in the aircraft providing patient care?

AAMS mandates that at least one registered nurse be on the aircraft when critical care (advanced life support) is to be provided. The qualifications required of other members of the crew will depend on the patient's condition and the philosophy of the flight program. Table 20-3 contains a current summary of flight teams in the United States.

Several studies have been published that have evaluated the role of physicians and flight nurses as the flight team (Baxt, 1986; Carraway et al., 1984; Kaplan, Walsh, & Burney, 1987; Rhee, Willits, Turner, & Ward, 1987; and Snow, Hull, & Severns, 1986). The general consensus of the research is that the role for flight physician is based on skills and medical judgment. Skills include intubation, tube thoracostomy, and pericardiocentesis. Medical judgment includes the identification of missed diagnoses (referring to more complicated medical problems) and the recognition of changes in the patient's condition that require medication. The physician does not require medical control protocols on which to operate.

Shea (1985) points out that a nurse/nurse or nurse/paramedic flight team are more cost effective than the nurse/physician team. In addition, others argue that skills can be learned with practice and judgment can be acquired with experience (Campbell, 1987). The availability of sophisticated communication systems, such as cellular phones, allows for quick consultation by

Table 20-3 Current flight team composition

Team composition	Percentage in service
Physician/Nurse	15%
Nurse/Nurse	15%
Nurse/Respiratory therapist	3%
Nurse alone	7%
Nurse/Paramedic	49%
Other (EMT, paramedic/ paramedic, nurse/EMT)	10%

Note. Data collated from *1988 Membership Directory* by Association of Air Medical Services, 1988, Pasadena, CA: Author.

National Flight Nurses Association recommendations for flight nurses

- Registered nurse with current licensure in state or states where practicing
- Graduate of an NLN-accredited program of nursing, preferably with a baccalaureate or higher degree
- Minimum of 2 years of experience in emergency or critical care nursing
- Advanced Cardiac Life Support certification
- Able to meet the physical requirements of the air medical program in which the flight nurse practices

---

flight nurses and/or medics when a physician is not on board the aircraft.

More research is needed before the appropriate flight team composition can be determined. However, recent legislation may contribute to some rethinking of flight team composition. In August 1986, COBRA (Public Law 99-272) went into effect. This law makes the transferring hospital and emergency physician responsible for the type of care that the patient receives during transfer. Hospitals and emergency physicians will now need to carefully weigh the type of team they choose to use when sending patients to other institutions or risk severe financial penalties if the optimal level of patient care has not been provided (Frew, Roush, & LaGreca, 1988).

Whether flight nurses should have prehospital care certification (emergency medical technician, paramedic) remains an issue. Many leaders in flight nursing believe that the depth of knowledge implicit with registered nurse status qualifies them to provide appropriate care for the patient in the prehospital area (Campbell, 1987). In 1986 the National Flight Nurses Association published "Practice Standards for Flight Nursing," which contains detailed recommendations for the education and training of flight nurses. The box (upper right) contains a summary of these recommendations.

In 1988 the "Air Medical Crew Standards" were completed and made available. These standards were developed with a grant from the United States Department of Transportation and with the collaboration of Samaritan Air Evac and AAMS. These standards provide a basic curriculum for both the basic and advanced air medical crew member.

The Emergency Nurses Association has also published a curriculum that can serve as a basis for the education of the nurse who practices in the prehospital care environment, such as the flight nurse. The "National Standard Guidelines for Prehospital Nursing Curriculum" (Emergency Nurses Association, 1991) was developed with input from several organizations who practice in this setting.

In summary, the most common type of flight team at present is the nurse/paramedic, though little research has been published about the use or effectiveness of this team. The most researched team composition has been the physician/nurse. Table 20-4 compares the American College of Surgeons' guidelines for differentiating aeromedical staff capabilities. The research demonstrates that the flight physician does play a role in patient transport, but the question remains—could this role be assumed by the flight nurse?

The Flight Nurse

Batterman and Markel (1986) described what they found to be the average flight nurse. By using a survey, they collected data from 127 flight programs in the United States. The box on p. 630 contains the "profile" they discovered.

The 1986 NFNA standards provide an excellent framework for the education and training of flight nurses. Both the "Air Medical Crew National Standard Curriculum" and the "National Standard Guidelines for Prehospital Nursing Curriculum" can also serve as resources for flight

Table 20-4 Guidelines for differentiating aeromedical staff capabilities

Training and skills	Crew member level			
	I (EMT-I)	II (EMT-P)	III (RN)	IV (MD)
Aeromedical physiology	R	R	R	R
Patient assessment skills	R	R	R	R
Recognition of lethal dysrhythmias and proficiency with defibrillation	R	R	R	R
Nasogastric tube placement	R	R	R	R
Urinary catheter placement	R	R	R	R
Oxygen therapy	R	R	R	R
Aircraft orientation	R	R	R	R
Aircraft safety	R	R	R	R
Emergency aeromedical procedures (crash and survival)	R	R	R	R
Aviation communication	R	R	R	R
Endotracheal intubation/ventilation	X	R	R	R
Needle thoracostomy	X	R	R	R
Pediatric trauma management	X	R	R	R
Insertion of central IV lines	X	X	R	R
Insertion of thoracostomy tubes	X	X	R	R
Ventilatory management (respirations)	X	X	R	R
Administration of appropriate pharmacology	X	X	R	R
Intracranial pressure monitoring	X	X	R	R
Insertion of intraosseous lines	X	X	R	R
Cricothyroidotomy	X	X	R	R
Basic overview of critical care categories	X	X	R	R
▪ obstetric				
▪ neonatal				
▪ pediatric				
▪ burn (including radiation)				
▪ cardiac trauma				
▪ central nervous system emergencies				
▪ toxicology				
▪ infectious diseases				
▪ psychiatric patients				
International rules	X	X	R	R
Medical/legal considerations	X	X	R	R

Note: From *Resources for Optimal Care of the Injured Patient* by American College of Surgeons, Committee on Trauma, 1990.
R, Required; *X,* not required.

nursing education. As flight nursing continues to evolve, so will the concept of flight team composition. More research is needed to ascertain the appropriate and most effective flight team composition.

ETHICAL ASPECTS

Not unlike other areas of nursing practice, some distinct ethical issues are faced by the flight nurse. These include pronouncing patient dead, deciding when to transport, and determining who should be transported by helicopter. Unfortunately, guidelines are limited and insufficient research is available to make these decisions. These decisions vary from program to program.

Wright, Dronen, Combs, and Storer (1989) evaluated the autopsy records of 67 patients transported by helicopter who had sustained a traumatic arrest at the scene. All of the patients eventually succumbed to their injuries, though two regained pulses in the ED. The autopsy reports demonstrated that all of the patients had at least

---

Profile of a flight nurse

RN: 6 to 10 years of experience
Flight nurse: 1 to 2 years of experience
Nursing experience: ED and ICU
Certification: ACLS
Flight data:
- crew consists of pilot, nurse, paramedic
- average flight less than 1 hour
- program completes 300 to 600 flights/yr
- transports one patient
Flight duties:
- keeps program statistics
- provides in-house staff education
- provides user-agency education
- conducts patient follow-ups
- makes rounds on flight patients
- assists in ED
Shifts: 12 hours

Note. From "Profile of a Flight Nurse" by K. Batterman and N. Markel, 1986, *Aeromedical Journal, 7,* p. 26.

---

two injuries incompatible with life and a majority of them had several injuries. These included atlantooccipital dislocations, severe head injuries, transected thoracic aortas, and ruptured heart ventricles. One of the conclusions drawn from the study is the need for flight programs to assess the safety issues of dispensing a flight team to a scene where the patient has no vital signs.

Programs in which physicians fly are better able to pronounce patients dead in the field. Most states do not allow the nurse or paramedic to make the decision to pronounce a patient dead. A policy should be available to guide the flight team when making that decision. The flight nurse should consider the feelings of the prehospital care providers or the personnel at the referring institution when making a decision whether to transport. Many times these people have been working long and hard trying to resuscitate the patient and feel strongly that more can be done if the patient is transported to a definitive care center. On occasion, the family of the victim may be there, and it can be very difficult for people to understand why their family member is not being transferred. Again, flight programs should develop and implement policies that provide guidelines for the flight nurse.

The protocol for deciding who is transported by helicopter varies from program to program. In

some institutions a physician may make the decision, and in others, rigid guidelines may already be in place that outline who is or is not transported by air.

Thomas and Jacobson (1991) noted that the ethical decisions made by the flight nurse should be made within a framework that considers four principles: (1) the principle of beneficence (will the transport be of benefit to the patient); (2) the principle of nonmaleficence (could the transport cause patient harm); (3) the principle of justice (assuring that patients are treated equally); and (4) the principle of autonomy (allowing patients to make their own decisions when possible).

The national AAMS and NFNA meetings have begun to provide a forum for the discussion of some of these issues. As flight programs continue to develop, it is hoped that some of the answers to these concerns will be discovered.

AIR TRANSPORT
Advantages

Multiple research studies, both published and unpublished, have been conducted to ascertain the usefulness of helicopters in the transport of critically ill or injured patients (Baxt, 1986; Boyd & Hungerpiller, 1990; Carraway et al., 1984; Gold, 1987; Johnson, 1981; Kaplan, Walsh, & Burney, 1987; Topol et al., 1987; Uhlhorn & Jacobs, 1982). The major advantages of helicopter transport include saving time, providing early and rapid accessibility to advanced care, providing advanced life support (crew configuration), enhancing communications, and as specifically noted by Boyd and Hungerpiller (1990, p. 54), the fact that receiving EDs that are familiar with helicopter transports may be better prepared to meet the needs of the traumatically injured patient.

Champion (1986) identified specific recommendations to help make the decision to use helicopters to transport the trauma patient. The box on p. 631 presents those recommendations.

In addition to recommendations for the use of helicopters to transport the multiply injured patient, Mattox (1988) advises that further guidelines be observed when using helicopter transport for the trauma patient. These include that (1) air ambulances be used for advanced life support only; (2) air ambulance service be under the same regional certification, review, and dispatch as existing emergency medical service vehicles; and (3) realistic time/distance guidelines for the use of

Recommendations for helicopter transport of the trauma patient

Urban/Suburban environment

Transport time to trauma center >15 minutes by ambulance

Ambulance transport impeded by access to or egress from the accident scene

Presence of multiple casualties

Rural environment

Time to local hospital via ambulance > time to trauma center via helicopter

Wilderness rescue

ground versus air ambulance be developed and used.

Baxt (1986) examined the use of helicopters to transport patients who had suffered blunt trauma. Seven hospital-based helicopter services from around the United States participated in the study. Crew composition was varied and included physician/nurse, nurse/nurse, and nurse/paramedic.

Using a statistical model that predicted the probability of mortality of the patient with blunt trauma, Baxt (1986) observed that patients transported by helicopter had a reduced mortality. Baxt (1986) posited two reasons that this reduction in mortality may have occurred. First, the helicopter can bring advanced medical skills directly to the injured patient, either at the scene or at another hospital. Second, hospital-based helicopter programs, similar to the concept of trauma centers, can bring an organized and coordinated approach to the care of the trauma patient. Because of the speed of the helicopter, this can be done in a timely manner.

The previously cited study by Baxt (1986) raises important issues related to the use of helicopter transport for the traumatically injured patient. What criteria should be used to determine if the patient should be transported by air? This issue continues to generate a great deal of controversy.

Baxt, Berry, Epperson, & Scalzitti (1989) looked at one of the criteria that has been used to determine whether a traumatically injured patient should be transferred by air. This specific criterion is *scoring*. Baxt et al. (1989) compared four

of the most frequently used scoring systems for classifying major and minor trauma: the PHI (prehospital index); TS (trauma score); RTS (revised trauma score); and CRAMS scale (circulation, respiration, abdomen, motor, speech). Data collected on 2400 patients from the Trauma Registry of San Diego were analyzed. The researchers found that the scores could predict whether the patients would live or die, but could not predict the extent of the patients' injuries and the hospital care required to treat them as reflected in the ISS (injury severity scale) score.

Kreis et al. (1988) examined the records of 8891 patients who were transported to trauma centers in Dade County, Florida. These researchers found that the TS predicted severe injury in 92% of the patients whose scores were less than 13. However, they also recognized a tendency of "overtriage" of patients. Many patients were transported by helicopter to trauma centers who did not need to be there.

Schiller et al. (1988) noted that there was little difference in patient outcomes for those trauma patients transported by helicopter or ground in a metropolitan area with advanced life support. The authors compared trauma patients transported by air and ground in the Phoenix area. Both the flight and ground crews in Phoenix can provide advanced life support.

When the need has been identified that the trauma patient must be transported, important components should be initiated before and during patient transport. The American College of Emergency Physicians (1990) recommends that the following guidelines be used:

- Health and well-being of the patient must be the overriding concern when any patient transfer is considered.
- The patient should be evaluated before transfer.
- The patient should be stabilized as much as possible before transfer.
- The patient and the patient's family should be informed about the reasons for and the risks of transfer.
- The patient should be transferred to a facility appropriate to the medical needs of the patient, with adequate space and personnel available.
- The receiving facility must agree to accept the patient.
- Economic reasons should not be the basis

for transferring or refusing a patient at a receiving facility.

- Communication about the patient's condition and initial care to the receiving facility must occur.
- The patient should be transferred in an appropriately equipped vehicle that is staffed by qualified personnel.
- When possible, written protocols and transfer agreements should be in place.

Crippen (1990) noted that critical care transport services must provide the expertise necessary for safe initial stabilization of the patient. In addition, the transport service should have the expertise to deal with the advanced technology that may be required by the patient, such as pulse oximeters and infusion pumps. The transport of the patient should be of potential benefit for the patient. Finally, it should be demonstrated that patient transport will result in financial savings because of improved medical care.

Disadvantages

The disadvantages of helicopter transport consist of problems related to weather, cost, and safety. Weather restrictions, such as poor visibility, ice, and thunderstorms, may make helicopter transport impossible. Even though the number of hospital-based helicopter programs has more than tripled since 1980, these services continue to be limited in some areas. Hodges (1989) noted that the cost of aeromedical services varied throughout the United States; the average cost was from $900 to $1550 for a round-trip transport. However, the question remains—how is the cost of human life measured?

Safety Issues

Since the first hospital-based helicopter transport program began in 1972, about 70 transport crashes have occurred. The worst year to date for fatalities was 1985. In that year 14 crashes and 13 fatalities occurred, the majority of whom were pilots and medical crew (Burney, 1987). In 1988, 7 crashes occurred in the United States. Of the 7 crashes, 2 involved fatalities. The preliminary crash rate for 1989 has been calculated at 5.3 crashes per 100,000 patients transported (Collett, 1991). In 1990 no helicopter crashes in the air medical industry were reported. Unfortunately, in 1991, 11 fatalities occurred.

Several situations have been identified that have contributed to accidents and injuries. These include pilot error, flying in less than optimal weather (minimal visibility), inexperienced flight teams, engine failure, and obstacle strikes (Collett, 1991).

Chin (1988) presented a survey carried out by the Pittsburgh Press that questioned 251 emergency medical services (EMS) pilots about what problems lead to EMS accidents. The pilots cited competitive pressures (being paid per flight completed, other programs operating in same area, and accepting flights when one program has turned them down), unfavorable weather conditions, malfunctioning equipment, fatigue, lack of regulations, and pilot error as the leading reasons air medical helicopter accidents occur.

In April 1988 the National Flight Nurses Association adopted a position paper, "Improving Flight Nurse Safety in the Air-Medical Helicopter Environment." The NFNA is the first organization intricately involved in air medical helicopter transport that has developed a position paper that directly addresses the safety issues related to providing critical care by using helicopter transport. Issues addressed in the safety paper include personal safety, aircraft familiarity, and physical and mental well-being. The variety of patients, the critical nature of patients, the physical environment, and the number of hours that a flight nurse may be required to work vary from program to program. However, all of these can serve as sources of stress and possibly contribute to safety problems. The NFNA safety paper provides guidelines for "safe" flight nursing practice. Table 20-5 summarizes the concerns addressed in the paper.

Safety should be the number one priority of all air medical transport programs. Hospital-based helicopter programs should provide in-depth safety presentations to the agencies that use their service. The presentations should include information about when to request the helicopter, how to set up a landing site, when to approach the aircraft, how to load and unload the aircraft, fire safety, and emergency landing. The box on p. 633 summarizes how prehospital, emergency, and other nonflight personnel should function around a helicopter to assure safety. Figures 20-1 and 20-2 illustrate helicopter hazards and safe approaches that can be made toward a helicopter.

Table 20-5 Summary of the NFNA safety
paper

Issue	NFNA position
Adequate physical maintenance	Adjust schedule so that flight nurses receive adequate rest, fluids, and nutrition.
Personal safety	Provide policy that supports flight nurse's refusal to participate in any flight he or she believes may be unsafe.
Patient restraint	Develop policies that cover the use of chemical restraints for the combative patient. Use hard restraints to secure patient before loading. Provide policy for transport of prisoners.
"Hot" loading and unloading (loading the aircraft when it is running)	Consider value of "hot" loading and unloading.
Helicopter configuration	Provide federal government–approved shoulder harnesses in the aircraft. Use crash-attenuating seats and crash-resistant fuel systems.
Flight nurse interaction with pilot	Hold recurrent safety briefings. Train flight nurses in position reporting, communication terminology, radio communications, and other related emergency procedures.
Protective gear	Use flight helmets, uniforms constructed of flame-retardant materials, and high-top, natural leather boots with cotton socks.
Physical and mental well-being	Provide formalized physical fitness programs and Critical Incident Stress Debriefing programs.
Aircraft familiarity	Ensure that back-up aircraft is of the same type as the primary aircraft.

Note. Modified from "National Flight Nurses Association Safety
Paper" by the National Flight Nurses Association, 1987, *National
Flight Nurses Association:* Thorofare, NJ.

Measures to ensure safety around a helicopter

1. Know what type of aircraft the flight program you work with has.
2. Always approach the helicopter from the front and where the pilot can see you.
3. Never approach the helicopter until signaled by the pilot or a member of the flight team.
4. **NEVER** walk around the back of the aircraft unless you are with a flight team member.
5. **DO NOT SMOKE** around the aircraft.
6. Do not carry objects above the level of your waist around the aircraft, and secure any loose objects.
7. Allow the flight team to direct loading and unloading of the patient.
8. When the aircraft is landing or taking off, protect your eyes by turning around or wearing eye protection.
9. When the aircraft is running, wear ear protection.
10. **NEVER** do anything around the aircraft that you believe may be unsafe.

As the research has illustrated, helicopter transport of the trauma patient can reduce mortality and morbidity, but placing the flight team, patient, and transferring personnel at any risk clearly defeats the purpose of air medical transport.

ANATOMIC AND PHYSIOLOGIC CONSIDERATIONS

When preparing the trauma patient for air medical transport, several things should be considered. The previous discussion explained when to use a helicopter for transport. This discussion will address the issues encountered when transferring the trauma patient by air. Multiple stressors have been identified that affect both the patient and flight crew in flight (Browne, Bodenstedt, Campbell, & Nehrenz, 1987). These include effects of barometric pressure, hypoxia, fatigue, noise, vibration, thermal stress, dehydration, and gravitational forces.

Barometric Pressure

The earth's atmosphere contains oxygen and carbon dioxide, which are gases vital to animal and plant life. Dalton's law and Boyle's law help ex-

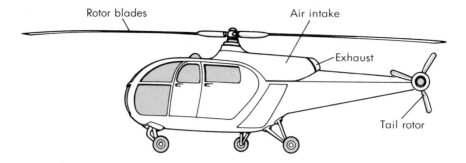

Figure 20-1 Helicopter hazard areas. (*Note*. From *Flight Nursing: Principles and Practice* by G. Lee, 1991, St. Louis: Mosby–Year Book, Inc.)

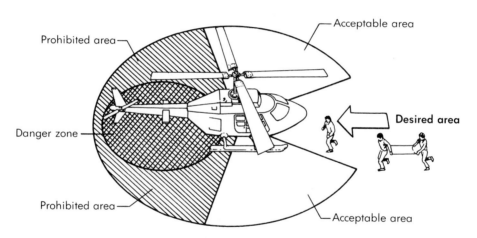

Figure 20-2 Safe approaches to helicopter. (*Note*. From *Flight Nursing: Principles and Practice* by G. Lee, 1991, St. Louis: Mosby–Year Book, Inc.)

plain the behaviors of gases and how they are affected by altitude.

Dalton's law states that the pressure of a gaseous mixture is equal to the sum of the partial pressures of its constituent gases. As barometric pressure decreases with increasing altitude, the pressure of each of the constituent gases decreases. Because oxygen is a gas, as altitude increases, oxygen will expand. Less oxygen, then, is available at higher altitudes. This helps explain why hypoxia develops at higher altitudes (NFNA, 1990; Waggoner, 1991).

Boyle's law states that at a constant temperature, the volume of a given gas is inversely proportional to the pressure to which that gas is exposed. As the altitude increases, barometric pressure decreases and the gas inside a closed space will expand.

Browne et al. (1987) noted that a combination of both Dalton's and Boyle's laws helps to explain the changes that occur as a result of changes in barometric pressure during flight. These changes in barometric pressure will affect such equipment as PASGs and endotracheal tubes. In addition,

Table 20-6 Expansion of gases at different altitudes

Altitude (1000 ft)	Barometric pressure (atm)	Barometric pressure (mm Hg)	Pressure change per 1000 ft (mm Hg)	Relative volume expansion
7	.771	586.4	22.6	1.297
8	.742	564.4	22.0	1.347
9	.714	543.2	21.2	1.400
10	.688	522.6	20.6	1.453
18	.500	379.4	15.9	2.000
28	.333	246.9	11.2	3.000
33	.250	196.4	9.4	4.000
42	.166	127.9	6.3	6.000
48	.125	96.1	4.7	8.000

Note. From *Flight Nursing Advanced Trauma Course* by T. Gregory, 1990, Thorofare, NJ: National Flight Nurses Association (NFNA).

Table 20-7 Blood gases at different altitudes

Altitude	Pao_2	Sao_2	$Paco_2$
Sea level	90-95	96	40
1,524 m (5000 ft)	75-81	95	32-33
2286 m (7500 ft)	69-74	92-93	31-33
4572 m (15,000 ft)	48-53	86	25
6096 m (20,000 ft)	37-45	76	20
7620 m (25,000 ft)	32-39	68	13
8848 m (29,029 ft)	26-33	58	9.5-13.8

Note. From *Management of Wilderness and Environmental Emergencies* (2nd ed.) by P. Auerbach and E. Geehr, 1989, St. Louis: Mosby–Year Book, Inc.
All values are for subjects ages 20-40 years who were acclimatizing well.

this will cause changes in the volume of gas in the sinuses, ears, and other hollow organs (NFNA, 1990). Table 20-6 illustrates the expansion of gases at different altitudes.

Flight nursing care based on the effects of altitude and pressure includes the assessment of the functioning of such equipment as PASGs, urinary catheters, endotracheal tubes, intravenous fluids, and gastrointestinal tubes. If urinary catheters, chest tubes, or gastrointestinal tubes are present, they should be left open to gravity or be connected to low suction. Glass bottles should be vented or replaced with plastic bags. Plastic IV bags also provide additional safety, because broken glass can be dangerous to both the patient and crew. Equipment should be frequently checked before and during flight.

Because gases do expand, a small pneumothorax may increase in size secondary to retention of gases in the pleural space. Placement of a chest tube may be required prophylactically before flight. In addition, the expansion of gastrointestinal gases could cause vomiting and aspiration. A nasogastric tube will help decrease the possibility of nausea and vomiting.

Occasionally, the expansion of gases in the sinuses and eardrums can cause discomfort for both the crew and patient, particularly if they have a cold or upper respiratory infection. Interventions to help decrease this discomfort include yawning, Valsalva maneuver if not contraindicated, pacifier or bottle for the pediatric patient to suck on, and

a topical vasoconstrictor, such as neosynepherine spray.

Hypoxia

The availability of oxygen decreases as altitude increases. Table 20-7 illustrates the effects of altitude on arterial blood gases. It is important to remember when looking at this table that these values are from participants who were between 20 and 40 years of age and who were acclimatizing well (Auerbach & Geehr, 1989).

Signs and symptoms of oxygen starvation are manifested in the central nervous system. Initially the symptoms include excitation, talkativeness, and hyperactivity. Secondary symptoms consist of depression (fatigue, decreased motor skills), impairment of reasoning, and deterioration of field and depth perception. Finally, the late sign of hypoxia is confusion, progressing to unconsciousness.

All trauma patients require oxygen, especially during transport. Depending on the extent and location of injury, patients may require intubation to protect their airway and decrease the risk of hypoxia. Oxygen by nasal cannula or face mask should be used when intubation is not required.

The altitude at which flight programs operate varies throughout the United States based on regional geography and flight distance. Fixed-wing transports are useful for flights where the distance of transport is over 150 miles (Hodges, 1989). Again, whether pressurized or nonpressurized aircraft is used depends on the program, type of patient, type of aircraft, and distance to be traveled (Hodges, 1989).

Many flight programs have begun to use pulse oximetry and CO_2 monitoring to assess the patient's response to altitude changes during flight. As more research becomes available, this type of monitoring equipment may be quite useful in preventing complications from hypoxia in already compromised patients (Dean, Bynoe, Castleman, Kudsk, & Fabian, 1988; Melton, Heller, Kaplan, & Mohan-Klein, 1988; Semonin-Holleran & Rouse, 1991; Taylor, Fallon, & Alexander, 1988; Waggoner, 1991). Pulse oximetry and CO_2 monitoring are particularly useful for the continued assessment of endotracheal tube placement during flight, since the noise generated by engines and rotors can make the assessment of breath sounds difficult, if not impossible. These devices provide additional safeguards that help decrease the risk of injury to the trauma patient during transport (Semonin-Holleran & Rouse, 1991).

Fatigue

The problem of fatigue affects both the patient and flight crew. The patient will fatigue easily because of his or her injuries. The flight crew may fatigue because of several variables, including:

- general unhealthiness of the individual crew members
- use of alcohol or cigarettes
- stress of the flight itself: demands on judgment; physical stress of flight
- rotating shifts (irregular work hours)
- presence of disease processes (e.g., cold, flu)
- poor diet, exercise, and rest habits

The NFNA Safety Position Paper contains recommendations to deal with the fatigue of flight (see Table 20-5).

Patients should be made as comfortable as possible. Keeping the patient warm, decreasing excessive stimulation, providing ear protection (even for the unconscious patient), and, in some cases, using sedation can help decrease patients' awareness of fatigue.

Thermal Stress

As altitude increases, temperature decreases. If the ground temperature is already cold, this may add additional stress to the flight crew and patient. When the body attempts to keep warm, oxygen demands increase.

Both the crew and the patient need to be protected. In winter, appropriate clothing should be worn. The patient should be wrapped in several layers to provide warmth. Space or reflective blankets may be useful. It is important to consider the chill factor and the wind's effect on exposed skin during patient transport.

Heat, as well as the cold, can be a source of stress. Equipment may get too hot and cause injury. The patient and crew may lose excessive fluid from perspiring. Water should always be carried on board the aircraft. Both the patient and crew need to be monitored for signs and symptoms of heat exhaustion or stroke.

Dehydration

As the altitude increases, water vapor decreases, so there is less humidity at higher altitudes. It is important to be aware of this stress and monitor the patient's response to fluid resuscitation. Humidified oxygen may be useful during a long flight to prevent irritation of the respiratory passages. As just noted, water should be kept on board the aircraft, particularly for long-distance flights.

Noise and Vibration

Many sources of noise exist around a helicopter. The engines, rotors, radios, and personnel are just a few. Noise interferes with patient assessment parameters, such as auscultating breath, heart, and bowel sounds and measuring blood pressure.

Observation and palpation become important skills for the flight nurse to use during flight to monitor the patient. Observing symmetrical chest expansion and abdominal distention and palpating systolic pressure and peripheral pulses can provide critical information about the trauma patient.

The flight nurse should furnish some type of ear protection for the patient. Blood pressure and pulse monitoring equipment is available for helicopters. Several companies are currently developing a stethoscope that may be useful in flight. Portable Dopplers may also be useful.

Vibrations may alarm the patient and thereby contribute to less effective body cooling in hot weather. Vibrations may trigger a fear response that can release catecholamines and cause blood vessel constriction and interfere with the body's attempt at vasodilation to cool itself. If the patient is alert, the source of vibrations should be explained to the patient and the patient should be closely monitored for signs and symptoms of heat exhaustion (Browne et al., 1987; Waggoner, 1991).

Constant vibration may have an effect on equipment in the aircraft. All loose equipment should be appropriately secured. Monitoring equipment may be affected by vibrations, and frequent evaluations by hospital clinical engineering are required to assure that the equipment is properly calibrated and functioning. Ensuring that this is done is an important responsibility of the flight nurse.

Gravitation

Gravitation forces affect the body during ascent and descent. Gravitation forces are influenced by weight distribution, gravity, and centrifugal force. Three effects of gravitation forces may impact the patient and flight crew during transport: increased intravascular pressure, stagnant hypoxia, and motion sickness. The most common problem that will be encountered in the majority of air medical operations is motion sickness. Interventions for motion sickness include high-flow oxygen, supine positions with limited head movement, visual fixation on a point outside of the aircraft, a flow of cool air onto the face, a cool cloth to the face, and medications such as scopolamine patches (transdermal) and promethazine (Phenergan) (IVFNA, 1990).

As the previous discussion illustrates, air transport physiology requires that the flight nurse be aware of the stresses and interventions that are needed in the air transport of the trauma patient. The patient has already been compromised by injury, and the means of transport should not be the source of additional stress or injury.

GENERAL ASSESSMENT AND INTERVENTIONS

During the transport of the trauma patient, the flight nurse is responsible for ongoing assessment, evaluation, and interventions. The size and internal configuration of the aircraft and the composition of the flight team help determine what initial stabilization will be needed in preparation for transport.

As with any trauma patient, airway with cervical spine immobilization, breathing, circulation, and neurologic deficit must be assessed and stabilized before transport. Specific interventions the flight nurse may need to perform will depend on whether the patient is brought from the scene or a hospital.

During transport, the trauma patient is continuously monitored and assessed. Anticipating and preparing for complications will help provide safe and effective care for the trauma patient.

Ineffective Airway Clearance

The airway should be evaluated and appropriately managed before the patient is loaded into the aircraft. If the patient is at risk for any airway compromise in flight, such as the patient with facial injuries, toxic inhalation, altered mental status, and flail chest, definitive airway management (endotracheal or nasotracheal intubation or cricothyrotomy) with cervical spine immobilization should be initiated before transport. Space limitations in some aircraft may make emergency airway management difficult. However, this varies from program to program.

Supplemental oxygen by nasal cannula or mask should be used when the patient is not intubated. If the patient cannot be intubated, a bag-valve-mask can be used.

To keep the cervical spine immobilized, a hard cervical collar should be placed on the patient. A backboard and head immobilizer will afford additional means of keeping the cervical spine immobilized.

Ineffective Breathing Patterns

The patient's chest should be exposed and the ventilatory status evaluated through observation of respiratory chest expansion. The presence of neck vein distention and tracheal deviation should be noted and appropriate interventions for tension pneumothorax performed. Breath sounds should be auscultated and the chest and neck palpated for subcutaneous emphysema.

Any life-threatening conditions must be treated by the flight nurse. Tension pneumothorax should be decompressed with needle thoracostomy. If medical protocols allow it, a chest tube may be inserted. If a chest tube is placed, its function must be evaluated in flight.

Gas Exchange

Because altitude may affect the compromised patient, constant assessment is needed for signs and symptoms of hypoxia. Changes in mental status, agitation, and lethargy are a few of the signs and symptoms that may be displayed by a hypoxic patient. If blood gas values are available before transport, oxygen delivery can be altered before transport. As stated, all trauma patients need some type of oxygen during transport.

Pulse oximetry and end tidal Pco_2 monitoring provide additional methods to assess gas exchange during flight. Volume-controlled ventilators are available for transport. However, these types of equipment are expensive and their use in air medical transport continues to be evaluated (Semonin-Holleran & Rouse, 1991).

Decreased Cardiac Output

The general appearance of the patient is evaluated. The flight nurse should observe for cool, clammy skin; tachycardia; hypotension; and the status of the jugular veins. The cause of any recognized shock state must be determined to differentiate a volume deficit from a restricted cardiac function. If the cause of the shock is from pericardial tamponade or tension pneumothorax, immediate treatment will be required.

When possible, two large-bore IV catheters should be placed. The fluid that is initiated will depend on the medical protocols. If the patient has suffered obvious blood loss and the flight team carries blood on board the aircraft, blood may be started. Blood is not routinely carried on most aircraft. Problems may exist with keeping the blood cool, especially during the hot summer months.

The use of PASGs is highly controversial. However, in transport they may serve additional functions (Lloyd, 1987; Mattox, Bickell, & Pepe, 1989; McSwain, 1988) If the patient has lower extremity injuries or a fractured pelvis, PASGs can help stabilize these injuries and provide some patient comfort. In the winter they will also help to keep the patient warm. If the aircraft is going to travel at an altitude above 8000 feet, the pressure in the pants should be closely monitored.

A cardiac monitor should be applied to the patient. During flight, frequent assessment of capillary refill can give information about the patient's circulatory status.

Altered Cerebral Tissue Perfusion

The patient's level of consciousness is evaluated during the primary survey. The Glasgow coma scale may be used. A quick pupil check and observation of extremity movement should be included. Changes in level of consciousness can be related to hypoxia, as well as to a head injury.

High Risk for Injury

Because safety is the number one priority for air medical transport, anticipating potential problems is extremely important. The NFNA Advanced Trauma Life Support Course (1990) provides a useful framework to use during the transport of the trauma patient. The box below contains these recommendations. This plan of care will enable the flight nurse to deliver the patient safe and competent care and will help protect the patient and crew from potential injury.

Assessment and management of the trauma patient during helicopter transport

1. Position belted members of the flight crew to facilitate effective management of the ABCs.
2. Have airway and suction equipment easily accessible.
3. Ensure all intravenous lines are accessible. Apply pressure bags or use in-line pumps (available on some types of blood tubing) in the event that fluid resuscitation is necessary and to facilitate fluid flow in the aircraft. Two large-bore lines should be in place.
4. Apply PASG (if indicated by protocol), and be prepared to inflate them during flight.
5. Immobilize the cervical spine with a rigid cervical collar, long backboard, and head immobilizer. Be sure that the airway is accessible.
6. Check that all tubes are secure.
7. Properly restrain a combative patient, either physically or chemically.
8. Place a cardiac monitor and have defibrillation equipment within visual field. Be sure that all equipment is secured.
9. Leave dressed wounds exposed for visual inspection.
10. Expose limb distal to fracture for observation of adequate circulation.

NURSING DIAGNOSES & EVALUATIVE CRITERIA	The trauma patient in flight	
Nursing diagnosis	**Nursing intervention**	**Evaluative criteria**
Impaired gas exchange	**Prevent patient hypoxia during transport** Monitor patient for signs and symptoms of hypoxia.	Patient will demonstrate no changes in mental status, agitation, and lethargy.
	Administer oxygen to patient and monitor patient with pulse oximeter.	O_2 saturations will read above 94%.
	Use CO_2 detector when patient is intubated.	CO_2 detector readings will indicate that tube is in the trachea.
High risk for injury	**Provide safe environment for both patient and crew during air transport** Secure all equipment during flight. Restrain patient as needed.	No injury will occur to patient or crew as a result of the flight experience.
	Position belted crew to facilitate effective management of the patient's ABCs.	Patient will be effectively monitored and managed during flight
Fear	**Decrease both the patient and family's fear about the transport** Provide information, including directions to receiving facility. Allow family member to accompany the patient.	Patient and family members will verbalize less fear regarding the transport Patient's family will be able to locate the patient.

Fear

As much as possible, the flight nurse should address patient and family fear about transport and patient outcome. Most people associate helicopter transport with critical illness, injury, or impending death, and still others may be afraid of flying.

Answering questions and providing information about what is to be expected during flight can help decrease patient and family fears. On certain occasions and if the aircraft is large enough, family members may be allowed to accompany the patient. The flight team must remember that the addition of another passenger, especially a family member, can put the patient and flight team at risk. The family member may object to treatment or may panic during flight. Whether family members or additional passengers can accompany the patient will vary from program to program, but it is an option the flight nurse may want to consider.

SUMMARY The specific assessment and interventions required before transporting the trauma patient by air include assessing and stabilizing the airway, cervical spine, ventilation, and circulation. Transport of the trauma patient in the helicopter demands that the flight nurse anticipate and be prepared to deal with any complications that may occur. The table above summarizes nursing interventions appropriate for the patient in flight.

During flight, the flight nurse continuously monitors and assesses the patient, as well as assures flight team safety and patient comfort. Aircraft size, noise, vibration, and the physiologic changes that may occur because of air transport make the transport of the trauma patient by air a challenge.

Research has demonstrated that air medical transport can make a difference in patient outcomes. The flight nurse plays an integral role in

COMPETENCIES The following clinical competencies pertain to care of the trauma patient during air transport.	☑	Identify the indications for the transfer of the trauma patient by air.
	☑	Evaluate the impact of flight on the traumatically injured patient.
	☑	Perform needed interventions to prepare the trauma patient for flight.
	☑	Apply safety behaviors when working around a helicopter.
	☑	Promote family involvement in the transfer process

these programs by providing a high level of knowledge, skills, and experience that contribute to the provision of safe and effective care for the transport of the traumatically injured patient.

Flight nursing practice allows nursing to go beyond the emergency and intensive care unit and demonstrate the difference that nursing can make. Flight nurses practice in an environment that requires them to have extensive education and preparation to provide the highest level of care possible. Flight nursing is exciting, challenging, and definitely different. Flight nurses can make a difference in the care of the patient who has been traumatically injured.

> But I desire to be the purple. That bright and shining part that makes the rest seem fair and beautiful. Why then do you bid me to become as the multitude? Then were I no longer the purple.
>
> *Author unknown*

RESEARCH QUESTIONS

- What is the best flight team composition for air medical transport?
- Does transport of the trauma patient from the scene make a difference in patient outcome?
- How can pulse oximetry be used during air medical transport?
- Should a traumatic arrest be transported?
- What criteria should be used by prehospital care providers to decide when to call a helicopter to transport the trauma patient?

RESOURCES

Association of Air Medical Services (AAMS)
35 S. Raymond Ave., Suite 205
Pasadena, CA 91105
Phone (818) 793-1232
FAX (818) 793-1039

Commission on Accreditation of Air Medical Services (CAAMS)
Box 1305
Anderson, SC 29522

Helicopter Association International (HAI)
1619 Duke St.
Alexandria, VA 22314
Phone (703) 683-4646
Hotline (703) 683-6488

National Flight Nurses Association (NFNA)
6900 Grove Rd.
Thorofare, NJ 08086
Phone (609) 384-6725
Fax (609) 853-5991

National Flight Paramedics Association (NFPA)
35 S. Raymond Ave., Suite 205
Pasadena, CA 91105
Phone (818) 405-9851

ANNOTATED BIBLIOGRAPHY

Baxt, W., Berry, C., Epperson, M., & Scaizitti, V. (1989). The failure of prehospital trauma prediction rules to classify trauma patients accurately. *Annals of Emergency Medicine*, 18 (1), 1-8.
Article that contains an evaluation of the most frequently used scoring systems that classify major and minor trauma and are used to help make transport decisions. These systems included the PHI (prehospital index), TS (trauma score), RTS (revised trauma score), and CRAMS. Data were collected on 2400 patients from the San Diego Trauma Registry. The researchers found that these scoring systems could predict whether the patient would live or die, but could not predict the extent of patient injuries and the hospital care that may be required to treat them as reflected in their ISS scores.

Carter, G., Couch, R., & O'Brien, D. (1988). The evolution of air transport systems: A pictorial review. *Journal of Emergency Medicine*, 6, 499-504.
Article that provides an historical perspective on the development and use of air transport for the critically ill or injured patient. Included are pictures and text that reflect the rapid development of this type of patient care transport.

Collett, H. (1989). Accident trends for air medical helicopters. *Hospital Aviation*, 8 (3), 6-11.
Article that provides an overview of the accidents that have

occurred in the aeromedical industry since its inception. It includes factual and statistical information about some of the causes. In addition, information about trends and possible interventions that may be used to decrease accidents, injuries, and death is presented.

Semonin-Holleran, R., & Rouse, M. (1991). Biomedical technology: Using it during patient transport. *Journal of Air Medical Transport, 10* (5), 7-12.

Article that presents information about current biomedical technology that can be used during patient transport. The article contains eight tables (pulse oximeters; CO_2 monitors; portable ventilators; intravenous monitors and pumps; cardiac monitors; multiple function monitors; blood pressure monitors; and CPR machines) and specific criteria (height, weight, width, display, accuracy, and battery life) that may assist in evaluating which biomedical technology may be of use during patient transport.

REFERENCES

American College of Emergency Physicians. (1990). Principles of appropriate patient transfer. *Annals of Emergency Medicine, 19* (3), 337-338.

Association of Air Medical Services. (1988). *1988 membership directory.* Pasadena, CA: Author.

Association of Air Medical Services. (1991). *1991 membership directory.* Pasadena, CA: Author.

Auerbach, P., & Geehr, E. (Eds.) (1989). *Management of wilderness and environmental emergencies* (2nd ed). St. Louis: Mosby–Year Book, Inc.

Batterman, K., & Markel, N. (1986). Profile of a flight nurse. *Aeromedical Journal, 8,* 26-29.

Baxt, G. (1985). Is there a role for flight physicians on EMS rotorcraft? *Trauma Quarterly, 1* (3), 39-42.

Baxt, G. (1986). Measuring the impact of rotorcraft aeromedical services. *Emergency Care Quarterly, 2* (3), 59-65.

Baxt, G., Berry, C., Epperson, M., & Scalzitti, V. (1989). The failure of prehospital rules to classify trauma patients accurately. *Annals of Emergency Medicine, 18* (1), 1-18.

Boyd, C., & Hungerpillar, J. (1990). Patient risk in prehospital transport: Air versus ground. *Emergency Care Quarterly, 5* (4), 48-55.

Browne, L., Bodenstedt, R., Campbell, P., & Nehrenz, G. (1987). The nine stresses of flight. *Journal of Emergency Nursing, 13* (4), 232-234.

Burney, R. (1987). Efficacy, cost and safety of hospital-based emergency aeromedical programs. *Annals of Emergency Medicine 16* (2), 227-229.

Burney, R., Rhee, K., Cornell, R., Bowman, M., Storer, D., & Moylan, J. (1988). Evaluation of hospital based aeromedical programs using therapeutic intervention scoring. *Aviation, Space, and Environmental Medicine, 6,* 563-566.

Campbell, P. (1987). Flight nurse practice: What is the governing body? *Journal of Emergency Nursing, 13* (4), 198-199.

Carraway, R., Brewer, M., Lewis, B., Shaw, R., Berry, R., & Watson, L. (1984). Life-saver: A complete team approach incorporated into a hospital-based program. *American Surgeon, 4* (50), 173-181.

Champion, H. (1986). Helicopter triage. *Emergency Care Quarterly, 2* (3), 13-21.

Chinn, J. (1988). Standardization, organization, and a responsible party. *Aeromedical Journal, 8,* 12-15.

Collett, H. (1991). Air medical accident rates. *Journal of Air Medical Transport, 10* (2), 14-15.

Crippen, D. (1990). Critical care transportation medicine: New concepts in pretransport of the critically ill patient. *American Journal of Emergency Medicine, 11,* 551-554.

Dean, M., Bynoe, R., Castleman, P., Kudsk, K., & Fabian, T. (September, 1988). *The effect of altitude on oxygen saturation (OS) during helicopter transport.* Paper presented at the Association of Aeromedical Services, Boston, MA.

Emergency Nurses Association (1991). *National standard guidelines for prehospital nursing curriculum.* Chicago: Author.

Frew, S., Roush, W., & LaGreca, K. (1988). COBRA: Implications for emergency medicine. *Annals of Emergency Medicine, 17* (8), 835-837.

Gold, C. (1987). Prehospital advanced life support vs. "scoop and run" in trauma management. *Annals of Emergency Medicine, 16* (7), 797-801.

Gregory, T. (1990). *Flight nursing advanced trauma course.* Thorofare, NJ: National Flight Nurses Association (NFNA).

Harless, K., Morris, A., Cenzig, M., Holt, J., & Schmidt, C. (1978). Civilian ground and air transport of adults with acute respiratory failure. *Journal of the American Medical Association, 28* (4), 361-365.

Hodges, J. (1989). Aeromedical transport. *Emergency Care Quarterly, 4* (4), 1-12.

Johnson, J. (1981). Medical care in the air. *Annals of Emergency Medicine, 10* (6), 324-327.

Kaplan, L., Walsh, D., & Burney, R. (1987). Emergency aeromedical transport of patients with acute myocardial infarction. *Annals of Emergency Medicine, 17* (8), 835-837.

Kreis, D., Fine, E., Gomez, G., Eckes, L., Whitwell, E., & Byers, P. (1988). A prospective evaluation of field categorization of trauma patients. *Journal of Trauma, 28* (7), 989-1000.

Lee, G. (1987). History of flight nursing. *Journal of Emergency Nursing, 4,* 212-218.

Lee, G. (1991). *Flight nursing: Principles and practice.* St. Louis: Mosby–Year Book, Inc.

Lloyd, S. (1987). MAST and IV infusion: Do they help in prehospital trauma management? *Annals of Emergency Medicine, 16,* 565-567.

Macione, A., & Wilcox, D. (1987). Utilization of helicopter emergency medical services. *Annals of Emergency Medicine, 16* (4), 391-398.

Mattox, K. (1988). Editorial comment. *Journal of Trauma, 8,* 1133-1134.

Mattox, K., Bickell, W., & Pepe, P. (1989). Prospective MAST study in 911 patients. *Journal of Trauma, 29* (8), 1104-1112.

Mayer, T., & Walker, M. (1984). Severity of illness and injury in pediatric air transport. *Annals of Emergency Medicine, 2,* 108-111.

Mc Swain, N. (1988). Pneumatic antishock garment: State of the art. *Annals of Emergency Medicine, 17* (5), 506-525.

Melton, J., Heller, M., Kaplan, R., & Mohan-Klein, K. (September, 1988). *Occult hypoxia during aeromedical transport: Detection by pulse oximetry.* Paper presented at the meeting of the Association of Aeromedical Services, Boston, MA.

National Flight Nurses Association (NFNA). (1986). *Practice standards for flight nursing*. Thorofare, NJ: Author.

Reddick, E. (1979). Evaluation of the helicopter in aeromedical transfers. *Aviation, Space, and Environmental Medicine, 50* (2), 168-170.

Rhee, K., Mackenzie, J., Conley, J., LaGreca-Reibling, K., & Flora, J. (1986). Therapeutic intervention scoring as a measure of performance in a helicopter emergency medical services program. *Annals of Emergency Medicine, 1,* 40-43.

Rhee, K., Willits, N., Turner, J., & Ward, R. (1987). Trauma score change during transport: Is it predictive of mortality. *American Journal of Emergency Medicine, 5,* 353-365.

Rhodes, M. (1986). A prospective study of field triage for helicopter transport. *Emergency Care Quarterly, 2* (3), 22-30.

Saywell, R., Woods, J., Rodman, G., Nyhus, A., Bender, L., Phillips, J., & Bock, H. (1989). Financial analysis of an inner-city helicopter service: Charges versus collections. *Annals of Emergency Medicine, 18* (1), 21-25.

Schiller, W., Knox, R., Zinnecker, H., Jeevanandam, M., Sayre, M., Burke, J., & Young, D. (1988). Effect of helicopter transport of trauma victims on survival in an urban trauma. *Journal of Trauma, 28* (8), 1127-1134.

Semonin-Holleran, R., & Rouse, M. (1991). Biomedical technology: Using it during patient transport. *Journal of Air Medical Transport, 10* (5), 7-12.

Shea, D. (1985). The role of nurses and paramedics in EMS rotorcraft. *Trauma Quarterly, 5,* 33-37.

Snow, N., Hull, C., & Severns, J. (1986). Physician staffing on a helicopter emergency medical service. *Emergency Care Quarterly, 2* (3), 40-45.

Taylor, V., Fallon, W., & Alexander, R. (September, 1988). *The effect of patient position during transport on oximetry and capnometry: A prospective study*. Paper presented at the Association of Air Medical Services, Boston, MA.

Thomas, F., & Jacobson, J. (1991). Applying ethical principles to air medical transport. *Emergency Care Quarterly, 6,* 1-6.

Topol, E., Fung, A., Kline, E., Kaplan, L., Landis, D., Strozeski, M., Burney, R., Pitt, B., & O'Neill, W. (1986). Safety of helicopter transport and out-of-hospital intravenous fibrinolytic therapy in patients with evolving myocardial infarction. *Catheterization and Cardiovascular Diagnosis, 12,* 151-155.

Trunkey, D. (1988). Trauma care at mid-passage: A personal viewpoint. *Journal of Trauma, 28* (7), 889-895.

Uhlhorn, R., & Jacobs, L. (1982). Helicopters: Extending the prehospital transportation system. *Medical Instrumentation, 16* (4), 202-203.

United States Department of Transportation (1988). *Air medical crew national standard curriculum*. Pasadena, CA: Association of Air Medical Services.

Waggoner, R. (1991). Flight physiology. In G. Lee (Ed.), *Flight Nursing: Principles and Practice*. St. Louis: Mosby–Year Book, Inc.

Wright, S., Dronen, S., Combs, T., & Storer, D. (1989). Aeromedical transport of patients with post-traumatic cardiac arrest. *Annals of Emergency Medicine, 18* (7), 721-726.

21 *Emergency Department Care of the Trauma Patient*

Christine May

OBJECTIVES
- ❏ Describe the evolution of emergency nursing as a specialty.
- ❏ Discuss typical roles for the emergency nurse in care of the multisystem trauma patient.
- ❏ Identify requirements for emergency departments and emergency nurses in trauma care delivery.
- ❏ Describe special circumstances that impact trauma care delivery by the emergency nurse.

INTRODUCTION Patients present to the emergency department (ED) with physical events ranging from acute, noncritical illness that occurs outside physicians' regular office hours, to episodic exacerbation of chronic illness in the absence of a primary physician, to life-threatening emergencies. These patients may arrive via emergency medical services (EMS) or in private vehicles. But in spite of the broad range of ill and injured patients seen in the ED, "emergency" physician coverage was at one time provided by physicians on staff whose rotating assignments included emergency room coverage. Among these physicians were dermatologists and radiologists, as well as surgeons, general practitioners, and internists. In some cases a variety of "moonlighting" physicians provided ER coverage. Nursing care was often provided by a house supervisor who responded when the patient arrived. Patients often met their private physicians at the "ER" for evaluation and treatment, and emergent patients were managed by the most readily available doctor on call.

In the mid-1960s, a number of factors such as implementation of Medicare and Medicaid programs, disconnection from family/primary care

physician, and preference for ED care, resulted in increased use of the ED (Pisarcik, 1980). As patient volume, acuity, and expectations increased, emergency *rooms* became *departments*, and "fill-in" nurses and doctors evolved to specialists. Physician availability improved when hospitals hired "ER" staff. More important, the acute care of a wide variety of ill and injured patients led to the identification of a new specialty: emergency medicine.

The American College of Emergency Physicians (ACEP) was established in 1968 and by 1991 comprised more than 15,000 members. The American Board of Emergency Medicine (ABEM) was established in 1976, and in January 1991 it comprised 9099 certified emergency physicians. To meet the educational preparation needs of this distinct specialty, residency training programs were developed; the first one began in 1970. By 1991 there were 83 established programs, which have prepared an estimated 3800 emergency physicians practicing in a variety of roles and settings (ACEP, 1991). Specific needs of EDs treating exclusively pediatric populations have also been recognized, and subspecialty training and certification are emerging (ACEP, 1990). As of 1991 there were 30 pediatric emergency medicine fellowship programs. Collaboration between the American Board of Emergency Medicine and the American Board of Pediatrics has resulted in the approval of subcertificates in pediatric/emergency medicine. The first examination should be available in late 1992 or early 1993.

Over the past 20 years, emergency nursing has also evolved to a distinct specialty with standards for preparation and practice (Rea, 1987); a 1989 survey estimated that there are 85,000 practicing emergency nurses (Lenehan, 1990a). Today's emergency nurse is a highly knowledgeable, skilled clinician with a unique combination of competencies that overlaps, draws from, and contributes to a number of clinical/functional areas. Whereas other nursing specialties are defined by body system (e.g., cardiovascular), disease process (e.g., diabetes), care setting (e.g., clinic, operating room, medical and surgical units), age group (e.g., pediatric), or population (e.g., women's health), emergency nurses respond to *all* patients' needs (ENA, 1989).

Not only does the emergency nurse care for a wide range of patient complaints, the emergency setting itself is unique in the hospital. There are no defined nurse:patient ratios or hours per patient day (HPPD) formulas. And although it is fiscally impractical to staff for the "busiest possible," ED managers must find a balance to assure safe conditions for an unpredictable flow of patients (ENA, 1991a). Careful tracking of times of day and days of week with the highest volume and/or acuity is useful for staffing to the average, but contingency plans must exist also, such as dedicated in-house resource nurses or nurses on call. Finally, it is important to realize that while in-patient units have finite census/bed availability, the ED in most cases is not permitted to divert patients. When the ED census reaches capacity, with patients awaiting disposition or in-patient admission, emergency nurses must adjust their pace and work pattern to incorporate admission orders.

The Emergency Department Nurses Association (EDNA) was founded in 1970 to recognize the special blend of knowledge and skills found among emergency nurses. By 1974 there were 65 chapters. By 1991 the number of chapters had increased to 228, with more than 20,000 members (ENA, 1991b). In 1980 EDNA became simply ENA, Emergency Nurses Association, to reflect

the expanding practice arenas, which include free-standing, urgent care centers; clinics; prehospital care; air rescue/transport; EMS agencies; business, educational, industrial, and correctional institutions; and trauma centers (Kelleher, 1990). Emergency nurses not only care for the patients who present to these diverse settings, but also are invaluable teaching resources in the classroom and clinical practice arena for a variety of emergency care providers.

The body of knowledge associated with emergency nursing was defined in the *Emergency Nursing Core Curriculum*, first published in 1975 and now in its third edition. Since 1975 the *Journal of Emergency Nursing* has provided substantive clinical information about this unique area of practice. The Board of Certification in Emergency Nursing (BCEN) was established in 1980, with the Certification in Emergency Nursing (CEN) examination designed to measure and declare competence in emergency nursing. By July 1991, 21,106 nurses had been certified (ENA, 1991b). Also, in 1983 the *EDNA Standards of Emergency Nursing* Practice was published, and a second edition (ENA) was published in 1991 (ENA, 1991c). Finally, the Trauma Nursing Core Course (TNCC) was introduced in 1986, and with 30,000 providers and 1500 instructors verified to date (ENA, 1992), it has become a standard for nurses involved in the initial care of trauma patients. Emergency nurses and the ENA are committed to trauma prevention, management, education, and research (MacPhail, 1989).

TRAUMA CARE AS A PART OF EMERGENCY NURSING

Trauma nursing has also been defined as a specialty, and emergency nurses have been at the forefront of its development (Beachley, 1989). The ED is recognized as the entry point to the hospital and is often the site of emergent resuscitation. The most critical role for the emergency nurse is in initial assessment, resuscitation, and stabilization of the injured patient. In addition, however, emergency nurses contribute to care before patient arrival and beyond resuscitation.

Relative to the prehospital setting, emergency nurses frequently are involved in training emergency medical technicians (EMTs) and paramedics (EMT-Ps) in the critical skills of triage, assessment, and resuscitation measures. Emergency nurses are often the hospital-based contact for prehospital providers, for advance notice of patients en route, for guidance in field care when radio protocols govern prehospital practice, and for feedback and follow-up on patients brought to the ED.

Similarly, the emergency nurse's practice extends beyond resuscitation as the patient is monitored and cared for in the ED and transferred to in-patient units or other facilities. The emergency nurse facilitates this transition by reporting to the receiving nurse, providing appropriate documentation, informing family, and often accompanying the patient.

And the emergency nurse even occasionally provides follow-up care: patients who return because of missed or worsening injuries; patients with recent or remote trauma identified as cause of a new complaint; and patients who present in the ED after missing a clinic appointment.

CARE OF THE TRAUMA PATIENT: AN EMERGENCY NURSE'S APPROACH

According to *Accidental Death and Disability: the Neglected Disease of Modern Society*, trauma is a disease with an epidemiology, characteristic presentation, and associated prevention potential (NASNRC, 1966). Injury is *not* considered random or "accidental," but rather, an interaction between agent (e.g., gun, knife, motor vehicle, bicycle, fire), host (the potential "trauma victim"), and environment (e.g., traffic, highway, drug and alcohol use by others). Knowing that predictable risk factors and mechanisms of injury exist, the emergency nurse works with the expectation that many of the emergent or urgent conditions that present to the ED might be the result of trauma. As discussed in Chapter 7, *potential* exists for severe injury when the patient's history includes mechanisms of injury, such as falls, assaults, bicycle or motor vehicle crashes, or penetrating wounds. Emergency care texts instruct the emergency clinician to "assume the worst" (Rosen et al., 1988), and this is particularly true of trauma patients.

A number of studies have correlated early recognition and management within a "golden hour" after injury with reduction of trauma-related mortality and morbidity. Because of the critical interface between identification of the trauma patient, entry into prehospital care delivery, and emer-gency care skills, emergency services have been identified by the committees on trauma of both the American College of Surgeons (ACS) (Appendix A) and the ACEP as essential to trauma care delivery systems (ACEP,1987; ACSCOT,1990). According to the ACEP position statement, the emergency physician is key in directing prehospital care, providing ED resuscitation and stabilization, and facilitating transition to in-hospital care, all of which have critical nursing components. Documents from ACEP that are pertinent to trauma include (1) the policy statement on Trauma System Quality Assurance approved in March 1990; (2) the Emergency Care Guidelines, which describe resources needed to serve the community for the prehospital setting, the emergency facility; patient disposition, and transfer issues; and (3) the Guidelines for Trauma Care Systems. Appendix C shows the suggested equipment and supplies for EDs and guidelines for providers in urban and rural settings.

The ACS document also identifies qualified emergency nurses as essential to the care of the trauma patients. Although these documents are used as guidelines for *systems*, which include designated trauma *centers*, the concepts of preparation and education, as well as evaluation of performance and quality of care, are applicable to all facilities receiving trauma patients.

Representatives of six major nursing specialty organizations established guidelines related to trauma nursing care in the *Trauma Nursing Resource Document*. This document addresses topics such as specialty nursing education, staffing, equipment, and general topics, including trauma research, quality management, system development, ethics, organ donation, and injury prevention (Proehl, Bires, Southard, & Tidwell, 1992).

Equipment and Supplies

A high-volume trauma center is expected to have a dedicated trauma resuscitation room, whereas in a smaller-volume or nondesignated facility, trauma patients may be evaluated and resuscitated in a general area used for emergent/urgent patient care. Basic resuscitation equipment for EDs is described in a number of texts and includes supplies for airway management, breathing support, IV access, fluid resuscitation, life-support medication, monitoring and defibrillation capability, and equipment for transport.

The ACS document describes additional needs for the care of trauma patients. Equipment and supplies specific to trauma patient needs include surgical trays, large-bore intravenous catheters and tubing, blood transfusion tubing, chest tubes, autotransfusion sets, and blood/fluid warmers (ACS, 1990).

As in other areas of the hospital, observation of Centers for Disease Control (CDC)–recommended universal precautions for contact with blood and body fluids must be provided for. In addition to moisture-proof gowns and gloves, trauma rooms should also provide goggles, masks, boots, and perhaps additional aprons to prevent soak-through of blood.

Trauma rooms must also have x-ray capability, which includes built-in or designated portable machines and lead shields or dividers for protection of staff and use between patients if the resuscitation area has multiple-patient capability.

Finally, consideration must be given to telephones, x-ray film view boxes, laboratory printers, computer terminals, provision for invasive and/or remote monitoring and so on.

Arrangement of equipment will vary considerably among EDs, but it is essential to develop a systematic and convenient organization with which all staff are familiar. Hospitals have used peg boards to hang equipment, modular storage units, and exchange carts from the central supply department. Diagrams, equipment check-off lists, orientation videotapes, and regular checks of equipment and function are all methods for assuring availability and staff familiarity. A suggested goal is to have sufficient appropriate equipment and supplies so that the nurse does not need to leave the resuscitation room. However, it is important to avoid clutter and unnecessary overstocking. Figure 21-1 illustrates an example of a trauma resuscitation room layout, but specifics are determined by the needs of each facility.

In addition to a dedicated and well-planned trauma room, plans must exist for multiple patient incidents and arrival of additional trauma patients when all spaces are filled. Back-up equipment carts, additional resuscitation areas that can be used for both critical medical as well as trauma patients, and timely movement of the noncritical patient out of the trauma room have all been effective means to ensure availability of resuscitation space. For hospitals to be appropriately prepared for patient arrival, prehospital protocols should include notification requirements.

Education and Team Development

The Emergency Nurses Association has described standards for emergency nursing practice, and the Core Curriculum provides guidelines for ongoing education (Kelleher, 1990; Lenehan, 1990a; Rea, 1987). In addition, the Trauma Nursing Core Course (TNCC) provides basic trauma knowledge and psychomotor skills (Rea, 1987). The systematic approach described by the TNCC is useful to identify the current level of staff skills, as well as learning needs. Hospitals might also choose to offer more detailed education specific to their own patient population or trauma program, in addition to or in lieu of the standard course.

Although it has not been clearly defined how often a nurse must perform a procedure or respond to a resuscitation to remain adept at both clinical decision-making and psychomotor skills, no trauma education program is complete with basic or one-time teaching. Methods to meet ongoing education needs of emergency nurses caring for trauma patients include in-service education programs, conferences, skills laboratories, and "mock codes" or drills. (Trauma-related competencies in which emergency nurses should remain proficient are provided at the end of this chapter.)

The most effective approach to trauma resuscitation is an organized team with a designated leader and specific assignments for each team member. The ACS emphasizes the potential need for urgent surgical intervention and therefore requires the team leader to be a surgeon. Emergency medicine includes a special expertise in rapid evaluation and resuscitation and suggests the emergency physician is the most appropriate team leader, with access to urgent surgical consultation. Although there still exists considerable controversy in this area, somewhat related to local and regional strengths of each specialty, all agree that a designated physician team leader is critical to an integrated approach to the trauma patient. Specific team composition varies with institutional needs and local/regional protocols. At a designated trauma center, the team includes a general surgeon, emergency physician, one to three nurses, and ancillary personnel from such areas as laboratory, radiology, and respiratory therapy. Other required specialties (anesthesia,

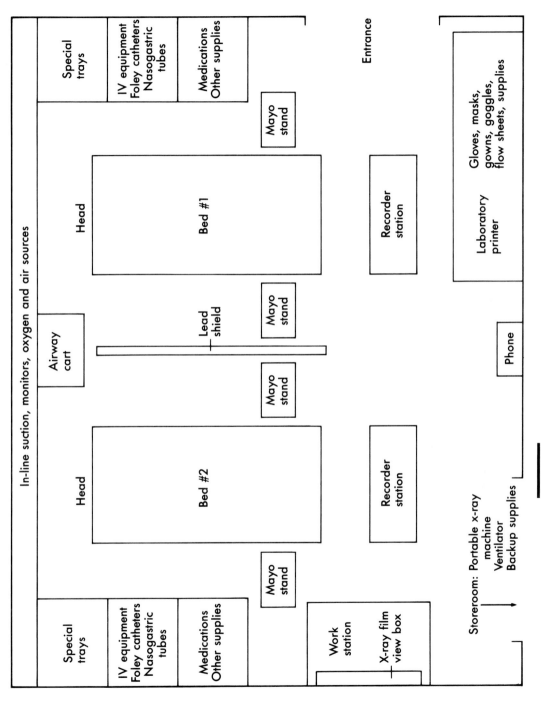

Figure 21-1 Example of trauma resuscitation room layout.

critical care, neurosurgery, orthopedics) may be included on the initial response team or may be consulted as needed. Nurses designated for initial response may be from the ED, ICU, OR, and resource pool or house supervisors.

On the other hand, in an ED of a hospital that is not a designated trauma center and that receives trauma patients with varying frequency, often there is one emergency physician, and the emergency nurse(s) fills the role of resuscitation nurse, recorder, and transport nurse. It is critical to have resources identified and roles assigned (May, 1987).

Additional support may include social services personnel, pastoral care personnel, registration/admission clerks, and security personnel for patient and staff safety. The incidence of violence directed at health care providers and retaliation against patients has increased. Strategies related to staff and patient safety include general hospital access issues, ED construction guidelines (bullet-proof glass, lock-out doors), identification badges, visiting policies and deterrants such as security "presence" and use of K-9 units (*ENA*, 1991d; Lenehan, 1991; Martin, 1991).

Models for team assignments

As noted, trauma team nurse roles vary with setting. Delineation of roles for emergency nurses might be that of a primary nurse who assesses the patient, anticipates and assists with procedures, and provides hands-on bedside care; and a secondary or circulating nurse, who documents critical data, accepts and routes specimens, and communicates with ancillary personnel and the family (May, 1987).

Rosen suggests a team captain, a procedure team, and a data team (Rosen et al., 1988). Building on this concept, roles are defined by tasks or procedures, such as (1) airway management, with responsibility for maintaining airway, providing supplemental oxygen, and anticipating/assisting with intubation and ventilation; (2) volume resuscitation, including setting up appropriate lines with warmed fluid, starting peripheral lines, assisting with invasive line placement, obtaining blood samples for type and crossmatch, and so on; and (3) recorder, who not only documents the resuscitation, but also might coordinate communication among the team, ancillary personnel, and significant others. This approach might be particularly effective when the number of nurses is limited, but other personnel are available. For example, the airway tasks might be assigned to a respiratory technician, or the recorder duties might be performed by a medical clerk.

When a number of physicians are available, as well as several nurses, nurse/physician teams can be considered. The physician who is placing a central line or performing a cutdown works with a nurse team member who prepares the fluid warmer, tubing, catheters, and sutures. Another nurse/physician team may anticipate and prepare for a thoracostomy, with the nurse premedicating the patient and then assembling the drainage system, while the physician places the chest tube. This model might be appropriate for unstable patients requiring many invasive procedures.

When nurses are pulled from elsewhere in the hospital, role assignments that utilize the skills from their primary area of practice are most likely to result in optimal staff effectiveness and comfort. Thus the emergency nurse is familiar with cervical spine immobilization, emergency lines, and airway assistance and might perform or assist with those interventions. The ICU nurse's expertise is in bedside care, monitoring for subtle changes, and perhaps administering Advanced Cardiac Life Support (ACLS) drugs if indicated. The OR nurse is invaluable when cricothyroidotomy or resuscitative thoracotomy becomes necessary. It is important to note, however, that when a number of nurses from throughout the hospital are drawn for trauma response, each must carry an assignment that can be temporarily suspended.

Finally, assignment of nurses on the trauma team may be simply practical or convenient, related to equipment location or expertise of the individual nurse.

In addition to immediate resuscitation assignments, a nurse should be identified who will accompany the unstable patient for further diagnostic studies, such as CT scan or angiography, and care for the patient until definitive care is assumed by the next team of caregivers, such as those in OR or ICU.

The models for nurse assignments described here have been used successfully, but the decision of what will work best for any institution depends on staff numbers and experience base, on frequency of need to assemble the team, on available education and practice opportunities, and on other available personnel resources.

Patient Management: Quality Performance

Expectations in the minimally staffed ED will differ from the multiperson team response in the designated trauma center, but the emergency nurse has responsibility for the initial assessment of the patient. The nurse may actually perform the primary and secondary surveys, may do *part* of the survey, or may function as recorder for the assessment done by another nurse or physician team member.

As described in other chapters, the primary survey includes assessment of the "ABCs" and life-saving interventions if indicated. **Airway** assessment includes position and patency and the ability of the patient to maintain both without assistance. Interventions might include improvement of position to open the airway, such as jaw-thrust or chin-lift, placement of an oropharyngeal or nasotracheal airway, and suction for emesis, blood, or debris. These interventions are within a nurse's scope of practice and should be applied if the patient airway is at all compromised. The impaired, obstructed, or unprotected airway might require more aggressive management, such as intubation, cricothyroidotomy, or tracheostomy, and the nurse should anticipate those procedures and assemble equipment and supplies. As noted in clinical chapters, it is critical to avoid hyperextension of the neck and to maintain adequate immobilization of the cervical spine when evaluating and managing the airway of a trauma patient.

Breathing is assessed by observation of the chest and auscultation of the lungs. High-flow oxygen is an independent nursing intervention and is indicated for all trauma patients (Rea, 1991). Inadequate respiration is assisted with a bag-valve-mask device, while steps are taken to identify and correct the underlying problem. Nurses should anticipate such procedures as needle and tube thoracostomy for pneumothorax; and thoracostomy and autotransfusion for hemothorax. Oxygenation may be assessed by pulse oximetry, although accuracy depends on adequate peripheral perfusion and hematocrit. Careful assessment of respiratory effort is ongoing, and ventilation is best evaluated by arterial blood gas.

Circulation is assessed by pulse, skin color and temperature, capillary refill, and blood pressure. The emergency nurse's role includes applying direct pressure to bleeding wounds, initiating large-bore intravenous lines, and obtaining bank blood for transfusion. Procedures to anticipate include

---

Resuscitation of the trauma patient
The emergency nurse's scope of practice

AIRWAY	**Cervical spine control** **Noninvasive airway (nasal/oropharyngeal)** **Suction** Intubation Cricothyrotomy/tracheostomy
BREATHING	**Oxygen** **Bag-valve-mask assist** Needle/tube thoracostomy
CIRCULATION	**Direct pressure** **Peripheral IV access** **Type and crossmatch** **Autotransfusion** **Monitoring ECG** **Serial vital signs** Venous cutdown Pericardiocentesis Thoracotomy
THERMO-REGULATION	**Fluid warmer** **Patient warming measures**

Boldface type represents interventions within the scope of nursing practice.

---

venous cutdown, percutaneous large-bore central lines, pericardiocentesis, and resuscitative thoracotomy.

A framework for the nurse's scope of practice in trauma resuscitation is outlined in the box above.

CASE STUDY   Sandra is a 19-year-old female involved in a moderate-speed automobile crash with extensive damage to the right front quarter panel and significant passenger space intrusion. The patient was an unrestrained front-seat passenger and was ejected from the vehicle, probably through the front windshield, which was noted by the paramedics to be missing. Her husband was the unrestrained driver and was also ejected. Their 12-month-old child was in an infant restraint in the right rear seat and was uninjured. The following case discussion will focus on Sandra.

Prehospital care   Three rescue units were on the scene, and the two adults were transported in separate ambulances to the closest adult trauma center. Radio report was as follows:

Two critical trauma patients, ejected from the vehicle, with major vehicle damage; probable significant head injury and other unknown injuries; female patient, history of brief loss of consciousness, now combative; blood pressure, unobtainable, but good pulses; pulse, 100; respiratory rate, 22; Glasgow coma scale score, 13.

What personnel would you assign to care for this patient?

In a trauma center, the probable severity of injury and instability of these two patients would result in activation of a full team, and perhaps back-up personnel as well. In an area without a trauma system or designated center, the emergency nurse would most likely be the one to identify and notify personnel resources and assemble equipment.

The plan would include assembling a separate team for each patient, with physician captain, at least one nurse, and clerical and ancillary help. As mentioned, the radio update is essential to prepare for the patient, especially as in this case, which included multiple victims. Decisions were made to move patients in the ED and to divide the trauma team between these two critical patients.

What interventions would you anticipate?

Because of the head injury, airway control is critical, and the emergency nurse would anticipate nasal or oropharyngeal airway and high-flow oxygen at the least, and most likely intubation and mechanical hyperventilation.

The trauma receiving area would be prepared for fluid resuscitation, with warmed crystalloid, large-bore tubing, large catheters, venous cutdown tray, and fluid warmer. Although caution is used with fluid administration in patients with head trauma, Sandra's hypotension, tachycardia, and agitation suggested clinical shock requiring volume resuscitation. Hypovolemia results in decreased cerebral blood flow, decreased cerebral perfusion pressure, and ultimately increased intracranial pressure.

In the field, Sandra was placed on high-flow oxygen via nonrebreather mask. She had an 18-gauge IV line placed, with lactated Ringer's solution infusing. A pneumatic antishock garment (PASG) was placed and inflated, presumably because of her unobtainable blood pressure, tachy-

cardia, and agitation. (Although the PASG is still seen, it is less and less in favor, as discussed in Chapter 9.)

Emergency department On arrival, the trauma team was divided between the two patients, with two nurses (one from the ICU) assigned to each team. Sandra arrived in full cervical spine precautions, with PASG inflated. She was tachycardic, tachypneic, and agitated.

Primary survey revealed the **Airway** to be unobstructed and atraumatic; **Breathing** was spontaneous, with equal bilateral expansion and a faster than normal rate; **Circulation** was compromised, with BP, 100/72; HR, 142; delayed capillary refill; and agitation. **Disability** was assessed as GCS score, 14, with spontaneous eye opening, some disorientation, and extremities moving appropriately to command. There were no complaints of specific pain, although the patient was extremely agitated. The pelvis was stable, and no significant abdominal findings were reported.

What intervention would you anticipate as a priority?

The patient's **shock** defined the priority. Because hypotension caused by head injury is generally a preterminal event encountered in a deeply comatose patient, other correctable causes must be identified. Clinical shock in this patient was more likely the result of hypovolemia, and so at least one more large-bore IV line was needed, warm crystalloid infusion was needed, and a clot was sent for type and crossmatch, anticipating surgery. In the absence of external bleeding or evidence of pelvis or long bone fracture, intracavitary hemorrhage was suspected. If a patient has potential for multiple sources of hemorrhage and can be stabilized with crystalloid, an abdominal CT scan is appropriate. If CT is not available or the patient is unstable, but without definite peritoneal signs, diagnostic peritoneal lavage is indicated.

How would you prepare for a diagnostic peritoneal lavage?

Once adequate venous access is assured with a minimum of two large-bore lines, an indwelling urinary catheter is placed to decompress the bladder and reduce risk of perforation with the lavage catheter. Drainage should be to a metered collection set so that output can be used as a measure of volume resuscitation. A gastric tube should be placed to decompress the stomach. The peritoneal lavage tray may be a commercially packaged disposable kit or assembled by central supply, and should be opened with sterile technique. There are several techniques for DPL incision, and description of the surgical technique is beyond the scope of this chapter. If gross blood is aspirated from the catheter, the lavage is considered positive. If gross blood is not present, the patient is lavaged with warmed isotonic solution via large-drip, nonvented tubing. Return is by gravity into the empty IV bag. Lavage fluid is evaluated by visual assessment (positive if newsprint not visible through fluid) or laboratory analysis, which includes cell count and Gram stain. When peritoneal lavage is positive, the patient is prepared for immediate laparotomy.

Sandra's peritoneal lavage was grossly positive, and she was transported to the operating room for emergency laparotomy. The source of her hemorrhage was a shattered spleen, and she underwent splenectomy and repair of a small liver laceration. Postoperatively, a CT scan of her head was performed, which showed no significant injury.

Sandra's husband also had an urgent head CT scan, which showed contusion and diffuse edema, without evidence of space-occupying lesion. Because the critical condition of both parents required all available nursing care, social services personnel assumed responsibility for follow-up of the uninjured child and other family support.

Beyond the ABCs

In addition to responsibilities related to the primary survey and life-saving interventions, the emergency nursing care includes completion of (or assistance with) the secondary survey, communication with family and significant others, pain management, and preparation of the patient for admission or transfer. Priority-setting and rapid decision-making are skills required of emergency nursing, which are never more applicable than in the care of the multiply injured patient.

As the first nurse encountered by the patient and family, the emergency nurse often assumes responsibility for reassuring the patient, contacting family and significant others, and initiating appropriate referrals, such as social services or pastoral care. Resources will vary considerably among EDs and trauma centers, and it is necessary for the emergency nurse to be familiar with referral patterns. Finally, the emergency nurse often coordinates follow-up with prehospital provid-

ers and law enforcement officials, including collection or preservation of evidence.

Nursing diagnoses

A number of nursing diagnoses are applied to the resuscitation phase of trauma care, i.e., those related to airway compromise, ineffective breathing, and fluid volume deficit. Expected patient outcomes for this phase include patent, protected airway with appropriate oxygen administration; adequate respiration and ventilation; and optimal perfusion as evidenced by clear mentation, normal heart rate, and sufficient urine output. In addition, the emergency nurse identifies the patient at physiologic risk for altered skin and tissue integrity, infection, and pain, as well as psychologic risk related to disturbance in personal identity, altered role performance, powerlessness, and variations in coping. Expected outcomes for nursing interventions are illustrated in the table on p. 652. Patient acuity and general condition will determine which diagnoses receive priority intervention from the emergency nurse.

SPECIAL CONSIDERATIONS
Triage

Triage, from the French word meaning "to sort," refers to setting priorities for patient care, personnel, equipment, and supplies. Although an extensive discussion is beyond the scope of this chapter, triage is a concept integral to both emergency nursing and trauma care.

Field triage criteria are used to identify the critical trauma patient, using such physiologic parameters as systolic blood pressure and respiratory rate; anatomic injuries, such as penetrating wounds or paralysis; and mechanism of injury, such as degree of vehicle damage and height of fall (ACS, 1986). In trauma systems, the goal of field triage criteria is to identify those patients who are likely to benefit from the dedicated resources at a trauma center and those who can be appropriately cared for at other facilities.

Within the ED, using data from the prehospital provider or gathered on initial encounter, the emergency nurse determines urgency. A number of different models for emergency departments have been used, and the professional nurse has been identified as the one most effective to perform triage (Sheehy & Barber, 1985). Nursing diagnosis provides a useful framework for setting

The emergency department patient

Nursing diagnosis	Nursing intervention	Evaluative criteria
Ineffective airway clearance	Provide chin-lift or jaw-thrust with cervical spine protection. Maintain position of jaw with cervical collar in place.	Airway will be patent. Respirations will be quiet.
High risk for aspiration	Remove debris with suction. Log-roll and/or suction if emesis occurs. Maintain position of tongue with oropharyngeal airway. Anticipate intubation, and assist with as needed.	Patient will not aspirate.
Ineffective breathing pattern	Provide supplemental oxygen.	Respiratory effort will be unlabored or supported.
Impaired gas exchange	Assist with ventilation. Anticipate and assist with procedures related to cause (e.g., pleural decompression, tube thoracostomy).	Ventilation will be adequate: • ABGs will be normal; • mental status will be clear.
Decreased cardiac output	Restore volume. Provide IV access. Administer crystalloid blood as ordered.	Blood pressure and heart rate will be within normal limits.
Fluid volume deficit	Anticipate and assist with corrective procedures (e.g., cutdown, pericardiocentesis, thoracotomy).	Perfusion will be adequate: • mental status will be clear; • urine output will be sufficient.
Ineffective individual coping	Offer appropriate information, reassurance, support.	Patient's behavior will be consistent with situation and condition.
Ineffective family coping	Allow visitation.	
Altered family processes	Refer to social services or other resources as indicated and available.	Family will respond appropriately and will be able to support patient.
High risk for hypothermia	Preserve body heat Control ambient temperature. Warm IV fluids and blood. Keep patient covered.	Patient will be normothermic.
High risk for infection	Maintain aseptic technique for procedures. Clean open wounds and skin of dirt, blood, debris.	Patient will not develop local infection related to ED procedures.
Pain	Administer analgesics as ordered. Provide reassurance.	Pain will decrease.

priorities in patient needs in terms of ineffective airway clearance; potential for neurologic deficit because of cervical spine injury; ineffective breathing pattern and impaired gas exchange; and alteration in cardiac output: fluid volume deficit (Kostic & Magaldi, 1989).

Triage categories vary among institutions, but the focus on determining the most critical patient needs and the most appropriate use of resources does not change. In general, patients' conditions are described as follows: needing minimal intervention (nonurgent); needing moderate intervention and ED capability, but are not a life threat (urgent); potentially life-threatening requiring immediate significant intervention (emergent); and immediately life-threatening, i.e., impending cardiac or respiratory arrest (Mancini & Cawley, 1986).

For trauma patients particularly, triage is critical. Identification of what interventions will be required depends on an experienced estimate or assessment of what the patient injuries will be. Because "trauma patients arrive at inappropriate times with unreasonable problems in unacceptable numbers" (Trunkey & Lewis, 1991), traditional staffing patterns often do not meet the needs of a severely injured multiple trauma patient, such as described in this chapter's case study. Although the ACS and ACEP guidelines provide a framework for essential and desirable resources, each facility decides how it will provide those resources. At a trauma center, arrival of the injured patient results in activation of a defined team. Response to a trauma patient in a non-trauma-designated hospital staffed for average patient volumes also requires a prearranged plan. Emergency nurses skilled in triage and involved in development of that response plan can make a significant contribution to trauma care.

Emergency Department Overload

Planning, preparation, and well-developed triage protocols facilitate effective use of resources. However, in all systems there is an endpoint to resource availability. Because of the wide variability among emergency medical services and trauma systems, a full discussion is beyond the scope of this chapter. Administrative protocols should be in place that consider predicted volumes of patients and specific local capability, including alternative sites of care and staff reserves.

Each emergency nurse should be familiar with these protocols.

A system that considers "bypass," or ambulance diversion, weighs and compares (1) the risks of turning patients away, which is the effect of bypass, and (2) the difficulty of caring for patients with less than optimal resources. Because of special trauma center requirements, such as surgeon availability, operating room capability, and 24-hour availability of CT scan, absence of any of those requirements may result in diverting patients to another trauma center. Other resources, such as intensive care unit beds, monitoring capability, and resuscitation personnel, impact all emergency patients.

Trauma system protocols range from "no diversion" to selective diversion of specific types of patients. These protocols are highly debated. Justification for diversion of trauma patients typically includes lack of OR capability, CT scanner malfunction, unavailable ED resuscitation personnel, space, or equipment ("ED overload"), and lack of in-patient critical care capability. It can be inferred from these criteria that a decision-making scheme could be developed. For example, patients with single-system head injury might be diverted from a center without CT capability; patients likely to need emergency surgery, such as those with penetrating wounds or rigid abdomen, might bypass a hospital with unavailable OR. The feasibility of implementing selective diversion depends on a number of factors, including (1) numbers and level of prehospital care, i.e., EMT or EMT-P—whether selective protocols can be adequately taught, implemented, and monitored; (2) injury mix of patients—whether patients predominantly have multisystem injuries; (3) number and location of trauma centers in the system—where the patients are diverted to; and so on.

A different approach, particularly in an area with a single trauma center, is that the trauma center is the *only* place that can rapidly evaluate and resuscitate the trauma patient. Therefore nontrauma patients should be diverted to other full-service hospitals with emergency and intensive care capability. Some systems require all trauma patients to be initially evaluated and stabilized at the trauma center, even if in-patient resources are limited. With this model, safety and feasibility of patient transfer must be considered.

Emergency departments may have protocols

for diversion when either ED or in-patient resources are overloaded or unavailable, but it must be remembered that when one facility is diverting patients, increased activity at another might result in overload of those resources, and so on. "When everybody's closed, nobody is closed" has become a slogan in today's healthcare atmosphere of all resources utilized to capacity. In addition, virtually all EMS systems have protocols for transport to the "nearest hospital" in cases of cardiac arrest or other *in extremis* conditions that are unmanageable in the field. It is important to know local protocols for diversion of trauma and other types of patients. It is equally important for the emergency nurse to have a plan for when the patients arrive despite system overload. When significant multiple casualty incidents occur, the hospital may need to initiate a phase of the disaster plan (see Appendix B).

Documentation

Trauma systems are charged not only with provision of optimal care, but also with review of that care for epidemiologic study and outcome analysis. The role of recorder often is assigned to the emergency nurse and requires careful attention to detail in the primary and secondary assessments. A number of flow sheets have been developed, and as with other equipment choices, each ED must decide what meets its specific needs. Data requirements are further discussed in Chapter 6.

Prevention

As discussed in Chapters 1 and 2, trauma is a disease, with identifiable and therefore frequently preventable causes. Data related to mechanism of injury, use of safety restraints such as seat belts and helmets, and risk factors such as drug and alcohol use should be included on the flow sheet. Emergency nurses have the opportunity to reinforce positive preventive behaviors, such as emphasizing the injuries the patient avoided by wearing a helmet. In addition, it is appropriate to assess the stable patient for referral to substance abuse rehabilitation or other high-risk behavior modification programs.

SUMMARY Emergency nursing has emerged as a distinct specialty over the past 20 years. Today's emergency nurse is a highly knowledgeable, technically skilled professional with a combination of competencies drawn from a variety of clinical areas. The ED is recognized as the entry point to the hospital; it is often the site of emergent resuscitation. The most critical role for the emergency nurse is in resuscitation, including assessment and stabilization of the injured patient. In addition, the emergency nurse contributes to care of the patient before arrival at the hospital and beyond resuscitation. See the table on p. 652 for a summary of emergency nursing diagnoses and interventions.

COMPETENCIES
The following clinical competencies pertain to **caring for the trauma patient in the emergency department.**

☑ Demonstrate proficiency in the following Trauma Nursing Core Course (TNCC) skills:
- assessment of the trauma patient;
- multiple trauma interventions (patient scenario);
- cervical spine immobilization;
- helmet removal;
- splinting, including traction splint application;
- airway device use and oxygen delivery.

☑ Describe indications, contraindications, and hypothesized effects of pneumatic antishock garment; demonstrate application, inflation, deflation, and removal.

☑ Anticipate need for chest drainage and autotransfusion; assemble equipment and provide appropriate pain control and support to patient.

☑ Implement use of rapid infuser and fluid warmer when indicated.

☑ Appropriately anticipate and assist with surgical procedures: sterile technique, instrument identification, nursing aspects of the procedure (venous cutdown, peritoneal lavage, cricothroidotomy, pericardiocentesis, resuscitative thoracotomy).

☑ Maintain familiarity with internal defibrillator: indications for use; how to assemble equipment; how to select voltage.

☑ Describe indications for invasive monitoring, assist with line placement and monitor set-up, assess parameters; intervene appropriately.

RESEARCH QUESTIONS

Education

- How often does a nurse need to practice trauma resuscitation skills to maintain proficiency; what is the optimal measure?
- Do nurses use information from multidisciplinary conferences to change their practice?

Clinical Practice

- Are there initial assessment findings in the apparently stable patient that correlate with significant injury:
  —head injury;
  —abdominal injury.
- Does follow-up with trauma patients discharged from the ED modify subsequent risk-taking behavior (e.g., unrestrained driver/passenger with minor injury; assault while intoxicated)?

System/Injury Prevention

- Are there factors related to mechanism of injury that can be correlated with injury severity, i.e., validation of triage criteria (can similar patients with similar mechanisms be expected to have similar injuries; when two like gender/age/physical condition patients sustain similar mechanism, why are their injuries different)?
- Is providing injury prevention information in the ED waiting room effective in improving safety practices?

RESOURCES

American College of Emergency Physicians
PO Box 619911
Dallas, TX 75261-9911
(214) 550-0911; (800) 798-1822

Emergency Nurses Association
Trauma Nursing Committee
230 E. Ohio St., Suite 600
Chicago, IL 60611
(312) 649-0297

Society of Trauma Nurses
888 17th St. NW, Suite 1000
Washington, DC 20006

International

Accident and Emergency Association of New South Wales
456 Shume Highway
Yagoona, Sydney, Australia
(01612) 708-3130

National Emergency Nurses' Affiliation (NENA) Canada
Box 100-217
2 Bloor St. West
Toronto, Ontario
Canada N4W3E2
(416) 291-0687

ANNOTATED BIBLIOGRAPHY

Kleeman, K.M. (1988). Family systems adaptation. In V.D. Cardona P.D. Hurn, P.J. Bastnagel Mason, A.M. Scanlon-Schilpp, and S.W. Veise-Berry, *Trauma nursing: From resuscitation through rehabilitation* (pp. 204-233). Philadelphia: W.B. Saunders.

Comprehensive discussion of family response to trauma provides theory and technique for family evaluation and crisis intervention. Using family systems theory, the chapter emphasizes the resuscitation nurse's ability and opportunity to assess and initiate appropriate interventions. Discussion of behaviors and effective approaches throughout the continuum from injury to recovery is particularly helpful.

Lenehan, G.P. (1991). Violence in the emergency department (theme issue). *Journal of Emergency Nursing, 17*(5).

Stimulated by events that have resulted in injury and death of emergency care providers, issue addresses the range of violence in EDs in urban, rural, and international settings. In addition, approaches and solutions are discussed.

Martin, L., Francisco, E., Nichol, C., & Schweiger, J.L. (1991). A hospital-wide approach to crisis control: One inner-city hospital's experience. *Journal of Emergency Nursing, 17*(6), 395-401.

Increasing incidence of violence within the ED and concern for staff safety led to development of a "disruptive patient task force." A crisis team composed of mental health, administrative, and security personnel may be called for potentially violent or disruptive situations. In addition, security measures and education programs related to rights and obligations of patients and staff have been designed and implemented. Staff are taught strategies for defusing and handling incidents while fulfilling their duty to treat and maintain a therapeutic environment. An excellent guide for EDs faced with these issues.

Mattox, K.L., Moore, E.E., & Feliciano, D.V. (1991). *Trauma.* Norwalk, CT: Appleton & Lange.

Although primarily a surgical text, this comprehensive review of trauma management is an excellent reference for most injuries encountered. Particularly interesting are chapters on history of trauma care, injury epidemiology, trauma scoring, management of battle casualties, and rehabilitation.

Sheehy, S.B., Marvin, J.A., & Jimmerson, C.L. (1989). *Manual of clinical trauma care: The first hour.* St. Louis; Mosby–Year Book, Inc.

Emergency nurses are most likely to care for trauma patients in "the first hour," and this basic manual addresses that time period. Although content is not particularly indepth, chapters are well referenced for further study of top-ics of interest. Photographs and drawings, as well as summary lists for assessment and therapeutic interventions, make the book helpful in planning orientation and in-service education for ED and prehospital providers. Compact in size and spiral bound, this manual might be useful in any ED that receives trauma patients.

REFERENCES

American College of Emergency Physicians (ACEP). (1987). Guidelines for trauma care. *Annals of Emergency Medicine, 16*(4), 459-63.

American College of Emergency Physicians (ACEP). (1990). The role of the emergency physician in the care of children. *Annals of Emergency Medicine, 19*(4), 435-436.

American College of Emergency Physicians (ACEP). (1991). Personal communication.

American College of Surgeons (ACS). (1986). Field categorization of trauma patients (field triage). Hospital resources document: Appendix F. *American College of Surgeons Bulletin, 71*(10).

American College of Surgeons Committee on Trauma (AS-COT). (1990). *Resources for optimum care of the injured patient* (pp. 28-30). Chicago: Author.

Beachley, M.L. (1989). Trauma nursing is a developing specialty. *Journal of Emergency Nursing, 15*(5), 372-73.

Emergency Nurses Association (ENA). (1989). Emergency nursing scope of practice (position paper). *Journal of Emergency Nursing, 15*(4), 361-364.

Emergency Nurses Association (ENA). (1991a). Nurse staffing in the emergency department (position paper). *Journal of Emergency Nursing, 17*(6), 28A.

Emergency Nurses Association (ENA). (1991b). Personal communication.

Emergency Nurses Association (ENA). (1991c). *Standards of emergency nursing practice* (2nd ed.). St. Louis: Mosby–Year Book, Inc.

Emergency Nurses Association (ENA). (1991d). Violence in the emergency department (position paper). *Journal of Emergency Nursing, 17*(6), 32A.

Emergency Nurses Association (ENA). (1992). Personal communication.

Kelleher, J.C. (1990). When dreams come true. *Journal of Emergency Nursing, 16*(1), 1-3.

Kostic, J. & Magaldi, M.C. (1989). Trauma triage: A nursing model. *Journal of Advanced Medical-Surgical Nursing, 2*(1), 19-25.

Lenehan, G.P. (1990a). The more things change, the more they stay the same. *Journal of Emergency Nursing, 16*(1), 4-5.

Lenehan, G.P. (1990b). ENA's 20th anniversary focus on members. *Journal of Emergency Nursing, 16*(3), 176-77.

Lenehan, G.P. (1991). Violence in the emergency department (theme issue). *Journal of Emergency Nursing, 17*(5).

MacPhail, E.R. (1989). Combatting injury: today and tomorrow. *Journal of Emergency Nursing, 15*(5), 365-66.

Mancini, M.E., & Cawley, K.A. (1986). Triage and classification in the emergency department. *Trauma Quarterly, 3*(1), 15-23.

Martin, L., Francisco, E., Nicol, C., & Schweiger, J. (1991). A hospital-based approach to crisis control: One inner-city hospital's experience. *Journal of Emergency Nursing, 17*(6), 395-401.

Mattox, K.L., Moore, E.E., & Feliciano, D.V. (1988). *Trauma*. Norwalk, CT: Appleton & Lange.

May, C.M. (1987). The emergency department nurse's approach to the trauma patient. *Trauma Quarterly*, 3(2), 31-40.

National Academy of Sciences National Research Council (NASNRC). (1966). *Accidental death and disability: The neglected disease of modern society*. Washington, D.C.: U.S. Department of Health, Education and Welfare.

Pisarcik, G. (1980). Why patients use the emergency department. *Journal of Emergency Nursing*, 6(1), 16-21.

Proehl, J., Bires, B., Southard, P., & Tidwell, K. (1992). Trauma notebook: Announcing the trauma nursing resource document. *Journal of Emergency Nursing*, 18 (1), 81-82.

Rea, R.E. (Ed.). (1991). *Trauma nursing core course*. (3rd ed.) Chicago: Emergency Nurses Association.

Rea, R.E., Bourg, P.W., Parker, J.G., & Rushing, D. (Eds.). (1987). *Emergency nursing core curriculum*. Philadelphia: W.B. Saunders.

Rosen, P., Baker, F.J. II, Barkin, R.H., Braen, G.R., Dailey, R.H., & Levy, R.C. (1988). *Emergency medicine: Concepts and clinical practice*. St. Louis: Mosby–Year Book, Inc.

Sheehy, S.B., & Barber, J. (1985). *Emergency nursing: Principles and practice* (2nd ed.). St. Louis: Mosby–Year Book, Inc.

Trunkey, D.D., & Lewis, F.R. (1991). *Current therapy of trauma*. St. Louis: B.C. Decker/Mosby-Year Book.

22 *Perioperative Care of the Trauma Patient*

■■

Jody Foss
Nancye Feistritzer

OBJECTIVES

❑ *Identify the role of the perioperative nurse in caring for the trauma patient during the preoperative, intraoperative, and postoperative phases of care.*

❑ *List nursing diagnoses that are appropriate during the perioperative period for a trauma patient.*

❑ *Identify the role of the emergency department (ED) trauma nurse in facilitating transfer of the patient to the operating room (OR).*

INTRODUCTION This chapter focuses on the role of the perioperative nurse in trauma care. Preoperative patient assessment data and intraoperative interventions for the trauma patient are addressed. Operative procedures are discussed briefly as they relate to the multiple injuries of the trauma patient. American College of Surgeons' guidelines for operative facilities are included.

CASE STUDY Marvin Garden is a 30-year-old man found stumbling at the scene of an auto crash. He is mumbling incoherently. His injuries include multiple head and facial lacerations; near enucleation of the right eye; compound fracture of the right wrist; and bruises over the right upper quadrant of the abdomen. His blood pressure is 88/60; pulse, 120; and respirations, 32. Paramedics dressed his head wounds and splinted his wrist. Lactated Ringer's solution is infusing through two 14-gauge intravenous catheters. He is receiving oxygen by mask at 12 L/min.

As the perioperative trauma nurse, you are the liaison between the OR and the ED.

What possible procedures might the OR team be alerted to prepare for? What injuries threaten this patient's life?

For a patient with multiple injuries, priority setting is essential. The facial and head lacerations do not seem life-threatening, and the near enucleation of the right eye may threaten this patient's vision, but probably not his life. Extremity fractures are considered a low priority. A major concern is Marvin's low blood pressure and rapid pulse rate. The inability to adequately perfuse vital organs is most certainly life-threatening and should be addressed. Therefore the OR team might be alerted to prepare a major abdominal or chest instrument set-up.

What are the most important aspects of this patient's history that should be communicated to the OR team?

The preoperative assessment includes all the necessary demographic data, as well as the physical assessment. Specifically, it is helpful if the OR team is informed about the nature of the procedure, any reactions to previous anesthetic, time of last meal, and current medications, vital signs, and fluid status.

Marvin tells the ED team that he takes medication for his blood pressure and has been on a diet to lose weight. He is 5 feet, 7 inches tall and weighs 300 pounds. Why is this information important to communicate to the OR team?

Obese patients do not tolerate the supine position used for exploratory laparotomy. Their efficiency of ventilation may be decreased, and blood volume to the heart and lungs increases. Close

659

monitoring of this patient's airway and blood oxygenation level is needed. Placing him in a lawn-chair position will facilitate respiration and cardiovascular status. Because Marvin has been taking medication for hypertension, the possibility of electrolyte imbalance exists. Especially important to assess is Marvin's serum potassium level—the surgical risk for Marvin increases if his serum potassium is abnormally low.

PERIOPERATIVE NURSING ROLE

When caring for the trauma patient, time is of the essence. Rapid action and successful intervention require aggressive treatment from a team of highly skilled professionals. Care begins at the prehospital site and continues through rehabilitation. The trauma team treats life-threatening injuries through the cyclic continuum of assessment, planning, implementation, and evaluation, until the threat to life no longer exists.

Systematic planning and preparation by all members of the trauma team ensure a smooth transition for trauma patients as they progress through the continuum of care. Because many traumatic injuries require surgical intervention, the perioperative (OR) nurse is an important member of the team.

The perioperative nurse who is a trauma team member is the liaison between the OR, ED, and inpatient units. The level of interdepartmental interaction varies among institutions. During the preoperative phase, the perioperative nurse visits the patient in the ED or contacts the ED nurse to assess the patient's readiness for surgery and to identify the proposed procedure(s) and any special needs for equipment or personnel. This information is then relayed to the surgical team so they can make preparations to receive the patient.

In some institutions the perioperative nurse assists the surgeon with resuscitative procedures performed in the ED. Chest tube insertion and tracheostomy are two such procedures in which the perioperative nurse's knowledge of aseptic technique and instrumentation is useful.

GENERAL ASSESSMENT AND INTERVENTIONS
Preoperative Assessment and Intervention

Systematic preoperative assessment and planning are applied to the surgical environment, as well as to the patient. A review of available surgical and personnel resources for handling the proposed procedure occurs during the initial assessment of the trauma patient. The classification of hospital EDs using the standards outlined by the American College of Surgeons, Committee on Trauma defines some of the operating room requirements, based on institution capabilities. The box on p. 661 presents a summary of these requirements.

Resource assessment

A level I status generally is found in a major trauma center or university hospital. Anesthesia and OR staff with specialty surgery capability must be immediately available 24 hours a day. Various types of specialized life-saving equipment and an operating room must be available at all times. A level II facility differs from a level I facility in that a level II is not required to have cardiopulmonary bypass oxygenator and operating microscope. A level III facility lists in-house OR staff as *desirable* versus *required*. No criteria are defined for a level IV facility OR. Undesignated facilities are required only to provide reasonable care if an emergency occurs and to give life-saving first aid. Personnel at these hospitals must know where to refer patients if necessary.

Patient assessment

Surgical care of the trauma patient is divided into three phases: preoperative, intraoperative, and postoperative. The perioperative nurse is concerned with all three phases and develops a patient plan of care that encompasses all of these phases. The goal of preoperative patient assessment and nursing care is to minimize operative risks and enhance the recovery process.

The head of a busy trauma service noted that a trauma patient has two assailants. The first assailant is the pavement, auto, or person that did the initial harm to the patient. The second assailant is the trauma team! Surgery is a planned assault on the body. The preoperative assessment helps identify factors that increase the risk of complications as a result of the planned assault. Figure 22-1 identifies a range of traumatic injuries that can result in the patient going to the OR for surgical interventions.

Nursing history The preoperative patient assessment begins with a nursing history. Collecting

---

Guidelines for differentiating operative capabilities

	Level I	Level II	Level III
I. Operating suite			
A. Personnel: operating room adequately staffed in house and immediately available 24 hours a day	E	E	D
B. Equipment: special requirements shall include but not be limited to the following:			
1. Cardiopulmonary bypass capability	E	D	—
2. Operating microscope	E	D	—
3. Thermal control equipment			
• for patient	E	E	E
• for blood and fluids	E	E	E
4. X-ray capability, including C-arm image intensifier and technologist available 24 hours a day	E	E	D
5. Endoscopes, all varieties	E	E	E
6. Craniotome	E	E	D
7. Monitoring equipment	E	E	E
II. Postanesthetic recovery room (surgical intensive care unit is acceptable)			
A. Registered nurses and other essential personnel 24 hours a day	E	E	E
B. Appropriate monitoring and resuscitation equipment	E	E	E

Note. From *Resources for Optimal Care of the Injured Patient* by American College of Surgeons, Committee on Trauma, 1990, Chicago: Author.
E, Essential; *D,* desirable.

---

elementary patient data enables the nurse to develop a therapeutic relationship with the patient and create an individualized plan of care. Obviously, when a patient is unable to communicate (e.g., comatose or head injured), obtaining patient data is more difficult. However, ideally the following data should be obtained and communicated to the OR team: drug allergies, time of last oral intake, current medications, and pertinent past medical history.

Information about previous surgeries and experiences with anesthetic agents is needed to determine if any tendency exists toward anesthesia complications. Malignant hyperthermia is a serious complication of anesthesia, and death occurs in more than 50% of the cases.

Family members can be helpful in eliciting a history if the patient is unable to communicate. It should be noted that family/significant others may be in shock over their loved one's injury. The perioperative nurse should be supportive, providing information on the patient's status as frequently as possible. It is sometimes difficult to think of the patient's family in the midst of an emergent or critical situation. Assistance may be provided through the hospital chaplain, social worker, or other staff. Family support still remains an integral part of the role of the perioperative nurse.

Preoperative planning

In the care of the trauma patient, the planning phase often occurs simultaneously with the assessment phase, since time is of the essence. Realistic patient goals should be based on the nursing diagnoses identified.

The potential for fluid volume deficit during the surgical procedure is high. Assessment of the preoperative fluid status determines intraoperative fluid replacement needs. Emergency/trauma staff should communicate to the OR staff the amount and types of fluids administered preoperatively. Labeling the IV fluids with numbers helps the OR team to estimate the amount of fluid infused during the prehospital and emergency phases of care. Intravenous lines and catheters placed in the emergency area are considered contaminated,

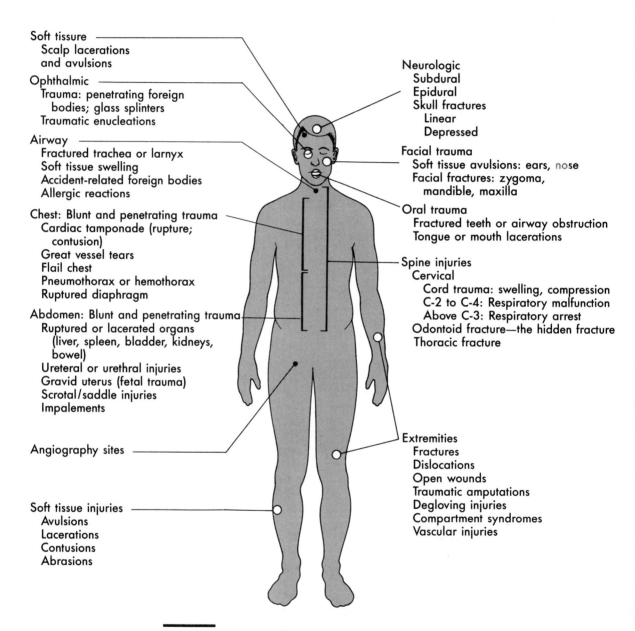

Soft tissue
Scalp lacerations and avulsions

Ophthalmic
Trauma: penetrating foreign bodies; glass splinters
Traumatic enucleations

Airway
Fractured trachea or larnyx
Soft tissue swelling
Accident-related foreign bodies
Allergic reactions

Chest: Blunt and penetrating trauma
Cardiac tamponade (rupture; contusion)
Great vessel tears
Flail chest
Pneumothorax or hemothorax
Ruptured diaphragm

Abdomen: Blunt and penetrating trauma
Ruptured or lacerated organs (liver, spleen, bladder, kidneys, bowel)
Ureteral or urethral injuries
Gravid uterus (fetal trauma)
Scrotal/saddle injuries
Impalements

Angiography sites

Soft tissue injuries
Avulsions
Lacerations
Contusions
Abrasions

Neurologic
Subdural
Epidural
Skull fractures
Linear
Depressed

Facial trauma
Soft tissue avulsions: ears, nose
Facial fractures: zygoma, mandible, maxilla

Oral trauma
Fractured teeth or airway obstruction
Tongue or mouth lacerations

Spine injuries
Cervical
Cord trauma: swelling, compression
C-2 to C-4: Respiratory malfunction
Above C-3: Respiratory arrest
Odontoid fracture—the hidden fracture
Thoracic fracture

Extremities
Fractures
Dislocations
Open wounds
Traumatic amputations
Degloving injuries
Compartment syndromes
Vascular injuries

Figure 22-1   Overview of injuries requiring operative intervention.

since ideal circumstances for placement often are not possible in a prehospital/emergent situation. They are usually replaced within 24 hours of admission. Lines placed for invasive monitoring purposes, (pulmonary artery, arterial, or central venous pressure monitoring lines) should not be used with flexible or long extension tubing, since this may alter the values during measurement. When blood or blood products are administered preoperatively in the emergency area, it is important to communicate this to the OR staff so the patient can be monitored for blood reaction. This is also true regarding antibiotic administration. It is advantageous to arrange a system for rapidly providing O-negative, uncrossmatched blood in the event of extreme blood loss. Type and crossmatch of the patient should be accomplished as soon as possible.

Planning the surgical procedure   The operative permit is an essential component of the preoperative planning phase. It is the surgeon's responsibility to have the operative permit signed after the proposed procedure and its risks have been explained to the patient. The hospital should have a policy for emergency situations on obtaining permission to operate on patients who are unresponsive or otherwise unable to sign a permit. The

signed permit should accompany the patient to surgery.

Before surgery, the patient's physical status is assessed by the anesthesiologist, using the American Society of Anesthesiologists' criteria outlined in Table 22-1 (Ripps, Eckenhoff, & Vendom, 1988).

Physical status classification is based on the patient's physiologic condition independent of the proposed surgical procedure. Intraoperative complications occur more frequently in patients who have a poor physical status classification. The elderly are especially at risk for intraoperative complications because of organ system changes that occur with aging. Table 22-2 describes those changes. When the intended surgery is emergent, any benefits gained by waiting for the patient's physical status to improve must be weighed against the hazards of waiting.

The final phase of preoperative planning is preparing the surgical environment to perform the proposed procedure. Often this area is overlooked, and chaos results when the patient is transferred to the OR. The perioperative trauma nurse team member performs a vital function in helping communicate environmental needs to the OR staff. Figure 22-2 provides an example

Table 22-1 American Society of Anesthesiologists' physical status classification

Status*	Definition	Description
1	A normal, healthy patient	No physiological, psychological, biochemical, or organic disturbance
2	A patient with mild systemic disease	Cardiovascular disease with minimal restriction on activity, hypertension, asthma, chronic bronchitis, obesity, or diabetes mellitus
3	A patient with a severe systemic disease that limits activity, but is not incapacitating	Cardiopulmonary or pulmonary disease that limits activity; severe diabetes with systemic complications; history of MI, angina, uncontrolled hypertension
4	A patient with an incapacitating systemic disease that is a constant threat to life	Severe cardiac, pulmonary, renal, hepatic, or endocrine dysfunction
5	A moribund patient not expected to survive for 24 hours, with or without operation	Surgery done as last recourse or resuscitative effort: major multisystem or cerebral trauma, ruptured aneurysm, or large pulmonary embolus

Note: From *Introduction to Anesthesia: The Principles of Safe Practice* (7th ed.) (pp. 15-16) by R. D. Ripps, J.E. Eckenhoff, and L.D. Vandam, 1988, Philadelphia: W.B. Saunders.
*For patients requiring emergency surgery, an "E" is added to the physical status.

Table 22-2 Organ system changes with aging and potential perioperative complications

Organ system	Physiological change	Perioperative complications
Cardiovascular	(−)Cardiac output with stress (and ? at rest)	Sensitivity to negative isotropy effects of general anesthesia (+); risk of pulmonary edema
	Autonomic dysfunction	Orthostatic hypotension exaggerated by postoperative bedrest, (+) risk of falls, (−) tolerance to postoperative ambulation; blood pressure liability
	(+) Rate of coronary artery disease	Myocardial infarction; ischemia-related arrhythmias; (−) cardiac output with intravascular volume depletion or vasodilation
Pulmonary	(−) Vital capacity	Additional decreased reserve if pulmonary function is affected by: <ul><li>lung resection</li><li>pulmonary complications</li><li>factors that diminish ventilation (e.g., CNS depression, diaphragm failure)</li></ul>
	(+) (Alveolar-arterial) oxygen gradient	
	(−) Maximal voluntary ventilation	
	(−) Clearance of oropharyngeal secretions	(+) Pulmonary infection, particularly with gram-negative organisms
	(+) Colonization of oropharynx with gram-negative rods	
Genitourinary	(−) Glomerular filtration rate	(+) Risk of acute renal failure (−) Drug clearance with toxic effects
	(−) Tubular function; reabsorption, concentration, and dilutional defects	Intravascular volume depletion; hyponatremia.
	(+) Atherosclerosis in aorta, renal artery	(+) Postprocedure atheroembolism
	(+) Bladder retention	Urosepsis
	(+) Bacteriuria	
	Urinary incontinence	Perineal skin breakdown
Gastrointestinal	(−) Colonic motility	Postoperative fecal impaction
	(+) Achlorhydria	Change in bowel flora; (+) infectious risk
Endocrine	(−) Beta-cell function	Postoperative hyperglycemia:
	(+) Insulin resistance	<ul><li>glycosuria with volume depletion</li><li>(−) neutrophil chemotaxis if blood sugar is uncontrolled</li></ul>
Musculoskeletal	(−) Muscle, bone mass	(−) Postoperative mobility with (+) deep venous thrombosis and atelectasis risk
	(+) Degenerative joint disease	(+) Risk of postoperative fracture with unsteady gait, orthostatic hypotension
Neurological	Autonomic dysfunction	Postoperative hypothermia
	(+) Rate of cognitive dysfunction	(−) Cooperation with postoperative therapies
	(+) Depressive symptomatology	(+) Postoperative depression
	(−) Thirst after water deprivation	Dehydration
Skin	(−) Number of dermal blood vessels	Increased risk of skin ulceration, infection
	(−) Reepithelizlization rate	(−) Rate of wound healing
	(−) Mucosal immunity	(+) Postoperative infectious risk
Immunological	Macrophage dysfunction	
	(−) In both antibody and cell-mediated immunity	

Note: From "Preoperative Considerations in the Geriatric Patient" by H.J. Keating III, 1987, *Medical Clinics of North America, 71*(3), pp. 575-576.
(+) = increased; (−) = decreased; ? = there exists suggestive but not definite evidence; CNS = central nervous system; postop = postoperative.

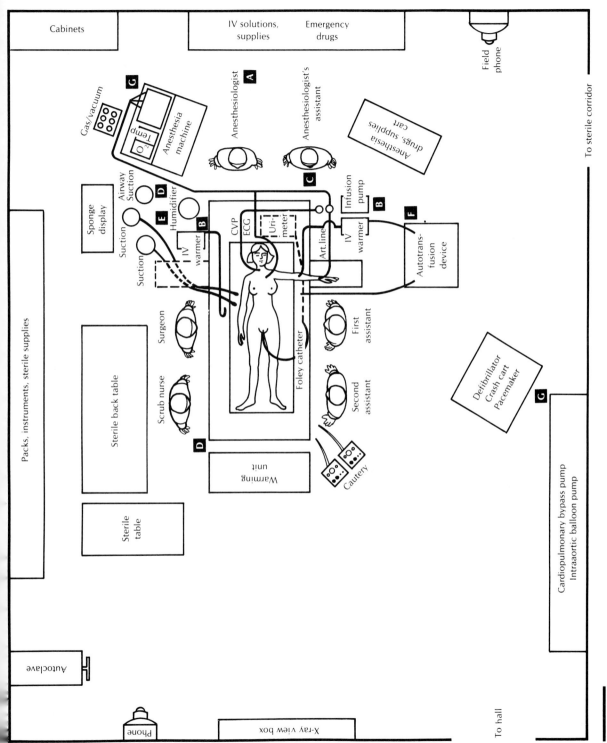

Figure 22-2 Operating room organization for trauma patient. (*Note.* From *Critical Decisions in Trauma* by E.E. Moore, B. Eiseman, and C.W. Van Way III, 1984, St. Louis: Mosby–Year Book, Inc.)

Table 22-3 Maintaining operating room availability

Method	Advantage	Disadvantage
Designated trauma room	Provides immediate access to surgical intervention	Not used except in trauma cases Costly to maintain
Next-room-out availability	Gives priority to the emergent trauma patient over other scheduled cases	Elective cases in that room may be delayed
	Allows all ORs to be used for scheduled cases More cost effective	Elective patients and surgeons may be upset at delay
Rotational list for emergency/trauma cases	Allows surgeon to know day on which he or she may be delayed	Elective cases in room may still be delayed
	Allows ORs to be used for scheduled cases if no trauma comes in More cost effective	Elective patients may be upset at delay

of a typical OR arrangement for the trauma patient.

Staff and room availability Most surgery departments do not have the luxury of having designated trauma operating rooms. Therefore room availability in a hospital with high operating suite utilization rate may be an issue. Preplanning by the OR nursing supervisor and the head of the trauma team alleviates many problems. Early warning of an incoming trauma is useful to the OR personnel. Many trauma centers have trauma alert systems, which inform key trauma team members of the need for their response. In a hospital where the OR team is not physically present, as in a level III facility, notification of personnel is initiated early in the resuscitation phase of care to ensure that the appropriate personnel are physically present when needed. The type and number of surgical instruments, the position of the operating table, the type of anesthesia used, and the general set-up of the OR suite depend on the procedure performed.

Operating room availability can be maintained through a variety of means. Table 22-3 describes several of these and presents the advantages and disadvantages thereof. Personnel availability can be achieved through both in-house staff and call team(s).

Intraoperative Assessment and Interventions

During the intraoperative phase, the perioperative nurse is responsible for monitoring and observing for signs of respiratory distress, dysrhythmias, and fluid and electrolyte disturbances. Continuous patient assessment and monitoring are necessary to ensure early detection of complications or to prevent complications.

Patient positioning

Planning the patient's position intraoperatively begins with the preoperative assessment. Information learned about the patient and existing medical conditions may affect the planned position. For example, obese patients do not tolerate the supine position. Their efficiency of ventilation decreases, since obese patients have a greater diaphragmatic excursion than normal patients.

Positioning a patient for a surgical procedure is based on specific criteria (Martin, 1987). The goal is to provide optimal exposure to the operative site and allow the anesthesiologist access for induction of anesthesia. The selected position promotes respiratory and circulatory function, avoids excessive pressure on a body part, and facilitates draping to maintain a sterile field and the patient's individuality, privacy, and dignity. Figure 22-3 provides an example of a typical thora-

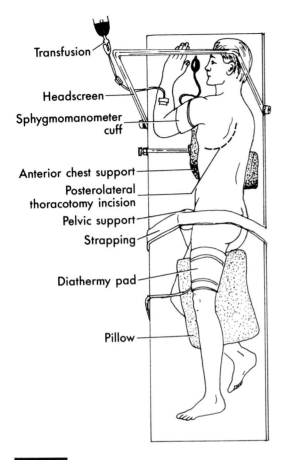

Transfusion

Headscreen

Sphygmomanometer
cuff

Anterior chest support

Posterolateral
thoracotomy incision

Pelvic support

Strapping

Diathermy pad

Pillow

Figure 22-3 Lateral position for thoracotomy incisions. (*Note.* From *Alexander's Care of the Patient in Surgery* [9th ed.] by M.H. Meeker and J.C. Rothrock, 1991, St. Louis: Mosby–Year Book, Inc.)

cotomy incision. The reader should note attention given to supporting and correctly positioning the entire body.

Often surgery on the trauma patient lasts several hours. Patients who are left lying on road gravel or in clothes develop pressure points and skin breakdown. The perioperative nurse is cognizant of this fact and plans the patient's position to prevent any damage that may result from the intraoperative position. Road gravel and dirt may be cleaned from the patient's back by using a portable vacuum. Bony prominences are padded, and limbs are positioned to prevent nerve damage. Antithrombolitic stockings are applied to facilitate venous return in the legs. When two surgical pro-

cedures are performed simultaneously, additional planning of patient position is needed to allow for access by both surgical teams.

Before incision and after induction and intubation, the patient is positioned to ensure adequate exposure of the operative site. All pressure points are padded and vulnerable nerve points relieved of pressure. Grounding pads for electrosurgical units are applied, and the site is prepped. Because reduction of fractures is a low priority, fractures are splinted and iced to prevent swelling. Fractures that are prone to develop compartment syndrome are monitored for signs of increasing pressure (see Chapter 11 for more information on compartment syndrome). When the pneumatic antishock garment (PASG) has been applied in the prehospital setting and placement covers a fracture, it is difficult to assess the circulatory status of tissue under the suit, which is also concealed by drapes during surgery. The condition of the skin and extremity at the time of application (prehospital or ED) should be reported to facilitate anticipation of complications.

Fluid maintenance

Planning maintenance of fluid and electrolyte balance is based on preoperative assessment information. The patient in shock or with a fluid volume deficit may need significant volume replacement. The perioperative nurse plans for autotransfusion and/or blood product replacement for these patients. Because the serum level of potassium is higher in blood that has been banked for longer than 3 days, the nurse must know how long the blood has been stored (Flever & Pendarvis, 1989). Blood and fluid warmers are prepared, so that the patient's body temperature is not lowered inadvertently (Burkle, 1988).

The perioperative nurse must work closely with the anesthesia and surgical personnel to estimate blood loss. This information is essential in knowing what volume of fluid and blood/blood product replacement should occur. Estimating blood loss is achieved through a variety of means, including the following:

- Measuring volume in suction cannister
- Measuring volume in cell-saver bowl; the blood can be readministered to the patient
- Weighing lap sponges
- Measuring area on floor that is covered by pooled blood

Temperature control

Controlling and monitoring the patient's temperature are other elements of the intraoperative planning phase. A cooling or warming pad is placed under the patient before surgery. Esophageal and/or rectal probes are placed for continuous temperature monitoring. Irrigation and intravenous fluids are warmed to body temperature. The room temperature may be adjusted to provide a warmer environment for the patient suffering from hypothermia.

Malignant hyperthermia Malignant hyperthermia is an inherited muscle disorder triggered by certain induction agents and anesthetics, such as succinylcholine and halothane. The incidence of malignant hyperthermia is 1 in 3000 to 15,000 for pediatric patients and 1 in 50,000 to 100,000 for the general population. In malignant hyperthermia, there is an abnormal transport of calcium across the cell membrane, resulting in an increased intracellular calcium. Normally, when muscles contract, calcium is released. When the muscle relaxes, the calcium is taken up again by the system. In malignant hyperthermia, the increased intracellular calcium causes generalized muscle contraction and fasciculation. Muscle oxygen consumption and lactate production increase, and increased aerobic and anaerobic metabolism occurs, which causes metabolic and respiratory acidosis. The acidosis affects the permeability of the cell membrane, impacting the movement of calcium and potassium across the cell membrane. The body temperature increases 1° C every 5 minutes (Rogers & Stugion, 1985).

The increase in the circulating catecholamines can lead to tachycardia, dysrhythmias, hypotension, and cardiac arrest. Prevention is the best treatment for this complication. However, if the complication does occur intraoperatively, it is treated with dantrolene sodium, a skeletal muscle relaxant that inhibits the release of calcium from the sacroplasmic reticulum. An initial dose of 2.5 mg/kg is given and repeated every 5 to 10 minutes until a maximum dose of 10 mg/kg is given or until the episode is controlled. The anesthetic agent is terminated, or changed if the situation precludes immediate termination. Immediate cooling measures are instituted.

Operative procedures

Planning for the procedure often occurs in a short time frame. Emergency procedures are generally classified as one of the following: a single operation procedure; multiconsecutive procedures; simultaneous procedures; and rapid resuscitation procedures (Campbell, 1987).

Single An example of a single operative procedure is the exploratory laparotomy. This should not be confused with the single procedure performed on a scheduled and prepped patient. Emergency surgery generally means the patient has sustained some sort of traumatic event and may be in a life-threatening situation. Understanding the mechanism of injury alerts the perioperative nurse to monitor for complications that may occur intraoperatively.

Multiconsecutive Multiconsecutive procedures are used when a patient has sustained two or more body system injuries. The chief trauma team surgeon and the operating room supervisor discuss and set priorities for procedures. Each surgical procedure is treated as a separate event. Instrument, sponges, and needles are counted for each procedure; used equipment and instruments are taken out after use. Constant monitoring of the patient occurs, since priorities may change. An example of multiconsecutive procedures are craniotomy followed by an exploratory laparotomy and placement of intramedullary rod in the femur.

Simultaneous Simultaneous procedures are used when a patient has two equally life-threatening of limb-threatening problems. Two separate OR teams perform surgery simultaneously. Careful planning of space and instrumentation is needed with this type of surgery. Both operative fields should be separated as much as possible to prevent cross contamination.

Rapid resuscitation Rapid resuscitative surgery is performed when a patient is so ill that emergency life-sustaining surgery is needed. Examples are burr holes to prevent brainstem herniation, tracheostomy, or repair of a ruptured descending thoracic aorta. Because the perioperative nurse has little time to plan for these procedures, it becomes a real challenge to anticipate the order of the surgeon's instrumentation, maintain sterile technique, and possess control of room events, all while serving as patient advocate.

One strategy to achieve advanced preparation for trauma procedures is through a case cart system. A case cart specific to abdominal, thoracic, neurologic, and orthopedic extremity injuries may be prepared and available at all times for immediate use. The case carts should include drapes, supplies, and sterile instrumentation that can be opened as rapidly as possible (see box below). Hospitals not using a case cart system can still develop a mechanism to have advanced availability of trauma supplies and instrumentation. When simultaneous procedures are performed, having a variety of case carts available is helpful to supply the needs of the different operating teams.

Supply counts The AORN Standards and Recommended Practices for Perioperative Nursing recommend that all sponges, sharps, and instruments be counted preoperatively, after closure of any body cavity, and immediately before completion of all surgical procedures. This is done to

---

Example of a trauma case tray system
Basic trauma OR supplies

Supplies	Number used	Suture	Number used
Case cart	_____	2-0 Silk #1032-51	_____
Trauma pack	_____	3-0 Silk #1017-32	_____
Extra-large gowns (2)	_____	2-0 Silk #1158-52	_____
Major basin set	_____	3-0 Silk #1158-42	_____
Prep tray	_____	2-0 Vicryl #J105T	_____
Sterile towels (6)	_____	3-0 Vicryl #J104T	_____
Grounding pad	_____	0 Chromic #641-63	_____
Stick sponges	_____		
Keutners	_____	**Trays**	
16 Fr. Foley catheter kit	_____	Trauma clamp tray	
Ioban drape #6651	_____	Trauma chest tray	_____
#15 Blade	_____	Trauma retractor tray	_____
#11 Blade	_____		
Sterile water (1000 ml)	_____		
Normal saline (1000 ml)	_____		
Suction canister	_____		
Hypothermia blanket	_____		

Trauma clamp tray

CVD Hartman	Lahey right-angle	7" Metzenbaum scissors
CVD mosquito	9" Fine right-angle	9" Metzenbaum scissors
STR mosquito	11" Right-angle	11" Metzenbaum scissors
CVD hemostat	Harrington right-angle	25 Deg Potts scissors
STR hemostat	Sponge stick	Short-angled fogarty clamp
6" Kelly	Allen bowel clamp	Short-straight fogarty clamp
8" Kelly	Dennis bowel clamp	Large-angled fogarty clamp
Hysterectomy peon	CVD shoestrings	Large-straight fogarty clamp
Scanlon	STR shoestrings	Nesting cooley clamp
Tonsil	Crilewood needleholder	Straight cooley clamp
Vanderbilt	6" Mayo Hager needleholder	Straight glover clamp
6" Kocher	8" Mayo Hager needleholder	Debakey aortic clamp
8" Kocher	11" Mayo Hager needleholder	Acutely CVD Debakey clamp
6" Allis	9" Sarot needleholder	Large Debakey aneurysm clamp
8" Allis	11" Sarot needleholder	Long medium hemoclip applier
10" Allis	CVD Mayo scissors	Long large hemoclip applier
6" Babcock	STR Mayo scissors	Small towel clamps
8" Babcock	9" CVD Mayo scissors	Large towel clamps
10" Babcock	9" STR Mayo scissors	

Continued.

Example of a trauma case tray system—cont'd
Basic trauma OR supplies

Supplies	Number used	Suture	Number used
Trauma chest tray			
8" Kocher	Adson brown forceps	Bone cutter	
Duval lung clamp	7" Martin forceps	Leksell rongeur	
Bronchus clamp	9" Diamond Debakey forceps	Lebsche knife	
Kidney pedicle clamp	9" Gerald forceps	Mallet	
Small Satinsky clamp 10"	#3 Knife handle	Scapular retractor	
Medium Satinsky clamp 10"	#4 Knife handle	Finochettio retractor w/screw	
Large Satinsky clamp 10"	Left Doyan elevator	Finochettio retractor w/small blades	
12" CVD Debakey aortic clamp	Right Doyan elevator	Finochettio retractor w/large blades	
12" STR Debakey aortic clamp	Alexander periosteal elevator	Small Allison lung retractor	
Wire twister	Rib approximator	Large Allison lung retractor	
Berry sternal needleholder	Rib shears	Rib spreaders	
25 Deg Potts scissors			
Trauma retractor tray			
#3 Knife handle	10" Potts tissue forceps	Narrow malleable retractor	
#4 Knife handle	10" Tissue forceps	Sweetheart retractor	
#7 Knife handle	10" Russian forceps	Wide Deaver retractor	
#3 Long knife handle	10" Tuttle forceps	Medium Deaver retractor	
Poole suction tip	11" Debakey forceps	Narrow Deaver retractor	
Pediatric Yankauer suction tip	Balfour retractor w/screw	Large Richardson retractor	
Adson dressing forceps	Short Balfour blades	Medium Richardson retractor	
Adson tissue forceps	Long Balfour blades	Small Richardson retractor	
7" Debakey forceps	Small bladder blade	Green goiter retractor	
Bonney forceps	Large bladder blade	Vein retractor	
9" Debakey forceps	Sharp Weitlaner retractor	Israel rakes	
7" Russian forceps	Gelpi retractor	Small Sharp rakes	
8" Tissue forceps	Army-Navy retractor	Large Sharp rakes	
10" Potts dressing forceps	Wide malleable retractor		

Complications of drugs used in anesthesia

Drugs used to induce unconsciousness: thiopental sodium (Pentothal), methohexital sodium (Brevital), diazepam (Valium), midazolam HCl (Versed), lorazepam (Ativan)

- Hypoxemia
- Airway obstruction
- Respiratory depression
- Tendency to produce laryngospasm
- Cardiovascular depression, especially in hypovolemic patients

Drugs used to induce analgesia: fentanyl (Sublimaze), droperidol (Inapsine)

- Respiratory depression
- Bradycardia
- Bronchoconstriction
- Hypotension
- Laryngospasm
- Hallucinations

Drugs used to produce muscle relaxation: succinylcholine chloride (Anectine), pancuronium bromide (Pavulon)

- Metabolized in liver (Pavulon) and excreted by kidneys
- Respiratory depression
- Bradycardia
- Hypotension

Volatile anesthetic agents: halothane (Fluothane), enflurane, isoflurane, nitrous oxide

- Myocardial depression; can cause dysrhythmias
- Cardiac output decreased
- Peripheral vascular resistance decreased
- Increased respiratory rate
- Depressed ventilation

---

ensure that foreign bodies are not left in the patient accidentally (AORN, 1991). Surgical counts are a major responsibility of the perioperative nurse. They are essential to providing quality patient care by protecting the patient from harm (Rowland & Rowland, 1990). In the event that the trauma patient's emergent condition does not allow time for a preoperative count, this should be documented and an x-ray film obtained at the end of the operative procedure.

Anesthesia

During induction of anesthesia, the trauma patient is at risk for cardiovascular and respiratory complications. The perioperative nurse assists the anesthetist or anesthesiologist with induction by applying cricoid pressure during intubation, because all trauma patients are considered to have full stomachs. Intubation can increase arterial pressure by 20 to 30 mm Hg and can increase heart rate. Patients with a history of hypertension or with increased intracranial pressure are at risk during this period. The box on the left describes some of the complications associated with agents commonly used in anesthesia.

Many anesthetic agents cause myocardial and respiratory depression, resulting in a decreased blood pressure. The causes of hypotensive episodes are the pharmacologic effects of anesthetic agents, the inhibition of sympathetic nervous activity, and the loss of baroreceptor control of arterial pressure. Patients who are hypovolemic as a result of hemorrhage are at high risk when given inhaled agents, such as enflurane (Ethrane). Continuous monitoring by an anesthetist or anesthesiologist and the perioperative nurse is vital to detect complications.

Postoperative Assessment and Interventions

During the immediate postoperative period when the patient is emerging from anesthesia, the perioperative nurse and the anesthesiologist evaluate the patient's respiratory and cardiovascular status. The patient is monitored continuously, including pulse oximetry, during transport to the post anesthesia care unit (PACU) or intensive care unit.

The goal of the immediate postoperative period is to ensure a safe and uneventful recovery. Recovery from general anesthesia usually takes longer than induction, and the patient's airway is especially vulnerable during this time. Once patients are in the PACU and their respiratory and cardiovascular status is stabilized, a full report is given to the post anesthesia nurse. The report should include the following information:

- Mechanism of injury
- Patient's injuries
- Patient status and surgery performed
- Respiratory and monitoring equipment needs
- IV lines, drains
- Anesthetic and other medications administered
- Estimated blood loss
- Intake and output during surgery

- Preoperative level of consciousness
- Unusual occurrences while in the OR
- Information about significant others

Often a delay occurs in treating certain injuries. For example, a patient who has sustained extremity injuries may not have the fractures reduced immediately; or the facial fracture may not be reduced until the swelling has decreased, if the airway is clear. Untreated traumatic injuries should be monitored closely for possible complications. Acutely ill patients may not have all injuries identified during the initial assessment. PACU nurses and critical care nurses who are responsible for recovering these patients should be alerted to look for undetected injuries.

Many hospitals are experiencing shortages of intensive care beds for a variety of reasons. This can mean that the trauma patient who would normally be transferred to an intensive care unit may stay in the PACU for an extended period. PACU nurses are being required to master the critical care skills of hemodynamic monitoring, ventilator care, and vasoactive pharmacology (Litwack, 1991). In addition, the PACU nurse must increasingly involve the family/significant others in postsurgical care, because they will continue to need support, comfort, and information.

SUMMARY The major goals of trauma care are to (1) prevent early death from failure to resuscitate, and (2) prevent late organ failure/death from inadequate or delayed resuscitation. The perioperative nurse as a trauma team member plans the patient's surgical experience with these goals in mind. Failure to maintain an adequate airway or fluid and electrolyte balance may have catastrophic results postoperatively for the trauma patient. Improper positioning during surgery that results in nerve or muscle damage has long-term effects, which may be irreversible. As a trauma team member participating in the continuum of trauma patient care, the perioperative nurse is the patient's advocate during the surgical experience. A well-organized and well-planned surgical experience helps to reduce the risk of complications and enhance the recovery process. See the table on p. 673-674 for a summary of nursing diagnoses and evaluative criteria for the perioperative patient.

**NURSING DIAGNOSES &
EVALUATIVE CRITERIA**   *Perioperative care of the trauma patient*

Nursing diagnosis	Nursing intervention	Evaluative criteria
High risk for ineffective airway clearance and impaired gas exchange Related to obstruction, local trauma, aspiration, loss of jaw position, effects of anesthetic, procedure, position	**Maintain clear airway** Ensure patent airway, and maintain cervical spine precautions. Provide high-flow oxygen. Ensure patent nasogastric tube, and empty stomach. Administer histamine receptor antagonists as ordered. Monitor airway and respirations during extubation, and transport to post anesthesia care unit, using pulse oximetry. Suction. Use artificial airway to maintain jaw position.	Pao_2 will be greater than 80 mm Hg on room air, and $Paco_2$ will be between 35 and 45 mm Hg; pH will be between 7.35-7.45. A patent airway will be maintained for the patient. Respiratory rate, rhythm, and depth will be in the patient's normal range. No aspiration will occur.
High risk for fluid volume deficit Related to hemorrhage, shock, previous illness	**Maintain normovolemia** Administer IV fluids and/or blood as needed to maintain blood pressure via large-bore needle or catheter. Consider PASG application. Insert urinary catheter, and monitor intraoperative output.	The patient will have a systolic blood pressure of greater than 100 mm Hg. Capillary refill will be 2 seconds or less. Urinary output will be 30 ml or more per hour.
High risk for electrolyte disturbance Related to the nature of the injury, medication, choice of resuscitative fluid	**Maintain electrolyte balance** Check electrolytes preoperatively. Replace depleted electrolytes. Administer blood that is less than 3 days old when giving more than 5 units.	Potassium, calcium, sodium, and chloride will be within normal range; cardiac rate and rhythm will be within normal limits.
High risk for anxiety Related to unfamiliar environment, concern for family/significant other, surgical procedure, planned anesthesia, belief that one will feel pain	**Promote coping strategies for anxiety** Orient patient to surroundings. Make patient aware of the plan of care. Keep patient, family, friends informed of patient status. Comfort and support family/significant other.	Physical and emotional factors increasing the patient's risk for surgery will be evaluated.
High risk for injury and impaired tissue integrity Neuromuscular damage, related to improper positioning, extended length of surgery Burns, related to improper grounding of electrocautery equipment Nosocomial infection, related to leaving a foreign object in wound	**Protect patient from environmental hazards** Pad all bony prominences. Position patient in a manner in which no pressure or abnormal stretching of nerves occurs. Apply grounding pads securely; perform safety check on electrosurgical equipment. Adhere to strict aseptic technique. Prepare surgical site with appropriate antiseptic.	Patient will be free of neuromuscular damage. Patient will be free of injury, as exhibited by correct needle, sponge, and instrument counts. Patient will be free of infection.

Continued.

Nursing diagnosis	Nursing intervention	Evaluative criteria
	Remove road gravel, dirt from patient's back before positioning supine. Place dry pads under patient after prepping skin.	
High risk for ineffective thermoregulation Related to a cool operating room environment, cool temperature of resuscitation fluids, surgical exposure	**Promote effective thermo-regulation** Provide warm irrigation fluid. Limit area of surgical exposure. Have warming pad in place. Adjust room temperature as needed. Monitor patient core temperature.	Patient will have normal temperature.
High risk for pain Related to surgical incision, untreated injuries	**Promote comfort** Observe patient for signs indicating pain, and give appropriate medication.	Patient will be reasonably comfortable and not overly sedated.
High risk for: fluid volume deficit Related to blood loss during surgery	**Maintain blood volume** Communicate and document estimated blood loss to surgical and anesthesia team. Communicate and document estimated blood loss to post anesthesia care unit so that fluid replacement may be planned. Monitor and document intake and urinary output.	Patient will be hemodynamically stable.

COMPETENCIES
The following
clinical
competencies
pertain to
**perioperative
care of the
trauma patient.**

☑ *Perform preoperative nursing assessment.*

☑ *Maintain patient safety in positioning, use of equipment, and transport.*

☑ *Monitor fluid loss and replacement in conjunction with other trauma team members.*

☑ *Perform surgical counts while recognizing potential urgent need for surgery.*

☑ *Provide appropriate instrumentation and supplies to the surgical field, based on type of patient injury.*

☑ *Recognize need for and provide emotional support to patient's family members/significant others.*

RESEARCH QUESTIONS

- Discuss the effect that a shortened and intesified preoperative teaching period has on the elderly trauma patient's recovery.
- Investigate the intraoperative and postoperative effects of trauma victims receiving hypertonic saline and dextran for resuscitation purposes in the prehospital setting.
- Identify the relationship and incidence of intraoperative cardiac arrest or electrolyte imbalance caused by hyperkalemia resulting from massive crushing injuries.

RESOURCES

American Association of Nurse Anesthetists (AANA)
216 Higgins Rd.
Park Ridge, IL 60069
(312) 692-7050

Association of Operating Room Nurses Inc. (AORN)
10170 E. Mississippi Ave.
Denver, CO 80231

Malignant Hyperthermia Association of the United States
(MHAUS)
PO Box 3231
Darien, CT 06820
(203) 634-4917
(Phone consultation in malignant hyperthermia emergencies—Medic Alert Foundation International, 1-209-634-4917, ask for INDEX ZERO)

ANNOTATED BIBLIOGRAPHY

Association of Operating Room Nurses (AORN). (1991). *AORN Standards and Recommended Practice for Perioperative Nursing:* perioperative. Denver: AORN.
Standards and recommended practice guidelines for perioperative nursing.
Foster, C.G., Mukai, G., Breckenridge, F.J., & Smith, C.M. (1979). *Effects of surgical positioning.* AORN Journal. 30(2), 219-232.

Discussion includes commonly used surgical positions and their effects on circulation, skin integrity, and postoperative pain.
Groah, L. (1983). Operating room nursing: The perioperative role. Reston, VA: Reston Publishing.
Good, overall reference to guide delivery of care to surgical patients.
Kneedler, J., & Dodge, G. (1987). *Perioperative patient care.* Boston: Blackwell Scientific Publications.
General, well-organized reference to care for the perioperative patient.
Rowland, H., & Rowland, B. (1990). *Operating room administration manual.* Rockville, MD: Aspen Publishers.
Checklists, guidelines, and forms for use in perioperative nursing practice.

REFERENCES

American College of Surgeons. (1986). *Bulletin,* 71, (10).
Association of Operating Room Nurses (AORN). (1989). *AORN standards and recommended practices for perioperative nursing.* Denver: AORN.
Association of Operating Room Nurses (AORN). (1991). *Standards and recommended practice for perioperative nursing.* Denver: AORN.
Burkle, N.L. (1988). Inadvertent hypothermia. *Today's OR Nurse,* 10(7), 26.
Campbell, S. (1987, September). *Trauma victim: OR challenge.* Paper presented at the Conference of Operating Room Nurses, Singapore.
Flever, L., & Pendarvis, J. (1989). Electrolyte imbalances. *AORN Journal,* 49, 992-1008.
Litwack, K. (1991). *Post anesthesia care nursing.* St. Louis: Mosby–Year Book, Inc.
Martin, J. (1987). *Positioning in anesthesia and surgery.* Philadelphia: W.B. Saunders.
McConnell, E. (1987). *Clinical considerations in perioperative nursing.* Philadelphia: J.B. Lippincott.
Ripps, R., Eckenhoff, J.E., & Vandam, L.D. (1988). *Anesthesia: The principles of safe practice.* Philadelphia: W.B. Saunders.
Rogers, A.L., & Stugion, C.L. (1985). *Malignant hyperthermia.* AORN Journal, 41, 369-378.

23 *Critical Care of the Trauma Patient*

■■■■■■■■■■■■■■■■■■■■■■■■■■■■■■■■■■■■■■■

Karen Johnson

OBJECTIVES

❑ State the nursing assessments made for the trauma patient in the ICU, using primary and secondary survey techniques and ongoing total body system assessments, including data from invasive and noninvasive monitoring devices.

❑ Discuss some of the considerations that impact nursing care delivery and trauma patient recovery in the ICU.

❑ Discuss the impact of technologic developments in caring for the trauma patient in the ICU, such as advances in mechanical ventilation; sophisticated monitoring systems; pharmacologic support; continuous arteriovenous hemofiltration; and pain management.

❑ Examine costs and patient outcomes associated with an ICU stay for the trauma patient.

INTRODUCTION Major advances in the care of traumatized patients have been made in the past few decades. Prehospital care, resuscitation measures, and timely operative intervention have made a significant impact on survival of the multiply injured patient. Consequently, trauma patients arriving into the intensive care unit (ICU) today tend to have multisystem organ injuries requiring complex nursing care. Although the events that take place before ICU admission usually determine survival, a significant number of trauma patients die in the ICU as a result of the late complications of trauma (Meyer & Trunkey, 1986).

The physical, personal, and cognitive demands of trauma nursing have been precisely described by Von Reuden (1991). The challenge of providing nursing care to trauma patients in the ICU generates a certain amount of excitement and stress. "It is probably no mistake that someone becomes a trauma nurse and not a librarian" (Lenehan, 1986). Care of the trauma patient in the

ICU places great cognitive, physical, and personal demands on the nurse.

The cognitive demands will be described throughout this chapter. Based on the Trimodal Distribution of Trauma Deaths, the ICU nurse knows that once a trauma patient arrives in the ICU, chances are the patient will suffer morbidity and mortality from the complications of trauma. The ICU nurse must (1) know the physiology of the healing process of specific organ injuries, (2) know which complications of trauma each patient is at risk for developing, and (3) perform astute assessments to identify complications. The ICU nurse must plan interventions in an "all out war" to prevent the complications associated with trauma. The ICU nurse must possess a knowledge of multisystem dysfunction and be able to collect and analyze a multitude of physiologic data to make quick, independent decisions. A multitude of complex skills and a diverse base of supporting knowledge are recognized as essential components of critical care nursing practice (Kennerly, 1990).

677

CASE STUDY V.W. is a 28-year-old man who was working in a coal mine when it collapsed. It took approximately 2 hours to dig him out. The paramedics at the scene appropriately immobilized him, intubated him, and placed two large-bore IV lines. His BP was 70/40; HR, 140; R, 32; and T, 97° F. A flight crew arrived at the scene shortly thereafter to transport him to the level I trauma center 120 miles away. On arrival to the emergency department (ED), his BP is 80/50; HR, 130; R, 22; and T, 97° F. He receives 6 liters of crystalloid and 2 liters of colloids while in the ED. His injuries include a superficial femoral artery tear and a fractured left femur. He is taken to the OR 45 minutes after arrival, for repair of his femoral artery tear and reduction of the femur fracture.

V.W.'s past medical history is significant for ETOH abuse (3 six-packs of beer a day). His wife, who is currently unemployed, and their two daughters (3 years old and 5 years old) arrive at the ED while V.W. is in the OR.

V.W. is now ready to be transported to the ICU. What aspects of the trauma resuscitation will impact on V.W.'s ICU presentation and ICU course?

Several aspects of V.W.'s resuscitation will impact on his ICU course. V.W's prolonged extrication time (2 hours) gives an indication to the ICU nurse of the length of time the patient was hypotensive and hypovolemic. V.W. was hypothermic on arrival. His superficial femoral artery tear and femur fracture indicate that he sustained a large volume of blood loss, resulting in a low hematocrit. These aspects of resuscitation measures help the ICU nurse to identify and quantify ischemic/hypoxic damage that V.W. received before the ICU admission. The ICU nurse can then modify nursing care in anticipation of hypoxic complications.

Assess factors that will impact on nursing care delivery and V.W.'s recovery in the ICU.

His history of ETOH abuse will complicate the assessment and management of V.W. in the ICU. ETOH abuse will impact his postoperative recovery and will place him at risk for postoperative complications. Within 2 days, he may show signs of withdrawl, including hypertension, fever, restlessness/agitation, and tachycardia. Other physiologic causes for these symptoms (e.g., sepsis, head injury, hypoxia) must first be ruled out.

V.W.'s family is now 2 hours from their home and their usual resources and support systems.

V.W.'s wife is unemployed and worried about finances, where to eat, and where to sleep. The ICU nurse assesses that the wife is at high risk for ineffective coping and incorporates a patient-family focus into the care plan.

Based on V.W.'s status, on what complications of trauma should the ICU nursing assessments focus?

Ongoing assessments in the ICU allow for early recognition of complications. V.W.'s crush injury and interruption of blood flow to distal tissues place him at risk for the development of myoglobinuria and subsequent renal failure. The ICU nurse should ensure that the development of hematuria after the ICU admission is investigated with urine myoglobin testing.

Using invasive and noninvasive hemodynamic data, the ICU nurse must assess the balance between oxygen supply and oxygen demand to prevent further system damage. Hemodynamic monitoring will allow manipulation of the physiologic determinants of cardiac output to ensure adequate oxygen delivery to tissues.

Monitoring V.W.'s respiratory status will be imperative because V.W. is at risk for developing respiratory insufficiency. A variety of factors is present that will contribute to tissue hypoxia, including reduced hemoglobin secondary to hemorrhage; increased metabolic demands associated with the stress response to injury; and shifts to the left of the oxyhemoglobin dissociation curve, caused by infusion of large volumes of banked blood and hypothermia.

V.W. is in a level I trauma center. What are the ICU requirements for a level I ICU according to the American College of Surgeons?

Required personnel are (1) a designated surgical director, (2) a surgeon credentialed in critical care on duty in the ICU 24 hours a day or immediately available in the hospital, and (3) a minimum nurse : patient ratio of 1 : 2 on each shift. Appropriate monitoring equipment and resuscitation equipment are required. Support services must be available—the patient must have immediate access to clinical diagnostic services.

ASSESSMENT
Initial Assessment

Critically ill trauma patients are admitted into the ICU as a direct admission either from the ED or from the operating room (OR) after emergency surgery. If emergency surgery was required, the trauma patient should enter the ICU directly from the OR (Boggs, 1989; Cardona, 1986; Meyer & Trunkey, 1986). Transport of critically ill patients has been shown to have a 13% morbidity (Insel, Weissman, Kemper, Askanazi, & Hyman, 1986). A stay in the post anesthesia care unit (PACU) after the OR would add another transport for the patient (from the PACU to the ICU), which may increase the incidence of morbidity. The ICU nurse recognizes this and facilitates a safe and timely transfer of the trauma patient into the ICU.

The ICU nurse, much like the ED and OR nurse, must prepare for the emergency admission of a multiply injured trauma patient. Orderly transition into the ICU begins with prior notice of the patient's arrival. The need for and importance of a timely, thorough nursing report from the referring area can not be overemphasized. Information the ICU nurse should receive about the patient is listed in the box below. This not only allows for preparation and procurement of needed personnel, supplies, and equipment, but also helps the ICU nurse to assess what impact the trauma resuscitation will have on the patient's presentation and prognosis in the ICU. ED and OR resuscitation measures can impact on the

---

Aspects of trauma resuscitation that impact on the patient's ICU presentation and ICU course

- Prolonged extrication time (gives an indication of the length of time the patient may have been hypotensive)
- Period of respiratory or cardiac arrest with a total loss of tissue perfusion
- Length of time the patient was hypotensive or hypovolemic
- Length of time the patient was hypothermic
- Blood loss and/or massive fluid resuscitation resulting in a low hematocrit
- Time on the backboard, which potentiates the risk of sacral and occipital breakdown
- Number of units of blood received (gives an estimation of the potential for development of ARDS)

---

trauma patient's ICU course, as summarized in the box above (Whitehorne, Cacciola, & Quinn, 1989). Many of these factors help to identify and quantify the ischemic hypoxic damage the patient experienced before admission to the ICU. The ICU nurse then modifies the nursing care in anticipation of hypoxic complications.

Immediately upon the patient's arrival to the ICU, the ICU nurse completes a rapid systems assessment of the trauma patient. The ICU assessment and management of the trauma patient are based on the Advanced Trauma Life Support and the Trauma Nurse Core Curriculum guidelines: rapid primary assessment, concurrently with the management of vital functions, and a secondary survey.

As in other settings, during the primary survey, the ICU nurse assesses airway, breathing, ventilation, circulation, and neurologic status. This assessment serves as a baseline for determining physical changes detected during the ongoing assessments. The endotracheal tube is assessed for placement, lung fields are auscultated, and the mechanical ventilator is checked for proper functioning and settings for effective ventilation. Heart sounds are auscultated. Pulse oximetry is initiated to assess oxygen saturation. Observation of capillary refill can indicate adequacy of peripheral cir-

---

Nursing report from referring area

- Name
- Age
- Injuries
- Allergies
- Surgical procedures performed
- Vital signs
- IV access
- Fluid intake (colloid and crystalloid)
- Fluid output (urine, all tubes and drains, estimated blood loss)
- Invasive hemodynamic values (if monitoring devices in place)
- Medications administered
- Past medical/surgical history
- Family members present (assessment of coping; assessment of knowledge of nature of injuries and treatment plan)

culation (Paul & Savino, 1987). Vital signs are taken. The patient's baseline ECG pattern is noted. A baseline neurologic assessment is made. The primary survey allows for a baseline assessment of the patient's vital functions upon arrival to the ICU.

Assessment and management of vital functions occur simultaneously during the primary survey. A pulmonary artery catheter and intraarterial catheter may be inserted by the physician at this time. A complete set of serum laboratory samples is drawn (e.g., electrolytes, ionized calcium, CBC, ABGs). Intravenous (IV) fluids are assessed for type of solution and rate. Patency of the IV catheters is checked as well. If required, vasoactive drugs are initiated or titrated. Urine output and drainage from chest tubes and all surgically placed drainage tubes are noted.

The secondary survey is conducted when the patient has been hemodynamically stabilized. The secondary survey begins with the reevaluation of airway, breathing, and circulation and continues with a neurologic and comprehensive head-to-toe assessment. The ICU nurse notes the location and condition of all abnormalities, such as abrasions, lacerations, and ecchymoses, throughout the physical assessment. The neurologic assessment is repeated and compared with the baseline admission assessment. Verification of nasogastric tube placement is made through auscultation. If a cervical collar is in place, proper cervical spine stabilization is assessed. Heart and lung sounds are reassessed and compared with the admission baseline. Based on ABG results, the mechanical ventilator settings are adjusted. Endotracheal suctioning is performed, noting color and amount of mucus. The color and amount of chest tube drainage are assessed and compared with the initial primary assessment. The nurse assesses for evidence of subcutaneous air and air leaks. If high levels of positive end expiratory pressure (PEEP) are needed to maintain oxygenation, the ICU nurse is aware that a previously placed chest tube does not eliminate the possibility of ipsilateral tension pneumothorax (Norwood, 1987a). Bowel sounds are auscultated. Drainage from all surgical wounds is assessed for amount and color. Urinary output is assessed for amount, color, and specific gravity, and a dipstick urine test is performed. The extremities are assessed for perfusion, including capillary refill, color, temperature, and pulses. Use of a Doppler device

may be required to assess peripheral pulses. Traction, if in place, is assessed for alignment. The patient is log rolled to facilitate the nurse assessing the patient's back for altered skin integrity. Any foreign objects (e.g., glass, grass, dirt) from the injury scene are removed. Some trauma protocols mandate that peripheral IV catheters placed in the field be removed, and if peripheral IV access is required, new catheters be inserted, using aseptic technique.

After the secondary survey, the patient is assessed for adequate pain control and then bathed. Frequent and ongoing assessments of vital functions are made. Once the patient is stabilized, the ICU nurse confers with the patient and family. If the patient is intubated and/or unconscious, the nurse completes the initial nursing history of the patient with the family. The patient and family are oriented to the ICU personnel and routines and to the various pieces of equipment used. Readiness to learn is assessed. Patient and family teaching is initiated. At this time the ICU nurse screens the trauma patient for inclusion and suitability for ongoing research studies.

Ongoing Assessment

The need for ongoing assessment of the trauma patient cannot be over-emphasized. Unlike other critical care patients, the trauma patient has multisystem dysfunction related to the initial injury and its sequelae (Von Rueden, 1989). For example, the patient with a crush injury may develop myoglobinuria, which may cause acute renal failure. The patient with long bone fractures is at risk for developing fat embolism syndrome. Prevention and early recognition of complications are imperative. (Assessment and management of complications of trauma is reviewed in Chapter 19.) The nursing care plan should focus on assessed needs, as well as anticipatory needs, related to specific injuries (Boggs, 1989).

In addition to assessing for life-threatening complications, another difficult problem the ICU nurse faces while caring for the trauma patient is assessment and recognition of "missed injuries." Missed injury may be suspected if the patient fails to show improvement despite appropriate management. Because the ICU nurse makes frequent, ongoing assessments, it is often the nurse who assesses that the patient is not appropriately responding to therapy. A sudden increase or change in character of drainage from wounds or catheters may suggest a missed abdominal injury or an anastomotic leak; a falling hematocrit without evidence of GI bleeding may occur with an expanding retroperitoneal or mediastinal hematoma; a diminishing of peripheral pulses with vascular injuries may indicate the presence of a missed arterial intimal flap; pelvic or peritoneal abscesses may develop in patients with missed rectal injuries (Langdale & Schecter, 1986). Ongoing assessments are imperative in detecting missed injuries. The ICU nurse should have a high index of suspicion when trauma patients are not appropriately responding to medical therapy.

Ongoing assessment and management of the trauma patient include the need for diagnostic tests that may require the transport of critically ill patients outside the protective environment of the ICU for prolonged periods. This may represent an additional risk to these patients. Indeck, Peterson, Smith, and Brotman (1988) examined the risk and cost of the transport of shock trauma patients out of the ICU for special diagnostic tests. They reported an average time away from the ICU of 81 minutes and required 3.3 personnel per trip. The average transport cost was $495. In this study, 68% of the trauma patients experienced serious physiologic changes of at least 5 minutes duration, as summarized in the box above. The ICU nurse must recognize that transporting the trauma patient to diagnostic procedures has a high occurrence of morbidity that may not be discovered, since monitoring and support are not as intensive as those in the ICU. Institutions should have guidelines and recommendations for transporting critically ill patients out of the ICU for diagnostic tests.

Essential to the management of the trauma patient in the ICU are ongoing assessment and monitoring with timely and adequate therapeutic interventions. Monitoring includes repeated physical assessments, laboratory data, diagnostic tests, and noninvasive and invasive monitoring. Monitoring of almost all body systems is usually indicated.

Monitoring
Hemodynamic monitoring

One of the most important responsibilities of the ICU nurse in the care of the trauma patient is to accurately assess the balance between oxygen supply and oxygen demand. Oxygen delivery is optimized to prevent further system damage (Whitehorne, Cacciola, & Quinn, 1989). Assessment of circulatory status includes ongoing assessments using the noninvasive techniques described in the primary and secondary surveys. Invasive monitoring includes the use of intraarterial and pulmonary artery catheters. Intraarterial blood pressure monitoring provides a continuous pressure tracing and allows for access to serum blood samples, including arterial blood gases. Placement of a pulmonary artery (PA) catheter allows for continuous monitoring and assessment of myocardial performance and oxygen delivery. The PA catheter enables the assessment of the preload and afterload components of stroke volume. Both the PA diastolic and pulmonary artery wedge pressures can assess preload to the left ventricle, whereas central venous pressure reflects preload to the right ventricle. Systemic vascular resistance can be calculated to assess systemic afterload. Pulmonary vascular resistance can be calculated to determine pulmonary afterload. The PA catheter is invaluable for directly measuring cardiac output. Continuous measurement of mixed venous oxygen saturation (SvO_2) can be obtained through the use of a PA catheter with oximeter capabilities. This allows for continuous observations of oxygen transport and cardiopulmonary function. If an SvO_2 PA catheter is not used, blood samples can be drawn through the PA catheter to assist in calculating oxygen transport and cardiopulmonary function. The advantage of this sophisticated hemodynamic monitoring equipment is that it provides rapid determination of myocardial performance and oxygen delivery and ultimately reduces mortality (Savino, 1987) (Figure 23-1). Hemodynamic monitoring

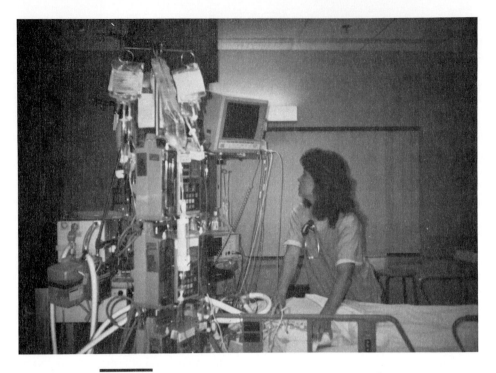

Figure 23-1 Hemodynamic monitoring can reduce mortality.

allows manipulation of the physiologic determinants of cardiac output to ensure adequate oxygen delivery to tissues.

Respiratory monitoring

Assessment of oxygenation and ventilation in the critically ill trauma patient is imperative. The trauma patient may have sustained injuries that directly affect pulmonary status (pneumothorax) or may be at risk for developing respiratory insufficiency. There is no substitute for frequent and thorough assessments by the nurse to detect subtle changes and to implement appropriate therapeutic interventions (Garg, Peck, & Savino, 1987). Breath sounds and chest tube drainage should be evaluated repeatedly and frequently for two reasons: (1) a hemothorax can occur after the initial evaluation in the ED; and (2) the rate of intrathoracic bleeding may be so slow that a significant deficit in blood volume is first detected in the ICU (Norwood, 1987a).

A trauma patient may or may not be intubated upon admission to the ICU. Aggressive pulmonary therapy with oropharyngeal suctioning, pulmonary physiotherapy, humidification, and in-

centive spirometry occasionally can obviate the need for mechanical ventilatory support (Garg, Peck, & Savino, 1987). The point at which initiation of mechanical ventilatory support is required is a critical decision. Ventilatory support should be initiated when the trauma patient shows early signs of respiratory failure. It is generally accepted that if the arterial oxygen pressure (PaO_2) falls below 60 mm Hg on room air or if the arterial carbon dioxide pressure ($PaCO_2$) rises above 45 mm Hg, endotracheal intubation and mechanical ventilation are required. The goals of ventilatory support are (1) adequate oxygenation with a safe fraction of inspired oxygen and (2) adequate oxygen delivery (Norwood, 1987a). Judicious monitoring of arterial blood gases is essential to manipulate the ventilator settings for treatment.

A fundamental goal in managing trauma patients in the ICU is to maintain adequate oxygenation in an effort to prevent hypoxemia. Prevention and treatment of hypoxemia require accurate assessment of adequacy of pulmonary gas exchange, oxygen transport, and cellular oxygen utilization (Von Reuden, 1989). The ICU nurse

---

> ### Factors that contribute to tissue hypoxia in the trauma patient
>
> - Shifts to the left of the oxyhemoglobin dissociation curve—can be secondary to (1) infusion of large volumes of banked blood, (2) hypocarbia or alkalosis, (3) hypothermia
> - Reduced hemoglobin (secondary to hemorrhage)
> - Reduced cardiac output (in the presence of cardiovascular insults)
> - Impaired cellular oxygen consumption (associated with metabolic alterations of sepsis)
> - Increased metabolic demands (associated with the stress response to injury)

---

must be cognizant of a variety of factors that contribute to tissue hypoxia in the trauma patient. The box above lists these factors, as summarized from Von Reuden (1989).

Neurologic monitoring

The clinical neurologic assessment performed by the ICU nurse at the bedside is the cornerstone of the neurologic evaluation of the trauma patient. The ICU nurse must recognize the difficult management of multiple trauma patients with head injuries, because treatments used to improve cardiopulmonary function and oxygen delivery (such as fluid resuscitation) often have detrimental effects on factors that determine optimal cerebral perfusion.

In the head-injured patient, an effective technique for neurologic assessment is continuous intracranial pressure (ICP) monitoring. Cerebral blood flow is assessed by calculation of cerebral perfusion pressure (CPP), which is the mean arterial pressure minus the ICP. At present, no reliable noninvasive indicators of ICP exist; thus it must be directly measured. Three devices that can mechanically monitor ICP are the subarachnoid bolt, intraventricular catheter, and epidural transducer. Using prescribed parameters, the ICU nurse can mechanically drain cerebrospinal fluid to reduce ICP. Maintenance of ICP below 15 mm Hg is the standard clinical end point. ICP monitoring has become well established and plays a vital role in the care of the head-injured patient.

Renal monitoring

The assessment and ongoing monitoring of renal functioning are critical to the survival of the trauma patient (Scalea, Phillips, Goldstein, Scalfani, & Duncan, 1987). These patients are at risk for nephrotoxic damage because of decreased perfusion, increased metabolic wastes, and the use of nephrotoxic antibiotics. Frequent measurement of urinary output serves as a guide to fluid replacement and as a monitor of the adequacy of renal tissue perfusion. Urinary flow of 0.5 to 1.0 ml/kg/hr is considered a satisfactory level (Paul & Savino, 1987).

Specific gravity should be assessed regularly, because it can be an early indicator of renal failure and will warn the ICU nurse of a problem hours before a rise in serum creatinine occurs (Whitehorne et al., 1989). Serum and urine osmolarity reflect the kidney's ability to concentrate urine. Urine should also be monitored for the presence of blood. Hematuria that develops within 6 hours after injury may indicate myoglobinuria. Trauma patients with muscle injury or interruption of blood flow to distal tissues are at risk for developing myonecrosis with the potential development of myoglobinuria and secondary renal failure. Prevention of this secondary renal failure is imperative. The ICU nurse should identify patients at risk and ensure that the development of hematuria after admission to the ICU is investigated. Early institution of a bicarbonate continuous infusion may help alkalinize the urine to prevent precipitation of myoglobin in the renal tubules (Langdale & Schecter, 1986).

One of the most serious complications affecting trauma patients in the ICU is oliguric renal failure (Norwood, 1987b). If the trauma patient becomes oliguric, the ICU nurse must assess for possible prerenal, renal, or postrenal causes of oliguria. Despite growing sophistication in ICU monitoring and therapeutics, posttraumatic renal failure continues to be a highly lethal condition, with a reported mortality of 60% to 75% (Butkus, 1983). It is for this reason that assessment of renal function in the critically ill trauma patient is imperative. The ICU nurse recognizes that the best treatment for renal failure in the trauma patient is prevention.

In addition to assessment of cardiovascular, pulmonary, neurologic, and renal status of the critically ill trauma patient, the ICU nurse also makes frequent total body assessments, including nutritional/metabolic, immunologic, integumentary, musculoskeletal, and gastrointestinal systems. It is imperative that the ICU nurse recognizes all components of individual organ system function and their interactions with other organ systems.

PLANNING CARE FOR THE ICU TRAUMA PATIENT

Critically ill trauma patients have a multitude of physical and emotional needs. When planning nursing care for the trauma patient in the ICU, the nurse must assess a variety of factors that impact on nursing care delivery and patient recovery, including the profile of the trauma patient; the profile of the family in crisis caused by the traumatic event; the physical and personal demands placed on the trauma ICU nurse; the complex ICU environment in which care must be delivered; and the complex ethical dilemmas stimulated by costly and sophisticated care.

Trauma Patient Profile

In addition to the complex physiologic care that trauma patients require in the ICU, these patients have complex psychosocial needs, which the ICU nurse must assess in planning nursing care.

The unique characteristics of the average trauma patient are well documented: a young adult, usually under the age of 35, under the influence of drugs or alcohol, who in the state of traumatic crisis suffers psychologic sequelae (Cardona, 1988). Nursing care of the trauma patient in the ICU creates some unique challenges as physiologic and psychosocial sequelae evolve that are not typical of those of other critically ill patients (Fontaine, 1989).

The use of alcohol influences the likelihood of virtually all types of injuries. Alcohol may be an important factor in 30% to 50% of all trauma cases (Schmidt, 1985). Substance abuse (alcohol and/or drug) complicates the assessment and management of the trauma patient in the ICU. The ICU nurse must care for a patient who is physiologically and psychologically labile and has multisystem effects of substance abuse, in addition to multisystem injuries and dysfunction.

Moderate levels of alcohol or drugs can mask pain and obscure physical signs and symptoms. Once the effects of the alcohol or drugs wear off, a previously drowsy patient may suddenly become violent and pull out invasive catheters. Postoperatively, the ICU nurse must continually assess the impact of drug or alcohol abuse on the patient's surgical recovery. Hepatic damage from chronic alcohol use can place the patient at an increased risk for many postoperative complications: altered nutritional and immunologic status; altered fluid and electrolyte balance; and hematologic disorders. In addition, drugs or alcohol may act synergistically with anesthetics, analgesics, and sedatives, which may cause unexpected depression of the central nervous system (Schmidt, 1985).

Between 7 and 48 hours after cessation of drinking, the patient may begin to show signs of withdrawl (Kelly, 1986). A mild increase in heart rate and blood pressure may be observed. However, these autonomic signs are usually present in the hyperdynamic trauma patient. The trauma patient in withdrawal may become increasingly restless, agitated, and disoriented. The astute ICU nurse also recognizes that these are signs and symptoms of hypoxia, which first must be ruled out. Patients may progress to delirium tremens (DTs) about 3 to 5 days after admission (Brown, 1983). The patient in DTs may have an elevated blood pressure, temperature as high as 103° F (40° C), a heart rate of 130 to 150 beats per minute, diarrhea, nausea, and vomiting. Again, many of these signs and symptoms complicate the assessment and care of the trauma patient in the ICU, because other physiologic causes for these symptoms must first be ruled out (e.g., sepsis, hypoxia). If seizures occur, physiologic sources of the seizures, especially in the head-injured patient, must be ruled out.

Nursing assessment of the trauma patient on admission to the ICU should include a history of the patient's substance abuse. Many nurses, however, believe this is an invasion of privacy. Obtaining a substance use history in a nonthreatening manner might be prefaced by such statements as, "To provide you with the best care, I need to know more about your drinking (or use of drugs), because this can influence your response to many of the medications we give you. I'd like to ask you some questions, and the more you are able to answer, the better we will be able to help you" (Zabourek, 1986). Unfortunately, many trauma patients in the ICU have an altered level of consciousness and the nurse cannot elicit an accurate substance abuse history. The patient's family may be able to provide information, but many substance abuse patients have not admitted to family or friends the use or abuse of substances.

Nursing interventions for the substance abuse trauma patient in the ICU may involve ethical decision-making. A dilemma exists about whether restraints are appropriate during acute alcohol withdrawal. Chemical restraints may be used. Chlordiazepoxide (Librium), when administered early in the withdrawal process, may eliminate the need for protection by physical restraint (Kelly, 1986). There is much debate on the administration of intravenous ethanol. Its use can postpone the withdrawal process until the trauma patient is over the acute life-threatening phase of recovery. However, the metabolic consequences are undesirable and may further impair liver function (Brown, 1983).

All injuries are associated with some type of psychologic reaction. Trauma patients' responses can be influenced by many factors. The manner in which an injury occurs, the nature of the rescue and injury, the parts of the body damaged, the emotional significance of the injury, the treatment procedures, the person's past general health, and personality factors influence the patient's psychologic response to injury (Schmidt, 1985; Bubulka, 1990). More so than the physical responses to trauma, the personal reactions distinguish each trauma patient and can not be predicted with certainty (Lenehan, 1986). Anxiety, fear, isolation, loneliness, grief, and sleep deprivation are just some of the many emotional effects the trauma patient may experience in the critical care setting (Fontaine, 1989). Unconsciously, the trauma patient begins to ward off threatening aspects of the experience by various means, such as regression, repression, denial, rationalization, fantasizing, and amnesia (Matteson, 1975; Schnaper, 1975). Regression, repression, denial, and rationalization are discussed in Chapter 15. When the trauma patient experiences a void in consciousness, the void is filled with retrospective fantasies. A predominant, almost universal, theme that trauma patients experience in the ICU is that of being held prisoner (Schnaper, 1975). This is understandable, because nursing care of the trauma patient in the ICU often includes physical and pharmacologic restraints. Studies have shown that patients remember very little about their stay in the ICU (Compton, 1991; Schapner, 1975). Trauma pa-

tients have described a phenomenon of "psychic numbing," in which they explain the emotional numbing as a subjective sense of not having feeling (Bubolka, 1990). Compton (1991) hypothesized that for periods of time, the critically ill person does not interpret or give meaning to his or her world and that critical illness and intensive care are defined as events that are neither pleasant nor necessary to think about.

The ICU nurse caring for a trauma patient must assess the individualized psychologic response to trauma and plan appropriate and therapeutic interventions (See Chapter 15 for specific nursing interventions for psychologic care of the trauma patient). Research suggests that the role of nurses is important in enhancing the psychologic well-being of trauma patients (Lenehan, 1986).

Family Profile

The family of the multiply injured patient experiences significant stress as a result of the traumatic event. *Family* in this chapter is viewed as the patient's *significant others*. The family's world stops as they are forced to deal with a sudden event for which they had no warning or opportunity to prepare. Patients may be flown to a hospital hours from their home. Families join the patients at the hospital, but they are hours away from their usual resources and support systems. Historically, ICU nurses have neglected needs of trauma patient families by using the excuse that they were too busy attending to the tasks necessary for maintenance of the patient's life (Kleeman, 1989). Recently, the involvement of families in ICUs has increased. Families play an important role in the physiologic stabilization of trauma patients and can make a positive impact on recovery and long-term adjustment (Dockter et al., 1988). Research has demonstrated it is necessary for ICU nurses to be well-prepared to deal therapeutically with families in crisis (Kleeman, 1989). A patient-family focus must be incorporated into the nursing plan of care. It is a responsibility of the ICU nurse to assess family members' psychosocial needs, identify families at risk for ineffective coping, and select interventions to support the family's emotional needs.

Families may feel vulnerable, helpless, and powerless (Caine, 1989; Coulter, 1989; Schlump-Urquhart, 1990). It is hard to predict how the family of the trauma patient will deal with the shock of what has happened. The box on p. 686

Factors that influence a family's response to trauma

Little or no time to prepare

Little or no experience with this type of stressor, either personally or with others

Little guidance regarding what is expected of them

Loss of control and feelings of helplessness

Amount of time spent in the crisis situation and its labile course

Description of family roles, responsibilities, and routine functioning

Perceived danger to and emotional impact of the injury on the family

Issues of responsibility, anger, guilt

Trauma sequelae (permanent physical/emotional damages)

Note. From Catastrophes: An Overview of Family Reactions by C.R. Figley. In C.R. Figley and HI McCubbin (Eds.), 1990, *Stress and the Family. Vol. II. Coping with Catastrophe,* New York: Brunner/Mazel; and from "The Family of the Trauma Victim" by D.S. Solursch, 1990, *Nursing Clinics of North America,* 25(1), p. 155-162.

Table 23-1 Family members' needs during ICU stay

Study	Identified needs of families of critically ill patients
Molter (1979)	To feel that there is hope To feel that hospital personnel care about the patient To be kept informed about the patient's progress
Bozzett and Gibbons (1983)	To gain relief from anxiety To obtain information To be useful To get help with family problems To be recognized for the significant role they play in the patient's recovery
Daley (1984)	To obtain information
Stillwell (1984)	To see the patient frequently To visit the patient whenever desired
Leske (1986)	To have visiting hours changed for special conditions To have a place to be alone in the hospital To talk about negative feelings To be encouraged to cry To have someone help with financial problems To have comfortable furniture in waiting rooms
Forrester, Murphy, Price, and Monaghan (1990)	To be assured that the best possible care is given to the patient To have questions answered honestly To know specific facts about the patient's condition To know how the patient is treated To be called at home about changes in the patient's condition To know the prognosis
Coulter (1989)	To gain relief from the stress of the ICU admission and sense of unreality To gain knowledge of critical illnesses To find ways of coping with the situation To gain information

---

lists factors that influence a family's response to trauma, as summarized by Figley (1983) and Solursh (1990). Six phases that families of trauma patients may experience are (1) high anxiety, (2) denial, (3) anger, (4) remorse, (5) grief, and (6) reconciliation (Coulter, 1989; Epperson, 1977). Families may experience these emotions simultaneously (nonlinearly).

The ICU nurse must be able to provide crisis intervention based on family needs. Several studies have been conducted to determine what family members' needs are during this crisis period in the ICU (Table 23-1). Three essential nursing interventions—informing, directing, and caring—are required to meet the needs of the family in crisis (Krozek, 1991).

Families are expected to absorb highly technical and potentially devastating information and make rapid decisions under a great amount of stress (Lenehan, 1986). Receiving information can help them to make sense of their situation (Coulter, 1989). When informing families, the ICU nurse should provide clear, simple, and accurate information on an ongoing basis. When communicating with families, a priority strategy is to provide effective, meaningful, open, and honest communication (Caine, 1989). Good eye contact and personalized communication should be used. The nurse should inform family members about the patient's condition and provide information and preparation for the many environmental stressors in the ICU. Expectations of the family should be explained to them. Families should know they have ready access to the medical and nursing staff who are immediately involved in the care of the patient. Research findings suggest that having the nurse present when the physician is explaining the patient's medical condition is valuable to families (Coulter, 1989). Coulter (1989) suggested that it may be appropriate to develop a nurse specialist role in which involvement would be specifically with the families of the critically ill. This nurse specialist role (Family Nurse Liaison) has been successfully implemented at the University of Kentucky Hospital in Lexington.

Family conferences and support groups are other ways to meet family needs for information and support. These group meetings can help in several ways: (1) help meet the emotional needs of families of trauma patients; (2) orient family members to the hospital and ICU environment; (3) explain medical terminology and information, and (4) provide a forum for discussion and to answer questions pertaining to other issues that arise (Boettcher & Schiller, 1990). It is possible with these group meetings to meet several families' needs simultaneously.

Families need direction. They need to know where the unit is, where the bathrooms are, where the waiting room is, how to get out of the hospital, and where they can get spiritual and/or financial counseling. A brochure can be given to the family that tells them about visiting hours, unit regulations, where to eat and sleep, and who the patient's physician and nurse are. Adaptation to the hospital can be enhanced when families are assisted in their search for information. Directing them to the best persons to talk with to get their information is helpful (Boettcher & Schiller, 1990). Families need to be told how they can participate in care of the patient and how they can help in the recovery process. For some relatives, the best way of coping with intense feelings of helplessness is to take part in the actual physical

care of the patient (Coulter, 1989).

Many frameworks exist from which the ICU nurse may practice a caring concern for families in crisis caused by trauma. A framework produced by Caine (1989) has been successfully demonstrated in a variety of critical care settings (Figure 23-2). By showing a caring, concerned attitude, the nurse can provide excellent care to the trauma patient's family. Touch should be used appropriately when communicating with families and patients. Individualized visiting hours recognizes the special needs of each family. Providing comfort to family members is as crucial as providing comfort to the patient. Using gentleness in speech and action, demonstrating respect for the patient's privacy, and exhibiting courtesy and compassion add to the family's sense of trust in the ICU nurse (Caine, 1989).

Several studies have demonstrated that family members want to visit the patient in the ICU regularly and frequently (Halm & Titler, 1990; Leske, 1986; Stillwell, 1984). ICU visiting policies have traditionally been restrictive in terms of the time, length, and number of visits and visitors allowed per day. In addition, visitor age and relation to the patient may be further restricted. Visiting policies are institutional-based or unit-based policies. The original purpose of restrictive ICU visiting policies is unclear. ICU visitation has become a major topic of discussion in critical care nursing for the following reasons:

- Consumer awareness of the importance of the family to patient recovery has prompted challenges to restrictive visitation policies.
- Families have described feelings of anger, frustration, anxiety, humiliation, and helplessness in relation to restrictive visiting hours (Chamel & Maddox, 1988).
- Liberal visitation practices in pediatric and maternity settings have produced physiologic benefits to patients (Heater, 1985).
- ICU nurses have found themselves "policing" hospital visitation regulations (Boetcher & Schiller, 1990).
- Restrictive visiting hours have become a source of frustration for nurses, patients, and families.

Reexamination of visiting policies requires a cooperative effort among patients, families, nurses, physicians, and hospital and nursing administration. This collaborative effort will help nurses

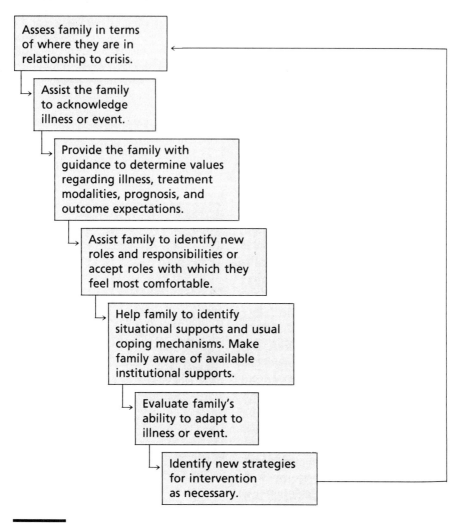

Figure 23-2 Suggested framework from which ICU nurse may practice caring concern for families of trauma patients. (*Note.* From "Families in Crisis: Making the Critical Difference" by R.M. Caine, 1989, *Focus on Critical Care, 16*[3], p. 188.)

identify and meet the needs of the trauma patient and the family. Decisions to alter ICU visiting policies should be based on research findings.

Physical and Personal Demands on the ICU Nurse

Strenuous physical demands are placed on nurses caring for trauma patients (Von Reuden, 1991). Many trauma patients in the ICU are in skeletal traction and require log rolling. Just trying to locate three to four additional nurses who aren't

busy to help with log rolling can be physically demanding! Working in tight quarters, the ICU nurse must maneuver in awkward positions. Many trauma patients cannot participate in self-care activities, requiring the ICU nurse to perform all of the patient's activities of daily living. Many patients have heavy drainage of bodily secretions and are diaphoretic. It is not uncommon for the ICU nurse to give a trauma patient several baths and complete bed linen changes a shift. Endurance is required, because the ICU nurse reor-

---

AACN position statement: Occupational hazards of critical care

Workplace hazards can be defined as the following:

- Biologic (bacteria, viruses, other microorganisms)
- Chemical (soaps, drugs, solvents, waste anesthetic gases)
- Ergonomic (lifting in awkward positions, working in tight spaces)
- Physical (noise, electricity, ionizing radiation)
- Psychologic (dealing with crises, death, abuse by patients, emotional stress, shift work)

---

ganizes and constantly resets priorities, since patients' needs and status may change hourly.

The ICU nurse is exposed to actual and potential health hazards. The American Association of Critical Care Nurses' position statement on occupational hazards of critical care identified health hazards of working in the ICU (see the box above). Exposure to these workplace hazards can produce acute symptoms or chronic disease states (AACN, 1988a).

Significant personal demands are placed on the ICU nurse when caring for a trauma patient. Tremendous emotional maturity and energy are required to deal with the unique psychologic aspects of caring for critically ill trauma patients (Von Reuden, 1991). Trauma care represents a crisis for nurses, as well as patients and families. The worst-case scenario is when the ICU nurse personally identifies with the trauma patient—seeing the patient as a brother, sister, mother, father, husband, wife, or child. Continuous exposure to patient and family crisis situations, day after day, takes an emotional toll on ICU nurses, even though they try to defend and harden themselves against it (Solursh, 1990).

Just as patients and families use coping mechanisms, so do ICU nurses. The coping mechanisms are as individualized as are the patients' and families' reactions to trauma crises. Common responses of ICU nurses caring for trauma patients include inadequacy, frustration, powerlessness, fear, guilt, insecurity, vulnerability, and sadness (Hogan, 1990). Solursh (1990) eloquently captures the coping used by ICU nurses when caring for trauma patients:

. . .trauma unit nurses often get reputations as being . . . hard . . . [in order] to survive the rigors of nursing in such environments, they *must* to some extent harden themselves . . . . This does not mean they should be unaware or indifferent to the psychic pain involved in trauma events. However, if they are too sensitive, too empathic, or identify too much with this aspect of the trauma situation, they will be unable to function effectively in dealing with the nursing tasks that must be performed. . .

Research is scarce that examines the chronic stress of the day-to-day exposure to crises that trauma nurses face. Lenehan (1986) offers two strategies for ICU nurses to cope with continuous exposure to trauma patients—assertiveness and trauma team meetings. Assertiveness promotes good communication of feelings, needs, and wants. Trauma team meetings can increase the team's spirit and purpose and can provide a forum for recognition of various team members. Mitchell (1983) studied the impact of critical incidents on emergency service personnel and developed the Critical Incident Stress Debriefing (CISD) program. The goal of the CISD program is to alleviate the acute stress response immediately after a critical event so that delayed stress reactions are eliminated. A CISD program for ICU nurses caring for trauma patients may be helpful (Hogan, 1990). These debriefings should be structured group meetings, held as soon after the incident as possible and led by a mental health care provider (i.e., psychiatric clinical nurse specialist). The session should allow ventilation of emotions and reactions. The end goal is to assist the nurse in understanding and dealing with the stress generated from the critical incident.

Levine, Wilson, and Guido (1988) studied the personality traits of 200 critical care nurses. They found that the personality traits of ICU nurses tended to be as follows: aggressive, assertive, competitive, persevering, moralistic, resourceful, and mechanical. There is a great need to study personality traits of ICU nurses who care for trauma patients. The goal of a study of this nature would be to identify nurses who could endure the demands of caring for trauma patients in the ICU.

The ICU Environment

Intensive care units have been defined in many ways, but basically, the ICU is a unit in which

Table 23-2 American College of Surgeons' trauma accreditation: Criteria for ICUs for trauma patients

	Level		
	I	**II**	**III**
Personnel			
Designated surgical director	E	E	E
Surgeon, credentialed in critical care by trauma director, on duty in ICU 24 hours a day or immediately available in hospital	E	E	D
Minimal nurse:patient ratio of 1:2 on each shift	E	E	E
Equipment			
Appropriate monitoring and resuscitation equipment	E	E	E
Support services			
Immediate access to clinical diagnostic services	E	E	E

E, Expected; *D,* desired.

maximal supportive care is given to limit injury or disease and prevent complications (Meyer & Trunkey, 1986).

The organizational structure of the ICU can affect the care the trauma patient receives. The American College of Surgeons' Trauma Center Designation criteria delineate ICU requirements for care of the trauma patient (Table 23-2). Based on the types of patients seen in level I trauma centers, a level I trauma center should have a level I ICU (Meyer & Trunkey, 1986).

The ICU environment is a stressful one for patients (Chyun, 1989; Cochran & Ganong, 1989; Williams, 1989). Research studies have revealed several stressors related to the environment, including presence of strange machinery, noises, noxious smells, continuous lighting, invasive procedures, lack of privacy, immobility, and separation from family (Gowen, 1979; Harris, 1984; Kleck, 1984; Noble, 1982; Stephenson, 1977). These stressors are thought to trigger sleep deprivation and an impaired psychologic state, often referred to as *ICU psychosis* or *ICU syndrome.*

Beginning on the third or fourth day in the ICU, patients may experience confusion, disorientation, hallucinations, and delusions (Cochran & Ganong, 1989). Research has indicated that 24% to 72% of ICU patients experience some degree of "ICU psychosis," and reversal of this condition corresponds directly with the time of transfer from the ICU to a general care unit (Kloosterman, 1991).

The nurse can modify elements in the ICU environment to decrease stressors. Noise levels should be decreased to prevent sensory overload and sleep deprivation. Noise levels can also exaggerate the hearing loss experienced by patients receiving aminoglycosides (Johnson & Kent, 1987). Noise levels can be decreased by promptly responding to bedside alarms (e.g., ventilators, volumetric infusion pumps). Noise emanating from personnel ("Who's got the keys?" or "X-ray!") has been found to be greater than noise generated by machines (Johnson & Kent, 1987). Shouting, calling across several beds, and unnecessary talk by the ICU nurses should be avoided. Calendars and clocks should be within the patient's line of vision. Keeping the patient's door closed maintains the patient's privacy and reduces external noise. Music for therapeutic purposes should be used with caution. No research has been reported that indicates what type of music is therapeutic for different patients under different illnesses and environmental conditions (Williams, 1989). Circadian rhythms can be maintained by closing the drapes and dimming the lights at night. Because nurses are a constant part of the ICU environment, they must manipulate these environmental stressors to produce a more therapeutic setting for the trauma patient's recovery. Further nursing research is needed to verify nursing interventions to prevent, reduce, or alleviate the impact of these stressors on the trauma patient's psychologic stability and recovery.

Ethical Issues

Unprecedented achievements over the past several decades have been made in trauma care. However, with these achievements have come perplexing ethical dilemmas, which are compounded by the fact that life-support techniques often render the patient unable to participate in treatment decisions. Two of the most common ethical dilemmas the ICU nurse faces when caring for trauma patients center around the issues of providing care

---

Criteria for determination of brain death

Any individual with the findings in section A (cardiopulmonary) or section B (neurologic) is dead.

A. Cardiopulmonary

An individual with irreversible cessation of circulatory and respiratory functions is dead.

   1. Cessation is recognized by an appropriate clinical examination revealing absence of responsiveness, heartbeat, respiratory effort.
   2. Irreversibility is recognized by persistent cessation of functions during an appropriate period of observation and/or trial of therapy.

B. Neurologic

An individual with irreversible cessation of all functions of the entire brain, including the brainstem, is dead.

   1. Cessation is recognized when evaluation discloses findings of a and b and c:
      a. The cause of coma is established and is sufficient to account for the loss of brain functions.
      b. The possibility of recovery of brain function is excluded.
      c. The cessation of all brain function persists for an appropriate period of observation and/or trial of therapy.

Note. From Transplantation (p. 445) by R.L. Simmons, R.J. Migliori, C.R. Smith, K. Reemtsma, and J.S. Najarian. In S.I. Schwartz (Ed.), 1989, *Principles of Surgery* (5th ed.), New York: McGraw Hill.

---

to the brain dead patient and providing costly and sophisticated care to severely traumatized patients whose prognosis is highly doubtful or whose future quality of life is debatable.

Advances in medical technology have produced the ability to sustain life in patients who have irreversible brainstem damage or who are "brain dead." Clinically, the patient with irreversible brainstem damage meets the following criteria: fixed, dilated pupils; absent reflexes; unresponsiveness to external stimuli; and the inability to maintain vital functions, such as respiration, heartbeat, and blood pressure, without artificial means (Simmons, Migliori, Smith, Reemtsma, & Najarian, 1989). The exact criteria for establishing brain death vary among institutions. The box above lists the guidelines for the determination of

brain death reported to the President's Commission for the Study of Ethical Problems in Medicine and Biomedical and Behavioral Research (1981).

Of brain death diagnoses, 95% are made in the intensive care unit (Walker, 1979). For indefinite periods of time, these patients continue to have a heartbeat and mechanically assisted respirations and are warm to the touch. They look and feel "alive." The nurse continues to deliver care, using highly technologic assessments and maintenance of hemodynamic and metabolic functions, in addition to basic nursing care interventions, such as hygiene, turning, suctioning, bladder and bowel care, and range of motion. The nurse also continues to deliver supportive care to the family (Borozny, 1990). The ICU nurse, who is intent on saving life, is called on to administer care to "dead" patients. Little is known about the experience of ICU nurses who provide this kind of care on a regular basis. Borozny (1990) studied the meaning that ICU nurses attach to their caring for the brain dead patient. Of interest, this study found that ICU nurses accept the concept of brain death, although they believe that there are two types of death—brain death and the traditional concept of death. Much more research is needed to understand the phenomenon of brain death and the ICU nurses' role in caring for the brain dead patient.

In addition to the complexities of caring for brain dead patients, the ICU nurse can face another ethical dilemma in caring for the trauma patient: providing highly technologic and costly care to a severely traumatized patient whose prognosis is highly doubtful or whose future quality of life is debatable. Quality of life must be discussed when deciding the degree and duration of continuing life-supporting interventions. Is the absolute *length* of life more important than the *quality* of the trauma patient's life? The answer is complex, because the trauma patient may be unable to participate in the decision-making process. Defining quality of life is a subjective process. What may be an unacceptable quality of life for one person may be acceptable for another.

Age is a factor in determining quality-of-life decisions. Differences in quality-of-life decisions exist among adults and young adults or children (Bell, 1990). Adults may have expressed their preferences about their wishes for life support in the event they were ever in an accident. They may have presented these views to a loved one or through a "living will" or "advanced directives." Through the living will document, the patient's preferences are specified in advance and serve as a guide to decision-making when the patient cannot function as an active participant (Widra & Pence, 1988). A young adult may not have a living will. When a child or young adult becomes a trauma patient, there is a reluctancy to "give up." Society's perception of a young death is that of a premature death. The temptation exists with younger patients to try a little longer or to be more aggressive (Bell, 1990).

When caring for trauma patients, the ICU nurse may be caught between the use of highly sophisticated technology and the ethical dilemmas inherent in its use. Successful patient management requires a multidisciplinary approach, including the nurse, physician, family, chaplain, social worker, and bioethicist. Although such committees will not eliminate the dilemmas, they can serve as a vehicle to educate, support, and, ideally, alleviate some of the stress involved in making very difficult life-and-death decisions that may be required while caring for the trauma patient in the ICU (Schaefer, 1989).

NURSING CARE OF THE ICU TRAUMA PATIENT

With the rapid pace of technologic development, the roles and responsibilities of the ICU nurse have become more complex. The ICU nurse has had to and must continue to provide nursing care to the trauma patient, using highly technologic skills. Highly technical skills are required for advances in ventilator therapy, sophisticated monitoring systems, pharmacologic support, continuous arteriovenous hemofiltration, and pain management. The ICU nurse faces a daily challenge to interface the "art" of nursing with the "science" of technology.

Advances in Ventilator Therapy

Pulmonary insufficiency associated with multiple system organ failure in the trauma patient has led to new advances in mechanical ventilation used in the ICU. Two advances in mechanical ventilation are simultaneous independent lung ventilation (SILV) and high-frequency ventilation (HFV). These nonconventional modes of mechanical ventilation are used for trauma patients with sig-

nificant pulmonary injury and/or adult respiratory distress syndrome (ARDS).

SILV is usually considered for the trauma patient with unilateral lung pathology. Specific criteria for initiation of SILV include (1) increasing hypoxemia despite increasing FIo_2 and PEEP, (2) decreased lung compliance with increased air resistance, and (3) failure to respond to conventional therapy (Smith & Glowac, 1989). SILV requires the insertion of a double-lumen endotracheal tube and the use of two synchronized mechanical ventilators.

SILV allows both lungs to receive individual tidal volumes, PEEP, and ventilation pressures. In the trauma patient with a unilateral pulmonary contusion, this may be especially advantageous, because the high ventilator pressures and PEEP necessary to ventilate the injured lung can cause barotrauma to the noninjured lung. SILV allows the injured lung to receive higher levels of PEEP required to overcome decreased lung compliance. Nursing care of the trauma patient receiving SILV includes assessment of endotracheal tube placement, frequent assessment of cuff pressures, humidification of the ventilatory circuit, and altered suctioning techniques (Smith & Glowac, 1989).

HFV is defined as ventilation frequencies at least 4 times greater than normal values and tidal volumes less than the patient's anatomic dead space (Smith & Glowac, 1989). In conventional mechanical ventilation, a bulk of gas (700 to 1000 ml) moves in and out of the lungs at slow rates (10 to 20 per minute). HFV supplies a small volume of gas at rapid rates. The turbulent gas flow that results from the rapid ejection of gases is thought to result in gas mixing throughout the tracheobronchial tree (Burns, 1990). Augmented dispersion of the gases, rather than simple diffusion alone, enhances gas transport. HFV decreases barotrauma, decreases intrathoracic pressure, and allows improved oxygenation and lower CO_2 levels (Smith & Glowac, 1989). HFV can be used in the management of acute respiratory failure. Advantages of HFV as described by Burns (1990) are summarized in the box on p. 693.

There are three methods of delivering HFV: high-frequency, positive-pressure ventilation (HFPPV), high-frequency jet ventilation (HFJV), and high-frequency oscillation. HFPPV uses tidal volumes equal to dead space, and ventilator rates of

---

Advantages of high-frequency ventilation (HFV)

- Less circulatory effects as compared with conventional mechanical ventilation (i.e., less effect on cardiac output)
- Lower transpulmonary pressures
- More positive intratracheal pressures
- Decreased risk of barotrauma
- Maintenance of negative intrapleural pressures throughout the ventilatory cycle

---

Nursing care of the patient receiving high-frequency ventilation (HFV)

1. Assess airway patency every 1 to 2 hours.
2. Suction. May use conventional hyperinflation, hyperoxygenation techniques. Some catheters have ports to allow suction catheter access without disconnecting the ventilator from the patient.
3. Accurately assess breath sounds. Turbulent gas flow makes auscultation of breath sounds difficult; therefore the HFV must be temporarily disconnected and the patient must receive manual ventilatory breaths.
4. Use ABGs judiciously. Pulse oximetry, SvO_2, and end tidal CO_2 monitoring can assist in monitoring oxygen delivery and utilization.

---

60 to 100 breaths/min. HFJV delivers small volumes of gas at rates between 100 and 600 breaths/min. The gas is delivered through a jet injector placed in the airway through a special endotracheal tube with a side port. The gas exits the jet catheter with high-velocity pulsations, causing negative pressure to develop. Gases are then diffused from higher to lower pressure areas. High-frequency oscillation uses rates of 900 to 3000 per minute. A small volume of gas is vibrated in the airways. Addition of fresh gases is provided by a circuit perpendicular to the airway ("bias flow"). Bias flow continually moves stale gases out of the airway while allowing adjustments in FIO_2 (Burns, 1990). The method of HFV used varies by institution. Nursing care of the patient receiving HFV as reported by Burns (1990) is summarized in the box, upper right.

SILV and HFV are two nonconventional modes of ventilation that may be used in the ICU in the care of the trauma patient. These modes of mechanical ventilation require different nursing care from that required for the patient receiving conventional mechanical ventilation. Consultation and collaboration with the respiratory therapy team are essential in managing patients receiving these ventilatory modes.

Sophisticated Monitoring Systems

Increasingly sophisticated computerized monitoring equipment has become commonplace in providing ICU trauma care. Computer technology provides accurate and precise physiologic data, which enable rapid interventions. Computers are invaluable to the care of the trauma patient—as long as the patient remains the primary focus.

The ICU nurse must use computer-generated data in conjunction with the clinical assessment of the patient's status.

Monitoring technology includes the use of computerized bedside components. The use of telemetry, once a revolutionary concept in care of patients with myocardial infarctions, is now standard practice. Most bedside components have arrhythmia monitors, which detect and diagnose arrhythmias. Advanced technology has enhanced the use of the bedside monitoring components to continuously monitor such physiologic parameters as SvO_2, end tidal CO_2, pulmonary artery pressures, cerebral perfusion pressure, intracranial pressures, SaO_2, respiratory rate, and arterial and mean arterial blood pressures. In addition, these monitors can calculate a number of derived hemodynamic and oxygenation parameters, including systemic vascular resistance (SVR), pulmonary vascular resistance (PVR), stroke work, A-a gradients, shunt fractions, oxygen delivery, and oxygen consumption. Before the advent of these bedside computers, nurses spent much time memorizing formulas and calculating these data. Now bedside computers calculate these parameters in a matter of seconds. As a "master of technology," the ICU nurse has become a manager of information, spending less time collecting data, but more time reviewing and analyzing more data than ever before (Sinclair, 1988). Advanced monitoring systems enhance the ICU nurse's ability to detect trends quickly and intervene early to prevent complications frequently associated with trauma.

Pharmacologic Support

Pharmacologic support has increasingly become important in the care of the trauma patient in the ICU. Vasoactive drugs and neuromuscular blocking agents are two such examples. These drugs affect the patient's oxygen delivery and consumption.

The patient's mean arterial pressure is closely monitored while the nurse titrates vasoactive drugs. It may be necessary to titrate vasoactive drugs every 5 minutes to achieve an acceptable mean arterial pressure. The ICU nurse must have a knowledge of prescription, loading dose, preparation, and appropriate dilution of a variety of vasoactive drugs. The nurse must be able to perform accurate dosage calculations in emergency situations and adjust infusion rates based on the trauma patient's clinical response to the infusion. A synthesis of available literature was made by Trujillo and Bellorin-Font (1990), which can serve as an excellent clinical guide to vasoactive pharmacologic support used in the ICU.

Neuromuscular blocking agents have been used in the ICUs since the 1960s. Only recently have they been used for prolonged periods in the management of critically ill trauma patients. The major action of neuromuscular blocking agents is to interrupt the transmission of nerve impulses at the neuromuscular junction between peripheral nerves and skeletal muscles. Neuromuscular blocking agents can be divided into two groups, based on their mechanism of action: depolarizing agents (succinylcholine) and nondepolarizing agents (d-turbocurarine, pancuronium, vecuronium and atracurium). Nondepolarizing agents are the agents most frequently used in the ICU for the management of the trauma patient. Conditions for the use of neuromuscular blocking agents include extreme agitation, high metabolic energy requirements, sepsis with respiratory insufficiency, seizures, and ARDS (Teres, Dawson, Roberts, & McDonald, 1989).

Nondepolarizing agents block the nerve impulse from reaching the muscle. Muscular paralysis decreases body oxygen consumption and metabolic energy expenditure. This facilitates adequate ventilation for trauma patients with respiratory failure. Continuous infusions of nondepolarizing neuromuscular blocking agents are es-

pecially helpful with controlling undesirable muscle activity (shivering, "bucking" the ventilator). The ICU nurse is responsible for monitoring the effectiveness of the neuromuscular blockade. These drugs are titrated to patient movement, using a peripheral nerve stimulator. The nurse stimulates a peripheral nerve (ulnar or facial), observes the muscle contraction, and assesses the degree of blockade. The dose is then titrated based on that response. The ICU nurse must also monitor for factors that increase the activity of nondepolarizing neuromuscular blocking agents, including the use of aminoglycosides and the presence of hyperthermia, hypokalemia, and renal and/or hepatic dysfunction.

All patients receiving neuromuscular blocking agents should concomitantly receive sedatives and analgesics (i.e., morphine and diazepam), because patients can still hear, think, and feel. Anecdotal reports demonstrate the need to constantly explain procedures to, talk to, reassure, and touch patients receiving these drugs (Parker, Schubert, Shelhamer, & Parrillo; Schnaper, 1975, 1984). Nursing research is needed to identify the needs and concerns of the trauma patient receiving neuromuscular blocking agents so that appropriate nursing interventions can have a positive impact on patients receiving these drugs.

Continuous Arteriovenous Hemofiltration

Complications of trauma frequently include renal failure and fluid volume overload. Conventional means of treating these conditions using hemodialysis or peritoneal dialysis may be contraindicated in critically ill trauma patients. Critically ill trauma patients often can not tolerate hemodialysis because of hemodynamic instability (hypotension), hypoxemia, or inability to tolerate the systemic anticoagulation required with hemodialysis. Critically ill trauma patients may not be candidates for peritoneal dialysis because this method reduces diaphragmatic compliance, can produce hyperglycemia, is inefficient in emergencies, and requires an intact peritoneum. Patients who may be candidates for continuous arteriovenous hemofiltration as summarized by Paradiso (1989), are described in the box on p. 695. Continuous arteriovenous hemofiltration (CAVH) or continuous arteriovenous hemodialysis (CAVHD) provides an alternative therapy for critically ill trauma patients in renal failure or with acute fluid overload.

CAVH is accomplished with the use of a hemofilter, which removes water and electrolytes from the vascular space. Blood moves from the patient's arterial circulation through the filter and is returned to the patient's venous circulation. In contrast to hemodialysis, CAVH does not use a pump to pull blood from the patient into the hemofilter. Rather, the patient's own arterial blood pressure drives the blood flow through the extra-

corporeal filter. A systolic blood pressure of 70 to 90 mm Hg or a mean arterial blood pressure greater than 60 mm Hg is needed for the blood to flow through the hemofilter (Palmer, Koorejiian, London, Dechert, & Bartlett, 1986; Price, 1989). As blood is pumped through the filter, hydrostatic pressure drives the filtrate across the filter membrane and out of the circulation (Paradiso, 1989). Extending from the filter is a port that drains the filtrate. The fluid that is removed is called the *ultrafiltrate*. Figure 23-3 demonstrates the CAVH system. CAVH is a slow, continuous process, often lasting days to weeks. CAVH is ideal for unstable hypotensive patients because it reduces the risk of rapid fluid and electrolyte removal, which can lead to further hypotension or dialysis disequilibrium syndrome.

CAVH systems are made by several manufacturers. Each type of system is accompanied by its own set of instructions. In addition, institutions using CAVH must have detailed nursing procedures that address preparation, attachment, monitoring the patient, monitoring the hemofilter, and termination of CAVH (Palmer et al., 1986). It is often the responsibility of the ICU nurse to

---

Ideal candidates for CAVH

Ideal candidates for CAVH may include patients with the following conditions:

- Oliguria despite diuretic therapy
- Pulmonary edema (with or without cardiogenic shock)
- Acute renal failure, especially in the presence of hemodynamic instability
- Traumatic recovery complicated by acute renal failure

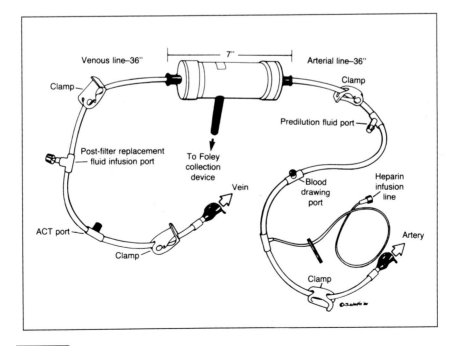

Figure 23-3   CAVH system. (*Note.* From "Continuous Arteriovenous Ultrafiltration: A Monitoring Guide for ICU Nurses" by C.A. Price, 1989, *Critical Care Nurse*, 9[1], p. 14.)

monitor the system and the patient receiving CAVH. For more detailed information on management of the patient and CAVH system, the reader is referred to references by Dirkes (1989); Palmer et al. (1986); Paradiso (1989); and Price (1989).

Pain Management

Major injuries, such as crushed or amputated limbs, multiple abrasions, lacerations, and open abdominal wounds, are visual reminders of the pain the trauma patient experiences in the ICU. Pain that goes unrelieved often affects the patient's behavior, physiology, treatment, and ultimate recovery (Smith & Glowac, 1989). Reasons that pain may go unrelieved in the ICU may include (1) the patient's inability to communicate pain; (2) the patient's assumption that the nurse knows he is in pain and is treating it; (3) the patient's being uninformed that pain relief is available; or (4) the nurse's insensitivity to nonverbal cues that pain exists (Fontaine, 1989).

The trauma patient must be assessed in a systematic way to evaluate pain. Physical mobility, facial expression, and hemodynamic changes should be assessed. A variety of pain assessment tools is available. Application of pain assessment tools to the trauma patient is difficult, but research has shown it is possible to use some form of pain management in the critically ill trauma patient (Mlynczak, 1989).

Traditional pain management therapies have been expanded to manage pain associated with traumatic injuries. Recent therapeutic modalities include the use of continuous intravenous narcotics, epidural analgesics with a local anesthetic, and patient-controlled analgesia (Smith & Glowac, 1989). Studies have shown that despite the availability of these treatment modalities, a considerable percentage of patients with pain are inadequately treated (Mlynczak, 1989). The ICU nurse must collaborate with physicians and pain management teams in selecting appropriate medications, route of administration, frequency of dose, and nursing interventions to enhance control of pain for trauma patients.

Analgesics can be administered in a variety of routes. However, all these routes may not be possible in the trauma patient. Oral administration is often hampered because of injury or surgery of the face or gastrointestinal tract. Intramuscular injections may have limited use in the trauma patient who is edematous or immobile, because these conditions interfere with medication absorption. Intravenous administration has the advantage of providing immediate pain relief and is more predictable and controlled for onset and duration of action (Mlynczak, 1989). Analgesics can be administered through an epidural catheter for multiply injured patients with pain poorly controlled by intermittent medication (Smith & Glowac, 1989). The level of analgesia provided by epidural narcotics is believed to be greater than that by IV narcotics, without significant depression of the central nervous system (Mlynczak, 1989).

Analgesics can be administered as the patient requests (PRN), on a regular schedule regardless of pain complaint, or by continuous infusion, or the patient may administer prescribed doses of medication with a patient-controlled analgesia (PCA) pump. The PCA pump is controlled by a hand-held button. When the patient experiences pain, the patient depresses the button and a prescribed dose of analgesic is delivered. The pump is programed to allow only a certain amount of analgesic to be delivered hourly. This on-demand administration, however, may provide erratic pain relief. Regularly scheduled doses may reduce the frequency of patient request for analgesic, but fluctuations in pain control can still occur. Continuous narcotic infusion has the advantage of constant pain control.

Optimal pain management of the trauma patient in the ICU requires ongoing assessments of the patient's response to the route and timing of administration of analgesics. Conventional and newer treatment approaches to relieve pain may be required.

In summary, when caring for a trauma patient, the ICU nurse must be sensitive, caring, technologically competent, and able to think analytically. The ICU nurse must be able to achieve a balance between the skills required in the use of technologic equipment and the "art" of caring.

IMPACT OF CRITICAL CARE ON THE TRAUMA PATIENT

ICU nursing care of the trauma patient must be evaluated in terms of cost and patient outcomes through research.

Cost

The costs associated with the management of traumatic injury (direct and indirect) are now thought to be $100 billion a year (Conn & McCabe, 1989). The direct costs resulting from motor vehicle crash injuries are approximately twice those resulting from heart disease (Injury in America, 1985). Increasing use of ICUs has been identified as a major factor in increasing hospital costs (Wagner, Wineland, & Knaus, 1983). ICU stays are estimated to account for almost 30% of hospital costs (Paino, Teres, Lemeshow, & Brown, 1982). Mean hospital cost per ICU patient has been estimated to be $20,942 (Muñoz, Josephson, Tenenbaum, Goldstein, Shears, & Wise, 1989). The mean total cost (hospital charges plus professional charges) per trauma patient requiring longer than 30 days in the ICU has been estimated at $136,546 (Goins, Reynolds, Nyanjom, & Dunhan, 1991).

With the advent of prospective payment systems, ICU nurses have increasingly become involved in controlling the cost of caring for critically ill trauma patients. Because cost is a major concern, every ICU must participate in determining financial implications of clinical decisions, evaluating and selecting capital equipment, and determining allocation of resources and expenditures used to provide nursing care. Also, the staff is held more accountable for the operation, function, and cost control of the services they provide (O'Grady, 1987).

Trauma also causes short-term and long-term disability, with indirect societal costs in terms of lost productivity. Additional, less-easily-measured costs include pain, grief, family/society disruption, psychosocial effects of disfigurement and long-term disability, epilepsy from head injury, mobility limitation from spinal cord injury, amputation, traumatic arthritis, and severe reduction in mental function as a result of trauma (Injury in America, 1985).

The direct and indirect costs of treating trauma patients in the ICU are staggering. Trauma prevention is the key in reducing these societal costs. ICU nurses can play an important role in community trauma prevention education programs, such as driver's education programs, and in influencing legislative issues, such as mandatory seat belt use, use of motorcycle helmets, drunk driving laws, and trauma systems development.

Patient Outcomes

The costs of treating trauma patients in the ICU are high, but the benefits of intensive care are poorly documented (Baggs, 1989). The impact of technology and resources used in caring for the trauma patient in the ICU needs further research. Collaboration among physicians and nurses in ICUs has shown to positively affect ICU patients' outcomes (AACN, 1988b; National Joint Practice Commission, 1981). White (1989) offers organizational efforts necessary for improving collaboration: implementing collaborative practice models; implementing joint practice quality assurance activities; and establishing joint professional activities. Collaborative practice models can be based on the AACN position statement, "Collaborative Practice Model: The Organization of Human Resources in Critical Care Units." Joint practice quality assurance activities can assess the cost-effectiveness of care, quality of care, and patient outcomes. Joint professional activities can include patient care rounds, joint projects, collaborative research, and educational activities. Using collaborative practice can result in improved quality of care, improved retention and satisfaction of nurses, increased patient satisfaction, and decreased costs of caring for the trauma patient in the ICU (National Joint Practice Commission, 1981).

SUMMARY Advances made in prehospital care, resuscitation measures, and timely operative intervention have impacted trauma patient survival. Now, more critically ill trauma patients are arriving in the ICU. A key responsibility of the ICU nurse is assessment of the trauma patient. Ongoing monitoring techniques using invasive and noninvasive data can detect missed injury and late complications of trauma. When planning care, the ICU nurse must assess a variety of factors that impact on nursing care delivery and trauma patient recovery, including the trauma patient profile, the family profile, physical and personal demands on the ICU nurse, the ICU environment, and ethical issues in the ICU. The role and responsibilities of the ICU nurse have changed with the rapid pace of technologic developments in the care of the critically ill trauma patients. These developments include advances in mechanical ventilation, sophisticated monitoring systems, pharmacologic support, CAVH, pain management, and infection control. ICU nursing care of the trauma patient must be evaluated in terms of cost and patient outcomes through research. For a summary of nursing care of the ICU trauma patient, see the table on pp. 698-700.

**NURSING DIAGNOSES &
EVALUATIVE CRITERIA** *Critical care of the trauma patient*

Nursing diagnosis	Nursing intervention	Evaluative criteria
Altered peripheral tissue perfusion Related to blood loss, fluid shifts. As evidenced by diminished/absent peripheral pulses, skin color changes (pallor/cyanosis), decreased arterial blood pressure, delayed capillary refill, edema, loss of sensory/motor function, hypotension, immobilization, orthopedic injury/devices, blood vessel trauma/compression, anesthesia, decreased cardiac output, decreased oxygenation/gas exchange	**Maintain tissue perfusion** Monitor vital signs hourly, and progress as per unit standards. Monitor hemodynamics hourly, and progress as per unit standards. Measure oxygen saturation by pulse oximetry hourly, and progress as per unit standards. Maintain patient on ordered mechanical ventilation settings. Suction q2hr/prn; TCDB q2hr. After extubation, TCDB/incentive spirometer q2hr. Arterial catheter to flush and monitor. Monitor arterial and venous blood gases, oxygen delivery/ consumption. Assess chest tubes hourly, and progress as per unit standards. Assess heart and lung sounds q4hr. Assess capillary refill and peripheral pulses q8hr. Assess organ functioning: renal, vital signs, sensorium, cardiac output. Monitor urine output per unit standards. Administer vasoactive/inotropic agents as ordered. Administer neuromuscular blocking agents/sedatives as prescribed to decrease metabolic/oxygen requirements. Apply pneumatic compression stockings as per unit protocol.	Patient monitoring will show the following: • SBP > 90, < 170; • HR > 50, <120; • PCWP > 6, < 18; • CO 4-8 L/min; • CI 2-4L/min; • ABGs WNL; • Sao_2 > 90%; • Svo_2 65%-80%; • audible breath sounds; • capillary refill <3 sec; • U/O .5-1.0 ml/kg/hr; • peripheral pulses present; • GCS score ≥ admission GCS score • BUN, Creatinine, SGPT WNL; • Hct > 28%; • Hgb >10 g; • No evidence of DVT or PE.
Fluid volume deficit Related to fever or increased metabolic rate, infection, abnormal drainage, peritonitis, high-solute tube feedings, diaphoresis As evidenced by dry skin and mucous membranes, increased serum sodium, increased pulse rate, decreased urine output, concentrated urine, decreased fluid intake, decreased skin turgor	**Maintain optimal fluid balance** Weigh patient per unit standards. Maintain NG tube to wall suction. Measure gastric output q8hr; assess NG aspirate for pH and guaiac q4hr. Replace fluid volume at prescribed hourly rate. Maintain patency of peripheral/ central IV catheters. Monitor urine output and specific gravity per unit standards. Monitor serum electrolytes, CBC. Monitor type and amount of all drainage.	Patient status will be as follows: • Weight within 5 lb of admit weight; • NG pH >4.0; • U/O .5-1.0 ml/kg/hr; • specific gravity 1.010-1.020; • electrolytes WNL; • PCWP WNL; • CVP WNL.

NURSING DIAGNOSES &
EVALUATIVE CRITERIA   *Critical care of the trauma patient—cont'd*

Nursing diagnosis	Nursing intervention	Evaluative criteria
Altered nutrition: less than body requirements Related to hyperanabolic/catabolic state (infection/trauma), chemical dependence, trauma, altered level of consciousness, surgery, wired jaw, stress, nausea/vomiting, inability to procure food, inability to chew, diarrhea As evidenced by inadequate food intake, actual/potential metabolic needs in excess of intake, weight of 10% to 20% or more below ideal for BSA, mental irritability/confusion, decreased serum albumin, decreased serum transferrin, decreased lymphocyte count	**Provide adequate nutrition to meet metabolic demands** Weigh patient as per unit standards. Administer enteral/parenteral feedings as prescribed. Assess tolerance of enteral feedings by assessing for residuals q4hr. Document when/why enteral feedings were not administered as ordered. Monitor serum albumin, lymphocyte count, transferrin, and iron-binding capacity.	Weight will be 10% to 20% of ideal. Serum albumin, lymphocyte count, transferrin, iron-binding capacity will be WNL. Indirect calorimetry will reveal adequate caloric intake to meet metabolic demands.
Impaired tissue integrity Related to metabolic/endocrine alterations, nutritional alterations, impaired oxygen transport, infection, NPO status, surgery, imposed immobility, trauma, therapeutic fixation devices, restraints, dressings, tape, solutions, urinary catheter, nasogastric catheter, endotracheal tube As evidenced by disruptions of corneal, integumentary, or mucous membranous tissue or invasion of body structure, edema, erythema, dry mucous membranes	**Maintain intact skin integrity; heal existing wounds** Assess wound for evidence of healing (granulation tissue) q shift. Assess for need for wound debridement (presence of eschar, slough) q shift. Assess skin, tissue integrity q shift. Turn patient q2hr. Assess need for specialty bed. Provide wound care as prescribed &/or per unit standards, using strict aseptic technique. Protect intact skin from wound/drain drainage. Provide oral care q2hr while NPO status, intubated. Maintain proper alignment/placement of all immobilizing devices (e.g., restraints, casts). Assess NG aspirate for pH and guaiac q4hr.	Existing wounds will heal without signs and symptoms of infection. Granulation tissue will be present. Wound cultures will be negative. No new skin or tissue breakdown will be evident. Mucous membranes will be intact, moist, pink.
Pain Related to musculoskeletal, visceral, vascular trauma, inflammation, diagnostic tests, invasive procedures, medications, immobility/improper positioning, pressure points (casts, bandages), stress	**Promote comfort** Assess for autonomic signs of pain. Medicate for pain as prescribed. Assess effectiveness of pain medication after given. Document effective pain control regimen for patient.	Patient will report or demonstrate comfort.

Continued.

Nursing diagnosis	Nursing intervention	Evaluative criteria
As evidenced by patient reports/ demonstrates discomfort, signs and symptoms of autonomic response in acute pain, guarded position, facial mask of pain	Use alternative methods of pain control as needed. Maintain proper body alignment with all therapeutic fixation devices. Assess pressure points on casts and bandages per unit protocols. Turn patient q2hr.	
High risk for infection Related to altered production of leukocytes, altered immune response, altered circulation, presence of favorable conditions for infection, chronic diseases, alcoholism, impaired oxygen transport, altered integumentary system, loss of consciousness, surgery, total parenteral nutrition, dialysis, tracheostomy, presence of invasive lines, prolonged immobility, trauma, contact with nosocomial infectious agents, increased hospital length of stay, malnutrition.	**Prevent infection** Provide oral care while NPO status/ intubated q2hr. Assess invasive line insertion site q shift. Provide invasive line care as per unit standards, using strict aseptic technique. Assess wound, drainage sites q shift. Provide wound care as prescribed/ unit standards, using strict aseptic technique. Provide wound drain care as prescribed/unit standards; maintain patency and strict aseptic technique. Assess VS and temperature as per unit standards. Monitor WBC. Notify MD of elevated temperature as per unit protocol. Obtain cultures as ordered. Administer antibiotics as ordered.	Temperature will be >97, $< 101.5°$ F. WBC will be > 5000 and $< 25,000/mm^3$. Wounds will show beefy-red granulation tissue. Mucous membranes will be pink, moist, intact. Sutured areas will be intact. No redness or purulent drainage will be evident from invasive catheters.

COMPETENCIES
The following clinical competencies pertain to **critical care for the patient with trauma injury.**

☑ *Perform continuous assessment of trauma patients to evaluate effectiveness of interventions to detect complications.*

☑ *Coordinate multidisciplinary services to improve patient outcomes.*

☑ *Include patient's family in the delivery of health services.*

☑ *Apply nursing process in meeting family members' needs.*

☑ *Promote nursing standards of care for the trauma patient.*

☑ *Evaluate the impact of intensive care services on trauma patient outcomes.*

CASE STUDY A.B. is a 17-year-old male who was involved in a single-car MVC. He was brought by ambulance to the nearest ED. On arrival, his BP is 120/60; HR, 90; RR, 44; and T, 98° F. His Glasgow coma scale score is 13. His injuries include closed head injury (mild), multiple facial fractures, bilateral rib fractures (4 through 7), bilateral pulmonary contusions, bilateral hemopneumothoraces, and a right femur fracture. Bilateral chest tubes are placed, and his femur fracture is reduced. He is transferred to the ICU for observation.

During the 12 hours after ICU admission, A.B.'s respiratory status continues to decline. He is complaining of difficulty breathing because of the pain of the rib fractures. His respirations are 46/min, and ABGs show a respiratory alkalosis. A.B. is intubated at this time. An epidural PCA catheter is placed for pain management. His ABGs and respiratory status improve after intubation.

Twenty-four hours after admission, A.B. is scheduled for a follow-up CT scan of his head. How will this impact on the nursing care A.B. will receive?

Transporting A.B. out of the ICU may present additional risks. The nurse should anticipate that she and A.B. will be out of the unit for longer than 1 hour. The nurse will review the nursing interventions and treatments scheduled during this time and complete them before transport (e.g., I&O, suctioning, dressing changes). The nurse brings the medications that will be due during the time away from the unit. A transport monitor will be needed to display ECG, arterial BP, and pulse oximetry. An emergency medication transport box is taken also. The nurse then locates at least three people who will be able to help with transporting A.B. to the radiology department. During transport and during the CT scan, the nurse anticipates changes in A.B.'s VS, including changes in BP, HR, RR, and possible oxygen desaturation.

While away from the ICU, the nurse tries to ensure that A.B. receives monitoring and support as equally intensive as that which he received in the ICU.

A.B.'s respiratory status continues to deteriorate. He continues to have a marked respiratory acidosis with worsening hypoxia. He has required increasing amounts of FIO_2 and PEEP to correct his hypoxia. The high levels of PEEP have caused significant barotrauma, necessitating six chest tubes. On ICU day 7, his ABGs are as follows: pH, 7.28; $\acute{P}CO_2$, 50 mm Hg; PO_2, 60 mm Hg; HCO_3, 28 mEq/L; Pao_2, 80%; on the following ventilator settings: FIO_2, 80%; TV, 1000 ml; IMV, rate 12; PEEP, 20 cm H_2O; and pressure support, 20. His pulmonary compliance is 16%, and peak airway pressures are 60. He has sustained another pneumothorax and now requires a seventh chest tube. At this point the physician decides to place A.B. on high-frequency jet ventilation (HFJV). How will this impact the nursing care A.B. receives?

The ICU nurse knows that HFJV will deliver a small volume of gas delivered at rates of 100 to 600 breaths per minute. The physician orders a TV of 200 with a rate of 120. The ICU nurse notifies the respiratory therapist to place the jet injector on the ventilator. The nurse prepares for reintubation of A.B. with the HFJV endotracheal tube. A.B. is reintubated successfully and the jet ventilator is applied. When assessing the impact of HFJV on A.B.'s cardiovascular status, the nurse notes that his cardiac output has increased. This is because the HFJV lowers transpulmonary pressures. When A.B.'s conventional mechanical ventilator settings include 20 of PEEP, the nurse assesses his lung sounds hourly because he is at an increased risk for barotrauma. While the patient is on the HFJV, the nurse knows that the risks of further barotrauma have decreased. Assessing his breath sounds will now be difficult because of the turbulent gas flow. The nurse must now take A.B. off the ventilator and have another person manually ventilate him while breath sounds are assessed. Because ABGs are costly and therefore used judiciously, the nurse attaches pulse oximetry and an end tidal CO_2 monitor to assist in monitoring gas diffusion and oxygen delivery.

RESEARCH QUESTIONS

As trauma nursing becomes a more widely recognized specialty, trauma nursing research will begin to receive concerted attention to develop a research-based nursing practice (Smeltzer, 1988). Unfortunately, the care of the trauma patient in the ICU is based on rituals, intuition, and traditions learned from caring for other types of critically ill patients. ICU nurses across the country need to participate in research to develop a scientific basis for care of the trauma patient in the ICU. The trauma patient in the ICU presents an abundance of questions in need of research.

Monitoring Ongoing Assessment

- What are the risks of transporting the trauma patient from the ICU for diagnostic tests?
- What are the effects of nursing care on other patients in the ICU when a nurse leaves the unit to transport a patient to diagnostic tests?
- What are "normal" hemodynamic parameters for the trauma patient in the ICU?
- How reliable and valid are hemodynamic waveform analyses made by ICU nurses caring for trauma patients?
- What are the most common "missed injuries" identified by the ICU nurse?

Nursing Care Delivery and Patient Recovery

- How much and for how long do trauma patients remember their ICU stay?
- What nursing interventions are most effective in protecting ICU trauma patients during substance abuse withdrawals?

Families in Crisis as a Result of Multiple Trauma

- What types of visiting policies promote satisfaction for ICU nurses caring for trauma patients?

Physical, Personal, and Cognitive Demands Placed On the ICU Nurse

- How does the day-to-day exposure to trauma crises affect ICU nurses?
- Is the CISD program effective in alleviating

acute stress responses in ICU nurses caring for trauma patients?
- What type of orientation program is most effective in terms of cost, safety, and long-term retention of ICU nurses caring for trauma patients?
- What are the personality characteristics of ICU nurses who care for trauma patients?

ICU Environment

- What nursing interventions are most effective in preventing ICU psychosis in the trauma patient?
- What nursing interventions prevent, reduce, or alleviate the impact the ICU environment has on trauma patients' psychologic stability and recovery?
- What effect does purposeful touch, music, or a soothing voice have on a trauma patient in the ICU?

Ethical Dilemmas

- What types of staff development programs are most effective in preparing the ICU nurse to cope with ethical dilemmas surrounding care of the trauma patient in the ICU?
- What guidelines may be most effective for dealing with ethical dilemmas that ICU nurses encounter in caring for trauma patients?

Technologic Developments

- What effect does range of motion in the ICU have on successful rehabilitation of patients with extremity trauma?
- What is the cost of ICU care for the trauma patient?
- What nursing interventions in the ICU enhance cost containment in the care of the trauma patient?
- How can collaborative practice in the ICU be facilitated and coordinated to positively affect trauma patient outcome?
- What ICU nursing interventions make an impact on trauma patient's physical and psychologic well-being?

ANNOTATED BIBLIOGRAPHY

Norwood, S.H. (1987). ICU management of the trauma patient. Part II. *Current Reviews in Respiratory and Critical Care, 10*(2), 11-16.
Excellent overview of the cardiovascular, renal, and neurologic care frequently required by trauma patients in the ICU.

Paul, B.K., & Savino, J.A. (1987). General monitoring techniques in the trauma patient. *Trauma Quarterly*, 3(3), 1-12.
> *Article that describes the monitoring techniques used in the care of the trauma patient in the ICU, including history, physical examination, laboratory data, radiographic examination, and noninvasive and invasive monitoring.*

Schlump-Urquhart, S.R. (1990). Families experiencing a traumatic accident: Implications and nursing management. *AACN Clinical Issues*, 1(3), 522-534.
> *Article that discusses the psychosocial impact of traumatic events on families and identifies strategies for critical care nurses to meet families' psychosocial needs.*

Von Reuden, K.T. (1991). The physical, personal and cognitive demands of trauma nursing. *Critical Care Nurse*, 11(6), 9.
> *Editorial that aptly describes the demands of nurses caring for critically ill trauma patients.*

Whitehorne, M., Cacciola, R., & Quinn, M.E. (1989). Multiple trauma: Survival after the golden hour. *Journal of Advanced Medical Surgical Nursing*, 2(1), 27-39.
> *Article that discusses critical care of the trauma patient and how the actual trauma resuscitation in the ED affects survival. A case study is used to emphasize aspects of management from the time of injury to eventual recovery.*

REFERENCES

AACN. (1988a). Position statement: Occupational hazards in critical care. *Focus on Critical Care*, 15(5), 70-71.

AACN. (1988b). Summary analysis of critical care nurse supply and requirement. Newport Beach, CA. Author.

Baggs, J.G. (1989). Intensive care unit use and collaboration between nurses and physicians. *Heart and Lung*, 18(4), 332-338.

Bell, N.K. (1990). Ethical dilemmas in trauma nursing. *Nursing Clinics of North America*, 25 (1), 143-154.

Boettcher, M., & Schiller, W.R. (1990). The use of multidisciplinary group meetings for families of critically ill trauma patients. *Intensive Care Nursing*, 6, 129-137.

Boggs, R.L. (1989). Multiple system trauma: Nursing implications. *Journal of Advanced Medical Surgical Nursing*, 2(1), 1-6.

Borozny, M. (1990). The experience of intensive care unit nurses providing care to the brain dead patient. *AXON*, September, 18-22.

Bozzett, F.W., & Gibbons, R. (1983). The nursing management of families in the critical care setting. *Critical Care Update*, 10, 22-77.

Brown, C. (1983). The alcohol withdrawl syndrome. *Western Journal of Medicine*, 138(4), 579-581.

Bubulka, G.M. (1990). Trauma patient reported recall. *Point of View*, 27(3), 6-7.

Burns, S.M. (1990). Advances in ventilator therapy. *Focus on Critical Care*, 17(3), 227-237.

Butkus, D.E. (1983). Persistent high mortality in acute renal failure. *Archives of Internal Medicine*, 143, 209-211.

Caine, R.M. (1989). Families in crisis: Making the critical difference. *Focus on Critical Care*, 16(3), 184-189.

Cardona, V.D. (1986). Nursing practice through the cycles of trauma. In V.D. Cardona, P.D. Hurn, A.J. Mason, & A. Scanlon-Schlipp (Eds.), *Trauma nursing: From resuscitation to rehabilitation*. Philadelphia: W.B. Saunders.

Chamel, E., & Maddox, J. (1988). Visiting in the ICU: Time for a change. *Critical Care Nurse*, 8(6), 2-3, 12.

Chyun, D. (1989). Patients' perceptions of stressors in intensive care and coronary care units. *Focus on Critical Care*, 16(3), 206-211.

Cochran, J, & Ganong, L.H. (1989). A comparison of nurses' and patients' perceptions of intensive care unit stressors. *Journal of Advanced Nursing*, 14, 1038-1043.

Compton, P. (1991). Critical illness and intensive care: What it means to the client. *Critical Care Nurse*, 11(1), 50-56.

Conn, A.K. & McCabe, C.J. (1989). New developments in trauma care systems. *Emergency Care Quarterly*, 5(2), 75-80.

Coulter, M.A. (1989). The needs of family members of patients in intensive care units. *Intensive Care Nursing*, 5, 4-10.

Craig, M.C., Copes, W.S., & Champion, H.R. (1988). Psychosocial considerations in trauma care. *Critical Care Nursing Quarterly*, 11(2), 51-58.

Daley, L. (1984). The perceived immediate needs of families with relatives in the intensive care unit. *Heart and Lung*, 13, 231-237.

Dirkes, S.M. (1989). Making a critical difference with CAVH. *Nursing '89*, 19 (11), 57-60.

Dockter, B., Black, D.R., Hovel, M.F., Engleberg, D., Amick, T., Neimier, D., & Sheet, N. (1988). Families and intensive care nurses: Comparison of perceptions. *Patient Education and Counseling*, 12, 29-36.

Epperson, M.M. (1977) Families in sudden crisis: Process and interventions in a critical care center. *Social Work in Health Care*, 2, 267-273.

Figley, C.R. (1983). Catastrophes: An overview of family reactions. In C.R. Figley and H.I. McCubbin (Eds.). *Stress and the family. Vol II. Coping with catastrophe*. New York: Brunner/Mazel.

Fontaine, D.K. (1989). Physical, personal and cognitive responses to trauma. *Critical Care Nursing Clinics of North America*, 1(1), 11-22.

Forrester, D.A., Murphy, P.A., Price, D.M., & Monaghan, J.F. (1990). Critical care family needs: Nurse-family member confederate pairs. *Heart and Lung*, 19 (6), 655-661.

Garg, V., Peck, M., & Savino, J.A. (1987). Respiratory monitoring in trauma. *Trauma Quarterly*, 3(3), 32-44.

Goins, W.A., Reynolds, H.N., Nyanjom, D., & Dunham, C.M. (1991). Outcome following prolonged intensive care unit stay in multiple trauma patients. *Critical Care Medicine*, 19(3), 339-345.

Gowen, N.J. (1979). The perceptual world of the ICU: An overview of environmental considerations in the helping relationship. *Heart and Lung*, 8, 340-344.

Halm, M.A., & Titler, M.G. (1990). Appropriateness of critical care visitation: Perceptions of patients, families, nurses and physicians. *Journal of Nursing Quality Assurance*, 5(1), 25-37.

Harris, J.S. (1984). Stressors and stress in critical care. *Critical Care Nurse*, 4, 84-97.

Heater, B.S. (1985). Nursing responsibilities in changing visiting policies in the intensive care unit. *Heart and Lung*, 3, 181-186.

Hogan, B.S. (1990). Caring for trauma victims: The emotional impact. *AACN Clinical Issues*, 1(3), 495-504.

Indeck, M., Peterson, S., Smith, J., & Brotman, S. (1988)

Risk, cost, and benefit of transporting ICU patients for special studies. *Journal of Trauma*, 28 (7), 1020-1025.

Insel, J., Weissman, C., Kemper, M., Askanazi, J., & Hyman, A. (1986). Cardiovascular changes during transport of critically ill and postoperative patients. *Critical Care Medicine*, 14(6), 539-542.

Johnson, S., & Kent, M. (1987). Noise in the recovery room and ICU. *Current Reviews in Respiratory and Critical Care*, 10(5), 35-38.

Kelly, F.M. (1986). Caring for the patient in acute alcohol withdrawl. *Critical Care Quarterly*, 8(4), 11-19.

Kennerly, S.M. (1990). Imperatives for the future of critical care nursing. *Focus on Critical Care*, 17(2), 123-127.

Kleck, H. (1984). ICU syndrome: Onset, manifestations, treatment, stressors and prevention. *Critical Care Quarterly*, 6, 21-28.

Kleeman, K.M. (1989). Families in crisis due to multiple trauma. *Critical Care Nursing Clinics of North America*, 1(1), 23-31.

Kloosterman, N.D. (1991). Cultural care: The missing link in severe sensory alteration. *Nursing Science Quarterly*, 4(3), 119-122.

Krozek, C.F. (1991). Helping stressed families in an ICU. *Nursing '91*, 21 (1), 52-57.

Langdale, L., & Schecter, W.P. (1986). Critical care implications in the trauma patient. *Critical Care Clinics*, 2(4), 839-852.

Lenehan, G.P. (1986). Emotional impact of trauma. *Nursing Clinics of North America*, 21(4), 729-740.

Leske, J.S. (1986). Needs of relatives of critically ill patients: A follow up. *Heart and Lung*, 15, 189-193.

Levine, C.D., Wilson, S.F., & Guido, G.W. (1988). Personality factors of critical care nurses. *Heart and Lung*, 17(4), 392-398.

Martin, M.T. (1988). Wound management and infection control after trauma: Implications for the intensive care setting. *Critical Care Nursing Quarterly*, 11(2), 43-49.

Matteson, B.I. (1975). Psychological aspects of severe injury and its treatment, *Journal of Trauma*, 155, 217-223.

Meehan, P.A. (1987). Neurologic monitoring in trauma. *Trauma Quarterly*, 3(3), 57-63.

Meyer, A.A., & Trunkey, D.D. (1986). Critical care as an integral part of trauma care. *Critical Care Clinics*, 2(4), 673-681.

Mitchell, J.T. (1983). When disaster strikes. *Journal of Emergency Medical Services*, 8, 36-39.

Mlynczak, B. (1989). Assessment and management of the trauma patient in pain. *Critical Care Clinics of North America*, 1(1), 55-65.

Molter, N.C. (1979). Needs of relatives of critically ill patients: A descriptive study. *Heart and Lung*, 8, 332-339.

Muñoz, E., Josephson, J., Tenenbaum, N., Goldstein, J., Shears, A.M., & Wise, L. (1989). Diagnosis related groups, costs and outcome for patients in the intensive care unit. *Heart and Lung*, 18(6), 627-633.

National Institutes of Health: Consensus conference on critical care medicine. (1983). *Journal of the American Medical Association*, 250, 798-804.

National Joint Practice Commission. (1981). *Guidelines for Establishing Joint or Collaborative Practice in Hospitals.* Chicago: The Commission.

National Research Council and Institute of Medicine, Committee on Trauma Research, Commission on Life Sciences. (1985). *Injury in America: A continuing health problem*. (1985). Washington, DC: National Academy Press.

Noble, M.A. (1982). *The ICU environment: Directions for nursing*. Reston, VA: Reston Publishing.

Norwood, S.H. (1987a). ICU management of the trauma patient: Part I. *Current Reviews in Respiratory and Critical Care*, 10 (1), 3-8.

Norwood, S.H. (1987b). ICU management of the trauma patient: Part II. *Current Reviews in Respiratory and Critical Care*, 10(2), 11-16.

O'Grady, T.P. (1987). Participatory management: The critical care nurse's role in the 21st century. *Dimensions in Critical Care Nursing*, 6(3), 131-133.

Paino, J.R., Teres, D., Lemeshow, S., & Brown, B.B. (1982). Hospital charges and long-term survival of ICU versus non-ICU patients. *Critical Care Medicine*, 10, 569-574.

Palmer, J.C., Koorejian, K., London, J.B., Dechert, R.E., & Bartlett, R.H. (1986). Nursing management of continuous arteriovenous hemofiltration for acute renal failure. *Focus on Critical Care*, 13, 21-30.

Paradiso, C. (1989). Hemofiltration: An alternative to dialysis. *Heart and Lung*, 18(3), 282-290.

Parker, M.M., Schubert, W., Shelhamer, J.H., & Parrillo, J.E. (1984). Perceptions of a critically ill patient experiencing therapeutic paralysis in an ICU. *Critical Care Medicine*, 12(1), 69-71.

Paul, B.K., & Savino, J.A. (1987). General monitoring techniques in the trauma patient. *Trauma Quarterly*, 3(3), 1-12.

President's Commission for the Study of Ethical Problems in Medicine and Biomedical and Behavioral Research. (1981). Guidelines for the Determination of Brain Death. *Journal of the American Medical Association*, 246, 2184.

Price, C.A. (1989). Continuous arteriovenous ultrafiltration: A monitoring guide for ICU nurse. *Critical Care Nurse*, 9(1), 12-19.

Savino, J.A. (1987). Hemodynamic monitoring in trauma. *Trauma Quarterly*, 3(3), 13-31.

Scalea, T.M., Phillips, T.F., Goldstein, A.S., Scalfani, S.J., & Duncan, A.D. (1987). Renal monitoring in trauma. *Trauma Quarterly*, 3(3), 46-56.

Schaefer, S. (1989). Patient advocacy: An ethical dilemma? *Focus on Critical Care*, 16(3), 191-192.

Schlump-Urquhart, S.R. (1990). Families experiencing a traumatic accident: Implications and nursing management. *AACN Clinical Issues*, 1(3), 522-534.

Schmidt, C.W. (1985). Psychiatric management of acute trauma. In G.D. Zuidema, R.B. Rutherford, and W.F. Ballinger (Eds.), *The Management of Trauma* (4th ed.). Philadelphia: W.B. Saunders.

Schnaper, H. (1975). The psychological implications of severe trauma: Emotional sequelae to unconsciousness. *Journal of Trauma*, 15(2), 94-98.

Simmons, R.L., Migliori, R.J., Smith C.R., Reemtsma, K., & Najarian, J.S. (1989). Transplantation. In S.I. Schwartz (Ed.), *Principles of Surgery* (5th ed.). New York: McGraw-Hill.

Sinclair, V. (1988). High technology in critical care: Implications for nursings' role and practice. *Focus on Critical Care, 15*(4), 36-41.

Smeltzer, S. (1988). Research in trauma nursing: State of the art and future directions. *Journal of Emergency Nursing, 14,* 145-153.

Smith, L.G., & Glowac, B.S. (1989). New frontiers in the management of multiply injured patients. *Critical Care Nursing Clinics of North America, 1*(1), 1-9.

Solursh, D.S. (1990). The family of the trauma victim. *Nursing Clinics of North America, 25*(1), 155-162.

Stephenson, C. (1977). Stress in critically ill patients. *American Journal of Nursing, 77,* 1806-1809.

Stillwell, S.B. (1984). Importance of visiting as perceived by family members of patients in the ICU. *Heart and Lung, 13,* 238-242.

Teres, D., Dawson, J.A., Roberts, C., & McDonald, W.A. (1989). *Indications for neuromuscular blockade in the intensive care unit.* West Orange, NJ: Health Education Technologies.

Trujillo, M.H., & Bellorin-Font, E. (1990). Drugs commonly administered by intravenous infusion in intensive care units: A practical guide. *Critical Care Medicine, 18*(2), 232-238.

Von Reuden, K.T. (1989). Cardiopulmonary assessment of the critically ill trauma patient. *Critical Care Nursing Clinics of North America, 1*(1), 33-44.

Von Reuden, K.T. (1991). The physical, personal and cognitive demands of trauma nursing. *Critical Care Nurse, 11*(6), 9.

Wagner, D.P., Wineland, T.D., & Knaus, W.A. (1983). The hidden costs of treating severely ill patients: Charges and resource consumption in an intensive care unit. *Health Care Financing, 5,* 81-86.

Walker, E.A. (1979). Advances in the determination of cerebral death. In R.A. Thompson and J.R. Green (Eds). *Advances in neurology: Complications of nervous system trauma* (Vol. 22) (pp 167-177). New York: Raven Press.

White, S.K. (1989). Bringing out the best in all of us. *Heart and Lung, 18*(6), 27A-30A.

Whitehorne, M., Cacciola, R., & Quinn, M.E. (1989). Multiple trauma: Survival after the golden hour. *Journal of Advanced Medical Surgical Nursing, 2*(1), 27-39.

Widra, L., & Pence, G. (1988). Ethical considerations. In E. Howel, L. Wildra, & M.G. Hill (Eds.), *Comprehensive trauma nursing: Theory and practice* (pp. 887-902). Glenview, IL: Scott, Foresman.

Williams, M.A. (1989). Physical environment of the intensive care unit and elderly patients. *Critical Care Nursing Quarterly, 12*(1), 52-60.

Zabourek, R.P. (1986). Identification of the alcoholic in the acute care setting. *Critical Care Quarterly, 8*(4), 1-10.

24 *Rehabilitation of the Trauma Patient*

■■

Karma Klauber

OBJECTIVES

❏ *Identify three mechanisms of injury that have potential for causing severe functional deficits and long-term disability.*

❏ *Differentiate between impairment, disability, and handicap.*

❏ *Recognize components of trauma nursing in the emergency and intensive care phases that contribute to outcome of persons with disabilities.*

❏ *Recognize the continuum of rehabilitation services and delivery systems required to maximize the recovery potential of a person with a head injury.*

❏ *Determine the rehabilitation focus of spinal cord injury care in the emergency and intensive care phases of recovery.*

INTRODUCTION The advanced technology of trauma care, coupled with the sophisticated communication systems that allow for rapid evacuation of trauma victims from accident scenes, has decreased mortality and created a population of seriously injured patients that did not exist 10 to 15 years ago (Haller & Buck, 1985; Klauber, Barrett-Connor, Hofstetter, & Micik, 1986; Silverstein & Lack, 1987). Human life changes with severe injury. Dramatic permanent alterations in the injured person's life-style and ability to function occur in many instances. Families and friends are impacted significantly. Roles change and life goals are put on hold or change directions, and relationships develop a different focus. *Trauma rehabilitation* is a broad term that is defined as the extensive process of helping injured individuals facilitate movement toward health and regain functional abilities. Rehabilitation is not a place, but a dynamic process of planned adaptive change that is imposed on the individual by the traumatic incident. The focus is not on cure, but on living with as much freedom and autonomy as possible at every stage in whichever direction the disability progresses.

Rehabilitation is recognized as a critical primary component in the designation of trauma centers in model systems of trauma care (American College of Surgeons, Committee on Trauma, 1986; Mansoory, 1986). Trauma nurses across the continuum of recovery contribute to and facilitate the long process of rehabilitation. Rehabilitation is an important component of nursing practice overall. It is also an area of specialized practice that is implemented within focused rehabilitation settings. It is difficult to concentrate on and fathom the long-term aspects and impact of the traumatic injury at the initial scene and emergency care stage. However, understanding the broad perspective of the recovery process after traumatic injury is essential. This understanding serves to enhance the skills of the trauma nurse in these early stages by recognizing the impact that early care and treatment have on the ultimate outcome of the injured person.

CASE STUDY Julie is a 22-year-old woman brought to the emergency department (ED) via helicopter after a motor vehicle crash. Her initial Glasgow coma scale

707

score is 6. BP is 96/60; HR, 120; and R, 28 and labored.

What clinical or diagnostic indicators can be used to most accurately predict head injury outcome in Julie's case?

The initial Glasgow coma scale score and posttraumatic amnesia are fairly strong predictors of outcome. The degree of brain stem injury, as demonstrated by ocular reflexes and auditory evoked responses, is also used as a strong predictor.

After initial stabilization in the ED and ruling out intracranial hematomas requiring surgical evacuation, Julie is transferred to the neurologic intensive care unit. What are the primary rehabilitation goals in this phase of care?

The two major focuses of rehabilitation in the critical care phase are eliciting meaningful responses from the patient and minimizing the potential for alterations in mobility and skin integrity.

SCOPE AND PHILOSOPHY OF REHABILITATION

Disability and chronic illness affect the physical, emotional, social, economic, and vocational status of individuals and their families. Severe traumatic injuries create disabled individuals and impact these broad functional areas. As a result, functional limitations and losses occur and changes in life-style often become necessary.

Rehabilitation is the process of maximizing the use of an individual's capabilities or resources to foster optimal growth and functioning. Rehabilitation is not an "end product" that comes after emergency care, intensive care, and acute care, but an integral part of all phases of care. If rehabilitation is viewed as "what comes after" other phases of care, the concept of illness to the injured person and family can be exaggerated. Elements of rehabilitation are begun from the onset of injury and focus throughout the recovery process on assisting the injured individual to maximize functioning and to begin the adjustment process to an altered self-concept and functional ability.

Impairment, Disability, and Handicap

The World Health Organization (1980) has outlined definitions and characteristics of conceptual differences between impairment, disability, and handicap.

An *impairment* refers to the loss or abnormality of psychologic, physiologic, or anatomic structure or function. Impairment reflects disturbances at the level of the organ.

Disability is any restriction or lack of ability to perform an activity in a manner or a range considered normal for a human being. Disability is concerned with abilities, in the form of composite activities and behaviors that are generally accepted as essential components of everyday life.

Handicap refers to a disadvantage for a given individual, resulting from an impairment or disability, that prevents the fulfillment of a role that is normal for that individual. Handicap is characterized by a discordance between the individual's performance or status and the expectations of the individual himself or of the particular group of which he is a member. It is the socialization of an impairment or disability. It reflects the consequences of impairment or disability for the individual from a broader societal perspective.

To illustrate the differences in the terms, consider a 27-year-old woman who sustained second- and third-degree burns to her face, upper trunk, and proximal arms. She received excellent burn care and rehabilitation and has minimal contractures that impact her functionally. She does remain with the characteristic scarring and discoloration of skin of the burned areas. Before her injury she worked as a flight attendant for a major airline. She greatly desires to return to her previous position, but her employer is reluctant to rehire her because of her changed appearance. This woman has an impairment in her integumentary system characterized by scarring of the burned areas. However, she does not have a disability. She can perform all of the functions she could before the burn injury. The impairment does, however, create a handicap for her because now she cannot perform a role that was normal for her. The handicap is imposed by societal values and reactions to an individual's facial appearance. The expected norms for someone in a public service position, such as flight attendant, are to be pleasing in appearance and not to have an obvious facial deformity.

Perceptions of disability

Wright (1960) emphasized the danger of shortcuts in language when referring to persons with disabling conditions. She supports using the slightly more involved expression of "a person with a disability" rather than stating "disabled person" or using the person's disability as a label, such as "quadriplegic" or "quad." This more positively stated format connotes that a person with a disability is first a person with many unspecified characteristics, in addition to a particular disability.

This perspective is one that applies to the healthcare field in general. For efficient communication, healthcare professionals often use "shorthand" labels to describe individuals with conditions and disease processes. Language is a powerful communicator of attitudes and perceptions. The reference to people as disease processes has the potential of communicating a devaluing statement to the persons who receive health care.

How visible a particular impairment or disability is becomes a contributing factor to societal response to an individual with the disability. Goffman (1963) refers to these visible characteristics as "stigma symbols." A person with a physical disability that is readily identified because of the use of a walker or wheelchair has a difficult time concealing the fact that he has the disability. Those with cognitive disabilities have a less difficult time passing as nondisabled individuals. The more visible the difference, the more information is available about the person's social identity. How that information is interpreted will depend on whether those observing know anything about the individual or the observable impairment. The obtrusiveness of the impairment and how it interferes with the flow of the interaction are other factors that impact society's reactions. Preconceived ideas about a visible impairment or disability also contribute to societal reactions (Goffman, 1963).

Spread is an important concept that is related to society's perception of an individual with an impairment or disability. Spread refers to the perception that if one disability is present, others must exist. For example, in meeting a person who is blind, one might assume that he or she also cannot hear. Often an individual with a physical disability is perceived as having a mental disability as well (Wright, 1960).

Trauma nurses and other specialists in the field of acute care and trauma rehabilitation are encouraged to honestly evaluate their own reactions to persons with disabilities. To facilitate optimal adjustment in the patient, this awareness from the interacting professionals can enhance the learning process of rehabilitation.

Basic Assumptions

Several basic beliefs about human beings contribute to the overall philosophy of rehabilitation:

- Each individual is a unique and complex being with unique assets, coping abilities, and goals.
- Each individual is valued and is deserving of respect and dignity.
- Each individual has the potential to regain self-esteem and has potential for growth.
- Each individual must satisfy many needs to enjoy and experience life.
- Individuals have in common the uniquely human need to hope.
- Each individual is whole and cannot be divided into parts.
- Each individual functions interdependently with the environment.

Basic Principles

Rehabilitation practice is based on a thorough assessment of the individual's abilities and life-style before the onset of the disabling condition, as well as the individual's current functional abilities. Rehabilitation focuses on the strengths and abilities the individual currently displays and which components of these abilities may be used to compensate for the limitations present. Approaching the process in a goal-oriented fashion assists the disabled individual, the family, and the professionals to measure progress and focus on movement toward independence in a manageable way. Rehabilitation planning is a dynamic process that involves the active participation of the individual and family. Quality of life is a central focus. It is critical that this be defined by the individual and family themselves and not from the perspective of the professionals. Rehabilitation promotes self-determination and self-responsibility. It is a dynamic learning process that focuses on the "why and how to" of change and adaptation to functional limitations, not on "doing for" the person. It involves facilitating the development of new or modified behaviors. The broad target goal is on preparing the person with the disability to return or move into a functional role within the family and community setting. In all settings and phases of the rehabilitation process, principles of treatment that prevent secondary disability are incorporated. Examples of secondary disabilities are (1) further limitations in mobility as a result of joint contractures and (2) pressure sores that further compromise skin integrity.

The long process of rehabilitation requires a balance between dependence and independence. Breaking down functional goals and objectives into measurable, manageable components is a key approach to achieving this balance. Creative problem solving, with an emphasis on flexibility and innovation, combined with common sense is a critical tool in rehabilitation. Interweaving psychologic adjustment issues and the disabled person's attitudes toward a changed life-style is an inherent treatment objective in the rehabilitation process. Rehabilitation is incorporating and adjusting to change.

Because of its broad and varied nature, rehabilitation requires a team approach. The needs of persons with impairments and disabilities are great, and many specialty areas are called on to contribute to the process. It has been an established practice of rehabilitation disciplines to work together to meet the physical, emotional, social, economic, and vocational needs of these individuals and their families.

The Rehabilitation Team

Ducanis & Golin (1979) outline the characteristics of a healthcare team. A team consists of two or more individuals. There is an identifiable leader, although the leader may shift. Teams function both within and among organizational settings. Roles of team members are defined according to the competencies of the team members, and collaboration occurs among team members. Specific protocols for operation assist in the accomplishment of tasks. Teams are patient-centered; that is, they function for the purpose of the patient and are task-oriented.

The concept of healthcare service delivery by way of a team approach is certainly not a concept unique to rehabilitation. Most forms of health care requiring the expertise of more than one provider typically use a multidisciplinary approach. Trauma teams are an excellent example of a highly orchestrated and highly skilled group of professionals who perform well-defined roles within the context of the trauma resuscitation room. In rehabilitation, providing services is em-

Table 24-1 Characteristics of multidisciplinary and interdisciplinary teams

Multidisciplinary	Interdisciplinary
Members of various disciplines	Members of various disciplines
Discipline-specific goals	Patient-oriented goals
Patient considered the recipient of care; not as significant contributor to goals and plan	Patient and family are core team members and contribute significantly to the goals and plan
Members primarily aware of and focus on their own individual goals	Members aware of all goals and actively work on all goals, as able
More limited communication and planning as a whole team	Extensive communication and planning as a whole team
Role definitions highly structured and usually less flexible	Role definitions structured, but remain more flexible to meet fluctuating needs of patient and team
Little cross-training of skills from one discipline to another	Extensive cross-training of skills from one discipline to another

Note. From "Informed Consent and Provider-Patient Relationships in Rehabilitation Medicine by A.L. Caplan, 1988, *Archives of Physical Medicine and Rehabilitating, 69*(5) pp. 312-317, and from "Ethical Issues in Teamwork: The Context of Rehabilitation" by R.B. Purtilo, 1988, *Archives of Physical Medicine and Rehabilitation, 69*(5), pp. 318-322.

phasized through the use of an interdisciplinary team approach rather than a multidisciplinary one. The characteristics of an interdisciplinary team approach are believed to promote a patient outcome in which the total is greater than the sum of its parts.

Table 24-1 compares and contrasts the characteristics of the two approaches.

Members of the rehabilitation team vary, depending on the needs of the patient and the setting in which the rehabilitation program is implemented. Members of the rehabilitation team who are typically involved in the intensive care and acute phases of recovery include physicians, nurses, physical therapists, occupational therapists, speech/language pathologists, nutritionists, psychologists, and social workers. Other team members may be added as patients' needs change, serving members of the core team or in consultant roles. They include the recreation therapist, audiologist, rehabilitation engineer, prosthetist, orthotist, vocational rehabilitation counselor, and clergy. Within the acute rehabilitation hospital or center setting, the members remain consistent with those who may be involved in the earlier recovery stages. However, the recreation therapist and vocational counselor are more likely to become more actively involved in the rehabilitation plan as the focus begins to shift to the development of leisure and vocational goals. In addition, within the rehabilitation center or hospital setting, rehabilitation nurses who are specifically trained in the care and rehabilitation process of persons with disability provide the nursing care.

Although rehabilitation principles and techniques are incorporated in all recovery phases of traumatic survivors, the emphasis within the focused rehabilitation setting is on improving and maximizing functional abilities through facilitation and restoration techniques or by teaching compensatory strategies that bypass limitations and promote functional performance. All team members contribute to and focus on treatment that promotes movement toward independence.

REHABILITATION CONTINUUM

The phases of recovery and rehabilitation after a severe traumatic injury can be divided into four broad categories: (1) emergency and intensive care; (2) acute care; (3) acute rehabilitation care; and (4) post-acute rehabilitation. The majority of individuals who survive severe trauma will require treatment in each of the four phases. The extent and type of rehabilitation within each phase will depend on the system affected and the severity of involvement.

Emergency and Intensive Care

Components of rehabilitation within the emergency and intensive care phases of the treatment of trauma victims focus on initial stabilization of the primary disability and prevention of secondary disability.

Acute Care

The acute care phase typically begins when the critical physiologic abnormalities have stabilized and the patient is moved from the intensive care

unit to the medical or surgical floor. Along with continuing treatment of the disruption of body systems, the focus gradually increases on the treatment of basic functional deficits that prevent an individual from living independently. This phase of treatment has been significantly shortened in recent years with the advent of prospective payment and the deemphasis on in-patient hospital care. The prevention of secondary disability is incorporated into this and each subsequent phase of rehabilitation.

Acute Rehabilitation

The acute rehabilitation stage is marked by the patient's movement to a structured rehabilitation setting. These exist as units within general community hospitals or trauma centers, as larger centers affiliated with a hospital, or as freestanding rehabilitation centers. The movement of a patient to a focused rehabilitation setting means that the primary focus of treatment is on improving functional abilities and facilitating the patient's adjustment to a changed self-concept. Acute rehabilitation settings focus primarily on improving basic self-care skills, such as mobility, elimination management, personal hygiene, feeding and swallowing, dressing, basic communication skills, and behavioral control issues. Most patients transferred to acute or in-patient rehabilitation programs have deficits in three or more of these functional areas. Teaching includes patient and family to facilitate recovery from injuries and a safe discharge to home (Figure 24-1).

Post-Acute Rehabilitation

Patients who are independent in basic self-care and those who make significant gains in acute rehabilitation are often treated in a post-acute rehabilitation setting. The design and services offered in post-acute rehabilitation are extremely varied and are driven by the specific disability population served. Out-patient rehabilitation is a more traditional and longer-standing model for service delivery. Patients return to a clinic setting to receive isolated rehabilitation services from individual discipline providers for fairly targeted functional areas. Treatment sessions are typically provided in hourly sessions two to five times per week. This form of rehabilitation lends itself to the treatment of physical disabilities, but is less effective for multiple disabilities and those disabili-

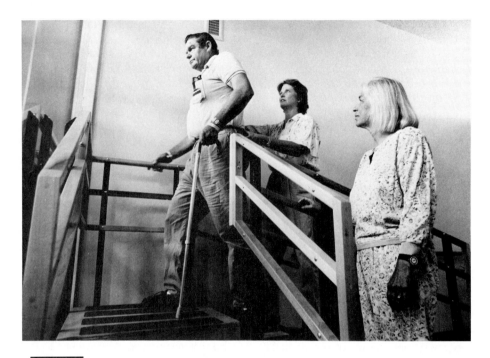

Figure 24-1   Safety training in use of cane for stair climbing and descent. Spouse or significant other should be instructed as well, and should participate in supervising and assisting patient. Critical goal in the case illustrated was for patient to be able to negotiate 40 steps to his mobile home. (*Note:* Photograph by Renee Burgard, Stanford University Hospital.)

ties that involve changes in cognition and behavior.

Day treatment programs

Day treatment programs are a relatively new method of rehabilitation service delivery. One impetus for their development was the increasing number of traumatically brain-injured individuals who had difficulty generalizing skills from the more isolated and fragmented services provided in the typical out-patient therapy model (Moore, 1986). Residential programs for the developmentally disabled population have been in existence for many years. The issues are dramatically different for the traumatically injured population as compared with those persons with developmental disabilities. Those with traumatic injuries must relearn skills, often basic ones, that were once second nature. Adjusting self-perceptions and goals in comparison with the functional levels that existed before the injury creates different psychologic adjustment issues. Residential-based pro-

grams for those recovering from traumatic injuries are a relatively recent development. These programs focus on these adjustment issues, as well as community reintegration and vocational goals for the newly disabled individual.

Special programs

Rehabilitation programs geared more specifically to the specialized educational and vocational needs of traumatically injured persons are another type of post-acute rehabilitation service. Public school systems provide special education programs to school-age children, as mandated by public policy. These programs typically group all disabled students together and do not differentiate between developmental disabilities and traumatic injuries. Some community college programs are beginning to address the specific needs of the traumatically disabled population and are developing specialized programs. Most colleges and universities have disabled student services that provide some services and advocacy for disabled students on campus. Vocational training programs targeted at specific disability populations are available in some areas. The rehabilitation program administered by the federal Rehabilitation Services Administration and locally by state departments of rehabilitation provides federal and state funds and services for counseling, training, and education (Bitter, 1979).

Service Delivery Models

A variety of service delivery models are used in rehabilitation. In the acute hospital and rehabilitation phases, most typically the medical model serves to organize the delivery of care. The focus is on the stabilization of illness and injury. Trauma nursing and the medical profession play a strong role in the delivery of care and contribute significantly to the decision-making process. As illness and injury stabilize and persons are left with functional changes that medical treatment cannot address, the medical model becomes less appropriate. Educational and vocational models become more appropriate means of service delivery. The emphasis is removed from the illness and disability itself. The focus is on bringing value to the social role that disabled individuals have in the community and providing culturally normative, age-appropriate activities and training methods to enhance the person's functioning and adjustment (Condeluci & Gretz-Lasky, 1987).

In 1975 and 1976 the model spinal cord injury systems were developed and supported as research and demonstration models by the Rehabilitation Services Administration. These models established a dedicated and coordinated system addressing the specific continuum of needs for the spinal cord–injured population. Seven model systems were developed, and all include a tightly coordinated, effective, field-based emergency medical and in-hospital trauma care capability. It was the first network that identified neurologic trauma of all kinds, including brain trauma. The model systems include the service components of emergency medical services; intensive/acute medical care; comprehensive, coordinated rehabilitation; psychosocial and vocational preparation; and long-term community follow-up. The model systems also include a coordinated, standardized data collection plan to allow for clinical research and epidemiologic studies. Model systems also promote education and training in the specialty

areas served. The improvements noted with the model spinal cord injury systems include a reduction in length of hospital stay, reduced complication rates, increased cost-effectiveness, and increased vocational and social productivity.

The first demonstration projects dedicated to traumatic brain injury were granted in 1978. These included a proposal for an appropriate delivery model for this population. Several research grants have been awarded since that time, and in 1987, five national demonstration projects were initiated for the development of model systems of care for traumatic brain injury. A national data base will be established as part of the research and demonstration activity (Thomas, 1988). The model systems' approach to spinal cord injury care has exemplified the rehabilitation effectiveness and cost-containment that categoric care makes feasible. As cost-effectiveness and clinical outcomes have been demonstrated, support for the system of care concept has increased and components and principles have been adopted in the management of other complex populations.

GENERAL ASSESSMENT: FUNCTIONAL LEVEL

The field of rehabilitation places a significant emphasis on the use of a functional assessment and diagnosis approach (Granger & Gresham, 1984). The language of disability and the terminology commonly used by professionals within the field focus on the functional changes that result from a disabling condition rather than the medical diagnosis. For example, an individual with traumatic spinal cord injury at the thoracic-4 (T4) level would be referred to medically as an individual with complete T4 paraplegia. The cause is important and gives additional information that should be factored into the overall rehabilitation planning process, but the initial consideration is the functional description of the person. *Functional assessment* refers to a method for describing abilities and activities to measure an individual's use of the variety of skills included in performing the tasks necessary for daily living, vocational pursuits, social interactions, leisure activities, and other required behaviors. Many efforts have been made to develop standardized assessment tools that objectively measure the level of performance in a variety of areas (Carey & Posavac, 1977; Katz, Ford, & Moskowitz, 1963; Mahoney &

Barthel, 1965; Schoening, Anderegg, & Bergstrom, 1965). A coordinated national effort to develop a functional assessment scale began in 1983 through the formation of a task force of the multidisciplinary professional organization, the American Congress of Physical Medicine and Rehabilitation, and the American Academy of Physical Medicine and Rehabilitation. The resulting tool is the Functional Independence Measure (FIM) (Task Force for Development of a Uniform Data System for Medical Rehabilitation, 1986). The intent of the FIM is to standardize the measurement of specific functional activities to allow for comparison of change within an individual rehabilitation setting, as well as compare large groups of individuals across centers.

The emphasis on functional assessment and diagnosis within rehabilitation closely parallels the nursing diagnosis framework. The North American Nursing Diagnosis Association (NANDA) uses nursing diagnostic categories (North American Nursing Diagnosis Association, 1988) based on human functioning. Although the terminology used by rehabilitation professionals may differ somewhat from nursing diagnosis terminology, trauma nurses who use nursing diagnoses are more likely to relate to some of the language of rehabilitation. To illustrate, consider an individual with a medical diagnosis of traumatic head injury with a left temporal subdural and intracerebral hematoma. In nursing diagnosis terminology, this person has the following diagnoses:
- Impaired verbal communication
- Impaired physical mobility
- Bathing/hygiene self-care deficit
- Dressing/grooming self-care deficit

Rehabilitation terminology may describe this individual as having the following:
- Impaired communication with receptive aphasia
- Impaired mobility with right hemiplegia
- Impaired self-care skills

Mechanisms of Injury

Trauma has the potential to create a variety of disabling conditions. The disability may be a relatively short-term condition, with functional capabilities temporarily altered and a strong potential for returning to premorbid functioning. Rehabilitation plays a critical role in assisting these individuals to return to a premorbid status. Severe trauma often alters functional abilities in permanent ways. Rehabilitation again plays a critical role in assisting individuals with permanent alterations in abilities to maximize their capabilities. This includes a major emphasis on a gradual psychologic adjustment to a changed self-concept. The remainder of this chapter focuses primarily on the role of trauma rehabilitation in the care of individuals with long-term disability.

ASSESSMENT AND INTERVENTIONS RELATED TO SPECIFIC INJURIES
Sensory/Perceptual Alterations and Responsiveness: Head Injuries

Traumatic injuries to the head and brain are the major cause of alterations in perception and cognition. The majority of injuries involve external trauma to the head. Another cause for alterations in cognition and perception is an injury that alters perfusion. This injury often causes hypoxic or anoxic injury to the brain. Functional changes similar to traumatic head injury can occur. Traumatic head injuries are the third-ranking cause of neurologic impairment and the leading cause of death and disability for individuals younger than 35 years. Twice as many males as females are injured. The primary cause of traumatic head injuries is motor vehicle crashes. The peak incidence occurs in the 15- to 24-year-old range (Kraus et al., 1984; National Head Injury Foundation, 1988). Of the approximately 700,000 persons with head injuries per year, it is estimated that 100,000 die; 50,000 to 100,000 survive with severe impairments that preclude independent living; and more than 200,000 suffer continuing problems that interfere with the skills of daily living (Jacobs, 1988).

Definitions of severity of injury

Severity of injury can be defined from a variety of perspectives. Jennett and Teasdale (1981) outline the severity classifications from the perspectives of administrative, clinical, and outcome measures. An administrative perspective is based on what happens to the patient—whether the person came to a hospital, was admitted, and if admitted, for how long. A clinical perspective refers to the response of the individual patient at the initial injury and during the initial course of care. The Glasgow coma scale (Teasdale & Jennett, 1974) is a measure commonly used in defining severity of injury at its onset. Severe injury is defined as a score of ≤8 for longer than 6 hours; moderate injury is a score of 9 to 12 for longer than 6 hours; and mild injury is defined as a score of 13 to 15 for longer than 6 hours. Posttraumatic amnesia, defined as the interval between the injury and the ability to lay down continuous memory of ongoing events, has been used as another common clinical measure of severity of injury (Russell, 1961; Russell & Nathan, 1946). Outcome measures of severity represent yet another perspective of severity. The Glasgow outcome scale is one example of a means of defining severity based on death or the functional characteristics of the survivor (Jennett & Bond, 1975). It was developed for use in studies with large numbers of subjects designed to research prognosticators of outcome and not for use on an individual patient basis (Table 24-2). Another scale that has been designed for use with the traumatic head injury population is the Rancho Los Amigos levels of cognitive functioning scale (Hagen & Malkmus, 1979). This is used primarily by rehabilitation professionals to describe the general progression of recovery and severity of an injury using behavioral descriptors of function (Table 24-3).

Because rehabilitation focuses on the broad span of disability recovery and adjustment, definitions of disability severity from the outcome perspective are used more often in the rehabilitation field. For example, a 24-year-old man with an initial Glasgow coma scale score of 7 indicates a severe injury. However, after a 1½ years of rehabilitation, he is placed in the "good recovery" category of the Glasgow outcome scale. In relation to more severely disabled persons, functionally he has a relatively minor injury. The functional description of "good recovery" is of most interest to rehabilitationists. Although far from exact, the initial severity definitions do become an important consideration when predicting ultimate functional levels in individuals.

Sequelae of head injury

Traumatic head injury has the capability of impacting every area of human functioning. The human brain is the ultimate initiator and regulator of functioning. Damage to this organ can result in a variety of deficits. The sequelae depend on the severity of injury, the location of injury (focal and diffuse), the degree of secondary brain

---

Table 24-2 The Glasgow outcome scale

Dead

Vegetative state	No evidence of psychologically meaningful activity, as judged behaviorally. Sleep/wake cycles present with periods of eye opening. Abnormal motor responses in all four limbs.
Severe disability	Conscious, but dependent on another person for some activities or supervision during all 24 hours daily.
Moderate disability	Independent in basic activities of daily living and may be capable of returning to work, but remains with some disability.
Good recovery	May have mild neurologic sequelae, but person is able to return to a normal social life and could return to work (although may not have done so).

Note. Modified from *Management of Head Injuries* (pp. 304-305) by B. Jennett and G. Teasdale, 1981, Philadelphia: F.A. Davis.

---

damage that occurs (ischemia, edema, destructive biochemical reactions, increased intracranial pressure, and potential brain shift and distortion), the early management of the patient, the provision of rehabilitation, and the premorbid abilities and characteristics of the individual.

Most severe head injuries cause initial changes in cognitive, physical, behavioral, and psychologic functioning. Patients usually exist within a family system. The head injury not only causes changes to the patient, but also may significantly impact the family system. See the box on p. 717 for the alterations that can occur in each of these areas of functioning.

The long-term studies of sequelae after traumatic head injury indicate that the cognitive and psychosocial effects are the most significant factors that create handicaps for survivors (Brooks,

Table 24-3 Rancho Los Amigos scale of cognitive levels and expected behavior

Level		Expected behavior
I	No response	Unresponsive to all stimuli.
II	Generalized response	Inconsistent, nonpurposeful, nonspecific reactions to stimuli. Responds to pain, but response may be delayed.
III	Localized response	Inconsistent reaction directly related to type of stimulus presented. Responds to some commands. May respond to discomfort.
IV	Confused, agitated response	Disoriented and unaware of present events, with frequent bizarre and inappropriate behavior. Attention span is short, and ability to process information is impaired.
V	Confused, inappropriate, nonagitated response	Nonpurposeful random or fragmented responses when task complexity exceeds abilities. Appears alert and responds to simple commands. Performs previously learned tasks but is unable to learn new ones.
VI	Confused, appropriate response	Behavior is goal-directed. Responses are appropriate to the situation with incorrect responses because of memory difficulties.
VII	Automatic, appropriate response	Correct routine responses that are robotlike. Appears oriented to setting, but insight, judgment, and problem solving are poor.
VIII	Purposeful, appropriate response	Correct responses, carryover of new learning. No required supervision, poor tolerance to stress, and some abstract reasoning difficulties.

Note. Modified from *Intervention Strategies for Language Disorders Secondary to Head trauma* by C. Hagen and D. Malkmus, 1979, Atlanta: American Speech-Language-Hearing Association, Short Courses.

1984; Brooks, Campsie, & Symington 1987; Goethe & Levin, 1984; McKinlay, Brooks, & Bond, 1981; Oddy, Humphrey, & Uttley, 1978; Thomsen, 1987).

Minor head injury*

Minor head injury represents the greatest percentage of head injuries that occur (Bijur, Haslum, & Golding, 1990; Kraus et al., 1984; Rimel, Giordani, Barth, Boll, & Jane, 1981). Minor head injuries were previously thought to be inconsequential with uneventful recoveries. Research done at the University of Virginia (Rimel et al., 1981) documented one of the first studies about the occurrence of disability in patients after a seemingly inconsequential head injury. Sequelae identified by patients at a 3-month follow-up included persistent headaches, difficulty with concentration, fatigue, and double vision.

*This section contributed by James C. Wilson, PhD, Director of the Neuropsychology Department, Kentfield Rehabilitation Hospital, Kentfield, CA.

The most significant finding was that 34% of the patients who were gainfully employed before their injury were unemployed at a 3-month follow-up. Pending litigation suggesting possible malingering was ruled out as a significant contributor. Only a small number of patients showed any clinically significant signs on neurologic examination. On initial evaluation at admission, 92% of the patients had normal neurologic examinations, and by discharge (48 hours or less later), nearly all the patients had normal results. However, the majority of a subset of patients given neuropsychologic tests were found to have significant cognitive deficits, involving attention, concentration, memory, and judgment. The role of alcohol in minor head injury was also highlighted by this study, which found that some alcohol was present in the blood of 43% of the total population.

Levin et al. (1987) used neuropsychologic measures to track recovery. Patients reported initial disturbances in attention, memory, and efficiency of information processing with minor head injury. Nearly all patients in this study reported

Potential sequelae of traumatic head injury

Cognitive

Reduced attention and concentration
Impaired memory (immediate and short-term)
Impaired problem-solving
Impaired planning and organization
Difficulty with concept (abstract) information
Impaired judgment
Impaired auditory processing
Impaired visual processing
Reduced processing speed
Inflexible thinking
Impulsive thinking

Physical

Paralysis/paresis
Impaired motor planning
Abnormal muscle tone
Impaired fine motor skills
Reduced endurance
Impaired mobility
Visual deficits
Motor speech disorders
Impaired swallowing

Behavioral

Inability to engage in purposeful activity
Disinhibition
Inability to respond appropriately to environmental cues
Socially inappropriate behavior
Social skills deficits
Impulsivity
Poor initiation
Restlessness

Psychologic

Emotional lability
Dependency and childlike behavior
Denial or unawareness of deficits
Reduced self-esteem
Depression
Exaggerated personality characteristics

Impact on family systems

Extensive role changes
Anxiety in family members
Depression in family members
Financial burden

Note. From Innovations in Head Injury Rehabilitation by P.M. Deutsch and K.B. Fralish, 1989, New York: Mathew Bender.

cognitive problems, somatic complaints, and emotional malaise initially, but most symptoms resolved at the 3-month follow-up.

Trauma nurses providing initial care to persons with minor head injury are in an excellent position to teach patients about potential sequelae that may be experienced early on after injury. A study designed to compare the effect of routine care, information, and information plus reassurance indicates a strong tendency for patients in the information plus reassurance group to return to work faster than those in the other two groups and to report fewer residual sequelae at a 3-month follow-up (Hinkle, Alves, Rimel, & Jane, 1986).

Evaluation and treatment Neuropsychologic testing is one of the few approaches that can detect the subtle cognitive deficits often associated with minor head trauma (Levin Eisenberg, & Benton, 1989). Although most patients (80%) eventually recover (by 6 months after injury), a significant minority continue to present with a complex array of symptoms—identified as the *post-concussion syndrome*. For those who have initially rather acute problems, as well as those who have persistent or lingering problems, neuropsychologic assessment (Figure 24-2) can be helpful in understanding cognitive and psychosocial dysfunction. Such testing can provide an important baseline measure, with which future recovery may be compared.

When the assessment is completed, test results, along with educational information, are shared with the patient. Treatment may include counseling, for both the patient and the family, compensatory cognitive retraining, and referral to a support group or head injury association familiar with minor head trauma.

Case example The effects of minor head injury are often subtle and frequently involve attentional ability (which interferes with concentration, memory, information processing, and reasoning). In the two contrasting cases illustrated in Figure 24-2, both individual A and individual B were given the Rey-Osterrieth Complex Figure test (see design at top of Figure 24-2) as part of a post-injury neuropsychologic assessment. Individual A, a 15-year-old female who suffered a concussion and received multiple trauma, did not sustain any lasting or significant cognitive deficits. Individual B, a 20-year-old female who also re-

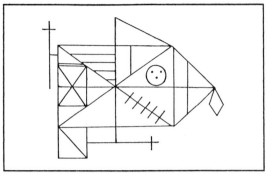

Rey-Osterrieth Complex Figure

Case "A"

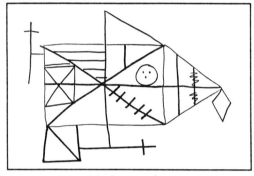

A1: Copy task

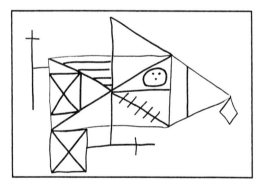

A2: Immediate recall

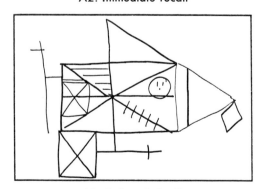

A3: Delayed recall

Case "B"

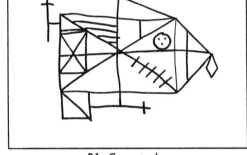

B1: Copy task

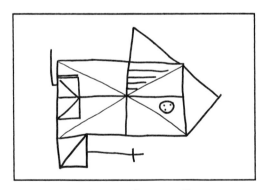

B2: Immediate recall

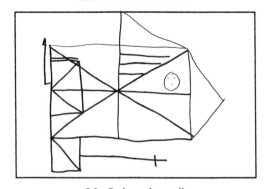

B3: Delayed recall

Figure 24-2 Neuropsychologic assessment testing with Rey-Osterrieth complex figure test. Case examples show patient drawings: initial copy of test figure (A1,B1); immediate recall drawings (A2,B2); and delayed recall drawings (A3,B3). (*Note*. Drawings courtesy James C. Wilson, PhD, Neuropsychology Department, Kentfield Rehabilitation Hospital, Kentfield, CA.)

ceived a concussion and was hospitalized briefly, had residual cognitive problems (attention/concentration) and subsequent psychosocial difficulties, including depression and disrupted educational and vocational adjustment. They were requested to copy the design (their efforts are shown in A1 and B1). Then, without being cued in advance, they were asked to recall the design by drawing it again from memory (immediate recall: see A2 and B2). Finally, again without advance cuing, they were asked to draw the design again from memory, 30 minutes later (delayed recall: see A3 and B3). The differences in their level of performance can be observed. Note the problems arising on the immediate recall task with individual B, whose performance was affected by her initially poor attention during the copy task. In contrast, individual A showed no such difficulty and scored above average in her immediate and delayed recall of the figure.

Rehabilitative focus

The management of head-injured patients in the emergency and intensive care phases includes surgical removal of mass lesions, control of intracranial pressure, and prevention of complications, such as respiratory insufficiency, hypertension or hypotension, hyperthermia, fluid and electrolyte imbalances, and seizures (Nikas & Tolley, 1982). Rehabilitation goals begin in the intensive care phase and can be interwoven into the primary focus of establishing and maintaining physiologic stability. The initial rehabilitation goal is to elicit and increase the frequency of meaningful responses to the environment. The second rehabilitation focus encompasses early treatment techniques that minimize the potential for alterations in mobility and skin integrity.

Rehabilitation protocols In some major trauma centers, rehabilitation protocols are established to assure that the early rehabilitation needs are incorporated into the intensive care phase of treatment. Boughton and Ciesla (1986) reported

guidelines using a Glasgow coma scale score of ≤ 12 as a criteria for initiating a rehabilitation assessment performed by a physical therapist. The components of an assessment in this phase include the patient's response to different forms of stimulation and an assessment of range of motion, muscle tone, reflexes, and isolated joint movement. Common members of the rehabilitation team to become involved in the intensive care phase are the physical therapist and the occupational therapist.

Sensory stimulation Sensory stimulation programs are designed to elicit responses from the patient during the early stages of head injury recovery. Little well-designed research has been done regarding the effectiveness of sensory stimulation programs, but reports from professionals support its usefulness (Whyte & Glenn, 1986). Trauma nurses and other professionals and family members interacting with the patient can implement sensory stimulation techniques. The program must be coordinated and must use a variety of sensory stimulation techniques (visual, auditory, olfactory, tactile, and kinesthetic). The stimulation should be presented only for brief periods, with adequate rest periods interspersed. Once a program is established, family members are ideal for assisting with the implementation—often patients will respond more consistently to familiar persons. In addition, assisting with the sensory stimulation program gives the family member a productive role in the patient's care and can help to ease the helplessness that family members experience (Buss, Chippendale, Hagen, Klauber, & Minteer, 1984).

Abnormal muscle tone Severe head injury often causes abnormal muscle tone. Joint contracture and decreased range of motion have been associated with abnormal muscle tone in head-injured patients (Booth, Doyle, & Montgomery, 1983; Sweeney & Smutok, 1983). Dynamic and static positioning can be used to achieve normal range of motion, as well as to facilitate normal movement patterns. The severely head-injured patient often assumes decorticate, decerebrate, or fetal positioning in bed. Proper bed positioning using reflex-inhibiting patterns may counteract these abnormal positions (Boughton & Ciesla, 1986).

Various side-lying positions have advantages over supine positioning. In the side-lying position, the weight of the body acts as the proximal point of control to maintain the arm beneath in a reflex-inhibiting posture. Trunk rotation, also a reflex-inhibiting position, is achieved by alternating lower extremity hip and knee flexion and extension (Figure 24-3).

To assist with decreasing intracranial pressure, supine positioning with the head of the bed elevated 15 to 30 degrees is common in the intensive care unit. To counteract the abnormal extensor posturing that is elicited with this position, modifications can be made. These include placing a sheet roll beneath the knees to create knee and hip flexion and placing rolls or sandbags at the hips to promote symmetrical external rotation.

The upper extremities can be positioned in full flexion, abduction, and external rotation, with

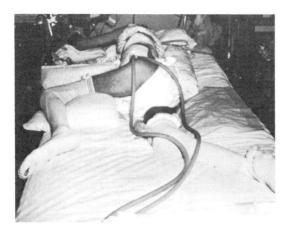

Figure 24-3 Side-lying posture as reflex-inhibiting position. Side-lying position can be achieved despite chest tubes, ventilator, nasogastric tubes, and intravascular lines. (*Note.* From "Physical Therapy Management of the Head-Injured Patient in the Intensive Care Unit" by A. Boughton and N. Ciesla, 1986, *Topics in Acute Care and Trauma Rehabilitation*, 1(1), pp. 1-18.)

the hands placed behind the patient's head. Consistent range-of-motion exercises are critical to prevent the formation of contractures. In patients with increased muscle tone, inhibitory positioning techniques used before the range-of-motion exercises can make them easier to perform.

Nurses in the intensive care unit or physical or occupational therapists are appropriate persons to implement range-of-motion exercises. Other positioning techniques can be extremely helpful for minimizing abnormal tone. Serial casting in the intensive care phase may be indicated for extremities that exhibit high tone. Neutral positions are considered inhibitory and therefore minimize abnormal tone (Booth, Doyle, & Montgomery, 1983). Other forms of static positioning aids may be appropriate for positioning of the hand and wrist. Resting hand splints can assist in promoting functional hand positioning, particularly in comatose or paralyzed patients with normal or low muscle tone.

Nursing interventions Early mobilization is an emphasis of rehabilitation. As soon as a patient can be moved out of bed and into a sitting position, this is encouraged. Proper positioning in the chair can be accomplished using bolsters and wedges.

Another area of nursing management in the intensive care phase that is important in promoting rehabilitation is the establishment of nutrition and bowel programs. Careful attention to maintenance of skin integrity is essential. Because of the many critical problems that are being managed in the intensive care setting such as increased intracranial pressure, the potential exists for minimizing the importance of skin care. From the perspective of rehabilitation, however, a breakdown in skin integrity can impact the patient's ability for early mobilization and prolong the rehabilitation process.

Agitation When the head-injured patient is stabilized physiologically, movement to the neurologic acute care floor occurs. Rehabilitation measures continue, and the establishment of a reliable communication system for the patient is emphasized (Hagen, 1983). Although the speech/language pathologist may already be involved from the intensive care phase, more often he or she becomes a more active member of the team at this phase. The patient's language at this stage

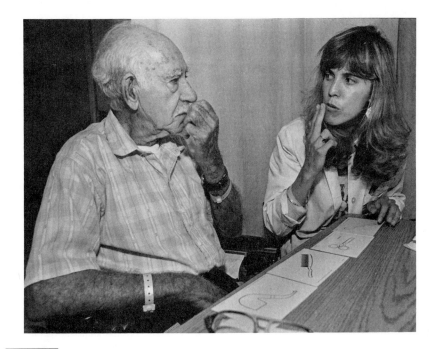

Figure 24-4   Speech pathologist coaching patient for improvement in speech and swallowing. Visual and auditory cues are used to improve receptive aphasia. (*Note.* Photograph by Renee Burgard, Stanford University Hospital.)

is usually confused, and cognitive abilities are grossly impaired. Basic orientation measures are instituted. Often the patient's behaviors are agitated. Unlike the early stages of promoting responses through additional planned sensory stimulation, the focus of treatment during periods of highly agitated behavior is one of minimizing environmental stimulation (Klauber & Ward-McKinlay, 1986).

If the patient is experiencing difficulty swallowing, an assessment of swallowing abilities performed by a speech/language pathologist or an occupational therapist is indicated (Ulrey & Woods, 1986), (Figure 24-4). If appropriate, swallowing therapy is instituted.

When further physiologic stabilization occurs, the patient moves to the structured rehabilitation setting. The patient may still be in a period of acute agitation. If so, the focus of the rehabilitation team is on minimizing the agitation and increasing the frequency of appropriate behavior. Patients are treated in quiet areas on a one-to-one basis. The use of restraints is minimized, and the environment is made as safe as possible to allow for the patient to work through the restlessness. As the patient moves beyond the agitated phase, the focus of treatment is on continued mobilization, maximizing independence in basic activities of daily living, establishing normal elimination patterns, and improving basic communication skills. The prevalent sequelae that impact all areas of functioning include the cognitive areas of attention, concentration, memory, and disorganized and delayed information processing. All members of the rehabilitation team incorporate strategies to address the cognitive impairments. Structure, consistency, and repetition are the hallmarks of head injury rehabilitation (Hagen, 1983). Team members who participate in the rehabilitation program include rehabilitation nurses, recreation therapists, psychologists, and neuropsychologists, in addition to those who are involved in the intensive care and acute neurologic phases.

Discharge from the acute rehabilitation setting is determined by a variety of factors. These include the level of independence the patient has achieved and the patient's ability to function in a less-structured setting, the discharge environment and support persons and their ability to manage the patient, and to a larger extent in recent years, the funding or lack of funding supports available to the patient. The majority of patients with moderate or severe head injuries require continued rehabilitation in the post-acute setting. The focus becomes the more complex issues of community reintegration. These include complex activities of daily living, such as home management issues, community transportation, educational pursuits, or return to work. Continued work on cognitive impairments and the development of compensatory strategies for remaining deficits are provided by the rehabilitation team. The development of adequate social and interpersonal relationship skills becomes of primary importance in this phase of rehabilitation. These factors create the greatest barriers to successful reintegration into the community (Brooks, 1984). The settings in which community reintegration issues are addressed include residential rehabilitation programs or transitional living centers, comprehensive day treatment programs, out-patient services, and home-based programs that focus on using the community for training purposes (Dixon, 1989). Rehabilitation team members who are actively involved in the post-acute phase include vocational rehabilitation counselors, neuropsychologists, and social workers, in addition to the other professionals who are involved in the acute rehabilitation setting.

Family education and involvement are critical at every phase of recovery from traumatic head injury. Most often it becomes the family who provides the long-term support and care for severely injured persons (Livingston & Brooks, 1988). Providing practical approaches for families, promoting respite, and providing resources for support and counseling are necessary.

Psychosocial considerations

As mentioned, the alterations that result from traumatic brain injury that create the most difficulty for survivors are in the social and emotional realms of functioning. Studies that include long-term follow-up of individuals with brain injury and their families consistently point toward these areas as the most troublesome (Brooks, 1984; Lezak, 1978; Lezak, 1987). Loneliness, boredom,

and feelings of worthlessness or uselessness are common complaints of head injury survivors. Anxiety, depression, and problems with significant relationships occur with increased frequency. A high percentage of survivors experience difficulty with handling anger, which may contribute to their decreased ability to sustain relationships (Lezak, 1987).

The significant "characterological" changes that occur with brain injury create significant financial and emotional burdens on family systems. They disrupt roles, relationships, communication patterns, and expectations and shared dreams. (Romano, 1989). Families constitute the primary care providers for most head-injured persons. Jacobs (1988), in the Los Angeles head injury survey, reported that significant stressors occur in most areas of family living, such as marital, parental, sibling relations, family activities, and the long-term goals of most family members. Most of the literature on family response to head injury has been written about adults. Few entries in the literature address the response of families to childhood injury (Waaland & Kreutzer, 1988). Common family reactions to head injuries in children identified in the literature include denial of the disability, overprotection of the child, anger, guilt, and blame directed toward professionals who cared for the injured child.

Functional outcome

Outcome predictors Three types of prognostic factors have been studied in relation to prognosis after head injury. These predictors are (1) preexisting factors, (2) clinical factors based on examination, and (3) medical or laboratory indicators (Mack & Horn, 1989). Most studies of predictors of outcome use the Glasgow outcome scale to describe levels of outcome (Jennett & Bond, 1975).

Preexisting factors include premorbid psychosocial background and age. Studies that have examined the personal and social resources before injury have supported the common-sense assumption that the greater one's personal and social resources, the better the outcome from head injury. Age has been identified as a significant factor in determining outcome (Jennett & Teasdale, 1981). The older the patient, the poorer the outcome. Children overall tend to fair better than adults with severe injury. However, one study (Filley, Cranberg, Alexander, & Hart, 1987) reported that children ages 1 month to 6 years had poorer outcomes than those ages 6 to 15 years.

Clinical factors identified as prognosticators include oculomotor reflexes, motor responses, the depth and duration of coma as measured by the Glasgow coma scale, and posttraumatic amnesia. The degree of brainstem involvement, as reflected by impaired ocular reflexes, combined with the Glasgow coma scale score, becomes a powerful predictor of outcome (Braakman, Habbema, & Gelpke, 1986). The length of posttraumatic amnesia (PTA) is correlated with outcome. The longer the period of PTA, the greater the disability (Russell, 1961).

Computerized axial tomography (CT) scanning as a single predictor of outcome is not very effective (Lobato & Cordobe, 1983), whereas evoked potentials are considered a powerful independent predictor of outcome (Braakman et al., 1986). Evoked potentials are a group of physiologic tests based on the observation that loss of myelin slows nerve conduction time. Brainstem auditory evoked responses demonstrate the integrity of the brainstem in a noninvasive manner (Earnest, 1983).

Complications Posttraumatic epilepsy is estimated to occur in 5% of persons with head injury (Jennett, 1983). Onset of the seizure disorder can occur at any time. Posttraumatic hydrocephalus is another potential complication. The incidence is estimated at 1% to 8% (Bontke, 1989). Heterotopic ossification (HO) occurs in 11% to 76% of head-injured individuals. Those with significantly abnormal tone and prolonged coma are at a higher risk. This type of ossification involves the depositing of ectopic bone around joints, causing limitations in joint motion and pain. Rehabilitation can be delayed or prolonged if this complication exists (Bontke, 1989). Educating the individuals with brain injury, as well as their families or long-term care providers, about the potential complications is a component of the entire educational process of rehabilitation.

IMPAIRED PHYSICAL MOBILITY

Alterations in mobility can greatly impact an individual's ability to perform basic and complex activities of daily living, as well as interact with society. Several mechanisms of traumatic injury can cause alterations in mobility. The specific causes discussed in this section include spinal cord injuries, peripheral nerve injuries, and traumatic amputations. A cause that does not immediately come to mind as a contributor to alterations in mobility is multisystem injury. The severely debilitating effects of prolonged immobilization during treatment of multisystem injury create yet another group of individuals who can benefit from rehabilitation services.

Spinal Cord Injuries

The incidence of spinal cord injury varies according to the source, but most reports indicate the annual rate as between 30 and 32 new spinal cord injuries per million persons in the United States (Stover & Fine, 1987). With this rate, it is estimated that 8000 persons receive spinal cord injuries per year. Of these, 5% are children younger than 15 years (Banta, 1984). The total number of individuals with spinal cord injuries is estimated at 906 per million. In the United States, spinal cord injuries occur most frequently in persons between the ages of 15 and 20 years. The average age is 29 years. There is a 4:1 ratio of males over females who sustain spinal cord injuries. Motor vehicle crashes cause 48% of spinal cord injuries. Refer to Chapter 11 for additional information on spinal cord injury statistics.

Specific spinal cord injuries

Quadriplegia is slightly more common than paraplegia (52% versus 48%) (Stover & Fine, 1987). From a rehabilitation perspective, a spinal cord injury is classified as either *complete* or *incomplete*, based on the residual neurologic functioning.

Complete injuries A complete injury is loss of all conscious motor and sensory function below the level of the lesion. An incomplete injury preserves or spares some motor or sensory function (Zejdlik, 1983). A significant decrease in the number of complete injuries has occurred from 1970 to present. This is primarily the result of the sophistication of emergency medical services and techniques for appropriate extrication and immobilization. The prognosis of complete injuries is less than 3% to 4% chance of spontaneous recovery, whereas in cases of incomplete lesions, the majority of patients experience at least some degree of neurologic recovery (Green, Eismont, & O'Heir, 1987).

Incomplete injuries With incomplete lesions,

several distinct patterns of neurologic deficit occur (Zejdlik, 1983).

Central cord syndrome is caused by damage to the central portion of the cord only. Because of the organization of the corticospinal tracts in the cord, arm movement and sensation are affected, but leg movement and sensation may not be.

Anterior artery syndrome is usually caused by infarction of the main anterior artery. The resulting injury causes damage to the anterior two thirds of the cord. The functional changes that result include loss of voluntary movement and major sensory tracts for pain and temperature. There is sparing, however, of the posterior column sensations of position, vibration, and touch.

Brown-Séquard's syndrome is caused by damage to one side of the cord only. Because of the arrangement of motor and sensory tracts in the spinal cord, the functional changes include loss of motor function below the level of the lesion on the same side as the lesion. However, pain and temperature sensations are preserved on the side of the lesion, but lost on the opposite side.

Conus and cauda equina injuries involve damage to the conus medullaris or the spinal nerves forming the cauda equina. Effects include variable patterns of loss of motor function, with sensory function not markedly impaired. The potential for a more favorable outcome is present because of the recovery potential of nerve roots. Because the bowel, bladder, and sexual functioning reflex centers are located in the conus (S2 through S4), these functions present with flaccid or areflexic involvement.

Sacral sparing refers to sparing of the sensation of the sacral area when the major part of the cord is damaged. This can occur because the vascular supply to the lateral cord is provided by the radicular arteries.

Sequelae of spinal cord injury

The functional changes that result from spinal cord injury depend on the level of the injury, as well as the completeness of the lesion. In general, the higher the level of injury, the more alterations in functioning occur. Table 24-4 lists the potential functional status as correlated with neurologic level of injury. This should be used as a guideline only, because many factors impact an individual's ability to function. Spinal cord injury impacts the individual in a wide range of physiologic and functional ways.

Alterations in bowel and bladder functioning, as well as changes in sexual functioning, result. Ineffective airway clearance can result because of the involvement of the muscles of respiration. The higher the level of injury, the more respiratory involvement there is. A person with respiratory quadriplegia has a C2 or C3 functional level and will require ventilator support on an ongoing basis. Partial preservation of the accessory muscles of breathing offers a potential to develop tolerance for being off the respirator for a few hours. Those individuals with respiratory quadriplegia require services provided by rehabilitation programs that specialize in this care.

Rehabilitation focus

Emergency and critical care phase   In the treatment of persons with spinal cord injury, trauma nurses working in emergency and critical care settings are in a unique position to influence the entire rehabilitation process, either in a positive or negative direction. The goals within the emergency and critical care phases include providing optimal critical and concurrent rehabilitative care, preventing or controlling secondary complications, and establishing a trusting relationship with the patient and family (Zejdlik, 1983).

Adequate management of the cardiovascular and respiratory functions of the individual with spinal cord injury is a priority of the trauma nurse. Monitoring and prevention of further neurologic damage through careful immobilization and continuous assessment of motor and sensory functioning are vital in the critical care and rehabilitation at this stage (Nikas, 1982).

A concurrent rehabilitation focus on the remaining physiologic needs of the person completes the emphasis of rehabilitative care during this early stage of treatment. Almost all patients with spinal cord injury will experience partial or complete loss of bladder function as a result of impaired neural control. Initial insertion of an indwelling catheter to prevent overdistension, followed by early implementation of an intermittent catheterization program will help to maintain optimal functioning of the urinary system (Metcalf, 1986; Nikas, 1982). Careful assessment of gastrointestinal functioning is important to prevent complications. Paralytic ileus and acute peptic ulcerations are common complications within the first days after injury. Careful attention to nutrition is critical, as well. Several authors support the initi-

Table 24-4 Potential functional status correlated to neurologic injury

Level	Motor ability	Sensory appreciation	Eating and grooming	Dressing	Bathing	Bowel and bladder care	Transfers	Mobility	Nonverbal communication
Quadriplegia									
C1-4	Limited movement of head and neck (C1-3) and some shoulder cap and diaphragm control (C4).	Limited sensation to head, neck (C1-2) and shoulder cap (C3-4).	Dependent on an assistant.	Dependent on an assistant.	Dependent on an assistant.	Dependent on an assistant.	Dependent on an assistant.	Requires electric wheelchair with breath, head, or shoulder controls. Likely dependent on a portable respiratory support system all or part of the time.	Independent with environmental controls (such as whistle to activate a phone dial tone, or a voice or head motion to activate an appliance)
C5	Full head, neck, shoulder, and diaphragm control. Add: Some elbow flexion.	Full head, neck, and shoulder cap sensation.	Independent with aids and setup.	Requires major assistance with aids.	Requires wheelchair shower with major assistance.	Requires major assistance with some aids.	Major assistance required; variable with type of transfer.	Requires electric wheelchair with adapted hand control and/or manual wheelchair with wheel rim projections.	Independent with aids and setup.
C6	Add: Some wrist extension (tenodesis).	Add: Sensation to the lateral aspects of forearm to include the thumb and first finger.	Independent with aids.	Requires minor assistance with aids.	Independent in wheelchair shower with aids.	Independent with aids.	Minor assistance required; variable with type of transfer.	Independent in manual wheelchair.	Independent with aids.

Note. Modified from Zejdlik, C.M. (1983). *Management of Spinal Cord Injury.* (pp. 456-459) by C.M. Zejdlik, 1983, Monterey, CA: Wadsworth Health Sciences.
Note. "Add" listed in motor and sensory columns means "in addition to levels above."

Continued.

Table 24-4 Potential functional status correlated to neurologic injury—cont'd

Level	Motor ability	Sensory appreciation	Eating and grooming	Dressing	Bathing	Bowel and bladder care	Transfers	Mobility	Nonverbal communication
Quadriplegia—cont'd									
C7	Full elbow flexion. Add: Elbow extension, wrist flexion, and some finger control.	Add: Sensation to the second finger.	Independent with or without aids.	Independent with aids.	Independent in wheelchair shower or tub with bath board and aids.	Independent with aids.	Independent with aids in all transfers.	Independent in manual wheelchair.	Independent with or without aids.
C8-T1	Moderate to full arm and wrist control. Add: Moderate to full finger control.	Add: Sensation to all the hand (C8) and the medial aspects of the upper and lower arm (T1).	Independent.	Independent.	Independent in tub with bath board and aids.	Independent with aids.	Independent with aids.	Independent in manual wheelchair.	Independent.
Paraplegia									
T2-12	Full upper extremity control. Add: Limited to full trunk control.	Full arm sensation. Add: Partial trunk sensation to the level of the injury.	Independent.	Independent.	Independent.	Independent with aids.	Independent.	Independent in manual wheelchair.	Independent.

L1-5	Full trunk control. Add: Some hip (L1-3), knee (L3-4), and ankle (L4-5) control and foot movement (L5).	Full trunk sensation upper leg (L1-3), anterior/posterior and laterall aspects of the lower leg and dorum of foot (L4-5).	Independent.	Independent.	Independent.	Independent with or without aids.	Independent.	Optional use of long leg braces for ambulation.	Independent.
S1-5	Moderate to full leg control. Add: Some foot control (disability can still be severe because of bowel, bladder, and sexual dysfunction).	Sensation to the lateral aspect of the dorsum and the sole of foot (S1); posterior aspect of the upper leg (S2); sacral area (S2-5).	Independent.	Independent.	Independent.	Independent with or without aids.	Independent.	Independent ambulation with or without short leg braces.	Independent.

ation of parenteral nutrition, followed by enteral nutrition as soon as possible. This contributes to the prevention of stress ulcers (Deitz, Bertschy, Gschaedler, & Dollfus, 1986; Dollfus, 1987; Laven et al., 1989). Appropriate management of neurogenic bowel during the critical care phase contributes to the maintenance of bowel tone, regularity, and ease in developing a reliable bowel program. Prevention of skin breakdown in these individuals is of paramount importance. Lack of sensation, the inability to move freely, and circulatory changes predispose this group to potential for breakdown (Martin, Holt, & Hicks, 1981).

Early implementation of physical therapy and occupational therapy while the patient is immobilized in the intensive care unit will assist with maintaining musculoskeletal system integrity. The treatment program for patients during this early phase includes chest physical therapy, range of motion and positioning, active exercises aimed at maintaining rather than improving muscle strength, and early activities-of-daily-living training. For patients with limited hand function because of quadriplegia, proper splinting of the hands in a functional position is of paramount importance. Opponens splints are used to keep the thumb in opposition to the first two fingers, maintain the web space, and slightly flex the fingers. A short opponens splint is used when wrist movement is present; a long opponens splint is used to support a flaccid wrist (Figure 24-5). In contrast to volar splints, opponens splints are used to promote thumb opposition. This splinting is performed in preparation for using the hands to their maximal functional ability.

Acute care When the patient is placed in a stabilizing orthosis, such as a halo brace for cervical injuries or total contact orthoses for thoracic or lumbar injuries, the rehabilitation therapists can assist with implementing a sitting program. Methods for pressure relief while sitting are instituted immediately. These methods include use of a proper wheelchair cushion, as well as a variety of weight-shifting techniques. (Imle & Boughton, 1987). A well-implemented sitting program is important during daily activities, as well as recreational sessions (Figure 24-6).

Acute rehabilitation In regional spinal cord injury centers (model spinal cord injury systems) and sophisticated trauma centers, persons with spinal cord injury often go directly to a spinal

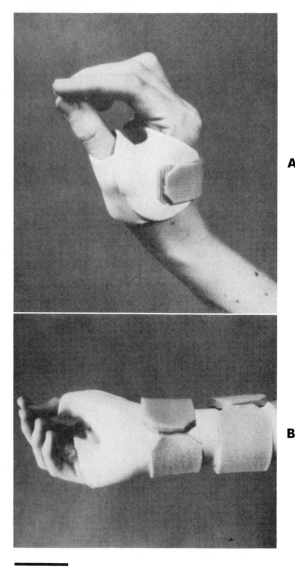

A

B

Figure 24-5 Opponens splints. **A,** Short opponens splint maintains thumb in opposition to preserve functional hand position. Good self-control of wrist movement is needed. **B,** Long opponens splint is used for same purpose when wrist movement is absent or weak. (*Note.* From *Management of Spinal Cord Injury* (p. 451) by C.P. Zejdlik, 1983, Monterey, CA: Wadsworth Health Sciences.)

cord injury rehabilitation center from the intensive care unit. The focus of rehabilitation within this acute rehabilitation phase is on teaching the individual with spinal cord injury to adjust to the

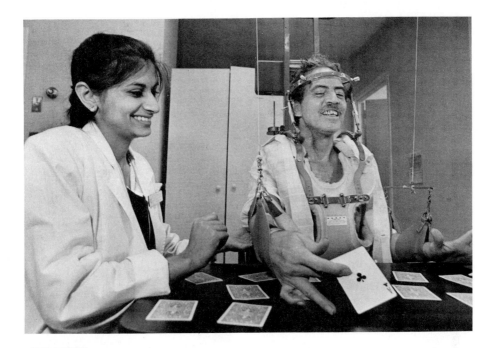

Figure 24-6   Patient in halo vest in recreational session. (*Note.* Photograph by Renee Burgard, Stanford University Hospital.)

alterations in mobility and self-care and assume responsibility for managing the functioning of his or her own body. Strengthening exercises and techniques for moving in bed and to and from different surfaces, maneuvering a wheelchair or walking with braces, and supportive devices are part of mobility training. Therapy aimed at maintaining muscle strength continues in the acute rehabilitation phase (Figure 24-7). Alternative techniques for personal care management (i.e., dressing, grooming, bathing, and feeding oneself) are focused on (Figure 24-8).

For individuals with complete high cervical lesions, the concept of independence is focused on more as a "mind process," because these individuals will be incapable of physical independence. The ability to direct one's own care and guide another person through the physical steps of performing the care is a viable rehabilitation goal (Frieden & Cole, 1985).

Patient teaching in the areas of nutrition, skin care, bowel and bladder management, sexuality, and respiratory care is included in the basic curriculum for individuals with spinal cord injury (Houston, 1984; Zejdlik, 1983). Those with injuries at the T6 level and above may have autonomic dysreflexia. This condition is created when the sympathetic division of the autonomic nervous system responds in an uninhibited manner as a result of lack of control from higher centers. The resulting emergent situation is one of rapidly increasing blood pressure and bradycardia. The primary treatment is removal of the stimulus causing the autonomic nervous system response. Patients must be taught what actions to take if they experience symptoms (Metcalf, 1986). The most common stimulus is a full bladder. Therefore patients are taught to perform intermittent catheterization as an initial step in identifying and managing the stimulus.

The in-patient rehabilitation program also focuses on teaching the disabled individual how others view disability. Assertiveness training to assist the person with spinal cord injury to communicate needs and to interact in society as a person with a disability is included. Peer counseling by others with spinal cord injury who are adjusting to the changes imposed on them can be helpful.

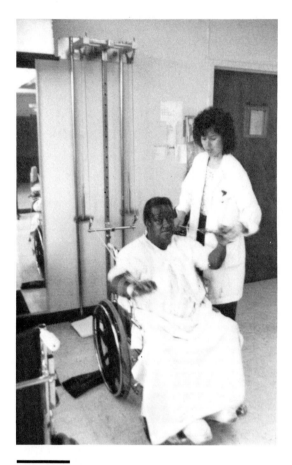

Figure 24-7 Strengthening exercises as part of acute rehabilitation allow use of mechanical aids and success with transfer techniques. (*Note.* Photograph courtesy of Stanford University Hospital Rehabilitation Unit, Stanford, CA.)

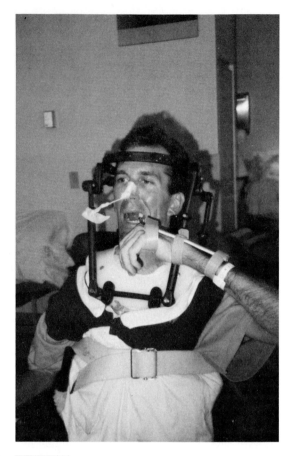

Figure 24-8 Patient with C5 quadriplegia using static splint with universal cuff to hold toothbrush. (Note. Courtesy Sharp Memorial Hospital Rehabilitation Center, San Diego, CA.)

Post-acute rehabilitation The post-acute phase of rehabilitation in spinal cord injury focuses on adjustment to the alterations imposed by the disability. Reestablishing life goals and looking at what type of productive activity is possible occur once the individual establishes patterns for meeting more basic self-care needs. Vocational rehabilitation counselors and psychologists can assist these individuals to continue adjustment and to consider alternative educational and vocational options. Assistance to meet the continued goals of community reintegration is provided through outpatient programs and independent living centers. Independent living centers are an outgrowth of the independent living movement that was initi-

ated in the late 1960s and early 1970s. These are community-based programs that have substantial consumer involvement. They provide directly or coordinate indirectly through referral those services necessary to assist severely disabled individuals to increase self-determination and to minimize unnecessary dependence on others (Frieden & Cole, 1985).

Psychosocial considerations

Adjustment to disability is a highly individualized process. A spinal cord injury affects all aspects of a person's life. It instantly imposes an overwhelming complex of losses. Some of the factors that affect adjustment include the person's self-esteem and self-concept, the degree of help-lessness felt by the person, the age of the person at the time of the injury, and the person's ability to acquire new roles as he or she goes through the rehabilitation process (Zejdlik, 1983). A strong support system promotes a higher level of independence. However, the effects of chronic disability on the family functioning can be wearing (McGowan & Roth, 1987).

Marital status of those with spinal cord injury is reportedly different from that of the general public. Brown and Geisy (1986) reported in their study that 21.9% fewer men were married and 39.1% fewer women were married. There were 13.2% more single men and 14.5% more single women with spinal cord injury. The percentage of men who were divorced was 8.8% higher than the average male population. Twenty-five percent more spinal cord–injured females were divorced. A study addressing marital adjustment after spinal cord injury indicates that the factors promoting positive adjustment in a marriage of one spouse with a spinal cord injury are very similar to those of able-bodied couples (Urey & Henggeler, 1987).

Functional outcomes

As mentioned, the functional outcomes of persons with spinal cord injury depend on many variables. Some of these variables are the level of injury, the completeness of the injury, and the support systems available to promote functional independence. Several studies support the efficacy of rehabilitation in this population and demonstrate the significant functional gains that are made (Burke, Burley, & Ungar, 1985; Yarkony et al., 1987). The employment rate for individuals with spinal cord injury seldom exceeds 50%. Factors that are identified as predicting employability include gender, motivation, whether ambulation was required in the last job, race, and education level (DeVivo, Rutt, Stover, & Fine, 1987).

Complications

Persons with spinal cord injury must be aware of the potential for continued problems with urinary tract infections, joint contractures, pulmonary problems caused by less efficient respiratory musculature, and skin breakdown. Significant advances in the rehabilitation and health care of individuals with spinal cord injury have greatly en-

hanced the outcome and life expectancy of these individuals. A 7-year survival rate study indicated that the probability of dying after a spinal cord injury was greatest within the first year, with the overall survival rate being 86.7%. Life expectancy is near normal in those who survive (Devivo, Kartus, Stover, Rutt, & Fine, 1987).

Peripheral Nerve Injuries

Acute peripheral nerve injury refers to damage resulting from sudden compression, transection, or stretching (Schaumburg, Spencer, & Thomas, 1983). Peripheral nerves have the capability of regenerating; therefore a significant opportunity exists for spontaneous recovery. Regeneration begins at approximately 1 month after injury, occurs at a relatively slow pace (approximately ½ inch per month), and depends on the type and severity of the injury (McGormack, 1981; Schaumburg, Spencer, & Thomas, 1983). The degree of peripheral nerve injury is ranked from first degree to fifth degree. First degree is least severe, and full spontaneous recovery is expected in weeks. Fifth degree is the most severe damage, with no motor or sensory conduction present and no recovery expected (Millesi, 1980).

Regardless of the origin of the injury, peripheral nerve lesions produce similar clinical manifestations. Muscle weakness or flaccid paralysis is the most obvious manifestation. Atrophy follows as a result of the denervation of the muscle, and deep tendon reflexes are diminished or absent. Sensation is also lost. Trophic changes, such as dry skin, hair loss, cyanosis, brittle fingernails, and slow wound healing in the involved area, occur with peripheral nerve injury.

Specific peripheral nerve injuries

The functional implications of peripheral nerve injuries depend on which nerve or groups of nerves are injured. Outcome also depends on the degree of nerve recovery. Omer (1980) reported that missile injuries had a 69% spontaneous recovery over a 3- to 9-month period.

Upper extremity Brachial plexus injuries can be caused by direct trauma causing an open injury or by foreign bodies thrust into the neck area during an accident. Most often the lesion is caused by traction in a longitudinal direction or by compression. Motorcycle accidents are a common cause of brachial plexus injury. The resulting functional disability causes complete paralysis of the arm; it hangs flail (flaccid) from the shoulder in slight internal rotation. Sensibility is completely lost with the exception of a small strip of the upper arm. Very often the patient suffers from severe pain and complains of phantom limb symptoms (Millesi, 1980).

Other upper extremity peripheral nerves that may be injured include the axillary nerve. Functional implications include the inability to raise the arm at the shoulder. The radial, musculocutaneous, median, and ulnar nerves are other upper extremity nerves that can be injured. Humeral fractures involve radial nerve paralysis 11% of the time (Omer, 1980). The median nerve may be injured in the region of the elbow and cause an inability to flex the index finger and the distal phalanx of the thumb, resulting in defective opposition of the thumb. This prevents any pincer-type movement and renders the hand useless (Schaumburg, Spencer, & Thomas, 1983).

Trunk and lower extremity Acute lesions of the lumbosacral plexus are uncommon, but may be involved in fractures of the pelvis. Injury to the femoral nerve causes weakness of knee extension, wasting of the quadriceps, loss of the knee jerk, and sensory impairment over the front of the thigh. This causes considerable difficulty with walking, because the knee cannot be locked into extension. If the sciatic nerve is injured, foot drop occurs. All muscles below the knee are paralyzed. Sciatic nerve injury can occur with fractures of the pelvis, as well as from gunshot wounds. The tibial and peroneal nerves in the lower portion of the leg can also cause problems with walking (Kopell, 1980). Nerve injuries are more common with dislocations than with fractures. The sciatic or peroneal nerves are injured in approximately 10% of patients with posterior dislocation or posterior acetabular fracture of the hip. Of knee dislocations, 25% to 35% cause peripheral nerve injuries (Omer, 1980).

Rehabilitation focus

Rehabilitation of peripheral nerve injuries is a long process. The initial approach is conservative as assessment of the potential for spontaneous recovery is made. When the patient is admitted to the intensive care unit or acute medical floor, consultation with occupational therapy and physical therapy initiates the rehabilitation process.

Splinting and surgery Splinting of the extremity combined with purposeful exercise provides the keystone of effective rehabilitation (Fess, 1986; McGormack, 1981). Splinting prevents secondary damage and preserves passive range of motion (Figure 24-9). In the treatment of brachial plexus injuries, conservative treatment is

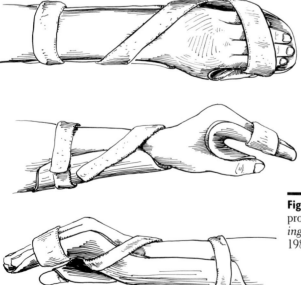

Figure 24-9 Volar splint maintains flaccid hand in proper alignment. (*Note.* From *Rehabilitation Nursing: Process and Application* (p. 379) by S.S. Dittmar, 1989, St. Louis: Mosby–Year Book, Inc.)

provided for the first 4 months. During the next 2 months, a decision is made regarding the appropriateness of surgical intervention for the purpose of neurolysis or nerve grafts. Potential for recovery from surgical intervention diminishes after the 6-month period. The projected recovery period is 2 years. If no improvement occurs during that period, amputation and fitting of a functional prosthesis are considered (Millesi, 1980).

Biofeedback   Another treatment modality for persons with peripheral nerve injury is biofeedback for learning to isolate specific muscle groups and sensory reeducation techniques to recognize "new" sensory patterns translated to them from partially innervated digits (Fess, 1986). Teaching compensatory techniques for activities of daily living is an important part of the rehabilitation plan (McGormack, 1981).

Vocational rehabilitation   Unless other disabling conditions are present, persons with peripheral nerve injury are provided rehabilitation services within the acute hospital and on an outpatient basis. If alterations in job performance are caused by the impairment, a vocational rehabilitation counselor may be involved in assisting the person to modify work approaches or to explore alternative vocational pursuits. Figure 24-10 shows the rehabilitative efforts by the patient to reclaim the use of his left hand. Psychological support is critical to persons with sudden alterations in functional abilities and self-concept.

Traumatic Amputations

The overall annual incidence of extremity amputations from all causes in the United States is estimated at 43,000. Trauma is a relatively small contributor to this number (Banerjee, 1984). The greatest number of amputations result from peripheral vascular disease. However, the incidence of traumatic amputations in the younger population is higher as compared with the elderly population. The mean age in a study of persons with traumatic amputation of the upper limb was 30 years (Sturup et al., 1988). A strong male preponderance exists for traumatic amputations. It is estimated that 85% of all persons with amputations in the United States have major lower extremity involvement (Banerjee, 1984). Traumatic amputations result primarily from work-related injuries and motor vehicle crashes. With trauma, the level of the amputation is determined by the ex-

tent of tissue injury. Amputation of an extremity is no longer considered a failure of treatment, but the beginning of a new phase in which most patients can be restored to high functioning through proper rehabilitation.

New approach: Rigid plaster dressings

The postoperative and rehabilitation treatment of amputations has changed significantly since the late 1970s, primarily because of the increased use of rigid plaster dressing applications in the operating room. Rigid dressings decrease pain, allow for earlier prosthetic use, reduce postsurgical edema, and decrease the healing time. A tendency exists for earlier psychologic adjustment, primarily related to earlier use of the prosthetic device (Banerjee, 1984; Dickey & Stieritz, 1981).

Rehabilitation focus

Physical and occupational therapists become actively involved in the rehabilitation process immediately after the surgical intervention. The focus of early rehabilitation is on preserving residual limb motions that will be used for prosthesis control, maximizing range of motion of the residual extremity, and strengthening and conditioning the person to maximize functioning. Wound healing and physical care of the stump are of primary importance to prevent complications. Trauma nurses can work in conjunction with the physical or occupational therapist to promote proper positioning and range-of-motion exercises with the patient. Depending on the patient's additional injuries, those with rigid dressings may be fit with temporary prostheses within 48 hours of the surgery. Depending on the extremity involved, adaptive techniques for accomplishing activities of daily living are taught by the occupational therapist.

The majority of patients with single limb amputations are provided continued rehabilitation in an out-patient setting after their initial acute hospitalization. Those with multiple amputations or other injuries may be treated in an in-patient rehabilitation setting before out-patient follow-up.

Prosthetics   In addition to continued work on strengthening and conditioning, intensive prosthetic training is provided for those who choose to use a prosthesis. A study performed in Denmark (Sturup et al., 1988) assessed the rejection rate of prostheses with upper extremity amputations.

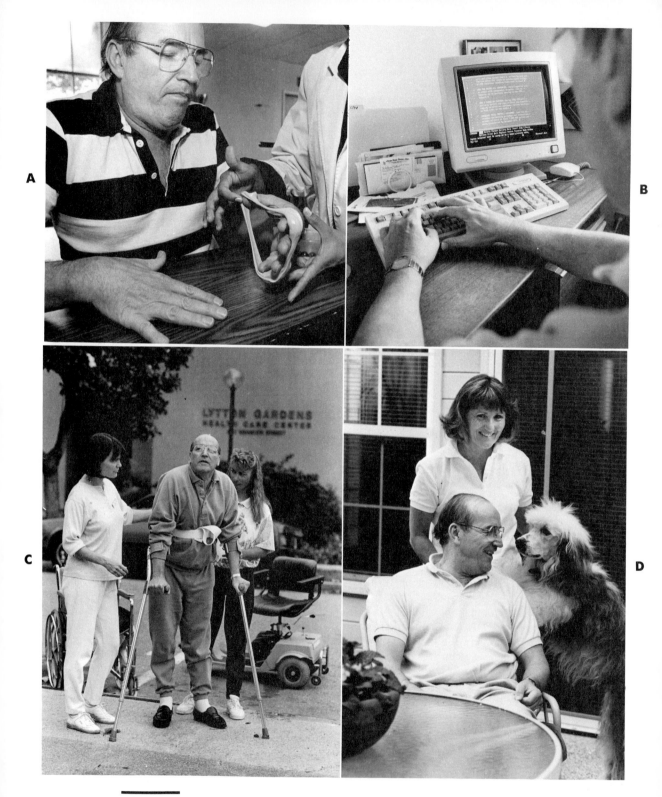

Figure 24-10 **A,** Rehabilitative exercise using putty to strengthen wrist, hand, and fingers. **B,** Regaining expertise on computer. **C,** Mobility training in community setting by physical and occupational therapists. **D,** Hard work resulted in successful return to vocational and family pursuits. (*Note.* Photographs by Renee Burgard, Stanford University Hospital.)

Two thirds of the patients used their prosthesis regularly. Use was highly correlated with the need from a vocational standpoint and if the amputation was of the dominant hand. Those with below-elbow prosthesis were a higher percentage of the users. The majority (98%) used the prosthesis for functional reasons. Only one individual used it only for cosmetic reasons.

Several different types of prosthetic devices are available. Myoelectric prostheses use the myoelectric potential of residual muscles to trigger the movements of the prosthesis. Switch-control prostheses use external switches that are activated to cause movement. The more recent developments in prostheses involve computer pattern recognition systems (Dickey & Stieritz, 1981; Gibbons, O'Riain, & Philippe-Auguste, 1987).

Personal and vocational adjustment

Adjustment to a traumatic amputation is an individual process, and adjustment to an altered body image may take a significant amount of time. Counseling from a professional, as well as peer counseling and support, is an important part of the rehabilitation process. Self-help support groups comprising individuals who function with amputations are available in larger cities. Vocational rehabilitation counselors are important team members because persons with amputations look at vocational goals. Assistance with job modification or vocational exploration can be provided.

Functional outcomes

Those persons with a unilateral, below-the-knee amputation can expect to function very closely to their preinjury level. Unilateral, above-the-knee amputations have a more functional impact. However, young persons can function very independently and can participate in sports that don't require extensive running. Elderly persons are impacted more significantly in mobility with an above-the-knee amputation. Those with bilateral, below-the-knee amputations can be ambulators, but ambulation is slower and endurance is limited. Those with bilateral, above-the-knee amputations are not functional ambulators, primarily because of the significant energy expenditure needed for ambulation (Banerjee, 1984). Those with upper extremity amputations have the capability of being very functional with the use of prostheses. However, the higher the amputation

in upper or lower extremities, the more difficulty with adaptation to the prosthesis (Pedretti, 1981).

Complications

Phantom sensations may create some difficulty for patients with amputations. These sensations usually diminish with time. A small percentage of patients have painful phantom sensations that cause burning, cramping, or shooting pains. A consistent inverse relationship has been demonstrated between stump temperature and that of the intact limb and complaints of burning, throbbing, and tingling pain (both phantom and stump). A correlation between stump muscle spasms and cramping phantom pain has been demonstrated (Sherman, 1989). In addition, it is hypothesized that denervation hyperactivity and hyperexcitability of central neurons follow injury to afferent pathways (Portenoy, 1989). Medications such as anticonvulsants and tricyclic antidepressants are prescribed for the treatment of phantom pain. These are selected to enhance the inhibition of the central neurons that have become hyperexcitable (Davar & Maciewicz, 1989). Bilateral exercises, massage, and desensitization techniques can assist in minimizing the sensations. Patients who continue to have severe pain that impairs functioning are referred to a pain service.

Continued care of the residual limb is an important consideration and educational need of persons with amputations. Breakdown in skin is a potential complication because of the continual pressure and weight-bearing on areas that normally don't receive such use. Equipment must be kept in good repair and replaced when needed (O'Sullivan, Cullen, & Schmitz, 1981). Growth in children, as well as weight loss or gain in adults, may create resizing needs.

Alterations in Tissue Integrity: Burns

Alterations in surface integrity can be caused by severe degloving injuries, as well as burns. This section discusses the rehabilitation of burns.

Advances in the care of persons with burns and the availability of new techniques for wound closure give even the most severely burned patient a chance for survival. Since the 1940s, the survival rate of those with extensive burns has increased dramatically (Salisbury & Petro, 1987). It is estimated that each year in the United States, 7500 to 12,000 persons die from burns. The elderly and young children are at the highest risk for death. The risk of fire injury is highest in the 18- to 25-year-old group (Antoon & Remensnyder, 1987; Silverstein & Lack, 1987). Thermal injury is the third most common cause of accidental pediatric death, with an estimated 1300 deaths and 3900 disabling injuries annually (Robinson & Seward, 1987). Refer to Chapter 14 for further information.

Thermal injury primarily results in destruction of skin and secondarily involves function of the musculoskeletal system. The degree of musculoskeletal impairment is determined by the depth and extent of the burn injury. The amount of tissue injury is determined by the extent of the burn surface and the duration of contact (Robinson & Seward, 1987). Chapter 14 explains the classification of burns and means of recovery.

Rehabilitation focus

Early intervention Burn injury treatment requires integration of the acute management with rehabilitation aspects from the first day of injury. In addition to the focus of fluid resuscitation, nutritional support, infection prevention, and surgical excision and coverage of the burn, the rehabilitation goals during the intensive care phase include limiting or preventing loss of motion, minimizing anatomic deformities, and preventing loss of body weight (Boswick, 1987a). Because of the frequently changing condition of the burn patient, flexibility of approaches is essential to maximize the rehabilitation goals. Physical therapists and occupational therapists become involved in the care of the burn patient from the first day of injury. Proper positioning techniques must be implemented within 24 hours to minimize contractures. Active motion to all extremities should begin the day of injury. Trauma nurses and therapists work together to ensure that appropriate positioning and frequent mobility occur throughout the day. Occupational therapists have expertise in designing and fabricating splints for use in positioning. Smith and Owens (1985) outline the benefits of a standardized protocol for use with the burn rehabilitation team. This ensures role clarification and communication of responsibilities in the rehabilitation process.

Pressure garments Early use of pressure garments on healed or grafted areas assists in preventing and controlling hypertrophic scar formation (Covey, 1987; Fowler, 1987; Smith &

Owens, 1985; Stern & Davey, 1985). Pressure maintains collagen in a parallel pattern, allowing intermolecular crosslinking to occur in a more favorable pattern with regard to underlying joints (Stern & Davey, 1985). Continued splinting and exercise also contribute to scar management. Early ambulation assists with joint mobility and flexibility and assists with maintaining cardiopulmonary fitness and increasing endurance. Adapted techniques for accomplishing activities of daily living are taught where needed.

Recurrent surgery When patients are stabilized physiologically, continued rehabilitation may occur in an acute rehabilitation center or through an out-patient setting. Additional surgeries may occur after the patient is initially discharged. These are performed to improve function or appearance. The focus on maintaining joint mobility, preventing contractures, and increasing strength and endurance continues. The proper care of the burned areas to prevent further breakdown and to minimize scarring is taught to the patient and family.

Psychosocial considerations

Fear and anxiety in the acute stages of burn recovery are the most common emotional responses seen. Persons have difficulty sleeping, often have nightmares, and are restless. Persistent pain contributes greatly to these feelings (Boswick, 1987b). Regression displayed by dependent and demanding behavior is a common reaction in the acute stages. This may be a substitute behavior for the grief the individual is experiencing related to perceived losses. Anger toward the healthcare staff and family members is also common. Feelings of helplessness, hopelessness, and depression are common during the first year after the injury. When survival is no longer an issue, anxieties and fears develop regarding appearance, ability to function and work, and family and social acceptance. The literature sites approximately 1 year as a point when psychologic adaptation begins to occur (Boswick, 1987b; Shenkman & Stechmiller, 1987). Major adjustments, particularly from the psychologic standpoint, can extend for years (Salisbury & Petro, 1987).

Functional outcomes

The percentage of total body surface area (TBSA) involved in the burn is an important parameter when considering return to work. Disfigurement is also a factor. Approximately three fourths of working adults return to work, but about half of them change jobs (Tate-Henderson, 1987). Elderly persons with burns have a significantly decreased functional level after injury. It is estimated that the majority of those with greater than 15% TBSA will not be able to return home independently (Salisbury & Petro, 1987).

SUMMARY   Trauma rehabilitation is a critical component in the continuum of trauma care and treatment. Elements of rehabilitation begin in the emergency and intensive care phases and continue in many cases for months and years. Trauma care has improved tremendously in the past 15 years, with mortality decreasing. As a result, more severely disabled individuals survive injuries and are faced with adapting and adjusting their lives to the limitations and changes that result.

Nursing diagnoses that are applicable to trauma patients depend on the type of trauma sustained and the resulting functional impairments. Three of the more common nursing diagnoses, with interventions and evaluation criteria, are outlined in the table on p. 738.

Trauma nurses are the healthcare professionals who initiate the process of rehabilitation by incorporating early rehabilitation techniques into the initial care of these individuals. An understanding of the entire rehabilitation process can provide an element of hope for the trauma nurse. Although a severely injured person may initially look unsalvageable for a return to any meaningful existence, the rehabilitation process can contribute significantly to the quantitative and qualitative aspects of the disabled person's life. This understanding gives a broader perspective to the trauma nurse of what lies ahead for the traumatically injured patient. This perspective can also contribute to the patient and family support that is initiated in the emergency and critical care stages of treatment (Figure 24-11).

Healthcare professionals are charged with developing healthcare delivery systems that can

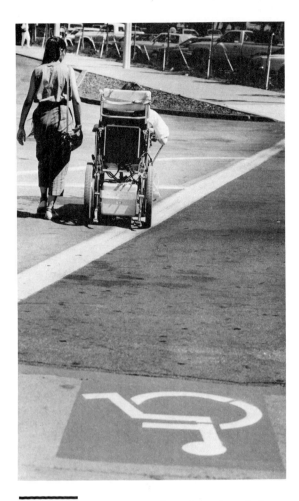

Figure 24-11   Maximizing independence is goal of rehabilitation. Here, although wheelchair is needed for mobility, community exploration and growing integration within society is evident. (*Note.* Photograph by Renee Burgard, Stanford University Hospital.)

meet the varied and complicated needs of the disabled population. Society in general is charged with providing expanded opportunities for those individuals with disabilities to function as productively and independently as possible. And finally, persons with disabilities have a responsibility to be contributors to society.

The trauma rehabilitation patient

Nursing diagnosis	Nursing intervention	Evaluative criteria
High risk for altered urinary elimination Related to nervous system deficit, limited concentration and awareness	**Promote adequate urinary elimination patterns** Initiate referral to urologist and urodynamic testing. Implement intermittent bladder program or other bladder program, as appropriate. Monitor I & O. Monitor number of incontinencies. Implement fluid intake schedule. Educate the patient about specific bladder program.	Urinalysis will show no WBCs; urine C&S will show no growth. Amount catheterized will remain less than 500 ml, or post-void residual will remain less than 100 ml. No incontinence will occur.
High risk for impaired mobility Related to structural deficit, physical restrictions during healing, pain	**Maximize mobility** Initiate referral to physical therapist. Obtain appropriate device to maximize current mobility status. Teach safe use of devices. Perform range-of-motion exercises, and encourage active range of motion, as appropriate. Assist patient with mobilizing, as tolerated.	Patient will mobilize at a maximal functional level, using appropriate mobilization device. Patient will practice safe mobilization techniques and avoid further injury.
High risk for self-esteem disturbance Related to changes in functional and cognitive ability	**Support productive coping mechanisms and reward progress** Refer to psychologist or social worker for disability adjustment counseling. Perform active listening and provide support to patient. Assist patient on a daily or weekly basis in outlining realistic short-term goals that are measurable. Provide successful daily experiences in self-care routines.	Patient will participate actively in rehabilitation program. Patient will be able to state some positive self-esteem comments that indicate feelings of hopefulness. Patient will engage in self-care activities.

COMPETENCIES
The following clinical competencies pertain to **mobilization in trauma patients with spinal cord injury.**

☑ Demonstrate proper bed-positioning techniques.
☑ Demonstrate proper transfer techniques, using the following transfer types:
  - standing pivot transfer;
  - slide board transfer;
  - Hoyer lift transfer;
  - two-person lift;
  - three-person lift.
☑ Apply immobilization and assistive devices correctly.
☑ Demonstrate knowledge of assistive device use and maintenance.

COMPETENCIES
The following clinical competencies pertain to **safety maintenance in trauma patients with head injury.**

☑ Demonstrate knowledge of managing the physical environment to minimize overstimulation.
☑ Demonstrate proper use of safety promotion devices.
☑ Demonstrate safe methods of physical management.
☑ Demonstrate knowledge of common cognitive impairments that alter the patient's own safety awareness and judgment.

RESEARCH QUESTIONS

- What differences are seen in patient outcome when rehabilitation services are actively started in the critical care phase as compared with initiating after the critical care phase?
- Does experience in working with disabled persons in the phases of trauma care after critical care impact the attitudes of emergency or critical care nurses toward trauma resuscitation? If so, in which ways?
- Do patients who receive planned sensory stimulation programs demonstrate responsiveness earlier than those patients who do not receive planned sensory stimulation programs?
- Do patients who receive care in a trauma system specifically designed to target the trauma diagnosis (such as the model spinal injury systems) have higher functional outcomes in a shorter time frame?

RESOURCES

American Association of Spinal Cord Injury Nurses
75-20 Astoria Blvd.
Jackson Heights, NY 11370-1178
(718) 803-3782

American Congress of Rehabilitation Medicine
5700 Old Orchard Rd., First Floor
Skokie, IL 60077-1057
(708) 966-0095

Association of Rehabilitation Nurses
5700 Old Orchard Rd., First Floor
Skokie, IL 60077-1024
(708) 966-3433

National Head Injury Foundation
1140 Connecticut Ave. NW
Washington, D.C. 20036
(800) 444-6443

National Rehabilitation Information Center
8455 Colesville Rd., Suite 935
Silver Springs, MD 20910
(800) 346-2742

ANNOTATED BIBLIOGRAPHY

Dittmar, S. S. (1989). *Rehabilitation nursing: Process and application.* St. Louis: Mosby–Year Book, Inc.
Comprehensive text addressing the assessment and treatment of the major nursing diagnoses seen in rehabilitation nursing.

Fisher, S. V., & Helm, P. A. (Eds.) (1984). *Comprehensive rehabilitation of burns.* Baltimore: Williams & Wilkins.
In-depth information about all aspects of burn rehabilitation and the various roles of team members in the rehabilitation process.

Rosenthal, M., & Griffith, E. R. (Eds.) (1990). *Rehabilitation of the head-injured adult* (2nd ed.). Philadelphia: F. A. Davis.
Broad perspective on the major aspects of head injury rehabilitation, with particular emphasis on assessment.

Trieshman, R. (1980). *Spinal cord injuries: Psychological, social, and vocational adjustment.* New York: Pergamon Press.
Comprehensive book exclusively devoted to the psychologic impact of spinal cord injury. Includes an exhaustive critique of the literature.

REFERENCES

American College of Surgeons, Committee on Trauma. (1986). *Optimal hospital resources for care of the seriously injured* (revised). Chicago: Author.

Antoon, A., & Remensnyder, J. P. (1987). Burns in children. In J. A. Boswick (Ed.), *The art and science of burn care* (pp. 255-262). Rockville, MD: Aspen Publishers.

Banerjee, S.N. (1984). Amputations. In J. V. Basmajian & R. L. Kirby (Eds.), *Medical rehabilitation.* Baltimore: Williams & Wilkins.

Banta, J. V. (1984). Rehabilitation of pediatric spinal cord injury: The Newington children's hospital experience. *Connecticut Medicine, 48* (1), 14-18.

Bijur, P. E., Haslum, M., & Golding, J. (1990). Cognitive and behavioral sequelae of mild injury in children. *Pediatrics, 86* (3), 337-344.

Bitter, J. (1979). *Introduction to rehabilitation.* St. Louis: Mosby–Year Book, Inc.

Bontke, C. F. (1989). Medical complications related to traumatic brain injury. In L. J. Horn & D. N. Cope (Eds.), *Physical medicine and rehabilitation: State-of-the-art reviews, 3* (1), (pp. 43-58). Philadelphia: Hanley & Belfus.

Booth, B. J., Doyle, M., & Montgomery, J. (1983). Serial casting for the management of spasticity in the head-injured adult. *Physical Therapy, 63,* 1960-1966.

Boswick, J. A. (1987a). Comprehensive rehabilitation after burn injury. *Surgical Clinics of North America, 67*(1), 159-166.

Boswick, J. A. (1987b). Emotional problems in burn patients. In J. A. Boswick (Ed.), *The art and science of burn care* (pp. 271-274). Rockville, MD: Aspen Publishers.

Boughton, A., & Ceisla, N. (1986). Physical therapy management of the head-injured patient in the intensive care unit. *Topics in Acute Care and Trauma Rehabilitation, 1*(1), 1-18.

Braakman, R., Habbema, J. D. F., & Gelpke, G. J. (1986). Prognosis and prediction of outcome in comatose head injury patients. *Acta Neurochirurgica, 36* (Suppl), 112-117.

Brooks, N. (Ed.). (1984). *Closed head injury; Psychological social and family consequences.* Oxford: Oxford University Press.

Brooks, N., Campsie, L., & Symington, C. (1987). The effects of severe head injury upon patient and relative within seven years of injury. *Journal of Head Trauma Rehabilitation, 2,* 1-13.

Brown, J. S., & Giesy, B. (1986). Marital status of persons with spinal cord injury. *Social Science & Medicine, 23* (3), 313-322.

Burke, D. C., Burley, H. T., & Ungar, G. H. (1985). Data on spinal injuries. Pt. II: Outcome of the treatment of 352 consecutive admissions. *Australian & New Zealand Journal of Surgery, 55,* 377-382.

Buss, P., Chippendale, J., Hagen, C., Klauber, K. W., & Minteer, M. (1984). *Sensory stimulation: A guide for families of brain-injured patients.* San Diego: Sharp Memorial Hospital.

Caplan, A. L. (1988). Informed consent and provider-patient relationships in rehabilitation medicine. *Archives of Physical Medicine and Rehabilitation, 69* (5), 312-317.

Carey, R. G., & Posavac, E. J. (1977). Program evaluation of a physical medicine and rehabilitation unit: A new approach. *Archives of Physical Medicine & Rehabilitation, 59,* 330-337.

Condeluci, A., & Gretz-Lasky, S. (1987). Social role valorization: A model for community reentry. *Journal of Head Trauma Rehabilitation, 2*(1), 49-56.

Covey, M. H. (1987). Occupational therapy. In J. A. Boswick (Ed.), *The art and science of burn care* (pp. 285-298). Rockville, MD: Aspen Publishers.

Davar, G., & Maciewicz, R. J. (1989). Deafferentation pain syndromes. *Neurologic Clinics, 7*(2), 289-304.

Deitz, J. M., Bertschy, M., Gschaedler, R., & Dollfus, P. (1986). Reflections on the intensive care of 106 acute cervical spinal cord injury patients in the resuscitation unit of a general traumatology centre. *Paraplegia, 24,* 343-349.

Deutsch, P. M., & Fralish, K. B. (1989). *Innovations in head injury rehabilitation.* New York: Matthew Bender.

DeVivo, M. J., Kartus, P. L., Stover, S. L., Rutt, R. D., & Fine, P. R. (1987). Seven-year survival following spinal cord injury. *Archives of Neurology, 44,* 872-875.

DeVivo, M. J., Rutt, R. D., Stover, S. L., & Fine, P. R. (1987). Employment after spinal cord injury. *Archives of Physical Medicine and Rehabilitation, 68,* 494-498.

Dickey, R. E., & Stieritz, L. (1981). Amputation and impaired independence. In B. C. Abreu (Ed.), *Physical disabilities manual.* New York: Raven Press.

Dixon, T. P. (1989). Systems of care for the head-injured. In L. J. Horn & D. N. Cope (Eds.), *Physical medicine and rehabilitation: State of the art reviews, 3* (1), (pp. 169-182). Philadelphia: Hanley & Belfus.

Dollfus, P. I. (1987). Initial hospital care of spinal cord injury. *Paraplegia, 25,* 241-243.

Drayton-Hargrove, S., & Reddy, M. A. (1986). Rehabilitation and long-term management of the spinal cord injured adult. *Nursing Clinics of North America, 21* (4), 599-610.

Ducanis, A. J., & Golin, A. K. (1979). *The interdisciplinary health care team.* Germantown, MD: Aspen Systems Corporation.

Earnest, M. P. (1983). *Neurological emergencies.* New York: Churchill Livingstone.

Fess, E. E. (1986). Rehabilitation of the patient with peripheral nerve injury. *Hand Clinics*, 2 (1), 207-215.

Filley, C. M., Cranberg, L. D., Alexander, M. P., & Hart, E. J. (1987). Neurobehavioral outcome after closed head injury in childhood and adolescence. *Archives of Neurology*, 44, 194-198.

Fowler, D. (1987). Australian occupational therapy: Current trends and future considerations in burn rehabilitation. *Journal of Burn Care and Rehabilitation*, 8(5), 415-417.

Frieden, L., & Cole, J. A. (1985). Independence: The ultimate goal of rehabilitation for spinal cord-injured persons. *American Journal of Occupational Therapy*, 39 (11), 734-739.

Gibbons, D. T., O'Riain, M. D., & Philippe-Auguste, S. (1987). *IEEE Transactions on Biomedical Engineering*, 34(7), 493-498.

Goffman, E. (1963). *Stigma: Notes on the management of spoiled identity*. New York: Simon & Schuster.

Goethe, K., & Levin, H. (1984). Behavioral manifestations during early and long-term stages of recovery after closed head injury. *Psychiatry Annals*, 14, 540-546.

Granger, C. V., & Gresham, G. E. (1984). *Functional assessment in rehabilitation medicine*. Baltimore: Williams & Wilkins.

Green, B. A., Eismont, F. J., & O'Heir, J. T. (1987). Prehospital management of spinal cord injuries. *Paraplegia*, 25, 229-238.

Hagen, C. (1983). Planning a therapeutic environment for the communicatively impaired post closed head injury patient. In S. J. Shanks (Ed.), *Nursing and the management of adult communication disorders* (pp. 137-169). San Diego: College-Hill Press.

Hagen, C., & Malkmus, D. (1979). *Intervention strategies for language disorders secondary to head trauma*. Atlanta: American Speech-Hearing Association, Short Courses.

Haller, J. A., & Buck, J. (1985). Does a trauma-management system improve outcome for children with life-threatening injuries? *Canadian Journal of Surgery*, 28(6), 477.

Hinkle, J. L., Alves, W. M., Rimel, R. W., & Jane, J. A. (1986). Restoring social competence in minor head injury. *Journal of Neuroscience Nursing*, 18 (5), 268-271.

Houston, J. M. (1984). Comprehensive education for those concerned with spinal cord injury patients. *Paraplegia*, 22, 244-248.

Imle, P. C., & Boughton, A. C. (1987). The physical therapist's role in the early management of acute spinal cord injury. *Topics in Acute Care and Trauma Rehabilitation*, 1 (3), 32-47.

Jacobs, H. E. (1988). The Los Angeles head injury survey: Procedures and initial findings. *Archives of Physical Medicine and Rehabilitation*, 69 (6), 425-431.

Jennett, B., & Bond, M. (1975). Assessment of outcome after severe brain damage. *Lancet*, 1, 481-484.

Jennett, B. (1983). Post-traumatic epilepsy. In M. Rosenthal & E. R. Griffith (Eds.), *Rehabilitation of the head injured adult*. Philadelphia: F. A. Davis.

Jennett, B., & Teasdale, G. (1981) *Management of head injuries*. Philadelphia, F. A. Davis.

Katz, S., Ford, A. B., & Moskowitz, R. W. (1963). Studies of illness in the aged. The index of ADL: A standardized measure of biological and psychosocial function. *JAMA*, 183, 914-919.

Klauber, K. W., & Ward-McKinlay, C. (1986). Managing behavior in the patient with traumatic brain injury. *Topics in Acute Care and Trauma Rehabilitation*, 1(1), 48-60.

Klauber, M. R., Barrett-Connor, E., Hofstetter, C. R., & Micik, S. H. (1986). A population-based study of nonfatal childhood injuries. *Preventive Medicine*, 15, 139-149.

Kopell, H. P. (1980). Lower extremity lesions. In G. E. Omer & M. Spinner (Eds.), *Management of peripheral nerve problems* (pp. 626-638). Philadelphia: W. B. Saunders.

Kraus, J. F., Black, M.A., Hessol, N, Ley, P., Rokaw, W., Sullivan, C., Bowers, S., Knowlton, S., & Marshall, L. (1984). Incidence of acute brain injury and serious impairment in defined population. *American Journal of Epidemiology*, 119, 185-201.

Laven, G. T., Huang, C. T., DeVivo, M. J., Stover, S. L., Kuhlemeier, K. V., & Fine, P. R. (1989). Nutritional status during the acute stage of spinal cord injury. *Archives of Physical Medicine and Rehabilitation*, 70 (4), 277-282.

Levin, H., Eisenberg, H., & Benton, A. (1989). *Mild head injury*, New York: Oxford University Press.

Levin, H. S., Mattis, S., Ruff, R. M., Eisenberg, H. M., Marshall, L. F., Tabaddor, K., High, W. M., & Frankowski, R. F. (1987). Neurobehavioral outcome following minor head injury: A three center study. *Journal of Neurosurgery*, 66, 234-243.

Lezak, M. D. (1978). Living with the characterologically altered brain injury patient. *Journal of Clinical Psychiatry*, 39, 592-598.

Lezak, M. D. (1987). Relationships between personality disorders, social disturbances, and physical disability following traumatic brain injury. *Journal of Head Trauma Rehabilitation*, 2,(1), 57-69.

Livingston, M. G. & Brooks, D. N. (1988). The burden on families of the brain injured: a review. *Journal of Head Trauma Rehabilitation*, 3(4), 6-15.

Lobato, R., & Cordobe F. (1983). Outcome from severe head injury related to the type of intracranial lesions. *Journal of Neurosurgery*, 50, 762-774.

Mack, A., & Horn, L. J. (1989). Functional prognosis in traumatic brain injury. In L. J. Horn & D. N. Cope (Eds.), *Physical medicine and rehabilitation: State of the art reviews* (pp. 13-26). Philadelphia: Hanley & Belfus.

Mahoney, F. I., & Barthel, D. W. (1965). Functional evaluation: The Barthel index. *Maryland State Medical Journal*, 14, 61-65.

Mansoory, A. (1986). Anatomy of a regional trauma center. *Delaware Medical Journal*, 58(12), 817-820.

Martin, N., Holt, N. B., & Hicks, D. (1981). *Comprehensive rehabilitation nursing*. New York: McGraw-Hill.

McGormack, G. L. (1981). Lower motor neuron dysfunction. In L. W. Pedretti (Ed.), *Occupational therapy: Practice skills for physical dysfunction* (pp. 246-256). St. Louis: Mosby–Year Book, Inc.

McGowan, M. B., & Roth, S. (1987). Family functioning and functional independence in spinal cord injury adjustment. *Paraplegia*, 25, 357-365.

McKinlay, W. W., Brooks, D. N., & Bond, M. R. (1981). The short-term outcome of severe head injury as reported by relatives of the injured person. *Journal of Neurology, Neurosurgery, and Psychiatry*, 44, 527-533.

Metcalf, J. A. (1986). Acute phase management of persons with spinal cord injury: A nursing diagnosis perspective. *Nursing Clinics of North America*, 21 (4), 589-598.

Millesi, H. (1980). Trauma involving the brachial plexus. In G. E. Omer & M. Spinner (Eds.), *Management of peripheral nerve problems* (pp. 548-568). Philadelphia: W. B. Saunders.

Moore, S. (1986). Treatment at Odyssey Ranch head injury program: An alternative to institutionalized rehabilitation. *Topics in Acute Care and Trauma Rehabilitation, 1*(1), 61-71.

National Head Injury Foundation (1988). *Head injury (fact sheet).* (Available from National Head Injury Foundation, 1140 Connecticutt Ave. NW, Washington, DC 20036).

Nikas, D. L. (1982). Acute spinal cord injuries: Care and implications. In D. L. Nikas (Ed.), *The critically ill neurosurgical patient* (pp. 107-124). New York: Churchill Livingstone.

Nikas, D. L., & Tolley, M. (1982). Acute head injury. In D. L. Nikas (Ed.), *The critically ill neurosurgical patient* (pp. 89-106). New York: Churchill Livingstone.

North American Nursing Diagnosis Association. (1988). NANDA-approved nursing diagnostic categories. *Nursing Diagnosis Newsletter, 15*(1), 1-3.

Oddy, M., Humphrey, M., & Uttley, D. (1978). Subjective impairment and social recovery after closed head injury. *Journal of Neurology, Neurosurgery, and Psychiatry, 46,* 611-616.

Omer, G. E. (1980). The results of untreated traumatic injuries. In G. E. Omer & M. Spinner (Eds.), *Management of peripheral nerve problems* (pp. 502-506). Philadelphia: W. B. Saunders.

O'Sullivan, S. B., Cullen, K. E., & Schmitz, T. J. (1981). *Physical rehabilitation: Evaluation and treatment procedures.* Philadelphia: F. A. Davis.

Pedretti, L. W. (1981). *Occupational therapy: Practice skills for physical dysfunction.* St. Louis: Mosby–Year Book, Inc.

Portenoy, R. K. (1989). Mechanisms of clinical pain. *Neurologic Clinics, 7* (2), 205-230.

Purtilo, R. B. (1988). Ethical issues in teamwork: The context of rehabilitation. *Archives of Physical Medicine and Rehabilitation, 69* (5), 318-322.

Robinson, M. D., & Seward, P. N. (1987). Thermal injury in children. *Pediatric Emergency Care, 3*(4), 266-270.

Rimel, R. W., Giordani, B., Barth, J. T., Boll, T. J., & Jane, J. A. (1981). Disability caused by minor head injury. *Neurosurgery, 9*(3), 221-228.

Romano, M. D. (1989). Family issues in head trauma. In L. J. Horn & D. N. Cope (Eds.) *Physical medicine and rehabilitation: State of the art reviews* (pp. 157-168). Philadelphia: Hanley & Belfus.

Russell, W. R. (1961). *The traumatic amnesias.* Oxford: Oxford University Press.

Russell, W. R., & Nathan, P. W. (1946). Traumatic amnesia. *Brain, 69,* 280-300.

Salisbury, R. E., & Petro, J. A. (1987). Rehabilitation of burn patients. In J. A. Boswick (Ed.), *The art and science of burn care* (pp. 265-269). Rockville, MD: Aspen Publishers.

Schaumburg, H. H., Spencer, P. S., & Thomas, P. K. (1983). *Disorders of peripheral nerves.* Philadelphia: F. A. Davis.

Schoening, H. A., Anderegg, L., & Bergstrom, D., (1965). Numerical scoring of self-care status of patients. *Archives of Physical Medicine and Rehabilitation, 46,* 689-697.

Shenkman, B., & Stechmiller, J. (1987). Patient and family perception of projected functioning after discharge from a burn unit. *Heart and Lung, 16* (5), 490-496.

Sherman, R. A. (1989). Stump and phantom limb pain. *Neurologic Clinics, 7*(2), 249-294.

Silverstein, P., & Lack B. O. (1987). Epidemiology and prevention. In Boswick, J. A. (Ed.), *The art and science of burn care* (pp. 11-17). Rockville, MD: Aspen Publishers.

Smith, K., & Owens, K. (1985). Physical and occupational therapy burn unit protocol: Benefits and uses. *Journal of Burn Care & Rehabilitation, 6*(6), 506-508.

Stern, L. M., & Davey, R. B. (1985). A team approach with severely burned children in a multidisciplinary rehabilitation setting. *Burns, 11,* 281-284.

Stover, S. L., & Fine, P. R. (1987). The epidemiology and economics of spinal cord injury. *Paraplegia, 25,* 225-228.

Sturup, J., Thyregod, H. C., Jensen, J. S., Retpen, J. B., Boberg, G., Rasmussen, E., & Jensen, S. (1988). Traumatic amputation of the upper limb: The use of body-powered prostheses and employment consequences. *Prosthetics and Orthotics International, 12,* 50-52.

Sweney, J. K., & Smutok, M. A. (1983). Vietnam head injury study: Preliminary analysis of the functional and anatomical sequelae of penetrating head injury. *Physical Therapy, 63,* 2018-2029.

Task Force for Development of a Uniform Data System for Medical Rehabilitation (1986). *Guide for use of the uniform data set for medical rehabilitation.* (Available through Project Office, Dept. of Rehabilitation Medicine, Buffalo General Hospital, 100 High St., Buffalo, NY 14203).

Tate-Henderson, S. (1987). Vocational rehabilitation: A new approach. In J. A. Boswick (Ed.), *The art and science of burn care* (pp. 285-298). Rockville, MD: Aspen Publishers.

Teasdale, G., & Jennett, B. (1974). Assessment of coma and impaired consciousness: A practical scale. *Lancet, 2,* 81-84.

Thomas, J. P. (1988). The evolution of model systems of care in traumatic brain injury. *Journal of Head Trauma Rehabilitation, 3*(4), 1-5.

Thomsen, I. V. (1987). Late psychosocial outcome in severe blunt head trauma. *Brain Injury, 1,* 131-143.

Ulrey, B. J., & Woods, N. M. (1986). The role of videofluoroscopy in the diagnosis and treatment of mealtime dysfunction in the brain-injured patient. *Topics in Acute Care and Trauma Rehabilitation, 1*(1), 19-31.

Urey, J. R., & Henggeler, S. W. (1987). Marital adjustment following spinal cord injury. *Archives of Physical Medicine and Rehabilitation, 68,* 69-74.

Waaland, P. K., & Kreutzer, J. S. (1988). Family response to childhood traumatic brain injury. *Journal of Head Trauma Rehabilitation, 3*(4), 51-63.

World Health Organization. (1980). *International classification of impairments, disabilities, and handicaps.* Geneva: World Health Organization.

Whyte, J., & Glenn, M. B. (1986). The care and rehabilitation of the patient in a persistent vegetative state. *Journal of Head Trauma Rehabilitation, 1* (1), 39-53.

Wright, B. A. (1960). *Physical disability: A psychological approach.* New York: Harper & Row.

Yarkony, G. M., Roth, E. J., Heinemann, A. W., Wu, Y., Katz, R. T., & Lovell, L. (1987). Benefits of rehabilitation for spinal cord injury. *Archives of Neurology, 44,* 93-96.

Zejdlik, C. M. (1983). *Management of spinal cord injury.* Monterey, CA: Wadsworth Health Sciences.

Epilogue

■■

In bringing this book to closure, the editors wish to address the artistic dimensions of trauma nursing. Throughout the book, the scientific aspects have been discussed as they relate to pathophysiology and interventions. As trauma nurses, each of us, however, recognizes that both science and art are essential in providing quality nursing care.

Trauma nursing is continuously evolving. As our knowledge requirements and technologic advances increase in number and complexity, we should not ignore the importance of personal experience in shaping nursing care. We thought that obtaining the views of a trauma nurse recently retired from practice would help illuminate changes in trauma nursing and provide some "words of wisdom" for those of us in practice.

FROM THE MEMORIES OF **Margaret Arnold** RETIRED NURSE
Victory Memorial Hospital
Emergency Care Unit
Waukegan, Illinois

As I look at nursing today and compare it to nursing 40 years ago, I can recount many changes. Today there is additional pressure placed upon the healthcare professional by state regulations, healthcare peers, patients, and their families. Nurses today have greater knowledge and responsibility than they did when I entered nursing in 1949. Today's nurses are supposed to be miracle workers; everything is expected to be as it is for the "glorified" nurse on television or in films. Today, as I recall my later nursing experience, I feel that the only glory one derives from nursing is what one feels in their heart. When you provide tender, loving care, you forget all the pressure imposed upon you by others. For nurses entering the field, I would advise them to always remember the internal gratification that comes from giving the best of their knowledge, skills, and understanding.

As a nursing instructor in Iowa once told me, "Nurses and physicians are not just educated, they are born to care for others." I believe that nursing is more than knowledge and skill; it requires compassion and love of your fellow human beings. The last 18 years of my career were spent in the emergency unit of a large hospital. I found joy in my job because I tried to assess each patient as if that patient was the only patient in our unit. Assessment requires listening and reassuring the patient, critically observing the patient, as well as assuring that all the medical details are followed. A holistic approach will encourage the nurse to remember that the patient is a human being who is asking for psychologic, spiritual, and emotional help, in addition to physiologic help.

In a typical trauma care setting, a nurse learns something new every day and the job is never boring. In spite of the exposure to diseases such as AIDS and the stress of specialized equipment and new procedures, the trauma setting remains one of the most exciting places to work in health care. No two days are the same, and each day is a new challenge. Perhaps this is why trauma nurses stay in trauma nursing.

My advice to anyone considering trauma nursing is, if you want to go into trauma nursing to help people, then do it. If that is not your purpose, don't do it. I have approached nursing as an opportunity to give of myself. Through this giving I have learned more about myself and I have received as much as I have ever given. I have learned to appreciate the input and advice of the other people who make up the health care team: physicians, aids, clerks, directors, security guards, paramedics, and all of the other people who play a role in the healing and comfort of the sick.

Trauma nurses see the results of crashes, gunshot and stabbing wounds, drug overdoses, heart attacks, strokes, burns, drownings, and much more. Yes, trauma nurses see it all. Because we see the ugly, the serious, and the sad, trauma nurses need to search for the joy that makes them unique. Trauma nurses must maintain this attitude and approach as they care for the sick and dying and comfort their families. We must never forget how lucky we are to be able to work with our minds, our hands, and our hearts to help someone else.

As I reflect back on my nursing career with all of its drawbacks and changes, without a doubt I would choose it again.

Margruete K Arnold

A Hospital Criteria

Resources for optimal care of the injured patient

The following table shows levels of categorization and their essential (E) or desirable (D) characteristics.

	LEVELS		
	I	II	III
A. Hospital organization			
1. Trauma service	E	E	D
2. Surgery departments/divisions/services/sections			
Cardiothoracic surgery	E	D	—
General surgery	E	E	E
Neurologic surgery	E	E	—
Ophthalmic surgery	E	D	—
Oral surgery (dental)	E	D	—
Orthopaedic surgery	E	E	—
Otorhinolaryngologic surgery	E	D	—
Plastic and maxillofacial surgery	E	D	—
Urologic surgery	E	D	—
3. Emergency department/division/service/section (see notes)[1]	E	E	E
4. Surgery specialties availability			
In house 24 hours a day:			
General surgery	E[2]	E[2,17]	—
Neurologic surgery	E[3]	E[3]	—
Orthopaedic surgery	E[4]	E[4]	—
On call and promptly available from inside or outside hospital (see notes)[5]			
Cardiac surgery	E	D	—
General surgery	—	—	E[6]
Neurologic surgery	—	—	D
Microsurgery capabilities	E	D	—
Hand surgery	E	D	—
Obstetric/Gynecologic surgery	E	D	—
Ophthalmic surgery	E	E	D
Oral surgery (dental)	E	D	—
Orthopaedic surgery	—	—	D
Otorhinolaryngologic surgery	E	E	D
Pediatric surgery	E	D	—
Thoracic surgery	E	E	D
Urologic surgery	E	E	D

Note. From "Resources for Optimal Care of the Injured Patient" by American College of Surgeons, Committee on Trauma, 1990, *ACS Bulletin, 75,* pp. 20-29.

Continued.

	LEVELS		
	I	**II**	**III**

A. Hospital organization—cont'd

5. Nonsurgical specialties availability

   In house 24 hours a day:

	I	II	III
Emergency medicine	E[7]	E[7]	E[10]
Anesthesiology	E[8]	E[8,9]	—

   On call and promptly available from inside or outside the hospital:

	I	II	III
Anesthesiology	—	—	E
Cardiology	E	E	D
Chest medicine	E	D	—
Family medicine	D[11]	D[11]	D[11]
Gastroenterology	E	D	—
Hematology	E	E	D
Infectious diseases	E	D	—
Internal medicine	E[11]	E[11]	E[11]
Nephrology	E	E	D
Pathology	E	E	D
Pediatrics	E[11,12]	E[11,12]	D[11,12] [2]
Psychiatry	E	D	—
Radiology	E	E	D

B. Special facilities/resources/capabilities

1. Emergency department (ED)

   a. Personnel

	I	II	III
1. Designated physician director	E	E	E
2. Physician who has special competence in care of critically injured and who is a designated member of the trauma team and is physically present in the ED 24 hours a day	E	E	E
3. A sufficient number of RNs, LPNs, and nurses aides to handle caseload	E	E	E

   b. Equipment for resuscitation and to provide life support for the critically or seriously injured shall include but not be limited to:

	I	II	III
1. Airway control and ventilation equipment including laryngoscopes and endotracheal tubes of all sizes, bag-mask resuscitator, pocket masks, oxygen, and mechanical ventilator	E	E	E
2. Suction devices	E	E	E
3. Electrocardiograph-oscilloscope-defibrillator	E	E	E
4. Apparatus to establish central venous pressure monitoring	E	E	E
5. All standard intravenous fluids and administration devices, including intravenous catheters	E	E	E
6. Sterile surgical sets for procedures standard for ED, for example, thoracostomy, venesection, lavage	E	E	E
7. Gastric lavage equipment	E	E	E
8. Drugs and supplies necessary for emergency care	E	E	E
9. X-ray capability, 24-hour coverage by in-house technician	E	E	D
10. Two-way radio linked with vehicles of emergency transport system	E	E	E
11. Skeletal traction device for cervical injuries	E	E	E
12. Swan-Ganz catheters	E	D	D
13. Arterial catheters	E	D	D
14. Thermal control equipment			
a. For patient	E	E	E
b. For blood and fluids	E	E	E

	LEVELS		
	I	II	III
2. Operating suite			
a. Personnel			
Operating room adequately staffed in house and immediately available 24 hours a day	E	E	D
b. Equipment: special requirements shall include but not be limited to:			
1. Cardiopulmonary bypass capability	E	D	—
2. Operating microscope	E	D	—
3. Thermal control equipment:			
a. For patient	E	E	E
b. For blood and fluids	E	E	E
4. X-ray capability including C-arm image intensifier with technologist available 24 hours a day	E	E	D
5. Endoscopes, all varieties	E	E	E
6. Craniotome	E	E	D
7. Monitoring equipment	E	E	E
3. Postanesthetic recovery room (surgical intensive care unit is acceptable)			
a. Registered nurses and other essential personnel 24 hours a day	E	E	E
b. Appropriate monitoring and resuscitation equipment	E	E	E
4. Intensive care units (ICUs) for trauma patients			
a. Personnel			
1. Designated surgical director	E	E	E
2. Surgeon, credentialed in critical care by the trauma director, on duty in ICU 24 hours a day or immediately available in hospital	E	E[17]	D
3. Minimum nurse-patient ratio of 1:2 on each shift	E	E	E
b. Equipment			
Appropriate monitoring and resuscitation equipment	E	E	E
c. Support services			
Immediate access to clinical diagnostic services	E[13]	E[13]	E
5. Acute hemodialysis capability	E	D	D
6. Organized burn care	E	E	E
a. Physician-directed burn center staffed by nursing personnel trained in burn care and equipped properly for care of the extensively burned patient			
or			
b. Transfer agreement with nearby burn center or hospital with a burn unit			
7. Acute spinal cord/head injury management capability	E	E	E
a. In circumstances in which a designated spinal cord injury rehabilitation center exists in the region, early transfer should be considered; transfer agreements should be in effect			
b. In circumstances in which a head injury center exists in the region, transfer should be considered in selected patients; transfer agreements should be in effect			
8. Radiological special capabilities			
a. Angiography of all types	E	E	D
b. Sonography	E	D	D
c. Nuclear scanning	E	D	D
d. Computed tomography	E	E	D
e. In-house CT technician 24 hours	E	D	D
f. Neuroradiology	E	D	—
9. Rehabilitation medicine			

Continued.

	LEVELS		
	I	**II**	**III**
B. Special facilities/resources/capabilities—cont'd			
a. Physician-directed rehabilitation and service staffed by personnel trained in rehabilitation care and equipped properly for care of the critically injured patient	E	—	—
or			
b. Transfer agreement when medically feasible to a nearby rehabilitation service	—	E	E
10. Clinical laboratory service (available 24 hours a day)			
a. Standard analyses of blood, urine, and other body fluids	E	E	E
b. Blood typing and cross-matching	E	E	E
c. Coagulation studies	E	E	E
d. Comprehensive blood bank or access to a community central blood bank and adequate hospital storage facilities	E	E	E
e. Blood gas levels and pH determinations	E	E	E
f. Serum and urine osmolality	E	E	D
g. Microbiology	E	E	E
h. Drug and alcohol screening	E	E	D[14]
C. Quality assurance			
1. Organized quality assurance programs	E	E	E
2. Special audit for all trauma deaths and other specified cases	E	E	E
3. Morbidity and mortality review	E	E	E
4. Trauma conference, multidisciplinary	E[15]	E[15]	D[15]
5. Medical nursing audit, utilization review, tissue review	E	E	E
6. Trauma registry	E[16]	E[16]	E[16]
7. Review of prehospital and regional systems of trauma care	E	D	D
8. Published on-call schedule must be maintained for surgeons, neurosurgeons, orthopaedic surgeons, and other major specialists	E	E	E
9. Times of and reasons for bypass must be documented and reviewed by quality assurance program	E	E	E
10. Quality assurance personnel—dedicated to and specific for the trauma program	E	E	D
D. Outreach program			
Telephone and on-site consultations with physicians of the community and outlying areas	E	D	—
E. Public education			
Injury prevention in the home and industry and on the highways and athletic fields; standard first-aid; problems confronting the public, medical profession, and hospitals regarding optimal care for the injured	E	E	D
	E	D	D
F. Trauma research program			
G. Training program			
1. Formal programs in continuing education provided by hospital for:			
a. Staff physicians	E	E	D
b. Nurses	E	E	E
c. Allied health personnel	E	E	E
d. Community physicians	E	E	D
H. Trauma service support personnel			
Trauma coordinator	E	E	D

Notes

1. The emergency department staff should ensure immediate and appropriate care for the trauma patient. The emergency department physician should function as a designated member of the trauma team. The relationship between emergency department physicians and other participants of the trauma team must be established on an individual hospital basis, consistent with resources but adhering to established standards that ensure optimal care.

2. Evaluation and treatment may be started by a team of surgeons that will include, at a minimum, a postgraduate year (PGY) 4 or senior general surgical resident who is a member of that hospital's surgical residency program. The trauma attending surgeon's participation in major therapeutic decisions and presence at operative procedures are mandatory and must be monitored by the hospital's trauma quality assurance program.

3. An attending neurosurgeon must be promptly available and dedicated to that hospital's trauma service. The in-house requirement may be fulfilled by an in-house neurosurgeon or surgeon who has special competence, as judged by the chief of neurosurgery, in the care of patients with neural trauma, and who is capable of initiating measures directed toward stabilizing the patient, as well as initiating diagnostic procedures.

4. An attending orthopaedic surgeon must be promptly available and dedicated to that hospital's trauma service. The in-house requirement may be fulfilled by an in-house orthopaedic surgeon or a surgeon who has special competence, as judged by the chief of orthopaedic surgery, in the care of patients with orthopaedic trauma, and who is capable of initiating measures directed toward stabilizing the patient, as well as initiating diagnostic procedures.

5. The staff specialists on call will be immediately advised and will be promptly available. This capability will be continuously monitored by the trauma quality assurance program.

6. Communication should be such that the general surgeon will be present in the emergency department at the time of arrival of the trauma patient.

7. In level I and level II institutions, requirements may be fulfilled by emergency medicine chief residents capable of assessing emergency situations in trauma patients and providing any indicated treatment. When chief residents are used to fulfill availability requirements, the staff specialist on call will be advised and be promptly available.

8. Requirements may be fulfilled by anesthesiology chief residents who are capable of assessing emergent situations in trauma patients and of providing any indicated treatment, including initiation of surgical anesthesia. When anesthesiology chief residents are used to fulfill availability requirements, the staff anesthesiologist on call will be advised and be promptly available.

9. Requirements may be fulfilled when local conditions assure that the staff anesthesiologist will be in the hospital at the time of or shortly after the patient's arrival. During the interim period, prior to the arrival of the staff anesthesiologist, a certified nurse anesthetist (CRNA) capable of assessing emergent situations in trauma patients and of initiating and providing any indicated treatment will be available.

10. This requirement may be fulfilled by a physician who is credentialed by the hospital to provide emergency medical services.

11. The patient's primary care physician should be notified at an appropriate time.

12. The pediatrician is not required in a system that has a designated pediatric trauma center to which all patients are taken.

13. Blood gas measurements, hematocrit level, and chest x-ray studies should be available within 30 minutes of request. This capability will be continuously monitored by the quality assurance program.

14. Toxicology screens need not be immediately available but are desirable. If available, results should be included in all quality assurance reviews.

15. Regular and periodic multidisciplinary trauma conferences that include all members of the trauma team should be held. These conferences will be for the purpose of quality assurance through critiques of individual cases.

16. Documentation will be made of severity of injury (by trauma score, age, ISS) and outcome (survival, length of stay, ICU length of stay), with monthly review of statistics.

17. The Committee on Trauma feels that the criteria outlined contribute to the optimal care of the injured patient. It is recognized that in certain level II hospitals, because of the size of the community, the surgeons can rapidly be available at the hospital on short notice. Under these circumstances, local criteria may be established that allow the general surgeon to take call from outside of the hospital, but with the clear commitment on the part of the hos-

Notes—cont'd

pital and the surgical staff, that the general surgeon will be present in the emergency department at the time of arrival of the trauma patient and be available to care for trauma patients in the ICU. Communications should be established to provide for advance notice, and the availability of the surgeon and compliance with this requirement must be monitored by the hospital's quality assurance program. In such hospitals, the requirement for initial neurosurgical and orthopaedic in-house coverage may also be fulfilled by the above-mentioned general surgeon.

B Disaster Planning

S. Marshal Isaacs

DEFINITIONS

Multiple casualty incident Any event that places an increased burden on the EMS system, yet can be handled by the local system in spite of a transient overload.

    EXAMPLE a multiple vehicle highway crash with a number of critically injured patients.

Limited disaster Any event that places an increased burden on the EMS system such that additional resources must be allocated from other systems to mount an appropriate response. Communication systems, utilities, shelters, transportation, and healthcare facilities are intact and undamaged.

    EXAMPLE an airplane crash at a local airport with many critically injured patients.

Generalized disaster An event with multiple victims with varying levels of severity of injury. There is damage or deficiencies in the communication systems, utilities, shelter, and transportation. Local healthcare facilities are nonfunctional or severely impaired, but hospitals in surrounding communities are able to absorb the increase in patient numbers. Water contamination, food shortages, epidemics, and psychologic problems are of major concern.

    EXAMPLE a major earthquake, hurricane, flood, or nuclear event.

■ ■ ■

It must be remembered that even in the setting of a "disaster," routine emergencies (e.g., asthma exacerbations, myocardial infarctions) still occur.

LEVELS OF RESPONSE

The four levels of response are as follows:
- Level 1   Hospital disaster plan
- Level 2   Local EMS disaster plan
- Level 3   National Disaster Medical System (NDMS)
- Level 4   Federal Emergency Management Agency (FEMA)

Level I: Hospital Disaster Plan

There will be differences for in-hospital versus out-of-hospital disasters. However, in all cases, a hospital disaster plan should do the following:

1. Establish a command post and the mechanism to activate the chain of command (Figure B-1).
2. Ensure that the activation of the system is simple and that a contingency exists should the telephone system be rendered nonfunctional (e.g., back-up portable radios stored in security and distributed to appropriate staff and locations if needed; phone access controlled via codes to ensure highest priority calls will go through; cellular phone back-up and a battery-powered television to keep abreast of outside information).
3. Restrict communications (radio, phone) to emergency use by authorized personnel.
4. Mandate the conservation of all water resources in the area.
5. Notify the senior administrator, trauma administrator, senior emergency physician, senior trauma physician, senior nursing ad-

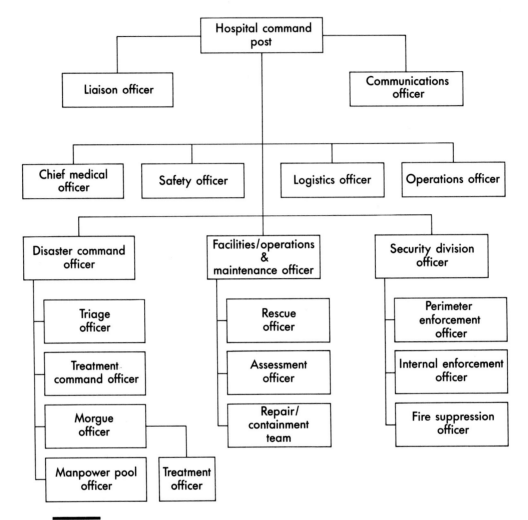

Figure B-I   Command organization structure algorithm. (*Note.* Courtesy Stanford University Hospital Disaster Mobilization Plan, Stanford, CA.)

ministrator, and person in charge of bed control/admissions.

6. Activate the chain of communication based on 'phase' activation of disaster plan:
   - Phase I   Limited response—local medical resources available and adequate.
   - Phase II   Moderate response—requires regional intervention.
   - Phase III   Complete response—local and regional resources overwhelmed. (ACEP, 1992)

7. Allow the disaster command officer to take charge of medically related hospital procedures and decisions in the acute phase of the response, after which the chief medical officer oversees all hospital care.

8. Designate a triage area in the ambulance bay and hallway outside of the emergency department, as well as a back-up site in case the ambulance/emergency area is damaged. A plan to investigate the immediate structural integrity of entrances, overhangs, and other areas within the disaster response units is necessary.

9. Designate specific treatment areas for the critically injured, the seriously injured but stabilized, the walking wounded, and a morgue.

10. Delineate specific roles and duties for all departments within the hospital.

■ ■ ■

Key points to consider relative to the hospital disaster plan follow:

1. Make the plan as simple as possible, to follow as closely as possible what happens under normal operating conditions—it should simply be an escalation of what would be considered a 'normal' response to a less resource-intensive situation.

2. Ensure that key personnel fully understand both the plan and their role in it. This may be made easier by (1) providing small printed cards (may be placed in vests) that list designated roles and responsibilities, (2)

providing disaster vests with bright colors and large print to designate appropriate key personnel, (3) maintaining a supply of pre-prepared disaster packets, and (4) facilitating continual day-to-day awareness of disaster areas by posting Velcro-backed disaster signs that designate disaster areas during drills or true disasters, but which flip over to specify the usual ED role of a specific area. Training of all personnel (including housestaff) and specifically all 'new hires' should include generic disaster preparation, as well as slide/sound programs concerning the specifics of the disaster plan. Figure B-2 shows a pocket card used for housestaff and medical students for quick access in the event of a disaster or a drill. Figure B-3 is a sample drawing of a quick reference to include in disaster manuals specific to the designated areas for each individual hospital plan.

TRIAGE CATEGORIES

Critical: (red) Salvageable. Patients needing major resuscitation or immediate surgical intervention

Urgent: (yellow)
   Casualties with major or serious injuries in whom a delay of several hours will not compromise life or limb
   Seriously injured but not salvageable without extensive efforts

Priority 3: (green) Minor injuries requiring care or those emotionally disturbed/distraught

Dead (black)

Disaster tag should be placed on the victim, NOT ON THE CLOTHING

BE PREPARED!!

Keep this card with you.

Know when to respond and where to go.

Know the role you will likely be asked to fill.

Know how to ensure your own safety so you'll be around to help others!

SUH

DISASTER

PLAN

(Medical Response)

Disaster Preparedness Committee

Ricardo Martinez, MD, Chairman

1991

A

Figure B-2   Pocket card delineating medical response to disaster. This copy is used for housestaff, but similar cards can be developed for nursing and other groups. **A,** Front. (*Note.* Courtesy Ricardo Martinez, MD, and Disaster Preparedness Committee, Stanford University Hospital, Stanford, CA.)

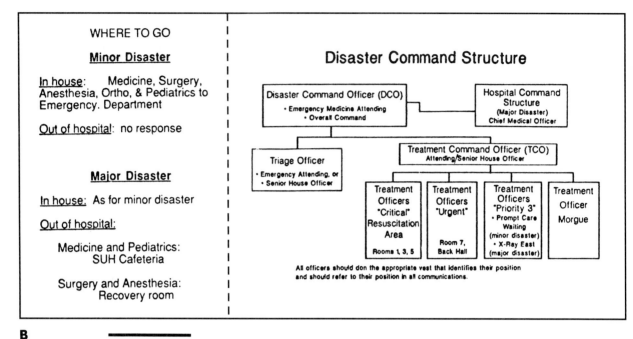

WHERE TO GO

Minor Disaster

<u>In house</u>: Medicine, Surgery, Anesthesia, Ortho, & Pediatrics to Emergency. Department

<u>Out of hospital</u>: no response

Major Disaster

<u>In house</u>: As for minor disaster

<u>Out of hospital</u>:

Medicine and Pediatrics: SUH Cafeteria

Surgery and Anesthesia: Recovery room

Disaster Command Structure

Disaster Command Officer (DCO)
- Emergency Medicine Attending
- Overall Command

Hospital Command Structure (Major Disaster) Chief Medical Officer

Triage Officer
- Emergency Attending, or
- Senior House Officer

Treatment Command Officer (TCO) Attending/Senior House Officer

Treatment Officers "Critical" Resuscitation Area — Rooms 1, 3, 5

Treatment Officers "Urgent" — Room 7, Back Hall

Treatment Officers "Priority 3"
- Prompt Care Waiting (minor disaster)
- X-Ray East (major disaster)

Treatment Officer Morgue

All officers should don the appropriate vest that identifies their position and should refer to their position in all communications.

B

Figure B-2, cont'd B, Back. Card folds over into thirds. (*Note.* Courtesy Ricardo Martinez, MD, and Disaster Preparedness Committee, Stanford University Hospital, Stanford, CA.)

3. Consider the need for back-up generators, lighting, and a hydraulic lift or stairway transport options should the elevators be rendered inoperative.
4. Assign disaster tasks in terms of positions rather than individuals.
5. Base the plan on what people are *likely* to do rather than what is thought they *should* do.
6. Schedule and implement **ongoing** mandatory disaster training, drills, and review.
7. Have available a current phone roster/call list.

Level 2: Local EMS Disaster Plan

1. Incidents call for a unified command structure to oversee the response of several agencies should they involve (1) more than one geographic jurisdiction, e.g., a flood; or (2) more than one functional jurisdiction, e.g., fire fighting, law enforcement, medical response, FAA.
2. Unified command serves to improve information flow and eliminates or reduces duplications of effort. It also serves to reduce functional and geographic complexities.
3. A disaster control facility should be designated and linked to other aspects of the system (including other hospitals).
4. A medical control officer should be appointed who is the senior medical person in charge.
5. Coordination with other agencies, e.g., fire, police, media, should be ensured.
6. Specific hospital resources, e.g., burn centers, trauma center, spinal center, should be considered.
7. Continual updates should be ensured concerning hospital, OR, ED, and ICU staff availability.
8. Normal EMS radio channels should be maintained, but brief reports and transmissions should be used. New technologies are available that use computers with uninterruptible power sources that can link hospitals, EMS systems, and providers in one or more counties, e.g., CHORAL, RediNett. Redundant sources, such as microwave phone lines, cellular phones, and access to

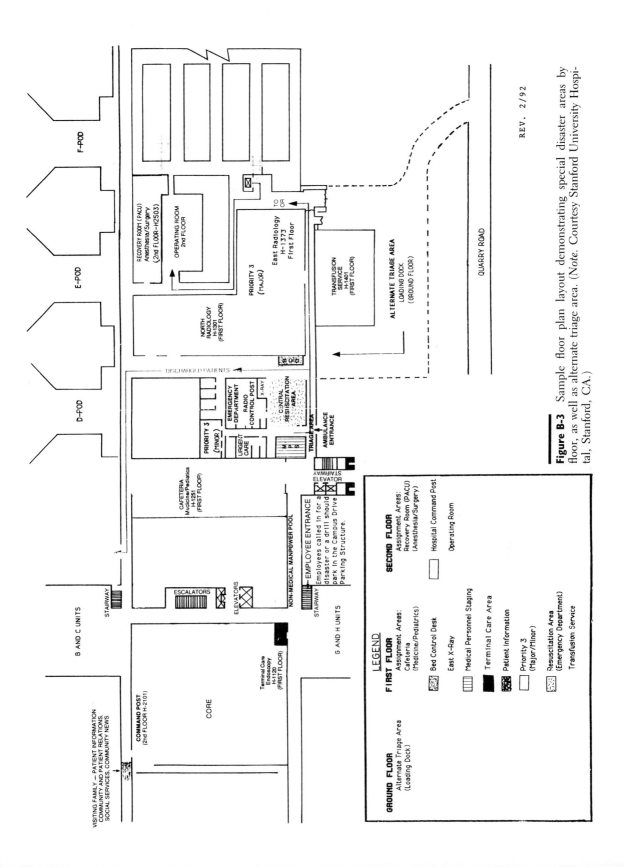

Figure B-3 Sample floor plan layout demonstrating special disaster areas by floor, as well as alternate triage area. (*Note.* Courtesy Stanford University Hospital, Stanford, CA.)

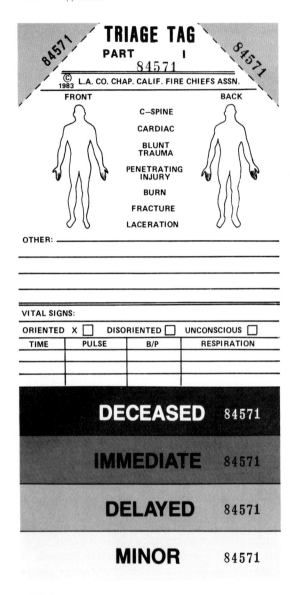

Figure B-4 Front half of triage tag with tear-off tracking numbers. (*Note*. Courtesy Los Angeles County Chapter of the Fire Chiefs Association.)

amateur radio frequencies, should be available.

Triage

Triage in the prehospital disaster setting is different from that within the hospital emergency department. It sometimes becomes necessary in the prehospital disaster setting to triage some critically ill patients to a "dead" category so as to maximize the number of salvageable patients when the number of casualties overwhelms the capabilities of the immediately available transportation resources. Triage should be provided by the most experienced medical care provider present at the scene.

Triage categories

I	patients requiring immediate surgical intervention or airway stabilization
II	patients with critical injuries that are not immediately life-threatening
III	patients with minor to moderate injuries, including the walking wounded.
IV	those victims who are dead; those who have obviously fatal injuries may be put in this category or may be put in category II until declared dead or resources become available to attempt to salvage them.

It has been suggested that priority status of patients be indicated through the use of triage tags with four categories that correspond to the triage categories just described (Figure B-4).

		Tag description	
Triage level	Color	Symbol	Category
I	Red	Rabbit	Urgent/immediate
II	Yellow	Turtle	Nonsurgical, delayed
III	Green	Ambulance crossed-out	First-aid only, minor
IV	Black	Cross/dagger	Dead/unsalvageable

Triage tags usually have prestamped numbers with detachable corners to help reconstruct each victim's progress through the disaster medical system. It also assists in helping family members and the media to identify patients. The receiving emergency department is responsible for recording the triage tag number in the ED admissions log. One limitation in a 'tear-off triage tag system

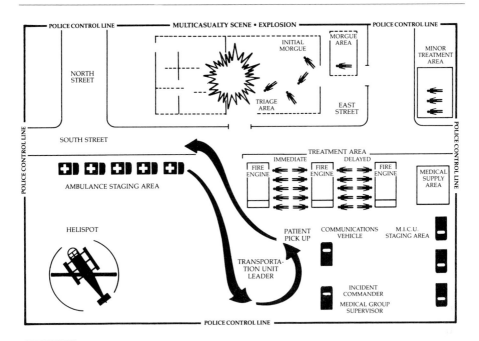

Figure B-5   Generic scene organization of multiple casualty incident. Flow of casualties and layout of triage, treatment, and transportation is shown. (*Note.* From *Disaster Response: Principles of Preparation and Coordination* (p. 181) by E. Auf der Heide, 1989, St. Louis: Mosby–Year Book, Inc.)

is that a patient's status can only be upgraded in urgency, and not downgraded. Another, more cumbersome, system uses color-coded cloths that can be changed if a patient's status changes.

Triage may be provided at the immediate site of injury if a large number of patients are grouped in one geographic area (Figure B-5). Otherwise, triage may be best provided by bringing patients to a central triage location.

Key point   Flexibility is the key in triage. If an adequate number of transport vehicles are available, rapid transport of all victims may obviate the need for systematic triage. However, some degree of triage is still necessary to divide the patients among receiving hospitals so that one does not merely "transport the disaster."

Debriefing

After each implementation of the disaster response, regardless of scale, debriefing sessions should be provided for all participants to determine how well the plan functioned, to consider

revisions, and to provide psychologic support for the EMS and hospital personnel.

Level 3: National Disaster Medical System (NDMS)

The National Disaster Medical System (NDMS) is a purely voluntary national system formed in 1980 whose primary objective is "to maximize the lifesaving potential in a mass disaster by mobilizing national resources when the resources of a stricken region are overwhelmed or destroyed" (Pretto & Safar, 1991). It is a cooperative effort under the aegis of the following:

1. Department of Defense
2. Department of Veterans Affairs
3. Department of Health and Human Services
4. Federal Emergency Management Agency (FEMA)

Key elements

The key elements of the NDMS are as follows:
1. To provide rapid medical responses via di-

saster medical assistance teams (DMATs) to support patient care within the disaster area

2. To evacuate patients and to assist communities to develop the capability to receive evacuated casualties

3. To coordinate the evacuation of casualties to sources of medical care outside of the region or even the state

Level 4: The Federal Emergency Management Agency

The federal administrative arm for disaster assistance, the Federal Emergency Management Agency (FEMA) provides financial and oversight assistance when directed to by members of the administration. Its functions include the following:

- Coordinates the federal response to the disaster
- Directs federal assistance to impacted communities after the event and during the recovery period

■ ■ ■

In conclusion, a disaster is a situation in which people may be trying to do quickly many activities that they are not used to performing, in an environment in which they are not familiar and which is highly stressful. This need not be the case; with good planning, practice, and revision, the unique problems posed by a disaster may be met with appropriate responses and favorable outcomes.

RESOURCES

American College of Emergency Physicians
Section of Disaster Medicine
1125 Executive Circle
Irving, TX 75038

Centers For Disease Control (CDC)
Section of Disaster Epidemiology
Atlanta, GA 30333

Disaster Research Center
University of Delaware
Newark, DE 19716

International Disaster Institute
1 Ferdinand Place
London, NW1, 8EE, UK

National Disaster Medical System
Parklawn Building, Room 16A-54
56000 Fishers Lane
Rockville, MD 20857

REFERENCES

American College of Emergency Physicians (ACEP), Disaster Committee. (1992). *Student manual for disaster management and planning for emergency physicians*, Emmitsburg, MD: Federal Emergency Management Agency, Emergency Management Institute.

Auf der Heide, E. (1989). *Disaster response: Principles of preparation and coordination*. St. Louis: Mosby–Year Book, Inc.

Federal Emergency Management Agency. (1981). *Disaster operations: A handbook for local governments*, Washington, DC: Author.

Kuehl, A.E. (1989). National Association of EMS Physicians: *EMS medical directors' handbook*. St. Louis: Mosby–Year Book, Inc.

Pretto, E.A., & Safar, P. (1991). National medical response to mass disaster in the United States: Are we prepared? *Journal of the American Medical Association*, 266 (9), 1259-1262.

Tierney, K.J. (1985). Emergency medical preparedness and response in disasters: The need for inter-organizational coordination. In W.J. Petak, *Emergency management: A challenge for public administration*, special issue, *Public Administration Review*, 45 (77).

C American College of Emergency Physicians (ACEP) Guidelines

Emergency department equipment, instruments, and supplies*

The equipment, instruments, and supplies listed below are suggested only. Each of the items listed should be either in, or immediately available to the area noted. This list does not include routine medical/surgical supplies, such as bandages, gauze pads, suture material, etc. It also does not include routine office items such as paper, desks, paper clips, chairs, etc.

General examination rooms

Examination tables or stretchers appropriate to the area. For any area in which seriously ill patients are managed, this should be a stretcher with capability for changes in position, attached IV poles, and holder for portable oxygen tank.
Stepstools
Chair/stool for emergency staff
Adequate lighting, including procedure lights as indicated
Oxygen supplies and equipment, including nasal cannulae, face masks, and venturi masks, as well as portable oxygen tanks
Suction capability, including both tracheal cannulae and larger cannulae

Oral and nasal airways
Wall-mount or portable otoscope/ophthalmoscope
Sphygmomanometer/stethoscope
Biohazard disposal receptacles
Masks, face shields, gloves, and other universal precaution materials
Adequate sinks for handwashing, including dispensers for germicical soap and paper towels

Miscellaneous—entire department

Security needs, including leather and soft restraints, and wand-type or freestanding metal detectors as indicated
Equipment necessary to assure adequate departmental housekeeping
Equipment for dictation of ED charts
Reference materials, including toxicology resource information
Nurse-call system for patient use
Separately wrapped instruments; specifics will vary by department
Availability of light microscopy for STAT procedures
Weight scales for both adult and infant
Tape measure
Radio or other device for communication with ambulances

---

*Note. From "Emergency Care Guidelines" by American College of Emergency Physicians, 1991, *Annals of Emergency Medicine*, 20, pp. 1389-1395.

Resuscitation room

All those items listed for general examination rooms

Direct communication with nursing station, preferably hands-free

X-ray equipment

X-ray viewboxes and hot light

Airway

  Endotracheal tubes, sizes 2.5 to 8.5 mm

  Laryngoscopes, including both straight and curved blades

  Laryngoscopic mirror and supplies

  Oral and nasal airways

  Suction apparatus, fixed

  Suction apparatus, portable

  Bag/valve/mask respirator, adult, pediatric, and infant

  Cricothyroidotomy instruments and supplies

  Tracheostomy instruments and supplies

  Fiberoptic laryngoscope

Breathing

  Closed-chest drainage device

  Chest tube instruments and supplies

  Emergency thoracotomy instruments and supplies

  Volume cycle ventilator

  Pulse oximetry monitor

  Peak flow meter

Circulation

  Monitor/defibrillator with pediatric paddles, internal paddles, appropriate pads and other supplies

  Temporary external pacemaker

  Transvenous and/or transthoracic pacemaker setup

  Automatic blood pressure monitor, noninvasive

  Cardiac compression board

  Blood/fluid pumps and tubing

  Blood/fluid warmers

  IV catheters, sets, tubing, poles

  Central venous catheter setups/kits

  Central venous pressure monitoring equipment

  Pericardiocentesis instruments and supplies

  12-lead ECG machine

  Cutdown instruments and supplies

  Intraosseous needles

Trauma and miscellaneous resuscitation

  Pneumatic antishock garmet, as indicated

  Cervical spine stabilization equipment

  Nasogastric suction supplies

  Gastric lavage supplies, including large lumen tubes

  Peritoneal lavage instruments and supplies

  Urinary catheters, including straight catheters, Foley catheters, Coude catheters, filiforms and followers, and appropriate collection equipment

  Lumbar puncture sets, both adult and pediatric

  Infrared infant warmer

  Emergency obstetrical instruments and supplies

  Hypothermia thermometer

  Warming/cooling blanket

  Vascular Doppler

  Wright spirometer

  Blood salvage/autotransfusion device

  Pediatric code cart, including appropriate medication charts

  Suture or minor surgical procedure sets (generic)

Guidelines for trauma care systems*

Trauma care systems entail three dimensions, incorporating four providers and 11 components in two settings [Figure C-1]. The following section describes individual components as either essential (E) or desirable (D) for each provider in each setting.

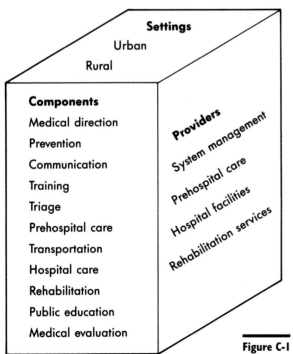

Figure C-1   Three dimensions of trauma care systems.

*Note. From "Guidelines for Trauma Care Systems" by American College of Emergency Physicians, 1987, *Annals of Emergency Medicine, 16*, pp. 459-463.

EXAMPLE

	Urban*	Rural†
I. Provider #1		
A. Component #1	E	E
B. Component #2	E	D
C. Etc		

	Urban*	Rural†
I. System management		
A. *Authority and responsibility.*		
Each system should establish its authority commensurate with its responsibility to provide trauma care, seeking enabling legislation when required.	E	E
B. *Central administrative agency.*		
Each system should identify a broad-based group of providers and consumers that is ultimately responsible for system management.	E	E
1. Master plan for system development, including criteria for each component, to be used for planning, implementation, operation, and evaluation	E	E
a. Prehospital criteria,[3] including triage, treatment, and transportation	E	E
b. Hospital criteria,[3] including facility numbers and levels, patient volumes, and staff/equipment standards	E	E
2. Medical director, familiar with and experienced in EMS and trauma system care	E	E
3. Administrative staff, familiar with and experienced in EMS and trauma system management	E	E
4. Prevention/public education		
a. Public education programs	E	E
b. Legislative advocacy programs	E	E
5. Training		
a. Clinical training for prehospital providers[4]	E	E
b. System utilization information for community physicians, nurses, and prehospital providers	E	E
6. Communications		
a. Regional plan	E	E
b. 911 access	E	D
c. Central control for medical direction and dispatch, including appropriate training for dispatchers	E	D
d. Linkage development	E	E
e. Equipment procurement	D	D
7. Data collection		
a. Adequate personnel	E	E
b. System registry participation	E	E
8. Medical audit		
a. Staff with expertise in quality assurance, statistics, and computers	E	D
b. Equipment and storage	E	D
c. Criteria for evaluating the system and its components	E	E
d. Quality assurance program, including feedback loop for demonstrated problems	E	E
9. Transplantation program coordination for potential donors	E	E
C. *Certification and decertification.* Each system should develop and implement policies and procedures for certifying and decertifying providers, including personnel, transportation, and facilities.	E	E
D. *Finance.* Each system should identify adequate resources, by line item, for planning, implementation, operation, and evaluation.	E	E
E. *Emergency/Disaster preparedness.* Each system should develop a regional disaster plan that integrates EMS, trauma care, and disaster management system resources.	E	E
1. Regional plan for all providers	E	E
2. Central control through local emergency management association	D	D

---

*System that encompasses at least one metropolitan area with 250,000 persons.
†System lacking any single population center.

	Urban*	Rural†
II. Prehospital care		
A. *Management agency.* Each system should identify an agency that is ultimately responsible for prehospital care. In some instances this function may be fulfilled by the central administrative agency.	E	E
1. Administration		
a. Medical director, familiar with and experienced in prehospital care	E	E
b. Support staff, familiar with and experienced in prehospital management	E	E
2. Training		
a. Sufficient experienced staff	E	E
b. Curriculum[4] integrated with system	E	E
3. Criteria		
a. Protocols[3] integrated with system	E	E
4. Certification and decertification		
a. Consistent with state and local criteria	E	E
b. Standardized clinical examination	E	E
5. Data collection integrated with system	E	E
6. Medical audit integrated with system	E	E
B. *Ambulance standards.* Each system should establish standards for land and air transportation, subject to legislative regulations.	E	E
1. Personnel	E	E
2. Equipment[3]	E	E
3. Process for ambulance certification and decertification	E	E
C. *Communication system.* Each system should develop a prehospital communication system that is fully integrated with the remainder of the EMS and emergency/disaster preparedness systems.	E	E
1. Central control for medical direction and dispatch	E	D
2. Equipment		
a. Minimize radio dead space	E	D
b. Equip all vehicles and aircraft	E	D
D. *Emergency/Disaster preparedness plan.* Each system should develop a prehospital emergency/disaster preparedness plan that is fully integrated with the remainder of the EMS system.	E	E
E. *Prevention/Public Education.*		
1. Injury prevention	E	E
2. First aid and CPR	E	E
III. Hospital facilities		
A. *Trauma hospitals.* Each system should identify an appropriate number of trauma hospitals to provide immediately available surgical care for seriously injured patients.	E	E
1. Standards[3]		
a. Emergency department	E	E
b. Surgery department	E	E
c. Nursing care	E	E
d. Laboratory/blood bank/x-ray	E	E
e. Computerized axial tomography	E	D
f. Trauma nurse coordinator	E	E
g. Treatment protocols	E	E
h. Integrated with EMS system	E	E
i. Documented institutional commitment	E	E
j. Current JCAH accreditation	E	E
2. Communication		
a. Integrated with EMS system	E	E
b. Base station hospital	D	D

*System that encompasses at least one metropolitan area with 250,000 persons.
†System lacking any single population center.

Continued.

III. Hospital facilities—cont'd	Urban*	Rural†
3. Helicopter landing capability		
a. On-site	E	D
b. Licensed by regulatory authority	E	E
4. Continuing medical education		
a. Physicians	E	D
b. Nurses	E	D
c. Prehospital providers	E	E
5. Protocols		
a. Prehospital bypass/rerouting, coordinated with other trauma hospitals through the central administrative agency	E	E
b. Treatment[3]	E	E
c. Transfer,[3] for all incoming patients regardless of origin	E	E
6. Prevention/public education		
a. Community-based programs	E	E
7. Data collection		
a. Adequate personnel	E	E
b. Hospital registry	E	E
c. System registry participation	E	E
8. Rehabilitation		
a. (See Section IV)	E	E
9. Medical audit		
a. Adequate personnel	E	E
b. Quality assurance program, including feedback loop for demonstrated problems	E	E
10. Emergency/disaster preparedness plan		
a. Internal plan	E	E
b. Integrated with remainder of emergency/disaster preparedness system	E	E
B. *Specialty care hospitals.* Each system should additionally identify specialty care hospitals for the small proportion of patients requiring such treatment. Access preferably entails prehospital transport, but also includes interhospital transfer when medically appropriate. If adequate facilities do not exist in the area, formal transfer agreements should be developed with nearby resources.	E	E
1. Standards		
a. Pediatric trauma[3]	E	D
b. Burns[3]	E	D
c. Spinal cord trauma[5]	E	D
d. Hand trauma/limb replantation	E	D
e. Eye trauma	E	D
2. Current JCAH accreditation	E	E
3. Communication		
a. Integrated with EMS system	E	E
4. Helicopter landing capability		
a. On-site	D	D
b. Licensed by regulatory authority	E	E
5. Training		
a. Physicians	E	D
b. Nurses	E	D
c. Prehospital providers	E	D
6. Protocols		
a. Prehospital bypass/rerouting, coordinated with other trauma hospitals through the central administrative agency	E	E
b. Treatment[3]	E	E
c. Transfer,[3] for all incoming patients regardless of origin	E	E

*System that encompasses at least one metropolitan area with 250,000 persons.
†System lacking any single population center.

	Urban*	Rural†
III. Hospital facilities—cont'd		
7. Prevention/public education		
a. Community-based programs	E	E
8. Data collection		
a. Adequate personnel	E	E
b. Hospital registry	E	E
c. System registry participation	E	E
9. Rehabilitation		
a. (See Section IV)	E	E
10. Medical audit		
a. Adequate personnel	E	E
b. Quality assurance program, including feedback loop for demonstrated problems	E	E
11. Emergency/disaster preparedness plan		
a. Internal plan	E	E
b. Integrated with remainder of emergency/disaster preparedness system	E	E
IV. Rehabilitation		
Rehabilitation planning, which should start with emergency department admission, may continue after hospital transfer or discharge. If adequate facilities do not exist in the area, formal transfer agreements should be developed with nearby resources.	E	E
A. *Special care facility.*		
1. Medical direction	E	E
2. Adequate staffing	E	E
a. Nursing care	E	E
b. Physical therapy	E	D
c. Occupational therapy	E	D
d. Psychosocial/substance abuse counseling	E	D
e. Family support services	E	D
f. Patient support groups	E	D
g. Orthotic/prosthetic services	E	D
h. Speech/language/hearing services	E	D
B. *Noninstitutional care.*		
1. Medical direction	E	E
2. Adequate staffing	E	E
a. Nursing care	E	E
b. Physical therapy	E	D
c. Occupational therapy	E	D
d. Psychosocial/substance abuse counseling	E	D
e. Family support services	E	D
f. Patient support groups	E	D
g. Orthotic/prosthetic services	E	D
h. Speech/language/hearing services	E	D
C. *Financial support.* Each system should identify adequate resources for rehabilitation.	E	E
D. *Data collection.*		
1. Adequate personnel	E	E
2. Provider registry	E	E
3. System registry participation	E	E
E. *Medical audit.*		
1. Adequate personnel	E	E
2. Coordinate with system audit	E	E
3. Quality assurance program, including feedback loop for demonstrated problems	E	E

*System that encompasses at least one metropolitan area with 250,000 persons.
†System lacking any single population center.

References

1. Institute on Medicine: *Injury in America: A Continuing Health Problem*. Washington, DC, National Academy Press, 1985.
2. National Safety Council: *Accident Facts*. Chicago, NSC, 1985, p 8.
3. American College of Surgeons: *Hospital and prehospital Resources for Optimal Care of the Injured Patient, and Appendices A-J*. Chicago, ACS, 1986.
4. American Academy of Orthopaedic Surgeons: *Emergency Care and Transportation of the Sick and Injured*, ed 4. Chicago, AAOS, 1987.
5. American Spinal Injury Association Foundation: *Guidelines for Facility Categorization and Standards of Care: Spinal Cord Injury*. Chicago, ASIAF, 1981.

D Organ Donation

Peggy Devney

INTRODUCTION Advances in the field of transplantation in the past 30 years have enabled thousands of individuals who would have otherwise died an opportunity for full and productive lives. In the past 2 decades the success rate of 1-year graft survival of transplanted organs has increased from 50% to more than 70%. Concomitantly, patient survival has also risen (the box on the right).

Although many transplants have been performed in the past few years, there remain many more patients on the waiting list than there are organ donors. Although the transplantation of a single kidney from a living donor has long been accepted medical practice, the 1990s have seen an increase in transplantation of partial livers and lungs from living related donors in an attempt to save lives (Figure D-1). There were 23,878 patients on the national waiting list on September 5, 1991 (18,924 waiting for a kidney; 2128 waiting for a heart, 1504 waiting for a liver; 602 waiting for a pancreas; 559 waiting for a lung; and 161 waiting for a heart and lung), and a new name is added every 30 minutes (UNOS, 1990). In 1992 it is estimated that 5 or 6 patients a day die while waiting for an organ transplant (National Kidney Foundation, 1992).

SUPPORT FOR ORGAN DONATION

Several studies performed in the 1980s and early 1990s show that the general public's attitude about organ donation and transplantation is favorable. The majority of the public surveyed knew about organ transplantation and overall would support the concept of donation of their own or a loved one's organs. The probability of donation of a loved one's organs increased when prior family discussion about donation had occured.

Along with public support for donation, the

One-Year recipient survival rates	
Kidney	92%
Pancreas	89%
Heart	83%
Liver	76%
Heart/Lung	57%
Lung	48%

Note: From United Network for Organ Sharing (UNOS). 1988. Richmond, VA.

United States government enacted several pieces of legislation that have facilitated the process of donation. The Uniform Anatomical Gift Act of 1968 was a key piece of legislation facilitating organ donation. This act established the legality of donating a deceased individual's organs for transplantation or other uses and protected healthcare personnel from potential liability arising from organ procurement (United States Congress, 1968).

The Uniform Determination of Death Act recognized that brain death is death: the irreversible cessation of all functions of the entire brain constitutes death in the same way as cessation of heartbeat and respiration. Many of the states have enacted brain death legislation that enables patients to be declared to be brain dead (United States Congress, 1974).

Required Request legislation was enacted in the mid-1980s on both the federal and state level. This law mandates that healthcare professionals identify and refer all potential donors to an organ procurement organization. The legislation further states that systems be in place that provide families of the potential donor information about the option for donation in order to make an informed decision. (United States Congress, 1986b). The Omnibus Budget Reconciliation Act of 1986 fur-

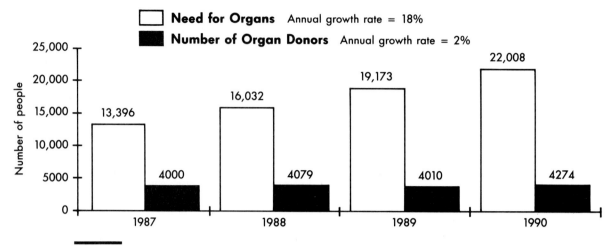

Figure D-I Need for organs compared with number of organ donors. (*Note.* From United Network for Organ Sharing [UNOS], September, 1991. Richmond, VA.)

ther requires hospitals participating in Medicare and Medicaid (virtually all hospitals in the United States) to establish written protocols for donation (United States Congress, 1986a).

ORGANIZATION OF THE DONATION AND TRANSPLANT NETWORK

The federal government has also played a major role in the organizational system for coordination of donation and distribution of organs for transplantation. In 1984 Congress passed the National Organ Transplant Act, which requires the establishment of the Organ Procurement and Transplantation Network (OPTN). The OPTN was contracted to the United Network for Organ Sharing (UNOS) to manage organ distribution and to establish a scientific registry. UNOS maintains a national computer network that provides a mechanism for matching available organs to the most desperately ill patients awaiting transplantation.

At the center of this distribution system are the organ procurement organizations (OPO). There are 70 regional organ procurement organizations nationally. These organizations provide a local link between the hospitals where potential donors are found and the transplant centers where potential recipients are transplanted. OPO staff are routinely available to provide local hospitals and healthcare professionals with a wide range of services. OPO staff are available to the hospitals to assist in approaching families about their option for donation after brain death has been estab-

lished. After the family has given consent, OPO staff oversee clinical management of the donor and coordinate recovery and placement of the donated organs. Additionally, the OPO staff follow up with the families of the donor to thank them and to inform them of the lives they have saved by their decision to donate. Currently, OPOs around the nation are establishing collaborative working relationships with hospitals and the medical communities to systematically address the issues related to developing and implementing donation protocols and procedures.

In spite of surveyed public opinion that reflects a positive attitude about donation and legislative mandates, a critical shortage of donors continues. It is now the responsibility of all healthcare providers to become familiar with the process of organ donation, recognizing that the offering of a choice (organ donation) in the death of a loved one benefits families and it is the right of every family to be provided an option for donation (Gallup Survey, 1990; Protas & Batten, 1986).

Where Donors are Lost

Several issues must be addressed before the organ shortage will be solved. According to a survey of OPO executive directors in 1989, donors are lost most often when families deny consent (estimated 38% of donor situations) (Association of Organ Procurement Organizations 1989). There are numerous reasons for families to deny organ donation, both societal and cultural. Families who consent to donation do so primarily for altruistic reasons. A number of studies show that families who donated believed that the donation benefited them in allowing them to cope with their loss. Many believed that donation made some good come from a tragic event—the fact that donation saved lives and that their loved one lived on in some manner. Additionally, families who declined donation were grateful to have been given an option (Protas & Batten, 1986).

An additional 12% of donors are lost by the lack of recognition and declaration of brain death by the medical and nursing professionals. Many times the declaration of death is perceived as a failure of the medical system to save the life. The declaration of brain death and its explanation to a bereaved family is time-consuming and uncomfortable for some health care providers. Some believe that confronting brain death will unduly burden the family.

Finally, 17% of potential donor families are not approached about their option to donate. The reasons for this are multifactorial. Some healthcare providers believe that offering information about donation at a time of grief is too much for the family. Some physicians worry about a perceived conflict of interest as the primary care giver approaching about donation. When healthcare providers fail to give families an option for donation, they are essentially making a decision for that family—a decision that is not theirs to make.

THE DONATION PROCESS
Recognition of a Potential Organ Donor

The donation process begins when the medical and nursing staff recognize that a patient has suffered a severe brain injury that either has resulted in or will soon result in the cessation of all brain activity. Over the past several years the general criteria for organ donors have changed dramatically. The current thought within the procurement community is to call the OPO early enough for assistance with determination of medical criteria. It is generally accepted that almost any patient may be a possible donor, excluding certain preexisting conditions (see the box on the right).

Additionally, the consideration for organ donors has been expanded to include individuals who are advanced in age (up to 70 years) and who have systemic illness such as hypertension and di-

---

Exclusion for organ donation

- Current intravenous drug abuse
- Preexisting untreated infection (septicemia, untreated; AIDS; viral hepatitis)
- Malignancy, except brain tumor
- Active tuberculosis

Note: From California Transplant Donor Network 1990. San Francisco.

---

abetes. In the past, these individuals had not been considered to be potential donors. More recently, such individuals have donated multiple organs, resulting in good function in the transplant recipient (Gruhen, 1989).

Declaration of Brain Death

Many potential organ donors are the result of vehicular injury, falls, abuse, or violence, leading to brain death. However, medical conditions such as cerebral vascular accidents, hypoxia, congenital vascular defects, and brain malignancy also contribute to the numbers of individuals who are pronounced brain dead. When brain death is suspected, the medical team will perform a number of neurologic tests that will be used to make the diagnosis of brain death. Currently, no uniform procedure is used throughout the nation to determine brain death; therefore it must be stressed that critical care nurses need to be familiar with state law and hospital policy used in their institution. Some policies may include special physician qualifications and timeframes for declaration. Most states have legislation that provides a framework for the diagnosis of brain death. The diagnosis of brain death may be made after three criteria are met: (1) the cause of the injury is known; (2) no CNS depressants are present, and the patient is normothermic; and (3) the condition is irreversible. The determination of brain death is made based on a clinical examination that determines the presence or lack of specific responses (see Table 10-8 in Chapter 10).

In some instances, a clinical examination will be enhanced by confirmatory tests, such as an EEG or perfusion studies, e.g., cerebral scan (using radioisotopes) or cerebral angiography to determine brain perfusion (see Table 10-9). The final diagnosis is made when cerebral and brainstem function are completely absent.

After brain death has been determined, the attending physician, nurses, and support staff (e.g., social workers, clergy) inform the family about brain death. All members of the healthcare team must use the same terminology when talking with the family, to give a consistent message. Use of the word "dead" (instead of "brain dead") and not making reference to the patient being on "life support" convey to the family that all agree that the individual is dead; that there is no hope for recovery. The concept of brain death is unfamiliar to many outside the healthcare profession. According to a 1990 Gallup survey, 59% of people surveyed said that brain dead meant that their loved one was dead, whereas 41% did not understand the concept. Families need time to process the information and may require explanations before they can understand.

OPO Involvement

The hospital staff, in conjunction with identifying and declaring an individual as brain dead, notifies the local OPO of the possibility of an organ donor. The OPO coordinator can offer suggestions as to management of the potential donor and in many instances can be available to come on-site to be part of the family conference. In a few areas of the country, the OPOs are notified early in the process; in other areas, OPOs are notified after the patient has been declared dead and the family has given consent.

Presenting the Option for Donation

After the family has been given time to process the information about brain death and **understands** that no chance of recovery exists, that their loved one is dead, the option for donation is presented. In most cases, families are presented with brain death information at the same time as information about organ donation. The challenge for families to comprehend brain death information while making a decision about donating organs is, in many instances, too much for families to deal with, making a positive choice for donation extremely unlikely. Recent studies have shown that when the information about brain death is sepa-

rated in time (decoupled) from the information about organ donation, families are better able to make informed decisions about donation. (Garrison et al., 1991).

Cultural Aspects of Donation

Although many public education efforts have been mounted throughout the United States, cultural constraints continue to affect donation. The major focus in the 1990s has been on current public education efforts that raise awareness and encourage commitment to donation within communities that are less likely to donate. For those families who are able, it is important that they be the messengers to the community at large. In a study done by Protas and Batten (1986), 86% of the families thought that donation provided a positive outcome of the death; 89% said that they would donate again; and 79% said that donation helped the grieving process.

The incidence of kidney failure is 4 times higher in African Americans than in Whites in the United States. Of those on the national waiting list for kidney transplants, 30% are African-descended. In 1990, 9% of the cadaver donor pool were African-descended, whereas 80% of the donor pool were White. Past studies by Dr. Clive Callender and more recent studies by Davidson and Devney (1991) reflect that obstacles to donation in the African American community are religious constraints, mistrust of the medical community, fear of premature death, and racism.

Hispanic Americans also donate at lower rates. Hispanics are also plagued by higher incidence of renal disease. A Gallup poll in 1985 suggested that a lack of understanding of the need for donation and language disparity may contribute to low donation rates.

Any approaches to families must consider the diversity of cultures present in the United States, and a sensitivity to these issues at the time of grief is especially important.

Donor Management

The clinical management of a potential organ donor involves the early treatment of hemodynamic instability, maintenance of systemic perfusion pressure, and prevention of systemic complications of brain death. The general guidelines for donor maintenance are to maintain a systolic blood pressure of 90 to 100 mm Hg; urine output of >90 to 100 ml per hour; a PaO_2 of >100 mm Hg; and pH of 7.4.

The brain-dead patient may be initially challenging to manage. Initial therapy for a brain-injured patient involves the administration of pharmacologic agents to normalize blood pressure, as well as osmotic diuretics to reduce the incidence of cerebral swelling. After the patient has been declared brain dead, therapy involves the treatment of hypotension with crystalloid and colloid, coagulopathy, diabetes insipidus, and hypothermia. Donor management involves compulsive aggressive medical and nursing management. Placement of arterial and central lines will allow for the assessment of cardiac filling pressures and volume status, an arterial line to measure arterial pressure and to provide easy access for frequent blood gas determinations. An indwelling urinary catheter will allow for easy evaluation of output. Throughout the donor process the following laboratory tests will be ordered to evaluate the individual as a potential donor:

- Serum creatinine and blood urine nitrogen
- ABO typing and complete blood count
- Electrolytes/liver enzymes
- Urinalysis
- Cultures of blood, urine, sputum
- Cardiac enzymes
- Chest x-ray examination
- ECG, echocardiography (ECHO), and sometimes for older donors, a cardiac catheterization
- Arterial blood gases

Continuous artificial ventilation must be maintained until the surgical recovery of the organs. Continued respiratory care is of the utmost importance to ensure good oxygenation and in the case of lung donation, clear, uninfected organs.

Maintenance of the donor's systolic blood pressure at 90 to 100 mm Hg or above is important to ensure adequate perfusion and oxygenation of vital organs. If this cannot be achieved by fluid resuscitation alone, use of a vasopressor agent is acceptable. Dopamine is preferred, because the use of other vasopressors may reduce renal blood flow.

Donor management requires the collective cooperation of the bedside nurse, transplant coordinator, laboratory staff, and consulting physician staff. All financial costs associated with donor evaluation (laboratory tests) and donor maintenance (ICU stay, nursing care, and OR time) are paid for by the organ procurement organization.

The critical care nurse is a vital link in the referral of donors, and because of this, he or she plays a part in determining who will receive organ transplants. For patients' families to be given the beneficial option for organ donation, the critical care nurse must play an integral role. It has been the goal of this appendix to facilitate this process (see the box below and Figure D-2).

Recommended process for successful organ donation

Early explanation of a grave prognosis. This will begin to prepare the family for the eventual outcome.

Notification of the local OPO. Early notification of the OPO will allow for evaluation as to the suitability of the potential donor.

Family counseling: grave prognosis. The team of healthcare professionals provide support and added explanations of prognosis after the physician has explained the prognosis.

Communication of brain death. After testing and diagnosis of brain death are made, the family is informed of the diagnosis. Simple, understandable language isused.

Family counseling around the issue of death. This is usually done by members of the team (e.g., social workers, clergy, nurses, and transplant coordinator).

First discussion of organ donation. A health care professional who is comfortable presenting the option for donation should approach the family. Ideally, the person talking with the family will have already established a rapport with the family.

Donation option and decision. If the OPO coordinator has not been previously involved, the coordinator will present specific expanded information about donation option. The family members must understand all aspects of organ donation, discuss the matter, and be in agreement with the decision before consent is given.

Note. Adapted from *Solving the Organ Donor Shortage* (pp. 23-24) by Partnership for Organ Donation, 1991, Boston: Author.

The Donation Process
Basic guidelines

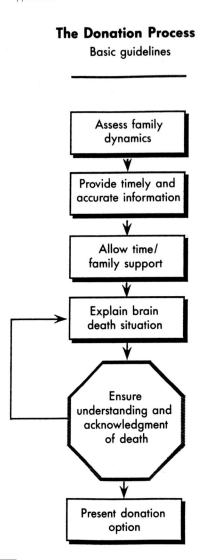

Figure D-2 Donation process: basic guidelines. (*Note.* From The Partnership for Organ Donation, Boston. 1991.)

REFERENCES

Association of Organ Procurement Organizations.

Corporate Decisions, Inc: Survey of OPO Directors: Fall, 1989.

Davidson, M. & Devney, P. (1991). Attitudial barriers to organ donation among Black Americans. *Transplantation Proceedings, 25,* 5.

Davis, F. (1990). *The injured brain book.* New York Regional Transplant Program.

Gallup Survey. "Americans and Organ Donation: Current Attitudes and Perceptions," Conducted for the Partnership for Organ Donation, Inc., Oct. 1990.

Garrison, R.N., Bentley, F.R., Raque, G.H., Polk, H.C., Jr., Sledac, L.C., Evanisko, M.J., & Lucas, B.A. (1991). There is an answer to the shortage of organ donors. *Surgery, Gynecology, and Obstetrics, 173* (5), 391-396.

Gruhen, C. (1989). Unpublished study of transplant results in recipients of organs from hypertensive donors in northern California.

National Kidney Foundation News Release for Community Meeting, San Francisco: January, 28, 1992.

Partnership for Organ Donation. (1991). *Solving the organ shortage:* Boston: Author.

Protas, J. & Batten H.L. (1986). Attitudes and incentives in organ procurement": Report to the Health Care Financing Administration: April. (1990).

United Network for Organ Sharing (UNOS). (1990). National Data Report.

United States Congress. (1986a). Omnibus Reconciliation Act.

United States Congress. (1986b). Required Request: AB 631.

United States Congress. (1968). Uniform Anatomical Gift Act: AB 1455.

United States Congress. (1974). Uniform Determination of Death Act: AB 2560.

Index

∎∎